NUTRITION
in Contemporary
Nursing Practice

NUTRITION
in Contemporary
Nursing Practice

MARILYN L. GREEN, RD, MS

Assistant Professor
Indiana University School of Nursing
Indianapolis, Indiana

JOANN HARRY, RN, BSN

Associate Director of Nursing, Education
Pontiac General Hospital
Pontiac, Michigan

Formerly, Lecturer
Indiana University School of Nursing
and Unit Director
Indiana University Hospitals
Indianapolis, Indiana

A WILEY MEDICAL PUBLICATION
JOHN WILEY & SONS

New York • Chichester • Brisbane • Toronto • Singapore

Sponsoring editor: Cathy D. Somer
Cover and interior design: Wanda Lubelska
Production editor: Eileen Tommaso
Copy editor: Janet S. Mais
Illustrator: Mel A. Dallas

Library of Congress Cataloging in Publication Data:

Green, Marilyn L   1945–

  Nutrition in contemporary nursing practice.

  (A Wiley medical publication)
  Includes index.
  1. Nutrition. 2. Nursing. I. Harry, Joann, joint author.
II. Title. [DNLM: 1. Nutrition–Nursing texts. WY150 G797n]

RT87.N87G73   612'.3   80-22426
ISBN 0-471-03892-X

Printed in the United States of America

10 9 8 7 6 5

To Dr. Shirley Karlson whose encouragement sustained me during my early years of university teaching

M.L.G.

To Ruth Woodham, a friend and confidante

J.H.

To Cathy Somer whose insight nurtured an idea into a reality

M.L.G.
J.H.

CONTRIBUTORS

Judith Bonner
Assistant Professor
Department of Pediatrics and
    Nutrition Science
University of Alabama in
    Birmingham
Birmingham, Alabama

Marlin C. Harmon, MS
Graduate Research Assistant
Department of Foods and Nutrition
The Food Science Institute
Purdue University
West Lafayette, Indiana

Patricia A. Harvey, BSN
Patient Care Coordinator
Indiana University Hospital
Indiana University Medical Center
Indianapolis, Indiana

Catherine Justice, RD, PhD
Associate Professor of Foods and Nutrition
Department of Foods and Nutrition
Purdue University
West Lafayette, Indiana

Cora Kurtz, RD, MS
Assistant Professor
Nutrition Division
Department of Epidemiology and Public
    Health
University of Miami School of Medicine
Miami, Florida

Josephine Novo Osborne, RN, MSN
Assistant Professor in Psychiatric
    Nursing
Indiana University School of Nursing
Indianapolis, Indiana

B. Swaminathan, PhD
Assistant Professor of Food Science
Department of Foods and Nutrition
The Food Science Institute
Purdue University
West Lafayette, Indiana

FOREWORD

The scope of health care is continually expanding. Given impetus by the recent Surgeon General's report *Healthy People,* the provision of care is no longer confined to the treatment of acute illness or the rehabilitation of patients with chronic disease but now directly addresses the various facets of health promotion and disease prevention, including increased emphasis on the nutritional care of clients.

Coupled with this enlarged sphere of health care action are ever-expanding roles for health care professionals. Recognizing that a person is more than a collection of organ systems, health care providers are expanding their care to include the "whole" person as he or she is affected by and, in turn, acts upon the environment. The World Health Organization's definition of health reflects this encompassing view: "Health is more than just the absence of disease; it is the state of complete mental, physical, and social well being."

To meet the diverse needs of clients in the health care system, a team approach is both vital and necessary. By blending their various levels and kinds of knowledge, skills, and approaches, members of the health care team can successfully accomplish the goal of comprehensive and continuous health care.

Central to this goal are constant communication and sharing between nurse and nutritionist/dietitian. With nutrition receiving increased attention as a primary contributor to health promotion in recent years, it is essential for the nurse to have a sound background in nutrition and to work with the nutritionist/dietitian in the delivery of nutritional service to clients.

This book is remarkable in that it accomplishes two key objectives in keeping with these current trends in health care: First, it gives equal attention to the professions of nursing and dietetics. Second, it emphasizes care of the "whole" client. Co-authorship of the text by a dietitian and a nurse lends a dual perspective that reinforces the concept of a team approach to nutritional care. The use of a nursing diagnosis framework, unique among nutrition textbooks, stresses the client's total well-being and provides a creative yet practical way of presenting nutrition content. Thus the text will serve as a fundamental source of nutrition information in a form that is particularly relevant to nursing students.

It is my hope that this book will have great impact on the delivery of care by the nurse–nutritionist team and will pave the way for even greater communication and understanding between the two professions.

Laura S. Sims, PhD, MPH, RD
Associate Professor of Nutrition
in Public Health
College of Human Development
The Pennsylvania State University
University Park, Pennsylvania

PREFACE

Since nutritional care is an integral part of the total nursing care of clients, the authors firmly believe that the principles and application of the science of nutrition are essential components of the basic nursing curriculum. Because of the large numbers of students enrolled in various types of nursing programs, we felt that a nutrition text should be available specifically for them, one that departs from the traditional approach of presenting a separate chapter on each of the major nutrient classes in favor of an approach that is more appropriate and useful for nursing students today.

This textbook is intended for all types of basic nursing students. It can be used in nursing programs that have a separate, basic nutrition course or a combined nutrition and diet therapy course. It can also be used as a reference in nursing programs that integrate part or all of nutrition into the nursing curriculum. The book can also serve as a reference for registered nurses and licensed practical nurses who are working in hospitals or doing private-duty nursing care.

The book is organized into two major parts. Part I presents the basic theory of nutrition, and Part II applies nutrition to nursing practice. The practical application of nutrition facts is emphasized throughout the text. Part I is divided into three units, each focusing on a particular aspect of nutrition. Unit I provides the basic facts and principles of the science of nutrition along with such nutritional

tools as the exchange system, the basic four, and the Recommended Dietary Allowances. Practical topics such as weight control, fast foods, vegetarianism, health foods, food production, and economical food purchasing are presented. In Unit II the functions of the nutrients are discussed using the nutritive process, which consists of the steps of ingestion, digestion, absorption, nutrient transport, metabolism, and excretion. The corresponding body systems are discussed in relation to these steps to demonstrate how the body makes use of the nutrients in food. Principles of physiology and chemistry are employed in this discussion to show the direct application of these sciences to nutrition. Unit III concludes Part I with a discussion of nutritional demands and eating patterns throughout the life cycle.

Part II is divided into two units that discuss the nursing and nutritive processes. In Unit IV the steps of the nursing process serve as a framework for discussing nutritional care. Two chapters are devoted to nutritional assessment, the initial step in the nursing process. A set of nursing diagnoses is then presented based on assessment of the nutritive process, and additional assessment data are provided for each alteration in this process. Following that, in Chapter 22, the steps of planning, intervention, and evaluation are discussed. The last chapter in this unit is concerned with the nursing aspects of medical interventions for nutritional support, such as intravenous therapy, tube feedings, test diets, hyperalimentation, and diet–drug interactions.

Unit V examines the dietary interventions for alterations in the nutritive process based on the nursing diagnosis classification. Dietary management is discussed in terms of objectives and rationale of the diet, general principles of the diet, and practical considerations. Throughout Unit V, it is emphasized that the dietitian is responsible for the initial diet instruction. The role of the nurse is to provide support, reinforcement, and practical suggestions about the diet to the client and the family. The nursing student is constantly encouraged to seek additional information from the dietitian.

Several pedagogical aids are provided throughout the text for both students and instructors. Each unit begins with a model that gives a visual overview of the content, followed by a list of behavioral objectives. Part II contains case studies to help students apply the principles of nutritional assessment and therapeutic diets. In Chapter 22, objectives, stated in terms of desired client behaviors, are given for each major nursing diagnosis affecting the nutritive process. These objectives can be used by nursing students or nurses for planning, intervention, and evaluation of clients' nutritional care. In each chapter of Unit V, the objectives are repeated along with the appropriate nursing diagnoses so that students can use them to focus on planning their clients' nutritional care.

The appendices contain several helpful tables including dietary standards, desirable weights, nutritive values of foods, and exchange lists for meal planning. Appendix J is an index of selected diseases and symptoms and associated nutritional nursing diagnoses. This index will be useful to students, since

pathophysiology is discussed in this text in terms of alterations in the nutritive process instead of specific diseases. It will also aid students in viewing certain diseases and disorders as alterations in one or more aspects of the nutritive process and in learning to predict what dietary interventions clients may need. An extensive glossary of nutrition, nursing, and medical terms, as well as selected terms from anatomy, physiology, and chemistry.

In this text, the authors have elected to use the word *client* to refer to those who are participants in their own health care. An exception has been made in cases in which the client is quite ill. In these instances, the word *patient* has been substituted. Some examples are the burned patient, the patient on hyperalimentation, and the surgical patient. For simplicity and clarity, the nurse or dietitian is always referred to as *she*. In some instances, the term *clinician* is used to designate the physician, nurse, or dietitian.

One of the authors of this text is a registered dietitian and the other is a registered nurse. Both authors have practiced in hospitals as well as taught nursing students for several years. Since the authors believe that nutrition is an essential part of the basic nursing curriculum and the nursing care of clients, we hope that this book will make a significant contribution to nursing education. It is our sincere expectation that this text will enable students to understand the role of nutrition in health maintenance and recovery from disease and to give more effective nutritional care to clients.

M.L.G.

J.H.

ACKNOWLEDGMENTS

Many people have been involved with the writing of this book, either directly or indirectly. First, Laura S. Sims, PhD, of Pennsylvania State University reviewed the entire manuscript. Her suggestions and constant encouragement were greatly appreciated. The authors also appreciate the helpful suggestions Richard G. Pflanzer, PhD, Department of Physiology, Indiana University School of Medicine made after a review of Unit II. Dr. David Allmann, Indiana University School of Dentistry reviewed the illustrations for Chapter 12 and offered many helpful suggestions. Individuals who contributed specific portions of the text were Josephine Osborne, Sara Porter, B. Swaminathan, Cora Kurtz, Judith Bonner, Catherine Justice, Patricia A. Harvey, and Marlin C. Harmon.

Jeff Collins assisted with photos, and Mel Dallas spent long and tedious hours on the illustrations for this text. Ann Van Camp, Librarian, Indiana University School of Medicine Library, conducted the many computerized literature searches for this book. The typing of most of the manuscript was faithfully done by Cecilia Overshiner. Her patience, forebearance, support, and attention to detail were greatly appreciated. Three other typists who assisted with the task were Lorna Moulton, Cynthia Allen, and Suzann Moes.

We would both like to acknowledge the constant interest, support, and encouragement of professional colleagues associated with Indiana University School of Nursing, the Department of Nutrition and Dietetics, and Indiana University Hospitals. Noted among these were Shirley Karlson, Connie Wesner, Freda Scales-Smith, and Ruth Woodham. Emily Williams, RD, provided assistance in countless ways. She assisted with the library research and spent many hours reading galley and page proofs. Her valuable suggestions and support during this task will never be forgotten. Betty Shalter, RD, of Indiana University Hospital and Emily Williams assisted in assembling and writing the therapeutic diets for Unit V.

We would also like to thank our personal friends for their support and encouragement. Some of those who assisted with proof reading and rewriting were Rebecca Sheckell, and Stephen and Susan Overstreet.

This book could not have been written without the professional guidance and skill provided by the staff of John Wiley. A special word of appreciation goes to Cathy Somer, former Nursing Editor, John Wiley & Sons, who was with this project from its beginning. Her professional abilities, enthusiasm, and patience guided the writing of this book from its conception until its realization as a completed manuscript. The authors also express appreciation to Linda Turner, Assistant Nursing Editor, for her efficient work and helpful suggestions concerning the manuscript. The transformation of the completed manuscript into an actual book involves the dedicated work of many people. Appreciation must be acknowledged for the excellent work done by Janet S. Mais, the copy editor, and Wanda

Lubelska, the designer. The production process proceeded smoothly under the skillful direction of Eileen Tommaso, the production editor.

Finally, a special word of thanks must go to our husbands, Rusty Green and Jack Harry. Not only did they allow us the time to work on the project, but they assisted with many household tasks. With the constant support of family, friends, and colleagues, the experience of writing this book has been well worth the effort and personal sacrifice.

M.L.G.
J.H.

CONTENTS

xv

NUTRITION
in Contemporary
Nursing Practice

PART I

THE THEORY OF
HUMAN NUTRITION

Part I presents an overview of nutrition. Both nursing and nutrition use principles from the basic physical sciences of physiology, chemistry, and microbiology and the social sciences of sociology, psychology, and economics to form their theories. Part I introduces the theoretical basis of nutrition in three units: Unit I, an overview of the science of nutrition; Unit II, a study of the functions of the nutrients in the nutritive process; and Unit III, a discussion of nutritional demands and eating patterns in the various stages of the life cycle. These three units provide nursing students with the scientific background they need for a general understanding of nutrition, knowledge that will help them integrate principles of nutrition into their care of clients.

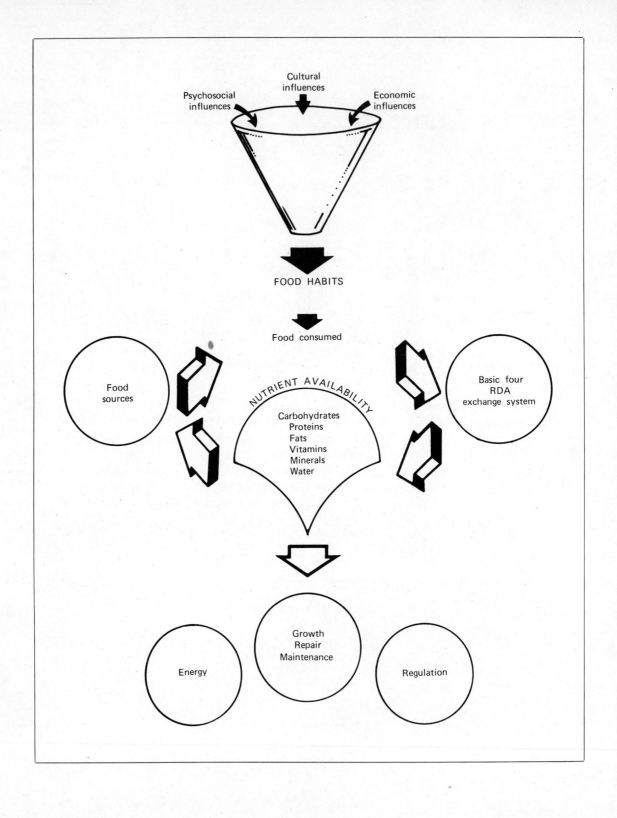

THE SCIENCE OF NUTRITION

Unit I, an overview of the science of nutrition, introduces the main concepts of nutrition, dietary tools, and some practical aspects of the subject. Its purpose is to present nutrition in an interesting way and to supply students with the basic facts and tools they need to understand current nutritional concerns fully. Chapter 1 discusses origins of food habits and helps students gain insight into their personal eating habits and those of their clients. Chapter 2 surveys the major classes of nutrients and their basic physiological functions. Chapter 3 examines the three classes of nutrients that provide Calories for the body and presents a method of classifying foods according to the content of these nutrients.

Chapter 4 describes how human energy requirements are estimated and measured. Chapter 5 examines the subject of weight maintenance and control by explaining the concept of energy balance and imbalance. The food sources of vitamins, minerals, and water are discussed in Chapter 6. Chapter 7 considers several major nutritional concerns in North America, such as the prevalence of malnutrition, the nutritive value of fast foods, food faddism, and vegetarianism. Chapter 8, which explores how the safety and quality of the food supply are maintained, includes information on food production, food processing techniques, and US food laws. The chapter ends with a discussion of family meal planning, economical purchasing of food, and safe storage and preparation of food in the home.

BEHAVIORAL OBJECTIVES

After completing this unit, the student will be able to:

1. Discuss the factors that influence food habits and consumption.
2. Identify food sources for the six major nutrients.
3. Discuss the major functions of the six major nutrients.

4. Given a specific client, identify the factors that determine energy requirements.
5. Discuss alterations in food habits that may lead to nutrient imbalance.
6. Assess factors in his own community that affect the safety and quality of the food supply.

Determinants of Eating Patterns

Josephine Novo Osborne

WHY YOU CHOOSE THE FOODS YOU DO

Food is necessary for survival. Human beings have learned to take in what food is readily available, passed on by their heritage and by their immediate surroundings. Often unquestioning, people eat what is "good for them" because their caretakers say so.

Foods have meaning to everyone and they are tied to each person's way of living. Culture and environment play a significant role in food habits. Beliefs, taboos, and prejudices about food are determined by a person's ethnicity. Both the socioeconomic status of family and community and the emotional makeup of the person also help determine food habits. All this learning occurs mainly in the context of the family.

Foods eaten are those easily obtainable because of their availability, price, and status position in a culture. For example, within a certain region or community, availability of resources (technology and geography) will determine the food that is consumed and thereby influence the food habits of the members of that region. Clams are eaten more on the East Coast than in the Midwest, and lobster is more readily available in Maine than in Utah.

I am indebted to Dr. Jill Armstrong, San Francisco State University, and Beverly Clinton, Department of Nutrition Education, Contra Costa County, Richmond, California, for their ideas and beliefs that are reflected in this chapter.

The *enculturating agents* (those that promote adaptation to a culture and assimilation of its values) of society—like family, religion, and schools—are all very complex and interrelated. It is difficult to say that one agent is more influential than another in determining food habits. Research has stated that the family, particularly the mother and father, play a most significant role in determining what is eaten (Armstrong, 1979; Burt and Hertzler, 1978; Hertzler and Vaughan, 1979). It is important to remember, however, that other aspects of a community influence the adjustment and lifestyle of the families living within it (Hanchett, 1979). Because of this complex interrelationship, nurses need to become aware of the consequences of their actions when they try to change clients' food habits. Nurses need to know what social and cultural changes may occur when food habits are changed within a system (individual, family, or community) (Cassel, 1957; Ritenbaugh, 1978). It is imperative to keep in mind that *no single factor* caused a client to develop his particular food habits. A multicausal approach to the study of the development of food habits is required.

Self-evaluation by the Nurse

To understand and accept their clients' food habits as valid for them, nurses need first to evaluate their own food habits by asking themselves: Why do I eat what I do and what do I feel is appropriate eating behavior for me and others? What are my own attitudes toward food and where did I get them? After

5

one answers these questions, increased self-awareness will occur. Failure to recognize and explore one's own food habits can lead to unwanted effects in the nurse-client relationships, such as labeling clients uncooperative or hard-core resistant when trying to modify their food habits. An *ethnocentric* attitude (believing that one's own way is best and should be desired) in nursing can result only in a breakdown in communication between nurse and client. The facilitative and advocative role of the nurse will be thwarted. Nurses should understand their clients; but they must first know themselves, which enhances their ability to change food habits or teach better ones.

Mills (1977) discussed how to determine one's food habits. She has carried out in the home economics classroom a structured procedure to determine food habits. The following is a modification of that procedure:

1. Write down the different foods that your family might eat almost every day and the reasons for doing so.

2. What foods would you be praised or scolded for eating, and who would administer this and why?

3. What does your family do for leisure times?

4. How is "extra" money spent in your family?

The answers to the questions can provide insight into one's food behavior, attitudes, and values. It is important to remember that there are no right or wrong answers. Everyone is unique. One's food habits are the result of adaptation to one's life events and circumstances.

Questions that are evaluative and provide directions for change ask: are your food habits nutritionally beneficial for you and do they promote an optimal level of wellness for you? Before nurses tell clients what is best, they need to look at what is best for themselves. It is difficult for a nurse to teach about

health and health-promoting ideas when she is not practicing what she is trying to teach. For example, it is difficult for a client to "hear" a nurse talk about obesity and heart disease when the nurse is obviously overweight. This conflict in the nurse can be communicated to the client in subtle and indirect ways (i.e., by nonverbal communication). Because awareness of self is very important in becoming an effective nurse, nurses need to develop healthy attitudes toward food and their own food habits.

Figure 1-1 depicts the interrelationships of the parts of society, the family, and the individual and how they influence food habits. The model shows that the individual is the center and that other factors influence him and his food habits. Those influences are hierarchically arranged, moving toward greater complexity. In assessing a client's food habits, the nurse first identifies the individual as a part of a family system. He is made up of physical, social, and psychological parts, which add up to a complex whole person with interrelated needs and emotions. The parts that determine his reactions to his environment are made up of his values, beliefs, and attitudes. The model moves outward from the self-concept to the family, group, community, and culture. Through the diagrammatic model the nurse can see a multidimensional approach to the development of food habits. The items listed are not all inclusive but serve as examples of the complex interrelationships that determine eating behavior.

Food Habits, Food Beliefs, and Foodways

Food habits are a product of one's food beliefs. These habits are derived from one's total life experience and are very resistant to change. Food habits are defined as what people eat, and the way in which they eat. *Food beliefs* are more complex and subtle and may be religious (e.g., Jewish food

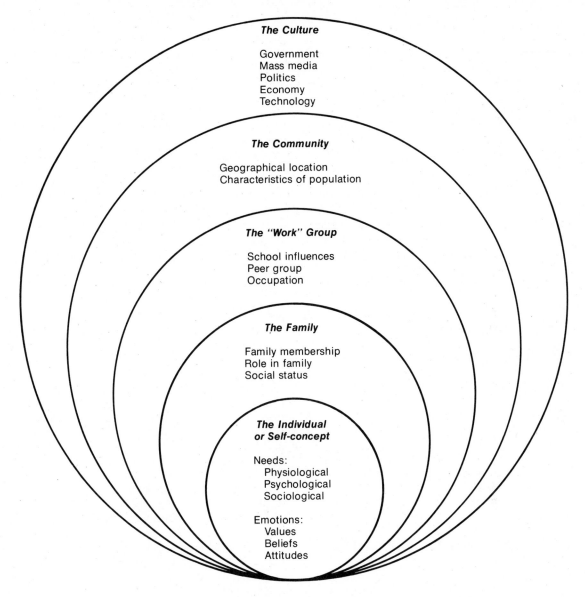

The Culture

Government
Mass media
Politics
Economy
Technology

The Community

Geographical location
Characteristics of population

The "Work" Group

School influences
Peer group
Occupation

The Family

Family membership
Role in family
Social status

The Individual
or Self-concept

Needs:
　Physiological
　Psychological
　Sociological

Emotions:
　Values
　Beliefs
　Attitudes

Figure 1-1. A multidimensional model of the development of food habits.

beliefs), traditional (turkey at Thanksgiving), or medicinal in origin. They are part of the why of what we eat and contribute in large measure to what we feel emotionally about food. This is poetically expressed in the lines from "Aunt Phoebe" by George Sands Bryan,

"What has upheld you on your way?
What has supported you when faint?
On what have you for strength relied?"
"My vittles," said the dear old saint.

Foodways have been defined as the behaviors that influence what people eat, and thus they play an important role in defining the culture of a community (Ritenbaugh, 1978).

The foodways of a culture are broad in scope. They determine both what is food and how it should be prepared. In the United States we do not eat dogs, but in China they were at one time a highly prized delicacy. Another example of a foodway was the practice in nineteenth-century France of permitting only the nobility to eat white bread. Foodways in a society tell a lot about the quality and quantity of life in that society. They tell about the culture of the people. Anthropologists study foodways in a society as a road map to the culture. Nutritionists study foodways to promote an optimal level of wellness among the population.

PSYCHOSOCIAL FRAMEWORK FOR THE STUDY OF FOOD HABITS

To know how psychosocial aspects of humans influence their food habits requires some basic assumptions about human nature. Man is an open system, constantly exchanging matter and energy between himself and his environment. Because of this exchange, he influences and is influenced by his environment. The way he affects his environment is determined by his self-concept. His self-concept is in turn influenced by his interactions with his environment, including those people with whom he comes in contact in his day-to-day

existence. When man reacts to his environment he reacts as a whole. If he breaks his arm, for example, his total being, both physical and emotional, is affected by his injury. If he loses his arm, thus changing a part of him, then he will have to change his whole way of seeing himself in the world and interacting with his environment. In summary, then, man reacts as a whole to stimuli; and if one part of him changes, the whole changes.

As a member of a family unit or similar group, he learns about himself and others. The individual, the family, and the community are all interdependent and interrelated systems within which he learns about his culture and acquires his spiritual and ethnical norms. These norms, or rules to live by, determine, among other things, his emotions about food. Food habits, too, are the result of total experience. Man is motivated to action by physiological needs and by the need for safety, love and affection, esteem (i.e., status and recognition), and *self-actualization* (i.e., creative growth) (Maslow, 1954). When those needs are not met, man is uncomfortable and seeks to meet them. When he is uncomfortable, he is described as in disequilibrium; tending toward comfort is described as moving toward equilibrium. Man tends toward the stabilization of experiences and does this in definable patterns or ways learned through experience with his present resources. For example, he has learned to go to the refrigerator when he is hungry and get some food, and he has learned to keep his hand off the burner of his electric stove while preparing his meal. He may have learned that certain foods are relaxing, so when he is tense he will choose the food that will relieve his tension. Because of this, food behavior has been called a *coping response*, one directed at meeting an unmet need.

Schafer and Yetley (1975) have proposed a model for food behavior. They state that internal factors like hunger, attitudes, and self-concept and external factors like family, friends, and education work together to determine food behavior. Their model is explained diagrammatically in Figure 1-2. The model demonstrates how food behavior is patterned behavior. A person absorbs stimuli from outside himself (external factors) and stimuli from inside himself (internal factors) and then acts toward food in a predictable way. Each person processes that information in a unique manner. Food behavior is, therefore, a response to both internal and external information, from a given situation at a given time, that has been processed by a person according to his previous experiences; and the response is carried out to meet a need.

Selective Perception

A person cannot tune in to all stimuli coming at him at a given time. If he does not filter out some stimuli, he will be overloaded and will have difficulty making decisions. Because of this he tends to develop a frame of reference for deciding what food is good for him, bad for him, or required. To remain in equilibrium (or stabilize his experience) he will tend to seek out information that fits this frame of reference and to avoid information that causes dissonance. Given the frame of reference that vegetarianism is the only way of life, for example, his behavior is likely to include seeking out information on the usefulness of vegetables for meeting body needs and rejecting information on how much meat the body needs daily. When the information that meat or essential amino acids are needed daily for good nutrition is comprehended, the vegetarian may need to restructure his behavior. When a behavior has been accompanied by a cognition (knowledge), then the new information is said to be integrated (Schafer and Yetley, 1975).

People reason about food according to their beliefs. They resist hearing new information or information different from their own because it makes them uncomfortable. Faulty or incorrect beliefs cause inappropriate behavior toward certain foods, and this behavior may be harmful nutritionally. For example, the Zulus of South Africa have held an ancient belief that women during pregnancy or during their menses would exert an evil influence on cattle, and so they were not

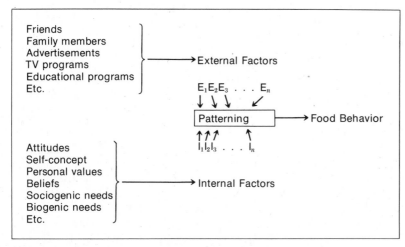

Figure 1-2. Model for observed food behavior. (Copyright The American Dietetic Association. Reprinted by permission from *Journal of the American Dietetic Association*, 66:129, 1975.)

allowed to drink milk during these times. Because men did not know when women were menstruating, they denied women milk most of the time (Cassel, 1957). This belief could be harmful because milk is an important source of calcium. The practice continues, however, because the information that contradicts it is rejected.

To understand people's unique food habits, nurses need to understand how clients have *cognitively* (intellectually) and *affectively* (emotionally) arrived at those food habits and beliefs. Further, nurses need to look at the relationship between clients' needs (what they want for themselves at a given time) and their goals (what they are motivated to do at a given time). Goals will be a reflection of values learned from past experiences. Needs will guide clients in a specific direction that also is a product of past learning. For example, if a person has learned that his anxiety is relieved by eating ice cream, he will tend to engage in that behavior when he feels anxious.

From the time that a baby is fed, food takes on many symbolic meanings to him. The baby will never be able to relate to food as only satisfying his physiological needs for satiety or for nutrients to build and maintain the body. Food has been called the crossroads of emotions, tradition, religion, and habit. Beyond its nutritional value, food is a means of expression and a means by which social relationships are maintained. (Armstrong, 1979)

Food as a Coping Response

Food is often used as reward or punishment. In the United States it is acceptable behavior to give children candy, sweets, or ice cream when they are good or in times of celebration. We can express love and approval by offering food, or we can express disapproval by withholding it. If a child has misbehaved, it is a common practice to withhold dessert or send him to bed without supper. We give a jailed prisoner only bread and water when he has broken prison rules. Adults may continue this symbolism established in childhood throughout their lifetime and, if they have been especially good or have been working hard, reward themselves with a special food or by going out to dinner.

Eating behavior continues when it is positively reinforced. Reinforcement may be physiological, as when hunger is eliminated. Eating may be situational, for example, always eating at a certain time of day or when arriving at Grandma's house or when guests come to visit. Emotional states, like boredom, anger, depression, or loneliness, can influence the quality and quantity of a person's eating.

Communication can occur through food. You can tell a lot about how people feel by observing how they eat. A hostile young woman may refuse to eat because she is angry at her parents, or an elderly patient in a nursing home may request bread and milk at bedtime, recalling the warmth of a mother in happier times. Patients or our significant others may talk back to us through food. The daughter that develops *anorexia nervosa* (a severe case of malnutrition because of a refusal to eat) or the son who feels unloved and tends to stuff himself at mealtime are communicating to us, and the nurse needs to recognize how they are coping with their frustration, anger, aggression or depression, or unmet needs for affection (Chappelle, 1972). Nurses need to be aware of behavior exhibited and understand the meaning of that behavior in relation to food.

People eat for many reasons. Socrates said, "Bad men live that they may eat and drink, whereas good men eat and drink that they may live." People do not always eat because of hunger. Sometimes people eat for emotional reasons. Kozlenko has stated "that the dictates of emotion overpower the subtle cues within signaling that the body has had enough" (cited in Keen, 1978, p. 80). Emotions can often lead to poor eating habits. Figure 1-3 is a survey created by Kozlenko on the emotional investment in food. The reader can use it to find out for himself how much emotional energy he places on food.

	Very Frequent 4	Often 3	Occasionally 2	Seldom 1	Never 0
Eat excessively when bored or depressed					
Insomnia					
Eat foods you know are "bad" for you					
Prefer eating alone					
Feel conspicuous or embarrassed when eating with others					
Parents used, made available, or encouraged sweets					
Fear weight gain					
"Hell with it all" feeling					
Will sneak or hide foods					
Alcoholic beverages					
Eat foods discouraged by parents					
Eat or drink in secrecy					
Drugs (tranquilizers, sleeping pills, appetite suppressants, etc.)					
Self-conscious of how my body looks					
I mistreat myself					
Wish I looked different					
Feelings (diet or otherwise) of being "rushed" or sense of time urgency					
Waves of anger or hostility					
Feelings of being in the midst of "struggle" (over diet or otherwise)					
Fatigue or "wiped out" feelings					
Uncontrollable hunger urges					
Gulp my food					
Stuff myself					
Indulge in sweets					
Eat when not hungry					

Figure 1-3. Emotional investment in food. (Reprinted from *Psychology Today Magazine.* Copyright © 1978, Ziff-Davis Publishing Company.)

Figure 1-3. (Continued)

	Very Frequent 4	Often 3	Occasionally 2	Seldom 1	Never 0
Eat and "run"					
Cravings for sweets					
Meals or heavy snacks after 7 PM					
Eat within an hour of retiring					
Eating binges					

Check the statements according to the appropriate frequency:

Very frequent   Roughly 50% to 90% of the time or almost every to every other day
Often   Roughly 20% to 50% of the time or 1 to 3 times weekly
Occasionally   Roughly 10% of the time or 2 to 3 times monthly
Seldom   Roughly 1% to 3% of the time or from 4 times yearly to once a month
Never   Essentially total avoidance

Scoring:

60 and below: Good relationship with your body, sensitive to physical needs.
61–80:   Average range, for normally healthy people.
81–95:   Eating is based somewhat too much on emotional directives.
96 and above: Excessive emotional interference in eating habits.

SOCIOCULTURAL FACTORS AFFECTING FOOD HABITS

Before exploring cultural influences on food habits, it is important to remember that man is a social being who spends most of his life in groups and plays roles according to norms within those groups. Man is unique because of his ability to communicate with others through symbols. Because of this phenomenon, his ideas, beliefs, attitudes, and values can become traditional ways transmitted across generations. Culture can thus be learned and it can become cumulative. Man's constant inquiry into the nature of things, his questioning and exploring, change his culture

constantly, even though its core identity remains the same. LeVine (1973) defines *culture* as an organized body of rules or norms that tell man how he should communicate, behave, or think about himself. Cultures are those expressions of human existence that are transmitted through the language of a group and its processes. As Armstrong (1979) puts it, "Culture is like a huge web; if you move any of its threads, you are also moving the whole fabric. A culture is an integrated whole; it is the totality of man's behaviors."

Certain generalizations can be made about the cultural influences on eating habits. The first is that most cultures will eat foods in complex mixtures with a preferred staple—

like potatoes for the Irish or the Russians, sometimes called "cultural superfoods"—forming the basis of the meal. Second, to make the food desirable or more palatable, the food is elaborated with spices or flavorings. Third, every cultural group tends to have its unique mixtures, such as the beef bourguignon of the French or the beef Wellington of the English. The continual use of certain foods and their combinations through cultural, technological, and geographical changes shows their value to that cultural group (Church and Doughty, 1976).

Foodways are considered adaptive when they have endured the element of time. Practices that are central to the culture and that have been in existence for generations are more likely to be nutritionally beneficial than are practices that are introduced as recently as this century. For example, the ability to digest milk was thought to be universal, a belief expressed in the advertisement that said, "Everybody needs milk." In the middle of the 1960s, physicians began to consider the possibility of lactose intolerance in people who developed symptoms like intestinal cramps, bloating, and diarrhea after ingesting milk. Researchers have shown a high correlation between the absence of dairying in a population and high rates of lactose intolerance. To introduce milk to certain groups may be detrimental (Ritenbaugh, 1978).

Subculture, Ethnicity, and Region

The United States is a melting pot of many different subcultural and ethnic groups. A *subculture* reflects the qualities of its culture but with some distinctive differences in role behavior and normative patterns (Cardwell, 1971). The subculture is closer to the individual members of society, and sometimes it can be at variance with the larger social group. Subcultures can be ethnic (such as Chinese), religious (e.g., Jewish), educational (academic), or economic (middle class) (Cardwell, 1971). People develop a distinct ethnicity through their interactions with their cultural and subcultural groups. Longstreet (1978) gives an innovative and distinct definition of *ethnicity* that is very relevant to the development of food habits and gives some understanding of why they are so ingrained in humans and so resistant to change: ethnicity is "that portion of cultural development that occurs before the individual is in complete command of his or her abstract intellectual powers and that is formed primarily through the individual's early contact with family, neighbors, friends, teachers and others, as well as with his immediate environment of the home and neighborhood" (p. 19).

Although people may have some control over their cultural, subcultural, and ethnic ways, some values may be so integrated that a complete awareness of their origin may be virtually impossible. How does all this influence our food habits or foodways? Food patterns and habits are one of the last cultural and ethnic traits to change. People retain their old ways, and a lot of inferences can be made about a specific subculture by studying its foodways. It can be concluded that early influences with significant others in the context of the family and community will greatly determine what foods we eat, what foods we believe are good for us or bad for us, how and where the foods should be eaten, and what foods should be eaten on what occasions. Steelman (1976) found that attitudes toward food vary with subcultures and that these subcultural variables are related to possible differences in value systems.

Individual subcultural groups are identifiable in the United States' pluralistic society, and the cultural pluralist works hard to maintain that individuality. For example, Chinese food is readily available; Mexican food has become more popular; and Soul Food is gaining wider acceptance. All of these are now part of the mainstream foodways of the United States, but there is still an "American" foodway which is common to all; it includes the "Big Mac" hamburger, the traditional fried chicken, corn on the cob in the summertime, and roast turkey for Thanksgiving dinner. Subcultural food patterns change because of the availability of foods, the prices, and the current food preferences of the group. The major identifiable cultural food patterns in the United States are shown in Figure 1-4.

Distinctive subcultural eating patterns are greatly influenced by the area in which people live, because of the availability of the food. The creole food of New Orleans is an example of the integration of the resources available to the people of the region with their cultural heritage. What they could grow and gather from their location determined the characteristics of creole food. This principle is illustrated in Figure 1-5. Readers can try to identify the reasons for the characteristic foodways of the different geographical regions from seeing the foods produced in each area.

Nurses need to recognize that eating habits and patterns vary with individuals and that characteristic cultural patterns can be observed among different nationalities and religious groups. A Jewish client might get deathly ill after eating pork, or a Seventh-Day Adventist might think he has done something very wrong after drinking an alcoholic beverage. A well-meaning nurse trying to help a client might find she has insulted him inadvertently. A story told by Fathauer (1960) at a time when cultural differences in food habits were not considered, serves as a good example. A well-meaning oil company felt sorry for its undernourished Arab workers and provided them with a nutritious meal at lunchtime—cafeteria style. The Arab workers were very angry and insulted because only beggars stand in line for food in their country.

Figure 1-4. Cultural food habits. (Adapted from *Cultural Food Patterns in the U.S.A.,* published by the American Dietetic Association, 1976.)

Chinese Food Habits

Milk: Considered luxury item, even disliked. Cheese rarely used, except in Northern China a cheese-type product from goat's or cow's milk.
Suggestions: Encourage use of milk in cereals or steamed eggs (pudding). Encourage milk cheese, ice cream, and bean curd.

Meat: Limited, mostly pork, fish and eggs, some chicken, shellfish; sometimes excluded from diet of children.
Suggestions: Encourage increased use of meat, fish, poultry, and eggs. Introduce "baby food meat" for children.

Vegetables and fruits: Spinach, broccoli, leeks, greens, bok toy (cabbage), carrots, pumpkin, sweet potatoes, mushrooms, soybeans, brussel sprouts, turnips, radishes, kohlrabi, white eggplant, yautia, eggplant, bambo shoots, and snowpeas.
Fruits considered a delicacy—snack food, some reserved for men. Fruits common: persimmon, peaches, plums, pears, large dates, apples, figs, winter melon, bananas, mango, red tangerines, papaya, pineapple, orange, litchee nuts, figs, small dates.
Suggestions: Increased use of fruits or vegetables high in vitamin C as snack or "dessert."

Breads and cereals: Millet and rice predominant; wheat products include noddles and steamed bread.
Suggestions: Encourage use of brown rice.

Miscellaneous: Soybean oil, peanut oil, and lard are used.
Suggestions: Affirm practice of limited use of fats but encourage liquid types.

Figure 1-4. (*Continued*)

Italian Food Habits

Milk: Adults use little except in coffee. Seldom thought of as food. Children may or may not get recommended amounts.

Cheese used frequently, and in preparation of cooked foods.

Suggestions: Encourage use of milk for all the family. Greater use of dry skim milk and evaporated can be encouraged. Encourage wider use of cheeses at end of meal with fruit and in cooking.

Meat: Veal, beef, pork, and chicken are most popular. All parts are eaten including organ meats. Highly seasoned meats are common. All kinds of fish, both fresh and canned, some fried in oil, used in stews or chowders.

Eggs are liked, the most expensive grades preferred.

Dried beans and peas are used in soups with pasta and served in salads.

Suggestions: Encourage cooking methods other than frying. Discourage the use of highly seasoned fatty and fried meats for small children.

Fish, eggs, dried peas and beans, and ricotta cheese make good meat substitutes.

Vegetables and fruits: Large quantities of escarole, swiss chard, mustard greens, dandelion greens, and broccoli are popular. Salads are part of most meals. Peppers and tomatoes are used in preparation of foods. Eggplant, zucchini, artichoke, mushrooms, and fava beans are favorites.

Fruits liked: Grapes, oranges, tangerines, figs, persimmons, and pomegranates.

Suggestions: Less cooking time and less use of oil. Encourage use of canned tomatoes when fresh are out of season.

Selection of fresh fruit in season and canned fruit juices when less expensive than fresh.

Bread and cereal: Pasta and rice are staples eaten each meal. Use of oatmeal and farina has increased.

Suggestions: Encourage use of whole grain bread.

Miscellaneous: Olive oil preferred for cooking. Lard and salt port are flavoring for soups and tomato sauce. Butter preferred for baking.

Suggestions: Urge families to use soybean, cottonseed, and corn oils.

Japanese Food Habits

Milk: Milk fresh and canned is used in small amounts, in coffee and milk desserts, such as ice cream. Cheese is used in only small amounts.

Suggestions: Encourage increased consumption of all forms of milk, including use of cheese.

Meat: Variety of salt and fresh water fish eaten, baked, boiled, and in soups. Raw fish consumed on occasion. Smoked, dried, and canned fish consumed. Beef, pork, and poultry preferred to lamb and veal, mixed with vegetables and seasoned with soy sauce. Eggs eaten raw, fried, boiled, scrambled, and in soups.

Suggestions: Encourage use of highly nutritious variety meats, hard and soft cheeses and cottage cheese for protein. Discourage eating raw eggs. Use of pea and bean dishes as well as peanut butter can be encouraged.

Vegetables and fruits: Commonly used vegetables are spinach, broccoli, carrots, green beans, peas, cauliflower, tomatoes, cucumbers, eggplant, peppers, and squash. May be prepared with meat, fish, and chicken. Fruits eaten are oranges, tangerines, grapefruit, apples, pears, and melons.

Suggestions: Encourage cooking procedures to preserve nutrients. Discourage par-cooking and draining of water. Emphasize use of fruits high in vitamin C.

Breads and cereals: Polished white rice is the staple. Consumption of wheat products is a post–World War II practice.

Figure 1-4. *(Continued)*

Suggestions: Encourage use of restored rice and discourage washing them prior to cooking. Suggest more frequent inclusion of potatoes cooked in skin in place of rice. Urge use of whole grain breads and cereals.

Miscellaneous: Butter used in small amount. Fat used in food only for deep fat frying. Simple cakes and cookies of sugar and rice flour contain little or no fat.

Seasonings are soy sauce or Miso sauce. Pickles with high salt content eaten in variety.

Suggestions: Seasonings and pickles should be used in moderation.

Jewish Food Habits

Milk: Dietary Laws prohibit using meat and milk at the same meal. (Six hours must elapse after a meat meal before dairy foods may be eaten; half an hour must elapse after a dairy food before meat may be eaten).

Cheeses—American, Muenster, and Swiss—well liked. Cottage cheese and pot cheese eaten plain or in blintzes and noodle puddings.

Suggestions: Encourage use of milk at breakfast and lunch times to insure adequate milk intake. Explain that cream cheese is a fat, not a milk substitute and encourage cheeses high in protein and calcium.

Meat: Separate dishes and utensils must be used for preparing and serving meat and dairy products.

Orthodox Jews use only the forequarters (rib section forward) of quadrupeds with a cloven hoof who chew their cud, i.e., cattle, sheep, goat, and deer. Animals and poultry must be slaughtered by a ritual slaughterer (shochet) according to specified regulations. Before cooking, meat is koshered by one of two methods: (1) soaking it in cold water for half an hour; salting it with coarse salt (koshering salt); and draining it to let blood run off. It is then thoroughly washed under cold running water and drained again before cooking. (2) Quick searing. Liver, for example, cannot be koshered by soaking and salting because of its high blood content. It is, therefore, rinsed, drained well, and broiled on a grill. It may then be fried, chopped, or combined with other foods. This second method is preferred for patients on salt restricted diets.

Meat is usually broiled, boiled, roasted, or stewed with vegetables added. Fish that have fins and scales may be used, such as whitefish (fresh and as gefilte fish); smoked sable; karp, lox (salmon); and caviar.

Shellfish (such as oysters, crab, and lobster) and scavenger fish such as sturgeon and catfish are not allowed.

Fish and eggs are considered "pareve" or neutral and may be eaten as dairy or meat.

Eggs are eaten in abundance. An egg with a clot of blood must be discarded.

Dried beans, peas, lentils are eaten liberally, especially as soup.

Suggestions: Discourage excessive use of delicatessen-type meats, such as corned beef, pastrami, and salami.

Urge use of fish, cheese, and other sources of protein.

Vegetables and fruits: Greens, spinach, sorrel leaves are used for Schav, a soup. Use is made of broccoli, carrots, chicory, sweet potatoes, and yams. Green peppers often stuffed with meat or dairy mixture. Green cabbage is cooked slightly and stuffed with beef and raisin mixture with tomato sauce. Root vegetables and potatoes are liberally used. Noodles as a potato substitute are preferred to rice. Beets are used in soup (borscht).

Orange or grapefruit used for breakfast. Cooked dried fruits (prunes, raisins, apples, peaches, pears, apricots) are commonly served with meat meal.

Suggestions: Stress more variety in use of dark green leafy and deep yellow vegetables, their correct method of cooking with small amount of water, covered pot and short cooking time.

Point out high caloric value of dried fruits.

Breads and cereals: Water rolls (bagel), rye bread, and pumpernickel are often used, as these do not have milk or milk solids and, therefore, can be eaten with meat or dairy meals. They are considered "pareve" or

Figure 1-4. *(Continued)*

neutral. Matzoth, also "pareve," is the only bread product allowed during Passover, but is commonly used throughout the year. Whole grains such as oatmeal, barley, brown rice, buckwheat groats (kasha) are used.

Suggestions: Encourage use of whole wheat bread at dairy meals. Matzoth, crackers, and saltines are not enriched and make little contribution to diet, other than Calories.

Miscellaneous: Sweet (unsalted) butter, usually whipped, is preferred to salted butter. Vegetable oils and shortenings are considered "pareve" or neutral. Chicken fat is often the choice for browning meats and frying potato pancakes.

Danish pastries, coffee cakes, homemade cakes and cookies may be eaten in large quantities. Honey cakes are served for various holidays.

There may be an overuse of relishes.

Soup may be used at every meal.

Soft drinks are served with meat meals when milk is forbidden.

Suggestions: The code "U" on a package indicates it is permissible. If in doubt check with local rabbinical authorities. Encourage greater use of vegetable oils.

Encourage desserts such as milk puddings, ice milk, ice cream, for dairy meals and fruit with meat meals.

Encourage soups high in daily nutrient needs. Discourage overuse of soft drinks.

Polish Food Habits

Milk: Children drink fresh milk, while adults may prefer buttermilk. Sour cream is also popular, used in soup, salad dressings, with berries, and raw vegetables.

Cheese is well liked. Cottage cheese is well liked and may be served with sour cream.

Suggestions: Encourage recommended intake of milk or milk products for whole family.

Meat: Meat commonly consumed—beef, pork, pigs' knuckles, sausages, smoked and cured pork, chicken, goose, duck and variety meats (liver, tripe, tongue, brains). Small amounts used in soups and stews. Fish, fresh, smoked, dried, or pickled, is used. Eggs well liked and also used in pancakes, noodles, dumplings and soups, along with legumes.

Suggestions: For economy greater use of meat substitutes and less expensive cuts of meat in the preparation of stews and soups. Greater amounts of meat may be desirable in mixed dishes.

Vegetables and fruits: Potatoes are a very important part of diet. Other popular vegetables include carrots, beets, turnips, cauliflower, kohlrabi, broccoli, sorrel, green pepper, peas, spinach, and green beans.

Vitamin C–rich fruits are not traditionally popular but citrus fruits may be used more today than in previous years. Dried fruits are liked.

Suggestions: Encourage retention of vitamin A in use of broccoli, kale, sorrel, green peppers, raw cabbage, fresh tomato in season, and canned and frozen citrus juices in off-season may be stressed for vitamin C.

Encourage proper cooking methods for retention of vitamin C in vegetables.

Stress use of root vegetables and fruits and vegetables in season.

Breads and cereals: Bread eaten with each meal. Pumpernickel, sour rye bread, and white bread are well liked. Sweet buns are common. Oatmeal, rice, noodles, dumplings, cornmeal, porridge and kasha are prominent.

Suggestions: Encourage whole grains.

Miscellaneous: Wide variety of fats and oils are used. Fond of candy, sweet cakes, and other sweets such as honey.

Coffee with cream and sugar is a favorite beverage. Tea is infrequent.

Polish foods are highly salted and seasoned.

Suggestions: Suggest more frequent use of fruits as desserts.

Figure 1-4. (Continued)

Puerto Rican Food Habits

Milk: Milk may be used in insufficient quantities due to economic conditions rather than because it is not liked. Although milk may not be consumed as such, a cup of cafe con leche may contain two to five ounces of milk.

The domestic American cheese is used in limited quantities. Native white cheese (resembling farmer cheese, but firmer and saltier) is used, but is expensive.

Suggestions: Use of milk as a beverage and in cooking may need to be encouraged, including evaporated milk, nonfat dry milk and in puddings and cereals.

Greater emphasis can be placed on use of cheese.

Meat: Chicken in combination with other foods is frequently eaten. Expensive cuts of pork and beef are usually fried. Ham butts and sausage used to flavor different dishes. The intestine of the pig is eaten either fried (cuchifritos) or stewed with native vegetables (salcocho) and chick-peas.

Fish is used in limited amounts, salt codfish is common. Eggs used in cooking and fried and scrambled eggs are popular.

Beans are eaten either cooked or served with rice daily. A sauce called "refrito" (green pepper, tomato, garlic, and lard) is served with beans and rice. Pigeon and chick-peas are popular.

Suggestions: Variety meats may be used in increased amounts. Emphasize lean, tender, and lower cost cuts with slow cooking methods.

Suggest that use of cuchifritos be limited to holidays. Encourage larger quantities of vegetables and meat as well as peas in salcocho.

More consumption of fresh, frozen, or canned fish.

Greater use of eggs as a main dish and meat substitute. Suggest larger amounts of beans than rice. Milk, meat, chicken, cheese, or fish should be eaten with the bean meal for protein. Pigeon peas are more expensive than chick-peas, and chick-peas protein is almost as good as that of the soybean.

Vegetables and fruits: Expensive imported vegetables, such as yautia, apio, malanga, name, plantain are frequently used. These viandas are high in starch and have fair amounts of B vitamins, iron, and vitamin C. Pumpkins, carrots, green pepper, tomatoes, and sweet potatoes are well liked. Pumpkin is used to thicken and flavor foods. Potatoes are eaten in small amounts in stews, soups, or are fried. Head lettuce, cabbage, fresh tomatoes, and onions are often salad ingredients. Long cooking of vegetables in stews is common.

Imported fruits are used often. Fruit cocktail, canned pears, and peaches are liked. Peach, apricot, and pear nectar are commonly used.

Suggestions: Encourage use of less expensive vegetables such as carrots, beets, yellow squash, turnips. Root vegetables may be prepared and served same way as tubers (plantain, yautia, yucca, name).

Urge use of more cooked and raw green leafy vegetables. Stress greater intake of other salad greens and cabbage. Emphasize correct cooking methods of vegetables, small amount of water, covered pot and short time.

Greater use of potatoes cooked in skin can be suggested.

Greater amount of citrus juices, fresh, frozen, or canned can be used. Encourage use of bananas and pineapple in season, also apples and pears. Recommend use of fruits canned in light rather than heavy syrup.

Breads and cereals: Bread used in only small amounts. Plantain is often eaten in place of bread. French bread, rolls, and crackers are most frequent choices.

Breakfast cereals—oatmeal, farina, cornmeal, and cornflakes are increasing. Cereals are often cooked in milk instead of water.

Suggestions: Encourage use of whole grain breads, enriched or brown rice. Encourage cooking cereal in milk. Use of sugar-coated cereals should be discouraged.

Figure 1-4. (*Continued*)

Miscellaneous: Butter is used in small amounts on bread. Lard and salt pork are used for flavoring in large amounts. Olive oil is favorite for salads.

Sugar is liberally used in beverages and desserts. Cakes, pies, guava, orange and mango pastes, and boiled papaya preserves are favored often between meals.

Black malt beer is a favorite beverage, and is combined with beaten egg for convalescents and pregnant women. It contains a fair amount of iron and some B vitamins and is high in Calories.

Canned soups are often served as main dish.

Suggestions: Suggest margarine in place of butter. Corn, cottonseed, or soybean oils in seasoning vegetables and other dishes rather than lard and salt pork.

Encourage less frequent use of sugar. Recommend use of other nourishing beverages such as milk and fruit juices.

Stress meal planning around a main dish made of a protein food rather than soups of low protein value.

Southern United States Food Habits

Milk: Limited amounts of milk are consumed. Buttermilk often preferred.

Cheese is well liked in sandwiches and baked macaroni.

Suggestions: Encourage use of evaporated and nonfat dry milk for both cooking and drinking, and greater use of cheese.

Meat: Chicken as "company" dish is enjoyed. Pork and variety meats are popular. Pigs' feet, hog jowls, ham hocks, cured ham, and heart are often eaten, stewed, boiled with vegetables, or fried. Spareribs are baked or barbecued. Lungs, kidneys, and brains are floured and fried. Chitterlings (intestines) are cut, dredged with cornmeal or flour, and fried crisp.

Beef is used in hash or stewed with vegetables. Cured tongue is also eaten.

Fish and shellfish, fresh, and canned, Swannee River catfish dipped in cornmeal and fried, boiled shrimp, fried scallops, and fried, stewed or raw oysters are popular.

Game—rabbit, squirrel, opossum—are usually used in a stew.

Eggs are usually fried.

Legumes and nuts—dried black-eyed peas and beans cooked with salt pork—are prominent part of meal. Peanuts and peanut butter are consumed.

Suggestions: Emphasize the lean, economical cuts of meat and stress that salt pork and bacon are fats not meats. Encourage stewing, baking, roasting, and boiling as methods of cookery.

Stress that white or brown eggs are equally nutritious, Grade B for cooking.

Urge that milk or cheese be served with the "bean meal."

Vegetables and fruits: Vegetables are liked but few eaten raw. Leafy greens, turnip greens, mustard greens, collards, cabbage, and green beans are cooked in water with bacon, ham hocks or salt pork. The cooking liquid may be eaten with cornbread. Tomatoes, fresh and canned, white potatoes, sweet potatoes, fried, baked, or candied with syrup are popular.

Fruits, although little citrus fruit, may be eaten. Fruits in season are eaten between meals and watermelon and lemonade are favorites in the summer.

Suggestions: Discuss quick-cooking of vegetables in little water to save vitamins. Note that addition of baking soda to water in which vegetables are cooked destroys the vitamins.

Stress that cooked or raw vegetables should be served in addition to potatoes or legumes.

Point out value of fruits. For limited budgets encourage serving citrus fruit or juice as well as cheaper grades of canned tomatoes, raw cabbage, "greens," and potatoes for vitamin C.

Figure 1-4. (Continued)

Breads and cereals: Few whole grain cereals are used. Hominy grits with gravy, hot biscuits with molasses, and cornbread are eaten.

White or polished rice cooked and combined with ham fat, tomatoes, onion, and okra is popular. Dumplings, pancakes, and hoecakes (originally baked on a hoe) are favorites.

Suggestions: Teach use of whole grain breads and cereals. Stress use of cooked cereals such as oatmeal. Emphasize inclusion of protein food such as meat or milk when casserole-is served.

Miscellaneous: Bacon and salt pork are liberally used. Lard used for baking and frying. Butter for preparing desserts. Gravies are used generously.

Sweets in cakes, cookies, pies, other pastries, and sweet breads are popular. Molasses and cane syrup are employed as sweeteners. Ice cream, jams, and jellies are eaten. Soft drinks consumed by children.

Suggestions: Discourage use of large amounts of bacon and salt pork where overweight and salt restrictions are factors. Suggest methods of cooking other than frying. Encourage use of margarine and oil.

Since rich desserts may tend to displace protective foods, especially in the low-income food budget, they should be used only in moderation. Excessive intake of sweets should be avoided, especially by small children.

Spanish American—Mexican Food Habits

Milk: Milk may be limited due to availability and economy.

Limited amounts of cheese are used.

Suggestions: Utilize various forms of milk in cookery, as a beverage—dried, evaporated or fresh milk. Increase use of cheeses to improve quality of protein in diet.

Meat: Chicken, pork chops, weiners and cold cuts and hamburgers usually used only once or twice a week.

Eggs used frequently fried. In rural areas, many have their own chickens.

Beans are usually eaten with every meal, cooked, mashed, or refried with lard.

Suggestions: Emphasis on variety of lower cost meats and cooking methods may provide more frequent use of meats.

Eggs are good meat substitute and daily consumption is encouraged.

Beans and lentils provide good source of protein and calcium. Their protein is enhanced when eaten with animal proteins such as milk, meat, eggs, or cheese.

Vegetables and fruits: Fried potatoes are basic, maybe three times a day.

Chilies from green and red peppers are popular each meal. These items are good sources of vitamin A even when dried. Green peppers are usually called "mangoes."

Fresh tomatoes are purchased the year around and most popular vegetable. Occasionally canned tomatoes are used.

Pumpkin, corn, field greens, onions, and carrots are used frequently.

Bananas, melons, peaches, and canned fruit cocktail are popular. Oranges and apples are used as snacks.

Suggestions: Encourage wide variety of vegetables. Different cooking methods could be used. Encourage use of peppers but stress caution in home canning methods.

Recommend a variety of fruit canned in light syrup as economical. Use of citrus fruits could be encouraged. Fruit drinks should not be substituted for fruit juices.

Melons (cantaloupe in particular) are encouraged due to high vitamin C content.

Breads and cereals: Bread is a popular item. Tortillas from enriched wheat flour are made daily. Sweet rolls are purchased. Purchased bread for sandwiches in sack lunches is a status symbol.

Breakfast cereals are usually prepared type with emphasis on sugar coated. Occasionally oatmeal is used.

Fried macaroni is prepared and served with beans and potatoes.

Figure 1-4. (*Continued*)

Suggestions: Continue use of enriched flour. In some sections where corn tortillas are used, encourage use of dried skim milk.

Encourage whole grain cereals. Cooked cereals more economical.

Encourage use of vegetables rather than excessive starch foods.

Miscellaneous: Lard, salt pork, and bacon fat are used liberally. Most foods are fried.

Soft drinks, popsicles, and sweets of all kinds are used liberally.

Suggestions: Encourage a variety of cookery procedures.

Purchased cookies, soft drinks, and sweets are expensive and do not contribute to nutritional needs. Utilizing more milk, ice cream, and juices would be helpful.

Food Habits as Role Modeling and Compliance

Strong rejections or desires for foods are learned either through role-modeling behavior (e.g., a model conveys the idea it is really masculine to eat a hearty steak) or through compliance (a strong desire to please the caretaker or food distributor, usually the mother). Frequently food preferences have more to do with associations with others and their attitudes toward food than with the nutrient value of the food. A person's associations tell him what to have an appetite for and when to have it. Somehow it does not seem right to have stew for breakfast or cornflakes for supper if it is customary not to eat those foods at that time.

Symbolic Meaning of Food

Because of its symbolic aspects food means more than satisfying hunger. To a young child, it can mean love. It may mean that one has been good and should be rewarded or that one has done something wrong and needs to be punished (e.g., go without dessert for misbehavior). Food's culturally determined symbolic meanings may be associated with mother love. For example, bread and milk given to a child at bedtime by his mother may symbolize affection and security. Turkey may be associated with Thanksgiving, or plum pudding or "special" cookies with Christmas. Ceremonial and social purposes of meals may be more important than nutrition in determining what people eat (Douglas, 1979).

Structure of Meals

According to Douglas (1979), meals have a consistent structure so people know what to expect. This is observed through what she calls *spatial layout,* whereby foods are arranged on a plate in a particular way or served in a particular order. In the United States at a dinner party, the appetizer is generally served first and the dessert and coffee last, for example. Therefore, when cultural barriers are crossed, the usual stop and start signals may be missed, leaving a person hungry or overstuffed. Douglas maintains that this may be the reason people often feel hungry shortly after eating Chinese food or overstuffed after eating in the European manner.

Mealtimes allow individuals and groups to communicate with one another in a unique way. Mealtimes, particularly those on special occasions with their distinctive foods, can be a time when social roles are observed, for culturally transmitted rules of conduct determine the behavior of the participants. Many inferences about a group's functioning and its participants can be made by watching their behavior at these times. The person with most

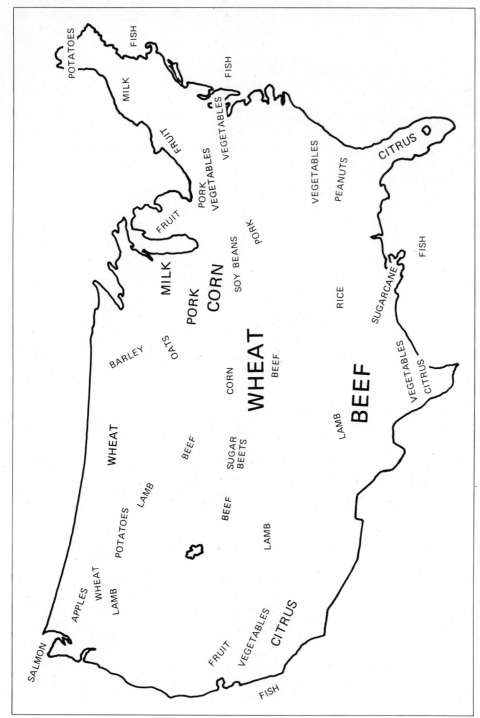

Figure 1-5. Typical food types grown in various regions of the United States.

influence may be served first. Children may be seen but not heard at mealtime. Power and authority can be observed.

Foods as Social Status

There are social influences on food choice such as foods for the rich and foods for the poor. An item that is expensive or difficult to obtain, such as escargots or crepes suzette, may be more prized. Refined sugar was once considered a luxury, but today it seems more fashionable to obtain the harder-to-get "natural" sugar. Upper-class Asians preferred polished white rice to the more nutritious unpolished variety, risking a vitamin B deficiency to remain identified with the upper class. Because French royalty at one time forbade white bread to commoners, white bread was for years more desired by that culture and ours. Now it seems to be in "better taste" to eat whole wheat bread or bread baked by one's own hands.

Steelman found in her study (1976) that foods that have a higher social status are more likely to be accepted by homemakers. To persuade more people to eat liver, its consumption must be viewed as more prestigious than it is in the United States today. Housewives will buy a steak for a special occasion because it is prestigious, not necessarily because it is nutritious or tasty. Corned beef and cabbage was once considered a "poor man's food," so it was not served on a special occasion. If needed dietary changes can be placed in a high-status category, they are more likely to be accepted.

Mass Media and Food Habits

Children in the United States spend a lot of time in front of the television set. What they see strongly influences their food habits. There they hear of special breakfast cereals they should eat. The sugar-coated variety may have the greatest appeal because it was "shot from guns" or because of its strong identification with some "hero." These young children may persuade the shopper to buy the special cereal although its nutritional value can be questioned.

Adults are enticed by advertisements for books that guarantee "weight loss in one week while you still eat your favorite foods." A large number of people buy them because who does not want to lose weight—painlessly? Looking in bookstores and discovering the number of books that tell people what they should or should not eat can be a very interesting experience.

Radio commentator Carlton Fredericks and others popularized the evils of sugar and suggested eating more protein would make it possible to avoid low blood sugar. This problem became for many people a rationalization for their real problems when they felt down (Keen, 1978a). Low blood sugar seemed both fashionable to have and plausible as an explanation for many problems.

The back-to-nature trend has been fostered by Madison Avenue, and they have "baptized everything from hair spray to potato chips with the magic words 'Natural—Nothing Artificial Added' " (Keen, 1978b, p. 62). How have *your* food habits been influenced by the media?

Jalso et al. (1965) studied nutritional beliefs and practices of 340 subjects and found that the aging population with a limited formal education and income were more likely to be influenced in their food habits by magazines and newspapers. Hence one way to combat food faddism is to present valid nutritional information to them in magazines and newspapers.

Economics and Eating Behavior

The literature frequently speaks of the cost of the item in determining food selection (Reaburn et al., 1979), and economics does play a major role in determining food habits (Mead, 1970; Queen, 1957). People suffering from poverty and resulting malnutrition frequently know how to eat better, but their eating habits are the result of lack of money to buy more expensive foods such as fresh fruits and meats.

Queen (1957) gave a most interesting argument for economics playing a more important role than cultural influences in determining food habits. He stated that in a relatively isolated, "primitive" society the people tend to eat the foods that are readily available, as, for example, olive oil on the Iberian Peninsula. Isolated from other groups, people develop customs and norms around their food. As they come into contact with other societies because of available transportation, they tend to vary their diet by making use of the greater variety of foods that transportation also makes available. Technology and transportation affect food availability; and ability to pay determines food usage and in turn promotes availability, which affects cost. At one time it was very rare to find artichokes or avocados from California in the midwestern supermarkets. Now they are more prevalent and less expensive than 20 years ago. In parts of the United States veal is less expensive and more readily available because of its higher consumption rate. Certain ethnic groups have devised special recipes for veal, such as scallopine or Parmesan, creating a greater desire to serve veal.

Social Problems and Food Habits

Because food habits are the result of a group's past history and its interaction with its present environment, it is best, when a client has a problem with a food habit to look for the meaning this food habit has for the client. Obvious social problems such as poverty, family breakdown, or alcoholism can influence food habits. Although poverty can cause a reduction in the variety of foods available to a group, and the resulting lack of many important foods in the diet (rather than preferred patterns of eating) may cause malnutrition, Cornely et al. (1963) found another reason people in poverty sometimes have malnutri-

tion. Studying the nutritional beliefs of low-income populations, they found a lack of sufficient information about the essentials of an adequate diet. It can be argued that this lack of knowledge occurred because of economic reasons and not because of a lack of motivation to learn. A third cause of malnutrition is family breakdown, which may lay the foundation for poor food habits because of an inadequate role model or the lack of a role model. Time schedules and roles may be diffused so that the eating habits of the family are irregular or inconsistent.

Alcoholism is another major social problem affecting food habits. It is a leading health problem in this country, to the extent that some authorities rank it fourth among major health problems (Nat'l Instit. of Mental Health, 1974). Alcoholics frequently have poor eating habits; because alcohol satisfies hunger, they tend to skip meals. This in turn tends to interfere with metabolism and the absorption of certain vitamins. If the alcoholic is married, economic problems can occur, particularly if the alcoholic is the breadwinner. If the alcoholic is the mother, children may lack the consistency of responses and patterning of the behavior essential to learning healthy eating habits.

Food Fallacies

Briggs and Calloway (1979) discussed common fallacious beliefs about certain foods. It is difficult to determine the origin of these beliefs, but many people tenaciously hold on to them, even today. Readers should see how many of the beliefs in Figure 1-6 they themselves hold.

PSYCHOCULTURAL EQUIVALENCES IN DETERMINING FOOD BEHAVIOR

Armstrong (1979) has an interesting and provocative term she has originated in relation to

Figure 1-6. Fallacies and facts about foods. (From *Bogert's Nutrition and Physical Fitness*, 10th Ed., by George M. Briggs and Doris Howes Calloway. Copyright © by W. B. Saunders Company. Copyright 1931, 1935, 1939, 1943, 1949, 1954, 1960, 1966, and 1973 by W. B. Saunders Company. Reprinted by permission of Holt, Rinehart and Winston.)

Fallacies	Facts
About certain foods	
Onions—cure a cold. Fish—is a brain food. Celery—is a nerve tonic. Oysters—increase sexual potency.	Foods in the same food group are more or less interchangeable, and the different tissues take up whatever nutritive elements they need from the blood stream, to which common reservoir of body-building materials all foods have contributed when they were absorbed after digestion. Special foods do not build special tissues.
Lemons—aid digestion. Oranges—cause acid stomach.	Acid fruits are supposed by some to be a cure for dyspepsia and by others to cause acid stomach. The stomach secretes a digestive fluid that contains hydrochloric acid, which is many times more strongly acid than lemons. If we did not have an acid stomach, conditions would be very abnormal and unfavorable for digestion.
Meats—necessary to build muscle and red blood. —extra amounts needed for muscular work. —poison the system.	Meats, especially organ meats, are excellent sources of iron, protein, and B vitamins, which are important for regeneration of red blood cells and plasma proteins. However, other foods, such as eggs and leafy vegetables, also furnish these nutrients. The energy for muscular work comes mostly from oxidation of carbohydrate and fat. If meats are inspected (free of bacteria and spoilage), kept refrigerated, and well cooked, they can have no harmful effects.
Combinations of foods	
Some food combinations are to be feared or shunned (fish and ice cream, tomatoes and milk).	Fear of certain foods or food combinations is psychologically bad and may lead to one-sided diets which do not provide essential nutrients in adequate quantity. When eaten in moderate amounts and under proper conditions, there are no foods that are incompatible. Selection of foods from all food groups, in the suggested number and size of servings, furnishes a better balanced diet, and thus one that is better for building health.
Nature cults	
Foods should be eaten in their natural state, mostly raw.	It is good to eat some foods raw, but others (such as whole grains and meats) are usually cooked to soften fiber, develop flavor, and promote their digestibility. If properly cooked, the loss of minerals and vitamins is moderate.
Natural sugars, such as honey and raw sugar, are better for one than refined sugar.	Although one may enjoy honey or raw sugar for the traces of impurities which give them flavor, they are no better as body fuel than refined sugar (cane or beet). The small amounts of minerals and vitamins in the unrefined products do not add appreciably to the whole day's quota, which must be furnished chiefly by other types of food.

Figure 1-6. (Continued)

Fallacies	Facts
Opposition to use of:	
Iodized salt	Adding small amounts of iodide to refined sea salt is simply replacing the iodine lost in the refining process. Use of iodized salt has proved a safe and effective way of preventing simple goiter in regions where both the water and soil are iodine-poor.
Fluoridated water	Addition of fluorine compounds to city water supplies in areas where water has less than normal amounts of this element represents regulating the naturally low fluorine content to a level that is entirely safe but sufficient to effectively reduce dental caries.
Pasteurized milk	Pasteurization of milk gives important protection against harmful bacteria and does insignificant damage to the nutrients in milk, except for some loss of vitamin C. The normal content of this vitamin in milk is too low and undependable to be counted on in the diet, so that it must be supplemented anyway by one or more rich sources of this vitamin.
Highly milled grains	
—should never be used.	Either whole or highly milled grains are good sources of energy and furnish some protein. However, the removal of the embryo and outer coats of the grain in milling involves loss of a relatively large proportion of the original content of higher-quality protein, of minerals, B vitamins, and all the vitamin E (in the embryo). Whole grain products tend not to keep as well in storage, and thus the highly milled products are favored by millers and bakers. If bread and cereals made with highly milled grain are used, they should be of the "enriched" variety—with several B-complex vitamins and iron added to replace amounts lost in milling, and other rich sources of the missing nutrients must be included in the diet.
	Although whole grains have a higher content of minerals and vitamins, bread and cereals made either from the whole grains or from highly milled ones, when enriched, are good food. White (patent) flour is not rendered poisonous by bleaching, as the faddists claim.
Devitalization by overprocessing	
The American food supply is devitalized by overprocessing.	Some processes do result in lowered nutrient content. Commercial firms take care to protect food flavor, color, and texture. This requires use of techniques that coincidentally tend to conserve nutrients better than home preservation does. Factories for canning or quick-freezing are located in the midst of areas where special crops are produced. Foods are canned in sealed tins from which air has been evacuated before the sterilization process. Dehydrated foods are processed at relatively low temperatures, under conditions (such as in vacuum) in which water is lost quickly. Special packaging also helps conserve vitamin content of foods before they reach the consumer.

Figure 1-6. (*Continued*)

Fallacies	Facts
Food additives are poison.	Substances added to foods must pass rigid tests that the foods themselves were never required to do, and the probability is that most are safer than some substances in casual food use (cassava, nutmeg, etc.). Some common additives are nutrients (vitamin C to prevent browning) and another can substitute for a vitamin (the antioxidant BHT for vitamin E).
Vitamin and mineral concentrates —are needed by most persons.	The federal Food and Drug Administration has stated: "According to the subclinical deficiency myth, anyone who has 'that tired feeling,' or an ache or pain in almost any part of the body, is probably suffering a 'subclinical deficiency' and needs to supplement his diet with some concoction. . . . Of course, no normal person can go through even a small part of his life without experiencing some of these symptoms. There is no basis for believing that they are usually due to subclinical deficiencies."

food habits: *psychocultural equivalences*. Her belief is as follows:

The people of any culture act the way they do because their culture has defined for them the limit within which meaningful behavior may occur. The people within the culture eat the way they do for the same reason. The behaviors that occur outside of these limits are within that one culture, considered bizarre or irrational. Imagine your response if you saw someone eating a caterpillar!

Those behaviors occurring within the limits are meaningful to the members of a culture and will evoke predictable behavioral resources from the group. That is to say that culture selects, out of a wide variety of possible food scources and food behavior, a narrow and specific set of food behaviors and assigns them meaning within its own framework. The culture, therefore, directs its members' behavior, sets limits on the kinds of food behavior (will you eat caterpillars?) and determines what food behaviors will be reinforced and learned (will sweets serve as a love or bribe food?). That is to say that an individual's range of food behaviors is established for him by his culture.

Culture also directs behaviors in specific situations. This is because some behaviors are appropriate to and have meaning in certain specific situations but not in others. These food behaviors appropriate at a barbecue are not appropriate at a formal dinner. People learn food behaviors for specific situations because their culture has defined only certain behaviors as having meaning in that specific situation.

Thus, culture exists in the mind of the individual and each member of a specific culture has a set of "psychocultural equivalencies." (Armstrong, 1979)

Psychocultural equivalencies is a term that refers to the commonly held beliefs, values, and symbols that exist in the minds of people sharing a similar culture. People of the same culture usually hold the same beliefs about food appropriate for a certain age group (like special foods for babies). For special occasions, ceremonies, or special seasons, certain foods are preferred; and these preferences are in the minds of all group members. So various cultures' beliefs, values, and symbols affect their food consumption patterns, which are therefore highly integrated into the total cultural framework.

These beliefs, values, and symbols system are transacted in childhood and they become integrated in the whole culture system. This makes them highly resistant to change in adulthood even though they are constantly being transacted throughout life. Since individuals of the same culture experience similar transaction experience with respect to food beliefs, value and symbols, we would expect that these same individuals would respond similarly to the same types of innovations.

Change may take place in adulthood, but usually cultural food consumption patterns take generations to change. Individuals are highly resistant to change or intervention with respect to food consumption patterns because of their emotional and symbolic attachments to food and food beliefs. The beliefs of individuals in a culture become more heterogeneous with each succeeding generation and as the number of external factors increases. Cultures are more apt to maintain their present system if homogeneity of the environment persists. (Armstrong, 1979)

This information is important for nurses when they are trying to change their client's food habits.

THE FAMILY AS AN AGENT IN DETERMINING FOOD HABITS

Most of us grow up in a family and it is there we learn about food and its meaning. During infancy the caretaker, usually the parents, introduces the child to his first experience of food. If the feeding process goes well and is associated with feelings of security and satisfaction, the infant will relate good feelings to food. If the food process is filled with confusion and inconsistencies, the infant may develop problems with eating later on (Bruch, 1978; Orbach, 1978). These attitudes established in early childhood affect what a person thinks, feels, and believes about food.

Schafer (1978) interviewed 116 couples from two midwestern cities and found that the immediate family was believed to have the greatest influence on food eaten. Influences outside the home, except for cost, were found to be less significant.

Kolasa (1978) discussed the mother's role in the transmission of food behavior. The mother is the primary transmitter of food habits. She is the pivot of family life. She teaches the child what foods are desirable, best for the child, and gratifying. She lets the child know either implicitly or explicitly what foods are to be avoided. In the US culture she is known as the repository of food lore (the moral and religious beliefs about food). She serves as an important link between the larger system and her family system because she is generally responsible for the preparation, purchasing, and distribution of food to the rest of the family; and her role in relation to foodways has its effect throughout the child's life (Kolasa, 1978). It is by example that children's food habits are most influenced. During 14 years of study and close observation of young nursery school children, Lowenberg (1974) became convinced that children's attitudes toward food are transmitted by those who guide them at mealtimes. Adult attitudes seem to carry more influence than adult words.

It is difficult to separate the individual from the family and its influences because more time is spent and more emotion invested there than in any other area. Nurses working with clients should consider them members of a family unit, and that whole unit should be observed when determining their food habits.

Family as a System That Influences Food Behavior

The family unit should be considered as a whole system in which all members influence one another. The family unit is also affected by its external environment. For each family unit, then, there is both an internal and external environment to consider. Internal environment is determined by such elements as family members' beliefs and values, family history, the moods of the family members, the roles they play or do not play, the culture of the family, finances, and resources. The external environment consists of the location of the family home, the political climate of the community, geographical location, and cultural system it is located in, and the community resources.

Within a family, there are characteristic ways of interacting that are governed by "rules," or norms. These rules can be made explicit (verbalized), like stating that mealtime is at 6 PM and everyone is expected to attend, or implied (not verbalized), in that we all know we will not have dog for dinner. These rules are ways in which family members are taught food habits with all their cultural, emotional, and social significance and symbolic meanings.

Everyone in a family has a role to play, for example, mom the food shopper and meal preparer and dad the breadwinner, or perhaps the reverse, for many role changes are occurring in US families. When everyone in a family knows what to expect from the others and all are fulfilling their roles, characteristic behavior patternings occur and the family is in equilibrium. Trouble occurs when change is introduced to the family and then expectations cannot be met as desired. Because of a tendency toward equilibrium, the family will attempt to keep things in the status quo. Yet families do change and need to change. Mom may need to go to work, so who will take over the job mom has vacated, or will mom have two jobs? New members may join the family, raising the questions of how they will be fed or how they will cause family food habits to change.

When a family is confronted with new problems, adequate resources to solve the problem may not be available to that family. If the family refuses to change its ways and tries to solve things in a set manner, never trying anything new, the family may be heading for trouble. This can be observed when a crisis situation occurs. Take for example a family in which the mother develops a chronic illness like multiple sclerosis. She will be going in and out of the hospital and may need to be in a wheel-

chair. Now if the family still continues to expect mom to do most of the cooking of the meals and shopping for the food, it will be difficult for mom to accomplish these tasks. The family will need to change their expectations of mom in order for the system to run smoothly. If they refuse to change, there will be a lot of strain on mom and the other family members.

From this perspective it is necessary to treat the family as a whole unit. If one family member needs to change food habits, then all other members will be affected by that change. It is important to remember that if you change one part of the family you change the whole family.

Families that tend to be flexible and willing to listen to new ideas and try them out are more adaptable. Families that believe there is only one way to cook meals or only one type of food (e.g., Portuguese food) will have trouble adapting to environmental and other changes that may occur either internally or externally. The food from the "old country" may be expensive in the new country and place financial stresses on the family; or the family may experience problems of poor nutrition because the food in the new country may not be of the same nutritional quality; or an important part of the meal consumption pattern may be missing in the new country. This can be demonstrated in the Polish dietary pattern in the "old country" of eating a lot of bread made from whole grain; in this country the bread was made of refined flour. Lacking the bulk in their new diet was associated with a higher incidence of cancer of the colon for the Polish immigrants in this country (Kolasa, 1978).

Decisions made about what foods are eaten and the manner in which they are eaten are generally made with the parents. Foley et al. (1977) found in their study that "children from families in which parents disagreed on child-rearing practices had poorer nutrient intakes and were relatively under or overweight" (p. 16). The mother, who is most often the shopper and food preparer, is influenced frequently by the foods preferred by the father or breadwinner, with children being the friendly persuaders. Parents who do not listen to the children's ideas and food preferences may run into difficulty, particularly when children become adolescents, a time when children like to assert their independence. The food they eat may become a way of being different from their parents (Hertzler and Vaughan, 1979).

Young (1968) has found that the most complex families have a greater diversity of eating habits, greater meal variety, more nutritional knowledge, and greater diversity of household pessimisms. This factor of complexity provides for more choices in decision making regarding eating behavior whereby families with fewer experiences tend to make fewer choices of food selection.

Haley et al. (1977) studied the relationship of food habits to age, sex, and selected family characteristics like parents' education, family size, and employment status of the mother. The authors stated that the relationship between food habits and family characteristics was not clear-cut. The educational background of the parents showed a strong influence on food habit, however; the greater the parents' education, the better their children's food habits would be.

Burt and Hertzler (1978) studied 46 families to determine who influenced kindergarten children's food preferences the most. Contrary to popular belief, they found that both parents influenced the child's food preferences equally. They indicated a need to look at the total family unit, rather than solely at the mother, to determine the food habits of clients and to facilitate change in food habits when change is needed.

Hertzler and Owen (1976) wrote about three major areas that need to be considered when determining food habits. The first is the level of *differentiation* of the family: the ability to process information and to understand the meaning of that information. This tells how

the process of learning and understanding better nutrition will occur. Take an example of a family who refuses to accept the fact that excess salt in the diet is harmful. The family may not understand the nurse's explanation of the reasons for the harm if she is too scientific. She may need to tailor the new information to their ability to understand. If the family is very knowledgeable about scientific data, however, and the nurse makes the information too simple, she may alienate them from her by insulting their intelligence.

The second consideration is *accessibility of information:* the networks of influence within the family and the degree to which the family interacts with the community, that is, its connections with the mass media and the number of community agencies the family has visited or been involved with. Looking at the structure of that information flow, there should be an evaluation made of the sort of group with which the family is in contact. Is the contact mainly with one ethnic group?

The third consideration is *solidarity* of the family: the amount of cooperation among its members. Cohesion and open communication can be examples of family solidarity. Family members that are communicating effectively with one another can share and accept useful information about health and healthy food habits and are more willing to accept the others' opinions. All these considerations underline the need to deal with the family as a total unit when determining food habits and to facilitate change in those habits.

Treating the Family as a Whole Unit to Achieve Dietary Changes

Nurses and nursing students are frequently called on to educate a hospitalized patient or an outpatient about a new diet plan. In the past, nurses have discussed the new diet regimen with the client and had difficulty understanding why the new diet plan failed soon after the client returned home. The reason for this problem may have been because the

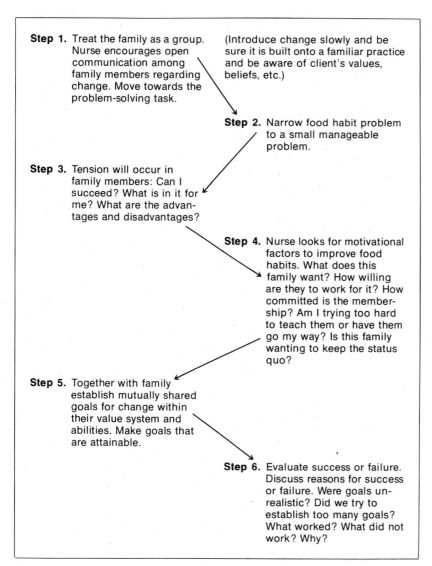

Step 1. Treat the family as a group. Nurse encourages open communication among family members regarding change. Move towards the problem-solving task.

(Introduce change slowly and be sure it is built onto a familiar practice and be aware of client's values, beliefs, etc.)

Step 2. Narrow food habit problem to a small manageable problem.

Step 3. Tension will occur in family members: Can I succeed? What is in it for me? What are the advantages and disadvantages?

Step 4. Nurse looks for motivational factors to improve food habits. What does this family want? How willing are they to work for it? How committed is the membership? Am I trying too hard to teach them or have them go my way? Is this family wanting to keep the status quo?

Step 5. Together with family establish mutually shared goals for change within their value system and abilities. Make goals that are attainable.

Step 6. Evaluate success or failure. Discuss reasons for success or failure. Were goals unrealistic? Did we try to establish too many goals? What worked? What did not work? Why?

Figure 1-7. Implementing dietary changes with a family.

cooperation and needs of the total family were not considered. To treat or educate a member from a family unit in isolation from other family members can set up the "identified patient" as different or uncooperative with the rest of the family. The following case study illustrates how the nurse can introduce dietary changes while working with the family as a total unit.

Johnnie, a 16-year-old boy, has been diagnosed recently as a diabetic. He needs to be taught a new way of eating. For his diet regimen to be successful, he will need the cooperation of the whole family and especially the cooperation of the food-buying and the food preparation channels in the household.

Another important determinant of the success of Johnnie's new diet plan is the economic situation of the family. Will the new change place an economic burden? Where poverty exists, those responsible for the dietary changes will need to seek out ways to provide meals within the food budget or to provide "welfare" foods to support the new diet regimen. Johnnie's new diet plan must be instituted within the existing values and past experiences of the family members. The degree to which new ideas are accepted will depend on how these values and past experiences fit the new dietary plan. The factors that influence the speed of adoption of the diet are:

1. Its relative advantages as seen by the family
2. Its compatibility with their lifestyle
3. Its simplicity (family may get discouraged if the plan seems difficult)
4. Its ability to be adopted in stages

Another factor to be taken into account in Johnnie's diet is the psychological aspect of family life. Recall from earlier discussion that people tend to pay attention to (perceive selectively) information that is in harmony with their personal values, attitudes, and beliefs and to ignore information that is not. New information should be presented in such a way that it reflects these values, attitudes, and beliefs. It has been demonstrated by research that information may be distorted to fit in with the client's frame of reference. To be an effective change agent, the nurse needs to know and understand her client-family.

Figure 1-7 illustrates how the nurse can implement dietary changes and treat the family as a whole unit. "One must see the reason for the proposed change, know how to go about achieving it, and receive group support" (Hertzler and Owen, 1976, p. 384).

GENERAL PRINCIPLES FOR CHANGE

Within the context of the family, the nurse needs to know the beliefs, attitudes, and knowledge about foods held by the client's family. What purposes do their beliefs serve and what subculture do they represent? Who makes the decisions about food habits—who is in charge? If changes need to be made, how long will it take to bring them about?

In summary, if general principles of good food habits are to be applied, the following recommendations can be made:

1. A study of family diet should be made. The food preferences of all family members need to be evaluated.
2. An interdisciplinary approach should be used to understand the family's food habits.
3. Recognize that eating is always an interpersonal experience that is charged with emotional complexity.

BIBLIOGRAPHY

Armstrong, J. Beliefs and culture patterns, personal communication, 1979.

Babcock, C. Attitudes and the use of food. *J. Am. Diet. Assoc.* 38:546, 1961.

Barlow, D., and Tillatson, J. Behavioral science and nutrition: A new perspective. *J. Am. Diet. Assoc.* 72:368, 1978.

Bennion, M. Food preparation in colonial America. *J. Am. Diet. Assoc.* 69:16, 1976.

Braden, C. J., and Herban N., *Community Health: A Systems Approach.* New York: Appleton-Century-Crofts, 1976.

Briggs, G. M. and Calloway, D. H. Food habits and beliefs. In Bogert's *Nutrition and Physical Fitness*, 10th Ed., pp. 380–381. Philadelphia: W. B. Saunders Co., 1979.

Brown, A. British food habits. *J. Hum. Nutr.* 31:41, 1977.

Bruch, H. Psychotherapy in eating disorders. *Can. Psychiatr. Assoc. J.* 22:102, 1977.

———. Obesity and anorexia nervosa. *Psychosomatics* 19:208, 1978.

Burt, J., and Hertzler, A. Parental influence on the child's food preference. *J. Nutr. Educ.* 10:127, 1978.

Calkins, A. Observations on vegetarian dietary practice and social factors. *J. Am. Diet. Assoc.* 74:353, 1979.

Cardwell, J. D. *Social Psychology: A Symbolic Interaction Perspective.* Philadelphia: F. A. Davis, 1971.

Cassel, J. Social and cultural implications of food and food habits. *Am. J. Public Health* 47:732, 1957.

Chappelle, M. The language of food. *Am. J. Nurs.* 72:1294, 1972.

Church, M., and Doughty, J. Value of traditional food practices in nutrition education. *J. Hum. Nutr.* 30:9, 1976.

Cornely, P., Begman, S., and Watts, D. Nutritional beliefs among a low-income urban population. *J. Am. Diet. Assoc.* 42:131, 1963.

Coughenour, C. M. Functional aspects of food consumption activity and family life cycle stages. *J. Marriage Family* 34:656, 1972.

Douglas, M. Accounting for taste. *Psychology Today,* p. 44, July, 1979.

Evans, R., and Hall, Y. Social-psychologic perspective in motivating changes in eating behavior. *J. Am. Diet. Assoc.* 72:378, 1978.

Fathauer, G. H. Food habits—An anthropologist's view. *J. Am. Diet. Assoc.* 37:335, 1960.

Fewster, W. J., Bastian, L., and Powers, R. Measuring the connotative meaning of foods. *Home Economics Research* 2:44, 1973.

Fleshman, R. Eating rituals and realities. *Nurs. Clin. North Am.* 8:91, 1973.

Foley, C., Hertzler, A., and Anderson, H. Food Habits and food belief. *J. Hum. Nutr.* 31:3, 1977.

———. Attitudes and food habits—a review. *J. Am. Diet. Assoc.* 75:13, 1979.

Gold, D. Psychological factors associated with obesity. *Am. Fam. Physician* 13:87, 1976.

Haley, J., Aucoin, D., and Rae, J. A Comparative study of food habits: II. Influence of age, sex, and selected family characteristics. *Can. J. Public Health* 68:301, 1977.

Hanchett, E. *Community Health Assessment.* New York: John Wiley & Sons, Inc., 1979.

Harris, M., and Ross, E. How beef became king. *Psychology Today.* 12:88, 1978.

Hecht, M. Children of alcoholics are children at risk. *Am. J. Nurs.* 73:1764, 1973.

Hertzler, A., and Owen, C. Sociologic study of food habits—a review. *J. Am. Diet. Assoc* 69:377, 1976.

Hertzler, A., and Vaughan, C. E. The relationship of family structure and interaction to nutrition. *J. Am. Diet. Assoc.* 74:23, 1979.

Jakobovits, C., Kelley, L., Roe, D., and Young, C. Eating habits and nutrient intakes of college women over a thirty-year period. *J. Am. Diet. Assoc.* 71:105, 1977.

Jalso, S., Burns, M., and Rivers, J. Nutritional beliefs and practices. *J. Am. Diet. Assoc.* 47:263, 1965.

Keen, S. Eating our way to enlightenment. *Psychology Today,* p. 62, October, 1978a.

———. The pure, the impure, and the paranoid. *Psychology Today,* p. 67, October, 1978b.

Kolasa, K. I won't cook turnip greens if you won't cook kielbasa: Food behavior of Polonia and its health implications. In E. Bouwens, Ed. *The Anthropology of Health.* St. Louis: The C. V. Mosby Co., 1978.

Lee, D. Cultural factors in dietary choice. *Am. J. Clin. Nutr.* 5:166, 1957.

LeVine, R. *Culture Behavior and Personality.* Chicago: Aldine Pub. Co., 1973.

Longstreet, W. *Aspects of Ethnicity.* New York: Teachers College Press, 1978.

Lowenberg, M. Development of food patterns. *J. Am. Diet. Assoc.* 65:263, 1974.

Lowenberg, M., and Lucas, B. Feeding families and children. *J. Am. Diet. Assoc.* 68:207, 1976.

MaHoney, M., and Caggiula, A. Applying behavioral methods to nutritional counseling. *J. Am. Diet. Assoc.* 72:372, 1978.

Maslow, A. H. *Motivation and Personality.* New York: Harper & Bros., Pubs., 1954.

Mead, M. Changing significance of food. *J. Nutr. Educ.* 2:17, 1970.

Mills, E. Psychosocial aspects of food habits. *J. Nutr. Educ.* 9:67, 1977.

Mindlen, P. E. The meaning of food. *J. Am. Diet. Assoc.* 30:576, 1954.

Nat'l Instit. of Mental Health, Nat'l Instit. on Alcohol Abuse and Alcoholism. *Alcohol and Health.* Publ. No. 72-9099. Washington: U.S. Govt. Printing Office, 1974.

New, Kong-Ming, P., and Priest, R. Food and thought: A sociologic study of food cultists. *J. Am. Diet. Assoc.* 51:13, 1967.

Orbach, S. Social dimensions in compulsive eating in women. *Psychotherapy: Theory, Research and Practice* 15:180, 1978.

Pangborn, R., and Bruhn, C. Concepts of food habits of "other" ethnic groups. *J. Nutr. Educ.* 2:106, 1971.

Queen, G. Culture, economics, and food habits. *J. Am. Diet. Assoc.* 33:1044, 1957.

Reaburn, J., Krondl, M., and Lau, D. Social determinants in food selection. *J. Am. Diet. Assoc.* 74:637, 1979.

Ritenbaugh, D. Human foodways: A window on evolution. In E. Bouwens, Ed., *The Anthropology of Health*. St. Louis: The C. V. Mosby Co., 1978.

Schafer, R. Factors affecting food behavior and the equality of husbands' and wives' diets. *J. Am. Diet. Assoc.* 72:138, 1978.

Schafer, R., and Yetley, E. Social psychology of food faddism. *J. Am. Diet. Assoc.* 66:129, 1975.

Schorr, B., Lanjur, D., and Erickson, E. Teenage food habits—a multidimensional analysis. *J. Am. Diet. Assoc.* 61:415, 1972.

Star J. The psychology and physiology of eating. *Today's Health*, p. 33, Feb. 1973.

Steelman, U. Attitudes toward food as indicators of subcultural value systems. *Home Economics Research* 5:21, 1976.

Wagner, M. The irony of affluence. *J. Am. Diet. Assoc.* 57:311, 1970.

Williams, S. R. *Nutrition and Diet Therapy.* 3rd Ed. St. Louis: The C. V. Mosby Co., 1977.

Wilson, C. Food habits—a selected annotated bibliography. *J. Nutr. Educ.* 5(Suppl.):41 1973.

Worthington, B., and Welch, L. *Nursing Clinics of North America.* Philadelphia: W. B. Saunders Co., 1979.

Young, F. W. The differentiation of family structure in rural Mexico. *J. Marriage Fam.* 30:154, 1968.

CHAPTER 2

Physiological Functions of Nutrients

In the previous chapter some of the social, cultural, religious, and psychological influences on food habits and eating patterns were examined. Besides these important influences on food habits, there is a much more basic reason for eating: survival. Food is one of the basic physiological needs, ranking in importance with air, water, sleep, and shelter. Food provides the necessary physiological function of nourishing the body and sustaining life.

PHYSIOLOGICAL REASONS FOR EATING

Energy

One of the primary reasons for eating is to meet the body's energy requirements (Fig. 2-1). *Energy,* the basic need of all living organisms, is the organism's capacity to operate. Capacity beyond that required for maintenance is required for participation in the events and experiences of life. Varying amounts of energy are required throughout the life cycle and in fluctuating states of wellness. Contrast the energy level of a 5-year-old child with that of a woman of 65 or the energy level of a teenager playing football with that of the same teenager recovering from surgery. The human body requires energy for muscular activity and for maintenance of body temperature and internal metabolic processes.

Growth

A second reason for eating is for growth and maintenance of body tissues. Everyone understands the important function of food in this regard when observing the rapid physical growth of a child during the first year of life (Fig. 2-2). In the adult where physiological growth has ceased, food functions to maintain existing body tissues for optimal body performance.

Resistance to Disease

Eating the proper foods helps promote resistance to disease and infection. You can probably recall your mother or grandmother encouraging you to eat balanced meals to avoid colds or flu during the winter. There is a known relationship between poor diet and increased physiological stress. An inadequate diet may lead to increased physiological stress and an increased incidence of the disease, although other good health habits such as sufficient rest, regular exercise, and adequate clothing to protect the body from exposure to the weather also contribute to disease resistance.

Recovery from Illness

Consumption of nutritional foods can also help a person recover from illness or disease. Illness produces a stress on the body that increases the overall nutritional requirements.

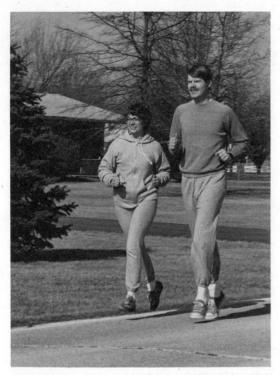

Figure 2-1. Food provides energy for jogging, and jogging helps to promote good health. (Photo by J. Collins)

During the acute phase of an illness, however, these increased nutritional requirements are often not met because of decreased ingestion of food due to decreased appetite, weakness, nausea, or pain associated with the disease state. During recovery, appetite and food intake increase; proper nutrition at this time can hasten rehabilitation.

Physical Appearance

Possession of a pleasant and acceptable physical appearance is another important reason for eating. Consuming adequate amounts of the recommended nutrients has a positive ef-fect on the physical appearance of all people regardless of their genetically determined physical features. Slenderness is a trait that is highly valued in the United States, as evidenced by the emphasis on weight reduction and the increased number of health spas. Specifically, males prize a well-developed, muscular physique, and females aspire to a well-proportioned figure. Heredity obviously plays a major role in determining physical characteristics, but proper nutrition can certainly help a person make the most of his physical appearance.

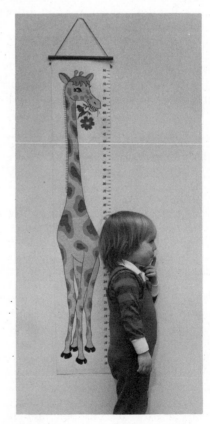

Figure 2-2. A balanced diet helps children grow strong and healthy. (Photo by J. Collins)

NUTRITIONAL STATUS

Nutritional status is the state of health related to the body's use of nutrients from food eaten. Nutritionally adequate diets can help provide improved physical appearance, healthy mental attitude, optimal functioning of the processes of digestion, and optimal use of the nutrients from food. Figures 2-3 shows examples of three basic good health practices for maintaining optimal nutritional status.

There is a positive relationship between good nutrition and health. Proper nutrition, however, does not guarantee that a person will be free from disease. The current focus of the health professions on health maintenance and preventive medicine has heightened the interest in the role of nutrition. In nursing there has been an increased interest in nutritional assessment as a tool for maintaining or improving the nutritional status of clients. The medical profession has also become more interested in the role of nutrition in the prevention and *etiology* of certain diseases such as heart disease, cancer, and colon disease. Physicians, nurses, and dietitians are all interested in indications of

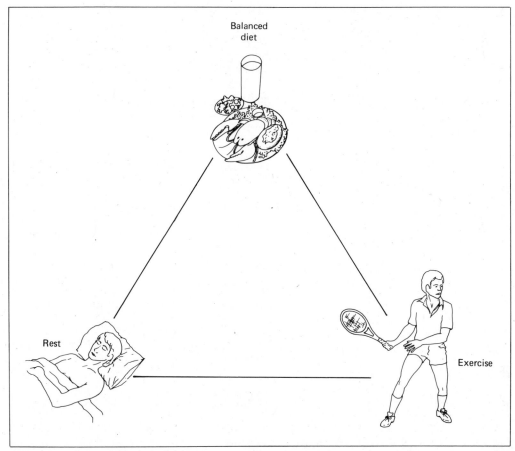

Figure 2-3. Good health practices.

TABLE 2-1. Clinical Evidences of Good Nutritional Status

General appearance	Alert, responsive; development appropriate for age.
Weight	Normal for height, age, and body build.
Integumentary system	
Skin	Smooth, slightly moist; color appropriate for race.
Hair	Shiny, firm, not easily plucked.
Muscular system	
Muscles	Firm and well-developed.
Posture	Erect, arms and legs straight, shoulders flat, abdomen in, chest up.
Skeletal system	
Bones	Straight, able to bear weight.
Teeth	Straight, white, no crowding, clean.
Nervous system	Appropriate attention span for age; senses intact.
Gastrointestinal system	
Mouth	Pink, moist, smooth.
Gastrointestinal function	Appetite appropriate for age; elimination regular.
Eyes	Bright, clear, shiny.

nutritional status. Table 2-1 is a list of clinical evidences of good nutritional status.

Not all people with good nutritional status will possess all the characteristics in Table 2-1 to the same degree. Each person should be evaluated against these criteria by considering what is optimal for that person in his state of health. Some of these criteria may not be consistently applicable to a given person on a nutritionally balanced diet because of genetic inheritance or a psychological or emotional problem.

NUTRIENTS

The food we eat contains *nutrients*, which are chemical substances needed by the body for its proper functioning. These nutrients are divided into six major classes: *carbohydrates, proteins, fats, vitamins, minerals,* and *water* (see

Fig. 2-4). Each class can be further divided on the basis of chemical characteristics or occurrence in the body. Details of this classification are presented in subsequent chapters.

All of the nutrients listed in Table 2-2 are essential for good health in humans. In nutrition the term *essential* has a special meaning; it designates those nutrients the human body cannot manufacture or synthesize and that therefore must be supplied daily by food. There are about 50 essential nutrients known at the present time to be required in varying amounts, many of which have been discovered in the past 40 years.

All the essential nutrients required by humans are present in the food we eat. *Food* may be defined as any substance which, when ingested, causes an organism to grow and maintain its health. *Nutrition* is the study of the processes (physiological and psychological) by

TABLE 2-2. Nutrients Essential for Man

Carbohydrate
Glucose

Protein
Essential amino acids

Leucine	Phenylalanine
Isoleucine	Threonine
Lysine	Tryptophan
Methionine	Valine
Histidine (for children)	

Fat
Essential fatty acid
  Linoleic acid

Vitamins

Vitamin A	B-complex vitamins	
Vitamin D	Thiamine	Folacin
Vitamin C	Riboflavin	Pyridoxine
Vitamin E	Niacin	Vitamin B_{12}
Vitamin K	Biotin	Pantothenic acid

Minerals

Major	*Trace*	
Calcium	Iron	Fluoride
Phosphorus	Copper	Selenium
Magnesium	Iodine	Chromium
Sodium	Manganese	Vanadium
Potassium	Cobalt	Tin
Chlorine	Zinc	Nickel
Sulfur	Molybdenum	Silicon

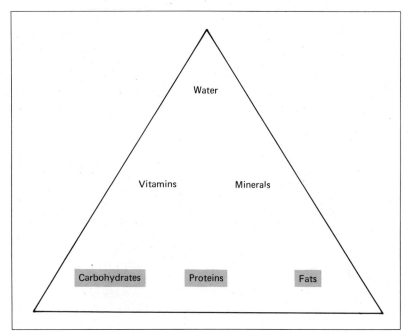

Figure 2-4. Classification of nutrients.

which a living organism receives and uses the nutrients from food for maintenance of its functions and growth of its tissues. The nutrients from food perform the three basic physiological functions of (1) providing energy, (2) building and maintaining body tissues, and (3) regulating numerous metabolic reactions. All six classes of nutrients perform each of these functions either directly or indirectly; all the nutrients are interdependent and interact in complex metabolic reactions. Table 2-3 is a summary of the direct and indirect functions of each class of nutrient.

Carbohydrates, proteins, and fats are collectively referred to as the *energy nutrients* because they contribute the energy value or *Calories* from food. Vitamins and minerals do not contribute to the caloric content of food, but they are substances vitally important to the building and maintenance of body tissues and the regulation of metabolic reactions. Minerals account for about 4% of the body

weight of an adult. Of the approximately 60 minerals that contribute to this weight, about 21 of them have been shown to be essential in human nutrition. Vitamins are substances that are required by the body in very small amounts, but without these small quantities serious nutritional deficiency symptoms develop. Vitamins are not an actual constituent

TABLE 2-3. Physiological Functions of Nutrient Classes

Major Function	Direct	Indirect
Provide energy	Carbohydrates, proteins, fats	Vitamins, minerals, water
Build and maintain body tissues	Proteins, minerals	Vitamins, carbohydrates, fat, water
Regulate body processes	Proteins, vitamins, minerals, water	Fat, carbohydrates

of the body tissue itself, but they play a role in the release of energy from carbohydrate, protein, and fat. Even though it is generally known that water is necessary for survival, it is often omitted in discussions of the nutrients. Water is in fact a very essential nutrient. It is a part of every cell. Most of the body's water is contained within the cells and the remainder bathes the cells and tissues. Water is an important solvent and it is necessary for digestion, nutrient transport to the cells, and removal of body wastes. Water is also a lubricant and it helps to regulate body temperature.

The daily inclusion of the proper amount of each of the essential nutrients in the diet may seem a monumental task; but, fortunately, many of these nutrients are required in very small quantities and are found in combination with other important nutrients in common foods. According to the National Dairy Council there are 10 nutrients of primary importance called *leader nutrients*. The supposition is that if these 10 leader nutrients are obtained in the recommended amounts in the daily diet, then the other 40 nutrients will also be consumed in adequate amounts. The 10 leader nutrients are carbohydrate, protein, fat, vitamin A, vitamin C, thiamine, riboflavin, niacin, calcium, and iron.

Physiological Functions of Nutrients

Providing Energy

The primary physiological function of the human organism is the production of energy for health and activity. Work, activity, and recreation, in fact life itself, would be impossible without energy. Even the concept of health involves not simply minimal levels of energy to accomplish necessary work but level and duration of energy to provide vitality and well-being. Carbohydrate, protein, and fat are the three nutrients that directly provide energy. Carbohydrate and fat are the two major contributors to energy; although protein does supply some energy, its primary

function is building and repairing body tissue. The body strives to conserve body protein for its primary function by using carbohydrate or fat ahead of protein as the source of energy.

The production of energy is a detailed chemical process discussed in Chapter 12. Vitamins, minerals, and water are all involved indirectly in the production of energy. The B-complex vitamins thiamine, riboflavin, and niacin are necessary components of *enzymes* and *coenzymes* required for the release of energy from carbohydrate, protein, and fat. Many are involved in the breakdown of carbohydrate, protein, and fat for energy. Iron as well as other minerals are required in the long series of complex chemical reactions necessary to release energy.

Building and Maintaining Body Cells

The physiological function of building and maintaining body cells is very important because growth and maintenance of all cells and tissues goes on throughout the life cycle. Proteins and minerals are the two major classes of nutrients specifically involved in building and maintaining body cells. Protein is the most abundant compound in the body after water. Protein, which composes about one-half of the dry weight of the body, is a major component in all body cells. Carbohydrate and fat are also constituents of every cell but to a much lesser extent than protein. Minerals, although comprising only about 4% of the body's weight, are also a constituent of every cell. Vitamins, though not actual components of the cell, assist in the formation of vital body substances or act as regulators of complex chemical reactions or body processes.

Protein as a constituent of every cell is essential for growth and maintenance of body cells throughout the life cycle. There is a constant turnover of protein within the body, for body cells are constantly being replaced by new cells. For growth and maintenance of body cells to occur, body protein must be replenished by adequate amounts of dietary protein, more specifically, the essential amino acids.

Protein is a particularly important part of blood, muscles, bones, hair, and skin. It is a basic component of many body compounds such as *hormones,* enzymes, and *pigments.*

Minerals such as sodium, chlorine, calcium, potassium, and magnesium are contained within the cell and in the fluid surrounding each cell. These minerals, although present in very minute amounts, perform specific physiological functions. Some minerals such as calcium and iron serve specific functions within certain tissues. Calcium is present in bones and teeth in combination with phosphorus and magnesium to give strength and rigidity to these structures. Iron is a component of the *hemoglobin* of blood, which transports oxygen to and carbon dioxide from the cells.

Regulating Body Processes

Another important function of the nutrients is the regulation of vitally important chemical reactions and processes in the body. Protein, vitamins, minerals, and water are the nutrients that assist in the *synthesis* (formation) of body substances or act as regulators of the utilization of carbohydrate, protein, and fat.

Protein is a component of many vital regulatory substances in the body including enzymes, hormones, body fluids, and *antibodies.* All enzymes are protein by nature and are vital for the complex chemical reactions of digestion, absorption, and *metabolism* to occur and for the formation of blood, bone, and other body tissues.

Functions of the Leader Nutrients

All nutrients work together to perform the three basic physiological functions. A closer look at each of the leader nutrients will provide a greater appreciation of the specific functions of each basic nutrient. A summary of the major physiological functions of the "leader nutrients" as developed by the National Dairy Council is found in Table 2-4.

Carbohydrate

The primary function of carbohydrate is energy production within body cells. The source of this energy is *glucose,* which is the end product of carbohydrate digestion. The glucose can either be used immediately by the cell for energy or converted into the short-term storage form, *glycogen,* or the long-term storage form, fat.

Some carbohydrate is needed in the daily diet for proper utilization of both protein and fat. The carbohydrate in the diet is said to be "protein sparing." This means that if there is adequate carbohydrate in the diet it will be used first for energy, thus sparing the protein for its important function of building and repairing body tissue. As little as 50 gm of carbohydrate is needed in the daily diet for normal utilization of fat. If an insufficient amount of carbohydrate is present in the diet, the body turns to fat as its next source of energy. With insufficient carbohydrate, the fat is broken down within the body at an abnormally rapid rate. As a result, large quantities of an acidic intermediate product, called *ketones,* accumulate and produce an abnormal physiological state known as *acidosis,* or *ketosis.* This is the danger that can result from the consumption of the very low carbohydrate diets used for weight reduction. This abnormal state of ketosis results in imbalances in the body. Thus following an extremely low carbohydrate diet is not sound physiologically and can be injurious to health.

Another important function of carbohydrate is the contribution that fiber makes to the diet. Because humans lack the digestive enzymes to digest fiber and cellulose, these portions of carbohydrate pass undigested into the large intestine, where they stimulate *peristalsis,* thus aiding in the elimination of waste.

TABLE 2-4. Nutrients for Health

Nutrient	Important Sources of Nutrient	Some Major Physiological Functions		
		Provide Energy	Build and Maintain Body Cells	Regulate Body Processes
Protein	Meat, poultry, fish Dried beans and peas Egg Cheese Milk	Supplies 4 Calories per gram.	Constitutes part of the structure of every cell, such as muscle, blood, and bone; supports growth and maintains healthy body cells.	Constitutes part of enzymes, some hormones and body fluids, and antibodies that increase resistance to infection.
Carbohydrate	Cereal Potatoes Dried beans Corn Bread Sugar	Supplies 4 Calories per gram. Major source of energy for central nervous system.	Supplies energy so protein can be used for growth and maintenance of body cells.	Unrefined products supply fiber—complex carbohydrates in fruits, vegetables, and whole grains—for regular elimination. Assists in fat utilization.
Fat	Shortening, oil Butter, margerine Salad dressing Sausages	Supplies 9 Calories per gram.	Constitutes part of the structure of every cell. Supplies essential fatty acids.	Provides and carries fat-soluble vitamins (A, D, E, and K).
Vitamin A (retinol)	Liver Carrots Sweet potatoes Greens Butter, margerine		Assists formation and maintenance of skin and mucous membranes that line body cavities and tracts, such as nasal passages and intestinal tract, thus increasing resistance to infection.	Functions in visual processes and forms visual purple, thus promoting healthy eye tissues and eye adaptation in dim light.
Vitamin C (ascorbic acid)	Broccoli Orange Grapefruit Papaya Mango Strawberries		Forms cementing substances, such as collagen, that hold body cells together, thus strengthening blood vessels, hastening healing of wounds and bones, and increasing resistance to infection.	Aids utilization of iron.
Thiamine (B$_1$)	Lean pork Nuts Fortified cereal products	Aids in utilization of energy.		Functions as part of a coenzyme to promote the utilization of carbohydrate. Promotes normal appetite. Contributes to normal functioning of nervous system.

TABLE 2-4. *(Continued)*

Nutrient	Important Sources of Nutrient	Some Major Physiological Functions		
		Provide Energy	*Build and Maintain Body Cells*	*Regulate Body Processes*
Riboflavin (B₂)	Liver Milk Yogurt Cottage cheese	Aids in utilization of energy.		Functions as part of a coenzyme in the production of energy within body cells. Promotes healthy skin, eyes, and clear vision.
Niacin	Liver Meat, poultry, fish Peanuts Fortified cereal products	Aids in utilization of energy.		Functions as part of a coenzyme in fat synthesis, tissue respiration, and utilization of carbohydrate. Promotes healthy skin, nerves, and digestive tract. Aids digestion and fosters normal appetite.
Calcium	Milk, yogurt Cheese Sardines and salmon with bones Collard, kale, mustard, and turnip greens		Combines with other minerals within a protein framework to give structure and strength to bones and teeth.	Assists in blood clotting. Functions in normal muscle contraction and relaxation, and normal nerve transmission.
Iron	Enriched farina Prune juice Liver Dried beans and peas Red meat	Aids in utilization of energy.	Combines with protein to form hemoglobin, the red substance in blood that carries oxygen to and carbon dioxide from the cells. Prevents nutritional anemia and its accompanying fatigue. Increases resistance to infection.	Functions as part of enzymes involved in tissue respiration.

SOURCE: Courtesy National Dairy Council.

Fat

Fat is also a source of energy, but it is a more concentrated source than carbohydrate. In fact fat provides more than twice the number of Calories per gram as carbohydrate. The storage form of fat is *adipose tissue*. All people have some adipose tissue, but some have more than others. Faced with a disaster with no food available for an indefinite time, a person with a large fat reserve may survive longer than one with only minimal fat reserves. Other factors that would, of course, influence survival are injury, the absence or presence of disease, and general nutritional status prior to the disaster.

Fat has an insulating effect in the body and therefore helps maintain a normal body temperature. A heavy person may find the temperature of a room too warm while a very slender person in the same room shivers.

Another important function of fat is padding and protection. All of the vital body organs such as heart, kidney, and lungs are surrounded by a protective layer of fat so that in the event of an accident or heavy blow to the body there is less danger of one of these organs being damaged.

Protein
The main function of protein is the building and repair or the growth and maintenance of body cells, processes that occur every second of the day all age groups. A large amount of growth of body cells is evident, of course, during childhood and adolescence, but even in the adult there is growth of new cells daily. Protein is also needed for the repair or growth of cells following disease or injury. In addition protein is needed in the formation of enzymes, hormones, hemoglobin, antibodies, and other vital body substances that play important roles in the regulation of the many complex physiological processes in the body. A secondary function of protein is energy production. A portion of all protein consumed may be converted into glucose to be utilized for energy.

Vitamins and Minerals
The vitamins are directly involved in regulating the metabolism of carbohydrate, protein, and fat. Of all the vitamins known to be essential in the human diet, the five counted among the leader nutrients are vitamin A, vitamin C (ascorbic acid), thiamine, riboflavin, and niacin. These vitamins are required by the body in the largest amounts. If foods containing them are included daily, the recommended amounts of the remainder of the vitamins will usually be obtained.

Vitamin A participates in two important functions within the body. It helps to regulate the formation and maintenance of the skin and the mucous membranes that line the body cavities. It also helps to regulate the vi-

sual process that causes the eye to adapt to dim light.

Vitamin C regulates the formation of *collagen,* the cementing substance that holds the body cells together. Collagen is important in imparting strength to blood vessels, assisting wound healing, and offering increased resistance to infection.

Thiamine, riboflavin, and niacin all function as components of enzymes required for efficient use of carbohydrate, protein, and fat. They are all needed for the release of energy from nutrients within the cell. Every cell of the body can be thought of as a tiny powerhouse where energy is continually produced to enable the cell itself to perform certain tasks and for the contraction of muscles to allow a person to perform activities.

The main function of calcium is to contribute to the formation of strong bones and teeth. Calcium also helps to regulate normal blood clotting, and it plays a vital role in the transmission of nerve impulses and in muscle contraction and relaxation.

Iron is part of hemoglobin and of the enzymes necessary for the final steps in the release of energy from carbohydrates, proteins, and fats within each cell.

Besides these seven vitamins and minerals many others are involved in regulating physiological processes. Vitamin D helps to regulate the absorption of calcium and phosphorous and thus indirectly influences the deposition of these minerals into the bones and teeth. Vitamin K, one of the important clotting factors, is necessary for the formation of *prothrombin* by the liver.

In addition to their many other functions, minerals act as regulators and activators. Calcium, sodium, and potassium each function in their own distinct way in regulating the transmission of nerve impulses and the resulting contraction of skeletal muscle. Some minerals such as calcium and sodium influence cell-wall permeability. Minerals also function as activators of enzymes and assist in chemical reactions; two that perform this function are magnesium and manganese. Some minerals are important constituents of enzymes themselves or of body hormones. Zinc is an important part of many of the enzymes required for digestion and absorption. Iodine is required in the formation of the hormone *thyroxine,* secreted by the thyroid gland and important in regulating the body's overall rate of metabolism. Some of the minerals are closely associated with each other either in terms of structure or function. For example, copper is found in close association with iron in the formation of hemoglobin. Cobalt is a constituent of vitamin B_{12} which is required for red blood cell formation. Fluorine is deposited in the bones and teeth along with calcium, phosphorus, and magnesium.

ADEQUATE DIET

From this brief introduction to the nutrients and some of their physiological functions, it can be seen that the science of nutrition, encompassing as it does all the physiological and chemical reactions that take place in our bodies, comprises a detailed body of knowledge. In actuality all of the six classes of nutrients could be said to function in some capacity in each of the three physiological functions. Fortunately, despite the complexity of the nutrients and their functions, there are simple guidelines for selecting food that will provide the proper proportions and amounts of nutrients to carry out all the physiological functions efficiently. A nutritionally adequate diet, or a *balanced diet,* is one that provides an optimal amount of each known essential nutrient to the body for the production of energy, for growth and maintenance of body cells, and regulation of body processes. A balanced diet provides an adequate intake of all nutrients and an avoidance of excesses.

Food Selection

An adequate diet involves more than simply eating the traditional three meals a day. The selection of individual foods to meet nutrient and caloric needs is the most important. It is also very important to remember that no one food provides all nutrients required in a diet and no one particular food is essential. A good example of these two principles is milk. Although milk is considered to be nature's most perfect food, and it contains most of the essential nutrients in the proper proportions, it is very low in two very important nutrients: vitamin C and iron. Even with all the beneficial qualities of milk, it is not mandatory that it be included in every person's daily diet. Calcium, protein, and the other essential nutrients in milk may be obtained from other food sources.

Some people are fond of popularizing findings from nutrition research. Their attempts to instill cautious attitudes about eating certain foods have left the average person not knowing what is considered "safe" to eat. Breakfast is a good meal to use as an example. The traditional farm breakfast in the United States used to reflect the abundance of this country. Picture for a moment a hearty breakfast of orange juice, hot cereal with cream, bacon and eggs, buttered toast with jelly, and coffee. With research in coronary heart disease and with other health discoveries and trends, these foods have gradually disappeared from the average breakfast table one by one. The egg was the first to go because of its high *cholesterol* content. Next went bacon, cream, and butter because of their high *saturated fat* content. Since then, the sugar on the cereal and jelly on the toast have been questioned because simple sugars have the effect of raising the *triglyceride component* in the blood, which is an added risk factor in heart disease. The harmful effects of the intake of refined sugars have also been questioned. The hot cereal has been replaced by the commercial dry variety, but some raise their eyebrows about the benefits of these dry cereals because of the addition of synthetic nutrients and numerous chemicals as food additives. So we are left with a piece of dry toast and a cup of black coffee. But wait a minute, the dry toast must not be white toast because of inadequate fiber, and coffee has been shown to raise *plasma-free fatty acids* and lower *blood sugar*. How about simply a glass of skim milk or orange juice for breakfast?

Some of the above statements do have a scientific basis; others depend on such factors as current body weight, age, activity level, and present physical health. There are no simple answers to what constitutes a good breakfast or any other meal. Additional research findings are regularly becoming available about the effects of diet on the state of health. Nutritionists cannot wait until all the dietary effects in health and disease are known to advise clients what they should or should not eat, anymore than a doctor can postpone treatment of a disease until a cure for that disease is known.

There are two groups of people who are the most prone to nutritional imbalances: those who are overconcerned with nutrition and those who are unconcerned. Overconcern about nutrition most frequently leads to food fads and the inclusion of high-potency vitamin and mineral supplements. Lack of concern about nutrition and eating habits is evidenced by the consumption of foods, often from vending machines, simply to satisfy present hunger pangs. Meal planning is not viewed as important, and food is usually eaten on the run.

Variety and moderation or just good common sense are most important when selecting foods for an adequate diet. Everyone needs a varied diet because no single food contains all the needed nutrients. A single food should provide no more than 10% of the total caloric intake (Winkler, 1976b). This principle supports the other general idea that what matters is not only which foods we eat but also the amounts of each.

Early Food Guides

Dietary standards have been available in the United States since 1921, when five food groups were published as a family food guide. Since that time discovery of specific nutrient needs has been paralleled by translation of these nutrient needs into food consumption guidelines. In 1941 the first *Recommended Dietary Allowances* were published by the Committee on Food and Nutrition of the National Research Council for the United States. These allowances included recommended daily intakes for Calories, protein, vitamins A and D, thiamine, riboflavin, niacin, ascorbic acid, iron, and calcium. Because the average person could not translate these recommendations into food requirements, a food guide called "Eat the Right Food to Help Keep You Fit" was published by the Bureau of Home Economics in 1941 when the first Recommended Dietary Allowances were accepted. In 1941, the National Dairy Council published their first "Guide to Good Eating," which was composed of seven food groups— the "basic seven" until about 1958—when the US Department of Agriculture released its leaflet based on four food groups. Since that time the *basic four food groups* have formed the basis for adequate food selection. Despite recent criticism of food guides in general and comments that the basic four may be oversimplified, some guide for nutritious eating is necessary and it seems that the lay person is more likely to remember four than seven food groups.

Four Food Groups

The basic four food groups generally familiar to the lay person today were developed by the US Department of Agriculture in 1958 and published in a guide called "Food for Fitness—A Daily Food Guide." An adaptation of this guide was made by the National Dairy Council and is called "Guide to Good Eating." Both of these guides contain the same recommended number of servings from each food group to meet the nutrient requirements for health. This widely used and publicized basic food guide is commonly known as "the basic four" or "the four food groups."

These four food groups are (Fig. 2-5)
- Milk group
- Meat group
- Vegetables and fruits
- Breads and cereals

The recommended number of servings from each group (see Table 2-5) to be included in the diet are easy to remember because the recommended daily servings from a group are either two or four for adults. Extra calcium and protein required for growing children or pregnant or lactating women are provided by increased recommended servings from the milk group.

The recommended number of servings from the milk group for adults of all ages is two cups a day. This quantity provides about three-fourths of the daily requirement for calcium. If this quantity of milk is not consumed, the calcium content of the diet will have to be obtained from other dairy products such as cheese, ice cream, or cottage cheese. These foods, however, do not contain, ounce for ounce, amounts of calcium comparable to the amount in fluid milk.

The meat group, which contributes protein to the diet, consists of meat, fish, poultry, eggs, and cheese. Dried beans, peas, and peanut butter may also be eaten as alternatives. The recommended number of servings from this group is a minimum of two 4 oz (113 gm) servings of cooked meat daily or the equivalent.

Vegetables and fruits provide many vitamins and minerals in the diet, especially vitamins A and C. A daily diet should include a total of at least four servings of vegetables and fruits. Within this group special attention should be given to including specific sources of vitamins A and C. Dark-green leafy vegetables or deep yellow or orange vegetables or fruits are excellent sources of vitamin A. A serving of these should be included in the diet at least every other day (three to four times a week). A good source of vitamin C, such as citrus fruit (oranges or grapefruit), should be part of every day's menu.

At least four servings of enriched or whole grain breads and cereals should be eaten daily to provide necessary vitamins, some protein, and minerals. This group also includes enriched grain products such as rice, macaroni, spaghetti, and noodles (see Figure 2-5).

Selecting foods from the basic four food groups is one approach to achieving a nutritionally adequate diet (Fig. 2-6). The four food groups are a guide to making intelligent decisions about food. Some people, including some nutritionists, consider the food groups antiquated, ineffective, overused, and badly in need of revision. The food groups originally developed for use with the general public have been used as the only basis for teaching nutrition for many years. In trying to be practical about nutrition and food habits, nutritionists have often overlooked the use of scientific facts and the motivational aspects of teaching nutrition. In this book the goal is not simply to provide knowledge about foods in a nutritionally adequate diet but to provide a framework that also includes scientific nutritional facts and motivation for changing or improving food habits.

Recommended Dietary Allowances

The Recommended Dietary Allowances (RDA) are guidelines for the daily intake of Calories and nutrients by people in the United States. These dietary standards are set by the Food and Nutrition Board of the National Research Council of the National Academy of Sciences. The definition of the RDA by this board states that "the Recommended Dietary Allowances are levels of intake of essential nutrients considered, in the judgment of the Committee on Dietary Allowances of the Food and Nutrition Board, on the basis of available scientific knowledge, to be adequate to meet the known nutritional needs of practically all healthy persons" (Food and Nutrition Board, Nat'l Research Council, 1980). The latest revision of the RDA (Food and Nutrition Board, Nat'l Research Council, 1980) lists recommended Calorie and nutrient levels

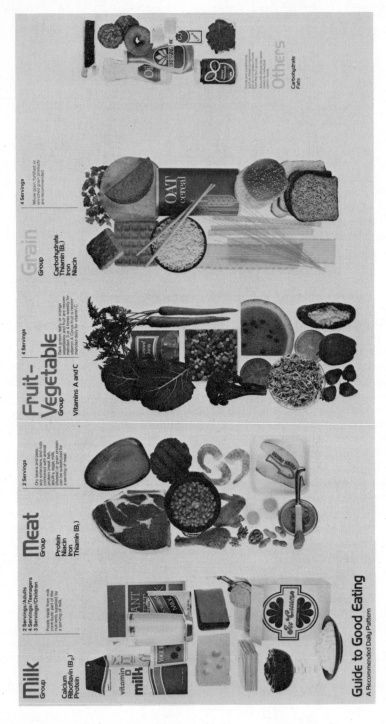

Figure 2-5. A guide to good eating. (Courtesy National Dairy Council)

TABLE 2-5. Guide to Good Eating: A Recommended Daily Pattern[a]

	Recommended Number of Servings				
Food Group	Child	Teenager	Adult	Pregnant Woman	Lactating Woman

Milk
1 cup milk, yogurt, OR
Calcium Equivalent
  1½ slices (1½ oz) cheddar
    cheese[b]
  1 cup pudding
  1¾ cups ice cream
  2 cups cottage cheese
	3	4	2	4	4

Meat
2 ounces cooked, lean meat, fish,
  poultry, OR
Protein Equivalent:
  2 eggs
  2 slices (2 oz) cheddar cheese[b]
  ½ cup cottage cheese[b]
  1 cup dried beans, peas
  4 tbsp peanut butter
	2	2	2	3	2

Fruit-Vegetable
½ cup cooked or juice
1 cup raw
Portion commonly served such
  as a medium-size apple or
  banana
	4	4	4	4	4

Grain, whole grain, fortified,
enriched
  1 slice bread
  1 cup ready-to-eat cereal
  ½ cup cooked cereal, pasta,
    grits
	4	4	4	4	4

SOURCE: Courtesy National Dairy Council.

[a] The recommended daily pattern provides the foundation for a nutritious, healthful diet. The recommended servings from the four food groups for adults supply about 1200 Calories. The chart gives recommendations for the number and size of servings for several categories of people.
[b] Count cheese as serving of milk OR meat, not both simultaneously.

"Others" complement but do not replace foods from the Four Food Groups. Amounts should be determined by individual caloric needs.

(protein; vitamins A, D, and E; ascorbic acid; folacin; thiamine; riboflavin; niacin; vitamin B_6; vitamin B_{12}; calcium; phosphorus; iodine; iron; magnesium;, and zinc) for 17 age groups, both male and female.

The RDA includes a margin of safety, or padding factor, to assure the dietary adequacy of most, if not all, healthy people. This margin of safety, however, does not allow for altered individual requirements under condi-tions of severe physical, emotional, or psychological stress or for prior dietary inadequacies. The RDAs are only estimates or recommendations of optimal physiological nutrient requirements. They are not requirements for individuals, only recommendations. A satisfactory intake of the RDAs provides for normal physiological function plus a nutrient reserve for many people. The RDAs are not intended to define the absence

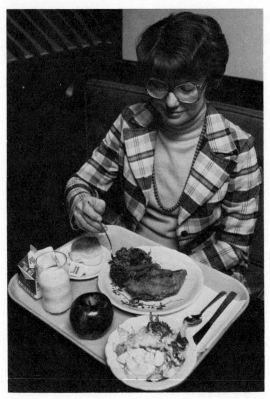

Figure 2-6. A basic four meal.

or presence of a deficient or malnourished state, nor are they intended to be used as the only basis for evaluating dietary adequacy. Calculation of nutrient intake and comparison within the RDA standard can reveal those areas of a diet that may need to be altered through better food selection.

EATING PATTERNS

In addition to eating the recommended quantities of food, the number of meals eaten daily and the presence or absence of snacks is important. It has been traditional in this country

as well as many others to eat at least three basic meals a day. It is important to include any snacks taken in addition to the basic meals when considering total dietary intake. A person's general lifestyle, economic status, and the importance he attaches to food as well as his individual food preferences do affect his dietary intake. Let us examine the effect some of these variables can have on obtaining adequate nutrients from the food consumed.

Frequency of Eating

There is a sound physiological reason for the habit of consuming three meals each day. The storage form of carbohydrate, the main energy nutrient, is the glycogen in the liver. Glycogen is continually converted to glucose, or blood sugar, to maintain an adequate level of glucose in the blood. These glycogen stores in the liver last for only about four hours after a meal, at which time the glucose level in the blood drops.

Also by four hours after a meal the stomach is completely emptied of food. Contractions of the stomach increase in frequency, creating a sort of gnawing sensation known as *hunger pangs*. This stimulates the flow of gastric juices, which further stimulates the contractions of the stomach. The end result of this sequence of events is that a person seeks food.

Breakfast

Eating breakfast, or at least eating something in the mornings, is particularly important for good health and maximum efficiency during the day. The word *breakfast* literally means to "break the fast" from the last time one has eaten, usually a time span of 12 hours or more. The classic Iowa breakfast studies of the 1950s highly substantiate the importance of eating breakfast for maximum efficiency and productivity throughout the day. These studies showed that the children who omitted breakfast had a poorer attitude toward their schoolwork and lower scholastic achievement than those who ate breakfast (Steele et al., 1952).

Number of Meals

Even though three meals a day is the standard pattern for eating, there is nothing magical about the number three. The important aspect is the food selection at the meals that are eaten. If the minimum number of recommended servings from the basic four food groups is consumed at only two meals or at two meals with snacks between, a person is just as likely to be receiving the recommended intakes of nutrients from the Recommended Dietary Allowances.

There is also evidence of the effectiveness of an increased number of smaller meals or the standard three meals with snacks between. For example some studies have found that people who are nibblers (those who eat small quantities more frequently throughout the day) are better able to either maintain their weight or lose weight. Also an increased number of meals or feedings during the day is beneficial to people with specific nutritional requirements resulting from disease or physiological stress. For example, a client with a peptic ulcer needs to receive small frequent feedings so that food is continually present in the stomach to have a neutralizing effect on the excess hydrochloric acid. Another good example is the client who has greatly increased nutritional requirements, especially for increased Calories, because of fever, surgery, or burns.

Standard Foods for Meals

Just as there is not an absolute fixed number of meals required during the day, so there are not specific foods that must be eaten at certain meals as long as the day's nutrient requirements are met. Certain foods or combinations of foods not commonly eaten at a certain meal may be quite nutritionally acceptable. For example, consider a piece of pizza or a toasted cheese sandwich eaten for breakfast, or bacon and eggs for dinner in the evening. There is nothing inherently wrong with these foods eaten at these meals. The important thing is the specific combination of foods eaten throughout the entire day.

Size of Meals

Because most people consume three meals a day, a general recommendation is to consume one-third of the day's allotment of food at each meal. Another suggestion is that breakfast contribute one-fifth of the day's nutrient requirements; each of the other two meals, two-fifths. This seems to be a workable suggestion inasmuch as many people in the United States prefer to eat a smaller portion of food at breakfast. Many people question the habit common in the United States of consuming little or no breakfast, a light lunch, and a large evening meal. A large meal eaten at the end of a busy day with little or no exercise following the meal may put an added strain on the heart and digestive system, but this large meal will not "turn into fat." The nutrients will be used during the night and the next day. A person consuming food in this manner will not gain weight unless the food consumed contains Calories that exceed that person's energy (Calorie) requirements over a 24-hour period.

The use of the names *lunch, dinner,* and *supper* for the noon and evening meals depends on the size of the meal, the time of the day when eaten, and the cultural heritage of the people.

Temperature of Foods

Some people prefer their food steaming hot, others lukewarm; some wait until all foods are room temperature; others do not even bother to heat their food. There is no physiological benefit to eating hot meals, but there may be considerable psychological impact related to the enjoyment of eating.

Snacks

The word *snack* brings to most people thoughts of crispy, crunchy, sticky, and bubbly high-Calorie foods consumed in front of the television, at the movie theater, during a break in routine, or at a friend's house. Snacks, for the most part, are thought of as high-Calorie and unnutritious additions to the daily food intake. It is true that many snacks do provide only *empty Calories,* that is, they contain a very low proportion of nutrients and a very high proportion of Calories. The word *snack,* however, means a light meal or a bite. There is no reason, therefore, why snacks carefully and thoughtfully selected from one or more of the four food groups cannot contribute significantly to a day's nutrient intake.

DIET VARIATIONS SATISFYING THE BASIC FOUR

Although the current food guide, the basic four, is composed of the four major divisions of foods that have consistently been included in food guides, personal diets that eliminate or restrict intake from one of these groups can still be nutritionally adequate with wise planning and selection. Servings of a specific food from another food group would need to be added to the diet.

For example, a client may not like to drink milk or may be unable to tolerate milk as a beverage. First, it would be necessary to determine whether the client likes other milk products and if he is able to consume milk in a cooked form. Ways of incorporating milk products into his diet using the milk equivalent on the basic four chart could be suggested. If, however, he does not like any type of milk product, he could be counseled to eat extra servings of such vegetables as spinach, kale, or broccoli, which supply fairly large amounts of calcium. He would be able to fulfill his protein requirement with a few

extra servings from the meat group, and his requirement for the other vitamins and minerals would probably also be met. It is possible to alter the recommended servings from the food groups in this manner because each food group contributes two divisions of nutrients. First, each food group contributes *some* of each of the nutrients, and second, each food group contributes specific nutrients that are higher in that group than in any other. Major nutrient contributions from each of the four groups are shown at the top of Figure 2-5.

Another modification of the use of the four food groups is in vegetarian diets. People who are true vegetarians select all their foods from the bread and cereal group, the fruits and vegetables group, and only the dried beans, peas, and peanut butter category of the meat group. A nutritionally adequate diet can be planned for vegetarians. An example of the distribution of foods from a lacto-ovo-vegetarian daily diet is shown in Figure 2-7. Also shown in Figure 2-7 is a daily intake for a person who prefers to snack.

One more thing needs to be mentioned about eating the recommended servings from the basic four. If a person is lacking one or even two servings from one or more of the food groups, this does not necessarily mean that the nutrients from his diet will fall below the RDAs for his age and sex category. His nutrient intake may still fall within the RDA standards because of an increased number of servings consumed from another food group, the incorporation of foods fortified with added vitamins and minerals, or the inclusion of a single food or foods especially high in vitamin and mineral content. For example, eating 3 oz of liver will greatly enhance a daily diet low in recommended servings, not only with protein but with iron, vitamins A and C, riboflavin, and niacin. In any case in which a person's daily intake falls below the recommended servings from the basic four, the actual nutrient content of foods consumed should be examined more closely. This may

Figure 2-7. Two diet variations that satisfy the basic four requirements. (From USDA *Yearbook of Agriculture,* 1974.)

Lacto-ovo-vegetarian Diet:

EARLY MORNING MEAL
Pineapple juice
Wheat flakes with milk
Doughnut (enriched)
Coffee

MIDMORNING
Peach

MIDDAY MEAL
Hard-cooked eggs—cream sauce
Whole wheat bread—butter or margarine
Brussels sprouts
Molasses cookies   Milk

EVENING MEAL
Vegetarian baked beans
Green pepper stuffed with rice and tomato sauce
Tossed green salad   French dressing
Raisin pie
Milk

Nutritional Foundation of This Day's Food

Milk Group 2 Cups	Fruit-Vegetable Group 4 Servings	Meat or Alternate 2 Servings	Bread-Cereal—4 Servings (Enriched or Whole Grain)
1 cup as beverage ½ cup with cereal ½ cup in cream sauce	1 serving—pineapple juice 1 serving—peach 1 serving—brussels sprouts 1 serving—green pepper	1 serving—2 eggs 1 serving—vegetarian baked beans	1 serving wheat flakes 1 serving doughnut 1 serving whole wheat bread 1 serving rice

Foods That Provide Additional Nutrients and Food Energy to Meet Individual Needs

From the 4 Food Groups	From Other Foods
Milk as beverage and in coffee Remaining ingredients in cream sauce Molasses cookies—enriched Tomato sauce Tossed green salad Raisin pie	Butter or margarine with bread Sugar in coffee French dressing

Figure 2-7. (Continued)

A Day's Food Intake for a "Snacker" Might Look Like This:

7:30 AM	Instant breakfast (instant breakfast powder + 1 cup milk)
10:00 AM	Two doughnuts (enriched) Milk
11:00 AM	Apple
12:30 PM	Hamburger (onion, relish, tomato slice), French fries, cola
3:00 PM	Plain Danish (enriched) Milk
4:30 PM	Hard-boiled egg Saltines
6:00 PM	Lasagna, coleslaw, iced tea
8:30 PM	Cheese dip with assorted raw vegetables (carrot strips, tomato wedges, cauliflower flowerets, broccoli flowerets)

Nutritional Foundation of This Day's Food

Milk Group 2 Cups	Fruit-Vegetable Group 4 Servings	Meat or Alternate 2 Servings	Bread-Cereal—4 Servings (Enriched or Whole Grain)
1 cup in instant breakfast 1 cup as beverage	Apple—1 serving French fries—1 serving Coleslaw—1 serving Raw vegetables—1 serving	Hamburger—1 serving Lasagna—1 serving (meat in it)	2 doughnuts—2 servings Hamburger roll—1 serving Danish—1 serving

Foods That Provide Additional Nutrients and Food Energy to Meet Individual Needs

From the 4 Food Groups	From Other Foods
Onion, relish, tomato Served on hamburger Hard-boiled egg Saltines—enriched Lasagna noodles (enriched) and sauce Cheese dip Milk in coffee	Instant breakfast powder Sugar in coffee Cola Dressing on coleslaw

be done by listing all foods and the amounts eaten for a 24-hour period, recording the nutrient value of each food from a table of food composition (see Appendix A), totaling the nutrient content of these foods, and comparing the total nutrients consumed with the person's RDA (see back cover). It must be remembered, however, that the RDA is not a *requirement,* only a *recommendation,* and that

failure to meet the RDA standard does *not* mean a person is deficient in one or more nutrients.

At the conclusion of this chapter the student is encouraged to record a typical day's food intake and compare his food intake to the recommended number of servings from the basic four food groups.

BIBLIOGRAPHY

Arlin, M. J. *The Science of Nutrition.* 2nd Ed. New York: Macmillan, Inc., 1977.

Breakfast—the martyred meal. *J. Am. Med. Assoc.* 198:1362, 1966.

Food and Nutrition Board, Nat'l Research Council. *Recommended Dietary Allowances.* 9th Ed., Washington, D.C.: Nat'l Acad. of Sciences, 1980.

Christakis, G. The case for balanced moderation, or how to design a new American nutritional pattern without really trying. *Prev. Med.* 2:329, 1973.

Guthrie, H. A. *Introductory Nutrition.* 4th Ed. St. Louis: The C. V. Mosby Co., 1979.

Hertzler, A. A., and Anderson, H. L. Food guides in the United States. *J. Am. Diet. Assoc.* 64:19, 1974.

Hicks, B. M. Food groups—where do they belong? *Food and Nutr. News* (Nat'l Livestock and Meat Board, Chicago) 48(3):1977.

Krause, M. V., and Mahan, L. K. *Food, Nutrition, and Diet Therapy.* 6th Ed. Philadelphia: W. B. Saunders Co., 1979.

McGlashan, A. Breakfast breakthrough. *Nursing Mirror* 134:13, 1972.

Mitchell, H. S., Rynbergen, H. J., Anderson, L., and Dibble, M. V. *Nutrition in Health and Disease.* 16th Ed. Philadelphia: J. B. Lippincott Co., 1976.

Robinson, C. H., and Lawler, M. R. *Normal and Therapeutic Nutrition.* 15th Ed. New York: Macmillan, Inc., 1977.

Steele, B. F., Clayton, M. M., and Tucker, R. E. Role of breakfast and of between-meal foods in adolescents' nutrient intake. *J. Am. Diet. Assoc.* 28:1054, 1952.

Ward, R. Understanding food. *Nursing Mirror* 144:57, 1977.

Williams, S. R. *Nutrition and Diet Therapy.* 3rd Ed. St. Louis: The C. V. Mosby Co., 1977.

Wilson, E. D., Fisher, K. H., and Garcia, P. A. *Principles of Nutrition.* 4th Ed. New York: John Wiley & Sons, Inc., Pubs., 1979.

Winkler, I. Importance of good nutrition. *Nursing Times* 72:1890, 1976a.

———. Moderation in all things. *Nursing Times* 72:1917, 1976b.

CHAPTER 3

Energy Components of Food

How often do we stop to consider what we are eating and, more important, whether it will meet the nutritional needs of the body? There is a familiar expression, "You are what you eat," which refers to the fact that the foods one eats become a structural part of one's body. One of the primary reasons nursing students study nutrition is to develop their own nutrition philosophy. Only with a clear idea of the importance of nutrition in health promotion and recovery from illness can nurses be enthusiastic and effective counselors concerning a clients' nutritional well-being. After examining the dietary standards for a nutritionally adequate diet, the next step in learning about nutrition is to turn to the classification of the three nutrients that contribute Calories to our diets (carbohydrate, protein, and fat) and to the food sources of these nutrients.

CARBOHYDRATES

There has been a recent trend to minimize the importance of *carbohydrates*. Some advocate eliminating carbohydrates on fad weight-reducing diets. Some severely restrict their intake of carbohydrates because they consider them to be "fattening." Others de-emphasize the importance of carbohydrates by referring to them as only "empty Calories."

Carbohydrates, contrary to these myths, are the substances that provide the primary source of energy for the body. Carbohydrates are inexpensive sources of many nutrients. They are easily digested and absorbed and are needed for effective use of other nutrients, especially protein and fat.

Classification

Carbohydrates are composed of the three elements carbon, hydrogen, and oxygen; hence the convenient abbreviation CHO for carbohydrate. The term *carbohydrate* comes from the fact that the ratio of hydrogen to oxygen is $2:1$, the same ratio as in water. Plants store the energy they derive from the sun in carbohydrate form through the biological process of *photosynthesis:*

Carbon dioxide + Water $\xrightarrow{\text{Sunlight}}$ Glucose (CHO) + Oxygen

This process is then reversed within plant and animal cells when energy is required and is called *respiration:*

Glucose (CHO) + Oxygen $\rightarrow$ Carbon dioxide + Water + Energy

These two processes are an oversimplification of the complex energy cycle. See Figure 3-1 for a representation of both of these processes.

The two basic components of carbohydrates in foods are *starches* and *sugars*. A more detailed scientific classification breaks the sugars down into single sugars, or *monosaccharides;* and double sugars, or *disaccharides*. The starches are referred to as complex sugars, or *polysaccharides*.

Monosaccharides

The monosaccharides, or single sugars, are the simplest of all carbohydrates. They are the end products of all carbohydrate breakdown and the building blocks from which all other more complex carbohydrates are constructed. There are three monosaccharides

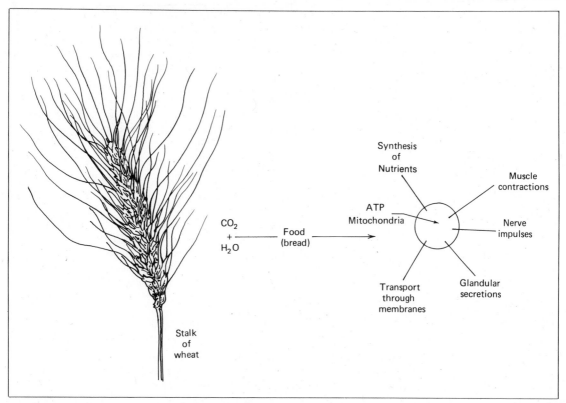

Figure 3-1. Photosynthesis and energy metabolism.

that are of nutritional significance: *glucose, fructose,* and *galactose.* All three of these are *hexoses,* which means they are each composed of a structure containing six carbon atoms (see Fig. 3-2). Two *pentoses* (five-carbon sugars), *ribose* and *deoxyribose,* are components of RNA (*ribonucleic acid*) and DNA (*deoxyribonucleic acid*), which are needed for protein synthesis. Both of these pentoses, however, can be synthesized in the body from glucose, so a separate dietary source is not required.

GLUCOSE. Glucose is the most important monosaccharide because it is the form of carbohydrate that circulates in the blood stream. It is the only source of energy that can be used

by the cells of the central nervous system and especially the brain. It is the chief end product from the digestion of all carbohydrates, and it is the substance most readily used by all cells for energy. Glucose is also commonly known as *dextrose* and is the monosaccharide most often given to patients on *intravenous* (IV) *therapy.* It is found in very concentrated form in honey, corn syrup, and molasses, but it is also found in sweet fruits such as oranges and grapes and in some vegetables.

FRUCTOSE. Another name for fructose is *levulose,* or more commonly, *fruit sugar.* It is found closely associated with glucose in honey and sweet ripe fruits. It is a product of the *hydrolysis,* or digestive breakdown, of the dou-

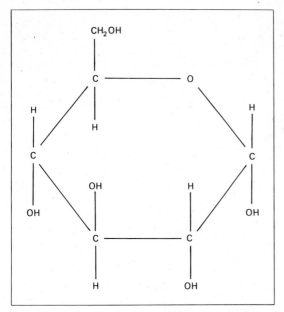

Figure 3-2. Chemical structure of glucose.

ble sugar *sucrose*. It is the sweetest of all the simple sugars. Honey is composed of almost equal proportions of glucose and fructose. Honey is a pure carbohydrate and does not contribute any health benefits other than being a source of energy like any other pure carbohydrate.

GALACTOSE.   Galactose is the one monosaccharide that does not exist by itself in nature; it is produced only after the digestion of the double sugar *lactose*. Lactose is milk sugar, so the only source of galactose in the diet comes from milk and other dairy products. During lactation, some glucose can be converted to galactose, and the two can be combined to form the lactose in human milk.

Disaccharides

The disaccharides, or double sugars, are composed of two of the monosaccharides linked together (see Fig. 3-3). The disaccharides are broken down (hydrolyzed) by the digestive enzymes into their component monosaccharides. The three disaccharides of nutritional interest are sucrose, lactose, and *maltose*.

SUCROSE.   Sucrose is common table sugar and is composed of one molecule each of fructose and glucose. Sucrose is manufactured either from sugarcane or sugar beets. Granulated sugar is almost 100% sucrose, whereas brown sugar, which has some molasses added back into it, is about 97% sucrose.

LACTOSE.   Lactose is the only common sugar that comes from an animal source. Com-

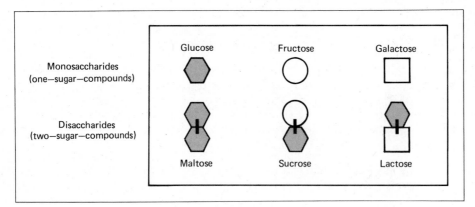

Figure 3-3. Monosaccharides and disaccharides.

monly known as milk sugar, it is composed of one molecule each of glucose and galactose. Human milk provides a slightly higher proportion (6.8 gm/100 ml) of lactose than cow's milk (4.8 gm/100 ml).

MALTOSE.   Maltose is composed of two glucose molecules and is always found in association with the breakdown of starch. In food, maltose is produced in malting and fermentation of cereal grains and is therefore present in malted milk, malted cereals, and beer. In the body, maltose is an intermediate product in the digestion of starch. Maltose is used with *dextrin*, a polysaccharide, as the source of carbohydrate in some infant formulas.

Comparison of Sugars

The various sugars studied thus far can be compared on the basis of their properties of sweetness and solubility (Table 3-1). Comparing all six of the common sugars for sweetness and considering sucrose (table sugar) as the standard, fructose is the sweetest and lactose the least sweet. All of the sugars in liquids with the exception of lactose are very soluble. All of the sugars contain 4 Calories for every gram. Because the caloric content is the same but the degree of sweetness varies, a dietitian or nurse could add a higher proportion (amount) of a less sweet sugar to a beverage to increase the Calories without the client being affected by excessive sweetness. Based on both the sweetening power and the solubility, the two sugars to be selected for such use should be maltose or galactose. These sugars are not generally found existing free in nature, however, so the other alternative up to this time has been to add glucose to a client's beverage. Intake of a large amount of simple carbohydrates, especially lactose, may irritate the gastrointestinal tract and lead to an *osmotic diarrhea*.

TABLE 3-1. Comparison of Physical Properties of Carbohydrates (Relative Values)

Monosaccharides	Sweetening Power	Soluble	Rate of Absorption
Hexoses			
Fructose	173	Yes	30
Glucose	74	Yes	100
Galactose	32	Yes	110
Mannose			10
Alcohol sugars			
Sorbitol	60	Yes	
Mannitol	50	Slightly	
Pentoses			
Ribose	—	Yes	
Xylose	40	Yes	15
Arabinose	—	Yes	9
Disaccharides			
Sucrose	100	Yes	
Maltose	32	Yes	
Lactose	16	Yes	
Polysaccharides			
Dextrin		Slightly	
Starch		No	
Glycogen		No	
Cellulose		No	

SOURCE: Reprinted with permission from Helen Andrews Guthrie, *Introductory Nutrition*, 4th Ed. St. Louis: The C. V. Mosby Co., 1979, p. 28.

Polycose

In 1974 Ross Laboratories developed a carbohydrate supplement called *Polycose*. This substance is produced by enzymatic hydrolysis, or breakdown, of cornstarch and is composed of units of both glucose and maltose. It has an excellent solubility in hot or cold liquids, is very low in sweetening power, and is relatively inexpensive to use. It is also very readily absorbed and utilized in the body. Polycose contains 4-Calories per gram like all other carbohydrates, but because of its low relative sweetness, large quantities can be added without making a product excessively sweet. For example, 50 gm of Polycose can be added to 1 cup of unsweetened orange juice, changing the caloric content from approximately 80 Calories to 280 Calories, without the client realizing the fact. The product comes in both powder and liquid form. If the liquid form is used, it must be remembered that the Polycose will dilute the nutrients in a given beverage unless the portion size is increased. The only use of this product is to increase the caloric content of foods. The product is a pure concentrated carbohydrate and should not be used by clients with diabetes mellitus or those who must restrict their intake of concentrated sweets. Polycose also has a low osmolarity and therefore minimizes the occurrence of osmotic diarrhea.

Polysaccharides

Polysaccharides, commonly known as starches, are more complex compounds composed solely of as many as 2,000 glucose units arranged as a long, straight chain (an *amylose* portion) or as a branched chain (an *amylopectin* portion) (see Fig. 3-4). These substances are not sweet; they are insoluble in water; and completeness of digestion for each one differs. The four polysaccharides of interest in nutrition are starch, *glycogen*, dextrin, and *cellulose* (i.e., fiber).

STARCH.   Starch is the storage form of carbohydrate in plants and is the most abundant

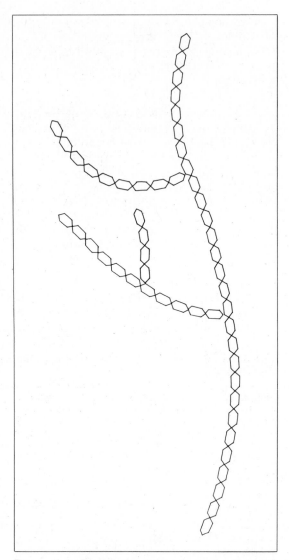

Figure 3-4. Partial structure of starch. Note the branched chains at regular intervals.

dietary source of carbohydrate in the world. The outer membrane of the starch granule is of a cellulose-type material. In order for the starch to be used by the body, this outer membrane must be broken by grinding or cooking. The starch molecule contains both an amylose (straight chain) and amylopectin (branched chain) portion. The amylopectin portion gives the starch molecule its gelling or thickening properties. Because starch granules have a great affinity for water and absorb it during cooking, there is a great increase in the volume of most starch products.

DEXTRINS. Partial breakdown of starch yields slightly soluble substances known as *dextrins*. This breakdown can occur either during digestion through the action of digestive enzymes, during cooking with moist heat, or through the long application of dry heat such as in the toasting of bread or browning during baking.

GLYCOGEN. Glycogen is the storage form of carbohydrate in animals. It is stored primarily in the liver and muscle. When extra quantities of glucose are available, the liver converts the excess glucose to glycogen. About $\frac{3}{4}$ lb ($\frac{1}{3}$ kg) of glycogen is generally stored in an adult. Muscle storage accounts for about $\frac{1}{2}$ lb (.225 kg) and liver storage for about $\frac{1}{4}$ lb (.113 kg). This stored glycogen can be broken down, or hydrolyzed, in the muscle or liver to glucose as needed by the body. Glycogen is not contained in animal muscle or liver tissue consumed as food by humans because the glycogen was converted to *lactic acid* during slaughtering.

CELLULOSE. Cellulose, or fiber, is an indigestible carbohydrate in our diets contributed by skins of fruits, coverings of seeds, and the structural parts of edible plants. Humans lack the digestive enzymes required to digest cellulose, so an undigested residue remains in the colon. Cellulose contributes bulk to the diet and aids in maintaining intestinal motility and therefore favors normal elimination.

OTHER POLYSACCHARIDES. There are additional polysaccharides that also cannot be digested, but they are used in various foods because of their ability to absorb water and to form a gel. One example is commercial pectin, which is available from apple peels and lemons and is used in making fruit jellies. Other polysaccharides are actually classified as food additives because they are added to foods to perform specific functions. Names of a few of these and their functions are:

- Agar, for thickening candy
- Alginates and carrageen, for giving body and smooth consistency to ice cream
- Vegetable gums (arabic, guar, xanthan), for water binding, thickening, and stabilizing in dairy desserts

Daily Carbohydrate Requirement

It should first be noted that there is no stated allowance contained in the RDA for carbohydrate. This is because the average person in the United States obtains more than adequate carbohydrate in his daily diet. There is, however, a general recommendation for carbohydrate intake. The minimum consumption of carbohydrate should be 50–100 gm/day to avoid the abnormal physiological symptom known as *ketosis*. About 50% of the Calories in the typical US diet are contributed by carbohydrate. This represents about 200–350 gm of carbohydrate consumed daily.

The daily requirement for fiber is 4–7 gm. This amount can be supplied by consuming one serving of whole grain bread or cereal, two servings of vegetables, and two servings of fruits.

PROTEINS

Protein is an important component of an adequate diet because protein is literally part of every cell in the body. Most fluids in the body contain protein, the exceptions being urine and bile. Basic knowledge about the food sources and requirements of protein will assist the nurse in assessing protein adequacy of a client's diet or identifying possible clinical symptoms of protein malnutrition.

Classification

Proteins are the most complex chemical substances known. They are composed of varying combinations of individual building blocks known as *amino acids*. The amino acids contain carbon, hydrogen, and oxygen (like carbohydrate), but in addition all amino acids contain the element nitrogen. All amino acids contain an amino group $(-NH_2)$, which explains how amino acids were originally named.

Plants and bacteria do not need individual amino acids to grow. They manufacture their own amino acids from carbon, hydrogen, and oxygen in the air and nitrogen either from the air or from simple compounds in the soil. Higher forms of life cannot manufacture all of their own proteins, so they must obtain part of their protein from the daily diet. In humans and animals, protein is digested and broken down into 22 amino acids and then rearranged into the many different proteins needed to maintain life and support growth. Protein digestion in people and animals produces the simple products needed by plants

and animals to build their own amino acids and proteins. The excrement of animals and the decaying products of plants and animals are returned to the soil to be recycled through the *nitrogen cycle*.

Of the 22 known amino acids, 9 are referred to as *essential amino acids* for the adult. This means that these 9 essential amino acids can only be obtained from foods in the diet. The remaining amino acids are referred to as *nonessential amino acids*. These nonessential amino acids are still essential to life, but it is not essential to eat protein foods to receive them; the body can manufacture or synthesize all of these amino acids.

Simple and Compound Proteins

The structure of a protein depends on the numbers of each amino acid present and the specific sequence in which the amino acids are linked (see Fig. 3-5). *Simple proteins* are substances that are composed only of amino acids. *Albumin* is a protein in egg; *zein* is a protein in corn; and *globin* is the protein in *hemoglobin*. It must be mentioned here that all

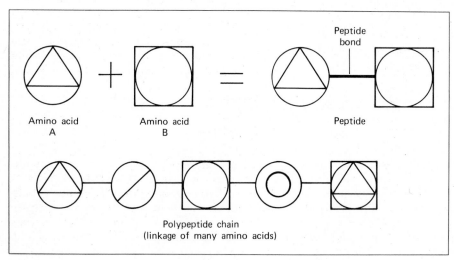

Figure 3-5. Amino acids linked together by peptide bonds form polypeptides, which then form proteins.

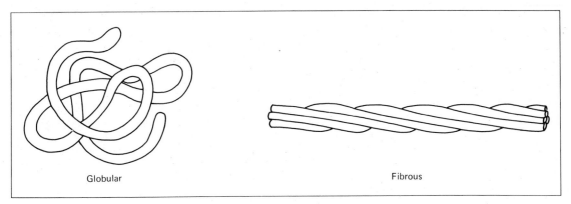

Figure 3-6. Globular and fibrous proteins.

protein foods contain more than one kind of protein; this is what makes them such very complex substances. Two basic types of proteins are *fibrous* and *globular,* a distinction based on the way the amino acids are bonded together (see Fig. 3-6).

The *compound proteins* are combinations of a protein with a nonprotein substance. Some examples of this type of proteins are hemoglobin (protein + heme) of blood and *casein* (protein + phosphoric acid) of milk.

Complete and Incomplete Proteins

A nutritionally useful classification of protein, based on the content of the essential and nonessential amino acids, is to categorize foods as either *complete, partially complete,* or *incomplete proteins.* A complete protein contains all the essential amino acids needed to maintain body tissues and support growth. Foods from animal sources, such as milk, meat, poultry, eggs, and fish, are examples of complete proteins. Of these foods human milk has the highest biological value; that is, it has the highest proportions of the essential amino acids. Eggs are next in biological value, followed by cow's milk.

A partially complete protein contains all nine of the essential amino acids, but it lacks a sufficient quantity of some of them. Partially complete proteins will maintain life, but they fail to support growth. Some examples of these proteins are dried beans and dried peas, soybeans, and nuts.

Incomplete proteins are deficient in one or more of the essential amino acids. These proteins will neither maintain life nor support growth when eaten alone. Examples of incomplete proteins are gelatin (even though it comes from an animal source), breads, cereals, and vegetables. These foods are sometimes classified as proteins of low biological value, referring to the fact that they contain a low proportion of essential amino acids.

LIMITING AMINO ACID. With the partially complete or incomplete proteins, the essential amino acid that is present in the smallest amount is referred to as the *limiting amino acid* of a specific food. For example, the limiting amino acid in wheat is *lysine,* and the limiting amino acid in corn is *tryptophan.* Gelatin is lacking in both tryptophan and lysine.

ALL OR NONE LAW. For best use by the body, some complete protein should be included with every meal. All the essential amino acids needed for the synthesis of a given protein must be present simultaneously and in sufficient amounts. If a single amino acid is missing, the amino acids will not be used for protein synthesis. In the case of all proteins except the complete proteins, if one of the essential amino acids is low in a food or a complete meal, the body will use the other essential amino acids at the rate of the limiting amino acid. The remainder of these amino acids will be used by the body as though they were only carbohydrates. This seems an extravagant way to waste expensive protein.

Protein Quality
Proteins differ in their ability to carry out maintenance and growth of body tissues according to the relative amounts of essential amino acids present. Two measurements of protein quality are based on nitrogen retention within the body.

BIOLOGICAL VALUE. The *biological value* of a protein is a measurement of protein quality of a food based on the retention of nitrogen within the body. The higher the proportion of nitrogen supplied by the essential amino acids, the higher the biological value of that food. The measurement is based on the percentage of nitrogen retained. A protein that contains a biological value of 70 or more is capable of supporting growth as long as the caloric content of the diet is adequate. Eggs have the highest biological value, followed by milk, fish, and beef.

NET PROTEIN UTILIZATION. *Net protein utilization* is a measurement that takes into account the differences in the digestibility of various proteins. It is a combination of the biological value and the *coefficient of digestibility*, which makes it a more useful measurement than the biological value. Both of these methods emphasize the high degree of desirability of a high content of essential amino acids.

Protein Requirements
There is an RDA for protein. The recommendation for a 154 lb (70 kg) male and a 120 lb (55 kg) female are 56 and 44 gm/day, respectively. Not everyone, of course, weighs

either 154 or 120 pounds, so the basis for this recommendation is 0.8 gm of protein per kilogram of ideal body weight for an adult. Protein requirements are higher during growth, pregnancy, and lactation and also with illness and surgery. Increased muscular activity does not increase a person's requirement for protein. The protein requirement of an athlete is the same as that of an office worker, although the athlete has a much higher caloric requirement than the office worker.

Protein quality also effects protein requirements. In general, the lower the quality of the proteins in the diet, the higher the protein requirement. The protein requirements are based on three different levels of protein quality. A pure vegetarian has a somewhat higher protein requirement than a person who eats mainly complete proteins.

Supplementary Effects of Protein

Vegetable proteins, even though they are incomplete proteins and lack certain essential amino acids, can be put together in certain combinations to yield a protein that has quality equal to or higher than meat. The reason for this phenomenon is that each vegetable protein is not low or lacking in the same essential amino acid. In this way, two vegetable proteins can complement or supplement each other. Also, small amounts of an animal protein can be combined with a larger amount of a vegetable protein to greatly increase the quality of the vegetable protein.

Large Amounts of a Single Food
When very large amounts of a single food are eaten daily, the total content of essential amino acids may be quite adequate. This is true in the case of rice when about 1 lb of cooked rice is consumed daily. Even though some of the essental amino acids are quite low in a regular size portion, inclusion of this large quantity daily increases their content until a comparably adequate intake of each is

obtained by comparison with the amino acid requirements. It should be remembered, however, that a diet consisting of only rice would be inadequate in many important vitamins and minerals.

Combining Animal and Plant Proteins

When a small amount of animal protein is fed with a larger amount of plant protein, the quality is as effective as when only animal protein is fed. We see examples of this principle very frequently in our daily experiences; putting milk on cereal or eating a cheese sandwich at noon are two very common ones. The favorite peanut butter and jelly sandwich eaten with a glass of milk also very effectively illustrates this point. Such simple casseroles or combined dishes as ham and beans, spaghetti, chili, and macaroni and cheese are good examples of combining plant and animal proteins. Note that macaroni and cheese is a complete protein, so a serving of meat does not need to be included to make the menu higher in protein quality. Generally the amino acid that is low in plant protein is found in high quantities in the animal protein, and the resulting combination is quite adequate in both amino acids and protein content.

Combining Vegetable Proteins

Certain vegetable proteins can be combined together quite successfully because not all plant proteins are deficient in the same amino acids. The amino acids that are low in one vegetable protein can be supplied by another vegetable protein that is high in that particular amino acid. The resulting combination will be higher in protein quality than when either are eaten separately. Successful combining of vegetable proteins requires knowledge of complementary protein combinations and, more specifically, knowledge of the amino acid content of foods (see Fig. 3-7).

In Central America, when corn and dried beans are eaten in the form of tortillas and refried beans, the combination provides a satisfactory protein quality. Another good ex-

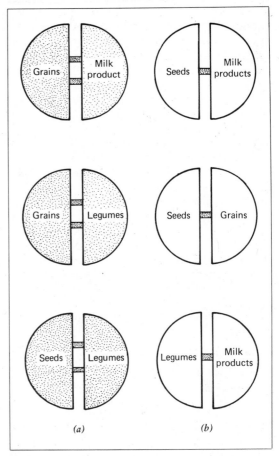

Figure 3-7. Protein complementarity: (a) several foods within each group demonstrate protein complementarity; (b) only a few items within each group demonstrate protein complementarity.

ample is the combination of baked beans and steamed brown bread served in New England. A third example is the traditional dish Quick Hoppin' John, served in the South on New Year's Day. This dish is composed of black-eyed peas, rice, tomatoes, green pepper, onion, and a small amount of bacon.

Vegetarian diets are also a good example of modifying the typical US diet by omitting certain protein foods. Vegetarian diets consist of grains, *legumes,* fruits, and vegetables. In addition to these foods some vegetarians consume milk products (lactovegetarian) or eggs (ovovegetarian) or both (lacto-ovovegetarian). Those vegetarians who include milk or eggs in their diet should not have any difficulty obtaining an adequate level of protein. Pure vegetarians, who consume no animal sources of protein, include legumes, whole grains, nuts, and vegetables to provide a balanced proportion of essential amino acids for an adequate protein intake. Legumes are a classification of foods not generally familiar to most people but widely used by vegetarians. They include peas, chick-peas, navy beans, lima beans, pinto beans, black-eyed peas, kidney beans, lentils, and soybeans. These foods, however, must be consumed in the proper combinations and proportions at each meal to receive the benefits of their supplementary relationships. Some basic food combinations that have a supplementary effect on each other are:

- Beans + Wheat
- Legumes + Rice
- Soybeans + Wheat + Rice

If carefully planned, vegetarian diets will be adequate in all nutrients except vitamin B_{12}, which is often lacking in pure vegetarian diets because it is found only in meat, eggs, and dairy products. The subject of vegetarianism and the nutritional adequacy of the diets is examined further in Chapter 7.

Improving Protein Quality

Considerable research is being conducted to improve the quality of plant proteins for use in underdeveloped countries. This may be accomplished through the addition of the limiting amino acid directly to the food or through the genetic improvement of cereal grains. Other special combinations of foods such as *Incaparina* (whole grain corn and sorghum, cottonseed flour, torula yeast, calcium carbonate, and vitamin A) and *Superamine* (hard

wheat, chick-peas, lentils, sugar, skim milk, and a vitamin-mineral mixture) have been developed by the World Health Organization, the Food and Agricultural Organization, and UNICEF. Other interesting sources of protein for the world currently under study are fish protein concentrate (FPC), soy protein concentrate (SPC), leaf protein concentrate (LPC), and single-cell proteins (SCP) from yeast, fungi, or algae.

FATS

Questions are being raised today by the public about the relationship of dietary fat to the incidence of coronary heart disease. To answer these questions adequately, the nurse must have a fundamental and yet practical understanding of such terms as *saturated fat, cholesterol,* and *polyunsaturated fat.*

Fats are a very concentrated source of energy in the body; they yield over twice as many Calories as carbohydrate. Fats add to the palatability or taste appeal of our diet through use of butter or margarine, frying of foods, dressings on salads, or sauces and gravies. Anyone who has had to severely restrict their fat intake realizes the inherent contribution fat makes to a meal.

Classification

Another term sometimes used for fat is *lipid,* although the term *lipid* actually refers to a broader group of substances than fat. *Lipid* is a chemical term that refers to a group of substances that have similar properties. They are insoluble in water and have a greasy feeling. Lipids include fats and oils but also such substances as *sterols,* cholesterol, *lipoproteins,* and the fat-soluble vitamins. Another way to define *lipids* is to refer to them as "fats and fat-related substances." The term *fat* in nutrition commonly refers to fats and oils. The classification of lipids is given in Table 3-2, but

TABLE 3-2. Classification of Lipids Important to Nutrition

I. *Simple Lipids*
   A. Fatty acids
   B. Neutral fats: Mono-, di-, triglycerides (esters of fatty acids and glycerol)
   C. Waxes (esters of fatty acids with high molecular weight alcohols)
      1. Sterol esters
      2. Nonsterol esters
II. *Compound Lipids*
   A. Phospholipids: Compounds of fatty acids, phosphoric acid and nitrogenous base
      1. Phosphoglycerides
         a. Lecithin
         b. Cephalin
         c. Sphingomyelins
   B. Glycolipids: Compounds of fatty acid combined with carbohydrate and a nitrogenous base
         a. Cerebrosides
         b. Gangliosides
   C. Lipoproteins: Lipids in combination with protein
III. *Derived Lipids*
   A. Fatty acids: Mono- and diglycerides
   B. Glycerol: Water-soluble component of triglycerides and interconvertible with carbohydrate
   C. Sterols
      1. Cholesterol, ergosterol
      2. Steroid hormones
      3. Vitamin D
      4. Bile salts
   D. Fat-soluble vitamins
      1. Vitamin A
      2. Vitamin E
      3. Vitamin K
      4. Coenzyme Q (ubiquinone)

SOURCE: Reprinted with permission from M. V. Krause, and L. K. Mahan, *Food, Nutrition, and Diet Therapy*, 6th Ed. Philadelphia: W. B. Saunders Co., 1979, p. 55.

only those lipids that are important components of dietary fat are discussed in this chapter.

Fatty Acids

Fatty acids are the major component of all food fats. The properties of food fats are determined by properties of the various fatty acids that they contain. Fatty acids are composed of the same three elements as carbohydrates, that is, carbon, hydrogen, and oxygen. Fatty acids in foods are composed of carbon chains that range from 4 to 24 carbon atoms. Some fatty acids contain the maximum number of hydrogen atoms that each carbon atom can hold. These fatty acids are called *saturated*, referring to the fact that the carbon atoms are "saturated," or filled, with hydrogen. Another type, *unsaturated fatty acids*, have some of the carbon atoms attached together by a *double bond*. This arrangement decreases the total number of hydrogen atoms in the fatty acid. Therefore, fatty acids can differ in both chain length and number of double bonds.

DEGREE OF SATURATION. The basic classification for fatty acids is based on the degree of saturation or the presence or absence of double bonds. The two general classifications of fatty acids are saturated and unsaturated fatty acids. Unsaturated fatty acids are further classified as either *monounsaturated* or polyunsaturated fatty acids. *Monounsaturated* means that the fatty acid contains only one double bond. *Polyunsaturated* refers to the fatty acids containing two or more double bonds (see Fig. 3-8).

CHAIN LENGTH. Saturated fatty acids vary in chain length from 4 to 24 carbon atoms, with the most common saturated fatty acids containing 14–18 carbon atoms. Unsaturated fatty acids have a longer carbon chain; they contain 18–22 carbons.

SATURATED FATTY ACIDS. Saturated fatty acids, which are commonly found in foods, originate from animal sources. Two short-chained saturated fatty acids that are found in butter and contain two and four carbon atoms, respectively, are *butyric* and *caproic acid*. The two most common saturated fatty acids found in foods are *palmitic* acid (with 16 carbons) and *stearic acid* (with 18 carbons). Fats composed mainly of saturated fatty acids

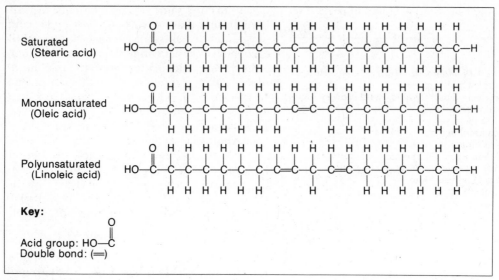

Figure 3-8. Common fatty acids.

are of a more solid nature at room temperature than are the unsaturated fatty acids.

UNSATURATED FATTY ACIDS. A monounsaturated fatty acid contains only one double bond. *Oleic acid* (with 18 carbons) is widely distributed in most food fats, and it is particularly high in olive oil. There are three polyunsaturated fats that are important in nutrition: *linoleic acid, linolenic acid,* and *arachidonic acid*. Linoleic acid generally occurs in foods in a higher proportion than the other two and is more often printed in tables of fatty acid composition of food fats.

As a general rule the longer the carbon chain and the higher the number of double bonds, the more liquid will be the nature of an unsaturated fat at room temperature. Thus a fat composed mainly of unsaturated fatty acids is of a more liquid nature at room temperature than fats containing primarily saturated fatty acids. Similarly, fats composed of a high proportion of polyunsaturated fatty acids are of a more liquid nature than fats composed mainly of monounsaturated fatty acids.

FATTY ACIDS IN FOOD FATS. Most food fats are composed of fatty acids from each of the major classifications. In other words, a common fat such as beef fat is composed of several saturated and several unsaturated fatty acids. What determines whether a fat is classified as saturated or unsaturated is the relative proportion of fatty acids it contains. For example, beef fat, because it contains a higher total proportion of saturated fatty acids than unsaturated fatty acids, is classified as a saturated fat. A comparison of the total fatty acid composition of several representative food fats is shown in Table 3-3.

Neutral Lipids
A *neutral lipid*, or a food fat, is composed of three fatty acids attached to a *glycerol* molecule. A food fat is also known as a *triglyceride*.

TABLE 3-3. Fat Content and Major Fatty Acid Composition of Selected Foods (in Decreasing Order of Linoleic Acid Content within Each Group of Similar Foods) (in Percentages)

Food	Total Fat	Saturated[b]	Unsaturated Oleic	Unsaturated Linoleic
Salad and cooking oils:				
Safflower	100	10	13	74
Sunflower	100	11	14	70
Corn	100	13	26	55
Cottonseed	100	23	17	54
Soybean[c]	100	14	25	50
Sesame	100	14	38	42
Soybean, specially processed	100	11	29	31
Peanut	100	18	47	29
Olive	100	11	76	7
Coconut	100	80	5	1
Vegetable fats—shortening	100	23	23	6–23
Margarine, first ingredient on label:[d,e]				
Safflower oil (liquid)—tub	80	11	18	48
Corn oil (liquid)—tub	80	14	26	38
Soybean oil (liquid)—tub[f]	80	15	31	33
Corn oil (liquid)—stick	80	15	33	29
Soybean oil (liquid)—stick[f]	80	15	40	25
Cottonseed or soybean oil, partially hydrogenated—tub[f]	80	16	52	13
Butter	81	46	27	2
Animal fats:				
Poultry	100	30	40	20
Beef, lamb, pork	100	45	44	2–6
Fish, raw:[f]				
Salmon	9	2	2	4
Mackerel	13	5	3	4
Herring, Pacific	13	4	2	3
Tuna	5	2	1	2
Nuts:				
Walnuts, English	64	4	10	40
Walnuts, black	60	4	21	28
Brazil	67	13	32	17
Peanuts or peanut butter	51	9	25	14
Pecan	65	4–6	33–48	9–24
Egg yolk	31	10	13	2
Avocado	16	3	7	2

SOURCE: Reprinted from *Fats in Food and Diet*, Agricultural Information Bull. No. 361, USDA, 1974.
[a] Total is not expected to equal total fat.
[b] Includes fatty acids with chains from 8 through 18 carbon atoms.
[c] Suitable as salad oil.
[d] Mean values of selected samples and may vary with brand name and date of manufacture.
[e] Includes small amounts of monounsaturated and diunsaturated fatty acids that are not oleic or linoleic.
[f] Linoleic acid includes higher polyunsaturated fatty acids.

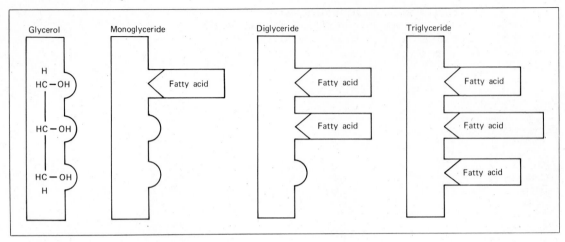

Figure 3-9. Structure of a food fat.

If the three fatty acids composing a triglyceride are all identical, the fat is called a *simple triglyceride*. If, however, at least two of the fatty acids are different, the fat is called a *mixed triglyceride*. The structure of a food fat may be seen in Figure 3-9.

Cholesterol

Cholesterol is a fat related substance that occurs primarily in foods of animal origin. It is a normal constituent of all body cells, and it is a precursor of many hormones. The body obtains its supply of cholesterol from food in the diet and from the body's own ability to manufacture (i.e., synthesize) cholesterol. Cholesterol is not an essential component of the daily diet because the body is able to make its own.

Requirement for Fat

There is no specific RDA for fat; the average diet supplies an adequate amount. In the average US diet 40–45% of the Calories come from fat. This represents a daily consumption of about 156 gm of fat.

FOOD EXCHANGE LISTS

A simple classification of foods, *Exchange Lists for Meal Planning,* is useful for discussing the carbohydrate, protein, and fat content of foods. The exchange lists were originally developed in 1950 by a joint committee of the American Dietetic Association, the American Diabetes Association, and the Public Health Service for use in planning diabetic diets; but they also have applications in planning any diet that requires modification of protein, fat, carbohydrate, or total Calories.

The exchange system consists of six lists of food from which a menu can be selected (see Appendix I). Each list or exchange group contains certain portions of food that are similar in their approximate content of certain combinations of carbohydrate, protein, or fat. Any food on one list can be "exchanged" or substituted for another food on that same list. Only the plain foods are included in these lists; there are no concentrated sweets, desserts, or fried foods. The six lists are:

List 1. Milk exchanges
List 2. Vegetable exchanges

List 3. Fruit exchanges
List 4. Bread exchanges
List 5. Meat exchanges
List 6. Fat exchanges

The student will notice a close similarity between these lists and the four food groups discussed earlier; see the end of the chapter for a comparison.

Food Sources of Carbohydrates

The food sources of carbohydrates come almost exclusively from plants. The one exception to this is milk, which is of animal origin.

Some foods, such as the common table sugars, are pure carbohydrate. This is essentially their only contribution to the diet. Other sugars, such as jams, jellies, honeys, and syrups, contain from 65 to 80% carbohydrates. These forms of carbohydrate may contain trace amounts of vitamins and minerals but not enough to make a significant nutritional contribution to the diet. Even though such foods as cakes, candies, and cookies do make a slightly higher nutritional contribution to the daily diet because they include other ingredients besides sugar, they are still 56–99% carbohydrate. The nutritional value would not even be considered "good" compared to that of a serving of vegetables or a slice of bread. A comparison of the percentages of carbohydrate contents of some common foods is presented in Table 3-4. Table 3-5 compares actual carbohydrate and caloric contents of some common foods. The student should note that fruits, vegetables, and grain products reveal a wide range of carbohydrate content. This variation in carbohydrate content has a direct effect on the caloric content of the food; the higher the carbohydrate content, the higher the number of Calories. When foods are categorized according to carbohydrate content, the effect on the groupings of foods will be more apparent.

Foods are considered as either starches or sugars on the basis of the predominance of the major classification of carbohydrates present. Many food sources of carbohydrate contain some monosaccharides, some disaccharides, and also some polysaccharides. Generally, if a food contains more polysaccharides, it is classified as a starch; if it contains a higher proportion of mono- and disaccharides, it is classified as a sugar. In the nutrition of carbohydrates the emphasis is mostly on total carbohydrate content and not on the individual components.

Bread and cereal products are high in starch and therefore high in total carbohydrate. Portions such as 1 slice of bread and $\frac{1}{2}$–$\frac{3}{4}$ cup of cereal, macaroni, noodles, or spaghetti each contain an average of 15 gm of carbohydrate. Milk is second to these foods in carbohydrate content. A cup of any kind of milk contains approximately 12 gm of carbohydrate. The three basic kinds of milk—whole, 2%, and skim—differ only in the fat content and therefore in total Calories.

Fruits and vegetables can be divided into those of low, moderate, or high carbohydrate content. This division can be made on the basis of water content. Those vegetables and fruits that contain a high proportion of water are lower in total carbohydrate and therefore lower in Calories. Conversely, those fruits and vegetables that are lower in water content are higher in carbohydrate content and total Calories.

TABLE 3-4. Carbohydrate Content of Major Food Groups

Food Group	Percentage of Carbohydrate
Sugars and concentrated sweets	70–99.5
Grain products	23–88
Fruits	8–31
Vegetables	3–26
Milk products	2–22
Meat	—

TABLE 3-5. Carbohydrate and Caloric Content of Some Common Foods

Food	Serving	Carbohydrate (gm)	Calories
Concentrated Sweets and Desserts			
Honey	1 T	17	65
Jellies	1 T	13	50
Jams	1 T	14	55
Milk chocolate	1 oz	16	145
Chocolate covered peanuts	1 oz	11	160
Cola beverage	12 oz	37	145
Angelfood cake	1 piece	32	135
Chocolate cake with chocolate icing	1 piece	40	235
Cherry pie	1 piece	52	350
Pumpkin pie	1 piece	32	275
Grain Products			
Popcorn, buttered	1 cup	5	40
Spaghetti	1 cup	32	155
Macaroni	1 cup	32	155
Rice	1 cup	50	225
Cornflakes, sugar coated	1 cup	37	155
Cornflakes, plain	1 cup	21	95
Oatmeal	1 cup	23	130
Bread, white (enriched)	1 slice	13	70
Milk Products			
Chocolate milkshake	10 oz	63	355
Ice cream	1 cup	32	270
Yogurt, fruit flavored	1 cup	42	230
Whole milk	1 cup	11	150
Fruits			
Applesauce, sweetened	1 cup	61	230
Applesauce, unsweetened	1 cup	26	100
Banana	one	26	100
Orange	one	16	86
Apple	one	20	80
Vegetables			
Peas	1 cup	29	150
Potato	1 medium	33	145
Corn	1 cup	31	130
Carrots, cooked	1 cup	11	50
Green beans	1 cup	7	30
Tomato	1 medium	6	25
Lettuce	1 cup	2	10

SOURCE: *Nutritive Value of Foods*, Home & Garden Bull. No. 72, rev., USDA, 1977.

In the exchange system all the fruits are listed together. Each fruit on that list contains 10 gm of carbohydrate per serving. A glance at the list will reveal that there are several differentiations in portion size. These differences exist because the individual fruits vary in carbohydrate contents. The fruits with a portion size of approximately ½ cup are classified as moderate-carbohydrate fruits. Those with a portion size of greater than ½ cup contain a higher proportion of water and a lower proportion of carbohydrate and are therefore classified as low-carbohydrate fruits. Also those fruits with a serving size of less than ½ cup are more concentrated in carbohydrate and therefore are called high-carbohydrate fruits. Examples of specific fruits in each of these classifications may be seen in Appendix I.

The carbohydrate classification of vegetables is very similar to that of fruits. The vegetables that are low in water content and high in carbohydrate content are referred to as starchy vegetables. They contain the same carbohydrate content (15 gm) as a serving of bread or cereal and are therefore listed with the bread exchanges. Corn, lima beans, peas, and potatoes are some examples of these starchy vegetables. The vegetable list is based on the moderate-carbohydrate vegetables in which one serving is considered ½ cup and the carbohydrate content is 5 gm per serving. Also included is a category of certain raw, leafy salad vegetables such as lettuce, parsley, and radishes that are high in water content and therefore very low in carbohydrate content. These raw vegetables may be used as desired in a diet.

Using this brief introduction to the carbohydrate content of foods as a basis, we can now discuss these foods in terms of a word meaningful to everyone—Calories. If the carbohydrate, protein, and fat content of a food is known, the caloric content of that food can be easily calculated. For use in the body, each gram of carbohydrate or protein will yield 4 Calories. Fat, a very concentrated source of energy, yields 9 Calories/gm. To determine the caloric content of a particular portion of food, multiply the grams of carbohydrate and protein in that food by 4 and the grams of fat, if any, by 9. Calculate, for example, the caloric content of 1 cup of whole milk, which contains 12 gm of carbohydrate, 8 gm of protein, and 10 gm of fat:

12 gm carbohydrate
× 4 Calories/gm
48 Calories

8 gm protein
× 4 Calories/gm
32 Calories

10 gm fat
× 9 Calories/gm
90 Calories

48 Calories from carbohydrate
32 Calories from protein
90 Calories from fat
170 Calories in 1 cup whole milk

A summary of the carbohydrate and caloric content of all the foods in the exchange system is given in Table 3-6.

Food Sources of Protein

As already stated, the two major classifications of protein are complete and incomplete proteins. Complete proteins are obtained primarily from animal sources and incomplete proteins from vegetable sources.

Animal Sources

Dairy products all derive their protein content from milk. Milk contains a good balance of the essential amino acids. The fact that human breast milk has a higher proportion of essential amino acids than even cow's milk gives credibility to the belief that breast feeding of infants supplies them with nature's most perfect food. Cheese is a concentrated source of protein because, through the action of either rennin or lactic acid on milk in the processing, the *casein* coagulates and the liquid portion, called the *whey,* separates. Most of the nutrients are available in concentrated form in the solid portion, or *curd.* According to the exchange method a cup of any kind of milk contains 12 gm of carbohydrate and 8 gm of protein, and the fat content varies depending on the type of milk used in processing.

Meat, poultry, and fish are all excellent sources of complete protein. The relative protein content of these meats depends on their content of moisture and fat. The higher

TABLE 3-6. Summary of Energy Nutrients and Calories in the Exchange Lists

Exchange List	Measure	Carbohydrate (gm)	Protein (gm)	Fat (gm)	Energy (Calories)
Bread Exchange		15	2	—	68
Bread	1 slice				
Cereal	½–¾ cup				
High-carbohydrate vegetables	varies				
Milk Exchange					
Whole	1 cup	12	8	10	170
2%	1 cup	12	8	5	125
Skim	1 cup	12	8	—	80
Fruit Exchange		10	—	—	40
High-carbohydrate	less than ½ cup				
Moderate-carbohydrate	½ cup				
Low-carbohydrate	more than ½ cup				
Vegetable Exchanges					
Moderate-carbohydrate	½ cup				
Low-carbohydrate	as desired, raw	5	2	—	28
Meat Exchanges					
Lean	1 oz	—	7	3	55
Medium-fat	1 oz	—	7	5	73
High-fat	1 oz	—	7	7	91
Fat Exchanges					
Butter or margarine	1 t				
Salad dressing	1 T	—	—	5	45
Other	varies				

the content of moisture, fat, or both, the lower the protein content. Fish and chicken are somewhat lower in fat content than beef and pork.

As mentioned before, eggs are the highest source of complete protein. The white and yolk each provide about an equal portion of protein.

Even though individual meats vary slightly in protein content, according to the exchange system the basic protein content of 1 oz of meat is 7 gm. The fat contents of different meats vary greatly, a difference discussed in more detail in the following section on fats.

Plant Sources

The two main groups of food from plant sources that contain protein are vegetables, and breads and cereals. Both these groups contain a low content of protein (2–3 gm) when consumed in the average ½ cup serving; yet for the true vegetarian who consumes much larger quantities from these two groups, the protein content can be quite high. The vegetarian, however, must exercise great skill in the way he combines these proteins for a certain meal. In the exchange system an average serving of vegetables contains 5 gm of carbohydrate and 2 gm of protein. Breads and cereals also contain about 2 gm of protein and 15 gm of carbohydrate. A listing of the foods from the exchange lists containing protein and fat may be found in Appendix I.

Food Sources of Fat

As previously stated, food fats are composed of both saturated and unsaturated fatty acids. The type of fatty acids that predominate determine whether the fats are classified as saturated or unsaturated.

Saturated Fats

Food fats from animal sources comprise the major portion of saturated fats in a diet. The meat and milk groups of the basic four comprise the largest number of examples. Beef, pork, and lamb are higher in saturated fat than are poultry and fish. The former meats are also much higher in fat content than the latter. In addition, the higher the fat content of the beef, pork, and lamb, the higher the saturated fat content. All milk products that are made from whole milk or those containing a large proportion of butter fat are high in saturated fat. Lard and butter are by-products from meat and milk, and they are also very high in saturated fat content.

Unsaturated Fats

Although unsaturated fats are contained mainly in vegetable fats, fish is one meat that contains a high proportion of polyunsaturated fatty acids. The other main source of unsaturated fats is margarines and oils manufactured from vegetable oils. A process in the manufacturing of margarines called *hydrogenation* is used to adjust the degree of hardness or softness in commercial margarines. In this process hydrogen is added to the double bonds of the unsaturated vegetable oils to make them more saturated and more solid in consistency. Margarines made from hydrogenated or partially hydrogenated vegetable oils are less expensive than those made from pure vegetable oils.

With the increased emphasis on the consumption of higher content of polyunsaturated fats, a margarine that is made from pure vegetable oil is more desirable than one made from hydrogenated or partially hydrogenated vegetable oil. Some vegetable oils contain a higher proportion of polyunsaturated fatty acids than others. Safflower oil is highest in polyunsaturated fat, followed by corn oil. Two vegetable oils, peanut and olive, are highest in the monounsaturated fatty acid, oleic acid. Another vegetable oil, coconut oil, is an exception to the rule that

vegetable oils are primarily unsaturated. Coconut oil contains primarily the saturated fatty acid, *lauric acid*.

Rancidity, a common problem with the use of lard and butter as primary sources of fat, changes flavor and odor, making the fat undesirable for use. Rancidity is the partial breakdown of fat caused by oxidation of the double bonds. Vitamin E is a natural *antioxidant* that occurs in high quantities in vegetable oils that are high in polyunsaturated fatty acids. Because of this high quantity of naturally occurring vitamin E, vegetable oils do not become rancid as rapidly as butter or lard.

The food lists from the exchange system that contain fat are the milk list, the fat list, and the meat list. Whole milk contains 3.5–4% butterfat, and so 2% milk contains half this amount of fat. Skim milk contains essentially no fat at all. Each serving from the fat list contains approximately 5 gm of fat or 45 Calories. The meat list in the exchange system is broken down into lean, medium-fat, and high-fat groups of meat and other protein foods.

Caloric Content of Exchange Lists

The exchange system is a simple and practical way to estimate quickly the caloric content of a few foods, a menu for one meal, or an entire day's intake. Placing foods containing similar contents of the energy nutrients (carbohydrates, proteins, and fats) into a particular list and using the average number of grams of carbohydrate, protein, and fat for these foods results in values that can be readily used to calculate the Calories in a given portion of food. The caloric content of each gram of either carbohydrate or protein is 4 Calories/gm and for fat is 9 Calories/gm. The calculation of the caloric content of a breakfast menu shown in Table 3-7 serves as an example. A student's breakfast consisted of ½ cup orange juice, 1 slice whole wheat toast, 1 t margarine, 1 poached egg, and 1 cup 2% milk.

TABLE 3-7. Caloric Calculation of a Breakfast

Food	Amount	Exchange List	Carbohydrate (gm)	Protein (gm)	Fat (gm)
Orange juice	½ cup	Fruit	10	—	—
Whole wheat toast	1 slice	Bread	15	2	—
Margarine	1 t	Fat	—	—	5
Poached egg	1	Meat (med.-fat)	—	7	5
2% milk	1 cup	Milk	12	8	5
		Total gm	37	17	15
			× 4	× 4	× 9
		Total Calories	148 +	68 +	135 = 351

The total Calories for the breakfast menu in Table 3-7 was 351 Calories. An alternate method for calculating Calories using the exchange system would be to calculate the Calories in each separate food item from its carbohydrate, protein, and fat content and total the Calories for each food. It must be emphasized that caloric contents of foods using the exchange system are only estimates, but this method is easier and more practical than looking up individual caloric contents of foods. This method can help a person calculate the caloric content of foods eaten by himself or by a client. It must also be remembered that the foods contained in the exchange lists are only plain, ordinary foods. No combined foods (such as casseroles or sauces) or concentrated sweets will be found in the lists. The caloric content of these foods and many others can be found in a table of food composition (see Appendix A).

A Comparison of the Basic Four and the Exchange System

Two systems for classifying foods have been introduced in this chapter. One system, the basic four food groups, categorizes foods into groups and specifies the number of servings per day for a nutritionally adequate diet. The other system, the exchange system, classifies foods containing similar quantities of the energy nutrients into six separate lists of foods. Although the two methods are used for different purposes, there are several similarities in the food groups. The two methods supplement each other in planning a nutritionally balanced diet. For example, a low-Calorie diet can be planned using the recommended servings from the basic four and calculating the caloric content of the day's diet using the exchange system.

Comparing these two methods, one notices that some foods, such as cheese, are placed in one group in the basic four but in a different group in the exchange system. This is because each of the two methods has a separate basis for categorizing the foods. The basic four categorizes foods according to specific nutrient content (including vitamins and minerals), and the exchange system uses only the average contents of carbohydrate, protein, and fat as a basis. The serving size also differs slightly between the two methods. A more complete comparison of the two methods is shown in Table 3-8.

Energy Nutrients and Caloric Content of the Basic Four

It is useful here to compare the minimum daily recommendations of the basic four food groups with the average contents of carbohydrate, protein, fat, and Calories in a typical meal pattern for one day. The calculations are given in Table 3-9 and were made

TABLE 3-8. Comparison of Basic Four and the Exchange System

Basic Four Food Groups	Exchange System
Milk group	Milk List
Whole, 2%, skim	Whole, 2%, skim
Yogurt	Yogurt
Cheese	
Cottage cheese	
Ice cream	
Fruit and vegetable group	Vegetable List
All fruits and vegetables	Low- and moderate-carbohydrate vegetables
	Fruit List
	All fruits and fruit juices
Bread and cereal group	Bread List
All breads and cereals	All breads and cereals
	High-carbohydrate or starchy vegetables
	Ice cream
Meat group	Meat List
All meats, fish, poultry	All meats, fish, poultry
Eggs	Eggs
Cheese[a]	Cheese
Cottage cheese[a]	Cottage cheese
Peanut butter	Peanut butter
Dried beans or peas	Fat List
Nuts	Fats
	Oils
	Margarine
	Dressings
	Bacon
	Nuts

[a] If not counted as part of milk group.

using the exchange values for carbohydrate, protein, and fat. These calculations using the basic four reveal many interesting facts. First of all the caloric content of the minimum servings of simply prepared foods is only 1,215 Calories. These Calories could be reduced even further by using skim milk instead of whole milk and choosing only lean meat instead of medium-fat meat. There is, therefore, no validity to the claim that if one ate the foods recommended by the basic four one would gain weight. It is not the actual foods in the basic four that contain so many Calories but the "extras" that are added (e.g., sauces, gravies, margarine, sour cream, etc.), the method of preparation (e.g., fried or deep-fat fried), and the addition of concentrated sweets and beverages.

Examination of the grams of carbohydrate and protein also reveals some interesting facts. First, the total grams of carbohydrate supplied by the minimum servings from the basic four (124 gm) is well above the minimum daily recommendation of 100 gm of carbohydrate. The most interesting comparison is that between the protein content of the basic four and the RDA for protein. The minimum servings of meat from the basic four is for two 2-oz servings (4 oz), or the equivalent, daily. When the grams of protein are combined with the protein contributed by milk and the small amounts of protein supplied by

TABLE 3-9. Energy Nutrients and Caloric Content of the Basic Four in One Day's Food Consumption

Food	Amount	Carbohydrate (gm)	Protein (mg)	Fat (mg)
Milk group				
Whole milk	2 cups	24	16	20
Meat group				
Medium-fat meat	4 oz	—	28	20
Vegetables				
Potato	½ cup	15	2	—
Green or yellow	½ cup	5	2	—
Fruit				
Citrus	½ cup	10	—	—
Other	½ cup	10	—	—
Bread and cereal group				
Cereal	½ – ¾ cup	15	2	—
Bread	3 slices	45	6	—
Margarine	3 t	—	—	15
Total gm		124	56	55
		× 4	× 4	× 9
Total Calories		496 +	224 +	495 = 1,215

vegetables and breads and cereals, the total daily protein supplied is 56 gm, which meets the RDA for protein for all adult males (56 gm) and all adult females (44 gm). Most Americans consume 4–8 oz of meat at each meal, which greatly and unnecessarily adds to the protein and caloric content of the diet. Extra protein will not harm a person, but the additional protein foods are expensive and the extra Calories may lead to a weight problem. Thus the basic four provides a daily meal pattern that, with sensible food selection and preparation, is adequate in protein and carbohydrate and still low in Calories. This daily meal plan can be easily increased in caloric content by the addition of other foods, primarily sources of carbohydrate and fat.

BIBLIOGRAPHY

Arlin, M. J. *The Science of Nutrition.* 2nd Ed. New York: Macmillan, Inc., Co., 1977.

Council on Foods and Nutrition, Am. Med. Assoc. The regulation of dietary fat. *J. Am. Med. Assoc.* 181(5):411, 1962.

Edelson, E. Sugar is not so sweet. *Family Health* 3:28, 1971.

Food and Nutrition Board, Nat'l Research Council. *Recommended Dietary Allowances.* 9th Ed. Washington, D.C.: Nat'l Acad. of Sciences, 1980.

Guthrie, H. A. *Introductory Nutrition.* 4th Ed. St. Louis: The C. V. Mosby Co., 1979.

Harding, M. G., Swarner, J. B., and Crooks, H. Carbohydrates in foods. *J. Am. Diet. Assoc.* 46:197, 1965.

Hertzler, A. A., and Anderson, H. L. Food guides in the United States. *J. Am. Diet. Assoc.* 64:19, 1974.

Hicks, B. M. Food groups—where do they belong? *Food and Nutr. News* (Nat'l Livestock and Meat Board, Chicago) 48(3), 1977.

Krause, M. V., and Mahan, L. K. *Food, Nutrition, and Diet Therapy.* 6th Ed. Philadelphia: W. B. Saunders Co., 1979.

Lachance, P. A. Points of view—food guides. *J. Nutr. Educ.* 4(2):46, 1972.

Mayer, J. The ABC's of protein. *Family Health* 5:24, 1973.

———. Protein—the master builder. *Family Health* 6:38, 1974.

Mitchell, H. S., Rynbergen, H. J., Anderson, L., and Dibble, M. V. *Nutrition in Health and Disease.* 16th Ed. Philadelphia: J. B. Lippincott Co., 1976.

Robinson, C. H., and Lawler, M. R. *Normal and Therapeutic Nutrition.* 15th Ed. New York: Macmillan, Inc., 1977.

Scheig, R. What is dietary fat? *Am. J. Clin. Nutr.* 22(5):651, 1969.

Williams, S. R. *Nutrition and Diet Therapy.* 3rd Ed. St. Louis: The C. V. Mosby Co., 1977.

Wilson, E. D., Fisher, K. H., and Garcia, P. A. *Principles of Nutrition.* 4th Ed. New York: John Wiley & Sons, Inc., Pubs., 1979.

Yudkin, J. Evolutionary and historical changes in dietary carbohydrates. *Am. J. Clin. Nutr.* 20:108, 1967.

CHAPTER 4

Energy Requirements

There is concern today about providing energy for our homes, offices, schools, and automobiles. In nutrition there is also concern about energy, but from a different perspective. We need to know (1) the energy, or caloric, value of foods and (2) the total energy, or caloric, requirements of a person. Because of evolving changes of lifestyle in industrialized countries in recent years, there has been a renewed interest in the energy expenditures resulting from various activities. More machines and labor-saving devices have resulted in a generally higher standard of living and less manual labor in both industry and the home. A shortening of the workweek has created more leisure time. All of these factors have led to a more sedentary lifestyle with decreasing energy expenditures and caloric requirements. Much of the American population has not, however, reduced caloric intake to correspond with the lower caloric requirements and expenditures. Therefore, this part of the population is considered to be overweight.

Many scientists and health professionals are interested in these aspects of energy for specific reasons. The physiologist is interested in the amount of energy expended during particular physical activity. The epidemiologist is concerned with the effects of a sedentary lifestyle and being overweight on the prevalence of degenerative diseases. The nutritionist recommends caloric intakes for weight loss, weight gain, or the maintenance of ideal weight and to meet energy requirements.

The purpose of this chapter is to present the factors that determine total energy requirements and show how to estimate those requirements. The results of an imbalance between caloric intake and energy expenditure, namely, the conditions of being overweight and underweight, are discussed in the following chapter.

TYPES OF ENERGY

The human body may be likened to a machine or engine that must constantly be refueled to enable it to perform work. The fuel for the body is, of course, food. Food provides the body with energy to do both external and internal work. The chemical energy available from food is converted in the body to electrical energy for the transmission of impulses through the brain and nervous system, to thermal energy for the regulation of body temperature, and to other forms of chemical energy for the synthesis of body compounds. This chemical energy from food is also converted into mechanical energy, which allows muscles to contract and work to be accomplished in the external environment. Figure 4-1 shows examples of the different types of energy.

MEASUREMENT OF FOOD ENERGY

Foods are quite frequently spoken of on the basis of the *Calories* they contain. Foods themselves do not actually contain Calories. They are composed of carbohydrates, proteins, and fats, which have their energy potential measured in Calories (i.e., kilocalories, or kcal). The Calorie used in nutrition can be defined

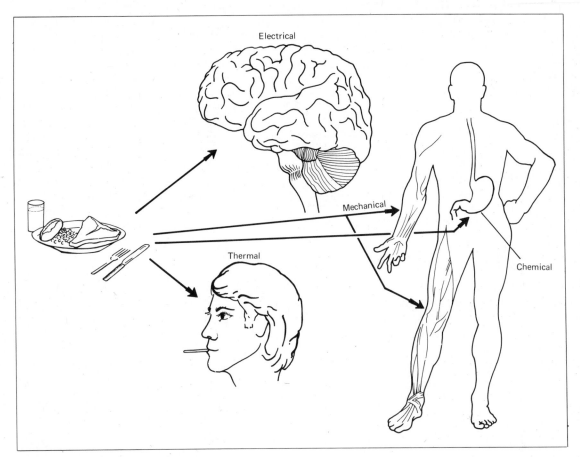

Figure 4-1. Energy transformation from food.

as the amount of heat needed to raise the temperature of 1 kg of water 1 degree centigrade. This unit (the kilocalorie) is 1,000 times larger than the calorie used in either biology or chemistry. In this text, *Calorie* is used to refer to the *kilocalorie,* which is the measure of the energy content of food.

Because of the eventual conversion of the United States to the metric system, there must be a change from the use of the familiar Calorie to a more precisely defined unit called the *joule.* The Calorie used in nutrition has not been rigorously defined and is not directly derived from the metric system. The *joule,* which is the unit of energy in the metric system, is defined as the energy expended when 1 kg is moved a distance of 1 m by a force of 1 newton. One calorie is equivalent to 4.184 joules; and a Calorie, or kilocalorie, is equivalent to 4.184 kilojoules or 4,184 joules. For an idea of the impact this will have on the thinking of the average person in the United States, consider a woman told by her doctor to go on a 1,000-Calorie diet. Imagine her surprise when on her next visit the doctor asks her how she is progressing on her 4,184-kilojoule diet and has she lost 2.2 kg yet? Obviously this change is not going to occur overnight, but it, as well as the gradual introduction of the rest of the metric system, has already begun. People in the United States will have to begin to "think metric" or continue to make the mathematical conversions from one system to the other. Despite the inconveniences and confusion the change to metric measurement will bring to an area such as nutrition, the field must make this change or it will be isolated from recent developments in physics and chemistry. The change should be integrated gradually into society by first using it in the scientific journals along with the Calorie. The first major step in this direction was the inclusion of kilojoules along with Calories in the 1974 edition of the *Recommended Dietary Allowances.*

ENERGY CONTENT OF FOODS

The energy content of foods, which is contributed by carbohydrates, proteins, and fats, can be determined both outside and inside the human body. The total energy content of a food can be determined outside the body by burning samples of food in pure oxygen in an instrument called a *bomb calorimeter.* This instrument, shown in Figure 4-2, is essentially a well-insulated sealed box that contains pure oxygen and the food sample to be burned. It is surrounded by a water bath. The heat produced by the combustion is measured and stated in terms of Calories. Food burned in this manner is completely oxidized to carbon dioxide, water, and nitrous oxide. The value obtained is called the *gross energy value,* or *heat of combustion,* of the food. Because the entire food sample is burned completely, a large amount of heat is released all at one time. This gross energy of foods (shown in Fig. 4-3) does not have much applicability. This type of heat production would not be practical in the human body because of the intensity of the heat produced and because all the energy available from the food would be produced

immediately after a meal. The body is more conservative in its production of energy. The transformation of chemical energy in the food into mechanical energy to perform work is never complete. The step-by-step breakdown of carbohydrates, proteins, and fats during digestion and metabolism into simple chemical substances insures the capture of about 55–60% of the potential energy in the form of the ATP (*adenosine triphosphate*), the form of energy used by individual body cells.

The practical information to have is the energy values available from burning food within the human body. All of the potential

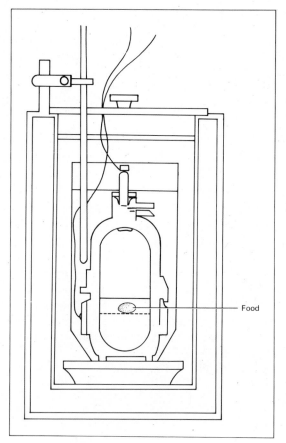

Figure 4-2. Bomb calorimeter.

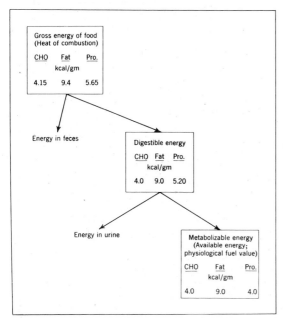

Figure 4-3. Energy value of food. (From R. L. Pike and M. L. Brown, *Nutrition: An Integrated Approach*, 2nd Ed., p. 853. Copyright © 1975, John Wiley & Sons, Inc. Reprinted by permission of John Wiley & Sons, Inc.)

energy in foods is not available for use in the body because food is not completely digested and absorbed. Some potential energy is lost in the urine and feces. In the typical US diet the coefficient of digestibility for carbohydrate is 98%; for fat, 95%; and for protein, 92%. When the gross energy values for carbohydrate, protein, and fat are multiplied by these coefficients of digestibility, the energy values are then:

Carbohydrate	4.0 kcal/gm
Protein	5.2 kcal/gm
Fat	9.0 kcal/gm

Some of the end products of protein metabolism, such as urea and uric acid, are excreted in the urine and their energy value is lost. This energy loss amounts to about 1.25 kcal/gm of protein. Subtracting this value from the figure given above for protein leaves 3.95 kcal/gm of protein. Rounding these figures off to the nearest whole number gives the *physiological fuel values* used in the last chapter:

Carbohydrate	4 kcal/gm
Protein	4 kcal/gm
Fat	9 kcal/gm

With the eventual use of the joule as the unit of energy in the metric system these values will be 17 kilojoules/gm of carbohydrate and protein and 38 kilojoules/gm of fat. Mental calculations of energy values of foods from grams of carbohydrate, protein, and fat will not be as simple as using the familiar and easy-to-use values of 4 and 9 kcal/gm.

It should be emphasized (1) that the physiological fuel values are based on pure samples of carbohydrate, protein, and fat, so that different energy values exist for the carbohydrate, protein, and fat in individual foods, and (2) that the coefficients of digestibility are also only averages. Table 4-1 gives the actual physiological fuel values and coefficients of digestibility of several common foods. Figure 4-4 is an example of the differences in energy value obtained by using the actual values and the average values. This information is presented to show that the physiological fuel values are only averages, but very useful averages, quite adequate for calculating Calories.

FACTORS DETERMINING TOTAL ENERGY REQUIREMENTS

Three major factors determine a human's daily energy requirement: the *basal metabolic rate,* the degree of *physical activity,* and the *specific dynamic action* of food. For infants and children growth is an additional factor. Energy requirements are stated in Calories because the energy potential of food is measured in Calories (or joules).

TABLE 4-1. Data Used for Calculating Energy Values of Selected Foods

Food	Protein			Fat			Carbohydrate		
	Coefficient of digestibility, %	Heat of combustion less 1.25,[a] kcal/gm	Factor to be applied to ingested nutrients, kcal/gm	Coefficient of digestibility, %	Heat of combustion, kcal/gm	Factor to be applied to ingested nutrients, kcal/gm	Coefficient of digestibility, %	Heat of combustion, kcal/gm	Factor to be applied to ingested nutrients, kcal/gm
Butter	97	4.40	4.27	95	9.25	8.79	98	3.95	3.87
Cane or beet sugar (sucrose)	—	—	—	—	—	—	98	3.95	3.87
Eggs	97	4.50	4.36	95	9.50	9.02	98	3.75	3.68
Fruits, all (except lemons, limes)	85	3.95	3.36	90	9.30	8.37	90	4.00	3.60
Immature lima beans, cowpeas, peas, other legumes	78	4.45	3.47	90	9.30	8.37	97	4.20	4.07
Macaroni, spaghetti	86	4.55	3.91	90	9.30	8.37	98	4.20	4.12
Margarine, vegetable	97	4.40	4.27	95	9.30	8.84	98	3.95	3.87
Mature dry beans, cowpeas, peas, other legumes, nuts	78	4.45	3.47	90	9.30	8.37	97	4.20	4.07[b]
Meat, fish	97	4.40	4.27	95	9.50	9.02	—	—	—
Milk, milk products	97	4.40	4.27	95	9.25	8.79	98	3.95	3.87
Other cereals, refined	85	4.55	3.87	90	9.30	8.37	98	4.20	4.12
Other vegetable fats and oils	—	—	—	95	9.30	8.84	—	—	—
Potatoes and starchy roots	74	3.75	2.78	90	9.30	8.37	96	4.20	4.03
Rice, white or polished	84	4.55	3.82	90	9.30	8.37	99	4.20	4.16
Wheat, 97–100% extraction	79	4.55	3.59	90	9.30	8.37	90	4.20	3.78
Wheat, 85–93% extraction	83	4.55	3.78	90	9.30	8.37	94	4.20	3.95
Wheat, 70–74% extraction	89	4.55	4.05	90	9.30	8.37	98	4.20	4.12
Wheat, flaked, puffed, rolled, shredded whole meal	79	4.55	3.59	90	9.30	8.37	90	4.20	3.78
Wheat bran (100%)	40	4.55	1.82	90	9.30	8.37	56	4.20	2.35

SOURCE: *Principles of Nutrition*, 4th Ed. E. D. Wilson, K. H. Fisher, and P. A. Garcia, Copyright © 1979 John Wiley & Sons, Inc. Reprinted by permission of John Wiley & Sons, Inc. Data from A. L. Merrill and B. K. Watt, *Energy Value of Foods*, Agriculture Handbook No. 74 rev., USDA, 1973, p. 25.
[a] The correction, 1.25 kilocalories, has been subtracted from the heat of combustion. This gives values applicable to grams of digested protein and identical with Atwater's factors per gram of available protein.
[b] Carbohydrate factor, 3.87 for brain, heart, kidney, and liver; 4.11 for tongue and shellfish.

	Carbohydrate (gm)	Protein (gm)	Fat (gm)
1 egg, poached	1	6	6

Method 1: *Using Calories per gram*
Considering the coefficient of digestibility and heat of combustion from Table 4-1.

Carbohydrate	Protein	Fat		
3.68 Calories/gm	4.36 Calories/gm	9.02 Calories/gm		
× 1 gm	× 6 gm	× 6 gm		
3.68 Calories	26.16 Calories	54.12 Calories	=	83.96 Calories

Method 2: *Using physiological fuel values*

Carbohydrate	Protein	Fat		
4.0 Calories/gm	4.0 Calories/gm	9.0 Calories/gm		
× 1 gm	× 6 gm	× 6 gm		
4.0 Calories	24.0 Calories	54.0 Calories	=	82 Calories

NOTE: Gram values for the egg are actual values, not values from the exchange system.

Figure 4-4. Two methods of calculating Calories from the energy nutrients.

Basal Metabolic Rate

Basal metabolism is the amount of energy required by the body during physical, emotional, and digestive rest, in other words, the amount of energy needed to maintain the involuntary activities of the body such as heart function, respiration, gastrointestinal peristalsis, secretion of glands, maintenance of muscle tone, and body temperature. The *basal metabolic rate* (BMR) may be thought of as the minimum amount of energy required by the body at rest in the fasting state to maintain physiological processes.

Although the BMR is the minimum amount of energy needed to sustain life, it nonetheless accounts for 50–70% of the total caloric requirement of people engaged in sedentary or moderate activity. For most people in the United States the BMR accounts for the major proportion of their energy requirement because their activity level is only sedentary to moderate. Only if a person is engaged in very active physical exertion does the energy requirement of his activity exceed his energy requirement for basal metabolism.

Contrary to popular belief, the student who studies diligently in the library all day or the executive solving daily business problems by vigorously pushing a pencil is expending very few Calories. Mental effort, no matter how intense, does very little to alter caloric requirements or BMR. The circumstances that do alter the BMR are body size and composition, age, sleep, endocrine gland secretions, and nutritional status.

Body Size and Composition

Body size has an effect on a person's BMR and also on the amount of energy expended in physical activity. The most frequently used formula for calculating an adult's BMR is based on *ideal body weight*. The BMR for men is 1 Calorie per kilogram of ideal body weight per hour, and for women it is .9 Calorie per kilogram of ideal body weight per hour. Ideal, not actual, body weight should be used in all BMR calculations because an actual weight that is over or under ideal weight will result in over- or underestimation. A more precise way to estimate BMR is to use a person's surface area, which reflects the rate of heat transfer from the body. Surface area takes into consideration both height and weight, and it corrects for body build. *Nomograms* have been developed for estimating surface area. The resulting surface area is then multiplied by a figure for Calories per square meter per hour for a specific age and sex category. A tall person has a higher BMR than a short stocky person because the tall person has a greater surface area. (See the section on estimating BMR later in this chapter.)

The BMR, however, is influenced by more than just size; the composition of the body plays an important role. The BMR is related to the proportion of active metabolizing cell mass in the body. The body skeleton and the *adipose tissue* are low in metabolic activity compared to organ and muscle tissues. The higher the proportion of muscle tissue, the higher the BMR; the higher the proportion of adipose tissue, the lower the BMR. A former athlete with a sedentary job would generally have a higher BMR than a man in poor physical condition with a sedentary occupation, because the athlete would have a higher proportion of muscular tissue. An obese person would have a lower BMR than either of these two men because of the high proportion of adipose tissue. For another example, compare two men, each weighing 190 lb (86.3 kg), but one man is 65 in (165.1 cm) tall and the other is 76 in (193 cm) tall. This comparison of a tall, slender man with a short, stout man reflects a large difference in body composition. The tall man has a much higher proportion of muscle to adipose tissue and therefore a higher BMR than the short man with too much adipose tissue. Body composition is also important to consider when comparing men with women. Most women have a higher proportion of adipose tissue than men and they therefore have lower BMRs. When calculating BMR, differences caused by body composition can be eliminated by using another measurement called *metabolic body size*, which is body weight in kilograms raised to the ¾

power ($W^{3/4}$), and it is based on fat-free body mass or lean body tissue.

Age

Age has an important effect on the BMR, especially during the growing years. The BMR increases from birth to age 2, at which time the BMR per unit of surface area is the highest during the life cycle. After age 2 the BMR decreases, but it increases again at puberty in anticipation of the final growth spurt. After age 20 there is a gradual decrease of BMR of about 2% per decade of adult life, although in many adults the decrease may be greater than 2% because of less physical activity, decreased muscle tone, and increased body fat. Fortunately, however, this greater decrease can be prevented by keeping physically fit and active and maintaining ideal weight.

Pregnancy is a period of rapid growth and development for the fetus. The mother's BMR increases 15–25% during the last trimester because of the high metabolic rate of the growing fetus and the weight gain of the mother.

Endocrine Secretions

The hormone *thyroxine,* produced by the thyroid gland, regulates the rate of metabolism, so alterations in the secretion of thyroxine necessarily have an effect on metabolic rate. When thyroid secretion is excessive (a condition known as *hyperthyroidism*), the BMR may be increased by as much as 75–100%. If, however, the activity of this gland is decreased, the BMR may be lowered by 30–40%.

Other endocrine secretions influence the metabolic rate, but to a much lesser extent than the thyroid secretion. An increased secretion of *epinephrine* from the adrenal glands during excitement or fear will increase the metabolic rate, but only momentarily. Whenever there is stimulation of the *sympathetic nervous system* there is an increase in the metabolic rate. The secretions of the pituitary gland also affect the metabolic rate; during growth the BMR of children and adolescents is increased by 15–20%.

The sex hormones also have an effect on the metabolic rate. The BMR in men is 10–15% higher than in women because of the presence of male sex hormones. The effect of the sex hormones combines with body composition to account for the lower metabolic rate in women. Also, in the menstruating woman metabolism is increased slightly before a monthly period but decreased somewhat during the period, changes that are so slight, however, that they are not usually considered in determining the energy requirement.

Sleep

During sleep, the BMR is about 10%/hr lower than in the waking state because of muscular relaxation and decreased activity of the sympathetic nervous system. The amount by which BMR is lower varies considerably among people because of differences in body movements during sleep.

Nutritional Status

A person's caloric requirement is directly related to that person's basal metabolism. Basal metabolism is by definition a measurement of people whose nutritional status is good. Malnourished and underweight people have lower BMRs because of decreased lean body tissue. In the underweight person the body seeks to conserve as much energy as possible by lowering the BMR. The more severe the undernutrition or starvation, the lower the basal metabolism. These people may also have a lower than normal body temperature and decreased muscle tone.

Some diseases increase the metabolic demands of the body and therefore increase basal metabolism. An elevation in body temperature above normal increases the BMR by 7% for each degree Fahrenheit (.55 C) rise above 98.6 F (37 C). The stress of surgery and burns also greatly increase the BMR because of the accelerated demands for re-plenishment of body tissue. Another disease that increases the metabolic rate is cancer; the accelerated rate of growth of the malignant tissue places high energy demands on the body, thus increasing the BMR. In all these medical conditions, increased Calories are needed to maintain the client's weight and prevent malnutrition. In contrast, any illness or condition that causes the client to lose weight or muscle mass will lower the BMR. The client confined to bed rest or in a wheelchair will lose valuable muscle tissue rapidly if not encouraged to do prescribed exercises. Consultation with a physical therapist concerning appropriate exercises may help minimize this problem.

Environmental Temperature

The variations in metabolic rate that occur because of changes in environmental temperatures are only slight. The human body protects itself against temperature changes by shivering when environmental temperatures are too low, or by perspiring when temperatures are too high. People living in the United States are protected from extremes of environmental temperatures by protective clothing and central heating in winter, and by lighter clothing and air conditioning during summer. A comfortable temperature range of 68–77 F (20–25 C) applies to the majority of living conditions in the United States.

There is evidence that prolonged exposure to either heat or cold without adequate protection will slightly increase the BMR. Although activity is generally decreased at high temperatures, the energy requirements of men performing specific work tasks at temperatures of 100 F (38 C) were higher than at lower environmental temperatures (Krause and Mahan, 1979). In environments where the mean temperature is below 0 F (−14 C), the energy requirement is about 5% higher, and there is also a small increase in energy expenditure caused by the extra weight of heavy winter clothing. These increased energy requirements only apply to prolonged exposure in these environments. Generally, no adjustments in energy allowances are directly warranted by environmental temperatures, but adjustments may need to be made because of the effect of the climate on the physical activity pattern of a particular person.

Activity

Added to the energy requirements for basal metabolic needs are energy requirements for daily activity. Although significant, they are usually less than those for maintaining basal metabolism. Only for very active people, such as lumbermen or athletes, do the energy requirements for activity exceed the basal energy needs. The energy required for physical activity depends on the type of activity, the length of time the activity is performed, and the size of the person performing the activity.

Several methods are used to estimate the energy requirements of activity. Activity levels are classified as sedentary, moderate, or heavy. One method estimates energy requirements for different activity levels as a specified percentage above basal requirements. A formula devised by the US Department of Agriculture has determined the average number of Calories required for four different activity levels for both men and women. Most people, however, participate in several activities in a day, some of which are sedentary and some of which are moderate. Tables have therefore been devised that list the energy cost of various activities as either kilocalories per hour or kilocalories per kilogram of body weight per hour. (More on these tables and their use is included in the later section of this chapter on estimating physical activity.)

It should be emphasized again that it is *physical* activity that requires most of the energy. The energy expended in mental effort studying or taking an exam adds very few

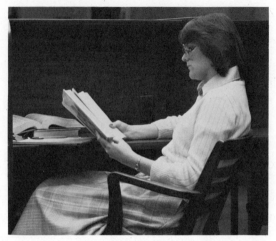

Figure 4-5. Studying uses only about 80 Calories an hour. (Photo by J. Collins)

Calories to the total caloric requirement (see Fig. 4-5).

Specific Dynamic Action of Food

It is a well-documented fact that the act of eating, followed by the general stimulation of the body's processes of digestion, absorption, and metabolism, requires energy. This increased heat production resulting from the ingestion of food is also known as the *calorigenic effect* of food or the *specific dynamic action* (SDA) of food. The increased heat production after a meal is useful in maintaining body temperature. The energy nutrients—carbohydrate, protein, and fat—are the nutrients that contribute to this phenomenon. Each energy nutrient when eaten separately has its own specific effect. Protein has an SDA of 30%; fat, 13%; and carbohydrate, only 4–5%. In the ordinary mixed diet this calorigenic effect is about 6% of the energy value of the meal. The calorigenic effect of a mixed diet has also been estimated to be approximately 10% of the energy required for basal metabolism and activity combined.

MEASUREMENT OF ENERGY EXPENDITURE

The basic methods for measuring energy expenditure were developed before 1920. These methods were initially very simple and have been refined in recent years.

Calorimetry

Because there is a direct relationship between heat and energy, the principle of *calorimetry* is used in the measurement of energy expenditure. *Calorimetry* is "the measurement of heat absorbed or given off by a system or body" (Lagua et al. 1974, p. 30). This measurement may be carried out by either direct or indirect means.

Direct calorimetry is the direct measurement of heat given off by a subject or produced by a food when it is combusted in an insulated chamber. This apparatus, called a *respiration chamber* or *respiration calorimeter,* is a well-insulated chamber surrounded by coils containing water. The animal or human subject is placed inside, and the heat given off by the subject is measured by the change in temperature of the surrounding water (see Fig. 4-6). Thus there is a direct measurement of heat exchange and, therefore, of caloric expenditure. This is the same type of method used to determine the physiological fuel values of the energy nutrients, described earlier in this chapter.

Indirect calorimetry measures the volume of oxygen consumed and sometimes the amount of carbon dioxide eliminated by a subject over a period of time. The amount of oxygen consumed is proportional to the amount of heat being produced and, therefore, to the number of Calories expended. The measurement is made by having the subject breath into one of several types of respiration devices (see Fig. 4-7).

Other methods of measuring energy expenditure, such as heart rate and pulse rate, have also been used, each with advantages and disadvantages.

BMR Measurement

Basal metabolism was previously defined as the amount of energy needed to maintain the involuntary activities of the body. Because it is the minimum amount of energy required by the body at rest, certain standard criteria must be fulfilled by the person who is going to have his BMR measured:

1. The subject must be in a fasting state; that is, he must not have eaten any food for 12–16 hours. This is necessary because the digestion, absorption, and utilization of food requires extra Calories. Because of this requirement, a basal metabolism test is usually performed in the morning.

2. The subject should be awake but in a reclining position.

3. The subject should be free from any emotional tension or fear.

4. Body temperature must be within the normal range.

5. The room where the test is to be performed should be of a comfortable temperature—70–75 F (21–24 C)—and humidity.

Measurement of the BMR may be accomplished by either direct or indirect means (see Figs. 4-6 and 4-7). The indirect method, which measures the subject's oxygen consumption, is ideal for medical diagnosis because the measurement can be made in a very short time.

Thyroid Function Tests

A third method for measuring the BMR is to measure the level of thyroxine production. *Thyroxine* is the primary hormone secreted by the thyroid gland. Because the thyroid gland has the greatest effect on metabolic rate, three different thyroid function tests have been used to assess metabolic rate. It must be re-

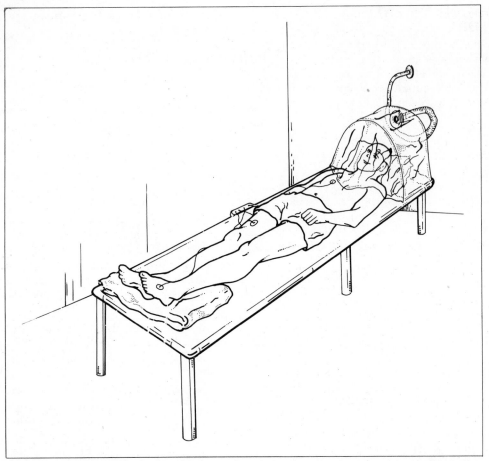

Figure 4-6. Direct calorimetry performed with subject in a respiration chamber. The subject may also be monitored by equipment that measures the exchange of oxygen and carbon dioxide and by thermocouples attached to the skin to measure heat exchange.

membered, however, that the thyroid function tests yield only relative, not exact, indications of energy requirements. The first thyroid function test is the protein-bound iodine (PBI) test. Iodine constitutes 65% of the weight of thyroxine, and there is a positive relationship between the amount of iodine bound to protein circulating in the blood and the level of thyroxine production. PBI levels in the blood that are either above or below established norms indicate the presence, respectively, of hyperthyoidism or hypothyroidism. Thus only a relative level of metabolic rate is revealed.

A more recent method of assessing metabolic rate by measuring thyroid function uses *radioactive isotopes* of iodine. Radioactive iodine is orally administered to the subject, and the rate of uptake by the thyroid gland and other tissues is measured. Still another

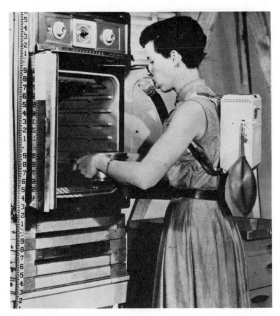

Figure 4-7. Subject wearing a Benedict Roth respirometer that measures the amount of energy in a task. (USDA photograph)

thyroid function test measures the blood levels of total serum thyroxine (T_4) and triiodothyronine (T_3).

Measuring Energy Expended in Activities

The activity levels of all living creatures, whether human or animal, vary in the course of a day. A person's activity level is determined by occupation, mode of transportation, leisure activities, and state of health. Interest in the amount of energy expended performing various physical tasks goes back to the end of last century. Energy expenditures for a variety of physical activities have been recorded. Passmore and Durnin (1955), two physiologists from Scotland, have measured and recorded considerable data on energy expenditures during various activities and occupations.

Measurement of the energy expended dur-ing physical activity may be accomplished by either direct or indirect calorimetry. Direct calorimetry necessitates placing the subject inside a special chamber called a *calorimeter* in order to measure the energy expended when a selected activity is performed. Some distinct disadvantages have precluded the general use of calorimeters for measuring the energy required for physical activities. One of the major disadvantages is that there are only a few of these large calorimeters available in the United States. Subjects must be persuaded to enter, alone, an insulated chamber about the size of a small room. The time that must be spent in this solitary chamber can be relatively short if energy expended during one particular activity is measured or up to 24 hours if total daily expenditure of energy is measured. The small number of these chambers, the limited number of willing subjects, and the high cost of chamber operation all combine to decrease the practicality of this measurement.

Although the primary means of measuring energy expenditure in the large calorimeters is heat loss from the subject, most of these large calorimeters are also equipped to analyze the air entering and leaving the chamber for oxygen and carbon dioxide content. Energy expenditure can be determined indirectly from oxygen and carbon dioxide exchange, but the indirect method of calorimetry is must less expensive and much more convenient than the direct method. The indirect method simply requires the subject to wear a portable apparatus called a *respirometer*. The subject breathes into the mouthpiece of the respirometer while performing the assigned task or activity. The oxygen consumption is related to the amount of energy liberated from the body as heat. From numerous scientific experiments it is known that the consumption of 1 liter of oxygen is equivalent to 4.825 kilocalories. The measurement is usually made for only a few minutes. The energy expended performing a specific activity for a longer period of time can then be calculated from the original data.

The advantages of this method over measurement by direct calorimetry are readily apparent. The measurement requires only a short period of time from the subject. The apparatus that is worn weighs only 8 lb (3.6 kg) or less. It is not necessary for the subject to be alone in an enclosed chamber. Most of the data of energy expenditure during physical activities and in selected occupations has been collected using the portable respirometer. With this method, however, the subject, must wear a face mask or mouthpiece and he is somewhat encumbered both physically and psychologically by the equipment.

There are a few other methods of measuring energy expended during physical activity that have been tried with varying degrees of success. One of these new methods is to use heart rate as an indicator of energy expenditure. The subject wears a small transmitter around the waist, which transfers the heart signals to a recorder. There is very little if any interference with work or activity using this method. Although there does seem to be a relationship between heart rate and metabolic rate, there is some question about the consistent correlation of heart rate and energy expenditure. The linear relationship holds only during moderate to heavy exercise. The use of net heart rate is not as precise as respiratory calorimetry because the heart-rate response is only valid when the total stress results from work load. Many other physical and psychological factors can affect heart rate, and the heart-rate response varies greatly with each person. The heart rate as a method of predicting energy expenditure is best used for those people engaged in moderate-to-heavy physical activity rather than those who are sitting or standing.

A similar method of predicting energy expenditure is the *average pulse rate*. The mean pulse rate for a person may be used to estimate energy expenditure over 24 hours. This method is useful only for tasks involving moderate-to-heavy physical exertion.

Of limited applicability is a method of estimating energy expenditure during activity by using an instrument called a *pedometer* that is worn suspended from the subject's waist. It measures the impulses occurring during each step; these impulses can be converted into physical activity. Human physical activity is seldom limited to walking; other bodily movements may move the instrument's balance arm and thus overestimate the distances walked, so the method is not often used.

The student should keep in mind these methods of measuring energy expended and their advantages and limitations as further examination of the sources of error in estimating energy expenditure are pursued in the following section.

ENERGY BALANCE

In its simplest terms, *energy balance* refers to an energy consumption (Calories) in food that balances an energy expenditure (BMR plus activity plus SDA) so that a person maintains ideal body weight. Energy balance results when energy intake exactly equals energy output (see Fig. 4-8). Casual observation of any group of people readily reveals that this balance is not as easy to maintain. Some are too thin, many are too fat, and only a very few are "just right." The multitude of weight-reducing diets in magazines, newspapers, and paperback books and the abundance of health spas and exercise salons point to an excessive energy consumption (Calories) relative to energy expenditure (activity level). Why is this energy balance so difficult for the average person to maintain?

The first part of this chapter stated that human energy requirements depend on four variables that are interrelated in a complex way: (1) body size and composition, (2) age, (3) physical activity, and (4) climate and other environmental factors. Caloric balance also depends on the four variables of (1) food intake, (2) energy storage, (3) loss of energy in

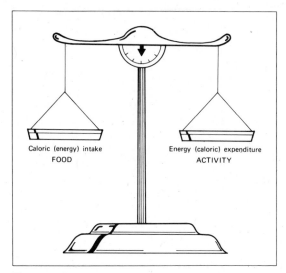

Caloric (energy) intake
FOOD

Energy (caloric) expenditure
ACTIVITY

Figure 4-8. Energy balance.

heat production, and (4) energy utilization during activity. The number of influences on both energy requirements and caloric balance serves to emphasize the complexity of the subject of ideal weight maintenance.

A few more general observations about how people vary serve to emphasize still more the complexity of the maintenance or attainment of ideal weight. There are many people who are able to maintain their weight over long periods of time despite very irregular patterns of activity and food intake. These are the people who seemingly can eat "anything" and never gain an "ounce." There are also some unfortunate people who cannot seem to lose any weight despite perpetual dieting. At the other extreme as a precious few people who desire to gain weight but, despite eating large quantities of fattening foods, are able to gain little or no weight. Because being overweight is the most common of the two kinds of caloric imbalance, most people can empathize with the overweight person struggling to lose weight but when confronted with an underweight person people may smirk and chuckle at his or her struggle. The un-

derweight person struggles just as much or more trying to gain weight as the overweight person trying to lose it.

Besides distinct differences in individual basal metabolic rates and levels of physical activity, two very basic explanations might be offered for general consideration. First, the human body may be thought of as analogous to a machine. Some people are simply endowed with more efficient bodies. This might be one explanation for the person who maintains his body weight despite erratic eating patterns and levels of physical exercise. Second, most nutrients are used with decreasing efficiency as their intake increases in the diet. If this fact also applies to Calories, it may be one of the reasons why the overweight find it so difficult to lose weight and also why they seem to add weight on such a relatively low intake of food. At this point, we can agree with Durnin, an expert on human energy requirements, and his associates (Durnin et al., 1973), that "the energy requirements of man and his balance of intake and expenditure are not known" (p. 418) There is a lack of adequate knowledge about the mechanisms by which energy balance is maintained in humans.

Lest all of this uncertainty plague the beginning student too much, there are a few known facts. One pound of body fat is equivalent to 3,500 Calories. This means that, to lose (or gain) one pound per week, the subject must adjust his caloric intake to a level 500 Calories below (or above) his daily energy requirement. The difficulty is not how much to adjust the daily intake of Calories but how to determine the actual energy requirement (daily Caloric intake requirement) of a specific person.

Ideal Body Weight

The first step in learning to calculate energy requirements is learning what ideal body weight is and how to calculate it. Ideal body weight is most simply and practically defined as that weight at which a person looks and feels best. The first height and weight tables that were available for adults were compiled by life insurance companies from data on their policyholders. Inasmuch as most adults continue to gain weight with advancing age, these higher weights were reflected in the tables. In recent years, the phenomenon of increased weight with advancing age has been reevaluated. The current thinking is that once growth in height has been completed, by about age 20, there is no physiological reason to gain weight with advancing age. Also, it is now known that people who have maintained their desirable body weight throughout their life have the best health prognosis. A general rule for adults is that the ideal weight of a person at age 25 should be maintained for the remainder of that person's life.

Body Frame

The major reasons for variations in body weight among individuals are variations in size of the body frame and in the proportion of fat to muscle tissue. People in the familiar Metropolitan Life Insurance Company height-weight tables (see Appendices E and F) are divided into either small, medium, or large body frame for given heights for both men and women. There is also a range of acceptable weights for each height and body frame. At the current time there are no good criteria for estimating frame size. Wrist diameter has been suggested as one criteria for frame size, but this measurement has been standarized on only a few subjects. This measurement is not fully reliable because some people have a prominent wrist bone but still have a small body build. The best decision about frame size comes from the person's realistic assessment of his own body frame.

Body Composition

Body composition, the other important reason for variations in body weight among individuals, is a function of the relative amounts of the two components, fat and muscle. It is

a well-accepted fact that muscle weighs more than fat. People who have a higher proportion of muscle tissue will weigh more than someone of the same height and body frame with more adipose tissue. Because of this phenomenon some athletes may even be classified as "overweight" by the standard height-weight tables because of their greatly increased muscle mass. Men have a higher proportion of muscle tissue to adipose tissue than women, so the suggested ideal weights for each frame size is about 10 lb higher for a given height for men than for women of the same height.

Calculating Ideal Weight

It is beneficial for the dietitian, nurse, or physician to have a convenient tool to use to assess a client's weight. There is a simple formula for estimating ideal weight that is easy to remember, that makes allowances for frame size, and that can be used for both men and women. The calculation begins with a base weight for the first 5 ft of height, which is 100 lb for women and 106 lb for men. For women, 5 lb is added to the base weight for each inch of height over 5 ft. For men, 6 lb is added for each inch over 5 ft. The resulting weight is for medium body frame. Adjustments for other body frames are made by adding 10% of the total weight for a large frame or subtracting 10% for a small frame (Am. Diabetes Assoc. 1977).

A female student who is 5 ft 6 in (167.6 cm) and has a medium body frame should ideally weigh 130 lb (59 kg). A girlfriend of this student who is also 5 ft 6 in (167.6 cm) but has a small frame should weigh only 117 lb (53.1 kg). A male student, also 5 ft 6 in (167.6 cm) and with a medium frame, should weigh 142 lb (64.5 kg). This formula is easy to use and easy to remember and provides the health professional with a quick assessment of a client's actual versus ideal weight. It should be reemphasized, however, that the formula provides only an estimate. The client may not agree that the weight obtained by the formula is his "ideal weight." The formula does not work equally well with all body frames and nutritional statuses. Despite its limitations, the student will find the formula useful in the initial assessment of a client's nutritional status.

Estimating Energy Requirements

From the preceding discussion of factors that determine energy requirements and the methods of measuring energy expenditure, it should be obvious that a person's energy requirement is not easily determined. Any level of caloric intake, whether arrived at by using a complex formula or a very simple one, is only a rough approximation of a person's daily energy requirements. Yet with all the current emphasis on weight reduction and maintenance of ideal body weight, it is useful to be able to estimate energy requirements. By comparing a person's estimated energy requirement with an average daily caloric intake of food, the nurse or dietitian is in a better position to assess the client's weight status and offer suggestions to bring the caloric balance back into equilibrium with the expenditure of energy. Daily energy requirements can be estimated either by figuring the Calories required for BMR and activity separately or by estimating total caloric requirements based on the general activity level of the client.

Estimating Basal Metabolic Rate

Because the BMR is the major portion of the total energy requirement for most people, an accurate estimate of the Calories required for BMR is necessary. The BMR may be estimated using ideal body weight, body surface area, or metabolic body size. One method is not necessarily more accurate or precise than another. Ideal rather than actual body weight in pounds or kilograms should be used for estimating BMR, as use of actual weight would produce either an over- or underestimation of caloric requirements.

IDEAL WEIGHT IN POUNDS. A simple rule of thumb for estimating BMR is explained by Deutsch in his book *Realities of Nutrition* (1976). Women are to add a 0 to their ideal weight in pounds and then add their ideal weight to the resulting figure. Men are to also add a 0 to their ideal weight in pounds but then add twice their ideal weight in pounds to the result. A 5 ft 4 in (162.6 cm) woman whose ideal weight is 120 lb (54.5 kg) should have a BMR of approximately 1,320 Calories/day (1,200 plus 120). A 5 ft 10 in (177.8 cm) man with an ideal weight of 160 lb (72.6 kg) would have a BMR of approximately 1,920 Calories/day, or 1,600 plus (2 × 160).

BODY SURFACE AREA. BMR may be estimated using surface area because heat is lost from the body and therefore energy is proportional to surface area. Body surface area is based on the relationship between weight and height. There is a formula for calculating body surface area, but it is more practical to use the nomogram shown in Figure 4-9. The body surface area is determined by plotting a person's height on the left and his weight in pounds on the right of the nomogram. A straight line is drawn connecting these two points and intersecting line III at the point of the person's body surface area (given in square meters). The person's basal metabolism may be estimated using Table 4-2, which gives the average number of Calories expended per square meter of body surface per hour according to a person's age. As an example, the body surface area for a 5 ft 4 in (162.6 cm) woman who weighs 120 lb (54.5 kg) is 1.6 sq m as shown in Figure 4-9. The Calories expended per square meter per hour for this 25-year-old woman are 35.70 (Table 4-2). Her basal metabolic rate of 1,371 Calories is determined by multiplying 35.7 Calories/sq m/hr by 1.6 sq m by 24 hours (1.6 sq m × 35.7 Calories/sq m/hr × 24 hr).

METABOLIC BODY SIZE. The BMR may also be calculated using metabolic body size (see

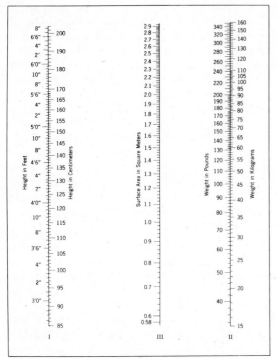

Figure 4-9. Nomogram for calculating surface area. (From R. L. Pike and M. L. Brown, *Nutrition: An Integrated Approach*, 2nd Ed., p. 829. Copyright © 1975, John Wiley & Sons, Inc. Reprinted by permission of John Wiley & Sons, Inc.)

Table 4-3). The BMR for both men and women may be calculated by multiplying metabolic body size by the factor 70. The BMR for the same women using this method is 1,414 Calories (70 × 20.2).

CALCULATING BASAL METABOLIC RATE. The BMR for adults can be calculated from the basic definition of BMR, which is 1.0 Cal/kg/hr for men and .9 Cal/kg/hr for women. As with all the other formulas, ideal body weight should be used in order to avoid an incorrect estimate. The BMR for the 5 ft 10 in (177.8 cm) 160 lb (72.6 kg) man would be 73 kg × 1 Cal/kg/hr × 24 hours = 1,752 Cal. The BMR for the 5 ft 4 in (162.6 cm) 120 lb (54.5 kg)

woman would be 55 kg × .9 Cal/kg/hr × 24 hours = 1,188 Cal.

ADJUSTING THE BMR. The two major variables that affect the BMR are sleep and age. The BMR is reduced during the hours the subject is asleep. On the average, sleep reduces the BMR by 10% for every hour of sleep. For example the BMR for the 5 ft 4 in

TABLE 4-2. The Mayo Foundation Normal Standards: Calories per Square Meter per Hour

Males		Females	
Age at Last Birthday	Mean	Age at Last Birthday	Mean
6	53.00	6	50.62
7	52.45	6½	50.23
8	51.78	7	49.12
8½	51.20	7½	47.84
9	50.54	8	47.00
9½	49.42	8½	46.50
10	48.50	9–10	45.90
10½	47.71	11	45.26
11	47.18	11½	44.80
12	46.75	12	44.28
13–15	46.35	12½	43.58
16	45.72	13	42.90
16½	45.30	13½	42.10
17	44.80	14	41.45
17½	44.03	14½	40.74
18	43.25	15	40.10
18½	42.70	15½	39.40
19	42.32	16	38.85
19½	42.00	16½	38.30
20–21	41.43	17	37.82
22–23	40.82	17½	37.40
24–27	40.24	18–19	36.74
28–29	39.81	20–24	36.18
30–34	39.34	25–44	35.70
35–39	38.68	45–49	34.94
40–44	38.00	50–54	33.96
45–49	37.37	55–59	33.18
50–54	36.73	60–64	32.61
55–59	36.10	65–69	32.30
60–64	35.48	a	
65–69	34.80		

SOURCE: *Nutrition: An Integrated Approach*, 2nd Ed. Copyright © 1975 John Wiley & Sons, Inc. Reprinted by permission of John Wiley & Sons, Inc.
[a] Obtained by extrapolation.

TABLE 4-3. Metabolic Body Size, $W^{3/4}$ for Body Weights from 1 to 100 Kg

W, kg	$W^{3/4}$ $kg^{3/4}$	W, kg	$W^{3/4}$ $kg^{3/4}$	W, kg	$W^{3/4}$ $kg^{3/4}$	W, kg	$W^{3/4}$ $kg^{3/4}$	W, kg	$W^{3/4}$ $kg^{3/4}$
1	1.00	21	9.8	41	16.2	61	21.8	81	27.0
2	1.68	22	10.2	42	16.5	62	22.1	82	27.2
3	2.28	23	10.5	43	16.8	63	22.4	83	27.5
4	2.83	24	10.8	44	17.1	64	22.6	84	27.7
5	3.34	25	11.2	45	17.4	65	22.9	85	28.0
6	3.83	26	11.5	46	17.7	66	23.2	86	28.2
7	4.30	27	11.8	47	18.0	67	23.4	87	28.5
8	4.75	28	12.2	48	18.2	68	23.7	88	28.7
9	5.19	29	12.5	49	18.5	69	23.9	89	29.0
10	5.62	30	12.8	50	18.8	70	24.2	90	29.2
11	6.04	31	13.1	51	19.1	71	24.4	91	29.4
12	6.44	32	13.5	52	19.4	72	24.7	92	29.7
13	6.84	33	13.8	53	19.6	73	25.0	93	29.9
14	7.24	34	14.1	54	19.9	74	25.2	94	30.2
15	7.62	35	14.4	55	20.2	75	25.5	95	30.4
16	8.00	36	14.7	56	20.5	76	25.8	96	30.7
17	8.38	37	15.0	57	20.8	77	26.0	97	30.9
18	8.75	38	15.3	58	21.0	78	26.2	98	31.1
19	9.10	39	15.6	59	21.3	79	26.5	99	31.4
20	9.46	40	15.9	60	21.6	80	26.7	100	31.6

SOURCE: *Nutrition: An Integrated Approach,* 2nd Ed. R. L. Pike and M. L. Brown, Copyright © 1975, John Wiley & Sons, Inc. Reprinted by permission of John Wiley & Sons, Inc.

(162.6 cm) 120 lb (54.5 kg) woman using the standard formula for calculating BMR was 1,188 Calories for 24 hours. To find how much this is reduced by sleep, her ideal weight in kilograms and the average number of hours she sleep per night must be known. Multiply 55 kg × .1 (for the 10% reduction) × 8 hours of sleep per night = 44 Calories. This is the amount of Calories by which her BMR is reduced because of the 8 hours of sleep. Her true BMR corrected for sleep is 1,144 Calories for a 24-hour period.

An adjustment in the BMR may also be needed for age. As stated earlier in this chapter, age is one of the circumstances that influences the BMR. The BMR per unit of body surface continues to increase until about age 2, after which it decreases throughout the remainder of the life cycle. Note that recommended caloric intake continues to increase until after adolescence, but this is because caloric requirements are based on the body size, which is continuing to increase until physiological growth is complete. For the adult, the BMR continues to decline at the rate of approximately 2% for every 10 years. At age 30 the BMR is only 98% of what it was at age 20; at age 40 it is only 96% of what it was at age 20; and so on. For example, the BMR of the 5 ft 4 in (162.6 cm) 120 lb (54.5 kg) woman at age 20 was 1,144 Calories per day; at age 30 it would be 1,121 Calories; and at age 50, 1,075 Calories.

Estimating Energy Costs of Activity
The expenditure of energy during life's activities is the second-largest contributor to the day's total caloric requirement. The calculation for BMR varies only plus or minus 15% among people with normal thyroid function inasmuch as it is based on ideal body weight. In contrast, amounts of energy expended

during physical activity vary greatly among individuals, depending on level of health, occupation, means of transportation, and leisure activities. For the average sedentary US adult the energy used for physical activity is less than their BMR for a recommended daily intake of less than 2,000 Calories. Contrast this with the average caloric intake of 5,600 Calories for Harvard football players. The US Army provides food rations supplying about 4,500 Calories daily for the troops engaged in strenuous work. Not only the type of physical activity but the efficiency and vigor with which it is performed affects energy expenditure.

The energy cost of activities is recorded in terms of Calories per hour or Calories per minute. The most useful tables, however, are recorded in terms of body weight and stated in the unit Calories per kilogram per minute or hour. Actual body weight is used to figure energy expenditure during activity because more energy is required to move a heavier body in the performance of a selected activity. For example, three people weighing 120 lb (54.5 kg), 160 lb (72.6 kg), and 200 lb (90.8 kg) will use 2.6, 3.2, and 3.8 Calories/min respectively while walking at a speed of 2 mph (3.2 km) (Passmore and Durnin, 1955).

Energy expenditure for activities are available in numerous tables. They are listed according to very specific activities, general activity levels, or occupations. The number of Calories expended during a day's activity can be obtained through very detailed record keeping of the activities performed or by simply adding a number of Calories for an activity level or by estimating a certain percentage above basal requirements for the appropriate activity level.

ACTIVITY RECORD. The most accurate method for determining the number of Calories expended for activity during a typical day is for the subject to enter a closed metabolic chamber where his energy expended can be measured under controlled conditions.

Another way would be for the subject to wear a portable respirometer as his daily activities are performed. Most subjects are not interested in being isolated in a closed chamber even for one day, nor are they interested in having their daily routine somewhat hampered by wearing a portable instrument, so a more practical yet accurate method is needed.

A more practical method is for the subject to keep a detailed record of all his daily activities listed and recorded in minutes. The subject must wear a watch (preferably with a second hand) and carry a small notebook to record each activity and the time spent. This method necessitates counting each stair climbed or recording the total time involved climbing stairs and keeping accurate records of the minutes spent in walking, running, or sitting. The more accurately and specifically each activity is recorded, the more accurate will be the estimate of the subject's energy expenditure. The best way to check accuracy in recording times is to total all the minutes recorded. The total number should be 1,440 minutes (the number of minutes in 24 hours).

An example of this method is found in Table 4-4, which records the energy requirements for both a male and female college student. As the table shows, the activities can be grouped and total hours in each category recorded. It will be noticed that the male subject weighs 143 lb (65 kg) and the female, 120 lb (55 kg). Because not every college student, of course, weighs exactly these amounts, a more accurate way would be to use a table that lists energy expenditures of a variety of activities in Calories per kilogram per minute. The resulting answer would be in Calories per kilogram. Multiplying this number by weight in kilograms would yield total number of Calories expended in one day. Using this method we see from Table 4-4 that the 120 lb female college student required 1,827 Calories per day.

A final point needs to be made about the way energy expenditure during activity is recorded. Most of the tables record gross values

TABLE 4-4. Energy Requirements of Sample Male and Female College Students

Activity	Man (65 kg)			Woman (55 kg)		
	Hours	Calories/kg/hr	Calories	Hours	Calories/kg/hr	Calories
Sleep (BMR corrected for sleep for 8 hours)	8	Cal/kg/hr .9(1 Calories ×65 Kg × 8 hr)	468	8	Cal/kg/hr .9(.9 Calories × 55 Kg × 8 hr)	356
Very light *Examples: typing, reading, writing, eating, watching TV, and listening to radio*	10	1.5	975	12	1.3	858
Light *Examples: walking 2.5–3 mph, preparing and cooking food, personal care, hand washing*	5	2.9	942	3½	2.6	500
Moderate *Examples: walking 3.5–4 mph, making bed, climbing stairs, walking with a moderate load of books*	½	4.3	140	½	4.1	113
Very active *Examples: jogging, swimming, playing tennis*	½	8.4	273	—	8.0	—
Total Calories			2,798			1,827

for energy expenditure rather than net values. This means that the values have the amounts for basal metabolism figured into them. If these values for activities were added to the already determined BMR, the person's energy requirement would be inflated. Table 4-5 is an example of the energy cost of activity that does not include basal metabolism and the Calories required to utilize foods. Another table, Table 4-6, contains energy expenditures that include both basal energy and specific dynamic action of food.

ACTIVITY LEVELS.   A much simpler and still fairly accurate way of estimating energy requirements is to use activity levels. Table 4-7 includes activity levels, common activities, and occupations classified according to activity level, with caloric expenditures given for each. To use this table, estimate the number of hours spent in each of the major activity levels. Using either Calories per kilogram per hour or simply Calories per hour, compute the energy expenditure on a 24-hour basis. Using the example of the female college student, all her activities can be grouped together under the major categories of sedentary, light, or

TABLE 4-5. Energy Cost of Activities Exclusive of Basal Metabolism and Influence of Food

Activity	Kcal/kg/hr
Bicycling (century run)	7.6
Bicycling (moderate speed)	2.5
Bookbinding	0.8
Boxing	11.4
Carpentry (heavy)	2.3
Cello playing	1.3
Crocheting	0.4
Dancing, foxtrot	3.8
Dancing, waltz	3.0
Dishwashing	1.0
Dressing and undressing	0.7
Driving automobile	0.9
Eating	0.4
Fencing	7.3
Horseback riding, walk	1.4
Horseback riding, trot	4.3

TABLE 4-5. (Continued)

Activity	Kcal/kg/hr
Horseback riding, gallop	6.7
Ironing (5-pound iron)	1.0
Knitting sweater	0.7
Laundry, light	1.3
Lying still, awake	0.1
Organ playing (30% to 40% of energy hand work)	1.5
Painting furniture	1.5
Paring potatoes	0.6
Playing ping-pong	4.4
Piano playing (Mendelssohn's songs)	0.8
Piano playing (Beethoven's "Apassionata")	1.4
Piano playing (Liszt's "Tarantella")	2.0
Reading aloud	0.4
Rowing in race	16.0
Running	7.0
Sawing wood	5.7
Sewing, hand	0.4
Sewing, foot-driven machine	0.6
Sewing, motor-driven machine	0.4
Shoemaking	1.0
Singing in a loud voice	0.8
Sitting quietly	0.4
Skating	3.5
Standing at attention	0.6
Standing relaxed	0.5
Stone masonry	4.7
Sweeping with broom, bare floor	1.4
Sweeping with carpet sweeper	1.6
Sweeping with vacuum sweeper	2.7
Swimming (2 mph)	7.9
Tailoring	0.9
Typewriting rapidly	1.0
Violin playing	0.6
Walking (3 mph)	2.0
Walking rapidly (4 mph)	3.4
Walking at high speed (5.3 mph)	9.3
Walking downstairs	[a]
Walking upstairs	[b]
Washing floors	1.2
Writing	0.4

SOURCE: Reprinted with permission of Macmillan Publishing Co., Inc. from *Rose's Laboratory Handbook for Dietetics*, 5th Ed., by C. M. Taylor, G. McLeod, and R. Rose. Copyright 1949 by Macmillan Publishing Co., Inc., renewed 1977 by Clara Mae Taylor, Corrine Robinson, Marilyn Lawler.
[a] Allow 0.012 kcal/kg for an ordinary staircase with 15 steps without regard to time.
[b] Allow 0.036 kcal/kg for an ordinary staircase with 15 steps without regard to time.

moderate activity. Her daily caloric requirement can then be figured using Calories per kilogram per hour or Calories per hour. Adjusting her BMR for 8 hours of sleep, totaling the number of hours spent in each activity category, and multiplying the number of hours by Calories required per kilogram per hour for the appropriate activity level, her caloric requirement is 2,102 Calories daily. Using only Calories per hour gives a very similar result of 2,000 Calories. Notice that even though three different methods were used to compute her caloric requirement, the three

TABLE 4-6. Energy Expenditure in Specified Activities, Including Basal Energy and the Effect of Food

Man (65 kg)	Calories/ min
In bed asleep or resting	1.08
Sitting quietly	1.39
Standing quietly	1.75
Walking 3 miles/hr (4.9 km/hr)	3.7
Walking 3 miles/hr (4.9 km/hr with a 10 kg load	4.0
Office work (sedentary)	1.8
Light Industry	
Printing	2.3
Garage work (repairs)	4.1
Laboratory work	2.3
Building Industry	
Laboring	6.0
Bricklaying	3.8
Farming (European, mechanized)	
Driving tractor	2.4
Feeding animals	4.1
Repairing fences	5.7
Forestry	
Planting	4.7
Felling with axe	8.6
Trimming	8.4
Sawing—hand saw	8.6
—power saw	4.8
Recreations	
Sedentary	2.5
Light (billiards, bowls, cricket, golf, sailing, etc.)	2.5–5.0
Moderate (canoeing, dancing, horse-riding, swimming, tennis, etc.)	5.0–7.5
Heavy (athletics, football, rowing, etc.)	7.5+

TABLE 4-6. (Continued)

Woman (55 kg)	Calories/ min
In bed asleep or resting	0.90
Sitting quietly	1.15
Standing quietly	1.37
Walking 3 miles/hr (4.9 km/hr)	3.0
Walking 3 miles/hr (4.9 km/hr) with 10 kg load	3.4
Office work (sedentary)	1.6
Domestic work	
Cooking	1.7
Light cleaning	2.5
Moderate cleaning, chopping firewood, etc.)	3.5
Recreations	
Sedentary	2.0
Light (billiards, bowls, cricket, golf, sailing, etc.)	2.0–4.0
Moderate (canoeing, dancing, horse-riding, swimming, tennis, etc.)	4.0–6.0
Heavy (athletics, football, rowing, etc.)	6.0+

SOURCE: J. V. G. A. Durnin and R. Passmore, *Energy, Work and Leisure*, London, 1967. As reported in *Energy and Protein Requirements*, FAO/WHO Technical Rep. No. 522, 1973.

answers are all within 200 Calories of each other. Estimating caloric requirements is not a precise computation; as a general rule, however, the simpler the method used, the greater will be the error of estimate. Even the detailed record of separate activities is only an approximation of caloric requirement.

PERCENTAGE ABOVE BMR. A method for estimating caloric requirements for energy is to add a certain percentage above the BMR. In this method, the percentages above the BMR are from 10% to 100%, depending on activity level. The specific percentages above basal for activities ranging from bed rest to such very active occupations as lumberjacking are shown in Table 4-7.

Estimating the Specific Dynamic Action of Food
One contributor to total caloric requirements is the SDA of food, also known as the *calorigenic effect of food*, which is perhaps more

TABLE 4-7. Caloric Expenditures in Various Activities and Occupations

Activity[a]	Occupation[b]	Percentage above Basal	Calories/ kg/hr[a]	Calories/ hr[c]
Sleeping				
Bed rest		10		
Very light		30	Men 1.5	100
Seated and standing activities, painting trades, auto and truck driving, laboratory work, typing, playing musical instruments, sewing, ironing. Also includes reading, writing, eating, watching television or movies, listening to the radio, playing cards, and other activities that require little or no arm movement.[c]			Women 1.3	
Light	*Light*	40–50	Men 2.9	160
Walking on level, 2.5–3 mph, tailoring, pressing, garage work, electrical trades, cannery work, washing clothes, shopping with light load, golf, sailing, table tennis, volleyball. Also includes preparing and cooking food; doing dishes, dusting; hand washing small articles of clothing; personal care, and other activities that require some arm movement.[c]	Men: Office workers, most professional men (such as lawyers, doctors, accountants, teachers, architects, etc.), show workers, unemployed men. Women: Office workers, housewives in houses with mechanical household appliances, teachers, and most other professional women.		Women 2.6	110
Moderate	*Moderately active*	60–75	Men 4.3	240
Walking 3.5–4 mph; plastering, weeding, and hoeing; loading and stacking bales; scrubbing floors; shopping with heavy load; golf; sailing; table tennis; volleyball. Also includes making beds, sweeping, light polishing and waxing, laundering by machine, and other activities that require moderate arm movement.[c]	Men: Most men in light industry, students, building workers (excluding heavy laborers), many farm workers, soldiers not on active service, fishermen. Women: Light industry, housewives without mechanical household appliances, students, department store workers.		Women 4.1	170
Heavy	*Very Active*	75–100	Men 8.4	350
Walking with load up hill, tree felling, work with pick and shovel, basketball, swimming, climbing, football.	Men: Some agricultural workers, unskilled laborers, forestry workers, army recruits and soldiers on active service, mine workers, steel workers. Women: Some farm workers (especially peasant agricultural), dancers, athlete.		Women 8.0	250

TABLE 4-7. (Continued)

Activity[a]	Occupation[b]	Percentage above Basal	Calories/ kg/hr[a]	Calories/ hr[c]
Vigorous Heavy scrubbing and waxing, hand washing large articles of clothing; hanging out clothes, stripping beds; walking fast, and bowling.[c]	*Exceptionally active* Men: Lumberjacks, blacksmiths, rickshaw pullers Women: Construction workers	over 100		350 and more
Strenuous Swimming, playing tennis, running, bicycling, dancing, skiing, and playing football.[c]				

[a] Adapted from Food and Nutrition Board, Nat'l Research Council, *Recommended Dietary Allowances*, 8th Ed. Washington, D.C. Nat'l Acad. of Science, 1974.
[b] From Food and Agriculture Org., *Energy and Protein Requirements*, Nutrition Meetings Rep. Ser. No. 52 of WHO Technical Rep. Ser. No. 522, Geneva, 1973.
[c] Adapted from L. Page and L. J. Fincher, *Food and Your Weight*. Home & Garden Bull. No. 74, USDA, 1960.

descriptive. A certain amount of the day's caloric intake is needed to digest, absorb, and metabolize our daily food intake. It may be somewhat comforting to some people that the body actually burns up some Calories during and after eating. Generally, this amounts to less than 150 Calories per day. The actual amount is about 6% of the day's total caloric intake when a mixed diet of carbohydrate, protein, and fat is consumed. Popular claims are made that protein has a higher calorigenic effect than the other energy nutrients and because of this more Calories are burned up when consuming a high-protein diet. It is true that protein does have a slightly higher SDA, but the amount is not high enough to make any significant difference.

Calculating Energy Requirements

Two main methods exist for calculating energy requirements. The first of these is a long method called the *factorial method*, and the second is actually one of several short methods.

Factorial Method

There are seven steps involved in this calculation. They are as follows:

1. Determine ideal body weight of the subject and convert from pounds to kilograms.

2. Determine BMR, using only *one* of the following methods:

a. Men: 1.0 Calorie per kilogram of ideal body weight per hour × 24 hours.
Women: .9 Calorie per kilogram of ideal body weight per hour × 24 hours.

b. Metabolic: Locate weight (kg) and metabolic body size (kg$^{3/4}$) in Table 4-3 and multiply by 70.

c. Locate BMR for weight and sex in an appropriate chart.

d. Body surface area: Locate body surface area in Figure 4-9. Locate number of Calories, according to age and sex, per square meter per hour for specific surface area × 24 hours in Table 4-2.

e. Use simple method for estimating BMR:
· Men: Add a zero to ideal weight in pounds

and add to this figure twice the ideal weight.

· Women: Add a zero to ideal weight in pounds and add to this figure the ideal weight.

3. Correct for sleep: Subtract. 1 Calorie per kilogram of ideal body weight × hours of sleep per night from the BMR.

4. Make other adjustments in BMR as needed.

a. Adjust for age.

b. Adjust for body weight:

· If slimmer than average add 5% to BMR.

· If pudgier than average (plump) subtract 5% from BMR.

· If overweight subtract 10% from BMR.

5. Add the number of Calories required for physical activity, using *one* of several methods:

a. Calculate Calories needed for activity from a personal activity record.

b. Estimate number of hours spent in each major activity category and calculate Calories required.

c. Select a general activity level and multiply by the appropriate factor. Use Table 4-8 or add the caloric requirement for the appropriate activity level (Table 4-9).

d. Figure Calories for activity as a certain percentage above basal according to a selected activity level.

e. Estimate Calories for activity in the following manner:

· Sedentary: Ideal body weight (pounds) × 3.

· Moderate: Ideal body weight (pounds) × 5.

· Strenuous: Ideal body weight (pounds) × 10.

6. Add the factor for specific dynamic action of food by multiplying the BMR plus activity figure by 10%. Add to accumulative answer.

7. The resulting Calories are the personal daily energy requirement for a selected person or client.

TABLE 4-8. USDA Factors for Activity Levels

Activity	Kcal per Lb per Day	
	Women	Men
Sedentary or light	14	16
Moderately active	18	21
Very active	22	26

SOURCE: M. V. Krause, *Food, Nutrition and Diet Therapy*, 5th Ed. Philadelphia: W. B. Saunders Co., 1972.

Short Methods

There are several short methods for estimating total caloric requirements in one easy step. The first of these was developed by the US Department of Agriculture and is referred to as the "Rule of Thumb." It is based on three activity levels for both men and women. The calculation involves taking the subject's ideal weight in pounds and multiplying by the suitable factor (see Table 4-8). The energy requirements for our female college student would be 120 pounds × 14 Calories per pound, or 1,680 Calories. This figure is quite low compared to the previous estimates, and it is probably incorrectly so because there is no separate activity level supplied for light activity. If the factor of 16 is used, which is midway between sedentary and moderately active, her caloric requirement would be 1,920 Calories, which is more realistic.

Another short method uses ideal body weight in kilograms. The ideal weight is mul-

TABLE 4-9. Caloric Requirements for Activity Levels

Activity	Kcal per Day	
	Men	Women
Sedentary or light	225	225
Moderate	750	500
Heavy	1,500	1,000
Very Heavy	2,500	

SOURCE: B. T. Burton, *Human Nutrition*, 3rd Ed. McGraw-Hill Book Co., 1976.

tiplied by one of three factors: 30 Calories per kilogram for sedentary; 35–40, for moderately active; and 45, for very active (Krause and Mahan, 1979). No differentiation is made for men and women, so this method produces only a crude estimate. With this method the female student requires 30 Calories/kg × 55 kg = 1,650 Calories per day.

Table 4-10 summarizes the energy requirements for moderately active adults at various ages.

Realities of Estimating Energy Requirements and Intakes

Some may find a discussion of the variables encountered in measuring or estimating daily energy requirements and expenditures and daily caloric intakes discouraging, but it is essential to emphasize the realities of the subject of energy balance. It is crucially important for the nurse to be aware of the complexities of this subject if she is to assist patients and clients in setting realistic goals for maintenance of energy balance. Actually, neither human energy requirements nor the precise number of daily Calories from food to maintain energy balance are known. Energy expenditures and caloric intakes can only be estimates of the actual requirements and intakes. When energy expenditure and caloric intake are in perfect balance, a person will be maintaining ideal body weight and energy

balance will be sustained. Energy balance is difficult, however, to maintain throughout the life cycle, as clearly evidenced by both underweight and overweight people of all ages. To attain ideal weight often becomes a process of "trial by Calorie," according to nutrition author Deutsch (1976). Attainment of ideal weight, however, is the subject of the next chapter. Let us consider some of the variables involved in measuring and estimating energy requirements and caloric intakes.

BMR

If the subject's BMR is within normal range, the measurement or estimate of the BMR will not vary nearly as much as an estimate of physical activity. If the secretions of the thyroid gland are abnormal, this hormonal irregularity can increase the BMR by as much as 100% or decrease it by 30–40%. The BMR is also influenced by body composition, age, and nutritional status; adjustments for these variables must be made. Ideal weight should always be used in calculating the BMR. The BMR varies with body surface area as it relates to height and ideal weight. Actual measurement of a subject's BMR by direct or indirect calorimetry or assessment of thyroid function will result in a more precise estimate than the use of a formula.

Activity

In contrast to the BMR, the energy expended in physical activity does vary with body size and body weight. This one variable alone makes assessment of energy expenditure even more complex and more difficult to estimate. Actual energy expenditure of a subject is measured by either direct or indirect calorimetry in only a very minute number of subjects who are generally part of energy metabolism research studies. Measurement by either of these methods contains some variables that cannot be controlled, such as the impact of isolation in a room or chamber during measurement and the impact of wearing a piece of equipment during the performance

TABLE 4-10. Average Energy Requirements of Moderately Active Adults

Age (Years)	65 kg Man (Calories)	55 kg Woman (Calories)	% of Reference
20–39	3,000	2,200	100
40–49	2,850	2,090	95
50–59	2,700	1,980	90
60–69	2,400	1,760	80
70–79	2,100	1,540	70

SOURCE: *Energy and Protein Requirements*, FAO Nutrition Meetings Rep. Ser. No. 52 of WHO Technical Rep. Ser. No. 522, Geneva, 1973.

of an activity. Even though measurements made in this way are very accurate, they are specific for one person for specific activities. On another day the same subject may have a very different level of energy expenditure. If the figures obtained are used on any one other than the subject, they become only general estimates of energy expenditure.

There are many tables of energy expenditure available, but these are only gross estimates when applied to individuals. The tables that list the energy expended per kilogram are the most accurate because the subject's body size will be reflected. Actual body weight should be used when estimating energy used for physical activity.

Stunkard (1960), in an article about physical activity, remarked that physical activity in humans is so irregular as to almost be considered random. The number of variables involved in estimating energy expended during physical activity are great, but the tools available are better than no tools at all. All those involved should simply be aware that the figures obtained are only estimates and are to be used that way.

Most physical activity does vary according to actual body weight—for example, running, walking, or participating in an active sport. Other activities—such as reading, writing, or knitting—are not affected by weight.

The length of time spent and the intensity of performance in an activity are very important in estimating energy requirements. It is quite true that playing football is a very strenuous sport that requires the expenditure of considerable energy. In observing any one football player, however, it is readily noticed that the intensity of his physical activity varies greatly throughout the game. The same is true with tennis or any other sport. Passmore and Durnin (1955) commented that for assessment of energy expended in an activity lasting more than 10–15 minutes, the metabolic measurement must be supplemented by accurate recording of activities and times. For

the football player the amount of time spent in the huddle, just standing, or involved in strenuous movements on the field is important. Whether a person is engaged in work or play, intensity affects energy expenditure considerably.

Another important variable is efficiency or training in the performance of a physical activity. A trained runner will use less energy running around a block than the neighborhood jogger, and of course the trained runner will be able to continue running much longer.

Another variable in estimating energy expenditure is characteristic movements of subjects. When sitting, does the person sit quietly or are there a variety of small movements, such as shaking a leg or tapping the toes or drumming the fingers? All of these movements during the day add to total caloric expenditure, but they are very difficult to estimate.

Sleep and SDA

It has been learned that sleep decreases the BMR by 10% during the hours of sleep. The manner in which a person sleeps during the night affects this amount. The more restless the sleeping pattern, the greater the number of Calories expended. Therefore, even when the BMR is corrected for sleep by 10%, the amount is still only an estimate. The value for the calorigenic or SDA of food is also only an estimate.

Food Intake

Beside the sources of error involved in estimating Calories required for BMR and especially Calories required for physical activity, there are also several sources of error in estimating daily food intake and actual daily consumption (Calorie intake) of Calories.

The dietitian or nurse must begin by obtaining from the client during an interview an accurate recollection of dietary intake for the previous 24 hours or a reasonable assessment of a typical day's eating pattern, a process that introduces error at the start. Most subjects asked to recall all food and approximate portion sizes eaten during the previous 24 hours will not be able to do this with 100% accuracy. The tendency is to omit some of the snack foods or beverages that were consumed or to underestimate amounts. The interviewee may not be able to give an accurate description of food consumed during a typical day because of the questions asked by the dietitian or nurse. Food intake may vary so much that there simply is no typical eating pattern. The best way to avoid these errors is to ask the client to record all food eaten for three days or, better yet, for seven. The daily caloric intake is calculated and a daily average is obtained.

The caloric intake of food consumed is determined by estimating Calories, either using the exchange system or looking up and recording the caloric content of foods from a reliable nutrition table. The Calories obtained using either method are still only estimates. Use of the exchange system involves rather large sources of error because not all foods on an exchange list contain the same number of Calories. Some foods contain more than the average number, some less. The use of a table of food composition is a more accurate way of estimating Calories, but several sources of error are also encountered in their use. Not all foods are listed in a table of food composition. Consumption of foods prepared by a home recipe or commercially prepared make estimation of Calories consumed only a little more accurate than guesswork. Sizes or portions of food are difficult to estimate and are often not the same as those listed in the food tables. Fruits and vegetables vary in caloric content with the specific variety and the season of the year. Meat, especially beef, differs in Calories depending on the fat content.

Even though there are many sources of error in estimating daily energy expenditure and the caloric content of a daily food intake, these estimates are necessary and useful as just what they are—estimates—which serve as guidelines. Additional research needs to be done in the field of energy.

BIBLIOGRAPHY

Am. Diabetes Assoc. and Am. Dietetic Assoc. *A Guide for Professionals: The Effective Application of Exchange Lists for Meal Planning.* New York or Chicago, 1977.

Ames, S. R. The joule—unit of energy. *J. Am. Diet. Assoc.* 57:415, 1970.

Arlin, M. J. *The Science of Nutrition.* 2nd Ed. New York: Macmillan, Inc., 1977.

Bray, G. A., Whipp, B. J., and Sankar, N. K. The acute effects of food intake on energy expenditure during cycle ergometry. *Am J. Clin. Nutr.* 27:254, 1974.

Conzolazio, C. F., Nelson, R. A., Daws, T. A., Krzywicki, H. J., Johnson, H. L., and Barnhart, R. A. Body weight, heart rate, and ventilatory volume relationships to oxygen uptake. *Am. J. Clin. Nutr.* 24:1180, 1971.

Deutsch, R. M. *Realities of Nutrition.* 1st Ed. Palo Alto, Calif.: Bull Pub. Co., 1976.

Durnin, J. V. G. A., Edholm, O. G., Miller, D. S., and Waterlow, J. C. How much food does man require? *Nature* 242:418, 1973.

Fulton, D. E. Basal metabolism rate of women. *J. Am. Diet. Assoc.* 61:516, 1972.

Groen, J. J. An indirect method for approximating caloric expenditure of physical activity: A recommendation for dietary survey. *J. Am. Diet. Assoc.* 52:313, 1968.

Guthrie, H. A. *Introductory Nutrition.* 4th Ed. St. Louis: The C. V. Mosby Co., 1979.

Hegsted, D. M. Energy needs and energy utilization. *Nutr. Rev.* 32(2):33, 1974.

Krause, M. V., and Mahan, L. K. *Food, Nutrition, and Diet Therapy.* 6th Ed. Philadelphia: W. B. Saunders Co., 1979.

Lagua, R. T., Claudio, V. S., and Thiele, V. F. *Nutrition and Diet Therapy Reference Dictionary.* 2nd Ed. St. Louis: The C. V. Mosby Co., 1974.

Mitchell, H. S., Rynbergen, H. J., Anderson, L., and Dibble, M. V. *Nutrition in Health and Disease.* 16th Ed. Philadelphia: J. B. Lippincott Co., 1976.

Passmore, R., and Durnin, J. V. G. A. Human energy expenditures. *Physiol. Rev.* 35:801, 1955.

Robinson, C. H., and Lawler, M. R. *Normal and Therapeutic Nutrition.* 15th Ed. New York: Macmillan, Inc., 1977.

Stunkard, A. A method of studying physical activity in man. *Am. J. Clin. Nutr.* 8:595, 1960.

Weaver, E. K., and Elliot, D. E. Factors affecting energy expended in homemaking tasks. *J. Am. Diet. Assoc.* 39:205, 1961.

Williams, S. R. *Nutrition and Diet Therapy.* 3rd Ed. St. Louis: The C. V. Mosby Co., 1977.

Wilson, E. D., Fisher, K. H., and Garcia, P. A. *Principles of Nutrition.* 4th Ed. New York: John Wiley & Sons, Inc., Pubs., 1979.

CHAPTER 5

Attainment and Maintenance of Ideal Weight

SOCRATES: *Beware of those foods that tempt you to eat when you are not hungry and those liquids that tempt you to drink when you are not thirsty.*

A startling fact is that, although the number one health problem in the developing countries is undernutrition and near starvation, a high percentage of people in the United States struggle with the problem of excessive body weight. It is impossible to know the full extent of undernutrition in the world, but an estimate has been made that about half of the world's population goes to bed hungry each night because they lack adequate food. In contrast, in the United States it is estimated that about 40% of the adults are overweight. This high percentage is not surprising if one takes a few minutes to observe people in a restaurant or shopping center. It is true that the person on a weight-reducing diet may also go to bed hungry, but not because of an inadequate food supply.

In the United States the population is almost obsessed with the attainment or maintenance of ideal weight. A casual glance at a current magazine usually reveals the latest weight-reducing diet or a new set of exercises to assist the slimming process. Though maintenance of ideal weight is a simple task for a fortunate few, attainment of ideal weight through weight gain or weight loss is quite difficult and the results are often discouraging. This chapter examines the causes, medical risks, and methods of treatment for both extremes of caloric imbalance, the condi-

tion of being overweight or obese that results when caloric intake exceeds energy expenditure, and the less frequent but still very important problem of being underweight, which results when energy expenditure exceeds caloric intake.

CALORIC INTAKE EXCEEDING ENERGY REQUIREMENTS

When caloric intake exceeds energy requirements over a period of time, the extra Calories are converted to fat and stored as excess body weight. Two terms commonly used in discussing this problem are *overweight* and *obesity*. Some confusion exists concerning their precise definitions, and they are often used interchangeably. *Overweight* simply means weight in excess of a standard or desirable weight for a given person. The standard desirable weights for adult men and women are the tables from the Metropolitan Life Insurance Company (Appendices E and F of this book). A person who is overweight is over his ideal body weight. The term implies nothing about what constitutes the excess weight; it may result from larger amounts of bony structure, muscles, or adipose tissue. The overweight condition spans weights from 10% to 20% above ideal body weight. The excess weight is not necessarily excess body fat; an athlete may be overweight by height-weight standards for his body frame but obviously in excellent physical condition. Being overweight does not always constitute a hazard to the person's health; yet, the client should be encouraged to lose a few pounds or at least to avoid gaining any more weight.

Obesity is a condition of being overfat in which a person is about 20% or more above ideal body weight. This condition refers to an accumulation of excess body fat, and it does represent a health hazard. The following discussion focuses on the development and maintenance of obesity as well as its prevention and treatment; the student should keep in mind that most of the same principles apply to the treatment of the overweight person.

Assessment of Obesity

The methods for assessing obesity are many and varied. They range from simple visual inspection to a complex method of calculating lean body potassium using a whole-body counter. Only those methods of practical use in a hospital or clinic setting are explained here.

Visual Inspection
The easiest way for a physician or nurse to assess a client's weight status is by visual inspection during a physical examination. Evidence of an excessive accumulation of body fat will be observed in the regions of the abdomen, buttocks, and upper thighs. The nurse or dietitian interviewing fully clothed clients should be alert for signs of the overfat or too thin person.

Height-Weight Relationship
Besides visual inspection the most common method of assessing weight status is to compare the person's actual weight with standard height-weight tables that list ideal weights according to frame size for men and women

(see Appendices E and F). The limitations in using these tables were explained in the previous chapter. When access to these tables is not possible, the evaluator can use the simple formula for estimating ideal weight also presented in the previous chapter.

Other Simple Tests
There are four other very simple tests that can be used to assess obesity (Thiele, 1976). The *pinch test* involves pinching up a fold of skin and *subcutaneous fat.* If the pinched fold of fat is greater than 1 inch (2.54 cm), the person is obese. In the *ruler test,* a ruler should lie perfectly flat when placed between the pubic bone and the rib cage. If it does not, the person is obese. The *girth test* is used for male subjects only. In the nonobese male the waist measurement should be equal to or less than the chest circumference. Another interesting test is called the *"perfect 36" index.* This test involves subtracting the person's waist measurement in inches from his height in inches. If the difference is somewhere between 36 and 40, the subject is considered to be of normal weight. A value of less than 25 may represent obesity.

Anthropometric Measurements
One common method for measuring subcutaneous fat is to measure skinfold thickness of the triceps or subscapular skinfolds with an instrument called a *caliper.* This is one example of an *anthropometric measurement. Anthropometry* is the scientific measurement of various parts of the body for comparing individuals. These measurements are useful tools to aid in assessing the nutritional status of individuals or groups. Other anthropometric measurements for assessing weight status are the circumference of the chest, abdomen, buttocks, thigh, calf, ankle, biceps, and forearm; measurements that are performed with a flexible steel tape measure. More detail about the use of these measurements in nutritional assessment is presented in Chapter 19.

Causes of Obesity

The cause of obesity in a client can no longer be viewed as merely overindulgence in food resulting from lack of self-discipline. The causes of obesity are now known to be complex and multifaceted. Although significant strides have been made toward a better understanding of the causes of obesity, there is still a great deal that is not understood. The causes of obesity have environmental, psychological, and physiological components that are complexly interrelated. The initial step in helping an obese client is to understand the interrelationships that have contributed to his obesity.

Environmental and Psychological Contributors

Many factors in the environment have a definite effect on a person's ability to maintain ideal body weight. Abundance of food and decreased physical activity levels in the United States have led to the increased incidence of obesity.

The increased use of labor saving devices in all areas of life has significantly reduced the energy requirement from that of 50 years ago, but in many instances the corresponding adjustment in caloric intake has not been made. The importance of adjusting caloric intake so it is more in line with energy expenditure is emphasized by considering that a consistent intake of 100 extra Calories a day represents an accumulation of 10 lb (4.5 kg) of weight in one year. The student can readily appreciate what an extra 200 or 500 Calories a day will produce in added body weight in one year. Calories *do* count, and an excess caloric intake above energy expenditure will produce excess body weight.

A closer look at a pattern of activities for a typical family in the United States reveals much about the level of physical activity. The following stereotyped illustration serves to emphasize some of the environmental and psychological influences contributing to obesity:

The family awakens and begins its activities for the day. Mother goes to the kitchen, plugs in the automatic coffee maker, and pours orange juice for the whole family. The father takes a shower and then shaves with his automatic shaver. By now the children are up and have settled themselves in front of the television to watch cartoons. Mother pours each member of the family a bowl of his favorite cereal and she puts a couple of pieces of toast in the automatic toaster for herself and her husband. The children eat their cereal in front of the TV, and father reads the morning paper. Mother sits sipping her coffee and prepares herself for the day ahead. Father is the first to leave. He drives his own car to his downtown office and parks the car in a reserved space in the lot directly next to the office building where he works. He reflects on how convenient this parking space is and on how, even though he has to pay "a bit" extra per month, it is really worth the extra cost. Inside the building he takes the elevator to the fourth floor, where he works. He is now ready to spend the morning behind his desk writing letters and making phone calls.

Meanwhile at home, mother puts a load of laundry into the automatic washer while the children dress for school. After they are dressed they return to the TV until mother announces its time to go outside and wait for the school bus. The mandatory use of school buses in the cities and suburbs for transporting children has deprived them of a pleasant form of daily exercise.

Mother runs the electric vacuum cleaner over the carpets before she drives to the shopping center. She automatically looks for the closest parking space. She rides the escalator to the floors of the department store and takes a break from her shopping by having a club sandwich and a piece of delicious cheesecake. Feeling refreshed, she completes her shopping and drives to a friend's home, where she plays bridge until 3 PM. Of course the hostess serves a high-Calorie dessert before allowing her guests to leave. Nuts, mints, and pretzels are also on the bridge tables all afternoon, and the dishes are kept full by the hostess.

Meanwhile, father and a client drive to a nice restaurant two blocks away for a luncheon meeting. They both order a "hearty" lunch, since they have been so busy all morning; each has beef stroganoff with a hot fudge sundae for dessert. They both drive back to the office and continue their meeting for the afternoon. About 3:30 PM, they have the secretary bring them each a large sweet roll and cola beverage from the cafeteria.

Mother arrives home five minutes before the school bus. While the children watch the afternoon cartoons on TV and have an afterschool snack of a cola and candy bar, mother relaxes with her favorite woman's magazine and a cola beverage. Father arrives home at 5:30 very tired, so he relaxes with the paper and a cocktail. At 6:30 the whole family drives to the grandparents' home because today is the youngest child's birthday. Grandma has fixed a wonderful roast beef dinner with all the family's favorite foods. Father dearly loves grandma's homemade cinnamon rolls and eats maybe one too many. After dinner comes the birthday cake and opening the presents. The boy blows out the candles, and then everyone watches him open his presents. Now it is time to eat the birthday cake. Everyone is really too full to eat the cake and ice cream, but no one will admit it so as not to hurt grandma's feelings after she worked so hard to bake and carefully decorate the cake. So everyone has a generous piece of cake and a dip of ice cream. The whole family sits around the TV and watches a special children's show. Then everyone thanks grandma for the lovely dinner and party and goes home. After such a "busy" day the children go right to bed, but mother and father stay up and watch the late show on TV. Mother prepares two cups of hot chocolate with whipped cream topping for them because the evening has turned quite cool. She believes that the hot chocolate will make them sleep more soundly after such a busy day.

Environmental and psychological contributors to obesity include:

1. Environmental contributors
   a. Decreased level of physical activity because of
   · Use of labor-saving devices.
   · Riding in an automobile or other means of transportation when walking or cycling might be feasible
   · Watching spectator sports events but not actively participating in any athletic events.

b. Failure to adjust caloric intake to meet lower energy requirement after age 25.
· Basal metabolic rate declines each year after age 25.
· Physical demands of an occupation may be less or entirely different from others.
· Some disabling illnesses may further reduce caloric requirement because of decreased physical activity.
c. Eating habits may add a significant number of Calories to daily food intake.
· Eating something sweet when drinking a cup of coffee.
· Eating between meals.
· Eating a snack before going to bed each night.
· Eating large amounts of food at each meal or snack.
· Feeling that a meal is not complete without a dessert.
· Snacking when watching TV.
· Drinking high-Calorie carbonated beverages to quench thirst.
· Consuming alcoholic beverages.
d. Use of food in entertaining and other social events.
· Food, beverage, or both are almost always offered to a guest.
· A guest to whom food is offered feels he must accept it to avoid hurting the hostess's feelings.
· Entertaining guests often includes serving a large quantity of rich food.
· Many holidays are celebrated with the consumption of large holiday meals.
· Food is present at almost any social gathering, reception, or open house.
2. Psychological contributors
   a. Eating in response to psychological states, for example:
   · To reduce tension or frustration.
   · To relieve boredom or depression.
   · To release anger.

b. Eating as a substitute for love and security.

These preceding psychological and environmental influences affect everyone at least to some extent, but one or more may be particularly relevant to a specific obese client. Determination of the environmental and psychological influences on a client's eating habits will bring the physician, nurse, or dietitian one step closer to counseling the client effectively about his weight.

Physiological Factors

The overweight client is affected not only by psychological and environmental influences but by the additional interaction of several physiological factors. Although only a very small percentage (less than 5%) of the obese have a definite medical problem with an underactive thyroid gland, there are several physiological factors that do influence obesity. Some are fairly well understood, but generally much more needs to be determined about complex physiological interactions.

GENETIC INFLUENCES. Evidence indicates that there are relationships between genetic factors and the incidence of obesity. As with other characteristics that are influenced by heredity, the obvious question that arises is the relative effect of environment and heredity on the development of the characteristic of obesity.

Although genetic obesity in humans has not been clearly identified, some human studies have yielded interesting observations. In families in which neither parent is obese, only 7% of the children will be obese. If, however, both parents are obese, the percentage of obese children rises to 80% (Mayer, 1959). Data available from twin studies show that identical twins that have been separated and raised in different homes have similar weights, whereas fraternal twins show greater weight differences. The weights of adopted children show only slight correlation with those of their parents, whereas the weights of

natural children show a high correlation with those of their parents (Newman et al. 1937; Withers, 1964).

Some other interesting studies involve physical body types. The *ectomorph* is slender, the *mesomorph* is muscular, and the *endomorph* is plump and round. Of these three body types (shown in Fig. 5-1) the endomorph is the most likely to become obese. The mesomorph may become obese if his build contains more endomorphic than ectomorphic components. This phenomenon does not mean that obesity is inevitable for the endomorphic person, but close monitoring of weight should be used to avoid it.

FAT CELL THEORY. A number of studies have shown that excessive weight gain in infancy leads to a higher incidence of obesity during childhood. Obesity in adolescence also tends to persist, and approximately 80% of all obese children remain so as adults. The most interesting breakthrough in the study of obesity in recent years has been the discovery of how fat cells develop. Fat is stored within the body, either by an increase in the number of fat cells (*hyperplasia*) or an increase in the size of the fat cell (*hypertrophy*). It is now known that there are critical periods in human development when fat cells may be deposited. During the last trimester of pregnancy, the first three years of life, and adolescence there may be an actual increase in the number of fat cells. If an excess number of fat cells is deposited during these critical periods, there is a greater likelihood that the person will have continual difficulty maintaining or losing weight for the rest of his life (Knittle, 1972).

In early obesity studies obese adults with a childhood history of obesity were compared before and after weight reduction to nonobese adults. The results showed that the increased fat storage in obese subjects was due primarily to a two- to threefold increase in number of fat cells. Some of the obese subjects also had an increase in cell size, but most had normal values for cell size. Weight reduc-

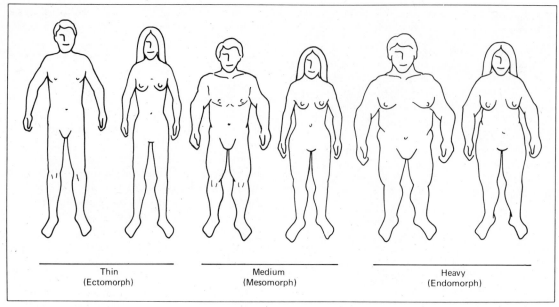

Thin
(Ectomorph)

Medium
(Mesomorph)

Heavy
(Endomorph)

Figure 5-1. Body types of men and women.

tion was associated with a decrease in size of the fat cell, but there was no significant alteration in cell numbers (Knittle, 1972).

Evidence exists that once adulthood is reached the number of fat cells is fixed. When an adult with no previous history of obesity gains weight, only the size of the fat cells increases, not the number. With loss of this excess body weight, the size of the fat cells returns to normal. In contrast, for the adult with a childhood history of obesity, loss of body weight reduces the size of the fat cells but not the number. Even after weight reduction has occurred, it appears to be easier for the person with a childhood history of obesity to regain excess weight than it is for the adult with no prior history, for these fat cells act as a reservoir waiting to be refilled with fat, which is what usually occurs.

Obesity, then, can occur through an increase in size of fat cells, number of fat cells, or both. Because an increase in number of fat cells is thought to occur during three critical periods of development and increase in the size of fat cells only can occur after adulthood is reached, weight reduction and maintenance are more difficult for the obese person with an increased number of cells deposited during one of the critical periods.

ENDOCRINE AND METABOLIC INFLUENCES. Many obese people try to blame their obesity on an endocrine malfunction. Though it is true that underproduction of thyroxine from the thyroid gland can lead to the development of excessive weight, this condition is present in only a very small percentage of obese subjects. It is not yet clearly understood what role the other endocrine hormones play in the development of obesity or on secondary influences on metabolism in the obese person.

Some obese people do have a decreased carbohydrate tolerance and a corresponding resistance to insulin, both of which are improved when the excess weight is lost. It is not clear whether these phenomena are a cause of the obesity itself or whether they are secondary to the obesity.

There may be a relationship between the increased secretion of growth hormone and the increased cellularity of adipose tissue. Although increased adrenal cortical function has been found in 30–60% of obese subjects, it is not clear how this fact relates to the obese state (Migeon et al., 1963).

An injury or tumor in the region of the *hypothalamus* that regulates eating may lead to excessive eating and obesity. This relationship between injury to the hypothalamus and excessive eating has been shown in animals but is not necessarily true in humans. Obesity resulting from this cause, however, would constitute a very small percentage of cases.

Classification of Obesity

Because obesity results from a complex interaction of social, environmental, economic, genetic, and physiological factors, some experts talk of the "obesities," and attempts have been made to classify the kinds of obesity. Obesity may be classified according to time of onset (juvenile versus adult), pathogenesis (regulatory versus metabolic), or psychological causes (reactive, developmental, and constitutional) (Bruch, 1957; Knittle, 1972; Van Itallie and Campbell, 1972).

The age of onset of obesity has an important effect on the success of a weight loss program. One classification divides obesity into either juvenile-onset or adult-onset obesity. Juvenile-onset obesity begins during developmental years when there is the potential for increasing the number of fat cells. Thus it could also be referred to as *hyperplastic obesity*, in which an increased number of fat cells is deposited. Adult-onset obesity is often characterized by a slow weight gain because of failure to adjust caloric intake to a lower energy expenditure or because of any other factors leading to an excess of intake of food during adulthood. In this type of obesity there is only an increase in the size of fat cells, and for this reason it is sometimes referred to as *hypertrophic obesity* (Knittle, 1972).

Another very interesting classification uses the "pull" and "push" concepts (Fig. 5-2). The "pull" theory suggests that excess food is pulled into the body because of a subtle *metabolic disorder* in the utilization of food, which may be based on an enzymatic, hormonal, or neurological defect. This type of obesity is basically the same as juvenile onset obesity. The "push" theory proposes that there is for nonphysiological reasons a *regulatory disorder* in feeding whereby the obese person force-feeds himself. This regulatory type of obesity corresponds fairly closely to adult-onset obesity (Van Itallie and Campbell, 1972).

A psychological classification of obesity has been developed by Bruch (1957). This classification involves distinguishing between reactive, developmental, and constitutional obesity. *Constitutional obesity* is due to physiological causes early in life. People with this type have been fat since early childhood or infancy. They generally have a healthy personal adjustment to their obesity, and they may even suffer some serious psychological problems if forced to reduce. *Developmental obesity* is common in children, especially those whose emotional development centers around eating as much as they want while at the same time avoiding social contacts and physical activity. *Reactive obesity* is most common in adults who overeat in response to psychological problems such as tension or frustration. These three types of obesities also fit into the juvenile and adult classifications. A summary of one classification of obesities is found in Table 5-1.

Maintenance of Obesity

Eating Habits

Because of the high level of interest in obesity and weight reduction, several studies have been conducted to investigate the eating

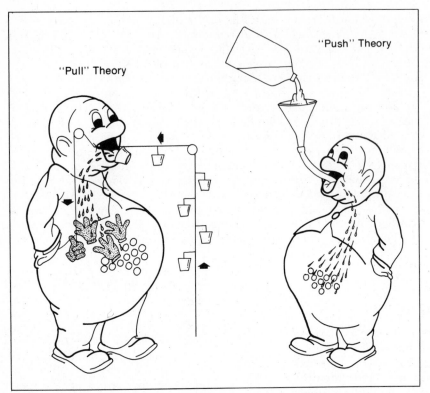

Figure 5-2. The "push" and "pull" theories of obesity. The "pull" theory of obesity proposes that a subtle metabolic disorder increases food intake either (1) by affecting hunger-satiety signals transmitted to a "satiety center" or (2) by altering the threshold of the satiety center to such signals. The "push" theory proposes that the obese person force-feeds himself, overeating for nonphysiological reasons. (Copyright The American Dietetic Association. Redrawn with permission from *Journal of the American Dietetic Association*, 61:385, 1972.)

TABLE 5-1. A Classification of Obesities

Basis of Classification	Juvenile Onset	Adult Onset
Fat cells[a]	Hyperplasia (increased number)	Hypertrophy (increased size)
Food intake[b]	Metabolic	Regulatory
Psychological origin[c]	Constitutional; developmental	Reactive

[a] J. L. Knittle, "Obesity in Childhood: A Problem in Adipose Tissue Cellular Development." *Journal of Pediatrics* 81:1048, 1972.
[b] T. B. Van Itallie, and R. G. Campbell, "Multidisciplinary Approach to the Problem of Obesity." *Journal of the American Dietetic Association* 61:385, 1972.
[c] H. Bruch, "Psychiatric Aspects of Obesity." *Metabolism* 6:461, 1957.

habits of obese people. It is generally observed that obese people respond more readily to any external stimuli associated with food. While the obese have a heightened response to many external stimuli associated with food, they seem to have a depressed reaction to the internal signals of gastric contractions, rumbling and gurgling, and *oral satiety*.

Because people are especially sensitive to external stimuli associated with food and eating, seeing a recipe for a cake with a taste-tempting color photo in a magazine may stimulate the obese person to bake and eat the cake without any reflection on internal feelings of hunger. Other examples of external stimuli that can stimulate overeating are the thought, appearance, smell, and taste of food. Anything associated with food acts as a stimulus to eating. Obese people might be referred to as "foodaholics" because of their intense reactions to the external stimuli associated with food.

It is quite interesting to note the obese subject's reaction to food when it is reduced to the bare essentials. In a study conducted by Campbell and associates (Campbell et al., 1971), both obese and nonobese subjects received a nutritionally complete diet in liquid form from a special automatically monitored "feeding machine." The liquid diet was dispensed by the subject to himself through a plastic tube. The nonobese adults consumed a sufficient number of Calories from the liquid diet to maintain their weight for several weeks. The obese subjects, however, spontaneously consumed far fewer Calories, and they lost weight rapidly. Obese subjects usually eat for nonphysiological reasons such as boredom, anxiety, habit, friendship, and of course the appearance, aroma, taste, and texture of the food itself. When these reasons for eating are removed and the subject is left with only the bare essentials of nutrition—that is, nutrients and Calories in a bland tasting liquid—he fails to regulate his intake (Van Itallie and Campbell, 1972).

In another study, Gates and his colleagues (Gates et al., 1975) observed the food choices of obese and nonobese subjects. They found that obese subjects selected not only larger quantities of food but also foods that were higher in Calories.

Obese subjects are almost always insensitive to the inner signals of hunger such as gastric distention, rumbling, and gurgling. They may not experience a true feeling of hunger, but they eat because it is time to eat or because the food is available. Some obese subjects also do not respond to *satiety*, the feeling of fullness and satisfaction following a meal. In an interesting study by Wagner and Hewitt (1975), the level of satiety in the obese and nonobese was assessed by recording the total time required to complete a meal, the number of mouthfuls or bites consumed during the meal, and the number of seconds each mouthful was chewed. The obese subjects finished eating their meal in less time and chewed each mouthful less than the nonobese subjects. There was too much variability in the number of mouthfuls among the subjects to reveal any clear-cut differences. That the obese eat rapidly and spend less time chewing their food seems to demonstrate that obese subjects do not take time to sense oral satiety. If oral satiety is present at all, it is a weak contributor to overall satiety. These observations again emphasize that the obese are affected more by external stimuli than by internal signals.

Psychological Implications

In the United States strong emphasis is placed on physical attractiveness, of which slenderness is a basic component. The overweight person is often viewed as gluttonous, self-indulgent, and lacking in willpower. The old adage Fat People Are Jolly is not necessarily true. Bruch (1957) wrote that for the fat person the psychological discomfort of relating to other people is a greater problem than any physiological discomfort or disease. The difficulty that the obese person has in relating to people often stems from the poor acceptance of the condition in the US sociocultural climate. In this situation the obese person suffers from severe self-doubt and a poor body image. The obese person has a preoccupation with weight and considers obesity itself and therefore his own body as objectionable and cause for shame (Bruch, 1972).

Medical Implications

Life insurance statistics reveal that there is a higher mortality rate among the obese from such medical conditions as cardiovascular disease. Obesity also increases susceptibility to certain diseases. In turn, the disabling effect of the disease leads to decreased physical activity, which of course has the effect of perpetuating the obesity. Chronic disease is more prevalent in the obese population, and mortality rates are higher for people who are 20–30% overweight (Guthrie, 1979).

Excess body weight imposes a greater load on the heart and circulatory system, especially during the stress of physical exertion. It is estimated that, for every pound of fat above ideal body weight, blood must be pumped by the heart through an additional two-thirds of a mile of blood vessels. This increased work by the heart may eventually lead to failure of the heart muscle itself. Also, there may be narrowing or complete *occlusion* (i.e., blockage) of an artery by the accumulation of fat and *cholesterol,* which may be due in part to a diet high in fat, cholesterol, and simple carbohydrates. *Plaque* formation within the artery reduces the diameter of the artery, causing the heart to work harder to pump the blood, thus increasing the arterial blood pressure. Statistically, obese people have higher levels of *triglycerides,* more cholesterol in the blood, and higher incidence of atherosclerotic heart disease than their counterparts. Obese people also generally have higher blood pressure than people of normal weight (Fig. 5-3). That the hypertension is due at least partially to excess body weight is

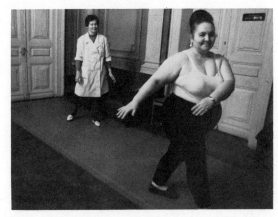

Figure 5-3. Diseases like obesity and high blood pressure may be directly attributable to the affluent society. (WHO photo by M. Jacot)

evidenced by the fact that blood pressure decreases as weight is lost.

Obese clients, particularly those with adult-onset obesity, often have some degree of carbohydrate intolerance with elevated levels of blood glucose and resistance of the tissues to insulin. It is these clients who are diagnosed as having adult-onset diabetes. When they lose weight, the carbohydrate tolerance often returns to normal. With the achievement of ideal weight, the cholesterol and triglyceride levels are also frequently reduced.

The obese also have a higher incidence of such conditions as gall bladder disease, gout, degenerative arthritis, and renal disease.

Besides influencing the incidence of certain diseases, obesity can be viewed as an added medical and surgical risk and as a physical handicap. The overweight person is at greater risk during and after surgery. The chances of developing complications during pregnancy and child birth are greater for the obese woman.

Obese people have decreased mobility and decreased agility, which makes them more susceptible to accidents and possible injuries.

They expend more physical effort to perform a given task because of their larger body size, and this increased physical effort often results in difficult breathing. They are often quite "winded" after climbing only a few stairs. Some obese people evidence the *Pickwickian syndrome,* characterized by an increased number of red blood cells, producing a flushed appearance to the face and *hypoventilation* (i.e., increased CO_2). The extra layers of fat may make the obese uncomfortable during warm weather and make them perspire quite freely.

Mann (1974) has suggested five general ways in which obesity may be detrimental to health:

1. The additional weight of the stored fat might overwork some of the body systems.

2. The greater food intake might increase the intake of harmful substances in food and damage the health.

3. The excessive intake of food increases glyceride transport and synthesis.

4. The decreased level of physical activity increases the incidence of chronic disease.

5. A genetic factor may exist between a tendency to obesity and metabolic disease.

Prevention of Obesity

Weight control programs are either preventive or corrective. In all the health professions the current emphasis is on health maintenance and prevention of disease states, but the average person does not think about his state of health when it is good, only when he has a particular disease or complaint. Most physicians, too, treat only a client's chief complaint or illness. Nonetheless, most health professionals would now agree it is more desirable to prevent obesity than to try to correct it after damage has already occurred. According to Sebrell (1958) the greatest hope for a solution to the problem of obesity lies in a program aimed at its prevention. Despite the need for continued research and study, health professionals and nursing and nutrition students must begin to consider what are essential components of a program for preventing obesity.

First, infants of fat mothers are not always overweight at birth. Widdowson (1955) found that fat mothers do have fat babies, but Wolff (1955) found that obese children were not obese at birth. Although some infants are born overweight as a result of excessive weight gain of the mother or the increased number of fat cells deposited during the last trimester of pregnancy, most infants are not born obese.

A program for the prevention of obesity should be aimed at establishing good eating habits during infancy and early childhood. A preventive program should be aimed toward nutrition education of mothers. Some mothers still believe that a fat baby is a healthy baby. This erroneous idea leads the mother to establish excessive eating habits in her child, even in infancy (Fig. 5-4). The mother may also tend to overemphasize the importance of food because of a strong desire to have a well-nourished child. What the mother is really doing is providing the child with over-

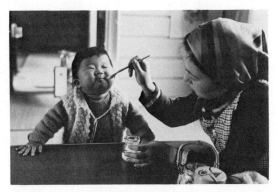

Figure 5-4. Overfeeding during infancy may lead to an increased number of fat cells and the development of obesity. (WHO photo by E. Schwab)

nourishment, which is leading to the development of obesity. Several years later the mother may finally realize that the child is overweight, but she hesitates to put the child on a diet because he is still "growing" and needs nourishment. She may rationalize that her child will outgrow his baby fat in a few years, anyway. The conclusion of this story is, however, that the child does not lose his baby fat but becomes an obese adolescent. As a teenager he now assumes major responsibility for his own eating habits. Unless the teenager is highly motivated and receives much psychological support from family and friends, the chances of his losing weight are very small.

Health and nutrition education should be directed primarily at young adults during the childbearing years, with primary emphasis on the establishment of nutritionally sound infant feeding principles and the development of good eating habits during childhood and adolescence. More nutrition education should be incorporated into the elementary school curriculum, along with other basic health habits and emphasis on the prevention of obesity. The need for regular physical exercise and its benefits should also be emphasized.

Early detection of a weight problem should be part of the routine physical examination performed by pediatricians on infants. All other health professionals such as nutritionists, hospital nurses, and school nurses who work with children and their mothers should be alert to changes in body weight so that appropriate weight-reduction advice can be offered. The old adage An Ounce of Prevention Is Worth a Pound of Cure is certainly true with obesity. Any weight gain of about 3 lb (1.4 kg) above a person's ideal body weight should be a signal to decrease caloric intake or increase energy expenditure to reduce the weight before the amount becomes any greater. Continual emphasis on this principle throughout life will help maintain good physical health. Two organizations that emphasize the importance of maintaining ideal weight and apply sound nutrition principles for weight reduction as part of their programs are the American Heart Association and the National Dairy Council.

Treatment of Obesity

The condition of being overweight develops over a period of several months to even several years. There is a gradual daily depositing of body fat resulting from an excess of caloric intake in relation to energy expenditure. This positive caloric balance gradually results in the accumulation of excess body fat. When a person finally realizes one day that he is overweight or finally decides to initiate a program of weight reduction, that person wants the excess weight to "disappear" almost immediately. There are basically two methods by which excess weight can be lost: decreasing caloric intake below energy requirements or increasing the level of physical activity.

Fad Diets

In response to the obsession with weight loss in the United States, more health and figure salons are springing up; more low-Calorie foods are available; more devices and aids for weight reduction are manufactured; and more authors are inspired to develop a new "low-Calorie" diet that will become the current best seller. Despite the many negative aspects of this phenomenon, there are some favorable outcomes. Foremost is increased awareness by the average person of the importance of personal weight maintenance within a few pounds of ideal body weight. There is also increased knowledge of the health risks associated with obesity and increased emphasis on staying in good physical condition through a regular program of exercise.

An interesting study was conducted in 1970 by Dwyer and Mayer to examine the percentage of the population who considered themselves overweight and to see how common dieting is within a population. Of the women answering the questionnaire, 27% said they were currently on a diet or that they diet from time to time, whereas only 13% of the men were or had been involved with diets. In the next part of the questionnaire 40% of the women but only 30% of the men stated that they omit or restrict their intake of certain "fattening foods," whereas 54% of the men and 30% of the women ate whatever they wanted with no concern about weight gain. Women were more concerned about being overweight than men. As a rule, the higher the social class the more concern there was about being overweight and the lower the incidence. This survey did reveal that large segments of the population are making attempts to control their weight.

The names selected for the popular fad diets are based on attracting the consumer's interest and immediately eliciting their support by getting them at least to try the diet for one or two weeks. The names appeal to the overweight person who wants to lose the excess body weight as quickly and as painlessly as possible. Most fad diets fit into one of the following general categories:

1. Famous people and places
2. Popular appeal
3. Emphasis on specific foods

A brief look back into the history of weight-reducing diets may help add some perspective to this topic. Over a century ago William Banting, a London undertaker, decided to do something about his obese state. He had become so fat that he could not even tie his shoes and he was forced to go downstairs backward because his center of gravity had moved so far forward as to make proceeding downstairs in the normal manner too hazardous. A surgeon, William Harvey, greatly restricted Banting's intake of carbohydrates but allowed him all the meat and dairy products he desired. Banting lost 85 lb in 38 weeks and wrote "A Letter on Corpulence, Addressed to the Public," in which he praised his doctor and the results of the diet (Banting, 1863,

p. 22). During the last 20 years there has been a renewed interest in similar diets all having the same basic features of low to very low carbohydrate content, no restriction of fat and protein, and unrestricted calories. Some of these familiar diets are the Air Force Diet, Dr Taller's Calories Don't Count, Dr Stillman's Quick Weight Loss Diet, and Dr Atkins' Diet Revolution.

A careful and objective evaluation should be made by health professionals of the fad diets to determine the source of their overwhelming appeal and whether they are medically safe. Popular appeal of fad diets is aimed at the emotions, de-emphasizing Calories and suggesting "easy" ways to lose weight. The diets emphasizing specific foods simply permit the dieter to select his favorite food(s) for a pleasant, painless way to reduce. Many of the diets are written by medical doctors or other people who are authorized to use "Doctor" before their name. Because doctors are highly respected members of society, it is difficult for the general public to believe that the diets they write about are only fads and in some cases may even be harmful. Diets bearing the names of such respected organizations as the US Air Force and the Mayo Clinic as part of their title also wield a lot of influence. It should be carefully noted, however, that both of these organizations have disclaimed any association with these diets (Hoffman, 1965; Pletcher, 1965). After a survey of weight-reducing diets offered in the United States, the US Senate Select Committee on Nutrition and Human Needs found that at least 51 were variations of the grapefruit-and-egg diet that has been discredited for many years.

There are some highly qualified "doctors" who are qualified to write about diets and weight reduction because they have their doctorates in nutrition, two of whom are Dr Phillip White of the American Medical Association and Dr Jean Mayer, president of Tufts University and author of his own book on being overweight. Mayer has for many years written extensively on basic nutrition and weight control in both professional journals and nonprofessional magazines besides conducting continued research on feeding regulations and obesity. Dr Frederick Stare of Harvard University is also a medical doctor with a practical knowledge of nutrition.

WEIGHT LOSS ON FAD DIETS.   Fantastic claims for weight reduction are made by the writers of the fad diets. One such claim, that "you can lose up to 20 pounds [9.1 kg] in 14 days without ever getting hungry;" is made by Dr Tarnower, author of the Scarsdale Diet, which is only a variation of the popular low-carbohydrate diet theme. Another fad is the use of liquid protein diets for weight loss. These diets have created severe electrolyte imbalances and some deaths have resulted. Use of these diets in research studies and responses from users do testify to the fact that these diets do effect weight loss during the time the subject follows the diet regimen (Worthington and Taylor, 1974). Is there some mysterious substance in food that dissolves fat or is there a fat-mobilizing hormone that converts stored fat to carbohydrate? The answer to both of these questions is no. There is no substance present in food that burns up fat. Fat is only "burned up" when caloric intake is less than physical energy expenditure. The acid in grapefruit was once alleged to have this magical property of dissolving fat, but this was disproved several years ago. No "fat-mobilizing hormone" has been identified in humans. *Growth hormone* is known to stimulate mobilization of fatty acids from fat deposits, but the existence and physiological function of a specific fat-mobilizing hormone remain to be established.

What then does account for the weight loss observed while the subject is adhering to one of these diets? To be effective *any* weight-reducing diet must provide for a decrease in caloric intake, an increase in energy expenditure or both. The reason for the weight loss is that the diet is low in total Calories (under

1,000). The low-carbohydrate diet is self-limiting in two ways. First of all, when overweight subjects drastically reduce their intake of carbohydrate, they are unable to make up the Calorie deficit thus created by increasing their intake of protein and fat. According to White all research shows that, when carbohydrates are restricted, people consume fewer Calories and less total food ("The Crash Diet Craze," 1973). The probable explanation is that proteins and fats tend to be more satiating (satifying) than carbohydrates. Also, even though protein and fat are not restricted, subjects quickly tire of a high-protein diet without accompanying carbohydrates and they voluntarily cut back their protein intake after a few days. As long as a group of volunteers remained on a low-carbohydrate diet, they did lose between 3 and 5 lb (1.35–2.25 kg) the first three-to-five days. Those continuing the diet beyond seven days lost at a rate of 2–3 lb (.9–1.35 kg)/wk. Once the diet was discontinued, however, the subjects regained 2–8 lb (.9–3.6 kg) the first week ("The Crash Diet Craze," 1973). The rapid loss of weight is due to changes in water balance. A large amount of fluid and sodium are initially lost from the body on any weight-reducing diet, but especially on a low-carbohydrate diet. The regaining of weight on discontinuation of the diet is due to regaining of fluids. This rapid loss of body weight followed by regaining several pounds on termination of the diet can be extremely discouraging to the person who really wants to lose. The excretion of sodium and water is minimized by increasing dietary carbohydrate somewhat.

PHYSIOLOGICAL EFFECTS OF FAD DIETS.   The real trouble with fad diets is that they are potentially dangerous to the health and certainly unnutritious. They cause abnormal physiological responses by the body as it attempts to maintain physiological equilibrium. Fad diets do not usually produce permanent weight loss. Weight is regained when the diet is discontinued and regular eating habits are resumed. The Yo-Yo syndrome of gaining, losing, regaining, and relosing weight can be more detrimental than maintaining excessive weight.

The Council on Foods and Nutrition of the American Medical Association (1973) critically reviewed the *low-carbohydrate ketogenic diets* and published a statement against Dr. Atkins' Diet Revolution. The physiological state produced by these low-carbohydrate diet regimens is the abnormal state of *ketosis,* a state similar to that of uncontrolled diabetes. In this physiological state the body turns to fat as its secondary source of energy because carbohydrate intake is so severely restricted. The body shifts into a faster rate of fat metabolism, breaking fat down for energy at an abnormally fast rate. Fat metabolism is proceeding so rapidly that the liver cannot detoxify all the intermediate products of fat metabolism. These intermediate products, called *ketones,* are strong acids and some accumulate in the blood and then spill over into the urine. The resulting state is called *ketosis.* The presence of ketosis leads to a depression of appetite, which further decreases the caloric intake from food.

The low level of dietary carbohydrate leads to a temporary loss of water and sodium from the body. The very high protein content of the diet imposes a greater strain on the kidneys by increasing the number of *solutes* (particles) that must pass through and bringing about an increased excretion of body water in an attempt to dilute these solutes. Both of these dietary adjustments may lead to excessive loss of body water and even dehydration.

Another potential hazard of these diets is *postural hypotension,* a rapid reduction in blood pressure brought about by a rapid shift from a supine to a standing position. Dizziness or even fainting may accompany this symptom. General fatigue and lack of physical energy during physical activity are also common occurrences.

Other undesirable effects are associated with increased levels of certain normal blood constituents. The increased levels of blood ketones increase the levels of blood *uric acid,* which may precipitate or exacerbate gout or gouty arthritis in certain subjects. Another great danger from the unrestricted protein and fat content of these diets is elevations in *serum lipids,* especially elevated levels of serum cholesterol and serum triglycerides. These rapid elevations in serum lipids could precipitate a heart attack in a susceptible person. Similar elevations in blood lipids are also found in perpetual dieters who lose, gain, and relose weight.

Fortunately most dieters who try these diets do not stay on them long enough to do themselves much harm, but it is the responsibility of health professionals to caution their clients about the potential health hazards of the ketogenic low-calorie diet regimens. A fitting conclusion to this section is a quote by a British physician, Dr. C. Stanford Read in 1908: "There seems to be an ever increasing number of individuals who for a time, will, believe any fresh dietetic rubbish that comes under their noses" (Wyden, 1965, p. 252). Fad diets will continue as long as people have a problem with weight control. Health professionals working with clients must take the time to evaluate new diets critically so they can advise their clients about possible health hazards.

Balanced Low-Calorie Diets

For a weight reduction program to be successful on a long-term basis there must be reeducation and retraining of a client's personal eating habits. If the person loses the desired amount of weight but then returns to his previous eating habits, the chances are the person will regain a large amount of the weight in a short period of time. This is especially true with adults who have been obese since early childhood because of their increased number of fat cells, which, though they do shrink in size during weight reduction, do not decrease in number. Thus they just wait to be filled up again when the person overeats.

A diet for weight reduction is one of the simplest modifications of a regular diet that can be made. In principle the diet need only contain a level of Calories below that required to maintain weight. The level of Calories should permit a weight loss satisfactory to both the person prescribing the diet and the client. A deficit of 500 Calories/day below maintenance level should result in the loss of about 1 lb (.45 kg)/wk. As a rule, the younger the person and the better the overall health status, the more weight could be lost each week by further increasing the daily caloric deficit. The difficulty in prescribing a weight reduction diet comes not in arriving at a caloric level but in considering a client's eating habits, nutritional needs, and psychological needs in devising an acceptable diet plan that is workable for that client. Simply handing the client a preplanned diet sheet will generally result in only short-term success. Taking the extra time required to become acquainted with the client and being willing to modify the diet plan with the client as weight reduction proceeds is worth the added effort for long-term success. White suggests that the best way to help the client keep his weight off is to help him develop good eating habits during dieting ("The Crash Diet Craze," 1973). He refers to dieting as an exaggeration of good eating habits, meaning that Calories are watched fairly closely. After the desired weight reduction has occurred, desserts are allowed in moderation.

The balanced low-Calorie diet that has proved successful for some people is a moderate-carbohydrate, high-protein, and low- to moderate-fat diet (see Fig. 5-5). The levels of vitamins and minerals, of course, should be adequate, or a vitamin and mineral supplement may be routinely prescribed. The level of Calories and also the amounts of carbohydrate, protein, and fat will vary for each client depending on age, sex, and physical activity level.

CALORIES. An adult man with a sedentary-to-moderate activity level will generally be

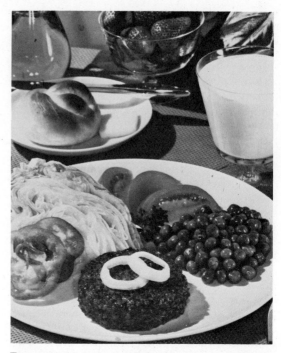

Figure 5-5. A balanced low-Calorie meal for weight reducing. (Courtesy National Dairy Council)

able to lose weight on 1,500–1,800 Calories. A woman with the same activity level will usually be able to lose on 1,000–1,500 Calories/day. If the diet is below 1,200 Calories, a vitamin and mineral supplement should be recommended.

CARBOHYDRATE. The amount of carbohydrate in a weight-reducing diet should be at least the minimum amount (50–100 gm) required to avoid ketosis. Many successful reducing diets provide about 45% of the Calories from carbohydrate. The level of carbohydrate can be adjusted to suit the client's preference as long as the minimum of 50–100 gm is provided.

PROTEIN. The protein content of a low-Calorie diet should be about 20% of the

Calories. Although .8 gm of protein per kilogram of ideal body weight is adequate for building and maintaining body tissues in the adult, it is usually desirable to increase the protein content of the reducing diet to provide 1.5 gm protein per kilogram, an amount that provides satiety value to the diet and decreases the hunger level between meals.

FAT. Fat comprises the remainder of the diet and contributes about 35% of the Calories.

ALCOHOL. It must be emphasized that alcohol also contributes Calories to the diet. Every gram of alcohol supplies 7 Calories. Carbohydrates are also provided in some alcoholic beverages such as wine and beer. If the client intends to continue consumption of alcoholic beverages, their caloric value must be figured into the total caloric content of the diet.

NUMBER OF MEALS. The number of meals or feedings included during the day should be based on the client's personal preferences and eating habits. All food and beverages consumed during the day should be figured into the basic diet plan. The preferable pattern is to include three main meals during the day. In human subjects there does not appear to be any increase in weight loss by taking in small, frequent meals rather than eating three main meals a day (Young et al., 1971). The pattern of eating that provides the most satiety and psychological satisfaction for the client is the most acceptable.

TYPES OF LOW-CALORIE DIETS. There are three approaches to weight reduction through low-Calorie diets:

1. Reduce portion sizes, omit desserts and concentrated sweets, or both.
2. Count Calories in all foods eaten in a 24-hour period, being certain not to exceed a set number of total Calories.

3. Plan daily menus and foods eaten around a diet pattern using the exchange system.

Some clients may be overweight because they are in the habit of eating at least two helpings of every food at a meal. Simply using their willpower and declining second helpings or decreasing the serving size of each food eaten may result in the desired weight loss. Other clients may need only to omit desserts for a period of time. Application and actual practice of these simple principles is, however, where the difficulties arise. People eat food for many more reasons than physiological nourishment. The pressures and influences from friends and family as well as personal, psychological, and environmental pressures often interfere with effective application of this method.

Another approach to effective weight reduction for some clients is to count Calories. A person restricted, for example, to no more than 1,200 Calories each day is allowed to eat whatever foods he desires as long as 1,200 Calories are not exceeded. There may be times when a combination of foods may be consumed early in the day that totals 1,200 Calories. Adhering to the rules of this regimen, the client will receive no additional food until the next morning. After this happens once, the client usually will be more careful to select foods of moderate caloric content so that his food intake is more evenly distributed throughout the day. The client should, of course, be instructed in the principles of a nutritionally adequate diet and its importance in maintaining good health. While consuming the entire 1,200 Calories from desserts may satisfy a psychological need and would theoretically result in weight reduction if the 1,200-Calorie limit was not exceeded, there would be no retraining of the person's eating habits. Even if excess weight was lost, once he resumed his regular eating habits, including both desserts and regular foods, he would obviously regain his excess weight quite readily. Clients using this method can greatly benefit from a few helpful suggestions of common substitutions that can be made to save considerable Calories throughout the day. A list of these substitutions and the Calories "saved" is presented in Table 5-2.

A third useful approach to weight reduction is through use of the exchange system (see Appendix I). The exchange lists provide for a wide variety of foods that can be included in a weight-reducing diet. The six separate lists of foods are grouped according to similar contents of carbohydrate, protein, and fat, and therefore Calories. A daily meal planned as closely as possible to the client's preferred eating habits by a dietitian provides the basis for the diet. The meal plan includes the number of food exchanges that are al-

TABLE 5-2. Substitutions to Reduce Caloric Intake

Food	Calories	Food	Calories	Calories Saved
Beverages				
Milk (whole), 8 oz	165	Milk (skim), 8 oz	80	85
Soft drink, 8 oz	105	Diet soft drink, 8 oz	1	104
Coffee with 2 lumps sugar and 2 T cream	110	Coffee with artificial sweetener and nondairy creamer	11	99
Cocoa (all milk), 8 oz	235	Cocoa (milk and water), 8 oz	140	95
Meats				
Loin roast, 3 oz	290	Pot Roast (round), 3 oz	160	130
Rump roast, 3 oz	290	Rib roast, 3 oz	200	90
Hamburger (moderate fat), 3 oz	240	Hamburger (lean), 3 oz	145	95
Pork chop (med), 3 oz	340	Veal chop, 3 oz	185	155
Eggs (scrambled), 2	220	Eggs (boiled or poached), 2	160	60
Cheddar cheese, 1 oz	105	Cottage cheese, uncreamed, 1 oz	25	80
Vegetables				
Baked beans, 1 cup	320	Green beans, 1 cup	30	290
Lima beans, 1 cup	160	Asparagus, 1 cup	30	130
Corn, 1 cup	160	Cauliflower, 1 cup	30	130
Succotash, 1 cup	260	Spinach, 1 cup	40	220
Fried potatoes, 1 cup	480	Baked potato, 2½ in dia	100	380
Mashed potato, 1 cup	245	Boiled potato, 2½ in dia	100	145
Salad w/1 T oil dressing	180	Salad w/1 T low-calorie dressing	40	140
Salad w/1 T blue cheese or dressing	105	Salad w/1 T low-calorie dressing	40	65
Soups				
Cream of chicken soup, 1 cup	210	Chicken noodle soup, 1 cup	110	100
Bean soup, 1 cup	190	Beef noodle soup, 1 cup	110	80
Minestrone soup, 1 cup	105	Beef bouillon, 1 cup	10	95
Chocolate cake w/icing	425	Sponge cake	120	305
Cupcake w/icing	230	Plain cupcake	115	115
Ice cream, 4 oz	150	Yogurt, fruit, 4 oz	60	90

SOURCE: *Are You Really Serious about Losing Weight?* 2nd Ed. Strasenburgh Laboratories, Rochester, New York, 1968.

lowed from each list for each meal. The client is then free to select foods from each exchange list for each meal. He is encouraged to substitute or exchange any food in a given list for any other food in that same list, being careful, of course, to adhere to the portion sizes.

The individual foods in the food exchange lists are the plain foods themselves; the method of preparation greatly affects the caloric content. Any method of preparation that does not include fat, sauces, and gravies will produce a food lower in Calories. The generally accepted methods of food preparation for low-Calorie diets are baking, broiling, grilling, roasting, and steaming. The use of exchange lists for meal planning need not be dull, monotonous, or unappealing. For the creative cook, use of exchange lists in meal planning often opens new aspects of cooking and eating. Many excellent, creative low-Calorie cookbooks are available to inspire the dieter.

The six exchange lists are grouped by milk, meat, fruit, vegetables, bread, and fat. All desserts and concentrated sweets are to be eliminated on the low-Calorie diet using the exchange lists. Concentrated sweets contain a large number of Calories in relation to the quantity of nutrients obtained. A piece of apple pie contains 350 Calories and a large apple, only 85 Calories. Besides containing considerably fewer Calories the apple contains a higher concentration of vitamins and minerals. A comparison of the Calories of basic foods prepared in different ways is shown in Table 5-3. An artificial sweetener should be used in place of regular sugar. There are several good ones on the retail market, and with encouragement most clients adjust well. Another important basic rule is to avoid eating fried foods and foods containing sauces and gravies.

The milk list consists of fluid milk and yogurt. There is a considerable difference in Calories between whole milk (170 Calories) and skim milk (80 Calories). The client who is

TABLE 5-3. Effect of Preparation on Caloric Content of Selected Foods

Food	Calories
Apples	
Fresh apple, one med	70
Applesauce, unsweetened, ½ cup	50
Applesauce, sweetened, ½ cup	115
Baked apple, 1 med	188
Apple crisp (brown Betty), ½ cup	211
Apple Pie (⅛ of 9-in pie)	410
Potatoes	
Boiled potato, med (without skin)	80
Baked potato, med (with skin)	90
Mashed with milk and butter, ½ cup	93
Potato chips, 10 med	115
French fries, 10 pieces	155
Grain products	
Saltine crackers, 4	50
Whole wheat bread, 1 slice	60
White bread, 1 slice	70
Macaroni, cooked, ½ cup	78
Spaghetti, cooked, ½ cup	78
Biscuit (home recipe), 1, 2 in dia	90
Noodles, egg, cooked, ½ cup	100
Pancake, 1, 4 in dia	104
Rice, cooked, ½ cup	113
Muffin	120
Cornbread muffin	125
Waffle, 5½ in dia	209
Milk	
Skim milk, 1 cup	90
2% milk, 1 cup	145
Whole milk (3.5% fat), 1 cup	160
*Cocoa (commercial mix) 1 cup	110
Cocoa (homemade), 1 cup	245
Chocolate milk, 1 cup	213
Malted milk, 1 cup	245
Milk shake, chocolate, 1 cup	268
Eggnog, 6 oz	233
Eggnog, Christmas type, 4 oz	335
Ice milk, 1 cup	200
Ice cream (10% fat), 1 cup	255
Yogurt (whole milk), 1 cup	150
Yogurt (partly skim milk), 1 cup	125
Yogurt, strawberry, 1 cup	225
Custard, 1 cup	305

SOURCE: Home & Garden Bull. No. 72, rev., USDA, 1977.
* Prepared with water.

really serious about losing weight should make a conscious effort to drink skim milk because of the large saving in Calories. If, however, skim milk is not acceptable, a compromise can be obtained by using 2% or low-fat milk (125 Calories).

All the vegetables listed in the vegetable exchanges contain approximately the same number of Calories per ½ cup serving. Some vegetables are missing from this list because they contain a higher proportion of carbohydrate and, therefore, of Calories; these vegetables are found in the bread list. Fresh, frozen, or canned vegetables can all be used. Frozen or canned vegetables that contain a special sauce or butter sauce should not be used because of the extra Calories. Butter, margarine, or bacon fat should not be added to vegetables during cooking. A small pat of butter or margarine may be added to the person's portion of vegetables at the table if that amount of fat is deducted from the meal plan.

The fruit list includes fresh or unsweetened canned or frozen fruit. The serving size for the fruits varies because the fruits vary in carbohydrate content. Any kind of fresh fruit may be used in the amount given in the list. Regular canned and frozen fruit should not be used because the fruit is packed in a sugar syrup or sugar has been added to the fruit. Some canned and frozen fruit, however, may be used if the label is read very carefully. Canned fruit that is packed in natural fruit juice or packed in water, unsweetened or artificially sweetened, may be used. Some frozen fruit such as cherries, strawberries, and other berries are frozen without the addition of sugar or sugar syrup. If added sweetness of the fruit is desired, an artificial sweetener could be used.

The bread list contains, of course all types of bread, but it also includes grain and cereal products and some starchy vegetables. Almost any kind of bread may be used except sweet rolls or doughnuts. All kinds of cereal may be used except the presweetened varieties. Notice that this list also includes such popular items as biscuits, cornbread, pancakes, waffles, French fries, and potato chips, but the consumer of these foods should omit

one-to-two servings of fat from the meal because of the higher fat content of these foods.

On the meat list there are three groups of meat based on fat content. The caloric content varies from 55 Calories/oz for lean meat to approximately 90 Calories/oz for high-fat meat such as beef brisket or spare ribs. Notice that these are Calories per ounce, not per serving. Approximately the same number of Calories are provided by 1 oz of meat as 1 slice of bread. Bread and starchy foods are often the first to be omitted on the weight-reducing diet, but a serving of meat contains more Calories than one of bread. The client on a weight-reducing diet should be encouraged to keep his protein intake fairly high because of the high satiety value of protein but not to omit bread and starchy foods in preference for meat. A good guideline to follow is to include not more than 3 oz of meat at the noon or evening meal. A well-balanced weight-reducing diet will include three meat exchanges (3 oz) at the noon and evening meal but also two-to-three servings from the bread list daily. The caloric content of this diet is still between 1,000 and 1,200 Calories. Selecting meats primarily from the low- and medium-fat categories is recommended. All the visible fat should be trimmed from the meat, and the meat should be prepared without the addition of fat. All meats should be baked, boiled, broiled, roasted, grilled, or steamed. The use of herbs, mushrooms, and low-Calorie sauces helps to enhance the flavor of baked meats.

The fat exchanges list servings of various foods that are equivalent to the Calories in 1 t of butter or margarine. The list includes all types of pure fat or oils, nuts, salad dressings, and different varieties of cream. Usually only one-to-two fat exchanges are allowed on a weight-reducing diet at each meal; the client is free to decide how to use those servings. Often there are three or four foods on which he would like to use butter or margarine, but he knows he is limited to only 1 t of margarine at that meal; so he must decide how to distribute the fat. Some overweight people are in the habit of using large quantities of margarine or other fats without realizing that every teaspoon of fat used contains approximately 50 Calories.

Other Methods of Treatment

Other techniques to assist with weight reduction include fasting or starvation regimens, exercise, medical interventions, self-help groups, and *behavior modification*. These techniques when used alone seldom produce significant long-term weight loss. When one or more of these methods is combined, however, with a balanced weight reduction diet the results are more enduring.

FASTING. Complete fasting may be used in some cases of obesity that are resistant to other forms of treatment, but it must be emphasized very strongly that fasting should always be undertaken only with proper medical guidance preferably in the hospital. Fasting may help convince the obese client that weight reduction is possible, that overeating is the cause of his obesity, and that he eats for reasons other than hunger.

Total fasting does require adequate fluid intake and also vitamin and mineral supplementation. The fasting may be short term, lasting up to three weeks; this type produces only minimal risk for the client but it has very little long-term effect on obesity unless a weight-reducing diet is followed after the fast is terminated. Intermittent fasting consists of a short-term fast of two weeks followed by one- or two-day fasts during the week until ideal weight is achieved; this type also produces a minimal risk for the client and must be coupled with a realistic diet for maintenance of ideal body weight. Prolonged fasting for several months may produce impressive weight losses, but it may also precipitate serious psychological disturbances such as irritability, depression, aggressiveness, and paranoia (Schneider et al., 1977).

Fasting may also produce some undesirable physiological effects. The ideal weight reduction program should produce weight loss without the breakdown of the body's lean body mass. Weight loss through starvation, however, produces 65% of the weight loss from lean body tissue and only 35% from adipose tissue. In some clients there may be an increase in the level of serum bilirubin, which is an index of liver malfunction. Other complications that may be noted are anemia, high levels of blood uric acid, ketosis, electrolyte imbalances, and postural hypotension. An inadequate amount of carbohydrate in the diet leads to increased excretion of water, sodium, potassium, and other electrolytes, which reduces plasma and extracellular fluid by 30%, resulting in decreased blood pressure and the symptom of postural hypotension. Hypertensive medications should not be administered during fasting because blood pressure is generally lowered.

Semistarvation diets of 300–600 Calories/day may also be used. Weight loss on these diets is also rapid, and men lose more rapidly than women because of their higher daily energy requirements.

Fasting should be used only where more traditional methods of weight reduction have not been successful or when weight reduction is recommended for medical reasons. The client who is on a fasting regimen should be under very close medical supervision and monitoring and even preferably admitted to the hospital. On completion of the fasting the client should be carefully refed and then instructed on a low-Calorie or maintenance-Calorie diet. If fasting is not used in conjunction with an educational program that develops new dietary habits, the client will regain the weight lost while fasting.

EXERCISE. The lack of regular physical exercise may promote the development of obesity in two ways: First, low physical activity and high quantities of Calories result in energy imbalance and the consequent accumulation of excess body fat (see Fig. 5-6). Second, the

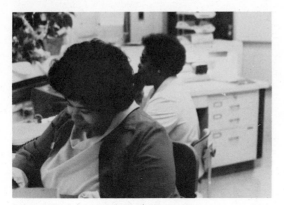

Figure 5-6. Calorie requirements are lower for those with sedentary occupations.

internal mechanism that regulates satiety and appetite may not function properly at low levels of physical activity (Natl Instits of Health, 1976).

Until recently the role of exercise in weight reduction did not receive much emphasis because it was believed that exercise served only to stimulate appetite. Regular physical activity may have a long-term effect on increasing the metabolic rate; an increase of 20% or more in the metabolic rate has been reported in several studies on the day following heavy exercise. For the sedentary person a moderate amount of physical activity tends to depress the appetite, not increase it as was commonly thought (Miller & Mumford, 1966).

MEDICAL INTERVENTIONS. Besides fasting, other medical interventions such as the administration of drugs and hormones and even wiring of the jaws have been attempted as measures for weight reduction. For the morbidly obese (at least 100 lb, or 45 kg, above ideal body weight), the physician might suggest intestinal bypass surgery or gastric stapling.

Some physicians have resorted to the use of drugs for treating obesity, but only a few of these drugs have been shown to be more effective than *placebos* in research studies with obese subjects. These drugs have different modes of action such as producing anorexia, decreasing absorption, increasing metabolism, or increasing excretion (i.e., laxatives and diuretics) of waste products. The classic "diet pills," the *amphetamines,* have been found to be useful along with a Calorie-restricted diet in some cases. They act by suppressing appetite and increasing activity level because of their stimulant effect on the central nervous system. The weight loss achieved does not justify the risk of the potential side effects that may result, some of which are insomnia, hypertension, cardiac arrhythmias, dry mouth, constipation, impotence, blood disorders, allergic reactions, and addiction (Thiele, 1976). The Food and Drug Administration states that the amphetamines have limited use and should be used only for a short period of time along with a low-Calorie diet.

Some overweight people resort to the use of diuretics and laxatives. *Diuretics* promote the loss of water and sodium from the body, and *laxatives* promote decreased absorption of food by increasing gastrointestinal motility and the bulk of fecal material eliminated from the colon. It is disturbing that some people resort to these means just to see their weight decrease by 1–2 lb (.45–.9 kg). Use of both of these types of drugs can result in serious fluid and electrolyte imbalances and psychological dependence.

A new appetite suppressant drug, fenfluramine, has a depressive effect on the central nervous system and produces drowsiness as a side effect. In one study 89% of the users of fenfluramine reported drowsiness and gastrointestinal symptoms. It seems to be an effective appetite supprsessant, but its effectiveness in producing long-term weight loss when used with a low-Calorie diet remains to be seen (Thiele, 1976).

Hormones such as progesterone, growth hormone, thyroid, and *human chorionic gonadotropin* (HCG) have been used. Administration of progesterone reduces the hypoventilation of the pickwickian syndrome, but its action is unknown. Human growth hormone is known to promote the breakdown of fat without increasing breakdown of lean body mass. An inadequate amount of this hormone, however, is available for comprehensive testing on obese subjects. The administration of thyroid hormone to some obese subjects has been practiced for a number of years. It does result in weight loss because of the effect of thyroxine on the metabolic rate, but the weight is easily regained once the hormone is discontinued.

A hormone that has been the subject of much controversy is HCG. It has been used by weight loss clinics during recent years. They claim that about six injections of HCG per week (or a total of 40 injections) help clients tolerate a low-Calorie diet without feeling weak and redistribute abnormal amounts of fat from the waist, thighs, hips, and so on. The client is also given a very low-Calorie diet to follow.

HCG is a hormone extracted from the urine of pregnant women, and its action on the body is relatively well understood. There is no scientific explanation, however of its usefulness in treating obesity. The American Medical Association has condemned use of this hormone for weight reduction. The weight loss from this regimen is due solely to the semistarvation diet of only 500 Calories. This diet was declared to be unsafe, especially with the minimal medical supervision frequently provided.

In recent years obese people have even resorted to having their jaws wired closed by bands connecting the upper and lower teeth. The medical term for this procedure is *dental splinting*, and it has been used in the treatment of hyperphagic obesity. A group of grossly obese persons who describe themselves as "compulsive eaters" go through periods of genuine concern about their excess weight, followed by diligent weight loss for several weeks or even months. Then there is a sudden collapse in their will to diet, usually precipitated by an emotional crisis, followed by a period of massive overeating and rapid regain-

ing of weight. Some of these subjects have been fitted with dental splints, and when crisis occurs, they have had to find an alternative response to overeating. The dental splints do not significantly effect their appearance and speech. After a period of several months of wearing the splints, two such clients were confident that they could now control this impulse to overeat.

Clients wearing these dental splints are instructed to consume some type of liquid diet through a straw. They prepare palatable liquid meals with the aid of a blender. It is of course necessary for them to carry wire cutters to be used if they experience nausea with impending vomiting. While such a drastic measure as this may produce weight loss, it does not retrain the client's eating habits. Unless a sensible low-Calorie diet is followed after the procedure is discontinued, the client is likely to regain much of the weight that was lost (Garrow, 1973).

A surgical method for treating the grossly obese subject is the intestinal bypass operation. This drastic procedure involves disconnecting a considerable portion of the small intestine, thus greatly decreasing the absorptive area of the small intestine and preventing complete digestion and absorption of all the food consumed. Because this surgical procedure is considered radical and carries with it certain medical risks, it is reserved only for clients who weigh more than 100 lb (45 kg) over their ideal body weight and whose excess weight is complicated by diabetes, hypertension, pulmonary alveolar hypoventilation, or serious orthopedic problems. Some medical conditions such as pulmonary embolism, myocardial infarction, and renal failure may become worse if intestinal bypass surgery is performed, so this procedure is performed on these clients only after very careful evaluation (Bray, 1976).

The medical term for this surgery is *jejunoileostomy*. Two types of this operation are currently being performed. One of these is the end-to-side bypass. In this procedure the end of the *proximal jejunum* is *anastomosed* to the side of the ileum 4 in from the *ileocecal valve*. In the other procedure, the side-to-side bypass, the proximal jejunum is anastomosed to the cut end of the *terminal ileum*. In both of these operations most of the 20 ft (600 cm) of the ileum and jejunum are bypassed, but they remain in the abdomen so that the entire small bowel may be restored in rare cases. Only 8–14 in (20–35 cm) of the jejunum and 2–4 in (5–10 cm) of the ileum remain for the absorptive area of the intestinal tract. This procedure effects removal of approximately two-thirds of the small bowel.

Oral intake begins about four days after the operation. Diarrhea will continue to be a problem during the first year following surgery, but it will continue to improve as the small bowel adapts. There is rapid weight loss during the first year, up to as much as 100 lb (45 kg). Weight loss after the first year continues but at a slower rate as the small bowel adapts and is capable of absorbing more nutrients. The weight loss following this procedure is permanent. The client's body image and self-esteem usually improve.

Important health benefits are a result of the surgery. Cholesterol and triglyceride blood levels may be lowered; insulin requirements for the diabetic may be reduced; blood pressure may be reduced; and pulmonary function improves. Many patients report that during the postoperative period their taste for sweet-tasting foods is reduced. They also become more responsive to the internal cues of hunger and satiety for regulating eating behavior (Bray, 1976).

Some of the complications that can result are death from liver failure or pulmonary embolus; the mortality rate is about 4–6%. Nausea and diarrhea are major problems during the first year. The long-term effects of this radical procedure are not completely known because the procedure is still relatively new. Even though this surgical treatment is quite radical, it can give the morbidly obese person the opportunity for a happier, more satisfying, and longer life through improved physical appearance and better health through weight loss (Bray, 1976).

Another surgical procedure for use with the morbidly obese is *gastric bypass surgery*. It limits the quantity of food that can be consumed at one time, but it allows for a more normal digestion and absorption. No hepatic or metabolic complications have been observed. The effects of this operation are still under investigation, but it may become more common as evaluation of its long-term results continues. The gastric resection appears to have a much lower incidence of side effects than the small bowel bypass and is therefore being used more frequently.

BEHAVIOR MODIFICATION.   A recent addition to the list of treatments for obesity is application of the theory of behavior modification. The principles of behavior modification have been used for many years in psychiatry and psychology, but they have more recently been applied to weight control. The ultimate goal of behavior modification puts a strong emphasis on the positive aspects of weight loss and maintenance. The goal is to help the client develop a permanent set of eating habits that will result initially in weight loss and then in maintenance of ideal body weight.

A basic assumption in behavior treatment of obesity is that the connection between environmental stimuli and the resulting response of eating is a learned behavior that can be unlearned and therefore altered. One of the aims of the therapy is to make the client more aware of the external cues in his environment that trigger his eating. The Mahoneys (1976), who are clinicians using behavior therapy to treat obesity, have described quite vividly what is wrong with the traditional weight-reducing diet:

Most diets are lists of do's and don'ts, but they usually tell us nothing about *how* to do the do's and avoid the don'ts. The implication is that the answer is will power; it's the dieter against the chocolate cream pie. Trouble is, as many dieters have discovered, the pie seems to get stronger as they get weaker. All too often, dieters resist temptation long enough to shed the unwanted pounds, and then go back to the old habits that put on those flabby ripples in the first place. (p. 39)

With behavior modification therapy, attention is focused on changing observable behavior instead of on such nebulous attributes as self-control, motivation, and willpower.

The first phase in a behavior modification program is the initial assessment of the client's eating patterns. The client is asked to keep a detailed food record of not only the foods consumed but also the time, place, degree of hunger, mood, and other environmental circumstances surrounding eating. From these records the therapist and client identify the major environments that stimulate the client to consume a higher caloric intake and reduce energy expenditure.

During the second phase, techniques are used that are aimed at altering eating behaviors that resulted in high caloric intakes. The client may be instructed to eat more slowly by chewing each mouthful a certain number of times, laying down the eating utensil between bites, or swallowing food before placing any more food on the utensil. Other suggestions might be to eat in only one particular place and not to talk, read, or watch television while eating. The aim is to make eating more of a "pure experience" by separating those times and places when and where one eats for non-physiological reasons, such as while watching television or between meals out of habit.

Another phase in behavior modification is the reprogramming of eating behavior. Emotional states such as boredom, anxiety, depression, and frustration are often associated with eating. This association between an emotional state and eating is learned through practice and can be changed. When the client feels bored or depressed and has the urge to eat, he is encouraged to engage in some other activity that he enjoys, perhaps listening to rec-

ords, watching television, playing the piano, knitting, or crocheting. Engaging in a pleasurable activity other than eating should serve to divert the client's attention away from food. Also, special errands, hobbies, reading, or work can be planned for the periods during the day when the client is most likely to be bored (Levitz, 1973).

Another tool of behavior modification is the use of *positive reinforcers*. For the overweight person food is a potent and immediate positive reinforcer. When the client practices new behaviors that result in decreased food and Calorie intake, a reinforcer can be used to strengthen the new behavior. These rewards ideally should be non–food related. Rewards that enhance self-image or lead to physical activity are emphasized. Examples might be new items of clothing or accessories, a trip to the beauty shop, or a gift membership to the local health spa, YMCA, or YWCA.

Although the major emphasis in behavior modification is on intake of food, the same principles can also be applied to increasing energy expenditure. The client should be encouraged to expend more energy in daily activities. One example is to suggest that the client park his car in the far corner of the parking lot because the time spent walking will be more productive than the time spent looking for a close parking space. Or if the client rides a bus, the suggestion might be made to get off the bus one or two blocks before the usual stop and walk the remaining distance.

Changing behavior by changing eating and activity patterns requires effort and a long-term commitment. Realistic changes in behavior for the client result in a more gradual loss of weight, but the well-established new behavior patterns will help keep the client from regaining weight. Weight reduction programs using behavior modification techniques have generally greater success than traditional methods.

Several commercial organizations have skillfully combined the principles of a nutritionally balanced Calorie-restricted diet with principles of group therapy to effect successful weight reduction and maintenance. Three of these organizations are TOPS (Take Off Pounds Sensibly), Weight Watchers, and Counterweight. Techniques practiced at the group meetings are group support and encouragement, competition among group members, and even ridicule by peer pressure if no weight was lost or a few pounds were gained during a week. A printed low-Calorie diet sheet is given to the client. Every week there is also a planned lesson on weight reduction followed by discussion and group participation. For the client who seems to benefit from group support and interaction, the dietitian or nurse can confidently encourage participation in any one of these organizations.

Counseling the Obese Client

Counseling the obese client concerning a successful program of weight reduction consists of four major areas of emphasis: providing sufficient motivation for losing weight, planning a realistic Calorie-restricted diet, supplying knowledge about the caloric content of foods, and providing support and encouragement during the dieting program. If any one of these areas is missing, the chances for successful and permanent weight loss are greatly reduced. The clinician or therapist counseling the client may be a physician, nurse, or dietitian or a combination of these professionals.

Motivation for Weight Loss

The proper motivation for weight loss precedes the planning of the Calorie-restricted diet because if the client lacks sufficient personal motivation to lose weight the best planned diet will be of absolutely no benefit. The best motivation for wanting to lose weight comes from within. The client may voluntarily inform the nurse or physician that he really desires to lose weight. Those who

are highly motivated have a specific reason: they get tired too easily; they are short of breath; or they simply do not feel well. Some clients will state that they desire to lose weight but when questioned further, they are unable to give reasons with any real conviction. This group of clients seldom pass beyond the stage of awareness that they should do something about their excess weight. They continually go on diets but never become involved in changing their eating habits.

The client who has a specific motive for losing weight is more successful at losing weight and keeping it off. The motivation might be improved physical appearance or improved health status. Clients with health problems related to obesity are often highly motivated to lose weight. A male client in his middle 40s with a successful business, a wife, and three children and who suffered a mild heart attack is highly motivated to lose weight, whereas six months before he may have only laughed at the suggestion. Sometimes a client in good health can be motivated to lose weight to prevent future trouble. This client, however, must understand that losing weight is hard work that demands determination and perseverance. He must also be convinced of the reasons why this decision is medically wise.

Following the decision to undertake weight reduction, it is helpful for the clinician to ask the client to agree to four basic premises about weight control:

1. Weight control requires a life-long commitment.

2. Weight control requires a thorough understanding of personal eating habits and a willingness to change.

3. Crash dieting or psychological or chemical crutches are ineffective.

4. Frequent moderate exercise is essential.

Besides motivation and commitment, the dieter needs to have a specific goal in mind. The clinician can help the client set a long-range but attainable goal of a weight to be reached in six months to one year. The client should be cautioned that the excess weight will not disappear rapidly. It took years to accumulate the excess poundage, so it will not disappear overnight. Initially the scales may show a drop of several (2–3) pounds (.9–1.4 kg) the first week, but much of this initial weight loss is loss of excess body fluid. Plateaus in weight loss should be expected. It is understandable that these will be discouraging, but having patience to continue on the diet will generally bring results the following week.

The favorite pasttime of many obese clients is eating. It is often quite helpful to find another activity or hobby that brings as much pleasure as eating. This activity should be substituted for eating whenever thoughts about food arise.

Realistic Diet

Once sufficient motivation is present for weight reduction, the next step is planning a realistic diet with the client. The common mistake often made by physicians, dietitians, and nurses is to hand the client a diet sheet and tell him to "follow this diet." This procedure is so impersonal that it discourages the client almost immediately, and he follows the diet for only a few weeks or not at all. The chances are the general food pattern and foods allowed are not even close to the client's food preferences and eating patterns. It is quite true that the obese client will be unable to include all his favorite foods, but the basic eating pattern and many of the food preferences usually can be retained.

The first step in arriving at a realistic diet plan is to ask the client to keep an accurate and complete record of all food and beverages consumed during one week. It is also helpful to have the client include the times when food was eaten, the location of eating, and whether he ate alone or with others. The client is told to follow his regular eating habits during that week and not to try to lose any weight. This food record will help document the eating habits that contributed to the weight problem, and it will be the basis for a realistic diet plan.

Discussion of the food record with the client involves compromises by both clinician and client. The resulting diet plan incorporates the client's basic eating habits but restricts the daily Calories to a level that will permit gradual weight loss. The resulting diet may be quite similar to the diet sheet that could have been handed to the client on the initial visit; the difference lies in the personal interest the clinician showed in the client's eating habits. From the client's viewpoint, he had a part in planning his own diet; because of this simple fact, he will better accept and adhere to the diet with consequent better chance for success. This personal diet should also help to retrain the client's past eating habits into healthier patterns.

Knowledge for Daily Dieting

At the beginning of the diet the client needs basic instruction in measuring or weighing portions of food, low-Calorie snacks, preferable methods of food preparation, and general caloric contents of common foods. Useful knowledge about the nutrients and Calories in food and helpful hints about low-Calorie food preparation will usually further increase the client's enthusiasm for the weight reduction program.

Most people are quite uninformed about the caloric content of foods; many foods they think to be low in Calories are actually quite high. One good example is a simple gelatin fruit salad; most dieters are quite surprised to learn that it contains 145 Calories. Recommending to the client an accurate Calorie book can increase the client's knowledge in the area as well as increase general enthusiasm for decreasing intake of high-Calorie foods. Calories should not be emphasized independently from the nutrient composition of foods. Vitamin and mineral content of foods can be emphasized using the basic four food groups.

Low-Calorie meal planning and preparation

basically involves reducing the fat and carbohydrate content of food. To reduce the Calories from carbohydrate, all concentrated sweets and desserts should be eliminated. An artificial sweetener should be substituted for regular sugar or honey whenever possible. Regular cola and soda beverages should be eliminated and the sugar-free versions substituted. Regular canned fruits should not be used because they are packed in a sugar syrup; however fresh fruit can be appreciated and enjoyed for its natural sweetness. Reducing the fat content of food can also greatly decrease the Caloric content of the food. The main way to accomplish this is not to fry foods. The leanest possible cuts of meat should be selected. Marbling is the visible fat within the meat. Highly marbled meats have a higher content of fat and therefore more Calories. When preparing chicken remove the fat pads under the skin. It is also recommended to remove the skin of the chicken before baking or at least before eating because the skin also contains fat. Refrigerating meat broths and drippings will cause the fat to rise to the top for easy removal. The delicious broth remaining can then be used to prepare fat-free gravy or in vegetables soups. Although regular butter or margarine is allowed on a weight-reducing diet but in small quantities, some clients may prefer to use a *diet margarine*. Diet margarine contains about one-half the Calories of regular margarine, so approximately twice the amount can be used. Substitute dairy products can be prepared that contain a much lower number of Calories. For example, mock whipped cream can be made from evaporated skim milk or nonfat dry milk solids. Creamed cottage cheese can be made by adding skim milk to dry cottage cheese. A substitute for sour cream can be made using either cottage cheese or buttermilk and a few other ingredients. Skim milk can be used to make cream soups and white sauces. A very acceptable low-Calorie salad dressing can be prepared from tomato juice, vinegar or lemon juice, and a blend of season-

ings. Other useful low-Calorie substitutes and recipes are found in *The American Heart Association Cookbook* (Eshleman and Winston, 1979).

Continuing to offer helpful cooking hints and information about Calories and nutrients in the form of minilessons or in conversation with the client should continue to stimulate his interest in weight reduction. It would also be helpful to have the client plan several snacks under 100 Calories, each of which could be enjoyed once or twice a day as they fit into the total daily caloric allotment.

Encouragement

A weight reduction regimen is not easy for anyone, and the obese client needs all the encouragement he can get. One very helpful source of encouragement is to suggest the client find either a fellow dieter or a sympathetic friend with whom to share feelings daily. When the dieter is craving a high-Calorie food, he should be instructed to *run* to the phone and call the friend. Just talking to a friend about the craving usually decreases the intensity of the craving and diverts the client from an unnecessary splurge.

The clinician should show positive reinforcement in the form of praise for the client's progress. Even if the client goes off his diet for a time, the clinician should tell him to forget about his failure and to start again. Obesity is not a moral issue, and the client should not be made to feel guilty about going off the diet for a short period of time. The clinician should remember that the obese client needs support, not chastisement.

It is important to learn how to eat sensibly in all situations. The client should be encouraged to eat out in restaurants or cafeterias. The food offered in cafeterias fits well into a low-Calorie meal plan because there are several entrees, one of which is often broiled, baked, or grilled, and a large selection of salads and vegetables. Eating in a restaurant poses a few more difficulties, but most of these can be avoided. If the client knows he will be eating dinner that evening in a restaurant, he can prepare for the event by eating a small but adequate breakfast and a small lunch. The client should be advised to order a la carte so he will not be tempted to eat the side dishes.

Weight Loss and Maintenance

The success of medical and dietary management of obesity has not been encouraging. Studies may be reported in which subjects have lost impressive amounts of weight, but if follow-up studies were conducted on these same subjects, it would be found that most of them regained the weight or a significant amount of it. About 60–75% of the overweight subjects who try to lose weight are able to achieve some measurable weight loss, but only 5% are able to maintain their new weight. Results are even more discouraging for the obese client who has a large amount of weight to lose. Only 25% of those who attempt weight reduction are able to lose 20 lb (9 kg), and only 5% are able to lose as much as 40 lb (18 kg) (Jordan, 1973). Why is weight loss and maintenance so difficult? Is it a problem of only insufficient motivation or are there other elements? The answer is that there are as many circumstances affecting the maintenance of obesity as there are foods affecting its development. Unlike many medical conditions that are treated by removing the offending agent, obesity cannot be treated by completely avoiding food. Eventually the dieter must again face food and a sedentary society that emphasizes food and de-emphasizes physical exertion. The obesity cycle is illustrated in Figure 5-7.

Defending Body Weight
Whatever the cause of obesity, once excess adipose tissue is deposited in the human body, it is extremely difficult to remove. Most people, including the obese, maintain stable body weights unless they are dieting. Obese

people gain weight and then stabilize at a higher weight level. This level of weight equilibrium is probably controlled by some mechanism that is still undiscovered. Equilibrium in any biological system is very resistant to change, and this seems to be quite true with respect to body weight. An attempt was made to induce excess body weight in normal-weight college students by feeding them two to three times their normal caloric intakes. After three to four months the investigators reached the conclusion that it was as difficult to increase the weights of these subjects as to remove excess weight. Three thin young men and two obese women were force-fed. The young men were underweight and they required an excess of 20,000 calories to gain $5\frac{1}{2}$ lb (2.5 kg), whereas the obese women required only 10,000 extra Calories to gain the same amount of weight. As evidenced by these and other studies, human beings resist alterations in energy balance in either direction, in effect defending their body weight. Once weight loss is achieved, how long must the new weight be maintained before a new equilibrium is established? The answer to this question is not presently known, but it is known that the longer a client has been obese, the more difficult losing weight and especially maintaining the desired weight becomes.

Reactions to Dieting
Because of the psychological, emotional, and physical stress involved in dieting, adverse reactions are sometimes experienced. On a balanced low-Calorie diet that allows for a gradual reduction of body weight by only 1–2 lb (.45–.9 kg)/wk, the physical difficulties experienced should be minimal and last only a few days. Some clients might experience a slight dizziness, weakness, abdominal cramps, or nausea the first few days. These physical symptoms usually disappear in a few days, and this group of clients continue to reduce and function well. Another group of clients may experience serious difficulties during dieting and even find it intolerable. These are

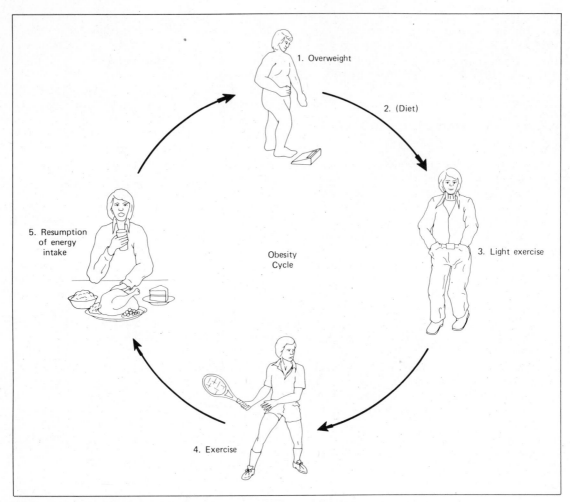

Figure 5-7. The obesity cycle.

the clients who because of a faulty adaptation use their obesity as a means of protection against more severe psychological illness.

Some obese clients during dieting become irritable, nervous, weak, preoccupied with food, and even depressed. Feelings of hostility and agression may increase as long as the clients remain on the diet. These psychological reactions are more likely to occur in clients whose obesity began in childhood; most clients with adult-onset obesity do not experience these reactions. The adult whose obesity began in childhood may experience more severe psychological symptoms from a severe Calorie restriction than from a total fast. Treatment as an outpatient may be more stressful than hospitalization during fasting or dieting.

Predicting Dieting Results

As the successes and failures of obese clients attempting to lose weight are studied, criteria are gradually becoming available to enable the clinician to predict the expected outcome for a client's weight reduction program. A list of predictors for successful weight reduction emerged from treatment of both private and clinic obese clients in a study by Shipman and Plesset (1963). A questionnaire was administered at the beginning to assess anxiety and depression states. The best prediction for success was the amount of weight loss between the first and second visit. Dieters with low levels of anxiety and depression lost more weight than those with high levels. A number of other indicators for success were:

- Age: people over 50 did poorly.
- Socioeconomic status: the well-to-do were more successful.
- Degree of obesity: those 60% or more above ideal weight did poorly.
- Marital status: widowed, separated, or divorced people did poorly; single women under 30 did very well, but single women over 30 did very poorly.
- Race: white people did much better than blacks.
- Referral source: clients referred by a specialty clinic or private doctor did better than those from a general medicine clinic.

Buskirk (1974) summarized the characteristics of the obese adult client most likely to experience success from a weight reduction program: (1) slightly or moderately overweight, (2) gained excess weight as an adult and has not previously attempted to lose weight, (3) sincerely desires to lose weight, and (4) is psychologically adjusted to undertake weight reduction.

Clinicians should accept the fact that not all obese clients should be placed on a weight reduction program. Perhaps someday there will be a set of well-established criteria to determine the clients who can safely be placed on a weight reduction program, but until then medical personnel must rely on the predictive information that is currently available and on a thorough and frank interview with the obese client.

CALORIC INTAKE BELOW ENERGY REQUIREMENTS

The condition of being underweight results when a client's caloric intake is below his energy requirements for an extended period of time. Being underweight is a form of malnutrition, and it is evidenced by a body weight of more than 10% below ideal body weight. The focus of attention on being underweight is often omitted from a discussion of maintenance of ideal weight because of the inescapable interest in obesity and weight reduction. The causes of being underweight are more readily apparent, but the resistance to a change in body weight is similar to the resistance found in obesity. It is often more difficult for the underweight to gain weight than for the overweight to lose.

Causes of Being Underweight

Being underweight may be the direct result of an inadequate quantity and quality of food selected to meet the energy requirements of metabolic and physical activities. This problem may also be due to poor absorption and utilization of food or to the presence of a wasting disease such as tuberculosis, hyperthyroidism, or cancer. Any medical condition that increases nutrient and Calorie requirements as a result of fever, infection, surgery, or the stress of the disease itself can result in being underweight if there is no parallel increase in Calories and nutrients.

Hazards of Being Underweight

Because being underweight is a form of malnutrition, it impairs health and general well-being. The underweight client frequently lacks the physical endurance to perform routine activities because he tires more easily and may even feel weak. Underweight people are often more sensitive to cold because of inadequate layers of fat to serve as insulation. The resistance to disease is lower in the underweight, especially in children. These hazards associated with being underweight all have an effect on food intake. Because the underweight client tires easily, he is often too tired to eat adequate meals. Being underweight lowers the client's resistance to disease. Frequent colds and flu may interfere with adequate ingestion of food. The hazards of being underweight decrease food intake and perpetuate the underweight state.

Treatment

The first step in the treatment of being underweight is to determine the basic cause. Is the underweight condition due primarily to the ingestion of inadequate quantities of food, or is there some medical condition present that is interfering with the normal absorption and use of nutrients from food? Is the inadequate ingestion of food due to an inappropriate selection of low-Calorie foods, or is the quantity of food purposely limited by the client to attract attention or elicit sympathy? Once the underlying psychological and physiological causes are identified and appropriate steps are taken to correct them, dietary counseling can be initiated to increase the daily caloric intake of food.

For a person to gain weight the caloric content of the diet must be increased by 500–1,000 Calories/day above the energy requirement for weight maintenance. In the diet for the underweight there are no actual restrictions on the foods allowed. The goal is to provide the greatest concentration of Calories and nutrients in the smallest volume of food. It is helpful to include foods the client particularly enjoys, provided they are also reasonably high in Calories. The diet should be planned using the basic four and including high-Calorie foods from each of the food groups. The use of sauces and gravies in the preparation of meats and vegetables can greatly increase the Calories. It is important, however, to reduce the intake of foods high in bulk that might have a tendency to depress the appetite. For example, serving an underweight client a large lettuce salad at the beginning of a meal may decrease the appetite for the rest of the meal. A better choice might be a gelatin fruit salad with whipped cream. Another word of caution is in order, however. Carbohydrate and fat do provide a large number of Calories, but the inclusion of very rich foods containing high proportions of either may depress the appetite too quickly. It is probably advisable to include very rich foods as desserts and not as the main entree. The underweight client should be encouraged to eat snacks between meals, and he should be supplied with a list of high-Calorie snacks. It is generally recommended to divide the food on a high-Calorie diet into three moderately large meals plus snacks or into six moderate meals. Additional ways to increase Calories follow:

MILK
• Always use whole homogenized milk.
• Add extra skim milk powder to milk to further increase Calories.
• Use heavy cream instead of light cream.
• Add whipped cream or ice cream to desserts.
• Serve cream soups instead of clear soups.
• Malted milk, milk shakes, or eggnogs can replace regular milk beverages to increase Calories.

MEAT
• Prepare meat with sauces and gravies.
• Fry meat whenever possible.
• Serve gravies on meat and potatoes.
• Include bacon, sausage, or ham with an egg for breakfast.
• Eat nuts between meals.

FRUITS AND VEGETABLES

• Eat canned or frozen fruit packed in a heavy sugar syrup.

• Serve cream or cheese sauces on vegetables.

BREADS AND CEREALS

• Eat bread with butter or margarine and jam, jelly, or preserves at every meal.

• Spread butter or margarine liberally on toast while hot.

• Place a tablespoon of butter or margarine on top of hot cooked cereal.

• Use both margarine and mayonnaise or salad dressing on sandwiches.

• Include potatoes, spaghetti, rice, macaroni, and noodles twice a day.

BIBLIOGRAPHY

Advising patients about fad diets. *Patient Care.* 10(11):100, 1976.

Arlin, M. J. *The Science of Nutrition.* 2nd Ed. New York: Macmillan, Inc., 1977.

Banting, W. *A letter on Corpulence, Addressed to the Public.* 2nd Ed., London: Harrison, 1863.

Bray, G. A. Intestinal bypass operation as a treatment for obesity, *Ann. Intern Med.* 85:97, 1976.

Bruch, H. Psychiatric aspects of obesity. *Metabolism* 6:461, 1957.

———. Psychological implications of obesity. *Nutrition News* (Nat'l Dairy Council) 35(3):9, 1972.

Buskirk, E. R. Obesity: A brief overview with emphasis on exercise. *Fed. Proc.* 33:1948, 1974.

Campbell, R. G., Haskim, S. A., and Van Itallie, T. B. Studies of food intake regulation in man: Responses to variations in nutritive density in lean and obese subjects. *N. Engl. J. Med.* 285:1402, 1971.

Council on Foods and Nutrition, Am. Med. Assoc. A critique of low-carbohydrate ketogenic weight reduction regimens. *J. Am. Med. Assoc.* 244:1415, 1973.

The crash diet craze. *Medical World News*, April 27, 1973.

Dep. of Drugs and Dep. of Foods and Nutrition. Am. Med. Assoc. Fallacy and hazard: Human chorionic gonadotropin 500-Calorie diet and weight reduction. *J. Am. Med. Assoc.* 230:693, 1974.

Dwyer, J. T., and Mayer, J. Potential dieters—who are they? *J. Am. Diet. Assoc.* 56:510, 1970.

Eshleman, R., and Winston, M. *The American Heart Association Cookbook.* 3rd. Ed. New York: David McKay Co., Inc., 1979.

Garrow, J. S. Dental splinting in the treatment of hyperphagic obesity. *Proc. Nutr. Soc.* 33:29A, 1973.

Gates, J. C., Huenemann, R. L., and Brand, R. J. Food choices of obese and non-obese persons. *J. Am Diet. Assoc.* 67:339, 1975.

Genuth, S. M., Castro, J. H., and Vertes, V. Weight reduction in obesity by outpatient starvation. *J. Am. Med. Assoc.* 230:987, 1974.

Gershberg, H. Use of drugs in the treatment of obesity. *Postgrad. Med.* 51:135, 1972.

Guthrie, H. A. *Introductory Nutrition.* 4th Ed. St. Louis: The C. V. Mosby Co., 1979.

Heydman, A. H. Intestinal bypass for obesity. *Am. J. Nurs.* 74:1102, 1974.

Hoffman, H. N. Mayo Clinic disavows "Mayo diet." *J. Am. Diet. Assoc.* 46:279, 1965.

Johnson, M. L., Burke, B. S., and Mayer, J. Relative importance of inactivity and overeating in energy balance of obese high school girls. *Am. J. Clin. Nutr.* 4:37, 1956.

Jordon, H. A. In defense of body weight. *J. Am. Diet. Assoc.* 62:17, 1973.

Keys, A., and Grande, R. Body weight, body composition, and calorie status. In R. S. Goodhart, and M. E. Shils, Eds., *Modern Nutrition in Health and Disease.* 5th Ed. Philadelphia: Lea & Febiger, 1973.

Knittle, J. L. Obesity in childhood: A problem in adipose tissue cellular development. *J. Pediatr.* 81:1048, 1972.

Konishi, F. Food energy equivalents of various activities. *J. Am. Diet. Assoc.* 46:186, 1965.

Konishi, F., and Harrison, S. L. Body weight gain equivalents of selected foods. *J. Am. Diet. Assoc.* 70:365, 1977.

Krause, M. V., and Mahan, L. K. *Food, Nutrition, and Diet Therapy.* 6th Ed. Philadelphia: W. B. Saunders Co., 1979.

Laurent, L. P. E. Obesity. *Nursing Mirror* 132(17):21, 1971.

Levitz, L. S. Behavior therapy in treating obesity. *J. Am. Diet. Assoc.* 62:22, 1973.

Mahoney, M. J., and Mahoney, K. Fight fat with behavior control. *Psychology Today*, p. 39, May 1976.

Mann, G. V. The influence of obesity on health. *N. Engl. J. Med.* 29:178m, 1974.

Mayer, J: Obesity: Causes and treatment. *Am. J. Nurs.* 59:1732, 1959.

Migeon, C. J., Green, O. C., and Eckert, J. P. Study of adrenocortical function in obesity. *Metabolism* 12:718, 1963.

Miller, D. S., and Mumford, P. Obesity, physical activity and nutrition. *Proc. Nutr. Soc.* 25:100, 1966.

Nat'l Instits. of Health. *Facts about Obesity.* Washington, D.C., 1976.

Newman, H. H., Freeman, F. N., and Holzinger, J. J. *Twins: A Study of Heredity and Environment.* Chicago: Univ. of Chicago Press, 1937.

Nutritive Value of Foods. Home & Garden Bull. No. 72, rev. Washington, D.C.: U.S. Dept. of Agriculture, 1977.

Pletcher, A. E. Air Force diet disclaimed. *J. Am. Diet. Assoc.* 47:200, 1965.

Robinson, C. H., and Lawler, M. R. *Normal and Therapeutic Nutrition.* 15th Ed. New York: Macmillan, Inc., 1977.

Rosenberg, B. A., Bloom, W., and Spencer, H. Obesity: II. Treatment and hazards. *J. Am. Med. Assoc.* 186(Suppl.):43, 1963.

Schneider, H. A., Anderson, C. E., and Coursin, D. B., Eds. *Nutritional Support of Medical Practice.* New York: Harper & Row, Pubs., Inc., 1977.

Sebrell, W. H. Weight control through prevention of obesity. *J. Am. Diet. Assoc.* 34:920, 1958.

Shipman, W. G., and Plesset, M. R. Predicting the outcome for obese dieters. *J. Am. Diet. Assoc.* 42:383, 1963.

Strasenburg Laboratories. *Are You Really Serious about Losing Weight?* 2nd Ed. Rochester, New York, 1968.

Stunkard, A. J., and McLaren-Hume, M. The results of treatment for obesity: A review of the literature and report of a series. *Arch. Intern. Med.* 103:79, 1959.

Stunkard, A. J., and Rish, J. Dieting and depression re-examined. *Ann. Intern. Med.* 81:526, 1974.

Thiele, V. F. *Clinical Nutrition.* St. Louis: The C. V. Mosby Co., 1976.

Van Itallie, T. B., and Campbell, R. G. Multidisciplinary approach to the problem of obesity. *J. Am. Diet. Assoc.* 61:385, 1972.

Wagner, M., and Hewitt, M. I. Oral satiety in the obese and non-obese. *J. Am. Diet. Assoc.* 67:344, 1975.

Widdowson, E. M. Reproduction and obesity. *Am. J. Clin. Nutr.* 3:391, 1955.

Williams, S. R. *Nutrition and Diet Therapy.* 3rd Ed. St. Louis: The C. V. Mosby Co., 1977.

Wilson, E. D., Fisher, K. H., and Garcia, P. A. *Principles of Nutrition.* 4th Ed. New York: John Wiley & Sons, Inc., Pubs., 1979.

Withers, R. F. J. Problems in the genetics of human obesity. *Eugenics Review* 56(2):31, 1964.

Wolff, O. H. Obesity in childhood: A study of the birth weight, the height, and the onset of puberty. *Qu. J. Med.* 24:109, 1955.

Worthington, B. S., and Taylor, L. E. Balanced low calorie vs. high protein low carbohydrate reducing diets: I. Weight-loss, nutrient intakes, and subjectives evaluation. *J. Am. Diet. Assoc.* 64:47, 1974.

Wyden, P. *The Overweight Society.* New York: Morrow, 1965.

Young, C. M., Scanlan, S. S., Topping, C. M., Simko, V., and Lutwak, L. Frequency of feeding, weight reduction, and body composition. *J. Am. Diet. Assoc.* 59:466, 1971.

CHAPTER 6

Regulatory Components of Food

Chapter 3 examined the food sources of carbohydrate, protein, and fat. These three nutrients, known as the energy nutrients, contribute to the caloric content of foods. Vitamins and minerals are essential regulatory components of the diet required in very small quantities daily. They do not, however, contain any Calories, nor does water, an equally essential nutrient. This chapter will examine the food sources of vitamins, minerals, and water.

VITAMINS

Until the first half of the twentieth century it was believed that the nutritional value humans obtained from food was due to the presence in the food of carbohydrate, protein, fat, and minerals. It was assumed that because almost 100% of all foods were some combination of these nutrients that these were all that were required for normal nutrition. It had been known for many years that certain diseases were cured by a change in dietary intake. As early as 1720 it was noted that consuming a small quantity of orange or lime juice would prevent the dreadful disease of scurvy, which had plagued British naval crews. In 1753 James Lind published his famous treatise on scurvy. At the end of the nineteenth century, a Japanese physician recognized the unbalanced rice diet as the cause of beriberi in the Japanese navy. Also during this time diseases of nutritional origin in animals continued to underscore the fact that there existed a substance in the certain foods that was a curative factor distinct from carbohydrate, fat, protein, or salt yet that was essential for health. A third phase in the search for these essential substances continued in animals fed synthetic diets. Confirmation of the existence of a substance of this nature was reported in 1881 by a Swiss biochemist, Lunin, when animals did not survive on a purified diet of carbohydrate, protein, fats, minerals, and water.

In 1912 the noteworthy "vitamine theory" was published by Casimir Funk and the word *vitamine* was coined to describe the components of natural foods that provided protection against such diseases as beriberi, rickets, scurvy, and pellagra. The final *e* on this word was dropped when it became evident that not all *vitamines* contained *amines* (chemicals containing nitrogen). One year later with the discovery of vitamin A by Elmer McCollum, the vitamin era in nutrition had begun. Discovery, isolation, and synthesis of each vitamin followed, with the peak of discoveries between 1930 and 1940. Since the discovery of vitamin A the vitamins have been classified according to an alphabetical system. Not all of the vitamins that have been discovered are essential substances for humans; some are only required by certain animals.

Definition

Vitamins are essential organic substances needed daily in very small amounts to perform a specific metabolic function. Plants can manufacture vitamins from the chemical elements available from the soil, but as a general rule animals cannot accomplish this task. One interesting example of this is vitamin C.

143

Rats, rabbits, and dogs can manufacture their own vitamin C, but humans, monkeys, and guinea pigs must rely on vitamin C from food.

The definition of a vitamin by Wagner and Folkers (1964) provides more information about composition and function:

The term vitamin is generally used to designate an organic compound which:

a. is a component of natural food but distinct from carbohydrate, fat or protein;

b. is present in normal food in extremely small concentrations;

c. is essential for normal health and growth;

d. when absent from the diet or not properly absorbed from the diet causes a specific deficiency disease; and

e. cannot be synthesized by the host and must therefore be obtained exclusively from the diet. (p. 6)

Vitamins do not provide energy nor are they an actual structural part of the body. Vitamins are required to help release the energy from foods through a series of metabolic reactions. They also assist in regulating the reactions by which the body tissues are maintained. The amount of vitamins required to regulate the chemical reactions releasing energy and maintaining body tissues is quite small. In fact, the total daily quantity of vitamins required for these chemical reactions would easily fit into an ordinary teaspoon (see Fig. 6-1). Yet if even one of these vitamins were missing from the daily diet on a consistent basis, a deficiency disease would become evident within a short time.

Nomenclature

The naming classification of vitamins is based on an alphabetical system. The first vitamin to be discovered was designated by the letter *A*. As each new vitamin was discovered the vitamin became known by the next alphabetical letter. Some of the common vitamins today originally had other letter designations. For example, thiamine (vitamin B_1) was originally named vitamin F, and riboflavin (vitamin B_2) was originally named vitamin G. Vitamins or nutrition factors have now been identified through the letter *Y*, but not all of them are essential for humans. At the present time there are 13 vitamins that have been identified as essential. Through research the functions of the vitamins have become better understood in recent years, and the nomenclature has become more and more complex. Although the alphabetical terminology is still used, the vitamins are becoming increasingly known by their chemical names. Common and chemical names of the essential vitamins are in Table 6-1.

Classification

Vitamins are grouped together on the basis of their solubility in either fat or water. This method of classifying vitamins was important in their initial isolation, and it continues to be relevant today. There are four fat-soluble and nine water-soluble essential vitamins that have been identified. The fat-soluble vitamins are vitamins A, D, E, and K; the water soluble

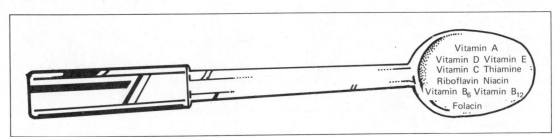

Figure 6-1. The daily requirement for all vitamins could fit into one teaspoon.

TABLE 6-1. Nomenclature of Vitamins

Common Name	Chemical Name	Discovery	Synthesis
Fat-soluble			
Vitamin A	Retinol	1913	1947
Vitamin D	Ergocalciferol (D_2)		
	Cholecalciferol (D_3)	1918	1936
Vitamin E	Tocopherol	1922	1937
Vitamin K	Phylloquinone (K_1)		
	Menaquinone (K_2)		
	Menadione (K_3) synthetic	1934	1939
Water Soluble			
Vitamin C	Ascorbic acid	1932	1933
Vitamin B complex			
Vitamin B_1	Thiamine	1921	1936
Vitamin G (B_2)	Riboflavin	1932	1935
Pellagra-preventive factor	Niacin (nicotinic acid, niacinamide)	1867	
Vitamin B_6	Pyridoxine	1934	1939
Vitamin B_{12}	Cyanocobalamin	1948	1973
Folacin	Pteroyglutamic acid	1945	1945
Pantothenic acid	Pantotheine, Pantothenol	1933	1940
Vitamin H	Biotin	1924	1942

ones are vitamin C (ascorbic acid) and eight members of the B-complex group. Knowledge of the general properties of the fat-soluble and water-soluble vitamins provides a better understanding of vitamin retention of foods, storage capacity in the body, daily supply in the diet, and rapidity with which deficiency symptoms develop.

The solubility properties of the vitamins are directly related to vitamin retention in foods during food preparation. The water-soluble vitamins are lost from foods into the cooking water. It is therefore recommended to use only a small quantity of water when cooking vegetables. For maximum nutritive benefit from foods cooked in this manner, the water used for cooking should be retained and used in soups, gravies, sauces, or simply consumed as an additional beverage with a meal. Using vegetable juices in gravies to replace some of the milk is also an excellent way to cut down on Calories. This same principle applies to the liquids of canned vegetables and fruits. When preparing fresh vegetables for cooking, they should be left as nearly whole as possible. The smaller the cut pieces of vegetables, the greater the surface area exposed and the more water-soluble vitamins will escape into the cooking water. The reason for cooking vegetables with the lid on the pan is to shorten the cooking time and allow retention of the liquids. Vitamins are not such an unstable nutrient that they disappear in the escaping steam. By contrast the fat-soluble vitamins are unaffected by cooking in water and they are very stable in the presence of heat under average food preparation conditions. The use of excessive heat such as in dehydration or sun drying or the use of rancid fats for frying may cause the destruction of the fat-soluble vitamins.

The body's storage capacity for vitamins has several applications to daily intake of fat-soluble and water-soluble vitamins. The body possesses the ability to store excess fat-soluble vitamins, but excess intakes of water-soluble vitamins are simply excreted in the urine. Because excess fat-soluble vitamins can be stored in such tissues as the liver, they do not absolutely need to be included in the diet every day. If an adequate supply of a fat-soluble vitamin, such as vitamin A, is included every other day, this is adequate. It is safest, however, to include a good source of the fat-soluble vitamins every day. Because excess quantities of the fat-soluble vitamins are stored, it usually takes many months for a dietary deficiency of a fat-soluble vitamin to become evident as a clinically recognizable deficiency symptom.

In contrast to this, an excess intake of the water-soluble vitamins will simply be excreted in the urine. An adequate intake of all the water-soluble vitamins, therefore, is definitely needed every day. Because excess amounts of the water-soluble vitamins are not stored by the body, clinical deficiency symptoms may appear within a few weeks or a few months with a consistently deficient dietary intake.

These principles should be applied to the practice of taking oral vitamin supplements. The excess quantities of the water-soluble vitamins present in the vitamin pill will simply be excreted in the urine. For the person who is already consuming an adequate diet, vitamin pills are a waste of money. This is also true for the person consuming large quantities of vitamin C to try to prevent the common cold. With the capacity of the body to store the fat-soluble vitamins, there is a danger of consuming too much of vitamins A and D and developing toxic symptoms. More on the need for vitamin supplementation comes at the conclusion of this chapter.

MINERALS

Definition

Minerals are inorganic elements present in food and are essential nutrients for humans. They constitute about 4% of the body's weight and are involved in numerous chemical reactions regulating the use of the other nutrients. In contrast to the vitamins, minerals are actual constituents of body tissues and fluids, and certain minerals are part of body compounds such as hemoglobin, thyroxine, insulin, and even some of the vitamins themselves. A few examples of compounds that include minerals are found in Table 6-2.

Classification

The classification of the minerals essential for humans is based on their occurrence in the body. Those minerals present in rather large amounts are called *major minerals,* and those present in small amounts are called the *trace minerals.* It should be noted that this classification does not imply anything about the importance of the major versus the trace minerals; it only refers to the actual content in the body. Two of the trace minerals, iron and iodine, are, respectively, very important parts of the hemoglobin portion of blood and of the hormone thyroxine. The major minerals are also known as *macronutrients;* the trace minerals, as *micronutrients.* The major minerals are calcium, phosphorus, potassium, sulfur, sodium, chlorine, and magnesium. The list of trace minerals required by humans continues to become longer as refined techniques for studying mineral metabolism become available. These advancements have made it possible to study smaller quantities of miner-

TABLE 6-2. Mineral Composition of Selected Body Compounds

Body Compounds	Minerals
Thyroxine	Iodine
Insulin	Sulfur, zinc
Hemoglobin	Iron
Myoglobin	Iron
Keratin	Sulfur
Carboxypeptidase	Zinc
Cytochrome oxidase	Copper, iron
Nucleic acids	Zinc
Amino acids (methionine, cystine, and cysteine)	Sulfur
Biotin	Sulfur
Thiamine	Sulfur
Vitamin B$_{12}$	Cobalt

als in living tissue and to determine essential roles for more and more of the trace minerals. Table 6-3 provides a classification of the mineral elements.

WATER

Water, the nutrient most often forgotten, is actually an astounding nutrient. Humans can survive for a month without food but only a few days when deprived of water. The human body is composed of approximately 55% water; in men the range is slightly higher than in women. This is because women generally contain a higher proportion of adipose tissue than men. Adipose tissue contains a lower proportion of water than does muscle tissue. The percentage of body water is also higher in an infant than in an adult.

Functions

Water has several important functions in the body. It serves as a solvent in which occur the body's chemical reactions, such as digestion and metabolism. Water composes the major part of blood and is therefore the solvent for transporting the water-soluble nutrients throughout the body. Water is also considered a building material, for it is a constituent of all types of body tissues—bone, muscle, connec-

tive tissue, and nervous tissue. Water also acts as a lubricant. Saliva helps lubricate a mass of food for ease in swallowing. The *synovial fluid* that lines the joints and allows the bones to move freely with very little friction contains a high proportion of water. Water is also a component of other mucus secretions throughout the body. Finally water serves to regulate body temperature. Some water is always lost from the skin and lungs by evaporation; this is called *insensible perspiration*. Physical exertion or high environmental temperatures also cause loss of body water through a process called *sweating,* or *sensible perspiration*.

Sources

The most common and most obvious source of water is water consumed as a beverage. Other liquids consumed as beverages are also sources of water. Most solid foods also contain some water. The percentage of water in solid food ranges from only 4% to 98%. A sampling of the water contents of some foods are found in Table 6-4. A final source of water is the metabolism of the energy nutrients within the cell. The metabolism of each energy nutrient produces a different amount of water. Each gram of carbohydrate will yield .60 gm of water; each gram of fat will produce 1.07 gm of water; and each gram of protein will produce .41 gm of water. It is interesting to note, therefore, that if the total number of grams of carbohydrate, protein, and fat are known from a daily diet the number of grams of *metabolic water* that will be formed can be calculated. This calculation, however, is not used very frequently because the range is fairly continuous.

Balance

The delicate balance of water intake and water loss is maintained with little or no thought in the healthy person. The kidneys and the thirst center in the brain are involved in maintaining this balance. In the

TABLE 6-3. Classification of Minerals

Major Minerals	Trace Minerals	Other Trace Minerals
Calcium	Iron	Nickel
Phosphorus	Zinc	Tin
Magnesium	Copper	Vanadium
Sodium	Manganese	Silicon
Potassium	Fluorine	
Chlorine	Chromium	
Sulfur	Iodine	
	Cobalt	
	Selenium	
	Molybdenum	

TABLE 6-4. Water Content of Common Foods

Food	Percentage Water
Lettuce	96
Celery	94
Watermelon	93
Green peas	92
Strawberries	90
Broccoli	91
Peaches	89
Grapefruit	89
Whole milk	88
Orange	86
Apple	84
Peas	82
Potatoes	80
Pears	77
Corn	76
Banana	76
Whole egg	75
Lean beef	62
Chicken breast	58
Cheddar cheese	37
Bread	36
Raisins	18
Butter	16
Popcorn	4
Crackers	4
Dry cereal	3
Sugar	1

healthy person, thirst is usually an indication that the fluid intake needs to be increased. In the young child or the ill person an indication of thirst may be absent or inadequate to allow replacement of body fluids that have been lost. This is especially the case with large losses of body fluids associated with vomiting, diarrhea, or a fever. More specific information about water balance is found in Chapter 11. A useful guideline for estimating water requirements is 1 ml (.03 oz) of water for every Calorie. This amount includes the water from beverages, solid food, and that produced during metabolism. Inasmuch as the caloric content of adults ranges from 1,400 to 2,300 Calories, the daily requirement for water would also be within this range.

RECOMMENDED INTAKES OF VITAMINS AND MINERALS

In chapter 2, the *RDA* was defined as a standard for evaluating dietary adequacy and making recommendations for food selection to improve a daily diet that appears to be low in one or more nutrients. Besides recommended intakes for Calories and protein, the RDA is composed of recommended intakes for 10 vitamins and six minerals for various age and sex groups. In the last 10 years, recommended intakes for vitamins and minerals have been established as a result of increased nutritional knowledge. As additional research and improved methods of studying the nutrients become available, it is quite probable that recommendations for additional nutrients will be added in future revisions.

Recommended Dietary Allowances

The recommended level for each nutrient in the RDA is established "to meet the nutritional needs of practically all healthy people living in the United States." Because the RDA is not a set of individual nutritional requirements, there is included for each recommended intake for a vitamin or a mineral a margin of safety that allows for individual variations. There is no way to know a person's personal requirement for any specific nutrient or even if the personal requirements are higher or lower than the RDA. The RDA is based on statistical probability. This means that the recommended intakes are set to exceed the requirements of most people (97.5%). An example of the application for a theoretical nutrient is shown in Figure 6-2. Even if a person consumes less than the RDA for some nutrients, it can not be said that his diet is necessarily inadequate in those nutrients. This is because the person's personal requirement cannot be known. It can, however, be said that the farther the intake for a given nutrient drops below the RDA and the longer this low intake continues, the greater is the

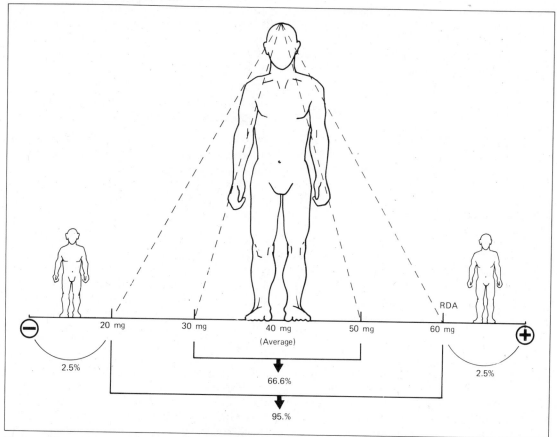

Figure 6-2. Variations in human nutritional requirements for a hypothetical nutrient: distribution of nutrient requirements over the population. The distribution curve emphasizes both the margin of safety and individual variations in nutritional requirements. The average (mean) requirement for the hypothetical nutrient is 40 mg; the RDA for it is 60 mg. Note that 66.6% of the population require 30–50 mg; 95% require 20–60 mg; 2.5% require more than 60 mg; and 2.5% require less than 20 mg.

risk for a nutritional deficiency. Notice that this is quite different from saying that intake of the nutrient below the RDA is proof that a nutritional deficiency exists.

The RDA are estimated by considering findings from reliable nutritional research. Ideally the recommendations should be based on nutritional experiments conducted on hu- mans, but often these studies are limited because human experiments are costly, of long duration, and have only a small number of subjects. Because of these limitations recommendations must be made based on studies of nutritional requirements of other mammals or from minimal quantities of a nutrient consumed by apparently healthy people. From the human studies available, requirements may be known for only one specific age category in the life cycle. The members of the Committee on Dietary Allowances of the Food and Nutrition Board of the National Research Council arrive at recommendations for the other stages of the life cycle through very careful interpretation and extrapolation from the available information.

The RDA is "designed for the maintenance of good nutrition of practically all healthy people in the United States." Nutritional needs change throughout the life cycle in relation to the demands for growth, changes in body functioning, or the added physiological demands of pregnancy and lactation. These changes are reflected in the recommended intake for various age and sex catagories within the RDA chart.

RDA's have not been established for all the essential nutrients for several important reasons. No RDA has been established for carbohydrate, fat, vitamin K, biotin, and pantothenic acid. Several of the major minerals such as sodium, potassium, and chlorine do not have an established RDA, nor do six of the trace minerals. RDA's are not necessary for carbohydrate and fat because most people consume more than adequate amounts of these nutrients. In some instances the quantity of the nutrient required, as for sodium or potassium, is very small and the amount supplied by the diet is quite adequate. The body is also very conservative with its sodium and potassium content. Deficiency symptoms may not have been observed in humans for some nutrients, such as the minerals. Recommended allowances are often established based partially on the minimum amounts of a nutrient known to prevent the development of a deficiency symptom. A margin of safety is then added to this amount. The synthesis of a few of the vitamins by the intestinal bacteria may also reduce the need for a specific allowance; this is the case for vitamin K and biotin. The revised edition of the RDA (Food and Nutrition Board, 1980), however, does give a

range of estimated safe and adequate daily dietary intakes for the nutrients just discussed. The RDA chart for the estimated safe intakes of selected vitamins and minerals are in Appendix C.

US Recommended Dietary Allowances (US-RDA)

The US-RDA stands for *US Recommended Daily Allowances*. This is a special set of nutrient allowances for protein and for 19 vitamins and minerals developed by the Food and Drug Administration for use in nutritional labeling. Stated most simply the US-RDA are "the amounts of protein, vitamins, and minerals that an adult should eat every day to keep healthy." The US-RDA are based on the RDA of the Food and Nutrition Board of the National Academy of Sciences and are actually a summary or composite of the RDA. There are four separate categories on the US-RDA for protein and for vitamins and minerals, the most commonly used of which is that for children over 4 years of age and for adults. For most nutrients the US-RDA is the highest level of recommended intake from the RDA within those age categories but excluding pregnancy and lactation. The other three categories are infants, children under age 4, and pregnant and lactating women. These groupings are used for foods or vitamin-mineral supplements specifically consumed by these age categories.

The US-RDA is used on food labels by stating the level of nutrients contained in food in terms of percentages of the US-RDA supplied by each nutrient. The required nutrient information that must appear on a nutrition label is the amount of protein, five vitamins (vitamins A and C, thiamine, riboflavin, and niacin), and two minerals (calcium and iron) expressed in terms of percentage of the US-RDA. Optional information may be included for 12 additional vitamins and minerals. The US-RDA for all nutrients except protein is shown in Table 6-5. Notice that there are

TABLE 6-5. United States Recommended Daily Allowances (US-RDA)

Nutrient	Unit	Infants (0–12 Mo)	Children Under 4 Yr	Adults and Children 4 or More Yr	Pregnant or Lactating Women
Vitamin A	IU	1,500	2,500	5,000	8,000
Vitamin D	IU	400	400	400	400
Vitamin E	IU	5	10	30	30
Vitamin C	mg	35	40	60	60
Folic Acid	mg	0.1	0.2	0.4	0.8
Thiamine (B_1)	mg	0.5	0.7	1.5	1.7
Riboflavin (B_2)	mg	0.6	0.8	1.7	2.0
Niacin	mg	8	9	20	20
Vitamin B_6	mg	0.4	0.7	2	2.5
Vitamin B_{12}	μg	2	3	6	8
Biotin	mg	0.05	0.15	0.3	0.3
Pantothenic acid	mg	3	5	10	10
Calcium	g	0.6	0.8	1.0	1.3
Phosphorus	g	0.5	0.8	1.0	1.3
Iodine	μg	45	70	150	150
Iron	mg	15	10	18	18
Magnesium	mg	70	200	400	450
Copper	mg	0.6	1.0	2.0	2.0
Zinc	mg	5	8	15	15

SOURCE: US Dept. of Health, Education, and Welfare, Public Health Ser., Food and Drug Admin., Office of Public Affairs, 5600 Fishers Lane, Rockville, Md. 20852. HEW Publication No. (FDA) 76-2042, revised January 1976.

US-RDA established for three nutrients that do not have RDAs (biotin, pantothenic acid, and copper).

It must be stressed that because the US-RDA uses the highest level from the RDA in establishing the US-RDA for specific nutrients, the US-RDA is higher than necessary for some people. Table 6-6 presents the percentage of the US-RDA needed to meet the RDA for individuals by age and sex. It will readily be noticed that most adults need only about 75% of the US-RDA to meet their own specific RDA and some children only need about 50% of the US-RDA to meet the RDA for their age category. Therefore, it can be seen that use of the US-RDA as a standard for nutritional adequacy results in an overestimation of nutrient needs, plus the fact that the RDA has an ample margin of safety inherent in its nutrient recommendations. The US-RDA however, is an easy and convenient *single* standard to use for *all* age groups. In interpreting nutritional adequacy of a specific food or a diet the point must be kept in mind that not all individuals need to consume 100% of the US-RDA for each nutrient for their nutritional intake to be considered adequate. On the other hand if a person consumes at least 100% of the US-RDA for each of the nutrients, this intake can be considered more than adequate nutritionally.

The FDA program for food labeling was developed to provide reliable but not absolutely precise information. The values for grams of carbohydrate, protein, and fat and for Calories and percentages of US-RDA for protein, vitamins, and minerals are rounded off to make the values easier to read and use.

With an understanding of the criteria used for establishing the US-RDA and reporting actual levels within foods on the labels, this new standard can be used successfully as a convenient way of assessing nutrient content of specific foods or meals. Conclusions about

TABLE 6-6. Allowances for Food Energy and Percentages of the US Recommended Daily Allowances Needed to meet the Recommended Dietary Allowances for Children, Men, and Women of Different Ages

Age (Years)	Food Energy[a] (Calories)	Percent of US Recommended Daily Allowance							
		Protein[b]	Vitamin A	Vitamin C	Thiamine	Ribo-flavin	Niacin[c]	Calcium	Iron
Child:									
1–3	1,300	35	40	70	50	50	30	80	85
4–6	1,800	50	50	70	60	65	35	80	60
7–10	2,400	55	70	70	80	75	50	80	60
Male:									
11–14	2,800	70	100	75	95	90	55	120	100
15–18	3,000	85	100	75	100	110	55	120	100
19–22	3,000	85	100	75	100	110	60	80	60
23–50	2,700	90	100	75	95	95	45	80	60
51+	2,400	90	100	75	80	90	35	80	60
Female:									
11–14	2,400	70	80	75	80	80	45	120	100
15–18	2,100	75	80	75	75	85	30	120	100
19–22	2,100	75	80	75	75	85	35	80	100
23–50	2,000	75	80	75	70	75	30	80	100
51+	1,800	75	80	75	70	65	25	80	60
Pregnant	+300[d]	+50[d]	100	100	+20[d]	+20[d]	35	120	100+
Nursing	+500[d]	+35[d]	120	135	+20[d]	+30[d]	35	120	100

SOURCE: US Recommended Daily Allowance, "Food Labeling," Federal Register, vol. 38, no. 49, part II, March 14, 1973. Recommended Dietary Allowances, 8th Ed. 1974, Natl Acad. of Sciences, Natl Research Council.
[a] Calorie needs differ depending on body composition and size, age, and activity of the person.
[b] US-RDA of 65 grams is used for this table. In labeling, a US-RDA of 45 grams is used for foods providing high-quality protein, such as milk, meat, and eggs.
[c] The percentage of the US-RDA shown for niacin will provide the RDA for niacin if the RDA for protein is met. Some niacin is derived in the body from tryptophan, an amino acid present in protein.
[d] To be added to the percentage for the girl or woman of the appropriate age.

the nutritional contribution of these meals to an entire day's dietary intake is left to the student to examine.

FOOD SOURCES OF VITAMINS AND MINERALS

Leader Nutrients

The National Dairy Council (1978) has stated that if an individual consumes adequate amounts of the 10 *leader nutrients* in the daily diet the other approximately 40 nutrients known to be needed for optimal health are likely to be present in sufficient quantities to meet the body's needs. These 10 leader nutrients are the same as the nutrients required to be listed on a nutritional label. Because the consumption of foods containing these nutrients forms the framework of a balanced diet, the food sources of these nutrients are presented here in terms of the percentages of the US-RDA for each vitamin or mineral.

A food-labeling rule was proposed by the Federal Trade Commission whereby to be mentioned as a source of a nutrient a food must contain 10% of the US-RDA for that nutrient. A second proposal was that, for a food to be considered a "good source" of a nutrient, it must contain at least 35% of the US-RDA. This proposal seemed very reasonable at first, but when lists were made of foods containing these level of nutrients, the results were unrealistic. The 35% entry level for nutrient content for a food to be classified as "good" was reasonable for vitamins A and C but unrealistic for thiamine, riboflavin, and niacin. This level was not workable for the B-complex vitamins because these nutrients, though present in fairly small quantities in foods, are present in a greater variety of foods. Therefore, although one food may not contain a very significant quantity of one of the B vitamins, it is still a significant source because of the additive effect from a number of foods consumed during the day. An alternative suggestion was to assume that if a person eats 15 different foods during the day a "fair share" of a nutrient per serving would be 6.67% of the US-RDA for that nutrient. Definite percentages have not officially been established, but for the purpose of discussion, important food sources of the leader nutrients in this chapter are based on the following percentages: 7.5%, 10%, 15%, 25%, 50%, and 75%. Use of this wide range of percentages reveals not only the best sources of a nutrient but the levels of vitamins A and C present compared to the levels of thiamine, riboflavin, niacin, calcium, and iron. A ranking system for food sources of the nutrients based on the percentage of the US-RDA supplied by that nutrient is shown in Table 6-7. Table 6-8 lists the percentage of the US-RDA for each leader nutrient in common foods.

The concentration of vitamins and minerals in any food is directly proportional to the portion size of the food being examined or consumed. Food sources of these nutrients are generally examined in one of two ways, each of which has advantages and disadvantages. The vitamin and mineral content of foods is compared using either a portion size com-

TABLE 6-7. Percentage of US-RDA for Food Sources of Nutrients

Nutrient	Food Sources			
	Excellent	Good	Fair	Poor
Vitamin A Vitamin C	75	50	25	10
Thiamine Riboflavin Niacin Calcium Iron	50	25	15	7.5

monly consumed or a standard 100-gm portion. Use of the common portion size provides analysis on the basis of quantities familiar to most people, but this method is not without some difficulties. Some foods are generally consumed in smaller quantities because of the nature of the food, making comparisons difficult. For example, a person who usually eats $\frac{1}{2}$ cup of applesauce is unlikely to eat $\frac{1}{2}$ cup of raisins when they are substituted. One slice of lunch meat or one frankfurter may be considered one serving, whereas 3 oz of pork, beef, or chicken is also considered one serving. Comparison of foods in this manner for their nutrient content is not totally accurate because comparisons are being made of products with unequal portion sizes.

Comparison of vitamin and mineral contents of foods is on the basis of a 100-gm portion for every food is more direct, but it has the disadvantage that it is highly unlikely that anyone would consume some foods in a 100-gm (approximately 3 oz or $\frac{1}{2}$ cup) portion at any given meal. Examples of foods that are very unlikely to be consumed in this amount at any given meal are butter or margarine, jelly, condiments, and spices. This method therefore overestimates the quantities of nutrients usually obtained from these foods. Although most meats, fruits, and vegetables are consumed in 100-gm portions, some foods, especially beverages, are generally consumed in amounts greater than 100-gm portions.

TABLE 6-8. Food Sources of Leader Nutrients

Food	Percentage of US-RDA	Amount of food	Food	Percentage of US-RDA	Amount of food
VITAMIN A					
Meat and meat alternates:					
Liver, beef	910	3 ounces	Broccoli, chopped, cooked from frozen	100	1 cup
Liver, calf	560	3 ounces	Apricots, canned	90	1 cup
Liver, hog	250	3 ounces	Broccoli, cooked	90	Medium stalk
Liver, chicken	60	1 ounce	Spinach, raw, chopped	90	1 cup
Chicken or turkey pot pie, home recipe	60	⅓ of 9-inch pie	Apricots, dried, uncooked	80	10 medium halves
Beef and vegetable stew	50	1 cup	Broccoli, cut, cooked	80	1 cup
Vegetables and fruit:			Melon balls, frozen, in syrup	70	1 cup
Carrots, canned	470	1 cup	Pepper, red	70	1 pod
Sweet potatoes, mashed	400	1 cup	Apricots, raw	60	3 fruits
Carrots, cooked	330	1 cup	Peaches, dried, cooked	60	1 cup
Spinach, canned	330	1 cup	Plums, canned	60	1 cup
Pumpkin, canned	310	1 cup	Carrots, strips, raw	60	6–8 strips (2½–3 inches long)
Sweet potatoes, pieces, canned	310	1 cup			
Collards, cooked	300	1 cup	Papaya, raw, cubed	50	1 cup
Peas and carrots, cooked	300	1 cup	Tomatoes, cooked	50	1 cup
Spinach, cooked	290	1 cup	Watermelon, raw	50	4 × 8-inch wedge (2 pounds)
Dandelion greens, cooked	250	1 cup			
Carrots, raw, grated	240	1 cup			
Sweet potatoes, boiled in skin	240	Medium potato	**Cereal and bakery products:**		
Turnip greens, canned, solids and liquid	220	1 cup	Pie, pumpkin	80	4¾-inch sector
Cress, garden, cooked	210	1 cup	Pie, sweet potato	70	4¾-inch sector
Chard, Swiss, cooked	190	1 cup	**Miscellaneous:**		
Mango, raw	190	1 fruit (⅔ pound)	**Soup:**		
Cantaloupe, raw	180	½ of 5-inch-diameter melon	Vegetable, with beef broth	60	1 cup
			Vegetable, vegetarian	60	1 cup
Kale, cooked	180	1 cup	Vegetable beef	60	1 cup
Mustard greens, cooked from frozen	180	1 cup	Apricot nectar	50	1 cup
Sweet potatoes, baked in skin	180	Medium potato	**VITAMIN C**		
Turnip greens, cooked	180	1 cup	**Meat and meat alternatives:**		
Vegetables, mixed, cooked	180	1 cup	Peppers, stuffed	120	1 pepper (6.5 ounces)
Squash, winter, baked	170	1 cup	Chop suey, with beef and pork, home recipe	60	1 cup
Mustard greens, cooked	160	1 cup	Liver, calf	50	3 ounces
Apricots, dried, cooked	150	1 cup	**Vegetables and fruit:**		
Beet greens, cooked	150	1 cup	Broccoli, cooked	270	Medium stalk
Cabbage, spoon, cooked	110	1 cup	Pepper, red, raw	250	1 pod
Sweet potatoes, candied	110	3-ounce piece	Collards, cooked	240	1 cup
			Broccoli, cut, cooked	230	1 cup

TABLE 6-8 (*Continued*)

Food	Per-cent-age of US-RDa	Amount of food	Food	Per-cent-age of US-RDA	Amount of food
Brussels sprouts, cooked	230	1 cup	Tangerine juice, from frozen concentrate	110	1 cup
Strawberries, frozen, sweetened	230	1 cup	Tomatoes, cooked	100	1 cup
Pepper, green, cooked	220	1 cup	Raspberries, red, frozen	90	1 cup
Orange juice, fresh	210	1 cup	Tangerine juice, canned	90	1 cup
Orange juice, from frozen or canned concentrate	200	1 cup	Cabbage, cooked	80	1 cup
Broccoli, chopped, cooked from frozen	180	1 cup	Cress, garden, cooked	80	1 cup
			Spinach, cooked	80	1 cup
Kale, cooked	170	1 cup	Strawberries, canned	80	1 cup
Turnip greens, cooked	170	1 cup	Cabbage, raw, finely shredded	70	1 cup
Orange juice, canned	170	1 cup	Cabbage, red, raw, shredded	70	1 cup
Peaches, frozen	170	1 cup	Rutabagas, cooked	70	1 cup
Pepper, green, raw	160	1 pod	Tomatoes, raw	70	3-inch diameter tomato
Grapefruit juice, fresh or from frozen unsweetened concentrate	160	1 cup	Turnip greens, canned, solids and liquid	70	1 cup
Cantaloupe, raw	150	½ of 5-inch-diameter melon	Tomato juice, canned or bottled	70	1 cup
Orange sections, raw	150	1 cup	Sauerkraut juice	70	1 cup
Strawberries, raw	150	1 cup	Grapefruit, white or pink, raw	70	½ medium fruit
Grapefruit sections, raw, white or pink	140	1 cup	Lemons, raw	70	1 lemon
Grapefruit juice, canned, unsweetened	140	1 cup	Asparagus, pieces, cooked or canned	60	1 cup
Grapefruit juice, from frozen sweetened concentrate	140	1 cup	Cabbage, common or savoy, raw, coarsely shredded	60	1 cup
Grapefruit sections, canned, syrup pack	130	1 cup	Okra, sliced, cooked	60	1 cup
Grapefruit juice, canned sweetened	130	1 cup	Peas, green, cooked	60	1 cup
			Sauerkraut, canned	60	1 cup
Papaya, raw, cubed	130	1 cup	Sweet potatoes, canned, mashed	60	1 cup
Grapefruit sections, canned, water pack	120	1 cup	Turnips, cooked	60	1 cup
Mango, raw	120	1 fruit (⅔ pound)	Coleslaw	60	1 cup
			Honeydew melon, raw	60	2 × 7-inch wedge (½ pound)
Cauliflower, cooked	120	1 cup			
Cauliflower, raw	110	1 cup	Loganberries, raw	60	1 cup
Mustard greens, cooked	110	1 cup	Melon balls, frozen, syrup pack	60	1 cup
Orange, raw	110	2⅝-inch-diameter orange	Beans, lima, Fordhook, cooked from frozen	50	1 cup

TABLE 6-8 (*Continued*)

Food	Percentage of US-RDA	Amount of food	Food	Percentage of US-RDA	Amount of food
Beans, lima, immature seeds, cooked	50	1 cup	Pork, fresh or cured, ham or shoulder, ground, lean	45	1 cup
Mustard greens, cooked from frozen	50	1 cup	Pork, loin chop, lean	40	2 ounces
Potato, baked in skin	50	Medium potato	Cashew nuts, whole kernels, roasted	40	1 cup
Spinach, canned	50	1 cup	Filberts, whole kernels, shelled	40	1 cup
Blackberries, raw	50	1 cup	Pork fresh or cured, ham or shoulder, sliced, lean	35	3 ounces
Raspberries, red, raw	50	1 cup			
Watermelon, raw	50	4 × 8-inch wedge (2 pounds)	Pork, cured, shoulder, sliced, lean and fat	30	3 ounces
Pineapple juice, from frozen concentrate	50	1 cup	Pork, fresh, ham or shoulder, sliced, lean and fat	30	3 ounces
Cereal and bakery products:			Kidney, beef	30	3 ounces
Spanish rice	60	1 cup	Peanuts	30	1 cup
Pie, strawberry	50	4¾-inch sector	Pork, cured, ham, sliced, lean and fat	25	3 ounces
Miscellaneous:			Spareribs	25	3 ounces
Orange juice, from dehydrated crystals	180	1 cup	Spaghetti (enriched) with cheese, canned	25	1 cup
Grapefruit juice, from dehydrated crystals	150	1 cup	Cowpeas, dry, cooked	25	1 cup
Cranberry juice cocktail	70	1 cup	Soybeans, dry, cooked	25	1 cup
Grape juice drink, canned	70	1 cup	Almonds, whole, shelled	25	1 cup
Orange-apricot juice drink	70	1 cup	Chestnuts, shelled	25	1 cup
			Pumpkin kernels	25	1 cup
Pineapple-orange juice drink	70	1 cup	Walnuts, English, chopped	25	1 cup
Pineapple-grapefruit juice drink	70	1 cup	Liver, hog	20	3 ounces
			Beef pot pie, home-prepared from enriched flour	20	⅓ of 9-inch pie
THIAMINE			Chicken or turkey pot pie, home-prepared from enriched flour	20	⅓ of 9-inch pie
Meat and meat alternates:					
Sunflower seeds	190	1 cup			
Pork, loin, chopped, lean	100	1 cup	Chop suey, with beef and pork, home recipe	20	1 cup
Brazil nuts, shelled	90	1 cup	Beans, navy (pea), dry, cooked	20	1 cup
Pork, fresh or cured, ham or shoulder, chopped, lean	60	1 cup	Peas, split, dry, cooked	20	1 cup
			Walnuts, black, chopped	20	1 cup
Pork, loin, sliced, lean only	60	3 ounces	Bacon, Canadian	15	1 slice
Pecans, halves	60	1 cup	Lamb, leg or shoulder, chopped, lean	15	1 cup
Pork, loin, sliced, lean and fat	50	3 ounces			
Pork, loin chop, lean and fat	50	2.7 ounces			

TABLE 6-8 (*Continued*)

Food	Percentage of US-RDA	Amount of food
Heart, beef, sliced	15	3 ounces
Liver, calf or beef	15	3 ounces
Polish sausage	15	2.4-ounce link
Pork sausage	15	1-ounce pattie or 2 links
Crab, deviled	15	1 cup
Macaroni (enriched) and cheese, home recipe	15	1 cup
Spaghetti (enriched) with cheese, home recipe	15	1 cup
Spaghetti (enriched) with meatballs, home recipe	15	1 cup
Beans, canned, with pork and tomato sauce	15	1 cup
Beans, lima, great northern, or kidney, dry, cooked	15	1 cup
Vegetables and fruit:		
Cowpeas, cooked	35	1 cup
Peas, green, cooked	30	1 cup
Peas and carrots, cooked	20	1 cup
Beans, lima, fresh, cooked	20	1 cup
Asparagus, pieces, cooked	15	1 cup
Collards, cooked	15	1 cup
Cowpeas, canned, solids and liquid	15	1 cup
Okra, sliced, cooked	15	1 cup
Soybeans, sprouted seeds, raw or cooked	15	1 cup
Turnip greens, cooked	15	1 cup
Vegetables, mixed, cooked	15	1 cup
Potato salad, with cooked salad dressing	15	1 cup
Orange juice, fresh or from unsweetened frozen or canned concentrate	15	1 cup
Pineapple, canned, water or syrup pack	15	1 cup
Pineapple, frozen, sweetened	15	1 cup
Cereal and bakery products:		
Hoagie roll, enriched	35	11½-inch-long roll

Food	Percentage of US-RDA	Amount of food
Cereal, ready-to-eat (check label)	25	1 ounce
Hard roll, enriched	15	1 roll (1.8 ounces)
Spoonbread	15	1 cup
Oatmeal, cooked	15	1 cup
Oat and wheat cereal, cooked	15	1 cup
Macaroni, enriched, cooked	15	1 cup
Noodles, enriched, cooked	15	1 cup
Spaghetti, enriched, cooked	15	1 cup
Rice, white, enriched, cooked	15	1 cup
Gingerbread, with enriched flour	15	⅛ of 9-inch-square cake
Pie, pecan	15	4¾-inch sector
Miscellaneous:		
Orange juice, from dehydrated crystals	15	1 cup
Soup, split pea	15	1 cup
Bread pudding, with enriched bread	15	1 cup

RIBOFLAVIN

Food	Percentage of US-RDA	Amount of food
Milk and milk products:		
Cheese, cottage	35	1 cup
Milk, partially skimmed	30	1 cup
Malted beverage	30	1 cup
Custard, baked	30	1 cup
Milk, whole or skim	25	1 cup
Milk, nonfat dry, reconstituted	25	1 cup
Buttermilk	25	1 cup
Chocolate drink	25	1 cup
Cocoa	25	1 cup
Ice milk, soft-serve	25	1 cup
Pudding, from mixes, with milk	25	1 cup
Pudding, vanilla, home recipe	25	1 cup
Rennin desserts	25	1 cup
Yogurt	25	1 cup
Ice cream, soft-serve	20	1 cup

TABLE 6-8 (*Continued*)

Food	Percentage of US-RDA	Amount of food
Pudding, chocolate, home recipe	20	1 cup
Tapioca cream	20	1 cup
Meat and meat alternates:		
Kidney, beef	240	3 ounces
Liver, hog	220	3 ounces
Liver, beef or calf	210	3 ounces
Almonds, whole	80	1 cup
Fish loaf	60	$4\frac{1}{8} \times 2\frac{1}{2} \times 1$-inch slice
Heart, beef, sliced	60	3 ounces
Almonds, sliced	50	1 cup
Liver, chicken	40	1 ounce
Beef, dried, chipped, creamed	30	1 cup
Welsh rarebit	30	1 cup
Lamb, leg or shoulder, chopped, lean	25	1 cup
Pork, fresh, ham or loin, chopped, lean	25	1 cup
Veal, stewed or roasted, chopped	25	1 cup
Braunschweiger	25	1 ounce
Chicken a la king, home recipe	25	1 cup
Macaroni (enriched) and cheese, home recipe	25	1 cup
Beef, chuck or rump, chopped, lean	20	1 cup
Lamb, leg or shoulder, chopped, lean and fat	20	1 cup
Pork, cured, ham, or shoulder, chopped, lean	20	1 cup
Pork, fresh, shoulder, chopped	20	1 cup
Pork, fresh, ham or shoulder, ground, lean	20	1 cup
Veal, loin, chopped	20	1 cup
Veal, rib, ground	20	1 cup
Turkey, dark meat, chopped	20	1 cup
Chicken or turkey pot pie, home-prepared from enriched flour	30	$\frac{1}{3}$ of 9-inch pie

Food	Percentage of US-RDA	Amount of food
Chop suey with beef and pork, home recipe	20	1 cup
Pepper, stuffed	20	1 pepper (6.5 ounces)
Spaghetti (enriched) with meatballs, home recipe	20	1 cup
Vegetables and fruits:		
Broccoli, cooked	20	Medium stalk
Broccoli, cut, cooked	20	1 cup
Corn pudding	20	1 cup
Collards, cooked	20	1 cup
Turnip greens, cooked	20	1 cup
Avocado, Florida, raw	20	$\frac{1}{2}$ fruit
Avocado, Florida or California, raw, cubed	20	1 cup
Cereal and bakery products:		
Cereals, ready-to-eat (check label)	25	1 ounce
Spoonbread	25	1 cup
Hoagie roll, enriched	20	$11\frac{1}{2}$-inch-long roll
Miscellaneous:		
Bread pudding, with enriched bread	35	1 cup
Oyster stew, home recipe	25	1 cup
Rice pudding	20	1 cup
Soup, cream of mushroom, with milk	20	1 cup

NIACIN

Food	Percentage of US-RDA	Amount of food
Meat and meat alternates:		
Peanuts	120	1 cup
Liver, hog	100	3 ounces
Chicken, light meat, chopped	80	1 cup
Turkey, light meat, chopped	80	1 cup
Liver, calf or beef	70	3 ounces
Chicken, breast	60	$\frac{1}{2}$ breast (3.3 ounces)
Chicken, stewed, dark meat, chopped	60	1 cup
Veal rib, chopped	60	1 cup
Tuna, canned in water	60	3 ounces

TABLE 6-8 (*Continued*)

Food	Per-cent-age of US-RDA	Amount of food	Food	Per-cent-age of US-RDA	Amount of food
Chicken, roasted, light meat, sliced	50	3 ounces	Pork, cured, ham, chopped, lean	30	1 cup
Turkey, canned	50	1 cup	Pork, cured, shoulder, ground, lean	30	1 cup
Rabbit, domesticated	50	3 ounces	Pork, loin, sliced, lean	30	3 ounces
Tuna, canned in oil, drained	50	3 ounces	Chicken fricassee, home recipe	30	1 cup
Tuna salad	50	1 cup	Turkey, dark meat, chopped	30	1 cup
Lamb, leg, chopped, lean	45	1 cup	Salmon, pink, canned	30	3 ounces
Kidney, beef	45	3 ounces	Beef pot pie, home-prepared from enriched flour	30	⅓ of 9-inch pie
Pork, loin, chopped, lean	45	1 cup			
Veal, stewed, chopped	45	1 cup			
Veal, rib, ground	45	1 cup	Beef, chuck, ground, lean	25	1 cup
Chicken, canned	45	1 cup	Beef, steak (club, porter-house, T-bone, or sirloin), lean	25	3 ounces
Chicken, stewed, light meat, sliced	45	3 ounces			
Turkey, light meat, sliced	45	3 ounces	Beef, steak (round)	25	3 ounces
Swordfish, broiled	45	3 ounces	Ground beef	25	3 ounces
Chicken, broiled	40	3 ounces	Lamb, leg, sliced	25	3 ounces
Goose	40	3 ounces	Lamb, loin chop, lean and fat	25	3.5 ounces
Lamb, shoulder, chopped, lean	40	1 cup	Lamb, shoulder, sliced, lean	25	3 ounces
Pork, fresh, ham, chopped, lean	40	1 cup	Pork, cured, ham, ground, lean	25	3 ounces
Veal, loin, chopped	40	1 cup	Pork, fresh, ham, sliced, lean	25	3 ounces
Turkey pot pie, home-prepared from enriched flour	40	⅓ of 9-inch pie	Pork, loin chop, lean and fat	25	2.7 ounces
Salmon steak, broiled or baked	40	3 ounces	Pork, loin, sliced, lean and fat	25	3 ounces
Sunflower seeds	40	1 cup	Veal, stewed, sliced	25	3 ounces
Beef, rump, chopped, lean	35	1 cup	Veal, loin or cutlet	25	3 ounces
Pork, fresh or cured, shoulder, chopped, lean	35	1 cup	Chicken, roasted, dark meat, sliced	25	3 ounces
			Chicken a la king, home recipe	25	1 cup
Veal, rib, sliced	35	3 ounces	Chicken pot pie, home-prepared from enriched flour	25	⅓ of 9-inch pie
Heart, beef, sliced	35	3 ounces			
Chicken, stewed, dark meat, sliced	35	3 ounces			
Chicken, roasted, dark meat, chopped	35	1 cup	Salmon, red, canned	25	3 ounces
Halibut, broiled	35	3 ounces	Salmon rice loaf	25	6-ounce piece
Mackerel, broiled	35	3 ounces	Sardines, canned, drained	25	3 ounces
Rockfish, oven-steamed	35	3 ounces			
Shad, baked	35	3 ounces			
Beef, chuck, chopped	30	1 cup			
Beef, rump, ground, lean	30	1 cup			

TABLE 6-8 (*Continued*)

Food	Percentage of US RDA	Amount of food
Beef and vegetable stew, home recipe	25	1 cup
Chop suey, with beef and pork, home recipe	25	1 cup
Corned beef hash, canned	25	1 cup
Peppers, stuffed	25	1 pepper (6.5 ounces)
Spaghetti (enriched) with cheese, canned	25	1 cup
Beef, chuck, sliced	20	3 ounces
Beef, rump, sliced	20	3 ounces
Beef, rib, sliced, lean and fat	20	3 ounces
Beef, flank steak	20	3 ounces
Beef, plate, lean	20	3 ounces
Beef, steak (club, porterhouse, T-bone, or sirloin), lean and fat	20	3 ounces
Lamb, rib chop, lean and fat	20	3.2 ounces
Lamb, loin chop, lean	20	2.3 ounces
Lamb, shoulder, sliced, lean and fat	20	3 ounces
Pork, cured, ham, sliced, lean	20	3 ounces
Pork, fresh, ham, sliced, lean and fat	20	3 ounces
Pork, fresh or cured, shoulder, sliced	20	3 ounces
Pork, loin chop, lean	20	2 ounces
Chicken, thigh	20	2.3-ounce piece
Turkey, dark meat, sliced	20	3 ounces
Chicken and noodles, home recipe	20	1 cup
Chow mein, home recipe	20	1 cup
Spaghetti (enriched) with meatballs, home recipe	20	1 cup
Lobster Newburg	20	1 cup
Crab, deviled	20	1 cup
Vegetables and fruits:		
Dates, pitted, chopped	20	1 cup
Peaches, dried, cooked, unsweetened	20	1 cup
Peas, green, cooked	20	1 cup

Food	Percentage of US RDA	Amount of food
Cereal and bakery products:		
Hoagie roll, enriched	25	11½-inch-long roll
Cereals, ready-to-eat (check label)	20	1 ounce

CALCIUM

Food	Percentage of US RDA	Amount of food
Milk and milk products:		
Cheese Parmesan, grated	40	1 ounce
Milk, partially skimmed	35	1 cup
Pudding, uncooked, from mix	35	1 cup
Milk, whole or skim	30	1 cup
Milk, nonfat dry, reconstituted	30	1 cup
Buttermilk	30	1 cup
Chocolate drink, made from whole milk	30	1 cup
Cocoa	30	1 cup
Malted beverage	30	1 cup
Custard, baked	30	1 cup
Pudding, vanilla, home recipe	30	1 cup
Rennin desserts	30	1 cup
Yogurt, made from partially skimmed milk	30	1 cup
Chocolate drink, made from skim milk	25	1 cup
Cheese, cottage, creamed	25	1 cup
Cheese, Swiss	25	1 ounce
Yogurt, made from whole milk	25	1 cup
Ice cream or ice milk, soft-serve	25	1 cup
Pudding, cooked, from mix, with milk	25	1 cup
Pudding, chocolate, home recipe	25	1 cup
Cheese, American, process	20	1 ounce
Cheese, Cheddar, natural	20	1 ounce
Cheese, cottage, uncreamed	20	1 cup
Ice cream or ice milk, hardened	20	1 cup

TABLE 6-8 (*Continued*)

Food	Percentage of US RDA	Amount of food	Food	Percentage of US RDA	Amount of food
Meat and meat alternates:			Beans, with pork and sweet sauce, canned	35	1 cup
Welsh rarebit	60	1 cup	Almonds, whole, shelled	35	1 cup
Sardines, canned, drained	35	3 ounces	Beef, chuck or rump, chopped, lean	30	1 cup
Macaroni (enriched) and cheese, home recipe	35	1 cup	Pork, cured, shoulder, chopped, lean	30	1 cup
Potatoes au gratin	30	1 cup	Pork, fresh, ham or loin, chopped, lean	30	1 cup
Beef, dried, chipped, creamed	25	1 cup	Heart, beef, sliced	30	3 ounces
Cheese souffle	20	1 cup	Clams, raw	30	4 or 5 clams
Lobster Newburg	20	1 cup	Beef pot pie, home-prepared from enriched flour	30	⅓ of 9-inch pie
Macaroni (enriched) and cheese, canned	20	1 cup	Beans, navy (pea), dry, cooked	30	1 cup
Vegetables and fruits:			Beans, white, dry, canned, solids and liquid	30	1 cup
Collards, cooked	35	1 cup			
Cabbage, spoon, cooked	25	1 cup	Cashew nuts, whole kernels, roasted	30	1 cup
Spinach, canned	25	1 cup	Beef, chuck or rump, ground, lean	25	1 cup
Turnip greens	25	1 cup			
Kale, cooked	20	1 cup	Pork, cured, ham, chopped, lean	25	1 cup
Mustard greens, cooked	20	1 cup	Pork, fresh, shoulder, chopped	25	1 cup
Rhubarb, cooked	20	1 cup			
Cereal and bakery products:			Pork, fresh, ham, ground, lean	25	1 cup
Spoonbread	25	1 cup	Veal, chopped	25	1 cup
Farina, enriched, instant	20	1 cup	Chicken or turkey pot pie, home-prepared from enriched flour	25	⅓ of 9-inch pie
Miscellaneous:					
Bread pudding	30	1 cup			
Oyster stew, home recipe	30	1 cup	Chile con carne with beans, canned	25	1 cup
Rice pudding	25	1 cup	Chop suey, with beef and pork, home recipe	25	1 cup
Soup, with milk:					
Green pea	20	1 cup	Corned beef hash, canned	25	1 cup
Cream of celery	20	1 cup	Beans, great northern or red kidney, dry, cooked	25	1 cup
Cream of mushroom	20	1 cup			
Cream of asparagus	20	1 cup			
			Beans, red kidney, dry, canned, solids and liquid	25	1 cup
IRON					
Meat and meat alternates:			Lentils, dry, cooked	25	1 cup
Liver, hog	140	3 ounces			
Pumpkin kernels	90	1 cup			
Liver, calf	70	3 ounces			
Kidney, beef	60	3 ounces			
Sunflower seeds	60	1 cup			
Liver, beef	40	3 ounces			
Walnuts, black, chopped	40	1 cup			
Clams, canned, drained, chopped	35	1 cup			
Beans, lima, dry, cooked	35	1 cup			

TABLE 6-8 (*Continued*)

Food	Percentage of US-RDA	Amount of food	Food	Percentage of US-RDA	Amount of food
Soybeans, dry, cooked	25	1 cup	Pork, cured, ham, sliced, lean	15	3 ounces
Beans, with frankfurters, canned	25	1 cup	Pork, fresh, loin or ham, sliced, lean and fat	15	3 ounces
Beans, with pork and tomato sauce, canned	25	1 cup	Pork, loin chop, lean and fat	15	2.7 ounces
Beef, chuck, sliced, lean	20	3 ounces	Pork, fresh, shoulder, sliced	15	3 ounces
Beef, flank steak	20	3 ounces	Veal, sliced	15	3 ounces
Beef, plate, lean	20	3 ounces	Veal, cutlet or loin	15	3 ounces
Beef, steak, sirloin, lean	20	3 ounces	Beef and vegetable stew, home recipe	15	1 cup
Pork, cured, ham or shoulder, ground, lean	20	1 cup	Chicken, dark meat, chopped	15	1 cup
Pork, fresh, shoulder, ground, lean	20	1 cup	Chicken, canned	15	1 cup
Pork, fresh, ham, sliced, lean	20	3 ounces	Spaghetti (enriched) with tomato sauce and cheese, canned	15	1 cup
Pork, loin, sliced, lean	20	3 ounces	Turkey, canned	15	1 cup
Turkey, dark meat, chopped	20	1 cup	Chow mein, chicken, home recipe	15	1 cup
Veal, rib, ground	20	1 cup	Chicken a la king, home recipe	15	1 cup
Peppers, stuffed	20	1 pepper (6.5 ounces)	Crab, deviled	15	1 cup
Spaghetti (enriched) in tomato sauce, with meatballs; canned or home-prepared	20	1 cup	Sardines, canned	15	3 ounces
			Shrimp, canned	15	3 ounces
Cowpeas, dry, cooked	20	1 cup	Tuna salad	15	1 cup
Peas, split, dry, cooked	20	1 cup	Vegetables and fruit:		
Beef, chuck, lean and fat, sliced	15	3 ounces	Peaches, dried, uncooked	60	1 cup
Beef, corned	15	3 ounces	Prune juice, canned	60	1 cup
Beef, plate, lean and fat	15	3 ounces	Dates, pitted, chopped	30	1 cup
Beef, rump, sliced	15	3 ounces	Raisins, seedless	30	1 cup
Beef, rib, sliced, lean	15	3 ounces	Spinach, canned	30	1 cup
Beef, steak (round)	15	3 ounces	Asparagus, pieces, canned	25	1 cup
Beef, steak (club, porterhouse, or T-bone), lean	15	3 ounces	Beans, lima, canned	25	1 cup
Beef, steak (sirloin), lean and fat	15	3 ounces	Beans, lima, fresh or frozen, baby, cooked	25	1 cup
Ground beef	15	3 ounces	Apricots, dried, cooked	25	1 cup
Lamb, shoulder, chopped, lean	15	1 cup	Peaches, dried, cooked	25	1 cup
Lamb, leg, chopped	15	1 cup	Cowpeas, cooked	20	1 cup
Pork, cured, shoulder, sliced	15	3 ounces	Cowpeas, canned, solids and liquid	20	1 cup
			Peas, green, canned	20	1 cup
			Spinach, cooked	20	1 cup

TABLE 6-8 (Continued)

Food	Percentage of US-RDA	Amount of food
Turnip greens, canned, solids and liquid	20	1 cup
Prunes, dried, cooked	20	1 cup
Beans, lima, Fordhook, cooked	15	1 cup
Beet greens, cooked	15	1 cup
Chard, Swiss, cooked	15	1 cup
Mustard greens, fresh or frozen, cooked	15	1 cup
Peas, green, cooked	15	1 cup
Sauerkraut juice	15	1 cup
Vegetables, mixed, cooked	15	1 cup
Boysenberries, canned	15	1 cup
Plums, canned, water or syrup pack	15	1 cup
Prunes, dried, uncooked	15	10 prunes
Cereal and bakery products:		
Farina, instant, enriched, cooked	90	1 cup
Farina, regular and quick-cooking, enriched, cooked	70	1 cup
Hoagie roll, enriched	40	11½-inch-long roll
Cereals, ready-to-eat (check label)	20	1 ounce
Cottage pudding with enriched flour and chocolate sauce	20	⅛ of 8-inch-square cake
Gingerbread, with enriched flour	20	⅑ of 9-inch-square cake
Pie, pecan	20	4¾-inch sector
Coffeecake, with enriched flour	15	2.5-ounce piece
Cottage pudding, with enriched flour and strawberry sauce	15	⅛ of 8-inch-square cake
Hard roll, enriched	15	1 roll (1.8 ounces)
Spoonbread	15	1 cup
Miscellaneous:		
Bread pudding, with raisins and enriched bread	20	1 cup

Food	Percentage of US-RDA	Amount of food
Oyster stew, home recipe	20	1 cup
Molasses, blackstrap	20	1 tablespoon
Apple brown Betty, with enriched bread	15	1 cup
Syrup, sorghum	15	1 tablespoon

SOURCE: B. Peterkin, J. Nicholas, and C. Cromwell, *Nutrition Labeling: Tools for Its Use*; Agric. Info. Bull. No. 382, USDA, 1975.

Milk is usually consumed in at least 1 cup (240 gm) portions so the 100-gm method greatly underestimates the level of nutrients usually obtained from a serving of milk. Both methods are presented here for comparison, but reference here is usually to portion size. The standard portion sizes selected are 1 cup for milk and other beverages; 3 oz for meats; 1 cup for a tossed salad or casserole; and ½ cup for fruits, vegetables, and most other foods.

Vitamin A

Vitamin A is present either in the preformed state in foods from animal sources or in the *provitamin* form of β-carotene from plant sources.

Preformed vitamin A is present in liver, kidney, eggs, whole milk, and butter. In these foods the vitamin A is associated with the fat because it is a fat-soluble vitamin. When the fat content of milk is lowered, the vitamin A content is also lowered. In the case of low-fat and skim milk, the vitamin A content is improved by fortification with vitamins A and D. *Fortification* means that additional nutrients are added to a food so that it contains more of these nutrients than were originally present. Most margarines are also fortified with vitamins A and D.

The vitamin A content from fruits and vegetables is directly proportional to the amount of carotene present. Carotene is a yellow-orange pigment, but it is sometimes masked by other colored pigments such as chlorophyll, the green pigment in many vegetables. It is interesting to note that, in the fall, cooler temperatures cause deterioration of the green chlorophyll, revealing the beautiful orange and gold colors that are actually carotenoid pigments. The darker the green and the deeper the yellow-orange color of fruits and vegetables, the higher the carotene and the higher the vitamin A content. Look at the list of foods containing significant quantities of vitamin A in Table 6.8 and picture the color of the food. Notice that even though such vegetables as green beans, peas, and corn contain some vitamin A the quantity is not nearly as high as in the darker green leafy vegetables. Although peaches contain some vitamin A, other fruits such as apricots and cantaloupe contain more because they are deeper in color.

Besides β-carotene there are some other red and yellow pigments in food that can be converted into vitamin A. *Cryptoxanthin* is such a yellow pigment found in yellow corn and oranges. Because of this a fresh orange surprisingly contains 260 IU of vitamin A, and 1 cup of orange juice contains 500 IU. An ear of yellow corn contains 400 IU of vitamin A, but white corn contains only a trace. One-half of a white grapefruit contains only 10 IU of vitamin A, whereas one-half of a pink grapefruit contains 440 IU. The red pigment in tomatoes also possesses some vitamin A activity; one fresh tomato contains 1,640 IU of vitamin A. For more food sources of vitamin A, see Table 6-8.

Vitamin C

The most common and best sources of vitamin C, or ascorbic acid, are lemons, limes, oranges, and grapefruits, the citrus fruits. An extremely high source of vitamin C is a tropical fruit called the acerola, or West Indian cherry. This fruit is also grown in Florida, Puerto Rico, and Hawaii. The raw fruit contains about 1,300 mg of vitamin C per $\frac{1}{2}$ cup. The common daily source of vitamin C, however, is citrus fruits, which contribute about 45–65 mg of this vitamin per average-size serving. For more food sources of vitamin C, see Table 6-8.

There are other fruits and some vegetables which are also excellent sources of vitamin C. An average serving of cantaloupe or strawberries contains almost as much vitamin C as $\frac{1}{2}$ cup of orange juice. Vegetables which are high in vitamin C are broccoli, brussels sprouts, cauliflower, and any of the dark green leafy vegetables such as collard greens, kale, and turnip greens. Other significant sources are fresh tomatoes, baked potatoes, and raw cabbage.

Thiamine

Thiamine is well distributed in many foods from both plant and animal sources, but it is found in large quantities in only a few foods. Because it is found in so many foods, the daily intake of a wide variety of foods from all food groups usually provides for an adequate daily thiamine intake. Brewer's yeast and wheat germ are the foods highest in thiamine content, but they are not commonly eaten in large enough quantities to make much contribution. Pork is the common food that contains the most thiamine. This vitamin is also found in significant quantities in meat, legumes, whole grains, and enriched cereals. Certain kinds of nuts when eaten in large quantities also make a significant contribution. Thiamine is present but to a lesser extent in fruits, vegetables, and milk. Table 6.8 lists more food sources.

Riboflavin

Another of the B-complex vitamins, riboflavin, is also well distributed in a variety of foods. Riboflavin content is the highest in Brewer's yeast and organ meats, but because of generally low consumption of these foods, they do not make a significant daily contribution. Milk and dairy products make the best single contribution of riboflavin to the daily diet. The next highest contributors are meats, poultry, and fish, followed by breads and cereals. Fruits and vegetables contain the lowest amounts of riboflavin. Table 6.8 lists more food sources.

Niacin

The best sources of niacin are organ meats, Brewer's yeast, and tuna fish. Other meats, poultry, fish, and peanuts are also good sources. There is an interesting relationship between protein and niacin. Niacin is available either preformed in foods or in the precursor form of *tryptophan*. Because some niacin can be derived from the essential amino acid tryptophan, which is present in nearly all foods, any food that is high in protein is also naturally high in niacin. Tables of food composition give only the amount of *preformed niacin* present in foods. To assess daily niacin intake accurately the amount of niacin contributed by the tryptophan must be taken into consideration based on the total protein content of the diet. The term *niacin equivalent* is used to refer to the total potential niacin of the diet, which consists of the preformed niacin plus the amount of niacin that could be derived from tryptophan. A *niacin equivalent* is defined as 1 mg of niacin or 60 mg of tryptophan. Considering both animal and vegetable sources, proteins contain about 1% tryptophan. Niacin equivalents can be figured using both preformed niacin and the niacin converted from the tryptophan of the protein. Most US diets contain adequate protein, so it is highly unlikely that the niacin deficiency disease, pellagra, will be seen.

Another interesting source of niacin is coffee. During the roasting process a derivative of niacin is actually converted to the vitamin, and during the brewing process the niacin is dissolved in the beverage. The stronger the coffee brew, the more niacin per cup. In some areas of the world where there is a low dietary consumption of niacin and protein, a high consumption of coffee may help to explain a low incidence of pellagra.

Calcium

The well-known sources of calcium, of course, are all milk and milk products. Milk is such an outstanding source of calcium that it is virtually impossible to obtain an adequate amount of calcium in a diet without any milk or dairy products. The dark, leafy vegetables are also considered good sources of calcium, but they are generally not eaten in a quantity that will make a very significant contribution to the daily intake. If the small bones in canned salmon are retained when preparing salmon patties or croquettes, the calcium content of the salmon is greatly enhanced. These bones have been somewhat softened by the canning process and are not usually too undesirable if allowed to remain.

Iron

Liver is the most excellent source of dietary iron. The other good sources are enriched breads and cereals, dried beans and peas, red meat (beef), and of course prunes and raisins. The level of iron, however, in an average-size serving of these foods is only about 10% of the US-RDA. Because the recommended daily intake of iron is set so high, especially for females of childbearing age (18 mg daily), it is generally not possible to plan daily menus that will meet this high recommended intake unless liver is included.

The iron contained in foods from animal sources is more readily utilized by the body than the iron from vegetable sources. Also, all iron from foods is better utilized when a good source of vitamin C is present in that meal. It is also interesting to learn that the use of iron utensils in food preparation results in an increased consumption of iron and that this iron is capable of being absorbed and used by the body.

Attendant Nutrients

The RDA also contain recommended daily intakes for several other vitamins and minerals besides the leader nutrients. Continued nutritional research into the functions and requirements of nutrients known to be essential to humans provides data to be used in the formulation of recommended daily intakes. The science of nutrition has continued to expand and RDA for several nutrients have been added since 1968. In the 1968 revision RDA were added for vitamin E, folacin, vitamin B_6, vitamin B_{12}, phosphorus, iodine, and magnesium. In 1974 a recommended intake for zinc was established. These additional vitamins and minerals for which RDA have been established can be referred to as *attendant nutrients*. This term refers to the fact that these vitamins and minerals are found in combination with the leader nutrients in common foods; consumption of food sources of the leader nutrients makes the attendant nutrients available to perform their physiological functions. There has been considerable research on the trace elements in recent years, and when sufficient information is known about their human requirements, RDA will undoubtedly be established for these as well. These attendant vitamins and minerals contained in the RDA are generally well distributed in many foods, and they are required in rather small quantities daily. Tables of nutrient composition for some of these vitamins and minerals are not as complete and widely available as those for the leader nutrients.

Even though they are widely distributed in foods, required in small amounts, and nutrient values of foods are somewhat limited, it is still important to know food sources of these vitamins and minerals inasmuch as RDA have been established. The vitamins are D, E, B_6, B_{12}, and folacin; the minerals are phosphorus, iodine, magnesium, and zinc. A good deal of similarity of food sources for these vitamins and minerals will be noted; this is because all of these nutrients are well distributed in several groups of foods.

Vitamin D

The major source of vitamin D is a nondietary source: the sun. Ultraviolet rays from the sun strike the skin and cause the conversion of a precursor of this vitamin into the form in which vitamin D can be used by the body. Foods are not a significant source of vitamin D except for those that have been fortified with it. Eggs, butter, liver, and fatty fish contain only small amounts of vitamin D. Adequate quantities of this vitamin cannot be obtained unless fortified foods are consumed and there is some exposure to sunlight. Because the ultraviolet rays of the sun cannot penetrate window panes and be used by the skin, people who are confined to a hospital or institution should receive a vitamin D supplement.

The requirement for this vitamin can be met by the healthy adult or child by ordinary exposure to sunlight. Exposure to ultraviolet rays can be greatly reduced by atmospheric smoke, fog, and general air pollution. In northern climates during the winter months, adequate exposure to the ultraviolet rays of the sun is not likely. Adequate penetration of the sunlight rays is greatly reduced in dark-skinned races. For all these reasons vitamin D is commonly added to milk, margarine, infant cereals, and prepared breakfast cereals.

It must be remembered that vitamin D is a fat-soluble vitamin that can be stored by the liver. Because of this storage capacity there is danger of excessive dietary intake. The condition of *hypervitaminosis D* manifested by elevated blood levels of calcium and calcification of the body's arteries and organs is usually the result of indiscriminate use of vitamin supplements. Because infants and young children are especially prone to this condition, pediatricians and mothers should be alert to all the foods their child is consuming that contain added vitamin D.

Vitamin E

Vitamin E is found primarily in plant sources. The best sources of this vitamin are the vegetable oils. A claim is often made by food faddists today that the higher intake of polyunsaturated vegetable oils has the effect of increasing the adult requirement for vitamin E and for this reason adults should take a vitamin E supplement. This statement contains only a half-truth. It is a fact that the higher intake of polyunsaturated vegetable oils does actually increase the vitamin E requirement. This does not, however, necessitate taking a supplement of vitamin E because the best single source of this vitamin is polyunsaturated vegetable oils.

Vitamin E is also found in high concentrations in whole grains and wheat germ. Other significant dietary sources are the dark-green leafy vegetables, nuts, and legumes.

Animal sources of this vitamin are somewhat limited; it comes from the organ meats (liver, heart, and kidney) and eggs.

Vitamin B_6

Vitamin B_6 is widely distributed in both plant and animal products. Pork and the organ meats have the highest content, followed by lamb and veal, and finally by fish and beef muscle. The best plant sources of vitamin B_6 are whole grains and wheat germ, but most of this vitamin is removed during processing and not replaced. One of the nutritional advantages that whole wheat bread has over enriched white bread is the presence of vitamin E, some of the B-complex vitamins, and some of the minerals. During milling of the wheat the outer portions of the wheat kernel are removed and with it many of the attendant nutrients. In the enrichment process only the thiamine, riboflavin, niacin, and iron are replaced. Other good vegetable sources of vitamin B_6 are legumes, potatoes, oatmeal, and bananas.

Folacin

The two most outstanding sources of folacin are the organ meats and dark-green leafy vegetables. The name *folacin* (*folium* meaning leaf) was selected because of the presence of this substance in green leaves. Folacin is also present in significant amounts in whole grains, legumes, and nuts.

Vitamin B_{12}

Vitamin B_{12} is present primarily in foods of animal origin. It is widely distributed in meat, fish, eggs, and dairy products. Fruits, vegetables, breads, and cereals contain virtually none of this vitamin. True vegetarians (those who consume no animal products at all) are likely to develop a deficiency of vitamin B_{12}, so many of them will consume a vitamin B_{12} supplement.

Magnesium

Magnesium is part of the chlorophyll of green vegetables; therefore green leafy vegetables are an excellent food source. Other good sources are dry beans and peas, soybeans, nuts, and whole grains.

Zinc

Foods high in protein are generally high in zinc. Meats and dairy products provide the best sources. Shellfish (especially lobster and Atlantic oysters) and red meats are the highest in zinc content. Turkey contains more zinc than chicken, and the dark meat of either is higher than the light meat. Nonfat dry milk and cheddar cheese are relatively high in zinc. Nuts and legumes are also good sources of zinc, as are whole grains. Because of the association between protein and zinc it should be noted that vegetarian and low-protein diets may be low in zinc content.

Iodine

The major food source of iodine is saltwater fish and seaweed. In areas where large amounts of seafood are consumed, an additional supply of iodine is not needed, but people residing inland where very little seafood is consumed and the iodine content of the soil varies need a dietary supplement. In the Midwest the best source of iodine in the diet is iodized salt.

The iodine content of plants depends on the iodine content of the soil, and the iodine content of eggs and dairy products depends on the diet of the animals. Because of these variables, tables listing the iodine content of foods are not very reliable.

Phosphorus

Phosphorus is more widely distributed in foods and less likely to be deficient in a diet. It is contained in meat, poultry, fish, and eggs, as well as in milk and dairy products. Phosphorus is also contained in cereal grains, dried beans and peas, and nuts. The major food sources of the attendant nutrients are summarized in Table 6-9.

INDEX OF NUTRITIONAL QUALITY (INQ)

A new measurement of nutritional quality developed by nutritionists at Utah State University is called the Index of Nutritional Quality (INQ) (Hansen et al., 1979). This measurement uses the concept of *nutritional density,* which is defined as a ratio of the nutrient content of a food to human nutrient requirements. The nutritional standard may be either the RDA or the US-RDA. The common denominator used in this ratio is Calories. A food that contains a high proportion of nutrients in a relatively few Calories is said to be high in nutrient density (Fig. 6-3). On the other hand, a food containing a large number of Calories but with a low proportion of nutrients is said to have a low nutrient density (Fig. 6-4). Inasmuch as the consumption of excess Calories leads to obesity and maintenance of ideal body weight is a concern among all age groups, the INQ is useful for selecting foods high in nutrient content but low in Calories.

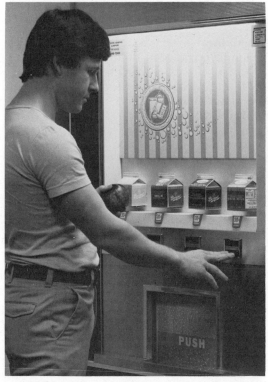

Figure 6-3. The apple and milk selected for a snack are low in Calories and high in essential nutrients. (Photo by J. Collins)

The INQ is a ratio of two percentages. It is defined as the ratio of the percentage of the standard of a given nutrient to the percentage of the standard of energy (i.e., Calories).

$$INQ = \frac{\% \text{ standard of nutrient}}{\% \text{ standard of energy (Calories)}}$$

A cup of whole milk, for example, contains 9 gm of protein and 160 Calories. The nutrient standard is 50 gm of protein to 2,000 Calories. These figures may be substituted in the equation as

$$INQ = \frac{9 \text{ gm}/50 \text{ gm}}{160 \text{ Calories}/2,000 \text{ Calories}} = \frac{18\%}{8\%} = 2.25$$

An INQ of greater than 1 for a given nutrient in a food means that the food supplies that

TABLE 6-9. Food Sources of Additional Nutrients

Vitamins		
Vitamin B$_6$	Vitamin B$_{12}$	Folacin
Bananas	(present in foods of animal	Liver
	origin only)	Dark-green vegetables
Whole grain cereals	Kidney	Dry beans
Chicken	Liver	Peanuts
Dry legumes	Meat	Wheat germ
Egg yolk	Milk	
Most dark-green leafy vegetables	Most cheese	
Most fish and shellfish	Most fish	
Muscle meats, liver and kidney	Shellfish	
Peanuts, walnuts, filberts, and peanut butter	Whole egg and egg yolk	
Potatoes and sweet potatoes		
Prunes and raisins		
Yeast		
	Vitamin D	
	Vitamin D milks	
	Egg yolk	
	Saltwater fish	
	Liver	
	Vitamin E	
	Vegetable oils	
	Margarine	
	Whole grain cereals	
	Peanuts	

Minerals		
Magnesium	Zinc	Phosphorus
Bananas	Shellfish	Meat
Whole grain cereals	Meat	Fish
Dry beans	Cheese	Poultry
Milk	Whole grain cereals	Wheat germ
Most dark-green vegetables	Dry beans	Whole grain products
Nuts	Cocoa	Dry beans
Peanuts and peanut butter	Nuts	Milk
		Milk products
Iodine		
Iodized salt		
Seafood		

SOURCE: Values from *Nutritive Value of Foods*, Home & Garden Bull. No. 72, rev., USDA, 1977.

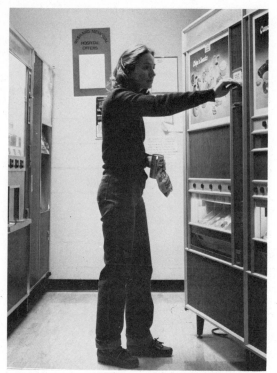

Figure 6-4. These snacks are high in Calories and low in essential nutrients. (Photo by J. Collins)

nutrient in adequate amounts compared to the number of Calories. Nutrients with INQs of less than 1 supply excess Calories in proportion to the nutrients. These nutrients would need to be supplemented in the diet by selecting other foods containing them. Foods that contain large amounts of fat and sugar do not supply high proportions of nutrients, and they therefore contribute to nutrient dilution. This means that a higher proportion of Calories is provided in comparison to nutrients.

This INQ can be used to show a composite picture of a single food, an entire meal, or an entire day's menu. Used in the form of a bar graph for a single food, the nutrients with INQs of less than 1 can be quickly identified

as nutrient deficits that must be made up by other foods in the diet.

The applications of the INQ are numerous. The INQ can be a useful tool in spotting low quantities of nutrients in specific foods. It can be used to evaluate the nutritional contribution of a single food, a group of foods, an entire meal, or a 24-hour dietary intake. It can be used with all groups of people from infancy to old age for nutritional education. The INQ is currently being considered as the new format for nutritional labeling.

VITAMINS AND MINERALS CONTRIBUTED BY THE BASIC FOUR

With the large number of vitamins and minerals required by humans, it is often difficult for the beginning student to recall food sources of the vitamins and minerals. Dividing the nutrients into leader nutrients and attendant nutrients and specifying their relative contribution to the basic four food groups can be helpful. Figure 6-5 provides a graphic picture of the relative distribution of the leader nutrients in the basic four food groups.

Milk Group

Milk has long been considered nature's most perfect food, and rightfully so, for it contains a remarkable blend of most of the essential nutrients. Milk is the first food available to many species of baby animals. It is the primary food of the human infant's diet for many months after birth. Milk is a complete protein that will not only maintain life but support growth. The only two nutrients in which milk is low are vitamin C and iron. For this reason dilute orange juice and an iron-fortified baby cereal are introduced early into the infant's diet.

The three leader nutrients present in the milk group in the highest proportion are protein, calcium, and riboflavin. Milk and dairy

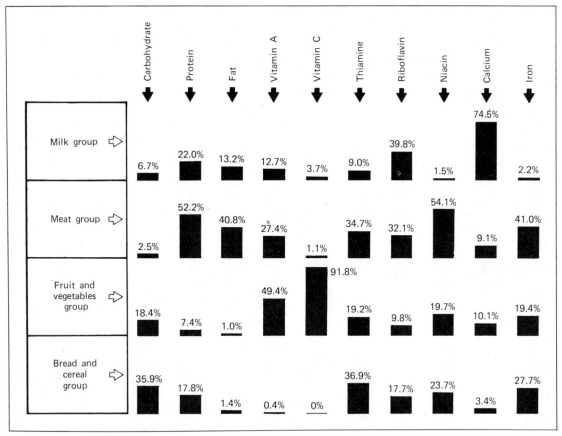

Figure 6-5. Relative distribution of leader nutrients in the basic four.

products are so high in calcium it is essentially impossible to obtain an adequate calcium intake without them. The best source of calcium is 1 cup of milk or yogurt. A larger portion of the other dairy products must be consumed to equal the calcium content of the cup of milk or yogurt. To equal the calcium content of 1 cup of milk, a person would have to consume 1½ slices (1½ oz) of cheese, 1¾ cups of ice cream, or 2 cups of cottage cheese. Milk is an outstanding source of the B-complex vitamin riboflavin, which is also found in each of the other food groups, but in lower amounts.

Milk is also a significant source of vitamins A, D, B$_6$, and B$_{12}$, and of phosphorus, magnesium, and zinc. Most of the milk available today in the market is fortified with vitamin D to the level of 400 IU/qt. Whole milk contains about 350 IU/cup; because of the removal of most of the fat from the low-fat (2%) and skim milks, these varieties usually have 725 IU of vitamin A added per quart. Since 1941, vitamin A has been added to margarine in the amounts of 15,000 IUs/lb.

Meat Group

The meat group contains all types of meat, fish, and poultry as well as eggs, legumes (dry beans and peas), and nuts. Cheese and cottage cheese can be considered in either the milk or the meat group. The leader nutrients that are contained in the highest amounts in the meat group are protein, niacin, iron, and thiamine. The meat group contributes over 50% of the niacin and protein in the diet and over 35% of the thiamine and iron.

Protein

Meat is a complete protein and supplies all the essential amino acids needed by humans to maintain life and support growth. The amino acid composition of an egg is so well balanced that it is used as a reference standard for comparing the protein quality of other foods. Each ounce of cooked lean meat, fish, or poultry, one egg, 1 slice of cheese, $\frac{1}{4}$ cup cottage cheese, $\frac{1}{2}$ cup dry beans or peas, or 2 T of peanut butter contains about 7 gm of protein.

Niacin

Meat is an excellent source of niacin in two different ways. First, meat is a natural source of preformed niacin. For example, chicken and tuna are the two highest content meat sources after the organ meats. Meat is also a good source of niacin because it is high in complete protein and contains the essential amino acid tryptophan, which has the potential for being converted to some niacin.

Thiamine

Thiamine is contained in fairly high amounts in all meats. It is extremely high in pork and pork products.

Iron

Meat is the major source of iron in the diet. Liver contains the highest proportion of iron (14.2 mg/100 mg). Red muscle meat contains considerably more iron than does white or light meat. This is because of the higher proportion of myoglobin, which contains iron, in red meats such as beef or pork. Chicken and turkey are considerably lower. The yolk of an egg is the part that contains the most vitamins and minerals, and it is here that iron is also found. Dried beans and peas are also high in iron, and they rank close in iron content on a 100-gm basis to the red meats.

Other Vitamins and Minerals

Many other vitamins and minerals are found in the meat group in lesser but still significant amounts. Other members of the B complex such as vitamins B_6 and B_{12}, folacin, and riboflavin are contributed by the meat group. Vitamin B_{12} is found only in foods of animal origin, that is, only in the milk and meat group. For this reason a true vegetarian who consumes foods from only the fruit and vegetable and grain groups is likely to have a dietary deficiency of vitamin B_{12}. Vitamin B_6 is well distributed in all foods but is particularly high in organ meats, pork, lamb, and veal. Vitamin A is very high in liver and other organ meats.

The other minerals that are relatively high in the meat group are phosphorus, zinc, and magnesium. All meat, fish, poultry, eggs, and dry beans and peas are rich in phosphorus. Zinc is particularly high in oysters, but it is also found in beef, pork, lamb, and the dark meat of chicken. The magnesium contribution by the meat group is not as high as its content in the other groups, but dry beans and peas and nuts are good sources of magnesium. Vitamin E and folacin are also particularly high in legumes and nuts.

Other minerals are found in certain foods in the meat group. Saltwater fish are excellent sources of dietary iodine. Meat is not known for its calcium content, but if the bones are retained in canned salmon its calcium content is greatly increased.

Fruit and Vegetable Group

The leader nutrients contributed by the fruit and vegetable group are vitamins A and C. This group contributes almost 50% of the vitamin A and 92% of the vitamin C to the daily diet. Citrus fruits are the best sources of vitamin C. The dark-green leafy vegetables or deep-yellow fruits or vegetables contribute the highest amounts of vitamin A.

The other vitamins provided are thiamine, niacin, folacin, vitamin B_6, and vitamin E. The minerals supplied by fruits and vegetables are phosphorus, magnesium, calcium, and iron. The dark-green leafy vegetables are a group of vegetables that contain a high proportion of several important vitamins and minerals. Not only are these vegetables high in vitamins A and C, but they contain very significant quantities of vitamin E, folacin, magnesium, calcium, and iron. Dark-green leafy vegetables should, therefore, be eaten regularly, not only for their content of vitamin A but for their contribution of these other vitamins and minerals.

Grain Group

The grain group contains all whole grains, enriched or fortified grain products including breads and cereals, and other grain products such as rice, macaroni, spaghetti, and noodles. This group contributes primarily carbohydrate, thiamine, niacin, and iron. The nutritive value of any food from this group depends on the amount of processing and the extent of enrichment or fortification.

Generally speaking the largest proportion of grain products in the United States undergoes a great deal of processing. It should be remembered that the processing of grain products was instituted in our country in response to a definite consumer preference for white bread and white rice. There is currently a definite trend back to the use of whole grain breads and cereals. Many people when selecting bread in the market faithfully read the labels, looking for a bread that is made from 100% whole wheat flour.

Structure of Wheat Kernel

To understand the differences in nutrient contents of the various types of grain products, the structure and nutrient composition of a kernel of wheat should first be understood. Figure 6-6 is a drawing of a typical kernel of wheat. The wheat kernel consists of three main parts: the *bran*, the *germ*, and the *endosperm*. The *bran* is the outer covering and is composed of indigestible cellulose or fiber; many of the B-complex vitamins; and such minerals as magnesium, zinc, and especially iron. The layers directly under the bran are rich in protein and phosphorus. The *germ* is referred to as the heart of the wheat because it is the sprouting section of the seed. This section contains fat and also the fat-soluble vitamin E; it also contains high-quality protein. Wheat germ is one of the best sources of thiamine available. The germ also contains carbohydrates; members of the B complex; and even higher concentrations of the zinc, magnesium, and iron that were found in the bran. The center portion of the wheat kernel is the *endosperm*, which is composed mainly of carbohydrates and protein and some of the members of the B complex and minerals. The endosperm is the part used in highly refined white flours. In the refining process the other two sections are not retained, so a large proportion of vitamins and minerals is lost. Enriched flours have four of the nutrients lost during processing replaced: thiamine, riboflavin, niacin, and iron. It is readily apparent, however, that, because only these four nutrients are replaced, refined white flour is lower in the remainder of the B-complex vitamins, vitamin E, magnesium, zinc, and probably some of the other trace minerals than whole wheat flour. The nutritional value of enriched flour can be viewed as deficient because lower levels of some of the essential nutrients are present; or it can be viewed as adequate given that these missing nutrients are required in only small amounts and are widely distributed in many foods, so that their dietary intake is probably still more than adequate. Whole grains themselves are important sources of vitamin B_6, folacin, vitamin E, magnesium, and zinc.

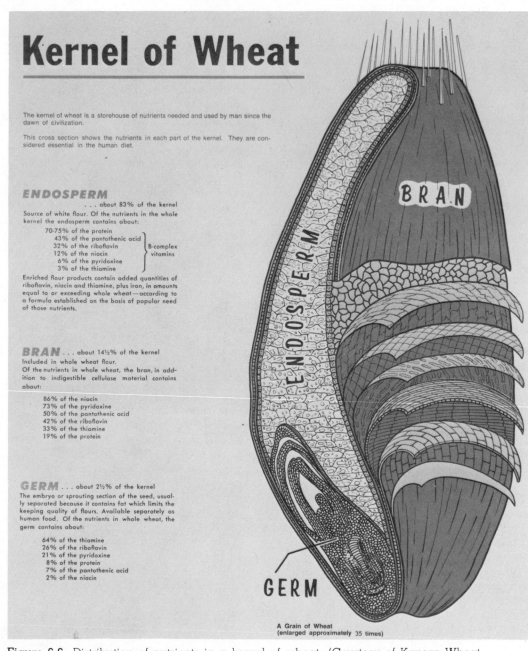

Kernel of Wheat

The kernel of wheat is a storehouse of nutrients needed and used by man since the dawn of civilization.

This cross section shows the nutrients in each part of the kernel. They are considered essential in the human diet.

ENDOSPERM

... about 83% of the kernel

Source of white flour. Of the nutrients in the whole kernel the endosperm contains about:

70-75% of the protein
43% of the pantothenic acid
32% of the riboflavin   } B-complex
12% of the niacin   vitamins
6% of the pyridoxine
3% of the thiamine

Enriched flour products contain added quantities of riboflavin, niacin and thiamine, plus iron, in amounts equal to or exceeding whole wheat—according to a formula established on the basis of popular need of those nutrients.

BRAN ... about 14½% of the kernel

Included in whole wheat flour.
Of the nutrients in whole wheat, the bran, in addition to indigestible cellulose material contains about:

86% of the niacin
73% of the pyridoxine
50% of the pantothenic acid
42% of the riboflavin
33% of the thiamine
19% of the protein

GERM ... about 2½% of the kernel

The embryo or sprouting section of the seed, usually separated because it contains fat which limits the keeping quality of flours. Available separately as human food. Of the nutrients in whole wheat, the germ contains about:

64% of the thiamine
26% of the riboflavin
21% of the pyridoxine
8% of the protein
7% of the pantothenic acid
2% of the niacin

BRAN

ENDOSPERM

GERM

A Grain of Wheat
(enlarged approximately 35 times)

Figure 6-6. Distribution of nutrients in a kernel of wheat. (Courtesy of Kansas Wheat Commission of Wheat Flour Institute)

Enrichment, though once a federal law, has been left to the state for enforcement. Although in 1971 only 30 states had enacted enrichment legislation, most of the bread sold in the United States has been enriched. Figure 6-7 shows a comparison of enriched bread and whole wheat bread. It can be seen that enriched bread is higher in some nutrients than whole wheat bread. Enriched white bread may surpass some of the wheat breads sold because these often are made from a combination of some whole wheat flour and unenriched white flour. If whole wheat bread is desired there must be careful reading of the labels to determine the type of flour used.

Although the enrichment of such products as rice, macaroni, spaghetti, and noodles is not required, these products usually are enriched. Some rolls and baked products sold in the food market may be prepared using un-enriched white flour, and only by reading the label will their content be known.

RELATIVE PROPORTIONS OF NUTRIENTS SUPPLIED BY THE BASIC FOUR FOOD GROUPS

To summarize all this information on the vitamin and mineral content of foods, let us turn again to the basic four food groups. Figure 6-5 shows the relative percentages of nutrients provided by each of the basic four food groups. From this figure it can readily be seen which groups contribute the highest percentages of a selected nutrient, and from that specific food sources can be recalled.

The nutrients provided by the minimum recommended servings from the basic four food groups can be evaluated using both the

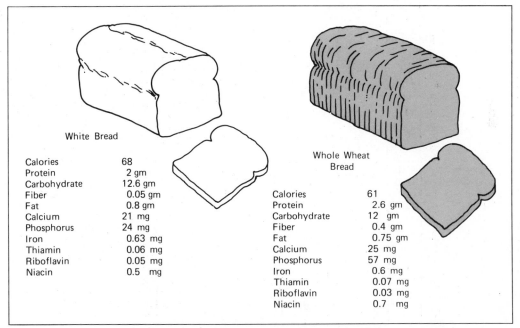

White Bread

Calories	68
Protein	2 gm
Carbohydrate	12.6 gm
Fiber	0.05 gm
Fat	0.8 gm
Calcium	21 mg
Phosphorus	24 mg
Iron	0.63 mg
Thiamin	0.06 mg
Riboflavin	0.05 mg
Niacin	0.5 mg

Whole Wheat Bread

Calories	61
Protein	2.6 gm
Carbohydrate	12 gm
Fiber	0.4 gm
Fat	0.75 gm
Calcium	25 mg
Phosphorus	57 mg
Iron	0.6 mg
Thiamin	0.07 mg
Riboflavin	0.03 mg
Niacin	0.7 mg

Figure 6-7. Nutrient comparison between enriched white bread and whole wheat bread. (Values from *Composition of Foods* (1963). Agriculture Handbook No. 8, rev. USDA, 1963.

TABLE 6-10. Leader Nutrients Supplied by Minimum Servings of the Basic Four

	Serving	Protein (gm)	Vitamin A (IU)	Vitamin C (mg)	Thiamine (mg)	Riboflavin (mg)	Niacin (mg)	Calcium (mg)	Iron (mg)
Ready-to-eat cereal	1 oz	3	1,180	9	0.29	0.35	2.9	44	2.9
Milk	1 cup	8	300	2	0.09	0.41	0.3	280	6
Orange juice	½ cup	0.5	135	57	0.075	0.01	0.01	10	0.1
Egg	1 lg	6	260	—	0.04	0.15	tr	28	1.0
Peanut butter	2 T	8	—	—	0.04	0.04	4.8	18	0.6
Bread, whole wheat	2 slice	6	tr	tr	0.18	0.06	1.6	48	1.6
Margarine	1 t	—	170	—	—	—	—	1	—
Jelly	1 T	—	—	1	—	0.01	tr	4	0.3
Apple, fresh	1	—	120	6	0.04	0.03	0.1	10	0.4
Cheese, Cheddar	1 slice	7	300	—	0.01	0.11	tr	204	0.2
Ham	2 oz	12	—	—	0.26	0.10	1.0	5	1.4
Broccoli	1 cup	6	4,500	162	0.16	0.36	1.4	158	1.4
Rice, enriched	1 cup	4	—	—	0.21	0.02	1.7	5	1.3
Pears	½ cup	0.5	5	1.5	0.015	0.025	0.15	6.5	0.25
Ice cream	½ cup	2.5	270	0.5	0.025	0.165	0.05	88	0.05
Totals		63.5	7,240	233	1.4	1.84	14.35	909.5	12.1
RDA for a woman 19–22		44	4,000 (800 R.E.)	60	1.1	1.3	14	800	18

SOURCE: Values from *Nutritive Value of Foods*, Home & Garden Bull. No. 72, rev., US Department of Agriculture, Washington, D.C., 1977.

RDA and the US-RDA. Table 6-10 shows a daily food intake based on the minimum recommended servings from the basic four. The minimum servings from the basic four do meet the RDA for all of the leader nutrients except iron. The minimum recommended servings from the basic four do not provide adequate quantities of several of the attendant nutrients, specifically magnesium, zinc, folacin, vitamin B_6, and vitamin E, but selecting a different variety of foods each day and eating dark-green leafy vegetables and whole grain breads and cereals will increase this intake. Also the RDAs for these nutrients have only recently been established, and they may be higher than necessary. Using vegetable oils daily for cooking or on a salad will greatly increase the intake of vitamin E.

Another interesting and practical way to evaluate the minimum servings from the basic four food groups is to use the US-RDA, the new standard for food labeling. Table 6-11 analyzes the minimum recommended servings from the basic four in terms of the percentages of the US-RDA for the leader nutrients supplied by the foods. It is readily apparent from the totals that the percentages for all the nutrients do not total 100%. To evaluate the adequacy of these percentages, the information in Table 6-6 must be used. Recall that the US-RDA is an optimal standard based on the highest RDA for any individual 4 years of age or older. The nutritional requirements of a woman aged 19–22 are not as high as those of a child or teenager, and therefore, she does not need to consume 100% of all the nutrients when the US-RDA is used as the standard. Table 6-6 provided the specific percentages for each nutrient for separate stages in the life cycle. Using the woman aged 19–22 as an example and comparing the percentages provided by the food with those needed by the woman, it is observed that the basic four provides the proper amounts of all the nutrients except for iron.

It will be noticed that a few percentages in Table 6-6 are over 100%. This is because the US-RDA standard was developed using the

TABLE 6-11. Percentages of US-RDA for Leader Nutrients Supplied by Minimum Servings from the Basic Four

	Serving	Protein	Vitamin A	Vitamin C	Thiamine	Riboflavin	Niacin	Calcium	Iron
Ready-to-eat cereal	1 oz	4	20	20	25	25	20		20
Milk	1 cup	20	6	4	4	24		30	
Orange juice	½ cup	1	5	100	8	1	2	1	1
Egg	1 lg	15	10		2	8		2	6
Peanut butter	2 T	16			4	1	2	1	1
Bread, whole wheat	2 slice	8			12	4	8	4	8
Margarine	1 pat		4						
Jelly	1 T			2					2
Apple, fresh	1		2	10	2	2			2
Cheese, cheddar	1 slice	15	8			8		20	2
Ham	2 oz	120			70	30	50	4	40
Broccoli	1 cup	8	90	270	10	20	6	4	40
Rice, enriched	1 cup	6			15	2	8		8
Pears	½ cup			2	1	1	1	1	1
Ice Cream	½ cup	8	6	1	2	8		10	
Totals		221	151	1,109	155	134	97	88	99
Goal for a woman 19–22		75	80	75	75	85	35	80	100

SOURCE: Values from E. Peterkin, J. Nicholas, and C. Cromwell, *Nutrition Labeling: Tools for Its Use*, Agricultural Information Bull. No. 382, USDA, 1975.

1968 revision of the Recommended Dietary Allowances. A few of the RDAs in the 1979 revision were increased, causing a few percentages to be over 100. The FDA will not make changes in the US-RDA until the changes in the RDA are enough to warrant it. This is quite understandable and practical when one considers the millions of labels that would have to be reprinted, just to update the US-RDA each time there was a revised edition of the RDA.

King and colleagues (1978) conducted a study in which 20 published full-day menus planned using the basic four food groups were analyzed for nutritional adequacy. These menus met or exceeded the RDA for most of the nutrients, although they provided only 60% or less of the 1974 RDA for vitamin E, vitamin B_6, magnesium, zinc, and iron. As a result these researchers proposed a modified basic four that recommended the inclusion of two servings of animal protein and two servings of legumes or nuts. They also recommended the inclusion of one serving of a dark-green vegetable daily instead of every other day. They also advised the inclusion of four servings of whole grain cereal products daily because whole grain products are slightly higher in some of the nutrients found to be low. Modifications of the basic four were also computed for special food preferences. For example, if milk were excluded, the servings of meat and dark-green vegetables were increased. Likewise, if no animal protein were to be consumed, the servings of milk should be increased. A special modification was made for low cost, which decreased the total servings from the milk and meat groups and increased the servings of whole grain cereal products to nine.

VITAMIN SUPPLEMENTATION

A fitting closing to this chapter seems to be a discussion of vitamin and mineral supplementation of the daily diet. People in the United States spend $500 million annually on vitamin and mineral supplements. Why do the people living in this country with the greatest variety and abundance of food on earth spend this incredible amount of money on vitamin preparations? Unfortunately, part of the reason may lie in the emphasis on vitamin and mineral requirements and specific functions of each nutrient. Because of a higher level of education, most people are exposed to information about nutrient functions and requirements in high school or college courses; but this knowledge is often not presented adequately and is usually not taught by a qualified nutritionist. People then believe that all these nutrients with their specific requirements and functions could not possibly be obtained from ordinary foods. So many people, encouraged in this thinking by food faddists, faithfully consume their vitamin pill, sometimes referred to as the "great American placebo." They take vitamin pills to play it safe or as a nutritional insurance policy against any possible nutritional deficiency.

Vitamin Supplement Myths

It is simply a myth that ordinary foods will not supply adequate vitamins and minerals to the diet. The foods, of course, must be consumed in amounts recommended by a reliable nutritional standard such as the basic four food groups.

Vitamin supplements have been said to improve one's immunity to illness. This may be true for an undernourished person, but there is insufficient reason to believe it is true for the well nourished. Contrary to popular belief, a vitamin supplement will not provide an extra amount of energy or help to "relieve that tired feeling." If a person experiences any of these benefits, it is probably because of the placebo effect of the vitamin.

Vitamin Preparations

First of all it must be pointed out that there is no difference between natural and synthetic vitamins. All vitamins are chemicals whether natural or synthetic, and the body cannot tell the difference. The only difference is that the natural vitamins cost a lot more.

The three major types of vitamin supplements available are the regular vitamin preparations, therapeutic supplements, and high-potency preparations of individual vitamins or special combinations of a selected few.

It is interesting to note that vitamins is all that vitamin supplements usually contain. Yet the analysis of the recommended servings from the four food groups in terms of the RDA showed that several of the minerals—iron, calcium, magnesium, and zinc—were low when compared to the RDA; most of the vitamins were present in the recommended levels except that small quantities of some of the B-complex group were low. From this analysis it seems just as important that minerals be present in the vitamin preparation. Many vitamin preparations do add iron, which is probably good because the RDA for iron for the woman of childbearing age cannot be met by the basic four.

The therapeutic vitamins often contain 5–10 times the recommended levels of the nutrients. For this reason these vitamin supplements should be classed as a drug and used in that manner. According to the new food-labeling law any product containing over 150% of the US-RDA for any nutrient must be considered a drug. These products are still available over the counter, but nutritionists long for the day when they will be sold by prescription only. These vitamins are very expensive and generally a waste of money except in special cases when prescribed by a doctor. The levels of nutrients contained are greatly in excess of the body's need. The excess of water-soluble vitamins will simply be excreted in the urine with generally no harm to the body; the excesses of fat-soluble vitamins, however, are stored. There are toxic symptoms that can result from excessive intakes, particularly of vitamin A and D.

Another important fact deserves close attention. The high quantities of some vitamins provided by supplements can alter the requirements for other nutrients. There is a delicate balance required among levels of nutrients. This delicate balance is present in foods, but with vitamin supplements man often creates an unnatural balance that might actually be harmful. Take as an example that the high level of one of the B-complex vitamins contained in the therapeutic vitamin supplement increases the requirement for one of the minerals that is already low in the average diet. This is going to increase the need for that mineral even more. A true-life example of this principle was seen in a man who lived in Florida for about a year. While he was there he consumed huge quantities of citrus fruit daily and therefore a large quantity of vitamin C. After he returned to live in one of the northern states, he developed scurvy (vitamin C deficiency) after a few weeks. He was now only consuming about one glass of orange juice daily. His very high daily intake of vitamin C while he lived in Florida temporarily increased his vitamin C requirement so that a lower intake that is adequate for most people and provides the RDA was inadequate for him because his nutritional requirement for this vitamin had been increased. Because enough is not known yet about imbalances in nutrient intakes, extreme caution should be exercised in using therapeutic vitamin preparations.

Indications of Need for Vitamin Supplementation

Lest the view of vitamin supplements be too negative, there are stages in the life cycle and circumstances when vitamin supplements are advisable. The times when a vitamin supplement is needed is during growth, when there is decreased food intake or poor food selection, and during the stress of certain illnesses or diseases.

Supplemental vitamins are needed during

infancy and often recommended during childhood. During the childbearing years women who are using the birth control pill may be advised to take a vitamin supplement, as the pill may increase the requirement for vitamin B_6 and folic acid in some women. The routine administration of a vitamin and iron supplement during pregnancy and lactation is quite common.

A vitamin supplement may be a wise choice for people with a reduced intake of food or poor selection of food. For those who are on a weight-reducing diet of less than 1,200 Calories/day, a vitamin supplement is generally recommended because it is quite difficult to obtain adequate nutrients in that reduced quantity of food. It *may* be desirable for college students to take a vitamin supplement, however this is not necessarily true. The student's own personal eating habits should first be examined carefully. If the student comes close to meeting the minimum servings from the basic four, a vitamin supplement is probably not needed. On the other hand, there are students, and others as well, who have no real interest in food, who eat sporadically from vending machines, and who give no thought to the kinds of foods they eat. These people, too, should be consuming a vitamin supplement.

Because the specific nutritional requirements of people undergoing the severe stress of disease and injury are not known, many patients or clients in these circumstances would benefit from a nutritional supplement. Examples would be clients recovering from surgery, those who are severely burned, and those with malabsorption disorders. Also the nutritional status of chronic alcoholics is often poor from the substitution of alcohol for food. More specific information about these conditions and the types of supplements recommended are found in Unit V of this book.

General Recommendations

Before deciding to invest in a vitamin supplement, a person should very carefully assess his own usual dietary habits. Recording all the food eaten for one week and placing the foods into the appropriate food group gives an excellent picture of overall food intake. Careful examination should also be made of all the enriched and fortified foods being consumed and the percentages of the US-RDA supplied by these foods. The person may find that he is consuming a cereal daily that has been fortified with vitamins and minerals to meet 100% of the US-RDA. Why take a vitamin pill that also supplies 100% of the US-RDA? The contributions that enriched and fortified foods and whole grain breads and cereals make to a daily nutrient intake may often be equivalent to a vitamin supplement.

After this careful assessment of dietary intake is made and before the final decision to take a vitamin supplement daily is made, three points should be considered: First, there is no need to select a vitamin supplement that contains more than 100% of the US-RDA for the nutrients contained. Excess intakes of vitamins and minerals above the RDA or over 100% of the US-RDA do not provide any additional beneficial effects; and if the content of vitamins A and D is quite high, toxicity symptoms may even result. Second, for women of childbearing age a vitamin that contains iron should be selected over one that does not contain iron because of the higher RDA for iron during these years. Third, for best utilization a vitamin supplement should be taken with a meal. Vitamins function as coenzymes or partners in the metabolism of carbohydrate, protein, and fat. If a vitamin supplement is taken in the morning with only a glass of water and no food, the vitamins will be poorly utilized.

BIBLIOGRAPHY

Arlin, M. J. *The Science of Nutrition.* 2nd Ed. New York: Macmillan, Inc., 1977.

Food and Nutrition Board, Nat'l Research Council. *Recommended Dietary Allowances.* 9th Ed. Washington, D.C., Nat'l Acad. of Sciences, 1980.

Guthrie, H. A. *Introductory Nutrition.* 4th Ed. St. Louis: The C. V. Mosby Co., 1979.

Hansen, R. G., Wipe, B. W., and Sorenson, A. W. Using the INQ to evaluate foods. *Nutrition News* (National Dairy Council) 42(1): 1979.

King, J. C., Cohensour, S. H., Corruccini, C. G., and Schneeman, P. Evaluation and modification of the basic four food guide. *J. Nutr. Educ.* 10(1):27, 1978.

Krause, M. V., and Mahan, L. K. *Food, Nutrition, and Diet Therapy.* 6th Ed. Philadelphia: W. B. Saunders Co., 1979.

Nat'l Dairy Council. *Nutrition Source Book.* Rosemont, Ill., 1978.

Peterkin, B., Nicholas, J., and Cromwell, C. *Nutrition Labeling: Tools For Its Use.* Consumer and Food Economics

Instit., Agricultural. Research Serv. Bull. No. 382. Washington, D.C.: U.S. Dept. of Agriculture, 1975.

Robinson, C. H., and Lawler, M. R. *Normal and Therapeutic Nutrition.* 15th Ed. New York: Macmillan, Inc., 1977.

Wagner, A. F. and Folkers, K. *Vitamins and Coenzymes.* New York: Interscience, 1964.

Williams, S. R. *Nutrition and Diet Therapy.* 3rd Ed. St. Louis: The C. V. Mosby Co., 1977.

Wilson, E. D., Fisher, K. H., and Garcia, P. A. *Principles of Nutrition.* 4th Ed. New York: John Wiley & Sons, Inc., Pubs., 1979.

Wittwer, A. J., Sorenson, A. W., Wipe, B. W., and Hansen, R. G. Nutrient density: Evaluation of nutritional attributes of foods. *J. Nutr. Educ.* 9(1):26, 1977.

CHAPTER 7

Nutritional Concerns in North America

During the last decade the word *malnutrition* has come to mean overnutrition as well as undernutrition. There has been an increased awareness of the relationship of nutrition to health and therefore a surging interest in the subject of nutrition, which has had positive effects. This heightened interest has, however, provided the food faddist with a susceptible audience for his half-truths.

This chapter examines the nutritional status of people in the United States and their nutritional practices. Nutritional status in Canada is also discussed.

NUTRITIONAL STATUS IN THE UNITED STATES

Nutritional status is the physical condition of the body resulting from the utilization of ingested nutrients from food. Nutritional status influences a person's level of health. Good nutritional status is evident when a person benefits from the consumption of all the essential nutrients from a well-balanced diet. Adequate body reserves of certain nutrients are also present. Poor nutritional status is evident when a person is deprived of an adequate proportion of one or more nutrients or of Calories over a period of time. Nutritional status is influenced not only by the ingestion of nutrients from food but by increased nutritional requirements or interferences with digestion, absorption, utilization, or excretion of nutrients.

Nutritional status is measured by a combined examination of dietary intake, physical signs, and laboratory measurements. Whether nutritional status is applied to individual subjects or to an entire population or nation, the assessment techniques are the same. A discussion of the components of nutritional assessment is presented in Chapter 19.

Poor nutritional status eventually results in a state of malnutrition. *Malnutrition,* simply defined, means poor or bad nutrition. It results from either a deficiency or an excess of nutrients. This broad definition of *malnutrition* includes not only nutritional deficiency diseases and starvation (undernutrition) but nutritional excesses such as obesity and certain vitamin toxicities.

Concern about the nutritional status of people living in the United States was aroused by the CBS television documentary "Hunger in America" broadcast during May 1968. During the preceding month a private group, the Citizens' Board of Inquiry into Hunger and Malnutrition, had released their report "Hunger U.S.A." estimating that 10 million Americans were malnourished or underfed. The criticism of this report was that it was based on testimony and opinion and not on hard facts. As a result of this report the US Senate Select Committee on Nutrition and Human Needs was formed, the White House Conference on Food, Nutrition, and Health convened in 1969, and three large nutritional surveys have been conducted.

Food Surveys

USDA Household Food Consumption Surveys
Since 1936 the US Department of Agriculture has conducted five surveys to evaluate

food consumption patterns in the United States. These surveys are based on a representative sample from the entire population. The adequacy of the diets is evaluated using the RDA as the standard. A diet was rated as good if it contained nutrient levels equal to or exceeding the RDA. A poor diet was defined as one that provided less than two-thirds of the RDA for one or more nutrients.

A comparison between the 1955 and 1965 surveys revealed that the quality of the American diet had not improved but had actually decreased. In 1955, 15% of all diets were considered poor, but in 1965 the proportion of poor diets was 20%. During these 10 years the changes in food consumption were that less milk and milk products, grain and cereal products, and fruits and vegetables were consumed while more meat, fish, and poultry; baked foods; and snack foods were consumed. The nutrients most often low were vitamins A and C, calcium, and iron (Adelson and Peterkin, 1968).

This decline in dietary quality raised some concern and seemed to support some of the findings of the Citizens' Board of Inquiry. It should be pointed out, however, that the USDA surveys use only dietary data and their criteria for a good or poor diet is based on the RDA. Diets containing nutrient levels below the RDA are not necessarily deficient because of the differences in nutrient requirements among people and the margin of safety included in the RDA to allow for these differences. When nutrient intakes are consistently below two-thirds of the RDA for a population over a prolonged period of time, the likelihood is greater that some people may manifest signs of deficiency.

The Nationwide Food Consumption Survey of 1977–78, conducted by the US Department of Agriculture, revealed some interesting findings. Caloric intakes of all age groups were lower between 1965 and 1977, with an accompanying decrease in the dietary intakes of carbohydrate, protein, and fat. Average intakes of vitamins and minerals met or exceeded the 1974 RDA with the exception of calcium, iron, magnesium, and vitamin B_6. The amount of calcium consumed decreased especially for infants, children, and teenagers. The average iron intakes were higher for infants, but about the same as for adult females in 1965. With respect to actual food consumed, there was a decrease in the quantity of vegetables used, primarily because of a decreased use of potatoes at home. The use of dark green vegetables increased as did the use of fruits, especially citrus fruits. The carbohydrate intake declined because of decreased consumption of breads and cereals, milk products, and concentrated sweets such as sugar, syrup, jelly, and candy. The intake of soft drinks, sugar desserts, and punches, however, increased. A decreased intake of fat was reflected by decreased use of fats, oils, milk products, bacon, and luncheon meats. The total quantity of protein foods consumed remained the same, but the amount of beef, poultry, fish, and nuts increased and the consumption of pork, luncheon meat, eggs, and dry beans decreased (Pao and Cronin, 1980).

Numerous studies of nutritional status were conducted between 1947 and 1967, but only a limited number had involved a sampling method to represent the entire population. Release of the data from the 1965 USDA Household Food Consumption Survey at approximately the same time as the Citizens' Board of Inquiry report pointed to the need for more comprehensive nutrition surveys that not only examined dietary intake but included a clinical examination and laboratory data. Three such surveys have been conducted since 1968. In December 1969 the White House Conference on Food, Nutrition, and Health was held out of concern for malnutrition among the poor and the concerns about food and nutrition in the entire nation. The US Department of Health, Education, and Welfare initiated the three nutrition surveys. The Ten-State Nutrition Survey and the Preschool Nutrition Survey were both begun in 1968. The Health and Nutrition Examination Survey (HANES) was conducted between 1971 and 1974. It is intended as an ongoing survey to monitor the nutritional status of the US population.

Ten-State Nutrition Survey

The purpose of the Ten-State Nutrition Survey was to determine the extent and location of malnutrition in the United States among the low-income segment of the population. The survey focused on families living below or slightly above the poverty level in 10 states (Kentucky, Louisiana, South Carolina, Texas, West Virginia, California, Massachusetts, Michigan, New York, and Washington). There were 40,000 participants in this evaluation of nutritional status. Half of those who participated were under 16 years of age. The largest percentage of the sample was white, followed by black, and the smallest percentage was Spanish-American. The four major assessments were (1) a detailed clinical examination including medical history, physical examination, *anthropometric measurements,* hand skeleton roentgenograms, and dental examination; (2) laboratory data on blood and urine samples to identify levels of nutrients; (3) detailed dietary data including actual foods consumed, frequency of use, dietary patterns, and food preparation facilities; and (4) socioeconomic factors.

The results revealed that a significant proportion of the population studied was malnourished or was at a high risk for developing nutritional problems. Evidence of malnutrition was found most commonly among the black population. There was also increasing evidence of malnutrition as income level declined, but there was a positive relationship between the number of years of education and nutritional status. Retarded growth and development were evidenced by the number of underweight and undersized children and adolescents. Adolescents had the highest prevalance of unsatisfactory nutritional status.

Male adolescents displayed even more evidences of malnutrition than females.

With respect to specific nutrients there was a high prevalence of iron deficiency anemia as evidenced by low hemoglobin and *hematocrit* values in all segments of the population, including adolescent and adult males. A large number of pregnant and lactating women had low levels of serum albumin even though dietary intake of protein seemed to be adequate. The Mexican-Americans in Texas had very low intakes of vitamin A as did the young people in all subgroups. Although there was no major problem with vitamin C intakes, low levels of vitamin C were more prevalent among men. The prevalence of poor vitamin C status increased with age (US Department of Health, Education, and Welfare, 1973).

Preschool Nutrition Survey

The US Preschool Nutrition Survey was conducted from 1968 to 1970. It involved 3,441 children aged 1–6 from 74 cities or residential areas in 37 states. There were 52% boys and 48% girls. The children were 80% white; 14% black; 5% Spanish-American; and 1% American Indian, Oriental, or other. The families of the children were classified into a socioeconomic rank, rank I being the lowest and rank IV the highest.

The data gathered and analyzed was dietary, biochemical (laboratory), and clinical. The methods for gathering the data were patterned after those in the Ten-State Nutrition Survey. Separate results were reported from the dietary, clinical, and biochemical data. It was not always possible to correlate the data from these three sources. A number of children had abnormal physical examinations, but there was essentially no correlation between these abnormal physical findings and the dietary or biochemical data. Only selected results from the dietary and biochemical data are presented here.

The protein intake per 1,000 Calories showed little difference with respect to age, sex, or socioeconomic status. The serum albumin levels remained essentially constant except that black children had slightly lower concentrations than white children. The black children's average iron intake was slightly higher than that of the white children, but the levels of iron stores (*transferrin saturation*) were generally higher in the whites than in the blacks. Average calcium intake of black children was less than that of white children. There was also a progressive decrease in the use of dairy products with increasing age in all socioeconomic groups, particularly in the lowest socioeconomic class and in black children. Also as socioeconomic level increased, fruits contributed more Calories and nutrients than vegetables to the children's diets. The intake of ascorbic acid (vitamin C) was consistently lower for black children than for white children. Plasma vitamin C levels were also consistently higher in white children than in black children. White children had consistently higher plasma levels of retinol (vitamin A) than black children, but these values did not correlate well with dietary intakes of vitamin A (Owen, et al., 1974).

Health and Nutrition Examination Survey

The most recent national nutritional survey is the Health and Nutrition Examination Survey (HANES). This survey is the United States's first attempt at continual nutritional monitoring of the nutritional status of its citizens. It is part of the National Health Survey Act of 1956, which is administered by the National Center for Health Statistics. Dietary data was obtained from a national sample of 20,749 civilian noninstitutionalized people aged 1–74 living in the United States. Nutritional status was assessed by physical examination, body measurements, laboratory data, and dietary intake information.

The dietary data is reported as mean nutrient intake expressed as percentages above or below the nutrient standard for various ages, sexes, and income levels. The nutrient standard was derived from consideration of daily allowances of the World Health Organization, the Interdepartmental Committee on Nutrition for National Defense, and the Recommended Dietary Allowances. The mean nutritive intake was recorded for Calories, protein, calcium, iron, thiamine, riboflavin, and vitamins A and C.

The nutrient reported most often to be below the nutrient standard in all population groups was iron. This was especially true in all age groups of white and black women through age 54. The only men in both races with iron intakes below the standard were boys aged 1–3, white men aged 15–19, and black boys aged 4–5 and 15–17 in the lower income groups. Black men aged 15–19 in the upper income groups were also below the standard.

As a whole, mean protein intake for all age groups of both races approached or exceeded the nutrient standard in all income groups. A few categories where intakes were below the standard were black men aged 55–64 in the lower income group and those over 65 in both income groups. Intakes of protein below the nutrient standard for women were found in the lower income groups of white women aged 15–17 and over 55. Black women aged 35–44 and over 55 years in both income groups had protein intakes below the standard (Abraham, Lowenstein, and Johnson, 1974; Abraham, Lowenstein, and O'Connell, 1975).

The other nutrients showed even less evidence of inadequacy. Only a few groups showed any deviation from the standard in mean intakes of calcium, vitamins A and C, thiamine, and riboflavin. It must be emphasized, however, that the HANES data reports only mean or average intakes for a population group. There is a much greater variability in individual intakes than is revealed by the mean. Some subjects have very high intakes and others very low intakes of each nutrient. The mean does not reflect these extremes but only the average intakes. The mean, however, is of some value in identifying certain population groups with low intake. The clinical data and laboratory data have been gathered, but they have not been analyzed in conjunction with the dietary data. Until all the data is analyzed and interpreted together, very little can actually be concluded about any relationship to malnutrition. The student is reminded that low dietary intakes do not necessarily indicate the presence of malnutrition.

Malnutrition in the United States

After this examination of the major nutritional surveys, what can be said concerning the existence of malnutrition in the United States? The broad definition of *malnutrition* simply is any disorder of nutrition resulting from either a lack or an excess of nutrients—either undernutrition or overnutrition. Malnutrition is either primary, resulting from an inadequate ingestion of the essential nutrients from food, or secondary, resulting from a physiological interference with digestion, absorption, or utilization of the essential nutrients. It must be emphasized that malnutrition develops over a period of time and in a well-defined series of steps. The three major sources of data used in the large nutrition studies were selected to determine the correlation between the data, if any, and the extent of malnutrition.

In the course of the development of malnutrition, the first level of detection is low dietary intake of one or more nutrients. If the low dietary intake is continued, the body's stores of the nutrient will become depleted. This reduction will be evident in reduced laboratory values for the specific nutrient. Some nutrients are depleted quite easily because they are not stored by the body; other nutrients are depleted slowly because they are stored; and a few nutrients remain at normal blood levels over a wide range of dietary intakes. The criteria for assessing blood and

urine is found in Chapter 19, where the process of nutritional assessment is discussed. The third and final stage in the development of malnutrition is the appearance of the physical sign or symptom. It is important to understand this sequence in the development of malnutrition for a better appreciation of the findings from the three major national nutrition surveys.

Undernutrition

To interpret the findings from the national nutrition surveys objectively, it is first necessary to notice the characteristics of the sample and the size. The USDA Household Food Consumption Survey was a representative sample of 15,000 subjects living in the United States. The Ten-State Nutrition Survey, by contrast, involved 70,000 subjects from low-income areas in 10 states. The Preschool Nutrition Survey included about 3,400 children aged 1–6 from several socioeconomic backgrounds. The most recent nutritional survey, the HANES, used a representative sample of about 30,000 people aged 1–74 from 34 states and the District of Columbia. Although the Ten-State Nutrition Survey is the largest survey attempted so far, the results were specifically for the poor. A comparable study has not been attempted on people living above the poverty level. Concern about the existence of malnutrition among the poor provided the impetus for this survey. The results should not be used in statements about the nutritional status of the entire population of the United States. The Council on Foods and Nutrition of the American Medical Association (1970) stated that there is actually no reliable estimate of the extent of hunger or malnutrition in the United States.

The USDA Household Food Consumption Survey and the HANES are both representative samples of the US population. Even though the sample size is considerably smaller the Ten-State Nutrition Survey, it is still large enough by statistical standards to provide a representative view of the nutritional status of the population. The Preschool Nutrition Survey used the smallest sample but was designed specifically to examine the nutritional status of the preschool population aged 1–6. Other factors determined the reliability of a research study, such as the methods of investigation selected and the training and consistency of the interviewers, though only the size and characteristics of the sample have been mentioned here.

The three major nutrition surveys all gathered dietary data, laboratory data, and clinical signs. When considering these results the student should keep in mind the stages in the development of malnutrition. A low dietary intake of a particular nutrient without the corresponding low laboratory value or the clinical sign is not too much reason for concern. A low dietary intake accompanied by reduced blood levels of the nutrient is more reason for concern. Low dietary intake accompanied by both reduced blood or urine levels and a clinical sign in a given population segment is reason for great concern.

An actual example may help to clarify these points. If the dietary intake of a specific population group is low in iron, that is, the intake of iron by that population does not meet the RDA, but neither low hemoglobin nor hematocrit blood values are evident and there are no physical signs of iron deficiency anemia, there is not much cause for concern. The conclusion that can be drawn from this data is simply that the dietary intake of iron is low in this population group compared to the RDA. If the situation remains the same, the population group *may* be in danger of developing iron deficiency anemia. Therefore, a careful consideration of all categories of data is needed with special attention to correlated findings between or among categories.

SPECIFIC POPULATIONS AT RISK. Although the Ten-State Nutrition Survey was biased toward those with low incomes, it did serve to identify specific populations at a nutritional risk. Schaefer (1977) identifies the very poor, the migrant workers, and the American Indians as groups most vulnerable to malnutrition. The specific stages of the life cycle at a greater nutritional risk are pregnancy, preschool, adolescence, and old age. People at any one of these life-cycle stages who are very poor, migrant workers, or American Indians are at an even greater nutritional risk. Some researchers also include infants in this high-risk category.

Identification of these high-risk groups through the national nutrition surveys has led to new or expanded nutritional screening programs and food assistance programs for these groups as well as to an increased emphasis on nutritional education. For example, the Federal Food Stamp program was expanded in 1971 to include the elderly. Also, the National School Lunch Program was expanded in 1966 to include breakfast for many children. A new federally funded program called Women, Infants, and Children (WIC) was begun in 1972 to supply commodity food to pregnant women and then to their newborn infants and young children until the age of 4. Many elderly citizens have been able to obtain a nutritional meal at least once a day through such programs as Meals on Wheels.

MALNUTRITION IN OUR HOSPITALS. Another group very vulnerable to malnutrition are hospitalized clients. This phenomenon had long been ignored, but it was dramatically brought to the attention of the medical profession by Butterworth in 1974 in his article "The Skeleton in the Hospital Closet." Since this announcement there has been an increased emphasis on identification of malnourished clients through improved methods of nutritional assessment (Blackburn et al., 1977).

Overnutrition

The United States is a nation of nutritional contrasts. There are nutritional deprivations of the poor and minority groups resulting from inadequate amounts and quality of food. There are the nutritional problems of obesity, overweight, and heart disease of many in the middle-to-upper income levels. There are the food faddists skilled at obtaining listeners and supporters for their exaggerated claims. It is by far the majority, however, who suffer from nutritional excesses (see Fig. 7-1). The high incidence of overweight, obesity, heart disease, diabetes, hypertension, and other chronic disabling diseases points toward various dietary excesses. There has been much publicity in recent years about the high incidence of these chronic diseases in our country and their relation to nutrition. A word of caution is necessary at this point: Diet is not the only factor contributing to these diseases. Heart disease, obesity, and diabetes are all multifaceted diseases with many complex precursors.

The US diet that leads to overnutrition has been labeled the "affluent diet" by Eckholm (1977). It is prevalent among those with incomes far above subsistence levels and access to a wide variety of food products. The diet contains excess Calories in relation to energy requirements, excess carbohydrate and fat, excess salt, and excess amounts of manufactured and processed foods. There may even be an excessive intake of vitamins and miner-

als, which may have a harmful effect on the body.

The fault of the affluent diet lies not in the kinds of foods eaten but in the excesses of certain foods and nutrients. No single food is necessarily hazardous, but excess amounts of many foods may be harmful over a period of time. The same is true of the nutrients of which food is composed. A certain amount of each nutrient is required daily to carry on the normal functioning of the body. The old adage If a Little Is Good, More Is Better is certainly not true with respect to nutrients. Excess amounts of some vitamins and minerals can lead to toxic symptoms, and excess amounts of fat (especially saturated fat), salt, and carbohydrates can be predisposing factors for chronic diseases.

EXCESS CALORIES.   The high percentage of the US population that is overweight or obese supports the fact that the daily caloric intake of the population is in excess of the energy expenditure in physical activity. It must be pointed out that excessive caloric intake and the resulting overweight condition plagues not only adults but a high proportion of children and teenagers.

EMPTY CALORIES.   The consumption of foods that contain high quantities of fat or sugar but very few if any other nutrients is a big problem in our society. Foods with these characteristics are referred to as containing *empty Calories;* some examples are carbonated beverages, cotton candy, candy bars, and potato chips.

Foods that contain a high proportion of either sugar or fat in relation to the other nutrients provide little to the diet except excessive Calories. Great concern over the high intake of foods with empty Calories, compared to foods with a high proportion of essential nutrients and lower Calories, prompted Jacobson (1975) to write an interesting book called *Nutrition Scoreboard* in which he pre-

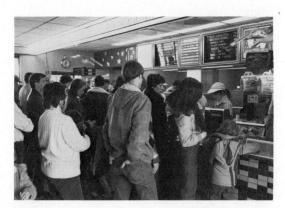

Figure 7-1. Overnutrition is the most common form of malnutrition in the United States. (Photo by J. Collins)

sents a numerical ranking system for foods based on their nutrient content. The system adds points to a food for protein content, naturally occurring carbohydrate, unsaturated fat, and essential vitamins and minerals. Points, however, are subtracted for sugar, fat, and saturated fat. The end result of this system is that each food is assigned a numerical value. Although this system has many shortcomings it does serve to emphasize the nutritional benefits of many foods over those composed primarily of empty Calories.

Another method of categorizing food is to use the concept of *nutrient density*, which is a ratio of food nutrient composition to human nutritional requirements. This concept was explained in the previous chapter using the INQ. The student will recall that foods high in fat and sugar suffer nutrient dilution and have a lower INQ (Hansen et al., 1979).

Consumption of foods containing empty Calories depresses the appetite for other more nutritious foods. If the intake of the empty-Calorie foods is high over a period of time, a person's nutritional status may be in danger because of a low intake of essential vitamins and minerals. If the total Calories contained in the daily intake is higher than the Calories required, the person will gain weight. Thus the person may be both undernourished (because of low intake of vitamins and minerals) and overnourished (because of excess Calories) at the same time.

EXCESS SATURATED FAT AND CHOLESTEROL. The relationship between high dietary intakes of *saturated fat* and *cholesterol* and the increased incidence of coronary heart disease has been the subject of much debate and publicity since the 1960s when the first reports of the classic Framingham Heart Study were published. Although all the necessary conclusive data is not in and some studies with conflicting results can still be found, there is enough data to show that there is a definite correlation between high dietary intakes of saturated fat and choles-

terol and an increased risk of coronary heart disease. Statements to this effect have been made not only by the American Heart Association but by the American Medical Association and the American Dietetic Association.

The US diet is characteristically high in saturated fats and cholesterol. Consider a favorite meal eaten out in a restaurant: a large steak with a large baked potato with lots of butter (possibly margarine), and sour cream. Adults who grew up on a farm became accustomed to large quantities of beef, pork, and bacon, dairy products containing high proportions of butter fat, and eggs. These foods of course have greatly influenced current food preferences. High intakes of saturated fat and cholesterol were not as harmful to the farm population 20 or 30 years ago because farm labor was strenuous work that required a great deal of energy. Excessive weight was not as prevalent at that time because the Calories consumed were used during the day of work. Studies have shown that physical exertion (exercise) has the effect of reducing serum cholesterol. Today the high dietary intakes of saturated fat and cholesterol are more crucial for both farmer and nonfarmer. The occupation of farming is much less physically demanding today with the more sophisticated equipment and the mechanization of tasks that used to be physically demanding.

EXCESS SALT INTAKE. The average US diet also contains an excessive amount of salt. A large proportion of the food supply is highly processed, and salt is used in processing because it acts as a preservative. Large quantities of salty snack foods such as potato chips, pretzels, and snack crackers are consumed. In the past, salt was even added to baby foods, primarily because mothers preferred the taste. Fortunately the level of sodium (salt) added to baby foods has been reduced in recent years. Many people automatically add additional salt to their food at the table even before tasting it.

In recent years several researchers have begun to link the high intake of salt with high blood pressure (hypertension). Epidemiological studies in populations with a high dietary intake of salt, such as the Japanese, reveal a higher incidence of hypertension (Dahl, 1972).

The average person consumes at least 10 times more salt daily than the body actually requires. People engaged in heavy physical labor and even athletes probably do not lose as much sodium as was once thought; the body's requirement for sodium is actually quite low. In fact it is so low that there is not even a recommended allowance established for it. Almost all people could obtain adequate sodium from just the natural sodium in their foods without ever picking up a salt shaker again.

EXCESS PROTEIN.   The one nutrient that was almost never low in the dietary intakes of subjects in the three major nutritional surveys was protein. Protein intakes were generally above the recommended allowance in almost all groups studied. In the 1965/1966 USDA Household Food Consumption Survey, protein intakes ranged from about 100% to 200% of the recommended allowances.

Inadequate dietary intake of protein is generally not a problem even among the poor. The high consumption of protein is related to a high consumption of animal protein, which also happens to contain high quantities of saturated fat and cholesterol. It is known that excessive intake of protein can lead to an increased requirement for fluid and to elevated levels of *protein metabolites* in the blood. It is interesting to note that Stillman strongly recommended that large quantities of water (8 glasses, daily) be consumed in addition to other beverages when following his high-protein Quick Weight Loss Diet (Stillman and Baker, 1967).

A quick look back at the basic four food groups will serve to emphasize the excessive protein intake of most people in the United States. The recommended intake from the meat group is two (2–3 oz) servings of meat daily for a total of 4–6 oz, or the equivalent, daily. Steaks available in most restaurants are at least 4 oz and most are 8–12 oz or more. Most customers order one of the larger ones and have no difficulty eating the entire steak. Of course a portion of the steak is bone and fat, but still the person is probably receiving more than his protein allowance in one meal. Quite probably an equal portion of meat has been consumed at the noon meal. All of this still does not take into account the protein that was quite possibly consumed at breakfast, such as eggs and bacon, ham, or sausage.

REFINED FOODS.   Concern has arisen in recent years about the use of highly refined and processed foods available in supermarkets. This concern springs from two major areas: the use of refined versus whole grain breads and cereals and the effects of food additives present in refined and processed foods. The concern with the use of highly refined foods is that some of the essential vitamins and minerals that were removed during processing were not replaced during the process of enrichment. Although this is true, most of the vitamins and minerals removed and not replaced are trace nutrients plentiful in a wide variety of foods. This concern may become more relevant if research reveals more about the functions of these nutrients and recommended allowances are established. The other criticism of refined breads and cereals is that they lack the fiber (roughage) that is present naturally in whole grain products. The highly refined diet has been blamed as being a causative factor in the development of colon disease. Although extensive research has been conducted in this area, no conclusions as yet have been reached. The requirement for fiber is approximately 5–6 gm/day. A high-fiber diet may be used as a preventive measure against intestinal disease. It is not necessary to go to the extremes of a high-fiber diet, however, as suggested by food faddists.

Another interesting use of the high-fiber diet may be as a means of lowering blood levels of serum cholesterol. Many questions, however, remain to be answered about its use, such as the optimal amount of fiber, the type of fiber that is most beneficial, and the long-term effect of using a high-fiber diet.

The other area of concern about the use of refined foods is the addition of food additives, which have been linked to *hyperactivity* and *hyperkinesis* in children. This topic is discussed further in the next chapter.

EXCESS VITAMINS AND MINERALS. Another concern about excesses in the US diet is possible overconsumption of vitamins and minerals through high-potency nutritional supplements. It was first believed that only excesses of nutrients that are stored in the body could be considered toxic. Excess intakes of several other vitamins and minerals not only may cause toxic symptoms but may actually alter the metabolism of other nutrients. For example, large doses of vitamin C decrease the amount of copper that can be absorbed from food. This imbalance in turn may lead to increased levels of cholesterol in the blood (Alfin-Slater, 1979).

It was pointed out in Chapter 6 that, if the daily diet is carefully selected from the basic four food groups, vitamin or mineral supplementation is not often necessary. If a person thinks a nutritional supplement is necessary, the supplement needs to contain no more than 100% of the US-RDA for the vitamins and minerals for any amount over the RDA is simply excess and a waste of money. For certain diseases or medical conditions a physician may prescribe a specific nutritional supplement. The supplement should be used as a temporary, corrective, or therapeutic treatment of a known nutritional deficiency. This therapeutic use of a nutritional supplement should not be confused with any claims a food faddist might make about the benefits of therapeutic doses of one or more vitamins or minerals.

National Concern for Nutrition

Three major developments in the past decade have increased government concern and participation in food, nutrition, and health matters in both the United States and the world (Lee, 1978). First, as previously discussed, national concern about the existence of malnutrition in the United States led to the initiation of the Ten-State Nutrition Survey and the Preschool Nutrition Survey and to the convening of the White House Conference on Food, Nutrition, and Health in December 1969. Second, the world food shortage of the early 1970s and sharply rising food prices intensified this concern. Third, the US Senate Select Committee on Nutrition and Human Needs issued the report *Dietary Goals for the United States*.

WHITE HOUSE CONFERENCE ON FOOD, NUTRITION, AND HEALTH. The major purpose of the White House conference was to evaluate the nutritional status of Americans and to plan the criteria for a national nutrition policy (Lee, 1978). The conference brought together people interested in the political and social issues of nutrition as well as the technical and scientific issues, and it was important because it brought the issues of hunger and malnutrition to the attention of the public. It was well attended by consumer groups who wanted to see action as well as discussion. The recommendations of the conference were extensive, and they centered on the four major areas: food assistance to the poor, nutritional education, nutrition and health programs, and the regulation of food production and supply.

US SENATE SELECT COMMITTEE ON NUTRITION AND HUMAN NEEDS. The Senate Select Committee on Nutrition and Human Needs was established in 1968 in response to concern about malnutrition in the United States. This bipartisan committee, first under the direction of Senator Robert Kennedy and then Senator George McGovern, has been an active one. Even when the president chose not to act on many of the recommendations of the White House conference, this committee continued to address the problems of poverty and malnutrition. After committee hearings, a congressional directive to the US Department of Health, Education, and Welfare resulted in the two surveys already discussed (Council on Foods and Nutrition, 1970), which in turn led the secretary of Health, Education, and Welfare to initiate the HANES ongoing surveillance of nutritional status.

In 1974, at the request of the Senate Select Committee on Nutrition and Human Needs, the National Nutrition Consortium (an organization representing the American Dietetic Association, the American Society for Clinical Nutrition, the American Institute of Nutrition, and the Institute of Food Technology) issued their Guidelines for a National Nutrition Policy (National Nutrition Consortium, 1974). In February 1977 the committee proposed the *Dietary Goals for the United States.* Although these goals generated considerable discussion and debate, they are the only document that addresses the other form of malnutrition in the United States, overnutrition (Lee, 1978). These goals were revised in December 1977, and in their final form they contained seven goals with seven recommended changes in food selection and preparation. A comparison of these dietary goals and the current US diet is shown in Figure 7-2.

1. US dietary goals:

a. To avoid overweight, consume only as much energy (Calories) as is expended; if overweight, decrease energy intake and increase energy expenditure.

b. Increase the consumption of complex carbohydrates and "naturally occurring" sugars from about 28% of energy intake to about 48% of energy intake to account for 55% to 60% of the (caloric) intake.

c. Reduce overall fat consumption from approximately 40% to 30% of energy intake.

d. Reduce saturated fat consumption to account for about 10% of total energy intakes; and balance that with polyunsaturated and monounsaturated fats which should account for about 10% of energy intake each.

e. Reduce cholesterol consumption to about 300 mg a day.

f. Reduce consumption of refined and processed sugars by about 45% to account for about 10% of total energy intake.

e. Decrease consumption of salt and foods high in salt content.

2. Recommended changes in food selection and preparation:

a. Increase consumption of fruits and vegetables and whole grains.

b. Decrease consumption of animal fat and choose poultry and fish, which will reduce saturated fat.

c. Decrease consumption of foods high in total fat and partially replace saturated fat with polyunsaturated fat.

d. Except for young children, substitute low-fat and non-fat milk for whole milk and low-fat dairy products for high-fat dairy products.

e. Decrease consumption of butterfat, eggs, and other high cholesterol sources.

f. Decrease consumption of refined and processed sugars and foods high in such sugars.

g. Decrease consumption of salt and foods high in salt content. (US Senate Select Committee, 1977)

Release of the US dietary goals generated a great deal of controversy among leaders in the medical, dental, and dietetic professions. On first glance the dietary goals look quite reasonable in light of the excesses of the US diet discussed earlier in this chapter. Proponents of the dietary goals focused primarily on this aspect. In many respects the efforts of the Senate Select Committee are quite commendable; the committee did work for more than five years examining the evidence about risk factors in the American diet. Some medical doctors credited the dietary goals with bringing the effects of overconsumption and their relationship to health into the national

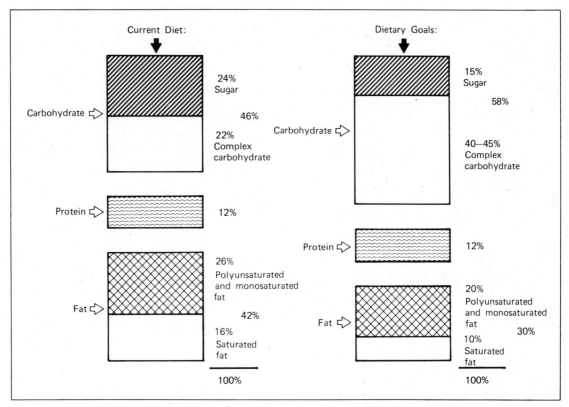

Figure 7-2. A comparison of the US dietary goals and the current US diet. (From *Dietary Goals for the United States*, 2nd Ed. Washington, D.C.: Senate Committee on Nutrition and Human Needs, 1977.)

debate ("Twenty Commentaries," 1977). The dietary goals may be a means of encouraging a more healthful daily eating pattern. Many proponents of the dietary goals endorsed them because they believe there are no identified health risks from complying with the stated recommendations of the goals: eating less meat, fat, sugar, salt, and cholesterol and eating more fruits, vegetables, unsaturated fat, and whole grain cereal products.

The opponents of the dietary goals are more concerned with the sweeping statements made about the relationship of chronic diseases (heart disease, cancer, hypertension, diabetes, obesity, and tooth decay) to dietary factors. The American Dietetic Association also came out with a somewhat more cautious statement in which they stated that, though inadequate data is available to assure that the entire population would benefit by following the dietary goals, there are many people, particularly those at risk for degenerative diseases, who would benefit. They pointed out, however, that dietary changes could not be brought about simply by governmental fiat (American Dietetic Assoc., 1977).

A select committee is formed to study a given subject, but it has no powers to initiate legislation. Usually such a committee is in existence for a two-year session of Congress, but the Committee on Nutrition and Human Needs was reestablished every two years until, despite some efforts to retain it, it was disbanded on December 31, 1977. This committee is to be commended for its accomplishments during the nine years of its existence; it generated interest, concern, and some healthy controversy.

The US consumer is confused about what is healthful to eat. The basic four food groups have been used for many years, but the consumer still has questions about what is healthful to eat. A set of general guidelines was published in February, 1980 (US Department of Agriculture and US Department of Health, Education, and Welfare, 1980). These guidelines are similar to the US dietary goals, but they are called "dietary guidelines for Americans." They should be helpful for food selection and preparation, while still allowing for flexibility within the diet. Each of the guidelines is described below:

1. Eat a variety of foods
   Include selections of
      fruits
      vegetables
      whole grain and enriched breads, cereals, and grain products
      milk, cheese, and yogurt
      meats, poultry, fish, eggs
      legumes (dry beans and peas)
2. Maintain ideal weight
   To improve eating habits
      eat slowly
      prepare smaller portions
      avoid "seconds"
   To lose weight
      increase physical activity
      eat less fat and fatty foods
      eat less sugar and sweets
      avoid too much alcohol
3. Avoid too much fat, saturated fat, and cholesterol
   Choose lean meat, fish, poultry, dry beans, and peas

Moderate the use of eggs and organ meats (such as liver)
Limit the intake of butter, cream, hydrogenated margarines, shortenings, and coconut oil, and foods made from such products
Trim excess fat off meats
Broil, bake, or boil rather than fry
Read labels carefully to determine both amount and types of fat contained in foods

4. Eat foods with adequate starch and fiber
   Substitute starches for fats and sugars
   Select foods which are good sources of fiber and starch, such as whole grain breads and cereals, fruits and vegetables, beans, peas, and nuts
5. Avoid too much sugar
   Use less of all sugars, including white sugar, brown sugar, raw sugar, honey, and syrups
   Eat less of foods containing these sugars, such as candy, soft drinks, ice cream, cakes, cookies
   Select fresh fruits or fruits canned without sugar or light syrup rather than heavy syrup
   Read food labels for clues on sugar content—if the names sucrose, glucose, maltose, dextrose, lactose, fructose, or syrups appear first, then there is a large amount of sugar
   Remember, how often you eat sugar is as important as how much sugar you eat
6. Avoid too much sodium
   Learn to enjoy the unsalted flavors of foods
   Cook with only small amounts of added salt
   Add little or no salt at the table
   Limit your intake of salty foods, such as potato chips, pretzels, salted nuts, and popcorn, condiments (soy sauce, steak

sauce, garlic salt), cheese, pickled foods, cured meats

Read food labels carefully to determine the amounts of sodium in processed foods and snack items

7. If you drink alcohol, do so in moderation

NUTRITIONAL STATUS OF CANADIANS

Between 1970 and 1972 the first national nutrition survey was conducted in Canada. This study was undertaken because of distinct changes in the Canadian lifestyle and eating habits during the past 10 years: increased urbanization, increased eating outside the home, and decreased physical activity. The two objectives of the survey were to estimate the prevalence of nutritional disorders and to identify the quality and quantity of food items consumed. The study examined 19,000 people. The survey procedure included a physical examination, dietary interviews, and an analysis of blood and urine constituents.

The general results were similar in many ways to the nutrition survey conducted in the United States. A large proportion of the Canadian adults were overweight. Elevated levels of serum cholesterol were common among adults. A deficit of protein, Calories, or both was found in some pregnant women and in a small proportion of children under age 5. Inadequate dietary levels of calcium and vitamin D were evident for many infants, children, adolescents, and pregnant women, though no clinical signs of rickets were seen (Sabry et al., 1974). There was evidence of a vitamin C deficiency among some of the general population, but particularly among the Eskimos and a considerable number of Indians. This was evidenced by low blood levels of vitamin C and also some clinical signs of vitamin C deficiency. There were, however, no cases of overt scurvy. A deficit of vitamin A was evidenced by low serum levels, but only a few clinical signs. Low levels of folate were also frequently observed.

The significance of these results remains under study (Sabry et al., 1974). As with any nutritional survey, release of the findings to the general population can result in overconcern and misinterpretation. The student will note that very few clinical symptoms or evidence of deficiency diseases were found. Low dietary intakes and low blood levels for some nutrients were found, which suggests marginal dietary intakes in some segments of the population. It is certain that nutritionists in Canada will take a close look at these low intakes and will plan nutritional education programs to reach these segments.

Nutrition Recommendations for Canadians

As a result of the Nutrition Canada nutrition survey, Canada is on its way toward the development of a national nutrition policy. In June 1977 four nutrition recommendations for maintaining and improving the health of the Canadian population were adopted by the Department of National Health and Welfare (Murray and Rae, 1979). These are much more general than the proposed *Dietary Goals for the United States,* but similarities may be noted. Also a study committee to define a nutrition policy for Quebec has formulated seven specific objectives to improve the health of the population (Blanchet, 1978). A comparison of the recommendations for Canadians, the objectives for Quebec, and the US dietary goals is found in Table 7-1.

NUTRITIONAL PRACTICES

Each person has his own nutritional practices influenced by the many factors examined in Chapter 1. Three nutritional practices are common enough to have an effect on the nutritional status of the population in general: the increasing consumption of food from

TABLE 7-1. Comparison of Nutritional Recommendations for the Populations of the United States and Canada

US Dietary Goals	Nutrition Recommendations for Canadians	Nutrition Objectives for Quebec
1. To avoid being overweight consume only as much energy (Calories) as is expended: if overweight, decrease energy intake and increase energy expenditure.	The prevention and control of obesity through a reduction in excess consumption of food and an increase in physical activity.	
2. Increase the consumption of complex carbohydrates and naturally occurring sugars from about 28% of energy intake to about 48% of energy intake.	The consumption of a diet that emphasizes whole grain products and fruits and vegetables and minimizes alcohol, salt, and refined sugars.	To increase the intake of dietary fiber.
3. Reduce the consumption of refined and processed sugars by about 45% to account for about 10% of total energy intake.		To reduce by 50% the intake of sugar (sucrose).
4. Reduce overall fat consumption from approximately 40% to about 30% of energy intake.	A reduction in the proportion of fat in the diet to about 35% of total energy intake.	To reduce by 25% the intake of fat.
5. Reduce saturated fat consumption to account for about 10% of total energy intake; and balance that with polyunsaturated and monounsaturated fats, which should account for about 10% of energy intake each.		
6. Reduce cholesterol consumption to about 300 mg/day.		
7. Limit the intake of sodium by reducing the intake of salt to about 5 g/day.	*Others:* The consumption of a nutritionally adequate diet, as outlined in Canada's Food Guide.	*Others:* To achieve both a 100% increase in the breast-feeding rate (from 28% to 56%) and to promote a more balanced diet for infants during the first year of life. To favor a change in daily food consumption so that well-balanced meals account for 80% of the daily caloric intake, with the remaining 20% coming possibly from snacks. To encourage the preservation of the nutritive value of foods. To achieve dietary variety by adopting a wide range of foods.

fast-food restaurants, the patronage of health food stores by those concerned about safety of the food supply, and vegetarianism. The object here is to separate fact from fiction about these practices.

Fast Foods

One of the United States's greatest success stories is that of Richard and Maurice McDonald, who opened in southern California a restaurant that featured a 15-cent hamburger, malt, and French fries. Just 10 years later there were 688 units, and by 1970 there were 1,592 (Goldberg, 1975). The largest segment of the food service industry is the fast-food industry. The fast-food restaurant is popular for many very practical reasons. It coincides with the fast pace of US life; and the food, compared to other restaurant food, is relatively inexpensive. The food is filling, generally satisfying, and served in a pleasant atmosphere if the patron chooses to eat inside. It has been estimated that by 1980, the US population will eat half their meals outside the home. Many of these meals will be at one of the fast-food chain restaurants (Consumer's Union, 1975). These restaurants have become so popular in the last few years that they are now found in downtown areas, in office buildings, on college campuses, and even in elementary and high school cafeterias, and in foreign countries. With all this popularity and enthusiastic public support, there is certainly justification for concern about the nutritional contribution made by foods consumed in these places.

A fast-food restaurant may provide a meal in the form of a hot dog, hamburger, fish, ham, or roast beef sandwich. Others offer a serving of specially prepared chicken or fish. Still others offer Mexican food or pizza. The accompaniments offered with these foods are French fries, onion rings, and in some places a lettuce salad, coleslaw, mashed potatoes, or corn on the cob. The beverages offered are malts, shakes, milk, carbonated beverages, coffee, and tea. A few serve breakfast, but most do not.

Several reports have been made in recent years about the nutritive content of fast foods and their contribution to the daily nutritive intake. As reported by Appledorf and Kelly (1979) only the nutritive content of fried chicken dinners and the typical hamburger, French fires, and milk shake have been determined by actual direct chemical analysis of the food. Most of the nutrient data on fast foods has been estimated from standard food composition tables. This latter method does not present as many problems as some would like to propose that it does. The nutritional analysis of a person's food intake is usually made using these accepted tables. More nutrient data from the fast-food chains about their specific products would be helpful, but it is not absolutely necessary to make a reasonable estimate of their nutritional value.

The food served in fast-food restaurants is sometimes called "junk food." Some people consider the fast food as having little or no nutritional value, and some actually experience guilt from eating an occasional meal at a fast-food restaurant. Because fast foods have become part of the US way of eating, they deserve to be put into nutritional perspective. One common criticism is that they contain too many Calories. This criticism deserves a closer look. A meal eaten at a fast-food restaurant may contain up to one-third of the daily caloric allowance provided snacks are not consumed indiscriminately between meals. According to the 1980 RDA, adult women can maintain their ideal weight on a daily caloric allowance of approximately 2,000 Calories. Adult men require approximately one-third more Calories per day (2,700 Calories). Teenage boys and girls require slightly more Calories per day. The caloric content of a fast-food meal, which ranges from 650 to 1,000 Calories, should be a reasonable number for maintaining ideal weight. The difficulty, however lies in the fact that a large proportion of adults, children, and adolescents are overweight. The caloric content of a typical fast-food meal may not allow for weight reduction. The Calorie content of a typical meal consisting of a large hamburger, French fries, and a chocolate shake is 993 Calories. The Calorie level is too high for all of the above groups of people except a teenage boy. These Calories can, however, be reduced significantly by changing the size of the hamburger and changing the beverage selection.

The one nutrient abundant in any fast-food meal is protein. The fast-food meal usually centers around some kind of a sandwich. Protein contents of these sandwiches range from 11 to 32 gm. Total protein content of all the foods selected for a meal typically ranges from 25 to 72 gm. The RDA for protein is 44–56 gm daily. Protein intake in fast-food meals is quite adequate, perhaps excessive. A smaller sandwich could safely be selected, reducing the number of Calories consumed. The meat used in the hamburgers of most leading hamburger chains is 100% beef.

Greecher and Shannon (1977) reported that a fast-food meal of a hamburger, French fries, and a carbonated beverage contained less than one-third of the RDAs for eight nutrients. The nutritive contribution of this meal was improved considerably by substituting a milk shake for the carbonated beverage. The nutrient most often found to be low in fast-food meals is vitamin A (Goldberg, 1975). Exceptions to this were that the foods from Pizza Hut and Taco Bell contained significant amounts of vitamin A (Young et al., 1978). Levels of Vitamin C were also generally low in fast-food meals unless French fries were selected. Even with the selection of French fries, the amount of vitamin C provided was still below the recommended level of one-third of the RDA.

The typical fast-food meal is also low in fiber, or roughage. The only fiber provided is the slice of tomato and the lettuce on the sandwich. This fiber deficit is made up by the salad bars offered by some fast-food restau-rants. This practice has the benefit of increasing not only the amount of fiber but the levels of vitamins A and C in the meal.

The sodium content of fast-food meals is also generally quite high. This poses a problem for people who must restrict their intake of salt (sodium) as part of their medical treatment. These people should refrain from using any additional salt and they should request their portion of French fries unsalted. Table 7-2 gives the nutritional composition of foods provided by several fast-food chains.

Fast food is definitely part of the US way of eating (see Fig. 7-3). These foods should not be referred to as "junk foods" because they can make a significant contribution to the daily food intake. Eating a hamburger and French fries for a quick lunch is certainly better than a cola beverage and a bag of potato chips or a candy bar. Although the caloric content of the foods selected may be too high for some people, the Calories can be reduced by a more prudent selection of food items. The selection of milk or a shake is always preferable to a carbonated beverage because of the higher nutrient content of the former two beverages. Because of the limited selection of food items, vitamin D and some minerals are low in fast-food meals. In Chapter 2 it was emphasized that the total amount and variety

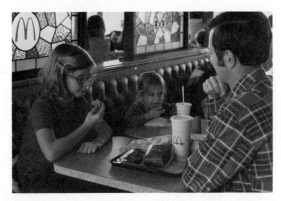

Figure 7-3. Eating in fast-food restaurants is a frequent practice of many Americans. (Photo by J. Collins)

TABLE 7-2. Nutritional Analyses of Fast Foods

Fast Foods	Food Chain	Calories	Protein (gm)	Carbohydrate (gm)	Fat (gm)	Vitamin A (IU)	Thiamine (mg)	Riboflavin (mg)	Niacin (mg)	Vitamin C (mg)	Calcium (mg)	Iron (mg)	Sodium (mg)
Egg McMuffin	McDonald's	352	18	26	20	361	0.36	0.60	4.3	1.6	187	3.2	914
Hot cakes with butter and syrup	McDonald's	472	8	89	9	255	0.31	0.43	4.0	<2.1	54	2.4	1,071
Sausage (pork)	McDonald's	184	9	tr	17	36	0.22	0.13	5.9	5.0	13	0.9	464
Scrambled eggs	McDonald's	162	12	2	12	514	0.07	0.60	0.4	<0.8	49	22	207
Hamburger, regular	Burger Chef	258	11	24	13	114	0.22	0.18	3.2	1	69	1.9	393
Cheeseburger	Burger Chef	304	14	24	17	266	0.22	0.23	3.2	1	156	2.0	535
Quarter Pounder	McDonald's	418	26	33	21	164	0.31	0.41	9.8	2.3	79	5.1	711
Big Mac	McDonald's	514	26	39	31	327	0.35	0.37	8.2	2.4	175	4.3	962
Big Shef	Burger Chef	542	23	35	34	282	0.34	0.35	5.4	2	189	3.4	622
Super Shef	Burger Chef	600	29	39	37	763	0.37	0.43	6.7	9	240	4.2	918
Whopper	Burger King	606	29	51	32	641	0.02	0.03	5.2	13	37	6.0	909
Brazier, regular	Dairy Queen	260	13	28	9	—	0.28	0.26	5.0	<1.0	70	3.5	576
Big Brazier, deluxe	Dairy Queen	470	28	36	24	—	0.34	0.37	9.6	<2.5	111	5.2	920
Hot Dog	Burger King	291	11	23	17	—	0.04	0.02	2.0	—	40	2.0	841
Brazier Cheese Dog	Dairy Queen	330	15	24	19	—	—	0.18	3.3	—	168	1.6	—
Brazier Chili Dog	Dairy Queen	330	13	25	20	—	0.15	0.23	3.9	11.0	86	2.0	939
Filet of fish	McDonald's	402	15	34	23	152	0.28	0.28	3.9	4.2	105	1.8	709
French fries	McDonald's	211	3	26	11	<52	0.15	0.03	2.9	11	10	0.5	113
Brazier onion rings	Dairy Queen	300	6	33	17	tr	0.09	tr	0.4	2.4	20	0.4	—
Original Recipe Dinner[a]	Kentucky Fried Chicken	830	52	56	46	750	0.38	0.56	15.0	27	150	4.5	2,285
Extra Crispy Dinner[a]	Kentucky Fried Chicken	950	52	63	54	750	0.38	0.56	14.0	27	150	3.6	1,915
Thin 'N Crispy Cheese Pizza[b]	Pizza Hut	450	25	54	15	750	0.30	0.51	5.0	<1.2	450	4.5	—
Thin 'N Crispy Supreme Pizza[b]	Pizza Hut	510	27	51	21	1,250	0.38	0.68	7.0	2.4	350	7.2	—
Thick 'N Chewy Cheese Pizza[b]	Pizza Hut	560	34	71	14	1,000	0.68	0.68	7.0	<1.2	500	5.4	—
Thick 'N Chewy Supreme Pizza[b]	Pizza Hut	640	36	74	22	1,000	0.75	0.85	9.0	9.0	400	7.2	—
Bean burrito	Taco Bell	343	11	48	12	1,657	0.37	0.22	2.2	15.2	98	2.8	272
Burrito Supreme	Taco Bell	451	21	43	22	3,462	0.33	0.35	4.7	16	121	3.8	367
Combination burrito	Taco Bell	404	21	43	16	1,666	0.34	0.31	4.6	15.2	91	3.7	300
Taco	Taco Bell	186	15	14	8	120	0.09	0.16	2.9	0.2	120	2.5	79
Tostada	Taco Bell	179	9	25	6	3,152	0.18	0.15	0.8	9.7	191	2.3	101
Cherry pie	McDonald's	298	2	33	18	213	0.02	0.03	0.4	1.3	12	0.4	456
McDonaldland Cookies	McDonald's	294	4	45	11	<48	0.28	0.23	0.8	1.4	10	1.4	330
DQ cone, medium[c]	Dairy Queen	230	6	35	7	300	0.09	0.26	tr	tr	200	tr	—
DQ chocolate dipped cone, medium[c]	Dairy Queen	300	7	40	13	300	0.09	0.34	tr	tr	200	0.4	—
DQ chocolate sundae, medium[c]	Dairy Queen	300	6	53	7	300	0.06	0.26	tr	tr	200	1.1	—
Banana split	Dairy Queen	540	10	91	15	750	0.60	0.60	0.8	18	350	1.8	—
Skim milk (8 oz)	Any	88	9	13	tr	10	0.09	0.44	0.2	2	296	0.1	127
Whole milk (8 oz)	Any	159	9	12	9	342	0.07	0.41	0.2	2.4	188	tr	122
Chocolate milk (8 oz)	Any	213	9	28	9	330	0.08	0.40	0.3	3.0	278	0.5	118
Coca Cola (8 oz)	Any	96	—	24	—	—	—	—	—	—	—	—	20
Fanta Root Beer (8 oz)	Any	103	—	27	—	—	—	—	—	—	—	—	23
Chocolate shake	McDonald's	364	11	60	9	318	0.12	0.89	0.8	<2.9	338	1.0	329
Chocolate malt, medium	Dairy Queen	600	15	89	20	750	0.12	0.60	0.8	3.6	500	3.6	—

SOURCE: Data compiled by E. A. Young, E. H. Brennan, and G. L. Irving, "Perspectives on Fast Foods." *Dietetic Currents* 5(5), 1978, Ross Laboratories, Columbus, Ohio.

[a] Dinner comprises mashed potatoes and gravy, coleslaw, roll, and three pieces of chicken.

[b] Based on a serving size of one-half of a 10-in pizza (three slices).

[c] Note that large and small sizes are also available.

of food eaten within the 24-hour period is what is important. If a fast-food meal is eaten at noon, care must be taken to eat adequate servings of fruits and vegetables at other meals to obtain adequate quantities of vitamins A and C and fiber, which are very low in fast-food meals. The two types of fast foods that have the highest percentages of most nutrients are pizzas and tacos. This is quite understandable because both products contain ingredients from each of the basic four food groups.

Restaurants and Cafeterias

Opponents of fast-food restaurants should take a closer look at the limited menus of other restaurants before judging fast foods too harshly. The standard restaurant menu includes a meat entree, choice of baked potato or French fries, a tossed green salad, and rolls or bread. The two nutrients usually low in a restaurant menu are also vitamins A and C because fruits and vegetables are generally not offered. Restaurants serve very large portions of meat (6–8 oz or more) in response to the customers' demand. Many people who must eat in restaurants are either trying to lose weight or adhere to a modified diet. Selection of food under these circumstances is very difficult. Restaurants should be encouraged to improve their menus of offering more fruits and vegetables, smaller portions of meat, and more menu items that have been baked, roasted, or grilled rather than fried and deep-fat fried.

Some restaurants have attempted to improve their menu selections. The practice of many restaurants of offering a salad bar with a wide variety of salads is a commendable step toward improving the nutritive content of their menus. Some restaurants also offer not only a choice of potatoes but a choice of two items from a selection that includes lettuce salad, coleslaw, applesauce, cottage cheese, corn, peas, and peaches. A few restaurants offer half-size or miniportions for customers who are trying to lose weight or who simply prefer smaller portions.

The best way to obtain a well-balanced meal at a reasonable cost is from a cafeteria. A wide variety of salads, entrees, vegetables, and desserts is offered. The extent of nutritional balance depends, however, on the combination of foods selected by the customer. The potential for well-balanced meals is always available at a cafeteria.

Food Faddism

In the United States there are many avenues of food selection available. The supermarket, with thousands of items, is but one of these. There are also fresh fruit and vegetable markets and roadside fruit stands. A wide variety of commercial eating establishments adds to the choices: cafeterias, ethnic restaurants, family restaurants, chain restaurants, and fast-food restaurants. Another option is patronizing health food stores. Lest the student be too quick to dismiss the health food store as a viable option, it should be pointed out that many of the products available in these stores are nutritious and healthful. It is important to examine carefully a person's motivation for visiting these stores as well as the pattern of daily food consumption when evaluating a person's total eating habits.

The purpose of this discussion is to provide the student with a basis for objectivity about food faddism, or health foods, by presenting a few comments about historical perspective, the general characteristics of food faddism, the types of people who patronize these stores, and the potential harm from food fads. It is not the authors' intention to critique individual fads or to discourage patronage of health food stores but to provide the student with a framework for understanding food fads as they relate to nutritional adequacy of diets and for counseling clients about fads. The discussion of the science of nutrition in the preceeding six chapters should already have equipped the student with some basic facts and tools for evaluating food fads.

Food faddism is not a development of the twentieth century. Claims about specific foods have special attributes have existed for centuries. Garlic was believed to provide physical strength, and cabbage was thought to cure certain illnesses. Special foods were advocated during the Middle Ages as cures for some diseases (Stare and McWilliams, 1977). Food faddists in the United States before 1930 were Sylvester Graham, Horace Fletcher, and Bernarr Macfadden. More recent names include Adelle Davis, Paul Bragg, and J. I. Rodale. Deutsch (1977) presents an interesting and entertaining survey and history of food faddism in his book, *The New Nuts among the Berries.* Because nutrition is a relatively new science, the facts are very susceptible to distortion. Also the emphasis placed on the association of good nutrition with health and poor nutrition with disease in teaching this subject has itself contributed to misconceptions (McBean and Speckmann, 1974). Because nutrition is associated directly with eating and because food intake is something most people can control themselves, the association of nutrition with prevention of disease and maintenance of health is here to stay. In other words, there have always been and always will be food faddists.

What are food fads? McBean and Speckmann (1974) define food fads as "favored or popular pursuits, diversion, or fashion in food consumption, prevailing for a short period of time" (p. 1072). There are generally considered to be three types of food fads: (1) including particular foods because they are believed to cure specific diseases, (2) omitting certain foods because they are believed to contain harmful constituents, and (3) eating "health foods" as an expression of lifestyle.

The prevalance of food misinformation in the US population was revealed in the results of *A Study of Health Practices and Opinions* (1972), some of which are:

- 75% believed that supplemental vitamins provide energy.
- 20% had the idea that arthritis and cancer were partly due to vitamin and mineral deficiencies.
- 26% used nutritional supplements without their doctor's advice.
- 10% had eaten organic or natural foods.

People *do* have questions and misconceptions about food. A study by Anderson and Standal (1975) inquired of the patrons of health food stores where they would go if they had a question about nutrition. The responses were: 45% would ask the health food store owner; 21% would go to health food books; 11% would ask their physician; 7% would ask other health food advocates; and only 6% would seek out a professional nutritionist. These responses reveal the high level of confidence in the health food store proprietor and the relatively low credibility of medical and nutritional professionals.

What type of people patronize the health food stores? The people and the philosophies they espouse are quite varied, but they can be divided into two main groups: the "general users" and the "unitary users" (Frankle and Heussenstamm, 1974). The general users are those who purchase a few popular "health foods" such as whole wheat bread, wheat germ, brown rice, and molasses. Wolff (1973) refers to these occasional patrons as "health foodists." The unitary users are the much more serious consumers who have a particular philosophy linked to eating. This group contains the food faddists and the serious vegetarians (Fig. 7-4). The latter group may include the extremists who go on bizarre diets such as the Zen macrobiotic dietary regimen.

A more detailed classification by Beal (1972) divides health food patrons into eight

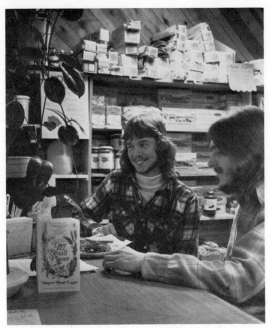

Figure 7-4. Vegetarians are frequent patrons of health food stores. (Photo by J. Collins)

categories based on their psychological motivation.

1. Miracle seekers
2. Antiestablishmentarians
3. Superhealth seekers
4. Distrusters of the medical profession
5. Fashion followers
6. Authority seekers
7. Truth seekers
8. Those concerned about the uncertainties of living

This classification includes, not only the casual and the serious patrons, but those who are seeking a quick cure for a disease or medical problem and those who have a basic distrust for modern food processing methods. Part of the interest in health foods seems to be a reaction against the eating habits of the previous generation, such as the almost exclusive use of white flour and processed foods. Wolff (1973) states that as the US environment and way of life become more artificial, the food becomes more artificial too. Perhaps this is somewhat true, and part of the health food fads are a reaction to this. Evidence that food manufacturers will produce the type of food demanded by the public is evidenced by the inclusion in the supermarket of both highly processed breakfast beverages and whole grain natural bread with no preservatives or additives (see Fig. 7-5). Both health foodists and food faddists have the desire for a healthier and simpler diet. There is nothing wrong with this motivation as long as it results in a diet composed of a variety of foods that are considered nutritionally adequate.

Many types of products available in a health food store are not harmful, but they are often unnecessary (see Fig. 7-6). The miracle claims made about a particular food, nutrient, or supplement, however, may be harmful if they cause a client to avoid seeking medical advise or to abandon a prescribed medical treatment. Claims that a certain food or nutrient possesses the ability to cure a disease or condition raise false hopes. People with terminal illnesses such as cancer are very prone to the lure of the food faddist. Bruch (1970) cites examples of educated people

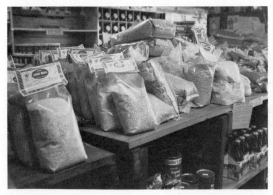

Figure 7-5. Many whole grain products are available in the health food store. (Photo by J. Collins)

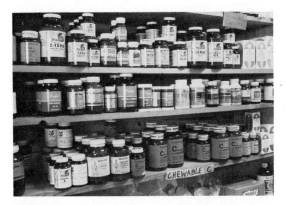

Figure 7-6. Health food stores offer a wide variety of nutrient supplements, most of which are unnecessary and very expensive. (Photo by J. Collins)

who, when faced with terminal illness, sought the advice of those with the latest medical knowledge and simultaneously turned to the advice of a food quack. Finding a remedy for a disease by consuming a certain food or nutrient supplement offers a glimmer of hope when the medical profession says there is none. The saddest situation occurs when a person delays or refuses medical treatment in preference to the cure offered by the health food product. No single food has any ability to cure a disease. A specific nutrient supplement will only relieve the symptoms of the specific nutritional deficiency disease associated with it (see Chap. 24). There are no known nutritional cures for cancer, heart disease, arthritis, and a host of other medical conditions.

Another potentially harmful aspect of health foods and nutritional supplements is the quantity of money spent for them. Health foods are big business, and most of the products available in health food stores are quite expensive. Some of the same or very similar products such as whole wheat bread, wheat germ, molasses, brown rice, and others can now be purchased in regular supermarkets for a fraction of their cost in health food stores. The same basic nutritional benefits are present in products purchased both places. The nurse or dietitian should make the client aware of these price differences in the process of counseling.

Finally, harm may result from the consumption of the many nutritional supplements available in the health food store. The harm that can result may be due to a nutritional excess in the case specifically of vitamins A and D or to a nutritional imbalance from incorrect proportions of nutrients consumed. Research increasingly indicates more harmful effects from nutrient imbalances, such as increased levels of one nutrient greatly decreasing the absorption of another. A diet that contains a variety of foods from the basic four food groups in the recommended amounts will usually contain adequate protein, vitamins, and minerals in balanced quantities. Any diet that contains only a few or a very limited number of foods is likely to be nutritionally inadequate. A good example of this is the Zen macrobiotic diet, in which the final stage is the consumption of only brown rice.

Counseling the food faddist or even the health foodist is not an easy task. Most of these people believe they have valid reasons for their food habits. They are not easily persuaded to change. The nurse or dietitian counseling one of these people needs to have a genuine concern about the nutritional adequacy of the client's diet. When counseling a client who regularly eats "health foods," information should always be gathered about the type and amount of nutrient supplements consumed daily. This nutrient supplementation regimen should be carefully reviewed for any harmful nutrient excesses. The nurse or dietitian should always attempt to explain normal recommendations for nutrients using the RDA. Charts, posters, and diagrams may be helpful to show relative quantities available in various foods. The attitude of the nutrition counselor should be one of basic acceptance of the client's selected eating habits. If it is stressed that they have a common goal in mind—that is, the consumption of nutrients from food to attain good health—the counseling may proceed with positive results.

One final caution: The average person has great difficulty separating nutritional fact from fiction. The writers of health food literature most often use half-truths and misquote or twist the results of scientific research to support their propositions although the average person has no way of knowing this. The books and literature available are written in an interesting, clear style that is generally easy to read and understand. With little or no scientific background, the average reader finds it easy to accept as true all that is written and claimed about a nutrient, product, or diet. Frequent patrons of a health food store run the risk of accepting more and more false information, perhaps ultimately succumbing to the lure of a foodquack.

Food Quack*

A *food quack,* often called a *health practitioner,* is a person who promotes a food, diet, food supplement, or special cooking utensils with exaggerated health claims. A quack uses misinterpretation and misinformation to play on the emotions of consumers. It is not uncommon for the quack either to own or to be a part owner in the product he is promoting. Quacks usually do not have the educational qualifications they claim.

A food quack will often:

• Claim the food or diet will cure an incurable disease.

• Pose as a health advisor or authority and often promote a food, book, food supplement, or piece of equipment such as a blender, slicer, or cooking utensil.

• Refer to membership in a professional-sounding scientific organization.

• Speak of or display a diploma of an unfamiliar but impressive-sounding school.

• Have testimonials to the food or product he is promoting.

• Use a title such as doctor, consultant, researcher, or nutritionist.

• State that modern food processing and chemicals added to food are slowly causing death.

• Claim his product has a secret formula.

• Claim diet, food, or product he is promoting is guaranteed to work.

• Appeal to emotions, especially fear of what will happen if the audience does not follow his advice.

• Refer to "unnutritious" foods and synthetic vitamins.

• Offer a quick way to lose weight, regain or enhance sexual potency, prevent gray hair, maintain youth, and indefinitely delay the aging process.

• Use scientific terminology fluently.

The food quack no longer needs to peddle his product and his misinterpretations from door to door, in a tent show, or on the street corner. Today he has a wide audience by way of radio, TV advertisements and talk shows, newspapers, and magazines. He can even be found at state fairs in a booth peddling his wares, reaching thousands of people every summer.

One can hardly read the newspapers or a magazine without reading about faddism in some form or about "scientific research findings." In a single copy of a magazine one could read about eliminating all dairy products to prevent and cure headaches, how eating acid foods with alkaline foods at the same meal will produce acidosis, the disparagment of scientific medicines, curing cancer, ways of preparing organic foods, organic gardening, testimonials, and curing obesity and disease by meditation. Newspapers as well as magazines publish scientific and nonscientific articles

---

* The rest of this section on food faddism and the following section on plant protein substitutes and extenders are by Sara Porter.

concerning the relationship of diet to cancer, diabetes, pregnancy, heart disease, and lung disorders. There is no wonder that food faddism is flourishing with an alarming rate.

As a response to these advertizing abuses and false claims, the Federal Trade Commission recommended rules for manufacturers' use in advertising "natural," "organic," and "health" foods: A food cannot be labeled "natural" if the food or any of its ingredients have been more than minimally processed to make it safe or edible or to preserve it. A "natural" food cannot contain any artificial ingredient. The term *organic* applies to food grown with organic fertilizers and minerals and without application of synthetic fertilizers. The term *health* food should be prohibited because it cannot be defined or qualified.

Health Foods

The term *health food* is a misnomer. Any edible food can be a healthy food. Nevertheless, health foods and health food stores are a very lucrative business. Organic or health food sales are currently estimated at $3 billion. They are sold by drug stores, supermarkets, department stores, and sales agents, with the largest selection being found in health food stores.

Because of misrepresentation of organically grown foods, a bill was introduced in Congress to establish definitions. The bill, HR 14941, May 11, 1972, states:

The term "organically grown food" means food which has not been subjected to pesticides or artificial fertilizers and which has been grown in soil whose humus contents has been increased by the addition of organic matter.

The term "organically processed food" means organically grown food which in processing has not been treated with preservatives, hormones, antibiotics, or synthetic additives of any kind.

Vegetarianism

Loosely defined, *vegetarianism* is any theory of diet advocating abstinence from meat and animal products in favor of a diet composed, in whole or in part, of plant matter and water. There are several types of vegetarian diets (Nat'l Dairy Council, 1979). The *strict,* or *vegans diet* excludes not only meat, poultry, and fish but animal products such as milk and eggs. The *ovovegetarian diet* includes eggs but excludes all other animal products. The *lactovegetarian diet* includes milk but excludes all other animal products. The *lactoovo-vegetarian diet* includes milk and eggs but excludes all other animal products. The *lactoovo-vegetarian* composed of raw fruits and nuts as well as honey and olive oil and generally excludes all other food. In addition one may speak of *pescovegetarian diets* and *pollovegetarian diets,* which include fish and poultry products, respectively, and which may or may not include milk and eggs.

There are many reasons why people may turn to vegetarian diets. Religion is one. The Seventh-Day Adventists are vegetarians, and their theology on the point is very specific regarding the exact diet to be followed (Deutsch, 1977). Various forms of the diet are recommended by the Hindu and Buddhist faiths, as well as by certain Islamic sects. Another reason for considering the vegetarian alternative may be a heightened regard for animal life and a belief that the domestication of food animals is both cruel and inhumane. Still another reason is the view that meat consumption is a luxury. Certain Christian monastic orders, such as the Trappist Order, take vows to abstain from meat in favor of a more plain or common fare. In a nonreligious context this view is the thesis for Lappe's (1975) dietary opinions presented in her book *Diet for a Small Planet.*

The vegetarian may give many other reasons for his diet, but as the reasons above show, vegetarianism cannot be dismissed as mere faddism. The vegetarian need not be an advocate of nutritional theories but, instead, a person reconciling his day-to-day living with deeply felt moral beliefs or economic principles. The antivivisectionist, the Trappist monk, and the struggling citizen depressed by the high cost of meat are all potentially vegetarians.

From a theoretical point of view it is tempting to regard plant matter as superior to animal products as a source of nutrients. This was the view of Sylvester Graham, W. K. Kellogg, and other prominent food faddists of the nineteenth and early-twentieth centuries, and it is still prevalent today. The idea is that, in the food chain, all animals must ultimately rely on plant matter. The cow eats the grass, and the farmer eats the cow. Perhaps if the farmer also ate the grass, he would spare himself (and the cow) all the problems attendant to dairy and beef farming.

Economically speaking, this argument is difficult to refute. Notes Lappe (1975), "An acre of cereals can produce 5 times more protein than an acre devoted to meat production, legumes . . . 15 times more" (p. 10). "In one year American livestock consumed the protein equivalent of six times the recommended protein allowance of our human population. . . . If we exclude dairy cows, the average conversion ratio for U.S. livestock is 7 pounds of grain fed to produce 1 pound of edible meat" (p. 13).

The chief question is—Can such a diet be nutritionally sound? It is true that cows and humans are both animals, but it is also true that as protein manufacturers they rely on very different means of production. Even though the protein matter created has a similar makeup, as in hair, bones, and hide, it is neither assembled in the same manner nor made from the same raw materials. The cow, because of its anatomy and physiology, can digest, for instance, the protein found in grass far more readily than humans can. It is protein quality, as well as quantity, that recommends a source of protein.

Lappe (1975) discusses the problem of protein quality in *Diet for a Small Planet.* Her solution is a diet that advocates the combining of vegetable and dairy protein sources in the meals according to the complementarity of each food's principal protein. The theory is simple but also nutritionally sound. She provides a calculation of the minimum protein; a factor for considering individual differences, both physical and lifestyle; and adjustments for "protein quality," or the usability of protein. As all the principal protein needs of humans are readily met by strictly lactoovo-vegetarian food choices, it is clearly possible that such a diet would be eminently suited to protein nutrition requirements. Figure 7-7 gives an example of a strict vegetarian diet.

The vegetarian diet may not in practice always prove nutritious for the person under its regimen, particularly the more restrictive diets such as the vegan's diet. Although many meat eaters in our society present classic patterns of malnutrition, vegetarians are nonetheless well advised to use special caution in assessing their individual nutrient needs.

A problem rather foreign to the conventional diet is eating insufficient quantities of food. Yet strict vegetarian diets are definitely characterized by reduced caloric intake because plant matter, particularly raw or unprocessed plant matter, is rather low in Calories relative to its weight. This is partially due to its water and fiber content. The problem is exacerbated by the additional time consumed in eating high-fiber foods. The desire to eat may cease well before sufficient caloric intake has been accomplished. Reduced caloric intake can mean reduced nutrient intake, and while the diet may prove excellent as a weight-reducing and maintenance program, it may also prove to be malnutritious over a period of time.

Dietary deficiency is particularly possible in the strict vegetarian diet, for plant matter is a poor source of minerals. Although certain green, leafy vegetables are high in calcium, this calcium may be unusable because the high fiber content of the diet may interfere with calcium absorption (or the absorption of other minerals). Then, too, the lack of a good source for vitamin D will hinder calcium absorption and utilization. For the lactoovo-

```
                 EARLY MORNING
Orange                         1 medium
Bulgur                         1 cup
   with brewer's yeast         1 tablespoon
Toasted wheat-soy bread        1 slice
   with honey                  1 tablespoon


              MIDMORNING SNACK
Shelled almonds                ¼ cup


                 MIDDAY MEAL
Split pea soup                 2 cups
Peanut butter sandwich:
   Peanut butter               2 tablespoons
   Whole wheat bread           2 slices
   Honey                       1 tablespoon
Fruit-sunflower seed salad:
   Apple                       ½ medium
   Banana                      ½ medium
   Sunflower seeds             ¼ cup
   Lettuce                     1 leaf


                    SNACK
Peach                          1 medium


                 EVENING MEAL
Soybeans                       1 cup
Brown rice cooked              1 cup
   fried in oil                2 tablespoons
   with chestnuts              2 tablespoons
   with sesame seeds           2 tablespoons
Collards                       1 cup
Pear                           1 medium


                EVENING SNACK
Raisins                        ¼ cup
```

Figure 7-7. Meal plan for a strict vegetarian. (Reprinted from USDA *Yearbook of Agriculture*, 1974.)

vegetarian these concerns may be ignored because milk and eggs are excellent sources for both calcium and vitamin D. In addition, exposure to sunlight will definitely alleviate the potential for vitamin D deficiency.

The vegan must also be concerned about iron deficiency and iodine deficiency, the latter completely alleviated by the use of iodized salt. The vegan diet has inadequate sources of vitamin B_{12}; yet followers of the diet rarely show overt signs and symptoms of deficiency. Those who do generally have a coexisting disorder, such as malabsorption. How long a person has been on the diet has a bearing on the problem, for the body may well store units exceeding the RDA by 1,000-fold. In addition, needs for this vitamin vary greatly. Further studies need to be done in this area.

The problem of evaluating the long-term effects of a vegetarian diet is generally that of evaluating the amount of stored nutrients in the body, as just discussed in connection with vitamin B_{12}. The person may well experience any number of dietary insufficiencies over an extensive period of time, unknowingly relying on stored nutrients. By the time a deficiency becomes evident, the person may have abandoned the diet that led to it. The vegan's diet in certain forms—in particular the so-called Zen macrobiotic diet, the Ehrets Mucousless Diet, and certain variations on these diets—has been studied and cases of malnutrition have been reported (Erhard, 1973). Nor were the reported deficiences technical or trivial in nature; deaths from extreme malnutrition have been reported.

The vegetarian can formulate a diet that is nutritionally sound (see Table 7-3). Lappe has been mentioned as one source; many other sources are available (Robertson et al., 1976; Smith, 1975). In addition, the diet plans of the Seventh-Day Adventists can be recommended, although they are completely unscientific in approach. The health history of the Adventist movement has established that the diet is sound in practice, if somewhat lacking in principle. The lactoovo-vegetarian diet is certainly nutritionally sound, for complete protein is provided by milk and eggs. An example of the modification of the basic four for this diet is found in Table 7-4. Sample menus for a lactoovo-vegetarian diet are given in Table 7-5.

TABLE 7-3. Complementary Plant Protein Combinations

Food	Amino Acids Deficient	Complementary Protein Food Combinations
Grains	Isoleucine; lysine	Rice + legumes Corn + legumes Wheat + legumes Wheat + peanut + milk Wheat + sesame + soybean Rice + Brewer's yeast
Legumes	Tryptophan; methionine	Legumes + rice Beans + wheat Beans + corn Soybeans + rice + wheat Soybeans + corn + milk Soybeans + wheat + sesame Soybeans + peanuts + sesame Soybeans + peanuts + wheat + rice Soybeans + sesame + wheat
Nuts and seeds	Isoleucine; lysine	Peanuts + sesame + soybeans Sesame + beans Sesame + soybeans + wheat Peanuts + sunflower seeds
Vegetables	Isoleucine; methionine	Lima beans Green beans Brussels sprouts ⎤ Cauliflower ⎬ Sesame seeds or + Brazil nuts or mushrooms Broccoli ⎦ Greens + millet or rice

SOURCE: From Bonnie S. Worthington, Joyce Vermeersch, and Sue Radwell Williams, *Nutrition in Pregnancy and Lactation*. St. Louis: The C. V. Mosby Co., 1977; modified from F. M. Lappe, *Diet for a Small Planet*. New York: Friends of the Earth, Ballantine, 1971.

TABLE 7-4. Recommended Daily Servings

Food Group	Number of Servings		
	Child	Teenager	Adult
Milk group	3–4	4–5	2
Protein, average grams	24–32	32–40	16
Meat alternate group	2	3	2
Protein, average grams	20	30	20
Fruit-vegetable group	4	4	4
Protein, average grams	8	8	8
Grain group	4	4	4
Protein, average grams	8	8	8
Total protein, gram average	60–80	78–86	52

SOURCE: Courtesy National Dairy Council.

TABLE 7-5. Sample Menus for Lactoovo-vegetarian Diet

Meal and Food Group	Menu 1	Menu 2
Breakfast		
Milk	Milk	Milk
Meat alternate		Scrambled egg or tofu (soy curd)
Fruit-vegetable	Orange	Prune juice
Grain	Oatmeal	Shredded wheat
	Date-nut muffin	Wheat soy bread
Others	Butter/margarine	Butter/margarine
	Coffee/hot cereal beverage	Coffee/hot cereal beverage
Lunch		
Milk	Cream mushroom soup (made with milk)	Cottage cheese for fruit plate
Meat alternate	Peanut butter, for sandwich	Lentil soup
Fruit-vegetable	Carrot sticks	Apricots, grapefruit, pineapple, grapes,
	Banana	lettuce leaves in fruit plate
Grain	Rye crackers	Whole wheat crackers
	Whole wheat bread	
Others	Beverage	Salad dressing
		Beverage
Dinner		
Milk	Yogurt	Milk
Meat alternate	Baked beans	Quiche—egg
Fruit-vegetable	Corn	Broccoli
	Collards	Spinach salad
	Sliced tomato salad	
Grain	Brown bread	Whole wheat roll
Others	Salad dressing	Salad dressing
	Butter/margarine	Butter/margarine
	Tea/hot cereal beverage	Tea/hot cereal beverage
Snacks	Cheese	Sunflower seeds
	Crackers	Apple

SOURCE: Courtesy National Dairy Council.

One claim often made for vegetarian diets is that they are health promoting. Generally speaking, this is a false claim in that no diet that is nutritious in every respect is anything less than health promoting. There have, however, been some scientific investigations that suggest the potential for lower colorectal cancer rates among lactoovo-vegetarians (National Dairy Council, 1979). The evidence is by no means complete or conclusive. Both Seventh-Day Adventists and Mormons, for instance, have significantly lower mortality rates from such causes as cancer and heart disease. Yet the Mormons do not abstain from meat, although they do preach moderation in meat intake. More important, perhaps, both groups forbid the consumption of alcohol and stimulants and the use of cigarettes. It is clear that good health and well-being are a product of a general lifestyle and not merely of its nutritional component.

The lactoovo-vegetarian diet is clearly satisfactory. The more restrictive diets need to be viewed with more caution, that caution increasing as the diet becomes more restrictive. Properly supplemented, however, even the vegans diet can be shown to be nutritious. The expertise of a nutritionist may be needed to develop adequate diet patterns using primarily foods of plant origin.

Many high schools and colleges are replacing typical snack foods with vegetarian foods. It is not uncommon to find vegetarian meals and snack bars in colleges. Numerous public eating establishments are offering meatless meals. Other countries are incorporating vegetarian combinations into the elementary school lunch program to help improve the nutritional status of children. India supplemented the school lunch with a mixture of sunflower meal, maize, roasted Bengal gram (chick-pea) flour, and sesame. Tests showed that the children had a significant increase in height and weight.

Plant Protein Substitutes and Extenders

That there is an economic need for increased plant-food substitutes in the traditional US diet can be seen in the recent development of protein substitutes in the food industry. Soy proteins, relatively new in popularity in the United States, have been used for thousands of years by Orientals in the form of *Tofu* (a soybean curd) and *miso* (a soy and rice fermentation product). Plant protein products are made by extracting protein from soybeans, cottonseed, wheat, peanuts, sesame, sunflower seed, or other vegetable products. At the present time more protein products are made from soy than any other plant source.

Protein content depends on the stage of refinement; the greater the refinement, the higher the protein content. Flour, grits, and granules, containing less than 65% protein, are made from plants after the removal of fat and water. Defatted soy flour contains about 50% protein and 50% nonprotein sources including fiber, carbohydrate, and minerals. As refinement continues, nonprotein components are removed. *Protein concentrates* are made by additional refining with the removal

of nonprotein products until protein content is between 65 and 90%.

Protein isolate is the most highly refined product, with at least 90%, and many are almost pure protein. The texture of many foods can be produced by different processing methods. Concentrates can be extruded under pressure to form chips, flakes, chunks, and other shapes. Other methods can produce the texture of shredded coconut, dried fruits, nuts, and meats. Protein isolates can be "spun" into long, thin fibers and then formed into shapes resembling meats. Protein concentrate, isolates, or flour, or a combination of these forms, are blended with other ingredients and fabricated into meatlike products. They are available in frozen, canned, or dried forms.

Extenders, usually in granular form, are used to extend flesh protein foods. The dry form must be rehydrated before use. Directions on the package should be followed as to the amount of water to use and length of time to allow for rehydration. After being rehydrated they should be treated as any other perishable food. The products sold in frozen form, after thawing, should be refrigerated and used within one or two days. It is important to follow package directions for cooking time and temperature, because some of the products become tough if cooked too long or at a higher temperature. Poultry, ham, bacon, ground beef, link sausage, and many other *meat analogs* are available in the stores today. Meat analogs can be used to supplement other plant protein, add variety to the meal, and replace the quantity of bulk normally consumed.

Plant proteins can be formulated to any carbohydrate, protein, or fat level. They can be blended to furnish favorable amino acid combinations with little or no cholesterol and low saturated fats. Some contain fewer Calories than comparable animal products. People with dietary restrictions in sodium, carbohydrate, or *gluten* should carefully read package labels. The plant proteins may contain more sodium than the natural foods; they also contain carbohydrate that would not be found in animal foods. Many contain wheat, but soy extenders are available for gluten-free diets. It seems likely that commercially prepared protein extenders for special diets will become more available in the markets.

Within the last few years many colleges, hospitals, restaurants, and other food institutions have been using food extenders to help cut food costs. The US Department of Agriculture has approved the use of 30% of textured vegetable protein in meat dishes served in the school lunch program.

Many convenience foods and often fresh ground meat contain extenders. Some analogs contain egg white or nonfat dry milk, which would prohibit their use by pure vegetarians. With the spiraling cost of meat and the dwindling supply of flesh foods, soy products will be used to a greater extent to help solve world food needs. Soy products will be needed both to supplement and to extend protein from flesh.

Companies who manufacture meat analogs and extenders have developed guidelines for menu planning, recipes, and Calorie-controlled diets. Different brands of egg substitutes are now found in the market. Recipe booklets usually available from the companies offer a wide variety of ways to prepare their product.

Recipes substituting green pea flour for 15% of the wheat flour in baking products has been developed by government scientists. Bread using the pea flour is high in both protein and fiber and low in fat. In one loaf of bread, the total protein value is boosted by 15%. The mixed flour has been used, and widely accepted, in Japanese noodles and doughnuts. Commercial-size loaves of bread made with pea flour are already being sold in one market. An Idaho seed company is developing pea flour to be used in commercially baked products. Pea flour has the potential to change the making of bread, for it does not effect either the taste or the baking quality, is superior to soy flour in baking qualities, and has little if any color.

NUTRITIONAL EDUCATION

Two simple but crucial contributors to poor nutritional habits emerge: first, an inadequate level of knowledge about nutrition principles because of inadequate education in this area, and second, most people's reluctance to change or even modify their food habits. The goal of nutritional education is to improve the level of nutritional knowledge and attitudes with the end result of changing or modifying dietary practices based on that improved knowledge.

Value clarification, identifying current lifestyles, awareness of eating habits, and health problems are not new in the educational curriculum. College courses that prepare teachers and state curriculum guides both show that these areas have been stressed for several years. Numerous seminars, workshops, and professional meetings centered around the needs of youth have been well attended. The National Nutrition Education Conference, 1971, held in Washington, D.C., emphasized the importance of understanding and ways of reaching youth to aid them in improving food habits. The conference was centered around three main themes: the youth in his environment; perceiving modern youth—his values, lifestyle, eating habits, and present state of health; and identifying and developing effective ways of aiding in the improvement of health.

Educators and health professionals need to know and understand the beliefs and psychological significance of food. There is a need to recognize and understand motivating forces associated with eating patterns. Educators should select subject matter and varied techniques to teach youth what they want and need to learn about diet and health. Educators and health professionals must become better informed about vegetarian diets and approach the subject with an open mind.

Nutritional education for the lay public has always existed through federal and state governmental agencies such as the state Cooperative Extension Services of the US Department of Agriculture, the home economists in the distrcit (or county) agricultural extension offices, and the public health departments. In addition, volunteer health agencies such as the American Heart Association and the American Diabetes Association provide nutritional education as part of their total educational program. Food industries such as the National Dairy Council, the National Livestock and Meat Board, the National Association of Fruit and Vegetables Growers, and the Bread and Cereal Institute provide useful nutritional information, films, and in some cases nutritional education programs. Professional associations such as the American Medical Association, the American Dietetic Association, and the National Dairy Council have initiated significant programs in nutritional education of the public in recent years.

National Dairy Council

The National Dairy Council has been quite active in nutritional education at the elementary and secondary school levels. They provide an extensive list of graded pamphlets, posters, films, and other visual aids for use in the classroom. Periodic nutrition workshops are provided for elementary and secondary teachers to learn to use the new nutritional curriculum material.

The National Dairy Council also has films, pamphlets, and posters that can be used in nutritional education of the public or for reference by professionals. The council began a nutritional education program in 1973 for the education of homemakers by nutrition educators. The objective is for these homemakers to train others in their localities. This

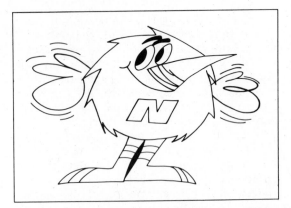

Figure 7-8. Nutribird. (Trademark, copyright by The American Dietetic Association. Redrawn by permission.)

method of education allows the principles of nutrition to reach a larger number of homemakers who, in response, will implement many of these nutritional principles with their families.

American Dietetic Association

In 1973 the American Dietetic Association instituted National Nutrition Week to be observed annually during the first week of March. The major purpose of National Nutrition Week is to educate the general public about the benefits of good nutrition. The state and district associations plan events for that week to be aimed at improving nutritional awareness and education of the public. Each year there is an attention-getting slogan for the week. A variety of materials including posters, bumper stickers, decals, and T-shirts, are available for members of the American Dietetic Association to order in advance. The nutrition and diet therapy departments of hospitals participate in some way to increase patients' awareness of nutrition during that week. Slogans used for National Nutrition Week since 1976 are:

1976 Improving Nutrition for the Nation
1977 Nutrition: Foodway to Fun and Fitness

1978	Nutribird says: Eat a Balanced Diet Everyday
1979	Set the Pace! Take the Food Way for Good Nutrition
1980	To Hit Your Stride, Eat Smart.
1981	Pep Up Your Prime Time. Exercise. . . Eat Right. . . Enjoy

In 1976 the association announced the development of an animated logo called Nutribird (Fig. 7-8). Its purpose is to symbolize good nutrition. It is used during National Nutrition Week and in television and radio spots for nutritional education. Also in 1976, in honor of America's Bicentennial, the American Dietetic Association framed its Nutrition Bill of Rights:

THE RIGHT TO GOOD NUTRITION

• Every American has the right to optimal nutritional health.

THE RIGHT TO FOOD CHOICES

• Every American has the right to access to a variety of safe foods that will promote good nutrition and improve resistance to disease.

THE RIGHT TO NUTRITION INFORMATION

• Every American has the right to nutrition education—to make informed choices from available foods; to have protection against food and nutrition misinformation.

BIBLIOGRAPHY

Abraham, S., Carroll, M. D., Dresser, C. M., and Johnson, C. L. Dietary intake of persons 1–74 years of age in the United States. In *Sourcebook on Food and Nutrition*, pp. 6–18. Chicago: Marquis Who's Who, Inc., Academic Media, 1979.

Abraham, S. F., Lowenstein, W., and Johnson, C. L. *Preliminary Findings of the First Health and Nutrition Examination Survey, United States, 1971–1972: Dietary Intakes and Biochemical Findings*. DHEW Publ. No. (HRA) 74-1219-1. Rockville, Md.: Nat'l Center for Health Statistics, U.S. Dept. of Health, Education, and Welfare, 1974.

Abraham, S. F., Lowenstein, W., and O'Connell, D. E. *Preliminary Findings of the First Health and Nutrition Exam-*
ination Survey, United States, 1971–1972: Anthropometric and Clinical Finds. DHEW Publ. No. (HRA) 75-1229. Rockville, Md.: Nat'l Center for Health Statistics, U.S. Dept. of Health, Education, and Welfare, 1975.

Adelson, S. F., and Peterkin, B. B. Quality of diets in U.S. households in spring 1965. *Family Economics Review*, March, ARS 62-5, 1968.

Alfin-Slater, R. B. Vitamins: Their use and abuse. In *Sourcebook on Food and Nutrition*. Chicago: Marquis Who's Who, Inc., Academic Media, 1979.

Am. Dietetic Assoc. Dietary goals: A statement by the American Dietetic Association. *J. Am. Diet Assoc.* 72:227, 1977.

Am. Med. Assoc. Dietary goals for the United States. *Rhode Island Med. J.* 60:576, 1977.

Anderson, M. A., and Standal, B. R. Nutritional knowledge of health food users in Oahu, Hawaii. *J. Am. Diet. Assoc.* 67:116, 1975.

Appledorf, H., and Kelly, L. S. Proximate and mineral content of fast food. *J. Am. Diet. Assoc.* 74:35, 1979.

Beal, V. A. Food faddism and organic and natural foods. Paper presented at the Nat'l Dairy Council Writers' Conf., Newport, R.I., May 1972.

Bernard, V. W. Why people become victims of medical quackery. *Am. J. Public Health* 55:1142, 1965.

Blackburn, G. L., Bistrian, B. R., Maini, B. S., Schlamm, H. T., and Smith, M. F. Nutritional and metabolic assessment of the hospitalized patient. *J. Parenteral Enteral Nutrition* 1:11, 1977.

Blanchet, M. Nutrition health of the Quebecois. *Nutrition Today* 13(4):6, 1978.

Bruch, H. The allure of food cults and nutritional quackery. *J. Am. Diet. Assoc.* 57:316, 1970.

Butterworth, C. E. The skeleton in the hospital. *Nutrition Today* 9(2):4, 1974.

Butterworth, C. E., and Blackburn, G. L. Hospital malnutrition. *Nutrition Today* 10(2):8, 1975.

Calvert, G. P., and Calvert, S. W. Intellectual convictions of "health" food consumers. *J. Nutr. Educ.* 7:95, 1975.

Christakis, G. The case for balanced moderation, or how to design a new American nutritional pattern without really trying. *Prev. Med.* 2:329, 1973.

Consumer's Union. How nutritious are fast food meals? *Consumer's Report*, p. 278, May 1975.

Council on Foods and Nutrition, Am. Med. Assoc. Malnutrition and hunger in the United States. *J. Am. Med. Assoc.* 213:272, 1970.

Dahl, L. K. Salt and hypertension. *Am. J. Clin. Nutr.* 25:231, 1972.

Deutsch, R. M. *The New Nuts among the Berries.* Palo Alto, Calif.: Bull Pub. Co., 1977.

Dietary goals for the United States. *Nutrition Today* 12(5):20, 1977.

Dwyer, S., Mayer, L., Kendel, R., and Mayer, J. The new vegetarians, who are they? *J. Am. Diet. Assoc.* 62:503, 1973.

Eckholm, E., and Record, F. The affluent diet. *The Futurist* 11(1): 1977.

Erhard, D. The new vegetarians: I. Vegetarianism and its medical consequences. *Nutrition Today* 8(6):4, 1973.

_____. The new vegetarians: II. The zen macrobiotic movement and other cults based on vegetarianism. *Nutrition Today* 9(1):20, 1974.

Frankle, R. T., and Heussenstamm, F. K. Food zealotry and youth: New dilemmas for professionals. *Am. J. Public Health* 64:11, 1974.

Goldberg, J. The fast food phenomena. *Family Health* 7(4):39, 1975.

Greecher, C. P., and Shannon, B. Impact of fast foods meals on nutrient intake of two groups. *J. Am. Diet. Assoc.* 70:368, 1977.

Hansen, R. G., Wipe, B. W., and Sorenson, A. W. *Nutritional Quality Index of Foods.* 1st Ed. Westport, Conn.: AVI Pub. Co., 1979.

Henderson, L. M. Programs to combat nutritional quackery. *J. Am. Diet. Assoc.* 64:372, 1974.

Jacobson, M. F. *Nutrition Scoreboard.* New York: Avon Books, 1975.

Lappe, F. *Diet for a Small Planet.* New York: Ballantine Books, Inc., 1975.

Latham, M. C., and Stephenson, L. S. U.S. Dietary Goals. *J. Nutr. Educ.* 9(4):152, 1977.

Lee, P. R. Nutrition policy: From neglect and uncertainty to debate and action. *J. Am. Diet. Assoc.* 72:581, 1978.

Loyd, F. G. Finally, facts on malnutrition in the United States. *Today's Health*, p. 32, Sept. 1969.

Mayer, J. One year later. *J. Am. Diet Assoc.* 58:300, 1971.

_____. *A Diet for Living.* New York: David McKay Co., Inc., 1975.

McBean, L. D., and Speckmann, E. W. Food faddism: A challenge to nutritionist and dietitians. *Am. J. Clin. Nutr.* 27:1071, 1974.

McNutt, K. W. An analysis of dietary goals for the United States. 2nd Ed. *J. Nutr. Educ.* 10(2):61, 1978.

Murray, T. K., and Rae, J. Nutrition recommendations for Canadians. *Can. Med. Assoc. J.* 120:1241, 1979.

Nat'l Dairy Council. Malnutrition in the United States. *Dairy Council Digest* 41(2):7, 1970.

_____. Nutrition and vegetarianism. *Dairy Council Digest* 50:(1):1, 1979.

Nat'l Nutrition Consortium. Guidelines for a national nutrition policy. *Nutr. Rev.* 32:153, 1974.

Owen, G. M., Kram, K. M., Garry, P. J., Lowe, J. E., and Lubin, A. H. A study of nutritional status of preschool children in the United States, 1968–70. *Pediatrics.* 53:597, 1974.

Pao, E. M., and Cronin, F. J. USDA's food consumption survey: nutritional implications. *Nutrition News* 43(2):5, 1980.

Robertson, L. C., Flinders, C., and Godfrey, B. *Laurel's Kitchen: A Handbook for Vegetarian Cookery and Nutrition.* Petaluma, Calif.: Nilgiri Press, 1976.

Sabry, Z. I., Campbell, J. A., Campbell, E., and Forbes, A. Nutrition Canada. *Nutrition Today* 9(1):5, 1974.

Schaefer, A. E. Malnutrition in the U.S.A.? *Nutrition News* (National Dairy Council) 32(4):13, 1969a.

_____. The National Nutrition Survey. *J. Am. Dietet. A.* 54:371, 1969b.

_____. Nutritional needs of special populations at risk. *Ann. N.Y. Acad. Sci.* 300:419, 1977.

Schafer, R., and Yetley, E. A. Social psychology of food faddism. *J. Am. Diet. Assoc.* 66:129, 1975.

Smith, E. A guide to good eating the vegetarian way. *J. Nutr. Educ.* 7:109, 1975.

Stare, F. J. and McWilliams, M. *Living Nutrition.* 2nd Ed. New York: John Wiley & Sons, 1977.

Stephenson, M. Textured plant protein products: New choices for consumer. *FDA Consumer,* May 1975.

Stillman, I. M., and Baker, S. S. *The Doctor's Quick Weight Loss Diet.* Englewood Cliffs, N.J.: Prentice-Hall, Inc., 1967.

A Study of Health Practices and Opinions. Final Report. Contact No. FDA 66-193. Washington, D.C.: Food and Drug Admin., U.S. Dept. of Health, Education, and Welfare, 1972.

Twenty commentaries. *Nutrition Today* 12(6):10, 1977.

U.S. Dept. of Health, Education, and Welfare. *Ten-State Nutrition Survey, 1968–1970.* DHEW Publ. No. (HSM) 72-8134. Atlanta, Ga.: Health Serv. and Mental Health Admin., 1973.

U.S. Dept. of Agriculture and U.S. Dept. of Health, Education, and Welfare. *Nutrition and Your Health: Dietary Guidelines for Americans.* Washington, D.C.: U.S. Gov't Printing Office, Feb. 1980.

U.S. Senate Select Committee on Nutrition and Human Needs, Dietary Goals for the United States, 2nd Ed. Gov't. Printing Office, Washington, D.C., 1977.

Wagner, M. G. The irony of affluence. *J. Am. Diet. Assoc.* 57:311, 1970.

White, P. L., and Selvey, N. *Let's Talk about Food.* Acton, Mass.: Publishing Sciences Group, Inc., 1974.

Wolff, R. J. Who eats for health? *Am. J. Clin. Nutr.* 26:438, 1973.

Worthington, B. S., Vermeersch, J., and Williams, S. R. *Nutrition in Pregnancy and Lactation.* St. Louis: The C. V. Mosby Co., 1977.

Youland, D. M., and Engle, A. Practices and problems in HANES. *J. Am. Diet. Assoc.* 68:22, 1976.

Young, E. A., Brennan, E. H., and Irving, G. L. Perspectives on fast foods. *Dietetic Currents* (Ross Labs) 5(5):23, 1978.

CHAPTER 8

Safety and Quality of the Food Supply

B. Swaminathan and Marlin C. Harmon

FOOD PRODUCTION*

World Food Production

The worldwide production of food, though not much in excess, is adequate, if managed properly, for the needs of the existing population. Increases in world food production are not keeping pace, however, with the tremendous increases in world population; if the current trends in population increases are not controlled, the world will face dire consequences by the turn of the century.

Great differences exist between the production of food in the developed regions of the world (North America, Western Europe, and Oceania) and in the developing regions (Africa, Latin America, Near East, and Far East). Figure 8-1 shows the total and per capita food production in the developed and developing countries for the period 1961–1976. It is evident that a 40% increase in the total food production of the developing countries did not result in a corresponding increase in the per capita food production because of significant population increases. During the period 1970–1976, population increased at an annual rate of 2.7% in Africa, while per capita food production increased only at 1.2%. In the Far East, which contains nearly

one-half of the world population, food production increased at an annual rate of 2.8% during 1970–1976, while population increased at an annual rate of 2.5% ("Growth of Food . . . ,"1977)

Food production in the Far East was able to keep pace with population increases during the early 1970s primarily because of improvement in agricultural methods and introduction of high-yielding varieties brought about by the Green Revolution. The impact of the Green Revolution has already peaked, however, and it would be unrealistic to expect food production to keep pace with the current rate of population increase in the Far East. Projected population levels for the year 2000 (Sukhatme, 1976) indicate that, even without an improvement in the current standards of diet in the developing countries, food supplies will have to be increased by 62% of the levels in 1980. Our ability to feed increasing numbers of people in the future is regarded as the most serious problem for which nations must seek an interdependent and global solution.

Diet Patterns of Developing and Developed Nations

Vast differences exist between the diet patterns in developing nations and those in developed nations. Cereals contributed approximately 65.4% of the total Calorie intake in the developing nations during 1972–1974, whereas the contribution of cereals to the total Calorie intake in developed nations dur-

---

* The following sections on *Food Production, Food Processing, Food Additives, and Food Laws* were written by B. Swaminathan and Marlin C. Harmon.

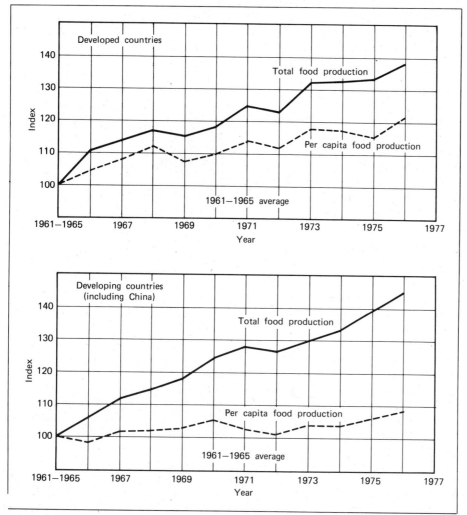

Figure 8-1. Total and per capita food production in developed and developing countries, 1961–1965 to 1976. (Courtesy of Food and Agricultural Organization of the United Nations, *Fourth FAO World Food Survey,* 1977. Redrawn by permission.)

ing the same period was only 26.4% In the developed countries cereals are used more for animal feed than for food. Animal products accounted for 33.4% of the daily per capita Calorie supply in the developed countries, whereas they accounted for only 6–10% of the daily per capita Calorie intake in the developing countries. As much as 58.6% of the total protein intake in the developed countries comes from animal sources, whereas only 14–28% of the total protein intake in the developing nations was from animal sources. The contribution of various types of food to the total per capita Calorie

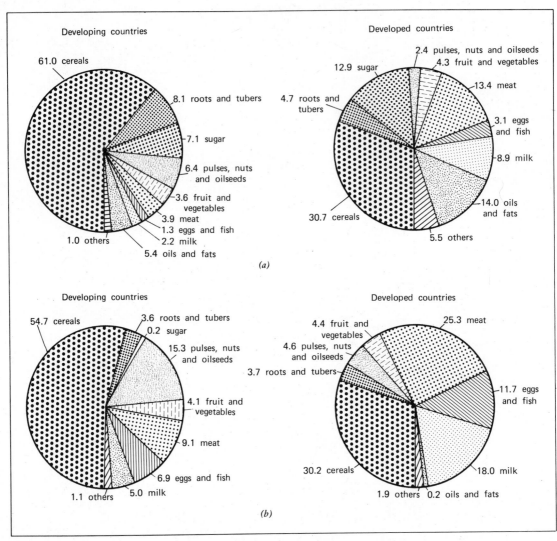

Figure 8-2. Dietary patterns in the developed and developing nations (1972–1974). (a) Percentage share of food groups in per capita *Calorie* supply. (b) Percentage share of food groups in per capita *protein* supply. (Courtesy of Food and Agricultural Organization of the United Nations, *Fourth FAO World Food Survey,* 1977. Redrawn by permission.)

intake and protein intake in the developed and developing nations is shown in Figure 8-2.

Food Production and Consumption in the United States

The United States produces a substantial amount of the total world food output. The total grain production in the world in 1977/1978 was estimated 1,316 million tons (1,184 tonnes), of which the United States produced 19.7% (Fig. 8-3). The United States produced more than 40% of the oil meal and edible vegetable oil output of the world in 1977/1978. Meat production in the United States in 1977 accounted for almost 25% of the world meat production (US Dept. of Agriculture, 1978). These figures assume great significance if we consider the fact that the population of the United States constitutes only 5.5% of the world population. The abundant production of food in the United States is reflected in the data on quantities of food nutrients available for consumption in the United States in 1977 (Table 8-1). In 1977 people in the United States consumed, on an

TABLE 8-1. Food Nutrients Available for Consumption in the United States (1977)

	Availability (per Capita per Day)
Food energy	3,380 Calories
Protein	103 gm
Fat	159 gm
Carbohydrate	391 gm
Calcium	.94 gm
Phosphorus	1.57 gm
Iron	18.6 mg
Magnesium	347 mg
Vitamin A	8,200 IU
Thiamine	2.09 mg
Riboflavin	2.50 mg
Niacin	25.6 mg
Vitamin B_6	2.29 mg
Vitamin B_{12}	9.7 mg
Ascorbic acid	116 mg

SOURCE: USDA, *Agricultural Statistics*, Washington, D.C., 1978.

average, 239.7 lb (107.9 kg) of meat, poultry, and fish; 34.5 lb (15.5 kg) of eggs; 350 lb (157.5 kg) of dairy products (including butter); 53.1 lb (23.9 kg) of fats and oils (exclud-

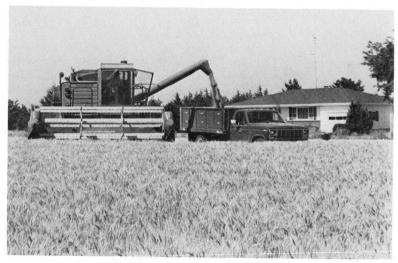

Figure 8-3. Wheat grown in the Midwest supplies the entire nation with bread. (Courtesy The Journal-Free Press, Osage City, Kansas)

ing butter); 137.2 lb (61.7 kg) of fresh and processed fruits; 206 lb (92.7 kg) of fresh, canned, and frozen vegetables; 129 lb (58.1 kg) of sugar and sweeteners; 139 lb (62.6 kg) of flour and cereal products; 86.4 lb (38.9 kg) of potatoes and sweet potatoes; and 17.2 lb (7.8 kg) of beans, peas, nuts, and soy products. Food accounts for less than 20% of the total consumer expenditure in the United States. In contrast, people living in countries of Western Europe spend 25–35% of their earnings on food, and people living in the Near and Far East may spend as much as 50% of their total earnings on food. The relatively low cost, abundance, and variety of food available in the United States is primarily due to the efficient growing, harvesting, preservation, storage, and distribution of food by the food industry.

FOOD PROCESSING

Food processing is primarily directed toward controlling deterioration and spoilage of food by applying the best available technology for handling and preservation. *Deterioration of food* is defined as those changes in food quality that are induced by physical, chemical, or biochemical reactions taking place within the food itself with or without the intervention of external environmental factors such as oxygen, carbon dioxide, water, heat, and light (Stewart and Amerine, 1973). *Spoilage of food* is caused primarily by biological agents such as insects and microorganisms. Spoilage caused by living organisms usually has a greater detrimental effect on food than deterioration. For example, putrefaction of meat left at room temperature for several days is brought about by spoilage microorganisms, whereas rancidity in meat (in particular, turkey and pork) stored for prolonged periods in the freezer is caused by deteriorative chemical reactions.

In addition to deterioration and spoilage, food infections and intoxications may occur

if food is stored under improper conditions or is handled under unsanitary conditions. Pathogenic bacteria are the major cause of foodborne disease outbreaks in the United States. In 1977 bacteria such as *Staphylococcus aureus, Salmonella, Shigella,* and *Clostridium perfringens* accounted for 64.2% of all confirmed foodborne disease outbreaks in the United States, whereas chemicals, parasites, and viruses were responsible for only 35.5% of the outbreaks.

Unit Operations in Food Processing
The processing of food is a collection of several operations, each one of which is contrived for a specific effect for the conversion of raw materials to finished product for the consumer. These operations can be divided into five basic types of processes: mechanical separations, physical-chemical separations, mixing operations, disintegrating operations, and forming operations. Within each of these five groups are found various techniques of accomplishing the specific type of operation. The nature of the raw product, the ultimate product desired, and the cost of the operation influence the choice of the techniques to be used in a particular situation. For example, the manufacture of mayonnaise involves the formation of an oil-in-water emulsion. This is achieved by the use of beating or dispensing equipment in some stage of the process to disperse the oil in aqueous solution. Egg yolk is used as the emulsifying agent in mayonnaise. The texture and uniformity of mayonnaise can be further improved by the use of colloidalizing or homogenizing machines. Finally, the product is packaged in glass or plastic containers and sealed.

Food Preservation by Canning
The process of canning as a means of food preservation was developed by Nicolas Appert in France around 1795. Appert recognized two important contributors to the preservation of food by thermal treatment: (1) the extent of heat processing required, which

varies with the type of food processed and size and type of containers, and (2) the need for hermetic sealing of containers after the heat treatment. Appert attributed spoilage of his canned foods to physical phenomena such as leakage of air into containers after processing. It was Louis Pasteur who showed that microorganisms were responsible for the spoilage and putrefaction of most improperly canned foods.

STERILIZATION AND COMMERCIAL STERILIZATION. *Sterilization* implies complete destruction of all microorganisms and spores. This can be achieved by exposing the material to moist heat at 121 C (250 F) for 15 minutes or the equivalent time-temperature combinations. Every particle of food in a container must be exposed to this treatment to render the product completely free of microorganisms and spores. Because the rate of heat transfer through food is very slow, it may take several hours to achieve a sterilizing environment in the coldest part of a can packed with a food product. Such a drastic treatment will lead to complete chemical deterioration of the product and will render it organoleptically unacceptable. Fortunately, sterilization, or complete destruction of all microorganisms, is not required for preservation of canned foods. Most of our canned or bottled food products are *commercially sterile*. This means that the degree of heat treatment given to the product is adequate to destroy all *pathogenic microorganisms* and reduce other microorganisms and spores to such a level that the product would not undergo spoilage. Commercially sterilized foods may contain a small number of heat-resistant spores that will not normally multiply in the food. Canned food products normally have a shelf life of about two years, after which there may be a perceptible deterioration in the flavor of the product as a result of chemical changes.

DETERMINATION OF THERMAL-PROCESSING REQUIREMENTS. An optimal thermal process is one that would achieve commercial sterility with the shortest exposure of product to heat. Three factors need to be considered in establishing a thermal process for a food product: (1) the nature and heat-destruction kinetics of microorganisms, (2) the nature and kinetics of inactivation of enzymes involved in food-quality deterioration, and (3) the nature and heat transfer characteristics of the food in the particular type of package to be used in the process.

The heat resistance of microorganisms varies with the type of microorganisms, the physiological state in which they are present (spores or vegetative cells) and the type of medium (food) in which they are present. The microorganism of greatest concern in canned foods is the pathogenic anaerobic sporeformer *Clostridium botulinum*, which produces a deadly neurotoxin (botulinal toxin) under anaerobic conditions. Other nonpathogenic spore-forming bacteria such as a putrefactive anaerobe and *Bacillus stearothermophilus* are even more heat resistant than *Clostridium botulinum*. Hence most thermal processes are based on the inactivation of the putrefactive anaerobe and *Bacillus Stearothermophilus*.

THERMAL PROCESSES. *Thermal death time* is the time required for destruction of microbes at a given temperature. The destruction of bacteria is known to follow a *logarithmic pattern*. That is, under constant heat conditions, the same percentage of bacteria will be destroyed in a given time period regardless of the size of the surviving population. For example, if a given temperature kills 90% of the microbial population in one minute, 90% of the remaining population will be killed in the second minute, and so on. The *D value*, or the decimal reduction time, is the time of heat treatment required to achieve one log reduction in the bacterial population. If a canned food product initially contains 10 million microorganisms and was given heat treatment equivalent to 7 D-values, it would still contain 1 surviving organism. Commercially canned foods are generally given a thermal treatment equivalent to 12 D-values. If a food product initially contained 10,000 spores of *Clostridium botulinum,* a 12-D process would render 99,999,999 of 100 million cans sterile.

The nature of the food influences the heat treatment to be given to render it commercially sterile. *Clostridium botulinum* does not grow in acid food (those with pH less than 4.5) such as tomatoes, pears, apricots, or cranberry juice. With acid foods, in many cases, heating at temperatures at or below 100 C (212 F) for a few minutes would constitute adequate heat treatment. *Clostridium botulinum* will grow, however, in low-acid foods (with pH greater than 4.5). Therefore, low-acid foods require more drastic heat treatment. A classification of foods on the basis of their pH and processing requirements is given in Table 8-2.

Food Preservation by Freezing or Refrigeration

Refrigeration and freezing are relatively recent introductions to the technology of food preservation. As late as the 1920s foods that were delivered by the manufacturer in frozen state completely thawed out before they could be brought home and were of poor quality (Potter, 1978). Today, freezing as a means of food preservation is increasing steadily in importance in terms of volume of food processed and is expected to grow in volume in the United States to approach and probably equal canning. *Refrigeration* generally refers to storage at a temperature range of 4.4–7.2 C (40–45 F), whereas *freezing* refers to storage at or below −18 C (0 F). Refrigeration and freezing prolong shelf life of foods by lowering rate of deteriorative chemical reactions. Refrigeration also aids in food preservation by lowering the growth rate of spoilage microorganisms and inhibiting the growth of pathogenic microorganisms. Freezing inhibits growth of all microorganisms. It must be emphasized that freezing does not result in complete destruction of microorganisms. As soon

as a frozen food is thawed, the microorganisms present in the food will begin to multiply and cause spoilage.

REFRIGERATION PRESERVATION. Refrigeration ideally of perishables should begin at the time of harvesting or slaughter and be maintained throughout transportation, warehousing, merchandising, and storage before use. The two requirements for proper refrigerated storage of foods are proper control of temperature and proper maintenance of air circulation and humidity. Adequately designed refrigeration units operating under optimal conditions should maintain the environment within ±1 C of the desired temperature. Factors that must be considered in the design of a refrigeration system are the kind and amount of food products to be stored, the frequency at which the doors to the refrigerated areas will be opened, the number of people that may be working in the refrigerated area (people generate heat), and the number of heat-evolving electric bulbs and electric motors that will be operating in the area (Potter, 1978). Fruits and vegetables respire and produce heat at varying rates. For example, it has been estimated that apples stored at 4.4 C (40 F) would respire and produce 590–840 Btu/ton in 24 hours. Broccoli, strawberries, and green beans have very high respiration rates (3,660–17,600 Btu/24 hr at 4.4 C). Therefore, special consideration needs to be given to design of refrigerators for bulk storage of fresh fruits and vegetables.

The air circulated within a refrigerator should not be excessively moist nor excessively dry. Excessively moist air will promote the growth of mold on food at refrigeration temperatures; very dry air will cause excessive drying of foods. Optimum relative humidities for the storage of various foods have been established, and those need to be taken into account in the design and operation of bulk storage for foods under refrigeration. Most foods store best at refrigeration temperatures when the relative humidity of the circulating

TABLE 8-2. Classification of Canned Foods on the Basis of Processing Requirements

Acidity Classification	pH Value	Food Item	Food Groups	Spoilage Agents	Heat and Processing Requirements
Low acid	7.0	Lye hominy Ripe olives, crabmeat, eggs, oysters, milk, corn, duck, chicken, codfish, beef, sardines	Meat Fish Milk Poultry	Mesophilic sporeforming anaerobic bacteria	High-temperature processing (115 to 121 C)
	6.0	Corned beef, lima beans, peas, carrots, beets, asparagus potatoes	Vegetables	Thermophiles Naturally occurring enzymes in certain processes	
Medium acid	5.0 4.5	Figs, tomato soup Ravioli, pimientos	Soup Manufactured foods	Lower limit for growth of Cl. botulinum	
Acid		Potato salad Tomatoes, pears, apricots, peaches, oranges	Fruits	Nonsporeforming aciduric bacteria	Boiling water processing (100° C)
	3.7	Sauerkraut		Acidic sporeforming bacteria Naturally occurring enzymes	
High acid	3.0	Pineapple, apple, strawberry, grapefruit Pickles, relish Jam-jelly	High acid foods High-acid–high-solids foods	Yeasts Molds	
	2.0	Cranberry juice, lemon juice, lime juice	Very acid foods		

SOURCE: Reprinted with permission from *The Technology of Food Preservation*, 4th Ed., p. 165, Norman W. Desrosier and James N. Desrosier (1977). AVI Publishing Co., P.O. Box 831, Westport, CT 06880, publisher.

air is between 80 and 95%. Celery and other crisp vegetables store best when the relative humidity of the air is 90–95%; nuts require a relative humidity of about 70% (Potter, 1978). Moisture loss from foods during refrigeration may also be prevented by proper packaging of food. Large cuts of refrigerated meat are usually protected from moisture loss by plastic wrappers or by spraying them with moisture-retentive coatings. Cheese is protected from moisture loss by wax coating. The loss of moisture and carbon dioxide from shell eggs during refrigeration is minimized by dipping the eggs in mineral oil, which coats and covers the pores of the shell.

FREEZING PRESERVATION. In 1977 over 20 billion lb (9 billion kg) of frozen foods with an estimated value of more than $18 billion were produced in the United States. It is estimated that the dollar value of frozen foods in the United States will further increase and come close to doubling by 1982. The per capita consumption of frozen foods in the United States is estimated to be 81.5 lb (36.7 kg) A plethora of convenience precooked frozen foods such as turkey dinners, chicken pot pie, breaded fish sticks, and other ethnic entrees are now available to the consumer.

Frozen foods are energy intensive and require low-temperature storage from the time of initial freezing to just before consumption. The commercial success of the frozen food industry in the United States owes much to the development of quick-freezing methods by Clarence Birdseye in 1920s.

THE PHENOMENON OF FOOD FREEZING. Water freezes at 0 C (32 F). The freezing point of most foods is below 0 C (32 F) because food is made up of water and other ingredients some of which are dissolved in the water. The temperature of a food undergoing freezing remains relatively constant at the freezing temperature until all the food is frozen, and then it approaches the temperature of the freezing

medium. Proponents of quick-freezing methods for foods advocate that a food undergoing freezing pass through the temperature of maximum crystallization (0–3 C, or 32–37 F) in less than 30 minutes. Hence the food industry does not use still-air freezing methods. Methods used for rapid freezing of foods include freezing in cold-air blast; direct immersion of food in a freezing medium; contact with refrigeration plates in a freezing chamber; and freezing in nitrogen, liquid air, or carbon dioxide (Desrosier and Desrosier, 1977).

In any given system freezing does not occur suddenly but takes place progressively. That is, all the food does not freeze at one time. When a milk bottle filled with milk is placed in a freezer, the liquid adjacent to the walls of the bottle will freeze first. Most of the liquid freezing initially will be pure water; thus the remaining liquid becomes more concentrated in minerals, protein, fat, and sugar. This concentrate, which gradually freezes also, becomes more concentrated as freezing proceeds. Finally, a central core of concentrate will remain unfrozen and will freeze if the temperature is lowered sufficiently. Such progressive freezing also occurs in the freezing of solid foods. Progressive freezing has serious ramifications for the quality of food. An unfrozen core or a partially frozen zone will deteriorate rapidly in texture, flavor, color, and other properties because of the high concentration of solutes in the remaining liquid phase. Thus, when milk is frozen slowly, the increase in concentration of minerals and salts in the unfrozen fraction can denature milk proteins and break up fat emulsions, which show up as curdling and butter granules (Potter, 1978).

The same kind of damage that occurs in foods undergoing slow freezing will occur if food is thawed slowly. Also, large volumes of frozen foods such as frozen roasts may take as long as 20–60 hours to thaw completely in air. During the slow thawing period there is considerable opportunity for bacterial multiplication, which may lead to spoilage of food or may cause foodborne illnesses. Thawing under cool running water (16–20 C, or 61–68 F) or agitated water at 16 C will greatly accelerate the thawing process and ensure the quality and safety of frozen foods.

Food Preservation by Drying

The use of *dehydration* for food preservation is based on the principle that chemical reactions and growth of microorganisms in food can be prevented by reducing the amount of moisture in food. The amount of available moisture (water) in a food is denoted by the term *water activity* (a_w). The water activity of pure water is 1.0 and of fresh foods such as meats, fruits, and vegetables is high ($a_w > 0.9$), and thus they are susceptible to chemical and microbial spoilage. The water activity of dehydrated foods such as dried milk, hamburger mixes, potato flakes, and juice crystals is much less ($a_w \simeq 0.2$), so that microbial spoilage is eliminated and rate of chemical reactions is lowered. The advantages of dehydrated foods are that the bulk is reduced by removal of water and they are stable at room temperature. The disadvantages of dehydrated food include the need for rehydration before consumption, loss of nutrients during processing, and deteriorative changes in food during the drying process. *Intermediate-moisture foods* are a separate class of food products that have a water activity below that of fresh foods and above that of conventional dehydrated foods. Intermediate-moisture foods may be consumed without rehydration. Examples of intermediate-moisture products are honey, jams, jellies, and preserves; fruit cakes; sweetened condensed milk; and cheese. Intermediate-moisture foods are not *readily* susceptible to spoilage; hence they do not require refrigeration and complex protective packaging. The product is more susceptible to mold once the package has been opened and the food exposed to air and moisture.

Because of the inherent advantages of intermediate moisture foods, considerable research effort is being expended on their development.

METHODS OF DEHYDRATION. Several methods are available for the dehydration of foods. Sun drying is the principal means of food dehydration in many developing countries even today. It is used even in developed nations such as the United States for the drying of grapes, raisins, and prunes. Sun drying has several disadvantages, however. It is dependent on elements beyond strict human control. It is also a very slow process during which spoilage of foods by microorganisms, insects, or rodents may occur. For example, in the African country of Chad, which has a large solar fish-drying industry, approximately 10% of the dry weight of the finished product is fly larvae deposited on the fish during drying (Labuza and Sloan, 1977).

The more common methods of dehydration used in the United States include drum drying, spray drying, vacuum-shelf drying, vacuum-belt drying, atmospheric-belt drying, freeze drying, fluidized-bed drying, rotary drying, cabinet drying, kiln drying, and tunnel drying (Potter, 1978). The choice of a particular type of drying method would depend on the nature of the material to be dried, the type of product desired, and the economic factors. Some methods such as spray drying are suitable for liquid products; other methods such as belt drying and tray drying are used for solid foods or mixtures containing food particles.

Freeze drying is the best dehydration process available at present, but it is not used to a very great extent because it is very expensive. The first step in freeze drying is the freezing of the water in the food; it is then directly removed by *sublimation* (direct change from solid state to vapor state). Frozen water will sublime at temperatures below 0 C (32 F) at pressures less than 4.7 mm. Controlled heat may be applied to the product during freeze drying to hasten drying if a sufficiently high vacuum is maintained (0.2–2.0 mmHg). Freeze drying is the method of choice for the preservation of delicate flavor and texture of sensitive, high-value foods such as coffee, juices, whole shrimp, and mushroom slices.

Preservation of Foods by Fermentation

Fermentation is one of the oldest forms of foods preservation. Even before it was known that microorganisms were responsible for fermentative reactions, the principles of fermentation were used in making foods such as bread, wine, and cheese. Today, fermentation is a major means of food preservation in developing countries, whereas it is used in developed nations to add variety to the diet. Because the process of fermentation is inherently an energy-efficient process, there is a renewed interest in the United States in exploring the potential for preparing new fermented foods.

The term *fermentation* is used to describe the breakdown of carbohydrates under anaerobic conditions. During fermentation, microorganisms partially use the nutrients in the food material and produce acids, alcohol, carbon dioxide, and other compounds that contribute to the flavor of the ultimate product. Carbohydrates are not the only constituents in foods that undergo changes during fermentation; proteins and fats are also broken down. Breakdown of proteinaceous materials is known as *proteolysis;* breakdown of lipids is known as *lipolysis.* Whether fermentative, proteolytic, or lipolytic changes occur in a particular fermentation process depends on the nature of the material, the type of microorganisms used, and the condition under which the fermentation is carried out. Some common fermented food products and the organisms involved in the fermentation processes are listed in Table 8-3.

The fermentation process needs to be strictly controlled to obtain the desired quality in the final product. Control over the process can be maintained by addition of salt (to inhibit salt-sensitive organisms and to encourage the growth of salt-resistant organisms), by controlling the temperature and level of oxygen, by reducing the bacterial load of the raw material, and by adding microorganisms that are most desirable in a particular fermentation process (starter cultures). Also, fermentation process itself is, to some extent, self-controlling. Many of the end products of bacterial growth and metabolism (acid, alcohol, etc.) are inhibitory to the growth of microorganisms.

Three major microorganisms are involved in the fermentation of cabbage to sauerkraut. In this fermentation microorganisms naturally present in cabbage are used. The process is controlled by adding and maintaining 2–2.5% salt and by carrying out the fermentation at a temperature near 21 C (70 F). Under these conditions, *Leuconostoc mesenteroides* grows first and produces acetic acid, lactic acid, alcohol, and carbon dioxide until the concentration of acid in the product approaches 1%. Further growth of *L. mesenteroides* is inhibited by 1% acid. *Lactobacillus cucumeris* takes over and carries on the fermentation and production of lactic acid until acid concentration reaches 1.5%. The final stage of fermentation is carried out by *Lactobacillus pentoaceticus,* which raises the acidity to above 2.5%.

The final products of food fermentations, such as acids and alcohol, are inhibitory to many common pathogenic bacteria such as *Clostridium botulinum.* Thus the safety of foods is enhanced by fermentation. The nutritional quality of foods is also improved by fermentation. Microorganisms involved in food fermentations break down the complex food materials and make them available in easily digestible forms. These microorganisms also synthesize several B-complex vitamins and other growth factors and enhance the nutritional quality of the final product.

TABLE 8-3. Microorganisms Used in Food Fermentations

Latic acid bacteria
  Vegetables and fruits
    Cucumbers → dill pickles, sour pickles, salt stock
    Olives → green olives, ripe olives
    Cabbage → sauerkraut
    Turnips → sauerruben
    Coffee cherries → coffee beans
    Vanilla beans → vanilla
  Meats → sausages such as salami, Thuringer, summer, pork roll, Lebanon bologna, cervelat
  Dairy products
    Sour cream
    Sour milk drinks—acidophilus, yogurt, cultured buttermilk, Bulgarian, skyr, gioddu, leban, dadhi, taette, mazun
    Butter—sour cream butter, cultured butter, ghee
    Cheese
      Unripened → cottage, pot schmierkase, cream
      Whey → mysost, primost, ricotta, schottengsied
      Ripened → Cheddar, American, Edam, Gouda, Cheshire, provolone

Lactic acid bacteria with other microorganisms
  Dairy products
    With other bacteria
      Propionic acid bacteria—Emmenthaler, Swiss, Samso, Gruyère cheeses
      Surface ripening bacteria—Limburger, brick, Trappist, Münster Port de Salut
    With molds—Roquefort, Camembert, Brie, hand, Gorgonzola, Stilton, Blue
  Vegetable products
    With mold—tempeh, soya sauce
Acetic acid bacteria—Wine, cider, malt, honey, or any alcoholic and sugary or starchy products may be converted to vinegar.

Yeasts
  Malt → beer, ale, porter, stout, bock, Pilsner
  Fruit → wine, vermouth
  Wines → brandy
  Molasses → rum
  Grain mash → whiskey
  Rice → sake, sonti
  Bread doughs → bread

Yeasts with lactic acid bacteria
  Cereal products → sour dough bread, sour dough pancakes, rye bread
  Ginger plant → ginger beer
  Beans → vermicelli

Yeasts with acetic acid bacteria
  Cacao beans
  Citron

SOURCE: Reprinted with permission from "Processing by Fermentation," p. 377, C. S. Pederson, in J. L. Heid and M. S. Joslyn, Eds., *Fundamentals of Food Processing Operations* (1967). AVI Publishing Co., P. O. Box 831, Westport, CT 06880, publisher.

FOOD ADDITIVES

Chemicals intentionally added to foods constitute a small but significant part of the many chemicals that human beings are adding to their environment. Food additives have become such a part of the way of life in the United States that it would be very difficult for us to put together a meal that contains no additives. A *food additive* may be defined as any substance that, when added either directly or indirectly, becomes a component of food or affects the functional characteristics of food. Additives are used in food not only to preserve them but to improve various functional properties such as flavor, odor, and texture and to improve the nutritional quality.

The use of additives in foods is not a recent development. Even before recorded history spices and salt were used to preserve meat and fish. The travels of Marco Polo were a consequence of the search for spices by tradesmen. Even the discovery of America by Columbus was the result of a serarch for new trade routes for tea and spices. Food colors were used by Egyptians as far back as 1500 BC.

Modern use of food additives has become necessary since technological revolution and industrialization have led to the concentration of the areas of food production and their separation from the areas of population. Food must be stored or transported under conditions conducive to spoilage. A class of food additives known as *preservatives* aid in retarding spoilage while food is transported from the production centers to consumers. Other additives such as antioxidants, colorants, and flavoring compounds are used to preserve and enhance the functional properties associated with food flavor, color, or texture.

It is possible to eliminate many additives from foods if a majority of our foods are prepared at home from basic raw materials. Yet most of us in the United States and other technologically advanced countries have come to accept convenience foods. We also demand more attractive foods of uniform quality and a wide choice of foods during all seasons of the year. Without food additives, it would be impossible to satisfy the demands of consumers for wholesome, appealing foods at a reasonable price. Desrosier and Desrosier (1977) suggest the use of additives in foods is justified to maintain or improve the nutritional quality of food, to enhance its keeping quality, or to make it attractive to the consumer in a manner that does not lead to deception.

Approximately 2,000 chemicals are intentionally added to foods to produce desired effects. In addition more than 10,000 chemicals may find their way into various foods during processing, packing, or storage. Examples of such incidental additives include extremely small amounts of pesticides used to treat crops, minute amounts of drugs fed to animals, and chemicals that migrate from packaging materials into the food. Natural and synthetic flavoring compounds constitute almost 85% of additives used in foods. It has also been estimated that functional food additives of natural and synthetic origin comprise less than 0.1% of the American diet.

Intentional food additives may be divided by function into several different categories. Desrosier and Desrosier (1977) have classified the functions of additives in foods as follows: acidifying, alkalizing, anticaking, antidrying, antifoaming, antihardening, antispattering, antisticking, bleaching, buffering, chill proofing, clarifying, color retaining, coloring, dough conditioning, creaming, curing, dispensing, dissolving, drying, emulsifying, enriching, firming, flavor enhancing, flavoring, flour maturing, foam producing, food-container lining, glazing, leavening, neutralizing, peeling, plasticizing, preserving (including antioxidizing), pressure dispensing, refining, replacing of air in food packages, sequestering, stabilizing, sterilizing, supplementing nutrition, sweetening, texturing, thickening, water retaining, whipping, and wrapper waterproofing.

Lehmann (1979) has classified currently permitted food additives into four major categories by function (Table 8-4). The nutrients (Group I) aid in improving or maintaining the nutritional value of processed foods. The additives in Group II serve to maintain product quality during processing, transportation, and storage. Additives in Group III are used to improve the organoleptic characteristics of food so that it becomes more appealing to the consumer, and those in Group IV enhance the appeal characteristics of food.

It is imperative that additives used in foods not pose hazards to the health of the consumer (Fig. 8-4). The present method of determining whether a chemical has undesirable effects is to feed animals, usually mice or rats, different levels of the chemical in their diet over their entire lifetime and sometimes through three or four generations. The highest test level is deliberately set high enough to

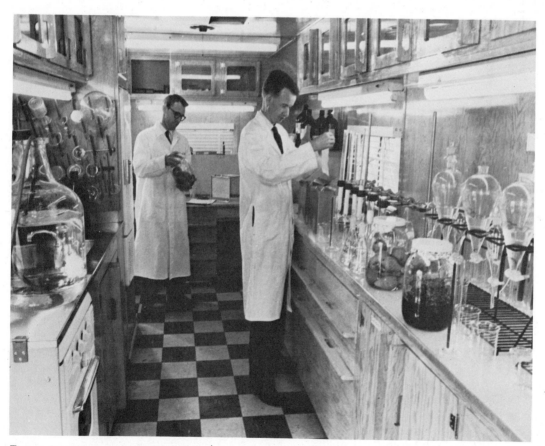

Figure 8-4. Chemists with the Food and Drug Administration monitor pesticide residues in food and examine the safety of food additives. (USDA photograph, courtesy Food and Drug Administration)

TABLE 8-4. Classes and Functions of Food Additives

Some Additives	Where You Might Find Them	Their Functions
	Group I (Purpose: To Improve or Maintain Nutritional Value)	
CLASS: NUTRIENTS		
B vitamins: thiamine, thiamine hydrochloride, thiamine mononitrate; riboflavin; niacin, niacinamide	Flour, breads, cereals, rice, macaroni products	Enrich: replace vitamins lost in processing
β-carotene (source of vitamin A)	Margarine	or
Iodine, potassium iodide	Salt	
Iron	Grain products	Fortify: add nutrients that may be lacking in the diet
Tocopherols (vitamin E)	Cereals, grain products	
Vitamin A	Milk, margarine, cereals	
Vitamin D, D_2, D_3	Milk, cereals	
Vitamin C (ascorbic acid)	Beverages, beverage mixes, processed fruit	
	Group II (Purpose: To Maintain Product Quality)	
CLASS: PRESERVATIVES (ANTIMICROBIALS)		
Ascorbic acid (vitamin C)	Fruit products, acidic foods	Prevent food spoilage from bacteria, molds, fungi, and yeast; extend shelf life; or protect natural color/flavor
Benzoic acid, sodium benzoate	Fruit products, acidic foods, margarine	
Citric acid	Acidic foods	
Lactic acid, calcium lactate	Olives, cheeses, frozen desserts, some beverages	
Parabens: butylparaben, heptylparaben, methylparaben, propylparaben	Beverages, cake-type pastries, salad dressings, relishes	
Propionic acid: calcium propionate, potassium propionate, sodium propionate	Breads and other baked goods	
Sodium diacetate	Baked goods	
Sodium erythorbate	Cured meats	
Sodium nitrate, sodium nitrate	Cured meats, fish, poultry	
Sorbic acid: calcium sorbate, potassium sorbate, sodium sorbate	Cheeses, syrups, cakes, beverages, mayonnaise, fruit products, margarine, processed meats	
CLASS: PRESERVATIVES (ANTIOXIDANTS)		
Ascorbic acid (vitamin C)	Processed fruits, baked goods	Delay or prevent undesirable changes in color, flavor, or texture—enzymatic browning or discoloration due to oxidation; delay or prevent rancidity in foods with unstable oils
BHA (butylated hydroxyanisole)	Bakery products, cereals, snack foods, fats and oils	
BHT (butylated hydroxytoluene)	Fruits, snack foods, cereals, instant potatoes	
Citric acid		
EDTA (ethylenediaminetetracetic acid)	Dressings, sauces, margarine	
Propyl gallate	Cereals, snack foods, pastries	
TBHQ (tertiary butylhydroquinone)	Snack foods, fats and oils	

CLASS: EMULSIFIERS

Substance	Foods	Purpose
Carrageenin	Chocolate milk, canned milk drinks, whipped toppings	Help to distribute evenly tiny particles of one liquid into another, e.g., oil and water; modify surface tension of liquid to establish a uniform dispersion or emulsion; improve homogeneity, consistency, stability, texture
Lecithin	Margarine, dressings, chocolate, frozen desserts baked goods	
Mono/diglycerides	Baked goods, peanut butter, cereals	
Polysorbate 60, 65, 80	Gelatin/pudding desserts, dressings, baked goods, nondairy creams, ice cream	
Sorbitan monostearate	Cakes, toppings, chocolate	
Dioctyl sodium sulfosuccinate	Cocoa	

CLASS: STABILIZERS, THICKENERS, TEXTURIZERS

Substance	Foods	Purpose
Ammonium alginate, Calcium alginate, Potassium alginate, Sodium alginate	Dessert-type dairy products, confections	Impart body, improve consistency, texture; stabilize emulsions; affect appearance/mouth feel of the food; many are natural carbohydrates that absorb water in the food
Carrageenin	Frozen desserts, puddings, syrups, jellies	
Cellulose derivatives	Breads, ice cream, diet foods, confections	
Flour	Sauces, gravies, canned foods	
Furcelleran	Frozen desserts, puddings, syrups	
Modified food starch	Sauces, soups, pie fillings, canned meals, snack foods	
Pectin	Jams/jellies, fruit products, frozen desserts	
Propylene glycol	Baked goods, frozen desserts, dairy spreads	
Vegetable gums: guar gum, gum arabic, gum ghatti, karaya gum, locust (carob) bean gum, tragacanth gum, larch gum (arabinogalactan)	Chewing gum, sauces, desserts, dressings, syrups, beverages, fabricated foods, cheeses, baked goods	

CLASS: LEAVENING AGENTS

Substance	Foods	Purpose
Yeast	Breads, baked goods	Affect cooking results, texture, and increased volume; also some flavor effects
Baking powder, double-acting (sodium bicarbonate, sodium aluminum sulfate, calcium phosphate)	Quick breads, cake-type baked goods	
Baking soda (sodium bicarbonate)	Quick breads, cake-type baked goods	

CLASS: PH CONTROL AGENTS

Substance	Foods	Purpose
Acetic acid/sodium acetate	Candies, sauces, dressings, relishes	Control (change/maintain) acidity or alkalinity; can affect texture, taste wholesomeness
Adipic acid	Beverage/gelatin bases, bottled drinks	
Citric acid/sodium citrate	Fruit products, candies, beverages, frozen desserts	

231

TABLE 8-4. (Continued)

Some Additives	Where You Might Find Them	Their Functions
Fumaric acid	Dry dessert bases, confections, powdered soft drinks	
	Cheeses, beverages, frozen desserts	
Lactic acid	Fruits/vegetables, dry/condensed milk	
Calcium lactate		
Phosphoric acid/phosphates	Fruit products, beverages, ices/sherbets, soft drinks, oils, baked goods	
Tartaric acid/tartrates	Confections, some dairy desserts, baked goods, beverages	
CLASS: HUMECTANTS		
Glycerine	Flaked coconut	Retain moisture
Glycerol monostearate	Marshmallow	
Propylene glycol	Confections, pet foods	
Sorbitol	Soft candies, gum	
CLASS: MATURING AND BLEACHING AGENTS, DOUGH CONDITIONERS		
Azodicarbonamide	Cereal flour, breads	Accelerate the aging process (oxidation) to develop the gluten characteristics of flour; improve baking qualities
Acetone peroxide	Flour, bread and rolls	
Benzoyl peroxide		
Hydrogen peroxide		
Calcium/potassium bromate	Breads	
Sodium stearyl fumarate	Yeast-leavened breads, instant potatoes, processed cereals	
CLASS: ANTICAKING AGENTS		
Calcium silicate	Table salt, baking powder, other powdered foods	Help keep salts and powders free flowing; prevent caking, lumping, or clustering of a finely powdered or crystalline substance
Iron ammonium citrate	Salt	
Silicon dioxide	Table salt, baking powder, other powdered foods	
Yellow prussiate of soda	Salt	

Group IV (Purpose: To Affect Appeal Characteristics)

Some Additives	Where You Might Find Them	Their Functions
CLASS: FLAVOR ENHANCERS		
Disodium guanylate	Canned vegetables	Substances that supplement, magnify, or modify the original taste and/or aroma of a food—without imparting a characteristic taste or aroma of its own
Disodium inosinate	Canned vegetables	
Hydrolyzed vegetable protein	Processed meats, gravy/sauce mixes, fabricated foods	
MSG (monosodium glutamate)	Oriental foods, soups, foods with animal protein	
Yeast-malt sprout extract	Gravies, sauces	
CLASS: FLAVORS		
Vanilla (natural)	Baked goods	Make foods taste better; improve natural flavor; restore flavors lost in processing
Vanillin (synthetic)	Baked goods	

Spices and other natural seasonings and flavorings, e.g., clove, cinnamon, ginger, paprika, turmeric, anise, sage, thyme, basil

No restrictions on usage in foods—found in many products

CLASS: NATURAL/SYNTHETIC (N/S) COLORS

N Annatto extract (yellow-red)	No restrictions	Increase consumer appeal and product acceptance by giving a desired, appetizing, or characteristic color—any material that imparts color when added to a food—generally not restricted to certain foods or food classes—may not be used to cover up an unwholesome food, or used in excessive amounts—*must* be used in accordance with FDA Good Manufacturing Practice Regulations
N Dehydrated beets/beet powder	No restrictions	
S Ultramarine Blue	Animal feed only 0.5% by weight	
N/S Canthaxanthin (orange-red)	Limit = 30 mg/lb of food	
N Caramel (brown)	No restrictions	
N/S Beta-apo-8' carotenal (yellow-red)	Limit = 15 mg/lb of food	
N/S Beta carotene (yellow)	No restrictions	
N Cochineal extract/carmine (red)	No restrictions	
N Toasted partially defatted cooked cotton-seed flour (brown shades)	No restrictions	
S Ferrous gluconate (turns black)	Ripe olives	
N Grape skin extract (purple-red)	Beverages only	
S Iron oxide (red-brown)	Pet foods only 0.25% or less by weight	
N Fruit juice/vegetable juice	No restrictions	
N Dried algae meal (yellow)	Chicken feed only	
N Tagetes (Aztec Marigold)	Chicken feed only	
N Carrot oil (orange)	No restrictions	
N Corn endosperm (red-brown)	Chicken feed only	
N Paprika/paprika oleoresin (red-orange)	No restrictions	
N/S Riboflavin (yellow)	No restrictions	
N Saffron (orange)	No restrictions	
S Titanium dioxide (white)	Limit = 1% by weight	
N Turmeric/Turmeric oleoresins (yellow)	No restrictions	
S FD & C Blue No. 1	No restrictions	
S Citrus Red No. 2	Orange skins of mature, green, eating-oranges; limit = 2 ppm	
S FD & C Red No. 3	No restrictions	Synthetic color additives certification: inspected and tested for impurities
S FD & C Red No. 40	No restrictions	
S FD & C Yellow No. 5	No restrictions	

CLASS: SWEETENERS

Nutritive sweeteners: Mannitol—sugar alcohol Sorbitol—sugar alcohol	Candies, gum, confections, baked goods	Make the aroma or taste of a food more agreeable or pleasurable
Dextrose Fructose Glucose	Cereals, baked goods, candies, processed foods, processed meats	
Sucrose (table sugar) Corn syrup/corn syrup solids Invert sugar	Cereals, baked goods, candies, processed foods, processed meats	
Nonnutritive sweeteners: Saccharin	Special dietary foods, beverages	

SOURCE: P. Lehmann, "More Than You Ever Thought You Would Know about Food Additives," Pts. II and III. *FDA Consumer* 13(4):18, 13(5):12. 1979.

produce a harmful effect. This is almost always possible inasmuch as nearly all chemicals including sugar, salt, starch, and some vitamins have harmful effects when fed to animals in megadoses ("The Risk/Benefit Concept . . .," 1978). At the completion of the feeding study, the lowest level of the chemical having a harmful effect is determined and the next lower level is designated as the *no-effect level*. The no-effect level is divided by a factor of 100 (generally referred to as the *100-fold safety factor*), and that level is used as the maximum permissible dietary level for the particular chemical. The 100-fold safety factor is used because there may be as much as a tenfold difference in sensitivity between humans and test animals, and there may be another tenfold difference in sensitivities among human beings. Each substance classified as a food additive must be tested for toxicological effects in laboratory animals before it can be approved for use in foods. Toxicological tests on one chemical may cost as much as $2 million and may take as long as three or four years to complete.

Food Additives and Cancer

Recently, public attention has been focused on the carcinogenic potential of certain food additives. Chemicals such as saccharin and nitrites that have been in widespread use for long periods of time are now suspected of being *carcinogens*. The Delaney anticancer clause of the 1978 Food Additives Amendment prohibits the use of any additive in food if the additive has been shown to cause cancer in any amount in laboratory animals. The absoluteness of the Delaney Clause may lead to some impractical situations. Trichloroethylene, a chemical used in the manufacture of decaffeinated coffee, has been shown to cause cancer in mice when fed at very high levels. Yet, to be exposed to the same level of trichloroethylene that caused cancer in mice, a human being would have to consume 50 million cups of coffee a day for 70 years. Similarly, the levels of the dye FD & C Red No. 2 that caused harmful effects in rats would be equivalent to a human dose of 1,600 lb (720 kg) of food containing 100 parts per million of the colorant. Our difficulties in determining the carcinogenic potential of food additives arise because we do not understand cancer completely. Our progress in determining the carcinogenic potential of food additives has not kept pace with our ability to detect chemicals in extremely small quantities. We do not yet have the capability of assessing the relative benefits and risks of chemicals added to food.

Perhaps the most widely publicized and debated issue today is the use of saccharin in foods. The FDA proposed a ban on the use of saccharin in foods and beverages after the completion of a study on saccharin by the Canadian government. The Canadian study involved feeding saccharin at 5% of the diet to two generations of laboratory rats. Among the first-generation animals, 3 of 100 developed bladder tumors. Among the second-generation rats, who were exposed to saccharin both prenatally and during their lifetime after birth, 14 of 100 developed bladder tumors. The proposed ban would have eliminated the use of saccharin in foods and beverages. In response to an unprecedented public protest, however, Congress passed an 18-month moratorium on the saccharin ban and later (June 1979) extended it until June 1981.

The alleged benefit of saccharin is that it aids in weight control. Cohen (1978) has estimated that substitution of saccharin-containing dietetic beverages for nondiet drinks would increase life expectancy by 100 times more than the cancer risk would reduce it. Others estimate that saccharin may be responsible for as many as 47,000 cases of bladder cancer in the United States each year and maintain that banning saccharin is the appropriate course of action. Opposition to the continued use of saccharin also stems from the fact that the beneficial role of saccharin in the control of obesity has not been firmly established. Some researchers indicate that saccharin may function as an appetite stimulant and may thus have negligible or no effect on the total Calorie intake of obese people. The case against saccharin appears to be gaining momentum at present. A study conducted by the National Cancer Institute of Canada on 480 men who had bladder cancer and a carefully selected control group has revealed strong correlation between saccharin consumption and incidence of bladder cancer. Saccharin has also been shown to be a promoter of carcinogenesis.

The use of nitrites in cured meat and poultry products has also come under criticism. Nitrites are used in meat, poultry, and fish products to obtain the characteristic cured-meat color and flavor. Nitrites also inhibit the growth of *Clostridium botulinum,* which produces the deadly botulism toxin in cured or canned meats. Recent research has shown that nitrites may react with secondary amines present in the food to form carcinogenic *nitrosamines.*

Consumers are justifiably apprehensive about the carcinogenic hazards from nitrosamines. Data from a recent research study conducted at the Massachusetts Institute of Technology indicates that oral administration of nitrites to rats increased the incidence of lymphatic tumors. It must be borne in mind while evaluating the risks of nitrites that the main sources of human exposure to nitrite is human saliva. Nitrate is a normal constituent of many vegetables and is present in large quantities in lettuce, beets, celery, and spinach. The nitrate consumed in the form of food is recycled through the saliva, and during this process it is partially reduced to nitrite by oral bacteria. It has been estimated that saliva supplies 9 mg grams of nitrites daily compared with 2.4 mg supplied by cured meats (Jukes, 1976).

Food Additives and Hyperactivity in Children

Hyperactivity is essentially a symptom. It may result from a child's basic personality, a temporary state of anxiety, or subclinical seizure disorders; or it may reflect a true *hyperkinetic state* ("Diet and Hyperactivity," 1976). The clinical manifestations of hyperkinesis are varied and may include short attention span and poor powers of concentration, impulsiveness and inability to delay gratification, decreased ability to experience pleasure, and frequent rejection of disciplinary measures. A child with hyperkinetic behavior will exhibit significant underachievement and classroom disruption in school and will disrupt family relations at home (Wender, 1973). It has been estimated that 3–10% of children in U.S. schools may be hyperkinetic, and the incidence may be as high as 25% in certain schools.

Feingold (1975) hypothesized that food additives may play a role in inducing or promoting hyperactivity in children. He claimed hyperactive (hyperkinetic) children with learning disabilities could be successfully treated by placing them on a diet free of artificial colors and flavors used in many processed foods. He proposed that the government should require full disclosures on food labels of the artificial colors and flavors used. He also suggested that food free of synthetic colors and flavors be designated by a special, easily recognized package symbol.

Recent studies conducted to test the validity of the Feingold hypothesis have failed to demonstrate a clear link between consumption of food additives and hyperkinesis in young children. A double-blind study conducted at the Food Research Institute of the University of Wisconsin on 36 boys between ages 6 and 12 showed no significant overall effect from the Feingold diet either as measured by classroom behavior or by parents (Larkin, 1977). The results of a study conducted at the University of Pittsburg on 15 children ranging from 6 to 12 years of age appeared to support the Feingold hypothesis.

It should be borne in mind that hyperkinesis is a symptom of a complex group of disorders and it would be simplistic to ascribe all hyperkinesis in children to food additives. An Interagency Collaborative Group on Hyperkinesis, working under the auspices of the FDA, has concluded that present studies have not conclusively established the Feingold hypothesis. The Committee on Nutrition of the American Academy of Pediatrics has concluded that there is no evidence that dietary modifications play a significant role in the treatment of children with hyperkinesis.

Food Additives and Allergy

The term *allergy,* or hypersensitivity, is generally used to determine altered immunological response to a material foreign to the body. The symptoms of immediate hypersensitivity appear almost immediately after exposure, whereas the symptoms of delayed hypersensitivity can appear from 24 to 96 hours after exposure to the *allergens.* The skin, the mucous membranes, the respiratory tract, and the gastrointestinal tract are the organs primarily affected by allergens. The manifestations of an allergic reaction may include eczema, hives, angioedema, rhinitis, asthma, abdominal pain, vomitting, diarrhea, dizziness, headache, joint swelling, and bladder inflammation (Catsimpoolas, 1979).

Food additives have been implicated as the cause of a large variety of unexpected food allergies. Such allergies usually have no relation to the nature of the food itself. Because allergies caused by food additives are difficult to identify, they pose a serious health hazard to the allergic people.

Among color additives permitted for use in foods in the United States, tartrazine (FD & C Yellow No. 5) has been incriminated as an allergen. It appears that aspirin-sensitive people may also be sensitive to tartrazine. A Swedish study conducted in 1972 in 52 patients with recurrent urticaria or angioedema showed that 7 of 8 aspirin-sensitive persons exhibited allergic symptoms after administrations of 1–2 mg of tartrazine. The FDA now requires label declaration on food products that contain tartrazine. Chemicals in other classes of food additives such as flavoring compounds, preservatives, antioxidants, emulsifiers, and stabilizers have also been implicated as causes of allergic responses in certain sensitive people. The Joint Food and Agricultural Organization–World Health Organization Expert Committee on Food Additives has recommended that n-octyl gallate, an antioxidant, should not be used in beverages liable to be consumed in large amounts. Recent reports indicate that the food preservative sorbic acid, which is being evaluated as a partial replacement for nitrite in cured meat products, may also have allergenic properties.

It has been estimated that less than 0.5% of the general population is likely to be allergic to a constituent of their diet. In evaluating the potential hazards of food additives, two factors need to be considered: Additives are necessary for the preservation, storage, and distribution of foods. They probably also account for only a small fraction of the total allergic responses associated with food. The total elimination of additives from foods on the basis of allergic reactions in some sensitive people would therefore be counterproductive.

FOOD LAWS

Law, Legislation, and Regulation

A *law* is a rule of conduct or action prescribed or formally recognized as binding or enforced by a controlling authority. *Legislation* is the exercise of the power and function of making rules (or laws) that have the force of authority by virtue of their promulgation by an official organ of state or other organization. A *regulation* is a rule or order having the force of law issued by an executive authority of a government. According to the Constitution of the United States, all legislative powers (at the federal level) are vested in the Congress. The authority to issue regulations based on the laws passed by Congress and to enforce compliance with the regulations is vested in the executive branch of the federal government, of which the president is the administrative head.

History of US Food Laws

When the United States established its independence in 1776, there were no federal food laws; consumers were their own food inspectors. Almost all food was sold in bulk. There were hardly any manufactured, processed, or packaged products. Because bread was the necessity for maintaining life, the first food laws passed by a few colonies dealt with the regulation of bread. A law enacted in 1646 by the General Court of Massachusetts states: "It is ordered by this Court and Authority thereof; that henceforth every baker shall have a distinct mark for his bread, and keep the true assizes, as hereafter expressed." A table followed, showing what a penny loaf of three qualities of bread—"white," "wheat," and "household"—should weigh when wheat was selling at a certain price. In 1720 the Massachusetts law was completely rewritten to prohibit adulteration. After independence the first general food law was passed in Massachusetts in 1784. It was designed to protect consumers from adulterated food, and it established criminal penalties for violators.

The country was undergoing an industrial revolution in the midnineteenth century. In the 1850s less than 50% of the general population was engaged in farming. As the production centers for food became organized and concentrated and as the distance increased between the areas of food production and food consumption, adulteration of foods became very serious. Poisonous substances such as copper sulfate, lead chromate, vermillion, and red lead were added to foods by unscrupulous merchants to cover up defects in foods and to deceive the consumer.

Dr. Harvey Washington Wiley, the chief of the Bureau of Chemistry of the US Department of Agriculture at that time (1883–1912) decided to convince Congress of the seriousness of the food adulteration problem. He organized a group of human volunteers (later known as Wiley's Poison Squad). Wiley fed massive doses of the chemicals used in foods at that time to his volunteers and documented the effects. At about the same time, Upton Sinclair published his book *The Jungle,* which described, in gruesome detail, the unsanitary and shocking conditions existing in Chicago's meat-packing plants. As a direct result of the above events, the Pure Food and Drugs Act and the Federal Meat Inspection Act (Fig. 8-5) became law in 1906.

The Pure Food and Drugs Act was not very effective because it did not lay down legal standards for foods. Also, the governmental regulatory agencies lacked authority to inspect warehouses. The burden of proof for showing that a chemical added to food was harmful was on the regulatory agency. To alleviate these shortcomings, Congress passed the Federal Food, Drug, and Cosmetic Act in 1938. At present the FDA is charged with the responsibility for administering the Food, Drug, and Cosmetic Act.

Federal Food, Drug, and Cosmetic Act

The Federal Food, Drug, and Cosmetic Act is the basic food and drug law of the United States. The law is intended to ensure that foods sold in the United States are pure and wholesome, safe to eat, and produced under sanitary conditions. It provides for truthful and informative labeling and packaging of processed foods. The FDA has several means of enforcing its provisions. Common enforcement actions are seizure of the product, obtaining an injunction against the sale or

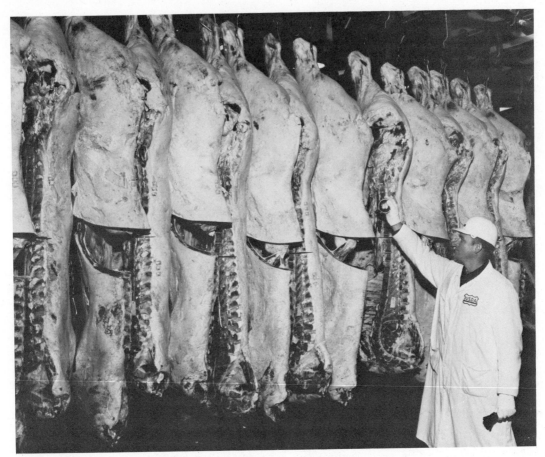

Figure 8-5. A USDA meat inspector applies a grade of quality to this meat carcass. (USDA photograph, courtesy Food and Drug Administration.)

manufacture of the product, and criminal prosecution of those responsible for the manufacture or distribution of products in violation of the law.

The Food Additives Amendment to the act was passed by Congress in 1958. This amendment is a very significant piece of legislation, for it shifts the burden of proving the safety of a food additive from governmental regulatory agency to manufacturer. The manufacturer or user of a food additive has to demonstrate its safety before it can be approved for use. The anticancer clause (com-

monly known as the Delaney Clause) is a proviso in the Food Additives Amendment that states that no food additive can be approved for use in foods if it has been shown to induce cancer in human or animal. The anticancer clause is absolute and does not permit risk-benefit evaluation of food additives by the regulatory agencies.

Exceptions to the Delaney Clause

Several classes of additives are excluded from the legal definition of a food additive. Substances *generally recognized as safe* (GRAS) by qualified experts are not considered food additives. Examples of GRAS substances are sugar, salt, citric acid, and many flavoring substances of natural origin. Also, pesticide chemicals used in or on raw agricultural commodities are not considered food additives, nor are chemicals introduced into food unintentionally. The Delaney Clause does not apply to such substances. For example, aflatoxins, which are potent carcinogens, are produced by the mold *Aspergillus flavus* growing on peanuts stored in humid environment. Peanut butter and other products may become contaminated with aflatoxins if they are prepared from moldy peanuts. Because aflatoxins are considered incidental rather than intentional additives, a maximum tolerance level for them in peanut butter can be set by the FDA. Similarly, tolerance levels in foods have been set for other toxic and carcinogenic incidental contaminants such as PCBs. The Delaney clause does preclude the FDA from setting any such tolerance levels for food additives. Hence, it has no choice but to ban food additives such as saccharin, cyclamates, and nitrites, although they may be only very weak carcinogens. Naturally occurring substances in foods are also not covered by the Delaney Clause.

The Color Additives Amendment (1960) applies to color additives and is very similar in scope to the Food Additives Amendment. The Delaney Clause also applies to color additives used in foods.

Meat and Poultry Product Regulation

The Food Safety and Quality Service of the U.S. Department of Agriculture (USDA) is charged with the responsibility of assuring the safety, quality, and wholesomeness of meat and poultry products sold in the United States. The agency conducts continuous inspection of meat and poultry products offered for sale in this country. The inspection entails antemortem inspection of animals to ensure their disease-free state, postmortem inspection of slaughtered carcasses, and inspection of further processed meat and poultry products. The cost of inspection is defrayed by charging an inspection fee based on the number of animals or birds inspected.

Grading of Food Products

In addition to meat and poultry inspection responsibilities, the Food Safety and Quality Service is also charged with grading meat and poultry products, eggs, dairy products, and fruits and vegetables. USDA grades are standards and are also measures of quality. For example, Grade AA and Grade A eggs are good for frying and poaching because they spread less in the pan and have firm yolk. US Prime and US Choice beef are more expensive grades of beef and are superior to US good and US commercial grades of beef in juiciness, tenderness, and other measures of quality. All grading services of the Food Safety and Quality Service are voluntary and are offered on a fee-for-service basis.

Other Federal Agencies Controlling Foods

Some other agencies involved in food regulation are the US Departments of Commerce and Treasury and the Federal Trade Commission. The National Marine Fisheries Service of the Commerce Department conducts inspection of fish and fish products and sets standards of sanitation, quality, grade, and identity for fish and fish products. Treasury's Bureau of Alcohol, Tobacco, and Firearms controls the production and sale of alcoholic beverages. The Federal Trade Commission safeguards the public by preventing the dissemination of false and deceptive advertising for food products. The Environmental Protection Agency regulates food industries by enforcing environmental antipollution laws.

FOOD TRANSPORTATION

After food production, food processing, and the regulation of food safety by enforcement of the food laws—the initial steps in what is sometimes called the *food chain* (Fig. 8-6), the next step is the safe transportation of food to a variety of outlets such as wholesale food companies, restaurants, schools, hospitals, and retail food stores. Unprocessed or fresh food goes directly from the producer to a roadside stand or a produce company and then to the retail store for purchase by a consumer. Food is transported within the United

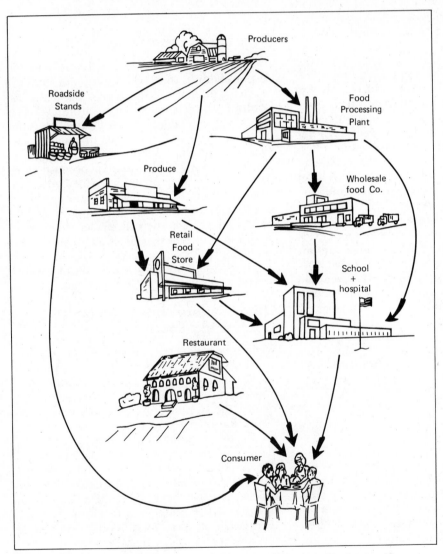

Figure 8-6. The food chain from producer to consumer. (Redrawn from *The Yearbook of Agriculture: Protecting Our Food.* USDA, 1966.)

States by airplanes, trucks, and trains equipped with modern refrigeration and freezing units. When food arrives at the retail food store, restaurant, school, or hospital, that institution is then responsible for the safe storage of the food. Supermarkets have a regular program designed to protect the safety of the food, which includes the rotation of stock on the shelves so that the oldest items are purchased first and the removal or price reduction of items with an expired freshness date. Other methods for insuring food safety include periodic checks of the refrigeration and freezing temperatures, a regular schedule for cleaning, and a periodic check for insects and rodents. Hospitals, restaurants, schools, and other institutions in which food is served are inspected for sanitation on a regular basis as defined by local laws.

FOOD USE IN THE HOME

The final step in the food chain is the purchasing of food by a consumer. The food may be purchased or obtained at a roadside stand, a retail food store, or a restaurant, school, or hospital. Nurses, dietitians, and home economists are constantly called upon to help families apply the principles of nutrition to food selection and preparation (Fig. 8-7). Two major concerns affecting food selection and preparation in many families today are the rising cost of food and the increased number of women working outside the home. There may be less money available for purchasing food and also less time available to prepare it. Each family has its own specific needs for help in menu planning, food purchasing, and food preparation. Dietitians and home economists are generally well equipped with such knowledge, and they are excellent resource people for nurses to use. Nurses so frequently encounter a need to counsel individuals and families about menu planning and food preparation that they require basic knowledge about menu planning economical purchasing

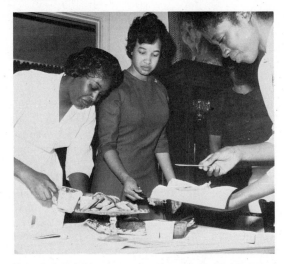

Figure 8-7. Nutrition aides help low-income families use commodity foods. (USDA photo by Kevin Shields)

of food, and methods of storing and preparing foods for safety and quality. This information should help nurses not only in counseling clients and their families but in planning and preparing better balanced meals for themselves or their families.

Meal Planning

Planning meals for a family involves many considerations, which can be grouped into four major topics: the food budget, the nutritive value of the meals, the appearance of the food served, and the time available for food preparation and eating. All these considerations depend on the particular family and their food preferences. Nutritious meals can be planned for the family using the basic four food groups as a guide. Economical purchasing of food is the subject of the next main section.

The appearance of the food served deserves attention. It is true that a food contains nutrients regardless of its appearance, but an attractively served meal does enhance appetite and enjoyment. This is one of the distinctions between the art and the science of nutrition. Variety is one of the keys to an attractively served meal. Consideration should be given in meal planning to including a variety of colors, flavors, textures, methods of preparation, and temperatures. Many examples could be given of menus containing foods of one basic color, flavor, or texture, but readers can easily construct some of these menus in their minds and immediately realize how unappetizing they would be. Variety in menu planning is sometimes difficult to attain because of therapeutic diet restrictions. For example, a prescribed bland diet may tend to result in menus quite similar in texture and color. On sodium-restricted diets, flavor needs to be enhanced with spices and herbs that are allowed. The planning of therapeutic diets and menus requires more creativity and planning to incorporate the desired variety.

The season of the year or the climate also requires consideration in meal planning. For example, hearty soups such as chili or homemade vegetable soup are more popular during the winter in a cold climate. In a tropical climate or during the summer, cold meals or sandwiches with fresh fruit and vegetable salads seem to be more acceptable.

In these times of rising food costs and unemployment, people at all income levels are interested in ways to save money on food purchasing. It is estimated that the average family in the United States spends 20% of its income for food. The lower the family's income, the higher the proportion spent for food. Families with a low income may be spending as much as 30 or 40% of their income for food. For the low-income family the challenge becomes how to eat better for less, thus stretching the grocery dollar to obtain maximum value. The USDA provides some help in the areas of food needs and food costs.

Food Needs

The components of a balanced diet were previously discussed in Chapter 2. A balanced diet can be obtained by eating regular meals and a wide variety of food. The daily food guide can be used for planning nutritious meals for the family (Table 8-5). The basic foods necessary for good health are the same for all the members of the family; the recommended quantities may vary. Daily menus can be checked against this guide to determine if the recommended number of servings are being included. It may be helpful to use a meal pattern based on the four food groups as a guide for planning daily menus. The meal pattern lists general categories of food for each meal (Table 8-6) and helps assure that a variety of foods will be included with each meal. It also permits a daily variety, since different foods may be included each day from the general food category.

Food Costs

The amount of money spent on food is influenced by the family's income and composition, the resources available for food preparation, and the actual food purchased. The USDA has developed four different food plans based on family income to assist consumers in setting up a food budget and planning menus: thrifty, low-cost, moderate-cost, and liberal (Peterkin, 1979).

The first step is to select a food plan that fits a given family. Table 8-7 shows how to determine the food plan for a specific family by using the family's income level and the number of members in the family. Table 8-8 shows the estimated food costs for a family or individual family members for each of the four food cost plans. This table can be used to estimate the weekly cost of feeding a family; however, some adjustments may have to be made. For meals eaten outside the home, subtract 5% from the cost for that particular person. For example, if the father eats lunch away from home five days a week, subtract 5% of the cost for each meal (a total of 25%) for a man 20–54 years old. For guests, add 5% for each meal for the age and sex category of the guest. Since this table is figured on the

TABLE 8-5. A Daily Food Guide

Servings Recommended		What Counts as a Serving[a]
Meat group 2 or more		2 to 3 ounces of lean cooked meat, poultry, or fish. As alternates: 1 egg, ½ cup cooked dry beans or peas, or 2 tablespoons of peanut butter may replace ½ serving of meat.
Milk group Child, under 9 Child, 9 to 12 Teenager Adult Pregnant woman Nursing woman	2 to 3 3 or more 4 or more 2 or more 4 or more 4 or more	One 8-ounce cup of fluid milk—whole, skim, buttermilk—or evaporated or dry milk, reconstituted. As alternates: 1-inch cube cheddar-type cheese, ¾ cup cottage cheese, ice milk, or ice cream, or ½ cup plain yogurt may replace ½ cup of fluid milk.
Vegetable—fruit group 4 or more, including: 1 good or 2 fair sources of vitamin C daily 1 good source of vitamin A— at least every other day		½ cup of vegetable or fruit; or a portion, for example, 1 medium apple, banana, or potato, a half a medium grapefruit or cantaloupe. *Good sources:* Grapefruit or grapefruit juice, orange or orange juice, cantaloupe, guava, mango, papaya, raw strawberries, broccoli, brussels sprouts, green pepper, sweet red pepper. *Fair sources:* Honeydew melon, lemons, tangerine or tangerine juice, watermelon, asparagus, cabbage, cauliflower, collards, garden cress, kale, kohlrabi, mustard greens, potatoes and sweet potatoes, cooked in the jacket, rutabagas, spinach, tomatoes or tomato juice, turnip greens. *Good sources:* Dark-green and deep-yellow vegetables and a few fruits, namely: Apricots, broccoli, cantaloupe, carrots, chard, collards, cress, kale, mango, persimmon, pumpkin, spinach, sweet potatoes, turnip greens and other dark-green leaves, winter squash.
Bread—cereal group 4 or more		Count only if whole grain or enriched: 1 slice of bread or similar serving of baked goods made with whole grain or enriched flour, 1 ounce ready-to-eat cereal, ½ to ¾ cup cooked cereal, cornmeal, grits, spaghetti, macaroni, noodles, or rice.
Other foods as needed To round out meals and meet energy requirements		Refined unenriched cereals and flours and products made from them; sugars; butter, margarine, other fats. Try to include some vegetable oil among the fats used.

[a] Amounts actually served may differ—small for young children, extra large (or seconds) for very active adults or teenagers.

TABLE 8-6. Meal Patterns Based on the Basic Four Food Groups

Meal Pattern	Meat	Milk[a]	Vegetable-Fruit	Bread-Cereal
Breakfast				
Fruit or juice (citrus, melon, strawberries)			X	
Main dish[b] and/or cereal with milk	X	X		X
Bread				X
Beverage		X		
Lunch				
Main dish[b]	X			
Vegetable or fruit			X	
Bread				X
Beverage		X		
Snack				
Beverage		X	X	
Other	X	X	X	X
Dinner				
Main dish[b]	X			
Vegetable			X	
Vegetable and/or salad (dark-green or deep-yellow vegetable at least every other day)			X	
Bread				X
Dessert		X	X	X
Beverage		X		

SOURCE: *Your Money's Worth in Foods.* Home & Garden Bull. No. 183, USDA, Washington, D.C., 1979.
[a] Enough milk is allowed for everyone at least once daily, and for children and teenagers more often, as suggested in guide, Table 8-5.
[b] Usually includes some meat, poultry, fish, egg, dry beans or peas, peanut butter, or cheese. It may contain other foods as well.

TABLE 8-7. The Food Plan for the Family

Income (before taxes)	1-Person Family	2-Person Family	3-Person Family	4-Person Family	5-Person Family	6-Person Family
$2,500 to $5,000	T[a] or LC	T[a] or LC	T[a]	T[a]	T[a]	T[a]
$5,000 to $10,000	MC	LC	T[a] or LC	T[a]	T[a]	T[a]
$10,000 to $15,000	L	MC	LC or MC	LC	T[a] or LC	T[a]
$15,000 to $20,000	L	L	MC	LC or MC	LC	T[a] or LC
$20,000 to $30,000	L	L	MC or L	MC	LC or MC	LC
$30,000 to $40,000	L	L	L	MC or L	MC or L	MC
$40,000 or more	L	L	L	L	L	MC or L

SOURCE: Peterkin, B. Consumer and Food Economics Instit., Agricultural Research Serv. *Family Food Budgeting for Good Meals and Good Nutrition.* Home & Garden Bull. No. 94. Washington, D.C.: U.S. Dept. of Agriculture, 1979.

T = Thrifty LC = Low Cost MC = Moderate Cost L = Liberal

NOTE: *To use this table,* locate the column that corresponds to the number of persons in the family. Then move down this column to the point opposite the family income before taxes are deducted. The plan shown there costs about the amount a typical household (of similar size and income) spends for food. It is the plan a family of that size and income can usually afford.
[a] Many families of this size and income are eligible for assistance through the Food Stamp Program.

TABLE 8-8. Estimated Cost (in Dollars) of One Week's Food at Home, United States Average, March 1979

Family or Family Member	Thrifty Plan	Low-cost Plan	Moderate-cost Plan	Liberal Plan
Family of two:[a]				
20–54 years	27.80	36.40	45.60	54.70
55 years and over	25.00	32.30	40.00	48.00
Family of four: Couple with—				
Children, 1–2 and 3–5 years	39.20	50.70	63.30	75.80
Children, 6–8 and 9–11 years	47.20	61.10	76.70	91.80
Family members:[b]				
Child:				
7 months to 1 year	5.60	6.80	8.30	9.80
1–2 years	6.30	8.00	9.90	11.80
3–5 years	7.60	9.60	11.90	14.30
6–8 years	9.70	12.40	15.60	18.70
9–11 years	12.20	15.60	19.60	23.40
Male:				
12–14 years	13.00	16.50	20.80	24.90
15–19 years	14.30	18.40	23.10	27.70
20–54 years	13.90	18.30	23.10	27.80
55 years and over	12.40	16.10	20.00	24.10
Female:				
12–19 years	11.60	14.80	18.40	22.00
20–54 years	11.40	14.80	18.40	21.90
55 years and over	10.30	13.30	16.40	19.50
Pregnant	14.30	18.20	22.40	26.70
Nursing	15.20	19.30	24.10	28.60

SOURCE: Peterkin, B. Consumer and Food Economics Instit., Agricultural Research Serv. *Family Food Budgeting for Good Meals and Good Nutrition.* Home & Garden Bull. No. 94. Washington, D.C.: U.S. Dept. of Agriculture, 1979.

[a] 10 percent added for family-size adjustment.
[b] Costs given are for individuals in four-person families. For individuals in other-size families, adjust costs as suggested in text.

basis of a family of four, the following adjustments should be made for families larger or smaller.

1 person	add 20%
2 persons	add 10%
3 persons	add 5%
4 persons	use as is
5–6 persons	subtract 5%
7 or more persons	subtract 10%

These dollar amounts are for food only. They do not include nonfood items that are purchased at the grocer store, such as soap, pet food, and paper goods. These items may account for over $0.25 of every dollar spent in the supermarket.

Table 8-9 shows the amount of food from each of the four food groups to serve individual family members each day for each of the four cost plans. Note that the thrifty and low-cost plans contain a larger amount of breads and cereals. The moderate-cost and liberal plans contain larger amounts of meat and fruits and vegetables. Note, too, that the servings meet or exceed the recommended servings from the basic four food groups. Each of these four food plans is therefore nutritionally adequate. Table 8-10 translates these quantities of food into sample menus for each of the four cost plans. Note the differences in the foods provided on each of the four food plans (Peterkin, 1979).

TABLE 8-9. Food Plans at Four Costs: Food to Serve Each Day[a]

Food Plan and Family Member	Milk[b]	Cooked Lean Meat or Alternate[c]	Vegetables and Fruit	Cereal and Bakery Products
Thrifty plan	(Cup)	(Ounce)	(½ cup[d])	(Portion[e])
Child:				
1–5 years	2	1½ to 2	2	3 or more
6–11 years	2 to 3	2½ to 3	2½ to 3½	6 or more
Male:				
12–19 years	3	3 to 4	3 to 4	7 or more
20–54 years	1½	4 to 5	3 to 4	7 or more
55 years and over	1½	4	3 to 4	7 or more
Female:				
12–19 years	3	3	3 to 4	5 or more
20–54 years	1½	4	3 to 4	5 or more
55 years and over	1½	3	3 to 4	5 or more
Low-cost plan				
Child:				
1–5 years	2 to 3	2 to 3	2 to 3	3 or more
6–11 years	2 to 3	3 to 4	3 to 4	5 or more
Male:				
12–19 years	3 to 4	5 to 6	4 to 5	6 or more
20–54 years	1½ to 2	6 to 7	4 to 5	6 or more
55 years and over	1½ to 2	5	4 to 5	6 or more
Female:				
12–19 years	3 to 4	4	4	5 or more
20–54 years	1½ to 2	4 to 5	4	5 or more
55 years and over	1½ to 2	3 to 4	4	5 or more

Many resources are available to the homemaker for assistance in meal planning. A wide variety of pamphlets and recipes are available from the USDA county extension agents, supermarkets, and large food companies. The homemaker in Figure 8-8 uses various cookbooks and the supermarket ads to plan her menus.

Food Purchasing

After the family menus have been planned, the next step is to write out a shopping list. This may be either a complete shopping list based on the menus or a partial shopping list. Using a complete shopping list may minimize the number of trips to the store, cut down on impulse buying, and be more economical. The menus that have been planned should be

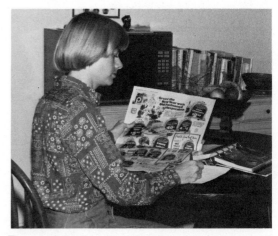

Figure 8-8. Careful planning of menus and shopping lists helps the homemaker cut food costs.

TABLE 8-9. (*Continued*)

Food Plan and Family Member	Milk[b]	Cooked Lean Meat or Alternate[c]	Vegetables and Fruit	Cereal and Bakery Products
Moderate-cost plan				
Child:				
1–5 years	2 to 3	2½ to 3	2 to 3	3 or more
6–11 years	3 to 4	4 to 5	4 to 5	4 or more
Male:				
12–19 years	4	5 to 7	4½ to 5½	6 or more
20–54 years	2	7 to 8	5 to 6	6 or more
55 years and over	2	6 to 7	5 to 6	5 or more
Female:				
12–19 years	3½ to 4	4 to 5	4 to 5	4 or more
20–54 years	2	5 to 6	4 to 5	4 or more
55 years and over	2	4 to 5	5	4 or more
Liberal plan				
Child:				
1–5 years	2½ to 3	3 to 3½	3 to 4	3 or more
6–11 years	3½ to 4½	5 to 6	5 to 6	4 or more
Male:				
12–19 years	4 to 4½	6 to 8	5 to 6	5 or more
20–54 years	2	9	6 to 7	5 or more
55 years and over	2	7 to 8	6 to 7	5 or more
Female:				
12–19 years	4	5 to 6	5 to 6	4 or more
20–54 years	2	6 to 7	5 to 6	4 or more
55 years and over	2	5 to 6	5 to 6	4 or more

SOURCE: Peterkin, B. Consumer and Food Economics Instit., Agricultural Research Serv. *Family Food Budgeting for Good Meals and Good Nutrition.* Home & Garden Bull. No. 94. Washington D.C.: U.S. Dept. of Agriculture, 1979.

[a] Amounts shown allow for some plate waste.
[b] As alternates: ¾ ounce of hard cheese or ¾ cup of cottage cheese, ice cream, or ice milk or ½ cup of unflavored yogurt may replace ½ cup of fluid milk.
[c] As alternates: 1 ounce of cooked poultry or fish, one egg, ½ cup of cooked dry beans or peas, or 2 tablespoons of peanut butter may replace 1 ounce of cooked lean meat.
[d] One-half cup of vegetable or fruit or a portion—one medium apple, banana, or half a medium grapefruit or cantaloupe. Smaller portions may be served, especially to young children.
[e] A portion is two slices of bread, one hamburger bun, one large muffin or cup cake, 1 ounce ready-to-eat cereal, or ¾ cup cooked cereal, such as oatmeal, rice, spaghetti, macaroni, or noodles. Smaller servings may be given, especially to young children, girls, and women; but the total daily amounts on the average should add up to portions listed.

flexible enough to allow for substitutions when discount coupons included with grocery ads appear in the paper. The homemaker should check the grocery ads weekly before going shopping, clip out useful coupons, and take along brand name coupons. Remember that a coupon is useful only when the product is one the family can use and its use helps to decrease the amount spent on food.

Some homemakers do not have an interest in planning menus in advance. They may prefer to shop from a partial list in which they write down general food needs. This type of food purchasing is a shop-now, plan-later list. An example of a partial list is shown below:

7 dinner meats (1 for company)
7 vegetables: canned, frozen, or fresh (1 for company)

TABLE 8-10. Sample Menus for a Day

Meal Pattern	Thrifty Plan	Low-cost Plan	Moderate-cost Plan	Liberal Plan
Breakfast:				
Fruit or juice	Orange juice (canned)	Sliced banana	Grapefruit sections (fresh)	Strawberries (fresh or frozen)
Main dish and/or cereal	Oatmeal with milk	Ready-to-eat cereal with milk	Omelet	Bacon and egg
Bread	Cinnamon toast	Corn muffin (from mix)	Toast	English muffin
Beverage	Coffee for adults	Coffee for adults	Milk (fresh) or coffee	Milk (fresh) or coffee
Lunch:				
Main dish	Peanut butter and jelly sandwich	Split pea soup	Sloppy Joe sandwich	Chicken, lettuce and tomato sandwich
Vegetable or fruit	Banana	Celery	Waldorf salad	Asparagus (frozen)
Bread	White bread (in sandwich)	Rye toast	Whole wheat bun (in sandwich)	Seeded roll (in sandwich)
Beverage	Milk (nonfat dry)	Milk (nonfat dry)	Milk (fresh)	Milk (fresh)
Other	Cookies (homemade)	Rice pudding	Potato chips	Sherbet
Snack:				
Fruit, cookies, etc.,	Cereal party snack	Orange	Ice milk, cookie	Cheese and crackers, peanuts
Beverage	As desired	As desired	As desired	As desired
Dinner:				
Main dish	Hamburger stroganoff	Fried chicken	Baked ham	Beef steak
Vegetable, pasta or rice	Noodles	Mashed potatoes (fresh)	Sweet potatoes	Corn on cob (fresh or frozen)
Vegetable and/or salad	Carrot-raisin salad (fresh)	Spinach (frozen)	Green beans (frozen)	Broccoli with butter sauce (frozen)
			Sliced tomato salad	Fresh fruit salad
Bread	Bread, white enriched	Bread, white enriched	Biscuit (ready-to-bake)	Dinner roll (bakery)
Dessert	Cookies (homemade)	Spiced cake (from mix)	Fruit gelatin	German chocolate cake (frozen)
Beverage	Milk (nonfat dry) or coffee	Milk (fresh) or coffee	Milk (fresh) or coffee	Milk (fresh) or coffee

NOTE: Milk for everyone at least once daily, and for children, teenagers, and pregnant and nursing women, more often. Spreads for bread and sugar for cereal and coffee may be added, if desired.
SOURCE: B. Peterkin, *Family Food Budgeting for Good Meals and Good Nutrition.* Home & Garden Bull. No. 94. USDA, Washington, D.C., 1979.

248

7 other vegetables, including potatoes, or rice,
macaroni, noodles, spaghetti (1 for company)
7 salad fixings: greens, raw vegetables, fruit,
cottage cheese (1 for company)
8 gallons milk
1 dozen eggs
2 packages cereal
1 package breakfast buns
Juice for breakfast
3 loaves bread
Cheese, peanut butter, tuna for sandwiches
Celery, carrots, pickles for lunches
Fruit for lunches
Canned fruit (4 large)
Cookies (2 boxes)
Cake mix (2 boxes)
Margarine
Coffee

Other items, such as salt, sugar, flour, salad
dressing, jelly, and mustard, are added as
needed. This partial type of list, however,
may necessitate additional trips to the store to
pick up miscellaneous items (US Department
of Agriculture Home and Garden Bulletin
No. 183, 1979).

Grocery Shopping

Many homemakers enjoy their weekly trip to
the supermarket. Some even look upon the
visit as a kind of adventure. Today's modern
supermarket with wide aisles, excellent lighting, and pleasant atmosphere presents a challenge to most homemakers. Some, however,
are bewildered and confused by the wide variety of products available. A modern supermarket contains 8,000 or more separate food
products. A single food may be available in 12
or more different forms. A given product may
be purchased fresh, frozen, canned, or dehydrated. A single product is available in several brands and sizes. There are also mixes,
imitation foods, and specially fabricated
foods.

Food purchasing demands time, energy,
and careful selection based on comparisons.
Grocery shopping should be done, if possible,
when the stores are not crowded. Food purchasing should not be attempted when the

shopper is hungry; this generally leads to impulse purchases. Where a person shops depends upon the availability of transportation
to the store. There are several types of food
stores: the local independent grocery, the
health food store, the quick-stop food chains,
the large supermarket food chains, and the
new discount warehouse food stores. The
shopper should select one or two stores in
which to shop instead of using extra fuel or
bus fare to shop for "bargains" at another
store. A grocery store should be selected on the
basis of its proximity to the home or office,
reasonable prices, and features such as variety
and quality of foods available and parking
facilities.

The purchase of certain foods, such as
meat, involves decisions based on economy
and quality. Some knowledge about the cuts
of meat and how they should be prepared will
help shoppers make wise selections (Fig. 8-9).
The best meat buy is not always the meat that
costs the least per pound. The unedible portion of bone, gristle, and fat should be considered. The number of servings per pound depends on the amount of bone and fat present.
The following may be used as a guide for
selecting meat and comparing the cost per
serving:

Three to four servings per pound from
items with little or no fat or bone, such as

Flank steak
Ground beef
Round steak
Stew meat, lean
Boned roast with little fat
Liver
Center cut of ham
Veal cutlet
Fish steaks and fillets

Two to three servings per pound from items
with a medium amount of bone, gristle, or fat,
such as

Most roasts
Some chops and steaks
Ham

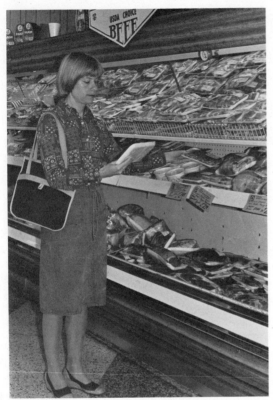

Figure 8-9. The purchase of meat requires the largest proportion of the food dollar.

Poultry
Dressed fish

One to two servings per pound from items with much bone, gristle, or fat, such as

Rib chops of lamb, pork, or veal
Plate and breast of lamb or veal
Spareribs
Shank
Porterhouse, T-bone, and club steaks
Chicken wings and backs
Short ribs (Home and Garden Bulletin No. 183, 1979)

The cost per serving for various cuts of meat can be compared by taking the cost per pound and dividing by the number of servings per pound for that particular cut.

Selection of fruits and vegetables also presents a challenge to shoppers. The number of servings per pound or container varies. Generally, fresh fruits and vegetables in season represent the best buy; however, if the crop was poor and the quantity available is limited, the price will be higher. Fresh produce must also be inspected for quality as well as price (Fig. 8-10).

Table 8-11 summarizes the nutritional bargains from the basic four food groups.

Consumer Aids

Food labeling, unit pricing, dating, and grading are types of information that can be used by the consumer to make wise decisions. Since

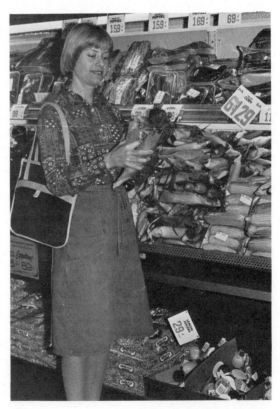

Figure 8-10. Fruits and vegetables in season are economical and have a high nutritional value.

the Fair Packaging and Labeling Act of 1966, the Food and Drug Administration requires that certain information be on every food label. This act requires that the name of the product appear on the principal display panel along with a statement of the net weight or net contents and name and address of the manufacturer or distributor. It also requires that the ingredients contained in the product be listed in the descending order of their prominence. A few foods do not require this listing of ingredients because a standard of identity has been established for them. A standard of identity is a basic recipe for a product, such as mayonnaise or salad dressing, established by the Food and Drug Administration. The standard requires that certain ingredients be used in the product. If optional ingredients are added to the "recipe," these must be stated on the label.

Several optional features may appear on food labels. A new format for nutrition labeling was instituted in 1974. Nutrition labeling is completely voluntary by the manufacturer unless a nutritional claim is made about the product or if any nutrient is added to a food. Under these two circumstances nutrition labeling is mandatory, and a specific nutrition labeling format must be used. The following information is required to be placed to the right of the principal panel:

1. Serving size and number of servings per container

2. Calories per serving

3. Grams of carbohydrate, protein, and fat per serving

4. Percentage of the US-RDA provided per serving for protein, vitamins A and C, thiamin, riboflavin, niacin, calcium, and iron

Optional information that may be provided is the fat and cholesterol content, including the percent of Calories from fat, the grams of polyunsaturated and saturated fatty acids per serving, the milligrams of cholesterol per serving, and the milligrams of sodium per 100 grams of the product. The percentage of

the RDA for other vitamins and minerals may also be included. The RDA as a nutritional standard was defined in Chapter 6. Examples of the nutritional labeling format are shown in Chapter 19.

Another consumer aid is the cost per unit of measure, as given in ounces, grams, liters, quarts, and so on. Many supermarkets are displaying the unit pricing on the edge of the shelf near the product. It can be used to directly compare the price among similar products. The number of servings per container on the nutrition label can be used to figure the cost per serving.

Grading of food by the USDA is also voluntary and is paid for by the processor or packer. The USDA grades are not a measure of nutritional quality. The grading system refers to such desirable qualities in food as tenderness, color, and uniformity of size. The nutritional quality of all the grades is comparable. The USDA grades are most commonly found on beef, veal, lamb, turkey, eggs, and butter. Other products that may contain grades are all types of fruits and vegetables, nonfat dry milk, and some cheese.

Open dating is a helpful guide to the consumer in deciding which perishable food products to buy. The four types of open dating commonly used are:

1. The *pack date* is the date the food was manufactured or packaged. This date is found on canned and packaged foods that have a long shelf life.

2. The *pull* or *sell date,* found on cold cuts and milk products, is the final date on which a product may be sold.

3. The *expiration date* is the last date the product should be consumed or used. Common examples of such products are infant formulas and yeast.

4. A *freshness date* may allow for normal home storage of the product following purchase. Bakery products are a common example. They are often sold at a reduced price after this date.

TABLE 8-11. Nutritional Bargains from the Basic Four

Food Group	More Economical	More Expensive
Milk	Skim and 2% milk	Whole milk
	Nonfat dry milk	Whole milk
	Evaporated milk	
Cheese	Cheese in bulk	Grated, sliced, or individually wrapped slices
	Cheese food	Cheese spreads
Ice cream	Ice milk or imitation ice cream	Ice cream or sherbet
Meat	Home-prepared meat	Luncheon meat, hot dogs, canned meat
	Regular hot dogs	All beef or all meat hot dogs
	Less tender cuts	More tender cuts
	U.S. Good and Standard grades	U.S. Prime and Choice grades
	Bulk sausage	Sausage patties or links
	Pork or beef liver	Calves liver
	Heart, kidney, tongue	
	Bologna	Specialty luncheon meats
Poultry	Large turkeys	Small turkeys
	Whole chickens	Cut-up chickens or individual parts
Eggs	Grade A eggs	Grade AA eggs
	Grade B eggs for cooking	
Fish	Fresh fish	Shellfish
	Chunk, flaked, or grated tuna	Fancy- or solid-pack tuna
	Choho, pink, or chum salmon	Chinook, king, and sockeye salmon (deeper
	(lighter in color)	red in color)
Fruits and Vegetables	Locally grown fruits and	Out-of-season fruits and vegetables or short
	vegetables in season	supply, exotic vegetables and fruits
	Grades B or C	Grade A or Fancy
	Cut up, pieces, or sliced	Whole
	Diced or short cut	Fancy-cut
	Mixed sizes	All same size
	Fresh or canned	Frozen
	Plain vegetables	Mixed vegetables or vegetables in sauces
Fresh		
Fruits	Apples	Cantaloupe
	Bananas	Grapes
	Oranges	Honeydew melon
	Tangerines	Peaches
		Plums
Vegetables	Cabbage	Asparagus
	Carrots	Brussels sprouts
	Celery	Cauliflower
	Collard greens	Corn-on-the-cob
	Kale	Mustard greens
	Lettuce	Spinach
	Onions	
	Potatoes	
	Sweet potatoes	
Canned		
Fruits	Applesauce	Berries
	Peaches	Cherries
	Citrus juices	
	Other juices	

TABLE 8-11. (*Continued*)

Food Group	More Economical	More Expensive
Vegetables	Beans	Asparagus
	Beets	Mushrooms
	Carrots	
	Collard greens	
	Corn	
	Kale	
	Mixed vegetables	
	Peas	
	Potatoes	
	Pumpkin	
	Sauerkraut	
	Spinach	
	Tomatoes	
	Turnip greens	
Frozen		
Fruit	Concentrated citrus juices	Cherries
	Other juices	Citrus sections
		Strawberries
		Other berries
Vegetables	Beans	Asparagus
	Carrots	Corn-on-the-cob
	Collard greens	Vegetables, in pouch
	Corn	
	Kale	Vegetables, in cheese and other sauces
	Mixed vegetables	
	Peas	
	Peas and carrots	
	Potatoes	
	Spinach	
	Turnip greens	
Dried	Potatoes	Apricots
		Dates
		Peaches
Breads and cereals	Day-old bread	Fresh bread
	Bread	Rolls, buns
	White enriched bread	Whole grain
	To-be-cooked cereal	Ready to eat cereals
	Regular cooking oatmeal	Quick cooking or instant oatmeal
	Plain rice	Seasoned rice
	Long-cooking rice	Parboiled or instant rice
	Graham or soda crackers	Specialty crackers

Another interesting addition to most food labels is the universal product code (UPC). A code consists of a set of numbered, parallel lines of varying widths. If the supermarket is equipped with a computerized checkout, the equipment can read the code and ring up the amount of the sale. Contrary to general belief, the lines do not contain the price of the food item. They contain information about name, manufacturer and product size only. The computer must be programmed with the current price of that item. One of the results of the UPC is the elimination of employee labor to stamp the price on each item. The price of the item is listed on the shelf and on the accompanying grocery receipt. The sales receipt from a computerized checkout system using UPC is usually more detailed than a regular receipt since an abbreviated form of the product name is printed out beside the price.

A couple of examples will illustrate how some of the consumer aids can be used to compare products as to nutritional quality, time required for preparation, and cost per serving. Two brands of beef stew could be compared. One can costs $1.39 and the other $0.99. Each contains three servings. The $1.39 beef stew lists beef as the first ingredient and it costs $0.46 cents per serving. The $0.99 brand lists beef as the third ingredient after water and potatoes. This beef stew costs $0.33 cents per serving. The decision to be made is whether the person purchasing the stew wants the higher protein content of the one product or the lower price of the other product. If other sources of protein are included in the meal, such as milk or cheese, the lower-priced stew is probably adequate. Another example concerns whether to buy long-cooking products or convenience foods. Long-cooking rice costs much less per serving (about $0.02) but takes about 20 minutes to prepare. Instant rice, on the other hand, takes only a few minutes to prepare but costs more per serving (about $0.08). So the question becomes, what does the consumer have more of—time or money? As a final example, one might compare the price per serving of a canned fruit or vegetable from a nationally advertised brand, a store brand, and a generic product. The cost savings of using the store brand or the generic product are often considerable, and the quality may not be noticeably different. In most cases the nutritional quality of these products is equal.

Food Storage

After food has been purchased, it is brought home to be stored until used. Nonperishable food is stored in the kitchen cabinets. Perishable food must be stored in the refrigerator or freezer or used immediately.

Nonperishable food should be stored in a relatively cool, dry place (preferably under 70 F (21 C), such as under the kitchen counter. The shelves should be clean and free from insects. All food should be covered for protection from insects. Many foods on the grocery shelf can be stored in the kitchen cabinet until they are opened; then they must be refrigerated (Fig. 8-11).

Select only high-quality fresh fruits and vegetables that are free from bruises and blemishes. Overripe or bruised produce will deteriorate rapidly and hasten the deteriora-

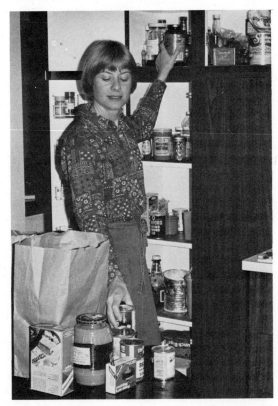

Figure 8-11. Staple foods may be safely stored for several months.

tion of other produce surrounding it. Though its price may be lower, it is not a good practice to purchase food in damaged packages or in cans that are dented or rusted. Never purchase a can that is bulged at the ends. Food is a delicate and highly perishable commodity, and it should always be purchased in the best possible condition.

Food should be stored in the refrigerator at a temperature of 40 F (4 C) or lower. This temperature will help to decrease quality losses and delay spoilage by retarding the action of enzymes and the growth of organisms that may be present. Foods vary in the amount of moisture and the temperaure required for storage. For example, green, leafy vegetables retain their crispness and nutrients better in cold, moist air. Meat and dairy products should be kept in the coldest part of the refrigerator. Fresh produce should be stored in the hydrator compartment or in plastic bags or plastic containers with tight-fitting lids (Fig. 8-12). A thermometer should be kept in the refrigerator so that the temperature can be closely monitored. For maximum cooling of the refrigerator, there must be adequate circulation of air. To maintain this circulation, the shelves should not be covered with foil or paper, and the unit should not be overcrowded with too many containers and food. The inside of the refrigerator should be cleaned regularly. A solution of baking soda and water may be used to freshen the interior. An open box of baking soda placed on a refrigerator shelf will help to absorb odors. Tables 8-12 to 8-14 give general guidelines for storing food in the refrigerator.

Frozen foods must be stored at 0 F (−18 C) or lower. Storage at temperatures above 0 F leads to a more rapid deterioration of the product. Freezer temperatures do not kill bacteria; they simply retard their multiplication. When purchasing frozen food, note the condition of the store's freezer cabinet and the condition of the freezer container. Do not buy frozen food in a torn, crushed, or juice-stained package. This condition indicates

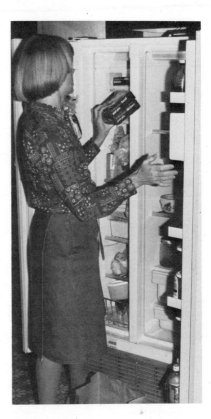

Figure 8-12. Most fresh foods are highly perishable and require proper storage in the refrigerator or freezer.

TABLE 8-12. Storage Guide for Milk Products and Eggs (in Refrigerator at 35–40 F)

Food	Storage Time
Eggs (store large-end-up)	7 days
Leftover yolks or whites	2–4 days
Milk	7 days
Cottage cheese	5–7 days
Soft cheeses	14 days
Hard cheese	Several months
Cheese spread or cheese food	7–14 days

SOURCE: Food Safety and Quality Ser., *Food Safety for the Family*. USDA, Washington, D.C., 1977.

TABLE 8-13. Storage Guide for Meats (in Refrigerator at 35–40 F)[a]

Food	Storage Time (Days)
Fresh meats	
Roasts (beef and lamb)	3 to 5
Roasts (pork and veal)	3 to 5
Steaks (beef)	3 to 5
Chops (lamb)	3 to 5
Chops (pork)	3 to 5
Ground and stew meats	1 to 2
Variety meats	1 to 2
Sausage (pork)	1 to 2
Processed meats	
Bacon	7
Frankfurters	7
Ham (whole)	7
Ham (half)	5
Ham (slices)	3
Luncheon meats	3 to 5
Sausage (smoked)	7
Sausage (dry and semidry)	14 to 21
Cooked meats	
Cooked meats and meat dishes	3 to 4
Gravy and meat broth	1 to 2
Fresh poultry	
Chicken and turkey (whole)	1 to 2
Chicken (pieces)	1 to 2
Turkey (pieces)	1 to 2
Duck and goose (whole)	1 to 2
Giblets	1 to 2
Cooked poultry	
Pieces (covered with broth)	1 to 2
Pieces (not covered)	1 to 2
Cooked poultry dishes	1 to 2
Fried chicken	1 to 2

SOURCE: Food Safety and Quality., *Food Safety for the Family.* USDA, Washington, D.C., 1977.
[a] Eating quality drops after time shown.

improper handling and partial thawing at some stage. Partial thawing will usually result in some deterioration of quality.

Remember that foods will not keep indefinitely in the freezer. Table 8-15 gives general guidelines for the length of time food can be safely stored in the freezer. The freezing unit of some refrigerators may not go as low as 0 F (−18 C). In these units, food should be stored only a few days. A refrigerator with a separate freezing unit will usually hold food at the desired temperature. If the refrigerator is not self-defrosting, it should be defrosted regularly to prevent the build-up of ice in the unit. Frozen food should be removed from the freezer during defrosting. It may be kept cold by placing it in cardboard boxes and covering it with newspaper. Run the freezer at least 10 minutes before replacing the food. If electric power is discontinued or if the freezer stops working, the food in a fully loaded freezer will stay frozen 1 to 2 days if the door is not opened (Home and Garden Bulletin No. 69, 1973).

Food Preparation

There are three basic methods for cooking foods: by moist heat, by dry heat, or by frying. Each one of these methods involves several special techniques that are encountered in following recipes.

MOIST HEAT

• *Boiling* is cooking in water or other liquid at boiling temperature (212 F or 100 C, at sea level). Bubbles rise continually and break on the surface.

• *Braising* is cooking meat or poultry slowly in steam from meat juices or added liquid trapped and held in a covered pan. Meat may be browned in a small amount of fat before braising.

• *Simmering* is cooking in heated air—usually in an oven—without water, uncovered.

• *Steaming* is cooking food in steam, with or without pressure. Food is steamed in a covered container on a rack or in a perforated pan over boiling water.

• *Stewing* is cooking in liquid, just below the boiling point.

DRY HEAT

• *Baking* is cooking in an oven or oven-type appliance in a covered or uncovered container.

TABLE 8-14. Storage Guide for Fruits and Vegetables

Hold at room temperature until ripe; then refrigerate, uncovered		
Apples	Cherries	Peaches
Apricots	Melons, except watermelons	Pears
Avocados	Nectarines	Plums
Berries		Tomatoes

Store in cool room or refrigerate, uncovered		
Grapefruit	Limes	
Lemons	Oranges	

Store in cool room, away from bright light		
Onions, mature	Rutabagas	Sweet potatoes
Potatoes	Squash, winter	

Refrigerate, covered		
Asparagus	Cauliflower	Parsnips
Beans, snap or wax	Celery	Peas, shelled
Beets	Corn, husked	Peppers, green
Broccoli	Cucumbers	Radishes
Cabbage	Greens	Squash, summer
Carrots	Onions, green	Turnips

Refrigerate, uncovered		
Beans, lima, in pods	Grapes	Pineapples
Corn, in husks	Peas, in pod	Watermelons

SOURCE: Consumer and Food Economists Institute, Science and Education Administration, *A Guide to Good Nutrition*, Home & Garden Bull. No. 1, USDA, Washington, D.C., 1978.

• *Broiling* is cooking uncovered on a rack placed directly under heat or over an open fire.

• *Roasting* is cooking in heated air—usually in an oven—without water, uncovered.

FRYING

• *Panfrying* or sautéing, is cooking in frypan in a small amount of fat, turning the food frequently.

• *Deep frying* or French frying, is cooking in a deep kettle, in enough fat to cover or float food.

It is important for the nurse to have an understanding of these methods for two basic reasons. First, knowledge of these cooking methods will assist the nurse in counseling clients about methods of cooking recommended for certain therapeutic diets. Any client who is on a low-Calorie, low-fat, diabetic, or bland diet should avoid eating and preparing fried foods. They should be instructed to prepare foods using moist or dry-heat methods that do not require the addition of any fat.

A second practical reason for understanding these cooking methods is to help clients obtain the most benefit from their meat purchases by explaining the optimal method of preparation for various cuts of meat. Meat cuts from beef, pork, and lamb may be divided into tender cuts and less tender cuts on the basis of the amount of connective tissue.

TABLE 8-15. Suggested Maximum Home-storage Periods to Maintain Good Quality in Purchased Frozen Foods

Food	Approximate Holding Period at 0 F (Months)
Fruits and vegetables	
Fruits:	
Cherries	12
Peaches	12
Raspberries	12
Strawberries	12
Fruit juice concentrates:	
Apple	12
Grape	12
Orange	12
Vegetables:	
Asparagus	8
Beans	8
Cauliflower	8
Corn	8
Peas	8
Spinach	8
Baked goods	
Bread and yeast rolls:	
White bread	3
Cinnamon rolls	2
Plain rolls	3
Cakes:	
Angel	2
Chiffon	2
Chocolate layer	4
Fruit	12
Pound	6
Yellow	6
Danish pastry	3
Doughnuts:	
Cake type	3
Yeast raised	3
Pies (unbaked):	
Apple	8
Boysenberry	8
Cherry	8
Peach	8
Meat	
Beef:	
Hamburger or chipped (thin) steaks	4
Roasts	12
Steaks	12

TABLE 8-15. (Continued)

Food	Approximate Holding Period at 0 F (Months)
Lamb:	
Patties (ground meat)	4
Roasts	9
Pork, cured	2
Pork, fresh:	
Chops	4
Roasts	8
Sausage	2
Veal:	
Cutlets, chops	9
Roasts	9
Cooked meat:	
Meat dinners	3
Meat pie	3
Swiss steak	3
Poultry	
Chicken:	
Cut-up	9
Livers	3
Whole	12
Duck, whole	6
Goose, whole	6
Turkey:	
Cut-up	6
Whole	12
Cooked chicken and turkey:	
Chicken or turkey dinners (sliced meat and gravy)	6
Chicken or turkey pies	6
Fried chicken	4
Fried chicken dinners	4
Fish and shellfish	
Fish:	
Fillets:	
Cod, flounder, haddock, halibut, pollack	6
Mullet, ocean perch, sea trout, striped bass	3
Pacific Ocean perch	2
Salmon steaks	2
Sea trout, dressed	3
Striped bass, dressed	3
Whiting, dawn	4

TABLE 8-15. (Continued)

Food	Approximate Holding Period at 0 F (Months)
Shellfish:	
Clams, shucked	3
Crabmeat:	
Dungeness	3
King	10
Oysters, shucked	4
Shrimp	12
Cooked fish and shellfish:	
Fish with cheese sauce	3
Fish with lemon butter sauce	3
Fried fish dinner	3
Fried fish sticks, scallops, or shrimp	3
Shrimp creole	3
Tuna pie	3
Frozen desserts	
Ice cream	1
Sherbet	1

SOURCE: *Home Care of Purchased Frozen Foods*, Home & Garden Bull. No. 69, USDA, Washington, D.C., 1973.

The less tender cuts of meat contain more connective tissue, and the collagen of the connective tissue can be softened by moist-heat cooking. If a less tender cut of meat such as a beef brisket is cooked by a dry-heat method such as roasting, the connective tissue will not soften and the meat will remain tough. The more tender cuts contain much less connective tissue, and they may be prepared using dry-heat cooking methods. Table 8-16 shows the recommended methods of cooking for common cuts of meat.

Cooking Equipment

The basic method for cooking foods can be accomplished using many different types of food preparation appliances. Technological development and advanced manufacturing processes, coupled with consumer demand, have helped to make a wide range of cooking appliances and utensils available on the market today.

The most common cooking appliance has been the gas or electric range, which uses conventional heating methods to cook and bake. In recent years, new appliances for cooking foods have been introduced that use less energy than gas or electric ranges. These include microwave ovens, convection ovens, and the new inductin range. Microwave cooking not only helps to reduce energy consumption and save time but also allows for greater nutrient retention because of the small amount of water that is needed in food preparation. Microwaved foods also cook in about one-fourth of the time required with conventional gas or electric ranges. Microwaves are produced with a wide variety of features such as electronic touch panels, memories, delayed-start functions, and temperature probes; some are equipped with turntables that rotate the foods to obtain a more even cooking pattern.

Another appliance available is the convection oven, which cooks by a high-speed fan that makes the hot air circulate, causing the food to heat quickly on the outside and sealing in moisture and natural juices. Convection ovens use more energy than microwave ovens but still considerably less energy than gas or electric ranges. Convection ovens are available in many sizes with many features and are now being combined with microwave ovens in one cooking appliance. The convection-microwave oven combines the best features of both to make a very versatile appliance.

Another cooking appliance that has been recently introduced is the induction range. The cookwave itself actually becomes the burner when cooking by this method, and the range top remains cool. Induction utilizes an electromagnetic coil that acts as the element and generates a magnetic field when steel cookware is placed on top. Induction ranges

TABLE 8-16. Meat Cooking Guide

Beef	Veal	Lamb	Pork
		DRY HEAT	
		Roasting	
Chuck or shoulder	Loin	Leg	Fresh and cured ham
Rib	Leg	Loin	
Round	Shoulder	Rib	Fresh and cured shoulder
Rump		Shoulder	
Sirloin			Loin
Sirloin tip			Spareribs
Tenderloin			
		Broiling	
Patties (ground)	Liver	Chops	Bacon
Thick steaks:		Liver	Canadian bacon
Chuck		Patties (ground)	Chops
Club			Cured ham slices
Porterhouse			
Rib			
Top round			
Sirloin			
T-bone			
		Panbroiling, panfrying	
Liver	Cube steaks	Chops	Bacon
Patties (ground)	Liver	Liver	Canadian bacon
Thin steaks:	Patties (ground)	Patties (ground)	Cured ham slices
Club	Cutlets or round steak		Liver
Cube steaks			Thin chops
Porterhouse	Loin and rib chops		Thin steaks
Rib			
Round			
Sirloin			
T-bone			
		MOIST HEAT	
		Braising, pot-roasting	
Chuck or shoulder	Cutlets	Breast	Chops
Flank	Loin and rib chops	Neck slices	Ham slices
Liver	Roasts:	Shanks	Liver
Round	Round	Shortribs	Shanks
Rump	Rump	Shoulder cuts	Spareribs
Shortribs	Shoulder		Steaks
Sirloin tip			Tenderloin
		Simmering, stewing	
Brisket	Breast	Breast	Cured ham
Corned beef	Riblets	Neck slices	Cured shoulder
Heel of round	Shanks	Shanks	Hocks
Neck			Shanks
Shanks			Spareribs
Shortribs			

SOURCE: *Family Fare: A Guide to Good Nutrition.* Home & Garden Bull. No. 1, USDA, Washington, D.C., 1978.

use less energy than gas or electric ranges because of instant heat response and the fact that the heat is confined to the pan. Since the top remains cool, spills are less likely to bake on. Children are also not as easily burned since the range top and handles of the pan remain cool.

The standard small appliances have been the electric skillet, percolator, toaster, can opener, and hand mixer. In recent years the market has been flooded with many specialty items for cooking and food preparation: food processors, juicers, blenders, mini-fryers, hamburger or hot dog cookers, egg cookers, pizza makers, doughnut makers, pressure-fryers, slow cookers, and hot-air popcorn poppers. The cost and versatility of small appliances should be considered in the process of selection. Some of these appliances have only one function, while others would be useful in many types of food preparation and cooking. Storage problems can occur when too many single-use appliances are purchased.

Cookware is composed of a variety of substances, including aluminum, stainless steel, cast iron, glass, pottery, stoneware, and plastics. Some of these substances are more suitable to one kind of cooking appliance, such as the gas or electric range, while others are versatile enough to be used in more than one cooking appliance. Metal cookware now comes in a variety of combinations, such as cast aluminum, aluminum, stainless steel with aluminum or copper bottoms, solid copper with tin linings, and cast iron. Today, much of the metal cookware is being made with nonstick coatings—T-Fal®, Silverstone®, and Teflon®. These coatings make it possible to fry foods with little or no oil or fat, and they make clean-up much easier. Most metal cookware is ideal for use with gas or electric ranges and convection ovens, and steel or iron cookware is suitable for the induction range. Glass or ceramic cookware, such as Corning® and Pyrex®, is very versatile and can be used in gas or electric ranges, microwave ovens,

and convection ovens. Glass and ceramics are ideal for storing leftover foods, are easy to clean, and are attractive enough to set directly on the table. Many items are now being made of stoneware or pottery that is suitable for gas or electric ranges, microwave ovens, and convection ovens. Often these items are more expensive, but they are generally easy to clean and are very attractive for use on the table. Unglazed and glazed clay products are also available. Generally these are soaked in water for a short period of time, emptied, then filled with the desired foods and very little additional moisture. These items can be used in gas or electric ranges and convection ovens, and they are suitable for the microwave oven. Meats tend to be more tender and to retain more nutrients when cooked in clay because little additional moisture has to be added. Plastics are now being developed that are durable enough for use in the microwave oven, and some can also be used in the oven of gas or electric ranges to about 300–400 F (148°–204 C). When plastics are being purchased, the versatility of the item should be taken into consideration. Plastics that can be used in both microwave and conventional ovens might be a better buy. Plastics are ideal for storage—many stack inside of one another. Some plastics are more difficult to clean than others. Light-colored plastics may stain or spot when in contact with certain foods.

Retention of Nutritive Value

Food is a delicate commodity that deteriorates rapidly and can be easily damaged during preparation and cooking. This damage or deterioration will lead to a reduced nutritive value. Care must be taken in selecting, storing, and handling food to ensure the conservation of nutrients in the food purchased. Careful consideration will result in high-quality food for the family.

As a general rule, fresh fruits and vegetables harvested directly are higher in nutritive value than produce that has been held in storage or transported long distances. For example, produce picked from a home garden may be higher in nutrients than produce that is available in the supermarket. Even frozen food that was packed immediately after harvesting may be higher in nutritive value than the fresh produce in the supermarket. Produce for use in the supermarket may be harvested at a point just below the peak of ripeness and allowed to ripen during storage, transportation, or display in the supermarket. The differences in nutritive value among fresh, transported, and frozen produce are only slight. Selection and preparation of a wide variety of fresh fruits and vegetables for the family is a more important consideration.

The nutritive value of a food may be damaged at any step in the food chain or in the home. A considerable loss of nutrients can occur during the food preparation process. In general, the less handling and manipulation of the food before cooking, the more nutrients will be retained. Preparation of fresh produce involves varying steps of washing, peeling, scraping, cutting, discarding, and sometimes soaking. As much as possible of the outer portions of foods should be retained and used. The amount of surface area exposed increases the loss of the water-soluble nutrients (Fig. 8-13). Foods should be left as whole as possible. Do not allow fruits or vegetables to soak in water before cooking. A loss of the water-soluble vitamins will occur. Usually this water is discarded either before or after cooking, and those nutrients are lost.

A practical rule to remember when cooking vegetables is to use only a small amount of water, cook in a pan with a tight-fitting lid, and cook the vegetables only until they are tender. Snapping the ends off green beans and soaking them in a large quantity of water several hours before cooking is a poor nutritional practice. The soaking water is then drained and the green beans covered with water and cooked on the range for several hours. Very few, if any, water-soluble nutrients probably remain in these beans. Make an

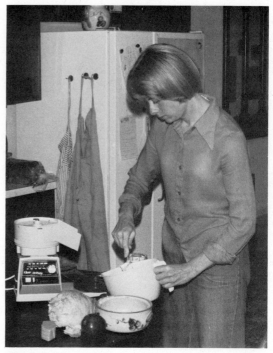

Figure 8-13. Proper food preparation and handling ensures the retention of nutrients and the safety of the food.

effort to learn to like cooked vegetables that are still crisp and have some texture. The stir-frying method of cooking is excellent, since the vegetables are cooked only a short time and they are still crisp (Home and Garden Bulletin No. 90, 1971). More specific suggestions for retaining nutritive value are found in Table 8-17.

Although it is true that cooking does reduce the nutritive content of food, cooking also provides some benefits. Cooking fresh vegetables and grains helps to soften the cellulose, thus decreasing the bulk and increasing the consumption of these foods. Cooking meat properly can increase the digestibility of the protein, although overcooking can decrease its value. Cooking can also increase the palatability of foods by changing their texture. Cooking also provides variety to the diet

TABLE 8-17. Retention of Nutritive Value

Food Group	Nutritive Losses			Retention
Vegetables				
Prepreparation	Vitamin A			Retain leafy parts of collard greens, turnip greens, and kale.
	Calcium, iron, and Vitamin A			Retain and use outer leaves of lettuce if not wilted or bruised.
	Vitamin C			Retain and use core and leaves of cabbage.
	Vitamin A			Retain and use broccoli leaves.
	Vitamins A and C			Use a sharp knife when trimming or shredding vegetables to prevent bruising.
Cooking	Vitamin C, B-complex vitamins, some minerals			Use a small amount of cooking water. Cover the pan with a light-fitting lid.
				Boil the liquid or cooking water for vegetables before adding the vegetable.
				Boil or bake potatoes, carrots, and sweet potatoes in their skins and peel after cooking.
Holding and reheating	Vitamin C			Use leftover vegetables within 1–2 days.
Fruits	Vitamin C			Well retained in citrus fruit juices, refrigerated either covered or uncovered.
		Storage temperature		
		65 F	80 F	
Canned foods	Vitamin C	10%	25%	Store canned foods at 70 F (22 C) for 1 year or less.
	Thiamine	Less than 10%	15–25%	Serve liquid off canned foods or use in some way.
	Vitamin A	Well retained	10%	
	Vitamin C, B complex vitamins			
Frozen foods	Vitamin C			Store at 0 F (−18 C) or lower for 1 year or less.
Meat, poultry, and fish	B-complex vitamins			Use drippings or meat stock in soups, casseroles, or gravy.
	Thiamine			Roasting beef rare to medium conserves thiamine.
Milk	Riboflavin			Protected by packaging in cardboard or plastic containers; exposure to light decreases riboflavin content.
Breads and cereals	Milling of grains removes the bran and the germ layers of the grain and also some B-complex vitamins and minerals.			Purchase whole grain, enriched, or fortified breads and cereals.
				Enrichment replaces thiamine, riboflavin, niacin, and iron.
				Fortification adds additional amounts of vitamins and minerals already present.
	Water soluble vitamins, especially thiamine			Use only a small amount of water to avoid draining.
				Do not wash rice before cooking or rinse after cooking.
				Baking conserves thiamine, but bake only until crust is light brown.
				Limit surface area exposed during baking.
				Toasting bread decreases the thiamine content.

SOURCE: *Conserving the Nutritive Values in Foods.* Home and Garden Bull. No. 90, USDA, Washington, D.C., 1971.

by allowing endless combinations of foods in recipes. A change in texture and taste can be experienced by eating a usually cooked food raw. For example, raw broccoli, cauliflower, cabbage, and carrots taste different from the cooked versions. Children may accept and eat these foods raw but reject them when cooked. Include a variety of both raw and cooked fruits and vegetables each day.

The nutritive value of food can be preserved by understanding some of the factors that influence the stability of the nutrients. Vitamins are the class of nutrients most easily destroyed during cooking. All uncooked foods contain enzymes that lead to the deterioration of the product and a reduction in the vitamin content. This process is hastened by destruction of the cell wall by bruises or cutting and by warm temperatures. Since the vitamins are organic chemical compounds, they have their own chemical properties. Vitamins are either stable or unstable under conditions such as an acid or alkaline medium, light, air, heat, or water. As a general rule, the water-soluble vitamins (the B-complex vitamins and vitamin C) are more easily destroyed by cooking. In fact, vitamin C is the most easily destroyed. Maximum conservation of nutrients can be obtained by using a small quantity of water, avoiding overcooking, and using the cooking liquid or juices in other food preparations such as gravies, soups, or fruit punches.

Safe Handling of Food

Whenever food is stored or handled, there is always the potential danger of foodborne illness. Poor food-handling practices that cause bacterial growth within the food may lead to illness. In one case the disease producing (pathogenic) bacteria may enter the food because of unsanitary food-handling practices by the food preparer. In *food infection,* the bacteria multiply in the contaminated food. When this food is eaten, the bacteria set up an infection in the digestive tract or the bloodstream. In another case bacteria that are already present in the food produce dangerous toxins. Eating this food leads to a serious type of food-related disease called *food intoxication* or *food poisoning.* The common foodborne illnesses and their causes, symptoms, and prevention are described in Table 8-18. A further discussion of these diseases is found in Chapter 24.

The prevention of these diseases involves safe food-handling practices. Bacterial growth thrives in an environment providing moisture, warmth, low acidity, and protein. Bacteria do not multiply rapidly at temperatures about 140 F (60 C), below 45 F (7 C), or in the presence of acid or large quantities of salt or sugar (Fig. 8-14). Knowing the most favorable and least favorable conditions for bacterial growth is important in the prevention of food-related illness. The foods that are the most suceptible to bacterial growth are eggs and products containing eggs; meat; fish and poultry; and low acid vegetables such as corn, green beans, asparagus, and peas.

The contamination of a food served in a family may affect some members of that family. Outbreak of illness from a contaminated food depends on individual susceptibility and the quantity of the food consumed. A food-related illness may affect many persons if the contaminated food is served at a church dinner, company picnic, or wedding dinner. An outbreak of a food-related illness also can be devastating in a school cafeteria, restaurant, hospital, or home for the elderly. For the healthy person the duration of a food-related illness will usually be brief. For the very young, the elderly, or those persons with serious illnesses, however, the consequences may be serious complications or even death. All persons involved with food preparation, especially those in institutions and those directly involved with the care of clients, should be conscientious not only to learn the rules of safe food handling but to practice them at home and at work.

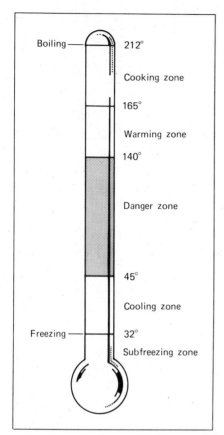

Figure 8-14. Temperature of food for control of bacteria. (Redrawn from *Protecting our Food, Yearbook of Agriculture,* 1966, p. 189.

The following are food-handling practices that will help to prevent foodborne illness.

CLEANLINESS OF FOOD PREPARER AND KITCHEN

1. Keep hands and nails clean and wear clean clothes when working with food.

2. Keep hands away from mouth, nose, and hair.

3. Wash hands with soap and water after using the toilet, smoking, sneezing, or blowing the nose.

4. Wash hands after handling raw meat, poultry, or eggs before touching other food.

5. Change dish cloths, towels, and sponges frequently.

6. See that work surfaces (counter tops and cutting boards), equipment, and dishes are clean before using.

7. Wash work surfaces and utensils with soap and water immediately after contact with raw meat, fish, poultry, and eggs.

8. Wipe off tops of jars and cans before opening

9. Use a utensil for handling food whenever possible.

10. Avoid using a spoon more than once for tasting during food preparation of service.

11. Avoid feeding a baby from a jar if the remainder of the food is to be stored.

FOOD STORAGE

1. Keep cold foods cold (below 40 F (5 C).

2. Make the grocery store the last stop when shopping and plan to go right home from the grocery.

3. After grocery shopping, refrigerate or freeze foods immediately after arriving home.

4. keep all foods containing eggs (cooked or uncooked) in the refrigerator. This includes cream, custard and meringue pies, custard fillings, cream puffs, eclairs, potato salad, meat salad, or sandwiches made with salad dressing.

5. It is safer to thaw meat in the refrigerator than at room temperature.

6. Do not place stuffing in uncooked meat or poultry and hold in the refrigerator. If stuffing is prepared in advance, refrigerate it separately and stuff the meat right before cooking.

7. Remove all stuffing from cooked meat and store it separately.

8. Refrigerate all leftovers immediately after a meal, including broth and gravy.

TABLE 8-18. Bacterial Foodborne Illness: Causes, Symptoms, and Prevention

Name of Illness	What Causes It	Symptoms	Characteristics of Illness	Preventive Measures
Salmonellosis Examples of foods involved: Poultry, red meats, eggs, dried foods, dairy products.	Salmonellae. Bacteria widespread in nature, live and grow in intestinal tracts of human beings and animals.	Severe headache, followed by vomiting, diarrhea, abdominal cramps, and fever. Infants, elderly, and persons with low resistance are most susceptible. Severe infections cause high fever and may even cause death.	Transmitted by eating contaminated food, or by contact with infected persons or carriers of the infection. Also transmitted by insects, rodents, and pets. Onset: Usually within 12 to 36 hours. Duration: two to seven days.	Salmonellae in food are destroyed by heating the food to 140 F and holding for 10 minutes or to higher temperatures for less time; for instance, 155 F for a few seconds. Refrigeration at 40 F inhibits the increase of Salmonellae, but they remain alive in foods in the refrigerator or freezer, and even in dried foods.
Perfringens poisoning Examples of foods involved: Stews, soups, or gravies made from poultry or red meat.	Clostridium perfringens. Sporeforming bacteria that grow in the absence of oxygen. Temperatures reached in thorough cooking of most foods are sufficient to destroy vegetative cells, but heat-resistant spores can survive.	Nausea without vomiting, diarrhea, acute inflammation of stomach and intestines.	Transmitted by eating food contaminated with abnormally large numbers of the bacteria. Onset: Usually within 8 to 20 hours. Duration: May persist for 24 hours.	To prevent growth of surviving bacteria in cooked meats, gravies, and meat casseroles that are to be eaten later, cool foods rapidly and refrigerate promptly at 40 F or below, or hold them above 140 F.

Staphylococcal poisoning (frequently called staph) Examples of foods involved: Custards, egg salad, potato salad, chicken salad, macaroni salad, ham, salami, cheese.	Staphylococcus aureus. Bacteria fairly resistant to heat. Bacteria growing in food produce a toxin that is extremely resistant to heat.	Vomiting, diarrhea, prostration, abdominal cramps. Generally mild and often attributed to other causes.	Transmitted by food handlers who carry the bacteria and by eating food containing the toxin. Onset: Usually within three to eight hours. Duration: one to two days.	Growth of bacteria that produce toxin is inhibited by keeping hot foods above 140 F and cold foods at or below 40 F. Toxin is destroyed by boiling for several hours or heating the food in a pressure cooker at 240 F for 30 minutes.
Botulism Examples of foods involved: Canned low-acid foods, smoked fish.	Clostridium botulinum. Sporeforming organisms that grow and produce toxin in the absence of oxygen, such as in a sealed container.	Double vision, inability to swallow, speech difficulty, progressive respiratory paralysis. Fatality rate is high, in the United States about 65%.	Transmitted by eating food containing the toxin. Onset: Usually within 12 to 36 hours or longer. Duration: three to six days.	Bacterial spores in food are destroyed by high temperatures obtained only in the pressure canner. More than six hours is needed to kill the spores at boiling temperature (212 F). The toxin is destroyed by boiling for 10 to 20 minutes; time required depends on kind of food.

SOURCE: Keeping Food Safe to Eat: A Guide for Homemakers. Home & Garden Bull. No. 162, USDA, Washington, D.C., 1978.

9. Store leftover foods in shallow containers to allow more rapid cooking.

10. Freeze a portion of cooked meat if there is more left than can be eaten in 2–3 days.

11. Keep all food covered during storage.

FOOD PREPARATION AND SERVICE

1. Keep hot foods hot (above 140 F, 60 C).

2. Use only fresh, clean, and unbroken eggs.

3. Cool custards or puddings containing eggs rapidly and refrigerate.

4. Do not hold foods in a pre-set (automatic) oven before cooking for more than 2–3 hours.

5. Do not partially cook meat one day and complete cooking the next.

6. If meat or poultry is to be stuffed, pack the stuffing lightly into the meat. Cook the stuffing to an internal temperature of 160 F (74 C).

7. Follow the temperature and timing directions for reheating frozen prepared foods.

8. Reheat leftovers thoroughly.

9. Food that is to be kept warm should be held above 140 F, 60 C).

10. Food held for more than 2–3 hours at 60–125 F (15–52 C) is very susceptible to bacterial growth and may not be safe to eat.

11. Food cooked in a slow cooker should reach a temperature of 140 F (60 C) in 4 hours or less to be safe. Check the temperature after 4 hours of cooking. It may be advisable to begin cooking on "high" for 1–2 hours if the cooker has a high setting (Home and Garden Bulletin No. 162, 1978).

FOOD PRESERVATION

1. Discard any canned food that shows signs of food spoilage, such as leaking, bulged ends, off-odor, or mold. Do not even taste it.

2. Low-acid vegetables, meat, and poultry, if home-canned, must be processed in a pressure canner to prevent botulism.

3. Tomatoes, pickled vegetables, and fruits may be safely home-canned using the water-bath method.

4. Boil most home-canned vegetables at least 10 minutes before tasting or serving. Boil home-canned spinach, corn, meat, or poultry at least 20 minutes.

5. If any home-canned food has an off odor or appearance, or foams, destroy it without even tasting (Home and Garden Bulletin No. 162, 1978).

Serving of Food

The final step in the food chain is the serving of economical, nutritious, and safe food to the family. If all the steps in the meal planning process have been carefully executed, the result is a well-balanced meal of nutritious, attractively prepared, and tasty food. The meal provides a pleasant atmosphere for the family to plan or discuss the day's activities.

The food preparer can assess the family's acceptance of the meal, assess the quantities of food eaten and leftovers, and make note of adjustments to be made the next time that menu or a similar one is served. Most food preparers who are in charge of feeding a family enjoy the challenge. There are, of course, many ways in which the entire family can become involved. Family participation becomes more common as more women are seeking careers and employment outside the home. The husband and wife may shop for groceries together, or the husband may be in charge of food purchasing. The husband or children may assist or be in charge of the food preparation and clean-up.

Planning and serving food to a family involves decisions about the time and money available for grocery shopping and food preparation. These involve further decisions about the types of foods to be purchased (home prepared or convenience foods) and the kinds of food preparation equipment to be used.

BIBLIOGRAPHY

Arlin, M. J. *The Science of Nutrition.* 2nd Ed. New York: Macmillan, Inc., 1977.

Catsimpoolas, N. Immunological aspects of foods and food safety. In S. R. Tannenbaum, Ed. *Nutritional and Safety Aspects of Food Processing,* pp. 399–409. New York: Marcel Dekker, Inc., 1979.

Cohen, B. L. Relative risks of saccharin and calorie ingestion. *Science* 199:983, 1978.

Consumer and Food Economics Instit., Science and Education Admin. *Keeping Food Safe to Eat: A Guide for Homemakers.* Home & Garden Bull. No. 162. Washington, D.C.: U.S. Dept. of Agriculture, 1978.

Consumer and Food Economics Research Div., Agricultural Research Serv. *Conserving the Nutritive Value in Foods.* Home & Garden Bull. No. 90. Washington, D.C.: U.S. Dept. of Agriculture, 1971.

Consumer and Food Economics Research Div., Agricultural Research Serv. *Storing Perishable Food in the Home.* Home & Garden Bull. No. 78. Washington, D.C.: U.S. Dept. of Agriculture, 1976.

Desrosier, N. W., and Desrosier, J. N. *The Technology of Food Preservation.* Westport, Conn.: AVI Pub. Co., 1977.

Diet and hyperactivity: Any connection? *Nutr. Rev.* 34:151, 1976.

Feingold, B. *Why Your Child Is Hyperactive.* New York: Random House, Inc., 1975.

Food and Drug Admin., Public Health Serv. *We Want You to Know about Foodborne Illness.* DHEW Publ. No. (FDA) 74-2044. U.S. Dept. of Health, Education, and Welfare, 1976.

Food Safety and Quality Serv. *Food Safety for the Family.* Washington, D.C.: U.S. Dept. of Agriculture, 1977.

Growth of food and agricultural production and food supply. In *The Fourth World Food Survey,* pp. 3–20. Rome: Food & Agricultural Org. of the United Nations, 1977.

Guthrie, H. A. *Introductory Nutrition.* 4th Ed. St. Louis: The C. V. Mosby Co., 1979.

Human Nutrition Research Div., Agricultural Research Serv. *Home Care of Purchased Frozen Foods.* Home & Garden Bull. No. 69. Washington: U.S. Dept. of Agriculture, 1973.

Jukes, T. H. Nitrates and nitrites as components of the normal environment. *Food and Nutrition News* 47(5):1, 1976.

Krause, M. V., and Mahan, L. K. *Food, Nutrition, and Diet Therapy.* 6th Ed. Philadelphia: W. B. Saunders Co., 1979.

Labuza, T. P., and Sloan, A. E. *Food for Thought.* Westport, Conn.: AVI Pub. Co., 1977.

Larkin, T. Food additives and hyperactive children. *Cereal Foods World* 22:582, 1977.

Lehmann, P. More than you ever thought you would know about food additives: II and III. *FDA Consumer* 13(4):18; 13(5):12, 1979.

Pederson, C. S. Processing by fermentation. In J. L. Heid and M. S. Joslyn, Eds., *Fundamentals of Food Processing Operations.* Westport, Conn.: AVI Pub. Co., 1977.

Peterkin, B. *Family Food Budgeting for Good Meals and Good Nutrition.* Consumer and Food Economics Instit., Agricultural Research Serv. Home & Garden Bull. No. 94. Washington, D.C.: U.S. Dept. of Agriculture, 1979.

Peterkin, B., Cromwell, C., and Vettel, R. *Food for the Family—a Cost Saving Plan.* Consumer and Food Economics Instit., Science and Education Admin. Home & Garden Bull. No. 209. Washington, D.C.: U.S. Dept. of Agriculture, 1978.

Potter, N. N. *Food Science.* Westport, Conn.: AVI Pub. Co., 1978.

The risk/benefit concept as applied to food. *Food Technology* 32:51, 1978.

Robinson, C. H., and Lawler, M. R. *Normal and Therapeutic Nutrition.* 15th Ed. New York: Macmillan, Inc., 1977.

Science and Education Admin. *Your Money's Worth in Foods.* Home & Garden Bull. No. 183. Washington, D.C. U.S. Dept. of Agriculture, 1979.

Stewart, G. F., and Amerine, M. A. *Introduction to Food Science and Technology.* New York: Academic Press, Inc., 1973.

Sikhatme, P. V. The world's food supplies. In *FAO Studies in Food and Population.* FAO Economic and Social Development Series 1. Rome: Food & Agriculture Org. of the United Nations, 1976.

U.S. Dept. of Agriculture. *Agricultural Statistics.* Washington, D.C., 1978.

Wender, P. H. Some speculations concerning a possible biochemical basis of minimal brain dysfunction. *Ann N.Y. Acad. Sci.* 205:18, 1973.

Williams, S. R. *Nutrition and Diet Therapy.* 3rd Ed. St. Louis: The C. V. Mosby Co., 1977.

Wilson, E. D., Fisher, K. H., and Garcia, P. A. *Principles of Nutrition.* 4th Ed. New York: John Wiley & Sons, Inc., Pubs., 1979.

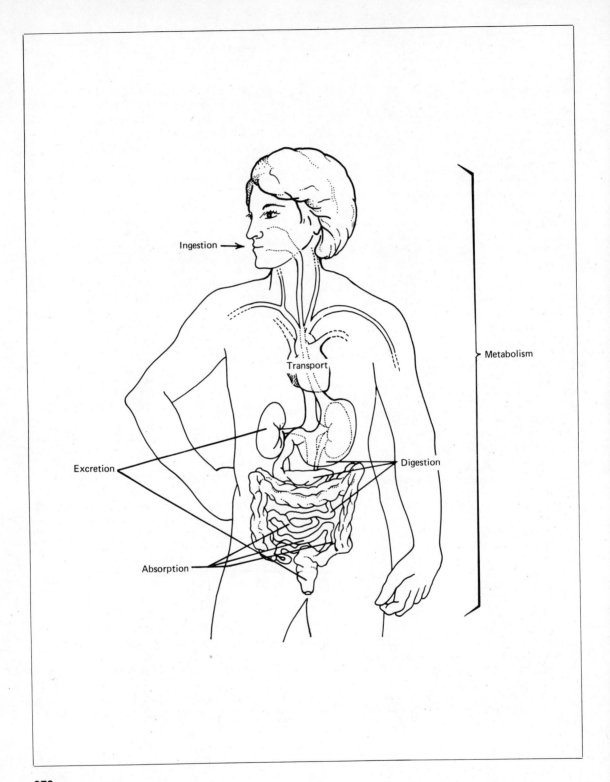

THE NUTRITIVE PROCESS

Nutrition is the process by which the living organism receives and uses the nutrients from food for the maintenance of its functions and the growth of its tissues. The process of supplying the organism with nutrients begins with the ingestion of food. The nutrients contained in food are made available to the body by the nutritive process, which consists of six separate steps: ingestion, digestion, absorption, transport, metabolism, and excretion. Incorporating principles from physiology and biochemistry, this unit examines the functions of the nutrients as they relate to the various steps in the nutritive process.

The ingestion of food and the regulation of food intake is the subject of Chapter 9. Chapter 10 describes how *motility* and secretions promote the digestion of food and the absorption of nutrients. Three important aspects of nutrient transport are discussed in Chapter 11: *vascular physiology, fluid* and *electrolyte balance,* and *acid-base balance.* The discussion of metabolism is divided between the next two chapters. Chapter 12 applies principles from biochemistry in considering the cellular metabolism of carbohydrates, proteins, and fats. This chapter concludes with a discussion of specialized cells, body tissues, and an introduction to the body systems. Chapter 13 covers the metabolism of the four structural body systems and the role of nutrition in the development and function of each system. This chapter ends with a brief explanation of the factors that influence nutritional requirements. The last chapter of this unit examines the role of the kidneys, colon, skin, and lungs in the excretion of nutritive wastes.

BEHAVIORAL OBJECTIVES

After completing this unit, the student will be able to:

1. Discuss the physiological factors that influence ingestion.
2. Identify the role of motility and secretions in the digestion and absorption of nutrients.
3. Discuss the maintenance of *homeostatic mechanisms* in the transport and storage of nutrients.

4. Identify the pathways that occur during metabolism of the energy nutrients.
5. Discuss *endocrine regulation* of metabolism.
6. Discuss the effects of nutrition on the development and maintenance of structural body systems.
7. Discuss the role of physiological mechanisms in the excretion of nutritive wastes.

CHAPTER 9

Ingestion

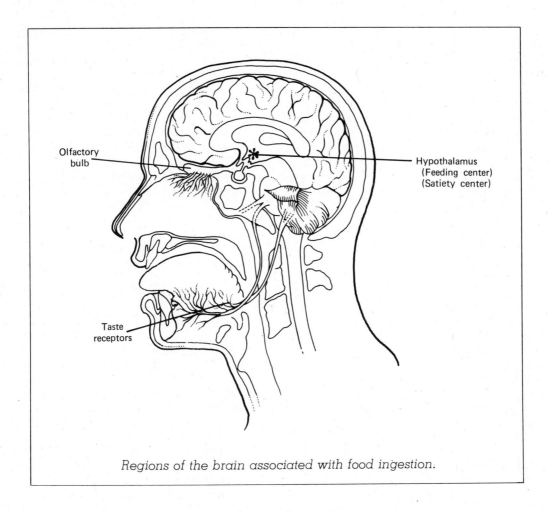

Regions of the brain associated with food ingestion.

Human beings depend on the environment for food, which must be ingested to sustain life. This chapter examines the events that affect the ingestion of food. Once food has been ingested the use of the food is influenced by numerous complex physiological and biochemical reactions and processes. The study of the use of the nutrients in food by the body is actually a study of the physiological and biochemical processes that occur. Major concepts from physiology and biochemistry are thus incorporated in this study of the nutritive process.

The benefits obtained from the nutrients in food can only be realized when the proper foods are consumed or ingested. Four major factors influence the process of ingestion of food: the desire to eat, the availability of food, the knowledge of nutrition, and the ability to ingest food. The availability of food and nutritional knowledge were discussed in Chapters 7 and 8; the desire to eat and the ability to ingest food are discussed here.

DESIRE TO EAT

The desire to eat is a complex blending of psychological, cultural, and physiological factors working together to produce the sensations of appetite, hunger, *anorexia*, and *satiety*. These sensations influence the quantity and sometimes the quality of the food ingested. The chemical senses of taste and smell also influence the ingestion of food. In addition to all these influences, hunger, satiety, and thirst centers located in the brain regulate food and fluid intake.

Appetite and Hunger

The two terms *appetite* and *hunger* are related to the psychological and physiological influences on food intake. Both, however, are misused in everyday conversation. *Appetite* is a psychological desire or craving for food based on pleasant past experiences with food. It is often a desire for a specific food independent of whether or not the person is actually hungry. *Hunger* is the physiological response of the body when its energy needs are not being met. It is also a craving for food, but it is more intense than appetite. It is characterized by the physical signs of brief, intermittent cramping sensations of tension in the abdominal region (*hunger pangs*), weakness and irritability, and a strong drive to secure food to eat. Mayer (1968) has defined *hunger* as "a complex of unpleasant sensations, felt after prolonged deprivation, which will impel a man to seek, work, or fight for immediate relief by ingestion of food" (p. 11, 12). Hunger is therefore instinctual and is the stimulus that initiates food intake. Appetite is a learned response and is based on past experiences with food.

A few short illustrations should serve to clarify these distinctions between hunger and appetite. A student who has been studying all evening for a nursing exam decides at 10 PM that she is hungry for a pizza. She tells her roommate and they phone in an order to have a pizza delivered. Both these students had a full-sized dinner at 6:30 PM, and they have been studying in their room since 7. These two students are probably not really "hungry." What they are experiencing is a craving, or "appetite," for pizza.

Hunger is sometimes equated with being malnourished. This, however, is not always the case. A person can be malnourished without being hungry or hungry without being malnourished. Malnutrition can be defined as either over- or undernourishment. Obese people may be malnourished from consuming an improper quality of food, but they are not hungry. Dieters may be quite hungry on their restricted food intake, but they are not necessarily malnourished.

Anorexia and Satiety

A good appetite is rightfully a measure of a client's health status. A healthy person has a natural desire to eat at regular times during the day. The times at which a person becomes "hungry" depend on his daily eating habits. A lack of appetite is called *anorexia*. With anorexia the normal desire for food is absent. This symptom may be due to fever, disease states, drugs, or psychological states. Anorexia is also a symptom of a deficiency of the vitamin thiamine. Increased levels of thiamine will restore a decreased appetite to normal levels but will not stimulate appetite beyond normal levels. Obviously if anorexia continues indefinitely, malnutrition will ensue ending in death.

The opposite of hunger is *satiety,* the feeling of fullness and psychological satisfaction after a meal. A person's hunger has been satisfied and his appetite gratified. From a physiological perspective satiety occurs following a satisfying meal when a person's nutritional stores have been replenished.

Appetite bears no relationship to the physiological need of the body for an amount of food; therefore the amount of food ingested is generally greater than is needed. The desire for food (appetite) and the palatability (appearance, aroma, taste, texture) of the food itself are the two major determinants of the amount ingested. Satiety has both a psychological and a physiological component. Most people do not eat simply to satisfy their hunger; they continue to eat until their appetite has also been satisfied. Eating beyond the point of physiological hunger is a major cause of overeating, and therefore of obesity, in the United States. Consider the traditional Thanksgiving dinner in which the family's favorite food is offered. In this situation no matter how full a person is, he can usually be enticed to eat more of a favorite food. This could be described as the *Thanksgiving effect.*

PSYCHOSOCIAL INFLUENCES

Though hunger is the main driving physiological force for securing food for ingestion, the psychosocial influences control food ingestion to a greater extent. A person's appetite, or psychological desire for specific foods, influences his ingestion of food to a greater extent than physiological hunger. These psychosocial influences are both environmental and psychological. Eating habits begin at the first feeding of a baby within the family. As the child grows, his eating habits and attitudes toward food are influenced more and more by the environment and his own psychological state, as shown in Chapter 1.

PHYSIOLOGICAL INFLUENCES

The regulation of food intake is not a haphazard process because most adults maintain a constant weight over a period of time. A person may be underweight or overweight, but left to regular eating habits, the tendency is to maintain this weight. The physiological regulation of ingestion can be divided into short-term and long-term mechanisms.

Short-term Regulation

Short-term regulation is acquired by ingestion of food at daily meals. Short-term regulation is primarily alimentary; that is, distention of the stomach after the ingestion of food suppresses the desire for food through the feeling of satiety. Also such events in the ingestion of food as chewing, salivating, and swallowing seem to "monitor" food intake, as do appearance, taste, and smell.

Sensory Regulation
The ingestion of food is closely related to the three senses of *vision, olfaction,* and *gustation,* senses quite useful in determining the desirability or palatability of food. The acceptability or palatability of food is related to such factors as appearance, color, smell, taste, temperature, and texture. A client's appetite is depressed if food served is lukewarm, tasteless, and looks uninteresting and if the por-

tions are too large. A pleasing combination of colors, flavors, and textures as well as food that is carefully seasoned and as hot as possible can, on the other hand, actually stimulate a client's appetite. Palatability is also conditioned by past experiences with food and the atmosphere in which the food is consumed.

The visual aspect of food is a major sensory influence on ingestion. Beautiful pictures of food in magazines or cookbooks can stimulate appetite and cause salivation. Sometimes even the thought of food can initiate secretion of gastric juices. A colorful, attractively served tray of food presented to a client in the hospital can actually stimulate the appetite and make the client feel more like eating. A messy tray that contains items of the same consistency and nearly the same color can certainly be an appetite depressant. Food served to a preschooler that is cleverly arranged to form a design or the face of a clown will usually be readily accepted even when the actual foods contained are not the child's favorites. When a person or client has been under much emotional or psychological strain or is very tired, food that is attractively served provides a real psychological lift and encouragement.

The two senses of olfaction and gustation are also important influences on ingestion, for the combination of smell and taste leads to the perception of flavor. Everyone would agree that one of the discomforts of the common cold is a temporary decrease in the sense of smell. This, of course, leads to a decreased ability to taste adequately and therefore to enjoy food. There are seven basic odors that can be detected: camphoraceous, musky, floral, ethereal, pungent, putrid, or pepperminty (Crouch and McClintic, 1976). Food may be either accepted or rejected by some solely on the basis of its aroma or odor. The sense of smell is 25,000 times more sensitive than the sense of taste. Sniffing enhances the sense of smell by directing the aroma or odor to a sensitive region of the nose for either acceptance or rejection. The sense of

smell also helps to protect a person against the ingestion of a harmful or spoiled food. Smell is an important component of flavor, and much of the pleasure of selecting and eating food would be lost if only the sense of taste were present.

The mouth is not only the port of entry for food but where the taste and texture of the ingested food is experienced. The sense of taste is the basic means of judging the palatability and, therefore, the acceptability of a food. Taste is a mixture of sensations, not only gustatory and olfactory, but *tactile, thermal,* and *kinesthetic* (involving hardness, toughness, and elasticity) (Bell et al., 1976). If a subject is blindfolded, has his nose held, and is told not to chew, it will be very difficult, if not impossible, for him to distinguish the tastes of such foods as apples, turnips, and onions. Some foods tend to have more flavor when they are hot. This is one reason for the decreased acceptance of food that has cooled off. Another reason is cultural conditioning; people become conditioned to eating certain foods hot, and when they are not at the desired temperature, the acceptability is impaired.

The basic sensations derived when food is placed in the mouth are sweetness, sourness, saltiness, and bitterness. Bitterness is perceived at the rear of the mouth; saltiness and sweetness, at the tip and edges of the tongue; and sourness more widely distributed. See Figure 9-1. Bitterness has the lowest threshold for detection, that is, the greatest sensitivity. This means that bitterness can be detected in a very weak solution. The other tastes in order of increasing thresholds are sour, salt, and sweet. The four basic tastes reflect specific constituents of food. A sour taste is produced by the hydrogen ion (H). Salty taste is due to the presence of ionized salts such as sodium, ammonium, calcium, lithium, and potassium. Hydroxyl groups (—OH groups) help cause a sweet taste. Sugars such as glucose and fructose contain these —OH groups. A bitter taste is contributed by alkaloids and

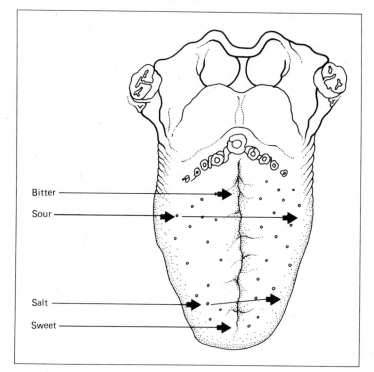

Bitter

Sour

Salt

Sweet

Figure 9-1. Regions of taste on the tongue.

organic molecules (Crouch and McClintic, 1976). The normal mucus secretions of the saliva serve as a medium for dissolving the taste components of food. A client who has a dry mouth has a decreased taste sensitivity and usually a loss of appetite.

Taste also arouses the experience of pleasantness or unpleasantness. Pfaffmann (1978) describes the sense of taste as "That specific chemosensitivity of the oral cavity, located on the lingual surface (tongue), but also on the palate, epiglottis, larynx, pharynx, and esophagus, which is normally stimulated by direct contact with chemical molecules or ions in solutions as they are taken into the mouth" (p. 1058).

Taste receptor cells reveal a *polarization* change following the chemical stimulation from food. The food chemicals do not pene-

trate the membrane of the taste cell, but they rapidly adsorb to the surface and cause depolarization. Peripheral nerves relay this information to the brain, where the message is interpreted in terms of past experiences with the same food. It is interesting to note that chemicals injected directly into the blood circulation can stimulate the taste cells. The sight or thought of a certain food may stimulate the taste center in the brain so that the food can almost be "tasted". If a person has set before him a dish that he is told contains vanilla ice cream, his brain and mouth are conditioned to the sweet taste of ice cream. Imagine his surprise and annoyance when the first bite reveals not ice cream but the bland and somewhat sour taste of plain yogurt.

An unpleasant sensation actually enjoyed by some people is called *gustatory sweating.*

Sweating occurs on the forehead and face of the person ingesting, for instance, the hot chilles served with Mexican food. Surprisingly, the taste receptors are not directly involved, but this is a reflex phenomenon initiated by the stimulation of pain receptors in the mouth.

Each taste bud is composed of 40–60 cells with the middle and lower portions of each in contact with nerve fibers. Taste buds are constantly growing, developing, dying, and being replaced. The average life-span of taste-bud cells is about 10 days. The number of taste buds not only differs among individuals but changes throughout the life cycle. An adult has 9,000 taste buds (Bell, et al., 1976). A toddler has an even larger number of taste buds and therefore a high degree of taste sensitivity. They even have taste buds in their cheeks. This is one reason a toddler may be observed holding a favorite food in the cheeks and just enjoying its taste. It is also because of the increased number of taste buds that toddlers prefer somewhat bland food to very spicy foods. In later life the number of taste buds declines, and this is the main reason why the elderly have a diminished taste sensitivity. The aged adult may prefer foods that are more highly flavored because of the decreasing taste sensitivity.

The condition of the oral cavity is also very important to the ingestion of food. The mouth and gums should be free from sores or abrasions for maximum enjoyment of food. The teeth should be in good repair. Teeth that are missing or broken or ill-fitting dentures can make the ingestion of food more difficult.

Gastrointestinal Tract Regulation

Increased contractions of the stomach are associated with the sensations of hunger, and these contractions cause a person to seek food for their relief. After the ingestion of food the stomach becomes distended as the walls stretch outward. There is a neural link between the stomach and the hypothalamus to inform the hypothalamus that the stomach is distended. The satiety center in the hypothalamus then sends out signals for the cessation of eating. Although these mechanisms are important in normal people, clients who have had their stomachs removed still experience hunger and satiety.

Long-term Regulation

Long-term regulation is metabolic and related to the nutritional status of the subject. The level of the body's nutrient stores is related to activity by the so-called feeding and satiety center of the brain, the *hypothalamus*. When nutrient stores are depleted, the feeding center of the hypothalamus becomes very active. Conversely, when the nutrient stores have been replenished, the satiety center of the hypothalamus exerts its activity. The purpose of long-term regulation is to protect nutritional status by maintaining adequate nutrient stores.

Although much has been learned about the regulation of food intake in the past few years, the specific event that initiates the ingestion of food has not been determined. Multiple physiological factors are believed to stimulate the ingestion of food. The brain, however, is the final integration point for the regulation of both the psychosocial factors.

Neural Regulation

Although there are several areas of the brain that are related to hunger and satiety, the hypothalamus has been studied extensively and is known to initiate both feeding and cessation of feeding. These responses of the hypothalamus were discovered through animal experimentation. Stimulating the *lateral hypothalamus* by an electrical impulse produced ravenous eating in animals that had previously been adequately fed. Stimulating the *ventromedial hypothalamus* produced satiety in the same animals. Even when presented with highly appetizing food, these animals would not eat.

In studies of laboratory animals, especially rats, lesions of both these areas of the hypothalamus have been created. Animals with lesions of the lateral hypothalamus produced complete loss of appetite and starvation. In contrast, lesions of the ventromedial hypothalamus produced the same ravenous appetite and overeating as occurred when the lateral hypothalamus was stimulated. Similar observations have been made in humans who have had disease or surgery in these areas of the brain.

The lateral hypothalamus serves as a *feeding center,* and the ventromedial hypothalamus is viewed as the *satiety center* that suppresses the activity of the feeding center. Thus the satiety center by its inhibition of the feeding center serves as a physiological cue to discontinue eating. Many people, however, either do not respond to this cue or ignore it completely, allowing their appetite to rule their food intake.

Other higher centers in the brain have important roles in the control of appetite. The *amygdala region* of the *limbic system* influences the ingestion of food because of its association with smell. Stimulation of this area also initiates the mechanical act of feeding. The cortical regions of the limbic system also have areas that when stimulated can either increase or decrease food intake. These regions seem to be particularly involved with the animal's drive to find food when it is hungry. Both the amygdala and the cortical regions as well as the hypothalamus are probably responsible for the quantity of food consumed (Guyton, 1977).

BRAIN NEUROTRANSMITTERS. Some recent evidence suggests that *brain neurotransmitters* may be involved in the regulation of food intake. The neurotransmitters *dopamine* and *norepinephrine* (noradrenaline) (which are catecholamines) are synthesized from the essential amino acid tyrosine; *serotonin* is synthesized from the essential amino acid tryptophan. Diets in which the source of protein is corn are characteristically low in the amino acid tryptophan, and decreased levels of brain serotonin have been recorded. Short periods of food deprivation, however, stimulate the synthesis of dopamine in the hypothalamus and of serotonin in the whole brain (Lytle and Messing, 1976). Noradrenergic neurons in the brain are required for initiation of ingestion and serotonergic neurons may be involved in its cessation (Stricker, 1978).

Two types of receptors in the ventromedial and lateral hypothalamus are sensitive to the catecholamine neurotransmitters, and they control appetite. The *α-noradrenergic system* plays a role in initiating feeding, whereas the *β-adrenergic system* is involved with satiety. Because these receptors are found in the ventromedial and lateral hypothalamus, this system is consistent with the dual-center theory of appetite regulation.

Metabolic Regulation

Another important means of regulating the ingestion of food lies in the supplies of usable fuels within the body. These fuels are derived from the ingestion of carbohydrate, protein, and fat and are, respectively, glucose, amino acids, and fatty acids and glycerol. This pathway to regulation is fairly slow because after ingestion the food must be digested, absorbed, transported into circulation, and either used directly or stored for later use.

GLUCOSTATIC HYPOTHESIS. It is generally known that a decrease in blood glucose is associated with the onset of hunger. The glucostatic theory proposed by Mayer, 1968 states that feeding is related more to the rate of glucose use than to the actual levels of blood glucose. A low rate of glucose use enhances feeding and vice versa. Food intake may be monitored by cells called *glucoreceptors* that are sensitive to glucose. These special cells are probably located in the brain, the gastrointestinal tract, or both places (Lytle and Messing, 1976).

LIPOSTATIC HYPOTHESIS. The physiological symptom of hunger is inversely proportional to the quantity of adipose tissue in the body; that is, as the amount of adipose tissue increases, the symptoms of hunger decrease. This is the main reason the obese person does not experience the physical symptoms of hunger. The amount of free fatty acids released each day within the body is proportional to the amount of stored adipose tissue. When these free fatty acids are released, they are thought to communicate information to the brain regarding hunger. Because the diet of the obese person contains ample sources of carbohydrate and fat for energy, only a very limited quantity of free fatty acids is released daily. These fatty acid levels are increased in the plasma only after deprivation of food, exposure to very cold temperatures, or exercise. This regulatory mechanism involving fat may be the most important long-term regulator.

AMINO ACID REGULATION. A decrease in the level of amino acids in the blood increases the ingestion of food and vice versa. Diets either excessive or deficient in amino acids tend to decrease appetite as measured by food intake (Lytle and Messing, 1976). It will be recalled that several of the brain neurotransmitters are dependent on amino acids for their synthesis. These neurotransmitters in turn exert an influence on food intake.

HORMONAL REGULATION. Because many of the endocrine hormones affect the use of carbohydrate, protein, and fat, they are indirectly involved in the regulation of food intake. Insulin secretion has the effect of lowering blood sugar and therefore depressing appetite after a meal. Many of the other hormones such as glucagon, epinephrine, the glucocorticoids, adrenocorticotropic hormone, and growth hormone increase blood glucose levels, which may stimulate appetite. For example, administration of growth hormone and glucocorticoids increases food intake. More detail on the hormonal regulation of metabolism is found in Chater 12.

ABILITY TO INGEST FOOD

A person's ability to ingest food depends on his ability to feed himself, the condition of the oral environment, and the ability to swallow. Impairment of any of these components will interfere with the actual ingestion of food.

Self-feeding

The act of feeding oneself requires muscular coordination. Absence of any of the previously discussed ingestion-stimulating mechanisms can hinder adequate self-feeding. There are four major groups of people who are generally unable to feed themselves: infants, some severely mentally or physically handicapped people, comatose clients, and some hospitalized clients. Feeding techniques are discussed in Chapter 24 under the topic inability to ingest food.

Oral Environment

The oral cavity is bounded on the outside by the lips. Inside the mouth are the teeth, the gums, and the tongue. Food ingested through the mouth remains in the oral cavity for a short time during the process of chewing. The ingestion of food depends on the condition of the mouth and oral structures, each of which has a specific function in preparing the food for being swallowed. The gums are continuous with the mucus membrane of the mouth; they also anchor the teeth in the upper jaw (*mandible*) and lower jaw (*maxilla*). Humans have four types of teeth specially adapted to a diet of both animal and vegetable sources. The four *incisor teeth* are used primarily for biting and shearing off food. The two *canine teeth* are adapted to tearing and shredding foods, especially meat. The *premolars* and *molars* function primarily in grinding food, especially that which is high in cellulose. The tongue has two sets of muscles. One set, the *extrinsic muscles,* is involved with the large-muscle movements of the tongue in and out of the mouth and sideways. The other set, the *intrinsic muscles,* is used for the finer movements that change the shape of the tongue and are involved in swallowing. The saliva in the mouth serves to moisten and soften the ingested food and to keep the mucus membranes moist. The secretion of saliva also helps to cleanse the mouth and teeth of excess particles of food. Another function of the saliva is to lubricate the food mass in preparation for swallowing.

An abnormality in any of the structures and functions of the oral cavity will alter a person's selection and ingestion of food. The mucus membranes of the mouth may be so dry there is interference with normal taste perception. Painful sores in the mouth will dictate food selection that will not irritate the sores. Decayed or missing teeth can also interfere with the ingestion of food. Management of these disorders is discussed in greater detail in Chapter 24.

Swallowing

Movement of a food mass from the mouth into the esophagus is called *swallowing,* or *deglutition.* Swallowing usually proceeds unconsciously and is considered a natural event in the act of eating; yet it is a complex series of actions that requires the coordination of many muscles and other structures in the head and neck. Before swallowing occurs, chewing moistens the food with saliva and decreases the particle size. The food is then formed into a mass as the tongue presses it against the hard palate.

During the act of swallowing, three openings must be blocked. In the first step the mouth is sealed by the jaw closing, and the tongue is elevated, moving the food back into the first part of the *pharynx* (throat). This event is under the voluntary control of the cerebral cortex. The next two steps are under involuntary control in the deglutition center in the medulla of the brain. (1) The *nasopharynx* is sealed by elevation of the soft palate and a temporary cessation of breathing. The *larynx* is also elevated, and a structure called the *epiglottis* closes over the opening, thus inhibiting speech temporarily. (2) Once inside the pharynx the mass of food stimulates the action of several cranial nerves, and after a complex series of actions, the *upper esophageal sphincter* relaxes and the mass enters the esophagus. Any obstruction, paralysis, or damage to a region in the brain that controls swallowing will result in difficult or painful swallowing and a modification in the type of food selected for ingestion. Techniques and foods that enhance swallowing are discussed in Chapter 24.

Sometimes a bite of food or a bone may gain entrance into the upper respiratory tract and cause a partial or total airway obstruction. This is possible because of the close proximity within which the digestive and respiratory functions occur in the neck region. The respiratory and digestive system share the *oropharynx* and the *laryngopharynx.* If food becomes lodged in the trachea and the airway is partially obstructed, the victim may cough and wheeze, possibly becoming cyanotic. Prompt assistance is vital to dislodge the food particle and restore breathing. The American Heart Association (1978) recommends that four sharp blows be delivered rapidly and forcefully to the victim's spine between the shoulder blades with the heel of the hand. The victim's chest should be supported with the other hand during this procedure. If this fails to dislodge the food, the second technique, called the Heimlich Maneuver, is to: (1) grasp the victim around the waist; (2) make a fist with one hand; (3) place the thumb side of the fist against the victim's abdomen, above the navel but below the *xiphoid process* of the sternum; (4) grasp the fist with the other hand and press the fist into the abdomen with a quick upward thrust. Repeat in a series of four blows to the back and four abdominal thrusts until the obstruction is cleared. These two techniques are part of cardiopulmonary resuscitation (CPR), the basic cardiac life-support method of the American Heart Association.

The following are some precautions that will help to prevent airway obstructions:

1. Cut food into small bites.
2. Chew food slowly and thoroughly.
3. Avoid laughing and talking with the mouth full.
4. Avoid excessive intake of alcohol before and during meals.
5. Do not allow children to walk or run with food or foreign objects in their mouths.
6. Keep small objects that might be swallowed away from infants and small children.

INGESTION THROUGHOUT THE LIFE-SPAN

Appetite and hunger fluctuate throughout the life cycle depending on rate of growth and level of physical activity. The healthy infant has a good appetite and consumes formula and baby food readily with little encouragement. A mother is well aware of her baby's hunger sensation when she is awakened several times during the night by demands for feeding. It is interesting that young infants are able to regulate their own intake of food to maintain a desirable weight, but mothers often encourage them to drink a little more formula or eat a little more food. This gentle form of encouragement by fondling and talking to the baby causes the inborn mechanism of self-feeding regulation to be soon lost. Between the ages of 9 and 18 months, the baby's appetite decreases in direct proportion to the growth rate. The child will eat a large amount at one meal and very little at the next or even completely refuse the meal. This sporadic pattern of eating occurs until age 4 or 5.

The school-age years represent a more steady growth rate accompanied by more regular eating habits. The period of adolescence is the final growth spurt of the life cycle; appetite is generally very good during this period. Snacks are important to the teenager because he is genuinely hungry due to the accelerated growth rate. Active sports and recreation also serve to increase appetite during these years.

In early adulthood, appetite for specific foods may remain the same, but the level of hunger is not as intense because the growth rate has gradually tapered off. Physical activity level has also declined, but in many cases daily ingestion of food remains the same. The adult is allowing his appetite to govern his food intake instead of the sensations of hunger and satiety. Without an adjustment in food intake, excess body weight will accumulate. Appetite remains generally good throughout the remainder of adulthood unless an illness or psychological disturbance depresses it temporarily.

In late adulthood (after age 60) appetite may be depressed because the senses of taste and smell are less acute. Other problems such as decreased salivary output, loss of natural teeth, or poorly fitting dentures may also interfere. Certain disease states and psychological disturbances such as loneliness and boredom also effect appetite. The activity of the older adult is generally greatly reduced, so there is very little to stimulate appetite. The physiological sensation of hunger may be experienced only slightly or not at all. Elderly clients frequently comment that they just do not get hungry.

BIBLIOGRAPHY

Am. Heart Assoc. *Cardiopulmonary Resuscitation (CPR)*. Tulsa, Okla.: CPR Pub., 1978.

Bell, G. H., Emslie-Smith, D., and Paterson, C. R. *Textbook of Physiology and Biochemistry*. 9th Ed. New York: Longman, Inc., Churchill Livingston, 1976.

Crouch, J. E., and McClintic, J. K. *Human Anatomy and Physiology*. 2nd Ed. New York: John Wiley & Sons, Inc., Pubs., 1976.

Friedman, M. I., and Stricker, E. M. The physiological

psychology of hunger—a physiological perspective. *Psychology Review* 83:409, 1976.

Guyton, A. C. *Basic Human Physiology: Normal Functions and Mechanisms of Disease.* 2nd Ed. Philadelphia: W. B. Saunders Co., 1977.

Lytle, L. D., and Messing, R. B. Appetite in the regulation of food intake for energy (animal and man). *Prog. Fd. Nutr. Sci.* 2:49, 1976.

Mayer, J. *Overweight: Causes, Cost and Control.* Englewood Cliffs, N.J.: Prentice-Hall, Inc., 1968.

Pfaffmann, C. Neurophysiological mechanisms of taste. *Am. J. Clin. Nutr.* 31:1058, 1978.

Stricker, E. M. Hyperphagia. *N. Engl. J. Med.* 298:1010, 1978.

CHAPTER 10

Digestion and Absorption

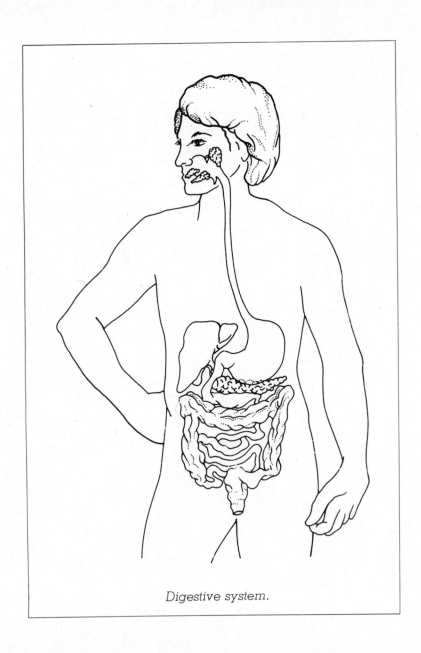

Digestive system.

During digestion food that has been ingested passes through a number of physiological processes to break the food down into simpler components that the body can use. The *digestive system* is presented with a variety of foods composed of combinations of carbohydrates, proteins, fats, vitamins, minerals, and water. All of these components must be separated in order to be absorbed, transported, and used for specific functions throughout the body. The energy nutrients (carbohydrates, proteins, and fats) must be broken down into the simpler units of monosaccharides, amino acids, fatty acids, and glycerol before they can be absorbed and used by the body. The other nutrients—vitamins, minerals, and water— can be absorbed with little or no change.

The purpose of the digestive system is to supply the rest of the body with a continual supply of nutrients from the food ingested. The only two activities of this system that are under voluntary control are *mastication* and *defecation*. The *autonomic nervous system* regulates the passage of food along the *digestive tract*, or *alimentary canal*, which may be viewed as one long tube extending from the mouth to the anus. These autoregulatory processes keep the food moving through the tract at a pace slow enough for adequate digestion and absorption to occur, but fast enough to supply nutrients to the rest of the body.

The digestive tract consists of several parts, each of which has a specific purpose: the mouth, the esophagus, the stomach (comprising *fundus, corpus,* and *antrum*), the small intestine (comprising *duodenum, jejunum,* and *ileum*), and the large intestine (including *ascending, transverse,* and *descending colon, sigmoid,* and *rectum*). Two accessory organs, the liver and the pancreas, produce secretions that are transported to the *gastrointestinal tract* (stomach and intestines) for use during digestion.

The digestive process is regulated by a number of mechanical, nervous, and hormonal controls. Following the swallowing of food, these mechanisms monitor the movement of the food mass along the tract, the secretion and action of the digestive enzymes, the acidity or alkalinity of the food mass, the absorption of the digestive end products, and the excretion of waste materials. In addition to all these functions, the digestive tract completely replaces its cellular structure every two to three days.

ALIMENTARY MOTILITY

The process of digestion involves both mechanical and chemical processes that occur simultaneously in each organ. The mechanical process that moves the food mass along the tract at an optimal rate for digestion and absorption is *motility*. The anatomical structure of the smooth muscle of the intestinal tract gives rise to the characteristic types of contraction and movement that occur.

Intestinal smooth muscle exhibits both *tonic* and *rhythmic contractions*. *Tonic contraction* is the state of continuous muscular contraction. It may increase or decrease in intensity, but it is always continuous. (Skeletal muscle as well has a certain degree of "tone.") The B-complex vitamin thiamine is important in helping to maintain muscle tone and normal functioning of the digestive tract. *Rhythmic contractions* produce a churning sort of movement that both aids in the continual mixing of the food and moves the food through the tract. This characteristic propelling movement is called *peristalis*. Peristalsis moves the food mass along the intestinal tract by a series of wavelike contractions at the rate of 1 cm (.4 in)/min (Guyton, 1977).

Several valves, or *sphincters,* help regulate food movement in the alimentary canal and prevent reflux into the preceding portion. The *cardiac* (esophageal) *sphincter* controls movement from the esophagus into the first portion of the stomach. The *pyloric valve* controls passage into the initial portion of the small intestine (duodenum); the *ileocecal valve* regulates passage from the ileum into the *cecum,* and the anal sphincter allows final passage from the body.

ALIMENTARY SECRETIONS

There are five important chemical secretions, each with a specific function in the digestive process: *mucus,* hydrochloric acid and *buffer ions,* digestive enzymes, hormones, and water and *electrolytes.* Mucus provides lubrication and protection of the tract itself. Water and electrolytes provide the fluid medium for the transport of the nutrients. The action of some of the digestive enzymes is dependent on the proper acidity or alkalinity provided by either hydrochloric acid or bicarbonate ions. Most of the secretion of digestive enzymes is controlled by the hormones produced by the stomach or small intestine.

DIGESTION

This unique interaction of the mechanical and chemical processes transforms nutrients in an orderly stepwise progression from more- to less-complex forms that the body cells can use. There are specific enzymes and hormones involved in each step of the process. For a closer look at this fascinating process of digestion, the mechanical and chemical events that occur in the mouth, stomach, and small intestine are presented in terms of the changes that occur after the ingestion of a specific meal:

Roast beef
Green beans
Baked potato with butter and sour cream
Lettuce salad with Italian dressing
Crackers
Canned peaches
Milk

The nutritive components of the foods in this meal that will undergo changes during digestion are shown in Table 10-1. The major events of digestion are summarized in Table 10-2. The student is encouraged to refer to both of these tables during the discussion of digestion that follows.

TABLE 10-1. Composition of Energy Nutrients in a Sample Meal

Nutrient	Roast Beef	Green Beans, Baked Potato	Lettuce	Crackers	Peaches	Milk	Italian Dressing
Monosaccharides							
Fructose		x	x		x		
Glucose		x	x		x		
Disaccharides							
Lactose						x	
Maltose				x	x		
Sucrose		x	x				
Polysaccharides							
Starch		x					
Fiber		x	x		x		
Protein	x	x		x		x	
Fat						x	x
Saturated	x					x	x
Monounsaturated	x					x	x
Polyunsaturated	x					x	x

TABLE 10-2. Summary of Digestion of the Energy Nutrients

Nutrient	Mouth	Stomach	Small Intestine	End Products
CARBOHYDRATES				
Monosaccharides				
Glucose				Glucose
Fructose				Fructose
Disaccharides			*Intestine*	Galactose
Sucrose			Sucrose $\xrightarrow{\text{Sucrase}}$ Glucose + Fructose	
Maltose			Maltose $\xrightarrow{\text{Maltase}}$ Glucose + Glucose	
Lactose			Lactose $\xrightarrow{\text{Lactase}}$ Glucose + Galactose	
Polysaccharides			*Pancreas*	
Starch	Starch $\xrightarrow[\text{(Amylase)}]{\text{Ptyalin}}$ Dextrins		Starch $\xrightarrow{\text{Amylase}}$ Dextrins → Maltose	
Fiber				Fiber
PROTEINS		Protein $\xrightarrow[\text{acid}]{\text{Pepsin Hydrochloric}}$ Polypeptides	*Pancreas*	Amino acids
			Proteins, Polypeptides $\xrightarrow[\text{Chymotrypsin}]{\text{Trypsin}}$ Dipeptides	
			Polypeptides, Dipeptides $\xrightarrow{\text{Carboxypeptidase}}$ Amino acids	
			Intestine	
			Polypeptides, Dipeptides $\xrightarrow{\text{Aminopeptidase}}$ Amino acids	
			Dipeptides $\xrightarrow{\text{Dipeptidase}}$ Amino acids	
FATS		Emulsified fat $\xrightarrow{\text{Lipase}}$ Fatty acids + Glycerol	*Liver and gall bladder*	Monoglycerides
			Fats $\xrightarrow{\text{Bile}}$ Emulsified fat	Diglycerides
			Fats $\xrightarrow[\text{Pancreatic lipase}]{\text{Intestinal lipase}}$ Glycerol, Mono- and diglycerides + Fatty acids	Glycerol
				Fatty acids

Digestion in the Mouth

Thought, sight, or smell of food initiates both *salivary secretion* and *gastric secretion.* This initial phase of digestion, known as the *cephalic phase,* occurs before ingestion. Although no food has actually been placed in the mouth, the digestive system is preparing itself for the possible and quite probable ingestion of food.

When food is placed in the mouth the mechanical process of mastication begins and chemical secretion of saliva occurs. The movement of the teeth produces a powerful cutting and grinding action. Thorough chewing of all food is important because it helps to increase the surface area of the food for maximum exposure to the digestive juices. Adequate chewing of raw fruits and vegetables is important because these foods contain outer cell membranes of indigestible cellulose that must be broken before the inside portions can be used.

Saliva contains both the enzyme *salivary amylase (ptyalin)* for the digestion of starch and a mucus secretion for lubricating the food before swallowing. Approximately 1,200 ml (36 oz) of saliva is produced daily. Besides the functions of starch digestion and lubrication, saliva also has the function of maintaining oral hygiene by helping to wash away pathogenic bacteria and by actually destroying some bacteria. Saliva contains a high proportion of potassium and bicarbonate ions; it is also composed of *mucin,* which is classified as a glycoprotein. A *glycoprotein* is a combination of a carbohydrate and a protein. When mucin is mixed with water it becomes known as mucus, the substance that imparts the lubricating characteristic to saliva.

Salivary amylase begins the initial digestion of starch. If the cracker is chewed thoroughly and held in the mouth for a few seconds, the small, chewed mass begins to taste somewhat sweet. This is because the salivary amylase has continued digesting some of the starch in the cracker into *maltose,* which is one of the *disaccharides,* or double sugars. This completeness of starch digestion usually does not occur because the food is swallowed rapidly; the length of time the food mass is exposed to the salivary amylase is simply not long enough for very much starch digestion to occur. Therefore starch digestion in the mouth is fairly insignificant. The most significant contribution of the mouth to the digestive process is the mastication of the food, which decreases the particle size and greatly increases the surface area in preparation for the remaining phases of digestion.

The voluntary act of swallowing moves the masticated mass of food out of the mouth and down the esophagus. The masticated food is at this point referred to as a *bolus.* The bolus of food is moved down the esophagus toward the stomach, partly by the force of gravity and partly by the wavelike peristaltic movements of the walls of the esophagus. The secretion of the esophagus is mucus, and it serves mainly as a lubricant for swallowing and for protection. The mucus secreted at the upper end of the esophagus protects it from excoriation by the food mass. At the lower end the mucus secreted serves to protect the esophagus from the possible reflux of the highly acid contents of the stomach. The cardiac sphincter also serves to prevent reflux of the acidic gastric contents into the esophagus.

Digestion in the Stomach

As would be expected digestion in the stomach is more complex, but the processes that occur still closely follow the basic principles of mechanical and chemical digestion. Only two major digestive enzymes are secreted in the stomach. One of these is *gastric lipase* to initiate the digestion of fat, and the other is a *protease, pepsin,* to initiate the digestion of protein. The functions of storage and mixing are important in the stomach. The delayed emptying of the stomach allows adequate digestion and absorption to occur in the small intestine.

When a bolus of food enters the stomach it remains in the upper portion (fundus) while the action of salivary amylase continues until the mixture becomes sufficiently acidic and the enzyme is inactivated. Because the walls of the stomach lack very much muscle tone, they continue to bulge outward to accommodate a quantity of food up to 1 liter at any one time. Remember that this is 1 liter (slightly more than 1 qt) of masticated, compressed food. The stomach can really stretch to accommodate a large amount of food at any one meal, but continual intakes of this quantity of food will lead to a serious overweight problem.

The bolus of food is gradually mixed with the gastric secretions until it becomes a semifluid mixture called *chyme*. The gastric secretions are secreted by three different types of cells in the stomach. The *mucus neck* cells secrete mucus; the *chief cells* secrete the digestive enzyme, *pepsinogen;* and the *parietal cells* secrete hydrochloric acid. Digestion in the stomach requires an acidic environment. The *proteolytic enzyme* pepsin is secreted in its inactive form, pepsinogen. Hydrochloric acid is needed to convert pepsinogen to pepsin. It is secreted in its inactive form so that it will not digest the stomach wall when no chyme is present. The *pyloric glands* near the lower end of the stomach also contain mucus-secreting cells. Large quantities of a thick alkaline mucus are spread over the entire stomach wall for protection against digestion of the stomach itself by the pepsin, which initiates the digestion of protein by hydrolyzing, or breaking, certain peptide bonds, thus splitting large protein molecules into somewhat smaller protein fragments called *polypeptides*. The initiation of some fat digestion may occur in the stomach because of the presence of gastric lipase, an enzyme that acts primarily on emulsified and butter fats.

Here in the stomach those foods from the sample meal that contain protein (roast beef, milk, and, in small amounts, crackers and vegetables) will be hydrolyzed to somewhat smaller protein fragments—polypeptides.

The small amounts of tributyrin fat in milk, butter, and sour cream will be broken down to fatty acids and glycerol inasmuch as gastric lipase acts mainly on the smaller short- and medium-chain triglycerides.

Gastric secretion is regulated by both nervous and hormonal stimuli. The sight, smell, and taste of food stimulate gastric secretion by way of the *vagus nerve.* The initial digestion of protein takes place during the gastric phase of digestion. These partially digested proteins as well as the bulk of food in the stomach serve to stimulate release of the hormone *gastrin* from the antral portion of the stomach, which in turn stimulates the parietal cells to produce hydrochloric acid and the chief cells to produce pepsin.

Food remains in the stomach from three to four-and-a-half hours depending on the composition of the chyme. The higher the fat content of the meal, the slower the gastric emptying time. This same sequence of events is initiated if the stomach contents are too acidic. Protein stimulates gastric secretion, but protein breakdown products retard gastric emptying to allow for adequate digestion of the protein. The carbohydrate portion of the food is the first part to be digested, followed by protein, and finally by fat. Fat and protein, therefore, contribute the so-called satiety to a meal because they remain in the stomach the longest period of time. The rate of stomach emptying is related to the amount of chyme the small intestine can process at one time (Guyton, 1977).

Digestion in the Small Intestine

Digestion in the small intestine is simply a completion of the steps already begun that convert carbohydrates, proteins, and fats into forms that can be used by the body cells. The major proportion of the digestion of all three energy nutrients occurs in the small intestine. The digestive processes and controls in each successive digestive organ are more complex than those in the preceding one. Digestion in the small intestine is the most involved of all. It occurs not only within the small intestine's interior channel (the *lumen*) but on its interior surface (the *intestinal mucosa*), the lining cells of which are covered with projections called the *brush border* (see section on "Absorbing Surface" later). The secretion of digestive enzymes arises, not only from the intestinal lumen and the intestinal mucosa, but from two other organs, the pancreas and the liver.

Intestinal Lumen

The mucous glands of the small intestine also produce mucus, especially in the first part of the duodenum at the location where the pancreatic digestive juices and the *bile* enter the small intestine. The function is protection of the intestinal mucosa from digestive juices.

The pancreas is located in close proximity to the duodenum, and it provides digestive enzymes for all three of the energy nutrients. These digestive enzymes enter the duodenum through the *pancreatic duct*. Pancreatic juice also contains large amounts of bicarbonate ions, which play an important role in buffering the acidic chyme that has been dumped into the duodenum from the stomach. The pancreatic secretions contain several different digestive enzymes for protein, carbohydrate, and fat. The proteolytic enzymes are synthesized in the pancreas in their inactive forms; only after they have been secreted into the duodenum do they become activated.

The presence of acidic chyme and polypeptides in the duodenum causes the secretion of two hormones from the intestinal mucosa. These hormones are absorbed into the blood, travel to the pancreas, and stimulate it to produce certain secretions. The hormone *secretin* stimulates the secretion of a large quantity of bicarbonate ions, which buffer the acidity of the newly arrived gastric chyme. These bicarbonate ions also provide the optimal pH for action of the pancreatic enzymes. The

second hormone, *pancreozymin*, stimulates the pancreas to secrete its digestive enzymes.

The presence of fat in the duodenum causes the intestinal mucosa to secrete the hormone *cholecystokinin*, which travels by the bloodstream to the gall bladder, where it initiates contraction of the gall bladder and the release of bile into the small intestine through the *common bile duct*. The purpose of the bile salts is to reduce the surface tension of the fat particles. The increased surface area of the fat allows greater exposure to the digestive action of the pancreatic lipase.

Carbohydrate and fat digestion are also continued by pancreatic enzymes. Pancreatic amylase continues digesting starch into disaccharides. These disaccharides will be further broken down into their component monosaccharides in the brush border of the intestinal mucosa. The major proportion of fat digestion is completed at this point by the action of pancreatic lipase, which converts mono- and diglycerides into the end products of fatty acids and glycerol.

Intestinal Mucosa

The final digestion of carbohydrate, protein, and fat is completed by specific digestive enzymes located within the brush border of the mucosa's epithelial cells. Final hydrolysis of each of the energy nutrients probably occurs on the outer surface of the *microvilli* that constitute the brush border, and absorption is almost immediate. There are at least two peptidases involved. One is *aminopeptidase*, which removes the terminal amino acid from the polypeptide by attacking the peptide bond. The other is *dipeptidase*, which converts dipeptides (proteins that contain two amino acids) into component amino acids. Three different *disaccharidases* split the disaccharides into the component monosaccharides. The name of the enzyme reveals the identity of the disaccharide it splits. For example, the enzyme *sucrase* splits sucrose into its components of glucose and fructose. The other disaccharide enzymes are *maltase* and *lactase*. There is also an intestinal *lipase* that splits neutral fats into glycerol and fatty acids. The final end products of digestion that are capable of being absorbed are glucose, fructose, galactose, amino acids, fatty acids, monoglycerides, and glycerol.

ABSORPTION

Nutrients can be absorbed in the stomach, small intestine, and large intestine. Small amounts of glucose, water, simple mineral salts, and alcohol are absorbed through the stomach, but most absorption occurs in the duodenum and jejunum of the small intestine. The structure of the small intestine is uniquely designed for this function. This amazing organ is a 24-ft (7.2-m) tube that is folded upon itself to fit within the abdominal cavity. An even more amazing fact is that the minute fingerlike projections along the entire length of the small intestine increase the absorbing surface to about 3,000 sq ft (272 sq m) (Pike and Brown, 1975), an area about the size of a small basketball court (Arlin, 1977). The absorption of water is the major absorptive task of the large intestine. Besides the absorption of water, however, other nutrients such as minerals, vitamins, and amino acids can be absorbed there. This is another example of the remarkable way the body conserves and uses the nutrients from food. The reabsorption of bile salts also occurs in the large intestine, allowing them to be reused in the digestive process. Other functions occurring in the colon are bacterial action, the accumulation of nondigestible residue, and the formation and elimination of feces. The whole absorption process is summarized in Figure 10-1. Maximum absorption of nutrients occurs when there is adequate secretion of digestive enzymes, normal motility, and a healthy absorbing surface.

Absorbing Surface

Because the major portion of absorption does occur in the small intestine, its absorbing surface and mechanisms require discussion here. The outer surface of the small intestine is smooth. It is the inner surface that is specially adapted for the maximum absorption of nutrients. The inner lining of the small intestine is gathered up into the *mucosal folds,* which greatly increase the exposed surface area. A closer examination of these folds reveals that they are covered with millions of small fingerlike projections from the region in the duodenum where the common bile duct empties to the ileocecal valve. These projections are called *villi* and they increase the absorptive surface an additional tenfold. Each villus is also covered with a layer of epithelial cells containing microvilli that collectively form the brush border. These microvilli increase the absorptive surface by another twentyfold (Fig. 10-2).

For a nutrient to be absorbed, it must first pass through the microvilli. The absorbed nutrients are channeled into either the *portal* or the *lymphatic circulation* depending on their solubility. The water-soluble nutrients enter the portal circulation; the fat-soluble nutrients, the lymphatic circulation.

Mechanisms of Absorption

The absorption of nutrients is an extremely complex process; the exact mechanics and actual events occurring during absorption still plague physiologists and biochemists. It is currently thought that absorption processes occur through *pores, carriers, pumps,* and *pinocytosis,* the mechanisms through which any substance gains entrance into any cell. These mechanisms are explained more fully in Chapter 11.

Pores

Some substances such as water and certain electrolytes move freely across membranes

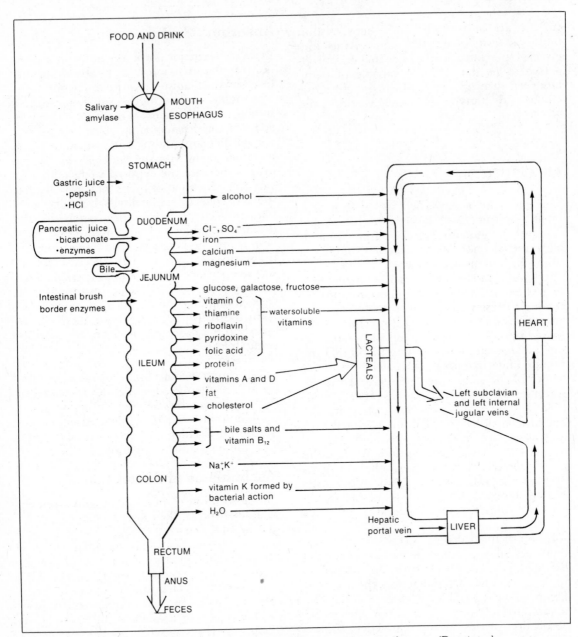

Figure 10-1. Sites of secretion and absorption in the gastrointestinal tract. (Reprinted with permission from M. V. Krause and L. K. Mahan, *Food, Nutrition, and Diet Therapy,* 6th Ed. Philadelphia: W. B. Saunders Co., 1979, p. 104.)

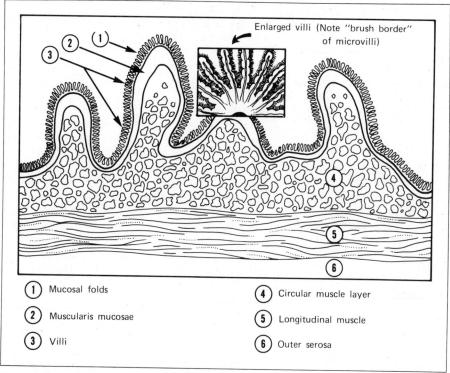

Enlarged villi (Note "brush border" of microvilli)

① Mucosal folds

② Muscularis mucosae

③ Villi

④ Circular muscle layer

⑤ Longitudinal muscle

⑥ Outer serosa

Figure 10-2. Intestinal villi and microvilli.

from a region of high concentration to a region of low concentration when no opposing pressure is present. These nutrients are thought to move through "pores," although these microscopic pores have never been seen. Substances can move in either direction depending on the concentrations, and thus this mechanism helps to maintain osmotic equilibrium.

Carriers

Most nutrient molecules are too large to pass through pores and must be helped through the membrane wall by a carrier. A water-soluble nutrient, like glucose or amino acids, cannot penetrate the cell membrane because it is high in lipid content. On one side of the membrane the nutrient to be transported

combines with a fat-soluble carrier such as a protein or a lipoprotein, making the nutrient soluble temporarily in the membrane. The nutrient-carrier complex moves across the cell membrane to the opposite side, where the carrier deposits the nutrient. The carrier acts exactly like a ferry or a shuttle bus in carrying out its function. This process is known as *carrier-mediated,* or facilitated *diffusion.* The movement is still from an area of high to one of low concentration, and no energy is required.

Pump

The mechanism through which most nutrients are absorbed is a pump. This process occurs from a region of low concentration to one of high concentration or when opposing pressure is present; therefore it requires energy. The *sodium pump* is important in the active transport of glucose and amino acids. The energy required to operate this pump is supplied by the cell. The cell also uses this energy for the transport of other nutrients. The advantage of this method is that the nutrients are rapidly moved into the cells and the general circulation.

Pinocytosis

Pinocytosis, a method of absorption necessary only for very large molecules, has been described as the cell engulfing or drinking in the molecule. The amount of nutrients absorbed in this manner is small, but it is interesting to note that intact proteins may be absorbed into the bloodstream by this mechanism and cause allergic reactions.

Influences on Absorption

Before discussing the absorption of each individual nutrient, it is important to examine some general influences on the absorption of all nutrients: the amount of the nutrient ingested, the physiological need of the body for the nutrient, the secretions and motility of the digestive tract, the absorptive surface of the small intestine, and the level of circulating hormones.

Ingestive Factors

The quantity of a nutrient that is finally absorbed is related both to the quantity of the nutrient ingested and to the body's physiological need for it. These two circumstances are especially pertinent when considering the ingestion and absorption of the water-soluble vitamins and the minerals. The greater the quantity consumed of one of these nutrients, the lower is the amount absorbed. Stress, low intakes, and growth spurts, however, increase the absorption rate.

The absorption rates for the three energy nutrients are much higher than those for any of the vitamins and minerals. Following digestion, 98% of carbohydrate is absorbed, 95%

of the fat, and 92% of the protein. Even though the rates of absorption of the vitamins and minerals are quite low compared to those of the energy nutrients, it must be remembered that vitamins and minerals are required by the body only in very minute quantities.

Digestive Factors

The adequate production of digestive secretions and the rate of motility along the tract both have important effects on the final absorption of the nutrients. Inadequate secretion of digestive enzymes will result in an insufficient breakdown of the energy nutrients so that, when they reach the small intestine and are presented for absorption, optimal absorption will not occur. An increased rate of motility through the digestive tract, such as occurs with diarrhea, decreases the time for exposure to both the digestive secretions and the absorptive surfaces.

Absorptive Surface

If the mucosal surface of the small intestine is inflamed or irritated, the absorptive area is decreased and maximal nutrients absorption will not occur. This may occur in inflammatory conditions of the small intestine or in certain medical conditions wherein the villi have actually been blunted. Medical conditions that affect both the digestion and absorption of nutrients are discussed in Chapter 25.

Absorption of Water-soluble Nutrients

Portal Circulation

The water-soluble end products of digestion are the monosaccharides, amino acids, glycerol, water-soluble vitamins, and minerals. These nutrients are absorbed from the small intestine into the portal circulation. The nutrients are transferred from the intestinal mucosa into the portal circulation through a network of capillaries. The portal circulation takes the nutrients directly to the liver, where they are further prepared for use by the body. The modified nutrients and nutritional substances then enter the general circulation and are delivered to the various cells for use. The events that occur in the liver and in the individual cells of the body are the subject of Chapter 12.

Location of Absorption

The water-soluble nutrients are absorbed at various sites along the entire length of the gastrointestinal tract from the stomach through the colon. The major portion of the absorption of these nutrients, however, occurs in the duodenum and jejunum. There is some selective competition for absorption sites between nutrients, meaning that an unusually high intake of one nutrient may actually decrease the absorption of another. Some of the nutrients, on the other hand, actually enhance the absorption of other nutrients. Some of the minerals require an acid media for maximum absorption, and so their absorption occurs in the upper portion of the duodenum. The electrolytes sodium and potassium are most readily absorbed along with water in the colon.

Monosaccharides

The three monosaccharides that are absorbed from the small intestine are glucose, galactose, and fructose. Final hydrolysis of these monosaccharides has previously occurred within the mucosal cell by the action of the enzymes sucrase, maltase, and lactase.

The monosaccharides are absorbed primarily in the lower duodenum and jejunum. There are also absorption sites in the ileum, and some monosaccharides may be moved on to this location for absorption. Glucose and galactose may be absorbed by passive diffusion when the concentration within the small intestine is greater than that in the general circulation. The more usual means of glucose and galactose absorption is by active transport involving the presence of sodium and the expenditure of energy. The energy required is supplied by the glucose already within the cell, and the energy required to pump the sodium out of the cell is the same as that required to transport glucose and galactose into the cell. Fructose is absorbed only by diffusion and only half as readily as the other monosaccharides.

Amino Acids

Most proteins are absorbed in the form of amino acids, but a small amount of di- and tripeptides may also be absorbed. The major portion of amino acids (60%) are absorbed in the proximal part of the small intestine (Guthrie, 1979). Competition exists for absorption among some amino acids, so receptor sites are also available in the stomach and colon. Amino acids are also absorbed primarily by active transport, which uses the sodium pump. Some of the amino acids may remain in the intestinal mucosa cells for the synthesis of intestinal enzymes and for making new intestinal cells. The liberation of amino acids during digestion is closely coordinated with the rate of absorption so that there is only a minimal loss in the feces (Robinson and Lawler, 1977). This is another excellent example of how the body conserves the nutrients it receives. Besides absorption of amino acids from dietary protein, there is also absorption of protein from intestinal secretions and from sloughed off epithelial cells (Krause and Mahan, 1979).

Glycerol and Short- and Medium-chain Triglycerides

A few of the end products of fat digestion are water soluble and can enter the portal circulation directly. These are the medium- and short-chain fatty acids and glycerol. The fatty acids that contain 10 or fewer carbon atoms are soluble in water. After final hydrolysis of the medium- and short-chain triglycerides has occurred within the intestinal mucosal cell by enteric lipase, the resulting medium- and short-chain fatty acids and glycerol can cross the epithelical cell and go directly into the portal circulation. Ingestion of fats containing medium- and short-chain triglycerides is especially helpful for clients who have malabsorption disorders (discussed in Chap. 25).

Water-soluble Vitamins

Most of the water soluble vitamins are absorbed in the upper part of the small intestine, either by active transport involving sodium or by passive diffusion. Thiamine is most readily absorbed in the acid media of the upper duodenum. Phosphorus is added to thiamine in the intestinal mucosa during absorption. This addition of phosphorus prepares thiamine for its important role as a cofactor in carbohydrate metabolism (see Chap. 10). Riboflavin is also easily absorbed. The addition of phosphorus to riboflavin in the intestinal mucosa enhances its absorption. During this process riboflavin is converted to the coenzyme *FMN* (*flavin mononucleotide*), which is important in many metabolic reactions. Niacin is also readily absorbed from the upper part of the small intestine.

All is not known about the absorption of the water-soluble vitamins, but the majority are believed to be absorbed in the jejunum. About one-fourth of the folacin found in foods is in a form that can be readily absorbed. The remainder of the folic acid must be freed by the enzyme *conjugase* in the mucosal cells of the proximal small intestine before it can be absorbed. Vitamin C aids in the conversion of folic acid to folinic acid, thereby facilitating its absorption.

The absorption of vitamin B_{12} is an interesting chain of events. Vitamin B_{12} is the only vitamin known to require exposure to a gastric secretion before it can be absorbed. This vitamin must come in contact with a *mucoprotein* called the *intrinsic factor,* which is present in the gastric secretion. Vitamin B_{12} is first separated from the peptide structure in which it naturally occurs in foods by the hydrochloric acid in the stomach and intestinal secretions. Vitamin B_{12} combines with the intrinsic factor and forms a complex that travels

on down toward the small intestine. In the ileum calcium helps bind the complex to the receptor sites. The absorption of vitamin B_{12} takes as long as three hours in comparison to the few seconds required for most of the water-soluble vitamins.

Minerals

Minerals are absorbed in all sections of the small intestine. The minerals with single charges are more easily absorbed than those with multiple ionic charges. For example, sodium, potassium, and chlorine with only one charge are more easily absorbed than calcium, magnesium, and iron, which have multiple charges.

CALCIUM. Calcium is absorbed by active transport from the acidic medium of the duodenum. It is also absorbed by passive diffusion across the intestinal mucosa from the jejunum and ileum. Only about 10–30% of the ingested dietary calcium is actually absorbed. Several conditions influence the amount of calcium absorbed. The absorption of calcium is regulated by the body's need for it. During times of temporary depletion and during growth, the absorption of dietary calcium is increased. Several nutrients also influence the absorption of calcium. When fat is present in moderate amounts the movement through the intestinal tract is slowed, allowing more time for calcium to be absorbed (Krause and Mahan, 1979). Yet when excess fat is consumed or general fat absorption is poor, the excess fat forms insoluble substances with the calcium so that its absorption is decreased. Calcium absorption is better when the dietary intake of protein is high than when it is low. The acidic effect of some of the amino acids on the intestinal tract increases the formation of soluble calcium–amino acid complexes and thus increases its absorption. Absorption of calcium is also enhanced by the presence of lactose, the carbohydrate in milk. Vitamin D has some effect on the intestinal mucosa that increases the active transport of calcium through the intestinal mucosa. The presence of ascorbic acid may also increase the absorption of calcium by increasing the solubility of the calcium salts in an acidic medium.

Under some conditions the absorption of calcium is inhibited. Two naturally occurring acids found in some foods combine with calcium in the digestive tract and form insoluble compounds that are not absorbed. Oxalic acid is found in large quantities in rhubarb, spinach, chard, and beet greens. Phytic acid is found in the outer layers of cereal grains, especially oatmeal. Even though foods containing these acids may be good sources of calcium, the calcium is not available to the body because it is not absorbed. An alkaline medium and increased intestinal motility also decrease the absorption of calcium. Immobilization and severe mental or physical stress can decrease ability to absorb calcium.

PHOSPHORUS.   About 70% of the phosphorus ingested is actually absorbed in the duodenum. Intestinal phosphatases release the phosphates from the organic complex in which they are found in foods. Phosphorus is most efficiently absorbed when ingested with equal amounts of calcium, which is why milk is such a good source of both calcium and phosphorus. Vitamin D also enhances the absorption of phosphorus.

IRON.   The absorption of iron involves a unique relationship among absorption, transport, and use. There is no mechanism for the excretion of iron; that is, plasma levels are not maintained by urinary excretion. The iron content of the body is regulated by the degree of absorption.

Most of the iron present in food is in the form of the *ferric* (Fe^3) *ion*. The *ferrous* (Fe^{12}) *ion,* however, is more readily absorbed by the intestinal tract, so the hydrochloric acid in the stomach acts on the ferric ion to convert it to the ferrous state. Vitamin C (ascorbic acid) also aids in this conversion to the ferrous state. Only about 10–30% of the daily iron

ingested is actually absorbed. This amount, however, is increased by the body during blood loss or iron deficiency. This absorption occurs mainly in the acidic environment of the stomach and duodenum.

The absorbed iron is carried into the cells of the intestinal mucosa, where it combines with the protein *apoferritin* to form *ferritin,* a temporary storage form of iron in the intestinal mucos and elsewhere in the body. Iron absorption is controlled by the amount of ferritin already present in the mucosal cells. When the content of ferritin is high because all available apoferritin has been combined with iron, additional iron arriving at the binding site is rejected and excreted in the feces.

OTHER MINERALS.   The other minerals are absorbed to varying degrees along the intestinal tract. For example, 90% of the fluorine ingested is absorbed into the bloodstream. Iodine is also readily absorbed, but its absorption is regulated by the level of circulating thyroid hormone. There is some competition for absorption among the minerals. For example, magnesium competes with calcium for carrier sites, and molybdenum competes with copper for absorption. Large amounts of calcium and iron tend to inhibit the absorption of manganese. This competition and inhibition of absorption among the minerals serves to reemphasize the importance of moderate intake of all nutrients through a wide variety of foods. It is also easy to see how an excess intake of any one or a combination of vitamins and minerals could upset the delicate regulation of absorption. A summary of nutrient absorption is provided in Figure 10-1.

Absorption of Fat-soluble Nutrients

Lymphatic Circulation

Nutrients that are too large to enter the portal circulation must gain access to the general circulation via the *lymphatic circulation*. The walls of the lymphatic capillaries are very thin and highly permeable to such large molecules as fat. Once the fat-soluble nutrients are rendered more water-soluble by specific steps, entrance into the lymphatic circulation is accomplished quite easily. Circulation by the lymphatic route to the liver may be thought of as "taking the long way home." The nutrients enter the lymphatic system in the abdominal cavity and drain into the *cisterna chyli,* which is the drainage reservoir for most of the body. It empties into the thoracic duct, which ascends the chest, enters the neck, and finally empties into the left brachiocephalic vein and thus into the heart. Now the contents can be pumped out of the heart and finally to the liver and other cells for use.

Fats

The absorption of the end products of fat digestion is a complicated but logical process in the intestinal wall in three stages. This stepwise process of absorption in necessary for every fatty acid with 14 carbon atoms or more; those with 12 or less may be absorbed as either a water-soluble or a fat-soluble product. Each stage of fat absorption can be followed in Figure 10-3.

STAGE 1.   The initial step in the absorption of long-chain fatty acids, monoglycerides, and diglycerides is the application of a *wetting agent*—bile—to make them more water soluble. The bile salts combine with the mono- and diglycerides and fatty acids to form a *micellar complex.* The micellar formation allows these fat products to come into closer contact with the absorptive surfaces of the brush border of the intestinal mucosa. In this way the bile salts act like a ferry to transport the fat products into the intestinal wall, thus facilitating their absorption. Once inside the intestinal wall, the bile salts are separated from the fat products. They travel via portal circulation to the liver, where they are recirculated in the bile.

STAGE 2.   The stage of fat absorption, which occurs within the intestinal mucosa, is continued hydrolysis of some of the fat products and also the synthesis or manufacture of new triglycerides. Some monoglycerides and diglycerides have reached this point without being completely hydrolyzed because the second and third fatty acids are removed from the glycerol molecule with increasing difficulty. An intestinal lipase completes the hydrolysis to monoglycerides, fatty acids, and glycerol. At this point all of the fatty acids and glycerol molecules available are synthesized into new triglycerides. Also there is some intestinal synthesis of cholesterol and phospholipid occurs at this time.

STAGE 3.   The final stage coats the newly formed fat products with a protein envelope, which enables them to gain entrance into the lymphatic system. The complex formed is a *lipoprotein complex* called *chylomicrons.* Chylomicrons are composed mainly of triglycerides with a small amount of cholesterol and phospholipids and a small amount of protein. The chylomicrons are only one of four types of lipoproteins that travel in the blood; the other three are produced by the liver and are discussed in the next chapter. These new triglycerides are now ready to be transported to the tissues for use.

Fat-soluble Vitamins

The absorption of the four fat-soluble vitamins requires the same substances that are required for fat digestion, that is, the bile salts and lipases. The vitamins, however, require only minor changes before they can be absorbed into the lining of the small intestine. Before it is absorbed by the intestinal mucosa, the various forms of vitamin A must be split by pancreatic lipase in the lumen of the small intestine into free *retinol,* the form of vitamin A that is almost completely absorbed. The retinol can then cross the mucosal wall with the aid of bile, which is a natural antioxidant and helps to stabilize the vitamin A and keep it intact. Within the intestinal wall retinol combines with a fatty acid, usually *palmitic,* and it

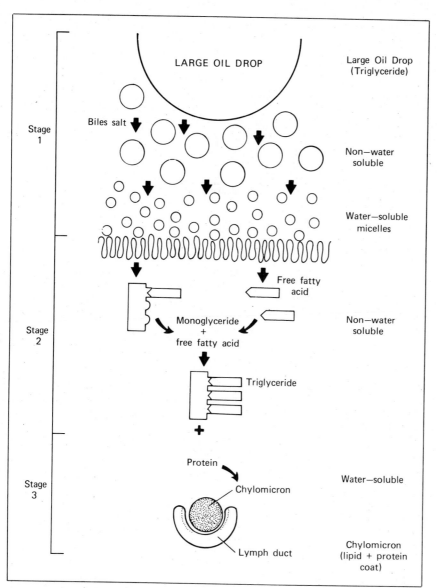

Figure 10-3. Absorption of fats.

is incorporated into the chylomicrons to be released into the lymphatic circulation. Most of the carotenoid form of vitamin A is converted to retinol in the intestinal mucosa, but only one-third of the carotenes are actually absorbed as such and carried into the bloodstream. It is these carotenoids that contribute to the yellow color of blood serum.

Vitamin D is absorbed along with other food fats from the jejunum and ileum with the aid of bile. It is also the only vitamin that can be absorbed through the skin into the bloodstream for transport to the liver and other organs for use. Vitamins E and K are absorbed with the aid of fat and bile in the small intestine. Vitamin E because of its antioxidant property helps to prevent the oxidation of vitamin A in the intestinal tract. Vitamin K is the only fat-soluble vitamin capable of being synthesized by the intestinal bacteria.

Absorption in the Large Intestine

The major absorption task for the large intestine is water absorption. Although the major portion of nutrients have been absorbed in previous sections of the gastrointestinal tract, there are secondary absorption sites for many of the nutrients in the colon. The colon also participates in extensive bacterial actions, acts as a reservoir for the accumulation of undigested residues, and is involved with the formation and elimination of feces.

Between 300 and 400 ml (10–14 oz) of water are absorbed through the walls of the colon each day, leaving only about 100–150 ml (3–5 oz) for the formation of feces. Large quantities of sodium and potassium are absorbed from the colon. A large amount of potassium is secreted into the intestine as a major component of digestive juices, but most of it is later reabsorbed—another example of how the body conserves and uses nutrients.

About 100 different species of bacteria have been identified in the human colon. This bacterial flora is involved with the synthesis of a number of vitamins. The daily requirement for biotin, folic acid, and vitamin K is provided by intestinal synthesis and absorption of these vitamins. (Note that RDAs for biotin and vitamin K have not been established.) Other B-complex vitamins such as vitamin B_{12} are synthesized by the colon, but not in nutritionally significant amounts.

BIBLIOGRAPHY

Arlin, M. J. *The Science of Nutrition.* 2nd Ed. New York: Macmillan, Inc., 1977.

Bruck-Kan, R. *Introduction to Human Anatomy.* 1st Ed. New York: Harper & Row, Pubs., Inc., 1979.

Freeman, H. J., and Young, S. K. Digestion and absorption of protein. *Annu. Rev. Med.* 29:99, 1978.

Guthrie, H. A. *Introductory Nutrition.* 4th Ed. St. Louis: The C. V. Mosby Co., 1979.

Guyton, A. C. *Basic Human Physiology: Normal Functions and Mechanisms of Disease.* 2nd Ed. Philadelphia: W. B. Saunders Co., 1977.

Krause, M. V., and Mahan, L. K. *Food, Nutrition, and Diet Therapy.* 6th Ed. Philadelphia: W. B. Saunders Co., 1979.

Pike, R. L., and Brown, M. L. *Nutrition: An Integrated Approach.* 2nd Ed. New York: John Wiley & Sons, Inc., Pubs., 1975.

Robinson, C. H., and Lawler, M. R. *Normal and Therapeutic Nutrition.* 15th Ed. New York: Macmillan, Inc., 1977.

Williams, S. R. *Nutrition and Diet Therapy.* 3rd Ed. St. Louis: The C. V. Mosby Co., 1977.

Wilson, E. D., and Fisher, K. H., and Garcia, P. A. *Principles of Nutrition.* 4th Ed. New York: John Wiley & Sons, Inc., Pubs., 1979.

CHAPTER 11

Nutrient Transport

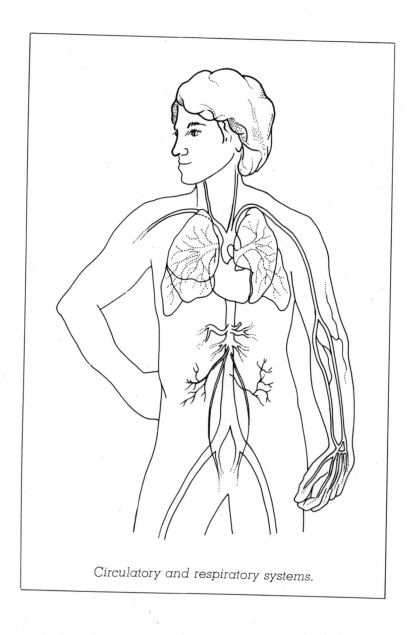

Circulatory and respiratory systems.

There are two major systems in the body that are responsible for the transport of nutrients: the *circulatory system* and the *respiratory system*. The circulatory system is composed of the heart, blood vessels, and lymphatic system. Nutrients absorbed from the gastrointestinal tract gain entrance into the blood. Blood is the transporting medium for the delivery of oxygen, nutrients, hormones, enzymes, and other substances needed by the cell. The blood also circulates through the kidney, where waste materials and excess nutrients and water are removed for excretion. The function of the kidney in removing nutrient waste is discussed in Chapter 14.

Oxygen and nutrients travel away from the heart and to the cells in vessels called *arteries*. The main arteries branch and terminate in smaller vessels called *arterioles*. The arterioles finally connect to *capillaries*, which allow the nutrients and oxygen to pass into the tissue fluid and finally into the cell itself. The tissue fluid surrounding the cells (*interstitial fluid*) is the final distance to be bridged before the nutrients enter the cell. At the same time, waste products and carbon dioxide are moving out of the cells into the tissue fluid into a capillary. See Figure 11-1.

The blood is composed of a fluid portion, called *plasma*, and the formed elements, red blood cells (*erythrocytes*), white blood cells (*leukocytes*), and platelets (*thrombocytes*). The primary function of the erythrocyte is to transport oxygen and carbon dioxide to and from the body cells. The erythrocyte derives its color from the respiratory pigment *hemoglobin*. The nutrients involved in the formation of both hemoglobin and erythrocytes are discussed later in this chapter. The leukocytes form the body's defense against viruses, bacteria, or foreign substances. The number of leukocytes, or the white cell count, is elevated during injury or infection as the body's normal response to these conditions. The platelets are involved primarily with the process of blood clotting. The nutritional com-

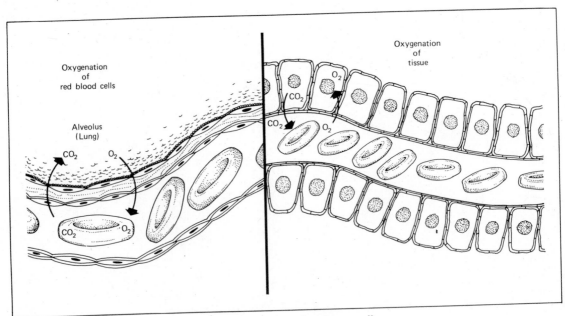

Figure 11-1. Delivery of oxygen by red blood cell to the tissue cells.

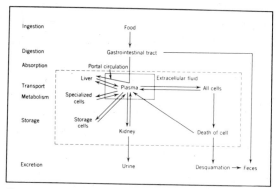

Figure 11-2. The pathways through which the nutrients in food become available and are transported to the individual cells in humans. (From R. L. Pike and M. L. Brown: *Nutrition: An Integrated Approach,* 2nd Ed. Copyright © 1975 John Wiley & Sons, Inc., p. 303. Reprinted by permission of John Wiley & Sons, Inc.)

ponents involved with blood clotting are also discussed later in this chapter.

Whereas the digestive system is considered an open system continuous with the external environment, the circulatory system is a closed system. The heart and blood vessels form a closed system through which blood is pumped throughout the body. The nutrients separated from food during the process of digestion gain entrance into the circulatory system through the process of absorption. These nutrients are absorbed either directly into the portal circulation traveling to the liver or first into the lymphatic circulation. Figure 11-2 shows an overview of nutrient transport.

Nutrients are transported through the blood to the liver for further metabolism or to individual body cells. The plasma is composed of approximately 90% water. The remaining 10% is composed of dissolved nutrients, hormones, and enzymes (Pflanzer, 1975). Of this 10% solid content the majority (7%) is the plasma proteins, composed of *albumin* and *globulins*. Small quantities of electrolytes, vitamins, fatty acids, glycerol, and

glucose are also present. Most nutrients, being water soluble, readily dissolve in the plasma. The fat-soluble nutrients such as triglycerides, fatty acids, and cholesterol are combined with a protein coat in the intestinal mucosa to make them more soluble (Arlin, 1977). These protein-wrapped lipids are called *lipoproteins.* There are four basic types of lipoproteins, which differ in the proportion of protein and fat substances they contain. Figure 11-3 is a summary of these lipoproteins. An evaluation of one or more of these lipoproteins in the blood may reveal the presence of a specific type of disorder called *hyperlipoproteinemia.* The fat-soluble vitamins, absorbed along with the fat products, also travel in the blood attached to an albumin fraction.

Carbohydrate travels in the blood primarily in the form of glucose from the liver. Protein is transported as albumin or globulin, in combination with carbohydrate (glycoprotein) or fat (lipoproteins) or as individual amino acids. Many of the other water-soluble vitamins and minerals readily dissolve in the plasma. Some vitamins and minerals, however, travel in the blood attached to a protein. Iron, for example, travels attached to a protein complex called *transferrin.* Table 11-1 is a summary of the forms in which nutrients are transported in the blood. The student should note that all of the nutrients known to be essential in human nutrition are found in certain levels in the blood. This is necessary because a supply of each nutrient should be readily available for immediate transport to cells as required.

STORAGE OF NUTRIENTS

Nutrients in the plasma are transported to cells for the production of energy, for the synthesis of new compounds, or for storage. Nutrients may be deposited within the body in the form of stores or reserves. Pike and Brown (1975) define a *nutrient store* as "an extra supply of a substance collected in specific cells or tissues that is available when

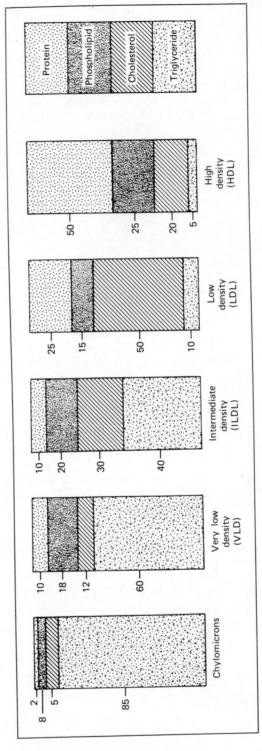

Figure 11-3. Relative composition of lipoproteins.

TABLE 11-1. Some Reported Plasma Constituents in Man

Minerals	Carbohydrates	Proteins	Lipids	Nonprotein Nitrogenous Substances	Vitamins	Enzymes	Hormones
Aluminum	Fructose	Prealbumin	Cephalin	Allantoin	Vitamin A	Adenosine polyphosphatase	Androgens
Bicarbonate	Glucosamine	Albumin	Cerebrosides	Amino acids	Carotenes	Acid	Chorionic gonadotropic hormone
Bromine	Acetyl glucosamine	α_1 Acid glycoprotein	Cholesterol	Alanine	Thiamine	Alkaline	Corticosteroids
Calcium	Glucose	α_1 Glycoprotein	Free	Aminobutyric acid	Riboflavin	Aldolase	Conjugated corticoids
Chlorine	Glucuronic acid	α_1 Lipoproteins	Ester	Arginine	Nicotinic acid	Amylase	Corticosterone
Cobalt	Glycogen	α_2 Glycoproteins	Cholic acid	Asparagine	Pyridoxine	Catalase	Hydrocortisone
Copper	Lactose	Ceruloplasmin	Fat, neutral	Aspartic acid	Pantothenic acid	Cholinesterase	17-Hydroxycorticoids
Fluorine	Pentose	Haptoglobins	Fatty acids	Citrulline	Pteroylglutamic acid	Dehydropeptidase	Epinephrine (adrenaline)
Iodine	Polysaccharides	α_2 Macroglobulins	Glyceride-	Cysteine	Vitamin B_{12}	β-glucuronidase	Estrogens
Iron	Nonglucosamine	Prothrombin	Phospholipid-	Cystine	Ascorbic acid	Histaminase	Estradiol
Lead	Protein-bound	β glycoproteins	Saturated	Glutamic acid	Vitamin D	Lactic dehydrogenase	Estriol
Magnesium		Transferrin	Lecithin	Glutamine	Tocopherols	Lipase	Estrone
Manganese		β_2 Globulin	Phospholipids	Glycine	Biotin	Phenolsulfatase	Insulin
Phosphate		Fibrinogen	Sphingomyelin	Histidine	Choline	Phosphatase	Norepinephrine (noradrenaline)
Phosphorus		β_1 Lipoproteins	Triglyceride	Isoleucine	Inositol	Acid	Progesterone
Inorganic P		β_2 Globulins		Leucine		Alkaline	Thyroid hormone (as protein-bound iodine)
Organic P		γ Globulins		Lysine		Phosphoglucose isomerase	
Adenosine triphosphate P				Methionine		Profibrinolysin	
Diphosphoglycerate P				1-Methylhistidine		Vitamin B_6 conjugase	
Hexosephosphate P				3-Methylhistidine			
Lipid P				Ornithine			
Nucleic acid P				Phenylalanine			
Potassium				Proline			
Rubidium				Serine			
Silicon				Taurine			
Sodium				Threonine			
Sulfate				Tryptophan			
Sulfur				Tyrosine			
Tin				Valine			
Zinc				Bilirubin			
				Creatine			
				Creatinine			
				Histamine			
				Imidazoles			
				Indican			
				Urea			
				Uric acid			
				Ammonia N			
				Polypeptide N			

Reprinted with permission from R. L. Pike and M. L. Brown, *Nutrition: An Integrated Approach*, 2nd ed. New York: John Wiley & Sons, Inc., 1975, pp. 306–307.

and if needed" (p. 311). Withdrawal from this store does not interfere with normal metabolism. In a *reserve* the nutrient is available for use in an emergency, but there is some impairment of health or physiological function (Passmore, 1965).

A true storage form exists for only a few nutrients. There are stores of carbohydrate in the form of glycogen in the liver, but they last only 3 to 4 hours and need to be continuously replenished by diet. The storage form of fat is adipose tissue. The length of storage time for adipose tissue is directly proportional to the quantity of fat stored. A true storage form of protein does not exist within the body. The major proportion of protein found in the body is in the muscle tissue. Muscle protein is not considered to be a true storage form because loss of muscle protein brings about some impairment of health or physiological function. Muscle tissue is therefore considered to be a reserve of protein.

There are true storage forms of the fat-soluble vitamins, A, D, E, and K. Vitamins A, D, and K are stored to a certain extent in the liver. Vitamin E is however stored in the muscle and adipose tissue. The B-complex vitamins are water soluble and are generally not stored, but reserves of these vitamins exist in certain tissues. Because these vitamins function as coenzymes in metabolism, they are present in their coenzyme forms in tissues where metabolic activity is high, such as in the liver and muscle. These reserves are very small and therefore these B vitamins need to be included in the diet daily. The body also does not actually store vitamin C, for it too is a water-soluble vitamin; but it has been estimated that a reserve of 1,500 mg exists. This reserve would last for about 90 days, after which time symptoms of a vitamin C deficiency are likely to occur.

The minerals may occur as either a store or a reserve. Iron is stored in the compound ferritin in the liver, spleen, intestinal mucosa, and all the reticuloendothelial cells. Ferritin is an iron protein complex. Additional iron may be stored in a similar compound called *hemosiderin* found in the liver. Some people with a genetic defect, especially men, store excess quantities of iron in the form of hemosiderin—a condition is known as *hemosiderosis.* Excessive amounts of this compound can cause damage to the liver tissue in a condition called *hemochromatosis.* In this condition the skin may even be bronze in color. The reserves of calcium, phosphorus, and magnesium are present in the bone; however continual dependence on this reserve will result in the development of brittle bones. When the body has enough calcium, the excess may be deposited in the trabeculae at the ends of the bones (Wilson, et al., 1979). Iodine is incorporated into the protein *thyroglobulin,* which is the storage form of iodine. The iodine is then incorporated into the thyroid hormones as needed. The secretion of thyroid hormones raise the basal metabolic rate. The sites of the major nutrient stores and reserves are shown in Figure 11-4.

VASCULAR PHYSIOLOGY

There are several important aspects of vascular physiology that are directly related to nutrition. Besides serving as a vehicle of transport, the formed elements of the blood have specific nutrition-related functions. The red blood cells contain hemoglobin, which combines with oxygen to transport it to the cells. Several specific nutrients are required for the formation of both hemoglobin and red blood cells. The platelets are involved in the important process of blood clotting. The white blood cells function in maintaining the body's immunity. Nutritional status influences immunity, as evidenced by decreased resistance to infection during malnutrition.

Erythrocyte and Hemoglobin Formation

The formation of hemoglobin and the formation of red blood cells are closely related.

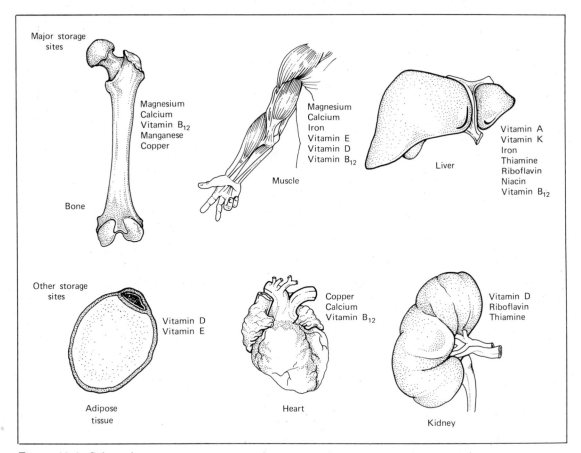

Figure 11-4. Selected common storage sites for nutrients.

Hemoglobin is an iron-containing pigment that readily combines with oxygen for transport to the tissues. Hemoglobin synthesis begins early in the development of the red blood cell and continues for a few days after the red blood cell leaves the bone marrow (Guyton, 1977). Hemoglobin is composed of a *heme* portion, which contains iron, and a protein portion, called *globin*. Adequate quantities of protein and iron are thus required for the production of hemoglobin, which occurs in four steps. The first two steps involve the formation of the *porphyrin ring*, which is the major framework of the heme portion. Pantothenic acid as a part of coenzyme A and pyridoxine (vitamin B_6) are needed for the synthesis of this ring structure. Zinc and magnesium are indirectly involved because they catalyze the formation of pyridoxal phosphate, which is a form of vitamin B_6 (Guthrie, 1979). Vitamin E and folacin are two nutrients involved in the next step, which is the formation of heme. The final step is the combininig of four heme molecules with one globin molecule to form hemoglobin.

Because the formation of red blood cells involves the formation of hemoglobin, many of the nutrients required are the same. The

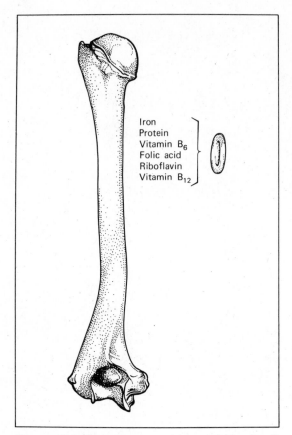

Iron
Protein
Vitamin B_6
Folic acid
Riboflavin
Vitamin B_{12}

Figure 11-5. Nutrients required for red blood cell formation in the bone.

B-complex vitamins, primarily pyridoxine, folic acid, and cobalamin (vitamin B_{12}), and also riboflavin (Pflanzer, 1975) are required for the formation of red blood cells. Copper is involved with the development of young red blood cells because of its association with iron (Wilson et al., 1979). Vitamin B_{12} is the nutrient needed for the maturation of red blood cells. See Figure 11-5 for a summary of the nutrients required for red blood cell formation. A deficiency of any of these nutrients will impair the production of adequate numbers of red blood cells and may lead to various kinds of anemias (discussed in Chap. 27).

Once a red blood cell has been formed, vitamin E helps to maintain the integrity of the membrane, thus preventing its *hemolysis,* or destruction (Williams, 1977). Premature infants may have a type of hemolytic anemia that results in rupture of the red blood cell membrane. These infants respond well to treatment with vitamin E.

Blood Clotting

The sequence of reactions in the clotting of blood is very complex. Although various theories of blood coagulation have been proposed, there is general agreement on the three major reactions that occur. Two nutrients play major roles in the blood-clotting mechanism, vitamin K and calcium. The factors necessary for the formation of a blood clot must be present in the blood at all times. The body has made provision for immediate availability of these nutrients. Vitamin K is one of the few vitamins synthesized by the intestinal bacteria; this assures its continual availability. The level of calcium in the blood is maintained within a normal range at all times. This is possible because of the reserve supply of calcium in the bones. Usually dietary calcium is used to replenish blood levels, but if inadequate calcium is available from the diet, it will be withdrawn from the bones.

One of the first steps in blood clotting is the synthesis of *prothrombin,* one of the clotting factors. The synthesis of prothrombin and other clotting factors occurs in the liver with the aid of vitamin K. A deficiency of vitamin K will interfere with the synthesis of prothrombin and therefore with the entire clotting mechanism. There are two good clinical examples where a vitamin K deficiency may exist. One is the newborn infant with a sterile gastrointestinal tract unable to synthesize vitamin K. Because of this deficit of vitamin K a condition known as *hemorrhagic disease* of the newborn could develop. This is characterized by massive internal hemmorrhaging, which could prove fatal to the infant. To prevent this condition the Committee on Nutrition of the American Academy of Pediatrics (1971) recommended that all newborn infants be given a parenteral dose of 0.05–1.0 mg of vitamin K as a prophylactic measure. Sometimes vitamin K is given to the mother before delivery, but there is doubt about how effectively vitamin K crosses the placenta. The other clinical example of a vitamin K deficiency is with prolonged antibiotic therapy. This type of therapy destroys the natural bacterial flora of the gastrointestinal tract and therefore inhibits the formation of vitamin K. Clients who are receiving anticoagulant therapy may also experience a vitamin K deficiency. Clients prone to developing blood clots are often directed to take anticoagulants such as heparin or dicumarol. While this therapy helps to reduce the formation of internal blood clots, it also interferes with the use of vitamin K. These clients should be taking a vitamin K supplement.

The second step is the conversion of prothrombin to *thrombin*. This reaction requires the presence of calcium ions and *thromboplastin*. The formation of thrombin is necessary because it acts as a cofactor in the final reaction. This final reaction is the conversion of *fibrinogen* to *fibrin*. Calcium is also needed in the conversion. *Fibrin* is the actual clot, and calcium helps to stabilize the fibers of the fibrin so that the clot is maintained.

Immunity

A subject of current interest is the impact of nutrition on immune function. *Immunity* is the resistance of the body to disease or infection agents. Every nutrient known to be essential to humans has some effect on immune function. Deficiencies of protein, folic acid, pyridoxine (vitamin B_6), pantothenic acid, iron, and vitamin A have been reported to impair the production of antibodies. The body's first line of defense is the skin and mucus membranes. The B-complex vitamins, protein, and vitamin A all function in the maintenance of the skin. The daily diet should therefore be adequate in these nutrients in order to maintain these structures and protect the body against direct invasion.

FLUID AND ELECTROLYTE BALANCE

The circulatory system provides the basic transport mechanism that supplies the cells with nutrients necessary for survival. An understanding of the composition, placement, and transport mechanisms of the fluids in the system is necessary to provide nutritional support for the patient.

Water is the most basic and abundant fluid in the body. In the average man, water accounts for 57% of his body weight. Women average slightly less water than their male counterparts, with about 51% of total body weight being water. In infants 75% of the body weight is water, with a progressive decrease in relative body water throughout the early development years. The water content of nonfat body tissue is 71 ml/100 gm of water. Fat, however, is relatively free of water, explaining why obese people may only have 43% of total weight as water. (See Table 11-2.)

Fluid Compartments

The body fluids are contained in two major compartments. The *intracellular fluid* is about

TABLE 11-2. Total Body Water (as Percentage of Body Weight) in Relation to Age and Sex

Age	Male	Female
10–18	59	57
18–40	61	51
40–60	55	47
Over 60	52	46

SOURCE: Reprinted with permission from Edelman, I. S. and Leibman, J., "Anatomy of Body Water and Electrolytes." *American Journal of Medicine* 27:257, 1959.

25 of the 40 liters of fluid volume in the body. The fluid within the cells varies somewhat from cell to cell but is generally seen as homogeneous. Each cell is a minute subsystem containing a myriad of substances necessary for cell survival. An explanation of these constituents is in the following sections on diffusion and osmosis.

The *extracellular fluid* contains the various ions and nutrients needed for maintenance of cell life. This fluid is constantly being moved throughout the body and is available for use by the cells. Extracellular fluid is transported in two ways, through the circulatory system and between the blood capillaries and cells.

The nutrients carried in extracellular fluid originate in the respiratory system, the gastrointestinal system, and the organs that have basic metabolic functions such as the liver, kidneys, and endocrine glands. The respiratory system allows oxygen to be placed into circulation and carbon dioxide to be excreted. Dissolved nutrients such as carbohydrates, fatty acids, and amino acids are absorbed from the gastrointestinal system into the blood. The kidneys remove from the plasma most substances not needed by the body. The liver alters some of the nonusable substances absorbed from the gastrointestinal tract into a form that can be absorbed and used by the cells.

Extracellular fluid can be divided into fluid contained within the plasma, interstitial fluid, cerebrospinal fluid, fluid in gastrointestinal tract, intraocular fluid, and fluid in what is called *potential spaces*. *Interstitial fluid* is the fluid between the cells of the body. Much of this water is bonded together in a gellike matrix that continuously allows dissolved substances to move through it. The *plasma* is the noncellular portion of blood. Plasma communicates constantly with the interstitial fluid through microscopic pores in the capillaries. Proteins in the plasma are the only constituents too large to move easily into interstitial fluid. The normal adult has approximately 3 liters of plasma. *Cerebrospinal fluid* (CSF) is in

most ways very similar to interstitial fluid with the exception that CSF contains more sodium and less potassium and glucose than the interstitial fluid outside of the central nervous system. There are about 140 ml of CSF in the normal adult. The eye is filled with *intraocular fluid*, which in many ways is similar to CSF. Spaces that normally contain little fluid but that under special conditions can be filled with large amounts are called *potential spaces*. Examples include the peritoneal cavity, the pericardial cavity, and the joint spaces. Under normal circumstances there are usually only moderate amounts of fluid in the gastrointestinal system. This fluid is similar in properties to interstitial fluid with the addition of specific glandular secretions that aid in the digestive process.

Blood

The blood is made up of plasma and cellular components. The average blood volume for a healthy adult is 5 liters, 3 liters being plasma, with red blood cells comprising the remaining 2 liters. The *hematocrit* is the percentage of red blood cells in the total blood volume. The normal hematocrit is approximately 40 for a man and 36 for a woman. The hematocrit at the capillary level is lower than the reading taken from a large artery or vein because the red blood cells tend to "stream" in the center of the large vessels, giving a higher concentration of plasma near the walls.

Composition of Body Fluids

The constituents of body fluids differ markedly in the two compartments. The extracellular fluid is high in sodium and low in potassium; exactly the opposite is true in intracellular fluid. The extracellular fluid contains significantly larger amounts of chlorine, bicarbonate, and glucose than intracellular fluid. The fluid within the cell has a higher concentration of phosphates, magnesium, and amino acids. These differences,

TABLE 11-3. Components of the Body Fluid Compartments

Substance	Intracellular	Extracellular
Na^+	10 mEq[a]/liter	142 mEq/liter
K^+	141mEq/liter	5 mEq/liter
Cl^-	4 mEq/liter	103 mEq/liter
HCO_3^-	10 mEq/liter	28 mEq/liter
Phosphates	75 mEq/liter	4 mEq/liter
Ca^{++}	over 1 mEq/liter	5 mEq/liter
Mg^{++}	58 mEq/liter	3 mEq/liter
Glucose	0–20 mg%	90 mg%
Amino acids	200 mg% (?)	30 mg%

[a] A milliequivalent (mEq) is used to measure the number of ionic charges of an electrolyte in solution and indicates the chemical combining power or activity of an electrolyte.

listed in Table 11-3, are extremely important to cell survival.

Movement Between Body Fluid Compartments

For the cells to use nutrients and oxygen, some means of transport must be available to get the substances from the plasma into the cell. Transportation into the cell occurs through two major processes: *diffusion* and *active transport*.

Diffusion

All molecules and ions in the body fluids are in constant motion, each randomly bouncing into other molecules and ions in the solution. This continual movement and bouncing is called *diffusion*. Each molecule is moving randomly, bouncing into millions of other particles each second.

If a dissolved substance is placed at one end of a container of solution, it will gradually diffuse throughout the entire container so that eventually there will be a relatively equal amount of the substance in all parts of the solution. This movement from an area of high concentration to one of low concentration is due to what is termed a *diffusion gradient*. In general, the greater the concentration difference, the greater the rate of

diffusion. To better understand this principle consider the addition of food coloring to water as an example. When you add food coloring to water, the food coloring itself is very concentrated. After a short time the entire glass of water will have turned a color, indicating that the food coloring has diffused completely through the solution.

Diffusion across the cell membrane occurs in much the same way. The membrane itself consists of a lipid matrix interlaced with a protein cover. Pores that are 8Å in diameter are also scattered throughout the cell membrane. Substances such as water and dissolved ions are small enough to pass through these pores easily. A few substances, such as oxygen, carbon dioxide, fatty acids, and alcohol, are lipid soluble. When one of these substances comes in contact with the cell membrane, it dissolves and moves through the lipid membrane in exactly the same way as other substances move through water. In order to be lipid soluble, particles must not be ionized.

Glucose is not lipid soluble; however, it is able to be transported across the cell membrane by using a carrier substance. The combination of glucose and this carrier substance is lipid soluble. When the combined glucose-carrier substance reaches the inside of the cell, the glucose is released unchanged for use by the cell. The specific substance that in this way facilitates the diffusion of glucose is unknown. Insulin appears to speed up the transport of glucose by the carrier seven-to-ten times. This mechanism, termed *facilitative diffusion*, is similar to *active transport*, discussed below. The primary difference is that facilitative diffusion only occurs from an area of high concentration to one of low concentration. For example, if the concentration of glucose inside the cell was significantly higher than that outside, glucose would not be diffused through the membrane.

Another form of movement is termed *filtration*. It is the selective passage of fluid through a semipermeable membrane under the force of hydrostatic pressure.

Osmosis

Cell walls are semipermeable membranes. Water and some other uncharged molecules are able to pass through the membrane, but larger molecules and most ions are prevented from passage. A net diffusion of water across a cell membrane occurs whenever there is a difference between the water concentrations on the two sides of the membrane. This movement of water across a semipermeable membrane is known as *osmosis*. Just as in simple diffusion, the concentration of the solute will tend to be equalized. If the dissolved substance is not able to pass through the semipermeable membrane, then water will move into or out of the compartments until both sides of the membrane have an equal concentration of solutes. The result is usually a swelling or shrinking of one compartment.

The tendency for movement of solvent molecules to a region of greater solute concentration can be prevented by applying pressure to the more concentrated solution. This pressure is termed *osmotic pressure*. In the body serum, osmotic pressure is primarily affected by sodium, bicarbonate, and chlorine concentrations.

The cell is an osmotic system with a highly elastic semipermeable membrane. The cell will shrink and expand when it is placed in media of different water concentrations. The importance of administering fluids that are of a similar concentration to intercellular fluids can be seen. If, for example, large amounts of *hypotonic* (of less concentration than body cells) *solutions* are administered, the body cells will swell and *lysis* will occur.

Pinocytosis

Minute quantities of substance can be transported through the capillary membrane by *pinocytosis*. What occurs during this process is that the endothelial cells of the capillary wall ingest small amounts of interstitial fluid or plasma, which then migrate to the other wall as small vesicles. The substance is then released intact. This is the only known means by which very large molecules, such as proteins, can be transported to the interior of cells.

Active Transport

As previously discussed, diffusion occurs when a substance moves from an area of high concentration to one of low concentration with a resulting equilibrium in solute concentration. *Active transport* moves a solvent against this concentration gradient, that is, from an area of lower concentration to one of higher concentration. For this to occur, energy must be expended. Active transport is similar to facilitated diffusion in that both need a carrier substance to move the solute across the cell membrane. The energy is used in the form of ATP, which is stored within the cell membrane. Examples of active transport occurring within the body include the absorption of glucose across the intestinal wall, transport of amino acids across various membranes, and reabsorption of some substances from the kidney tubules into interstitial fluids.

The most well known mechanism of active transport is the *sodium-potasssium pump*. During stimulation of a nerve cell, potassium moves outside the cell wall and sodium moves inside. As shown in Table 11-3 sodium exists in much greater concentration in extracellular fluid than in intercellular fluid, and potassium exists largely in intercellular fluid with much extracellular smaller concentrations. A carrier substance within the cell membrane combines with the sodium on the inside of the cell and transports it to the outside, there combining with a potassium ion and transporting it to the inside of the cell. This mechanism keeps the levels of intercellular electrolytes at appropriate concentrations.

Water Balance

Health depends on adequate regulation of intake and output of fluids and electrolytes. The average adult drinks about 1,200 ml (41 oz) of fluid in 24 hours, with an additional 1,000 ml (34 oz) absorbed from food. When nutrients are oxidized by the body, one of the end products is water. The amounts of water gained through oxidation vary with the kind of food used, but the normal adult usually gains between 300 and 400 ml (10–14 oz) daily. Fluid is lost through the kidneys in the amount of 1,500–1,800 ml (51–61 oz)/day. Adults loose approximately 500 ml of fluid through the skin each day. 300–600 ml (10–20 oz) is excreted through the respiratory tract, with the remaining 100 ml lost in the feces.

To preserve water balance, two compensatory mechanisms operate. The first is the adjustment of water intake by thirst; the second is adjustment of water output by renal mechanisms. *Thirst* is the desire to ingest liquids. It is not a simple sensation of dryness of the mucous membranes of the mouth and pharnyx but a much more widely perceived sensation similar to hunger. Thirst occurs when cellular dehydration is present, when extracellular fluid volume is decreased, or when thirst centers in the hypothalamus are stimulated. It has been suggested by certain research studies that thirst appears when the cell volume is reduced by 1–2%. The role of the kidney in water balance is discussed later in this chapter.

On the cellular level, two mechanisms are largely responsible for water balance. The first can be termed simply as the H_2O *pump*. Water is shunted from the inside of the cell to the outside in an effort to keep the cell hypertonic. If the cell is injured, this mechanism is the first to fail, leading to a swelling of the cell and eventual lysis. The other mechanism maintaining water balance within the cell is the osmotic pressure exerted by sodium within the cell. This mechanism stabilizes intracellular and extracellular pressures.

Excessive loss of fluids by any of the above channels can lead to a severe imbalance of water and electrolytes.

Dehydration

Dehydration is one of the common problems a nurse encounters in the clinical setting. The etiology of dehydration can be any one of a number of conditions or a combination of several. Common causes include a lack of water intake, which frequently occurs among the aged; excess sweating; excess fluid output, as in diabetes insipidus; and gastrointestinal fluid losses, as in excessive diarrhea or vomiting. If a large amount of extracellular fluid is lost, fluid and sometimes electrolytes move out of the cell into the extracellular fluid, resulting in cellular dehydration, the effects of which are easy to postulate.

Symptoms of dehydration include thirst, loss of skin *turgor,* lowered central venous pressure, increased blood viscosity, and hemoconcentration (elevated hematocrit, hemoglobin, and electrolyte values caused by a decrease in solvent). Skin and mucous membrane dryness occur first, then development of fever, mental agitation, and depression, finally, loss of consciousness. Therapy is replacement of fluid volume with the correction of any existing electrolyte imbalances. A solution of 2.5% or 5% dextrose in water is used to replace fluids. The solution is hypotonic, which will prevent red blood cell swelling and eventual hemolysis.

Hypovolemia is an abnormally decreased volume of circulating plasma in the body. One effect of severe *hypovolemia* is shock. *Shock* is an abnormal physiological condition resulting from an inadequate propulsion of blood and decreased tissue perfusion. Shock begins with a fall in capillary blood flow below the levels needed to maintain cellular function. Other causes that precipitate shock in addition to hypovolemia include cardiogenic failure, sepsis, neurogenic vasodilatation, and thromboembolism. The compensatory mechanisms that are initiated in response to shock are the same no matter what the cause. In general, the mechanism of shock can be outlined as follows:

1. The body responds almost immediately with reflex vasoconstriction. The blood pressure tends to stay in the normal range.

2. The progressive stage is entered when compensatory mechanisms are unable to cope with blood loss. *Tachycardia, dyspnea,* and *oliguria* occur.

3. Shock becomes irreversible when compensatory mechanisms break down, the total blood pH decreases, and vasodilatation occurs.

Water Intoxication

Water excess will create the problem of an abnormally low concentration of extracellular fluids. *Dilutional hyponatremia* occurs; it is a condition in which the total amount of sodium in the body is the same, but plasma concentration is low. Overhydration may result from excessive oral or IV fluid intake, inability of the kidneys to excrete water, or excessive antidiuretic hormone excretion. During overhydration, fluids shift to the intracellular space to equalize osmotic pressure until the excess water can be eliminated. Signs of overhydration include *polyuria,* symptoms of increased intercranial pressure (ipsilateral pupil dilatation, widening pulse pressure, deterioration in level of consciousness), and nausea or vomiting.

Water intoxication rarely occurs except in patients with severely impaired renal function. A hypertonic solution such as *mannitol,* may be given to cause an immediate decrease in intracellular fluid volume. Such an infusion produces an osmotic diuresis in which the patient will excrete larger and more dilute volumes of urine.

Edema

Edema results from abnormal compartmentalization of body fluids because of excess fluid in the interstitial space. It is due to disturbances in one or several factors involved in normal exchange of fluid between blood and tissue spaces. Causes of edema include high capillary pressure, which usually is caused by any condition having a sluggish venous return, as in congestive heart failure; a decrease in serum osmotic pressure, as in burns or other cases of albumin loss; blockage of normal lymph drainage channels, as in carcinoma or filarial conditions; and an increased capillary membrane permeability, which accompanies trauma or irritation. Treatment is aimed at correcting the cause of the edema.

One of the nurse's most important functions is the maintenance of fluid balance in the patient or restoration of such balance by the adequate and appropriate administration of fluids. To help the student anticiapte fluid imbalances, a summary of specific problems and alterations is presented in Table 11-4.

RENAL SUPPORT OF PHYSIOLOGICAL MECHANISMS

The kidneys have a primary role in maintaining homeostasis within the fluid systems of the body by excreting or retaining specific ions. The functional unit of the kidney is the *nephron.* Each kidney contains about 1 million nephrons, each forming urine independently. The nephron consists of a vascular component and a tubular component. The vascular component is known as the *glomerulus.* Its *afferent arteriole* supplies blood to the capsule, and its *efferent arteriole* moves it away. The tubular part of the nephron contains a series of tubes in which various components of the filtered serum are excreted or reabsorbed.

Usually about one-fifth of the total plasma is filtered through the glomerular membrane into the tubules of the nephron. As the filtered fluid flows through the tubules, water and many of the electrolytes are absorbed at various points back into the plasma of the *peritubular capillaries.* The unwanted portions fail to be reabsorbed and are excreted as a component of urine.

The kidneys regulate body fluid and electrolyte homeostasis through five major processes. The first is the maintenance of the op-

TABLE 11-4. Fluid Excesses and Deficits

	Excess	*Deficit*
General characteristics	Solute diluted	Solute concentrated
Potential causes	Cardiac insufficiency, cirrhosis, ascites, too rapid infusion of saline solutions, aldosterone secretion, renal disease	Gastrointestinal losses (vomiting, diarrhea, suctioning), diuretics, diaphoresis, lack of water intake
Symptoms	Pitting edema, dyspnea, neck vein distention, weight gain, increased intercranial pressure	Postural hypotension, poor skin turgor, anorexia, oliguria, vomiting, elevated temperature
Laboratory data	Low hematocrit, elevated central venous pressure, low serum sodium	Elevated hematocrit, elevated serum sodium, high urinary specific gravity, protein elevated, high serum osmolarity
Treatment	Diuretics, sodium and potassium deficits, water restriction, treatment of disease	Fluid replacement, treatment of underlying cause

SOURCE: Modified from Violet R. Stroot, Carea A. Lee, and Ann Schaper, *Fluids and Electrolytes: A Practical Approach,* 2nd Ed. Philadelphia: F. A. Davis Company, 1977.

timum level of extracellular fluids by varying the amount of urine output. Second, the kidneys maintain the osmolarity of body fluids at an isotonic level with intracellular fluids. Third and fourth, the renal system maintains blood volume and controls electrolyte concentration through the controlled reabsorption of water and through the selected reabsorption of electrolytes. Fifth, the kidneys are able to vary the pH of urine to aid in the maintenance of acid-base homeostasis.

ELECTROLYTE BALANCE

When chemical substances are placed in solutions, they either dissociate into ions or remain unchanged. *Electrolytes* are those that dissociate. Each ion carries an electrical charge, either positive or negative. Those that carry a positive charge are called *cations;* examples include Na^+ (sodium), K^+ (potassium), Ca^{++} (calcium), and Mg^{++} (magnesium). Negatively charged electrolytes are called *anions.* Cl^- (chlorine), HCO_3^- (bicarbonate), HPO_4^{--} (phosphate), and SO_4^{--} (sulfate) are among the anions in the body.

Regulation of body electrolytes is essential for the maintenance of body functions. The positive ions must be precisely controlled because of potentially drastic changes in body function. For example, a decrease in sodium concentration can cause severe muscle weakness; a potassium deficit may cause paralysis. An increase in sodium causes fluid retention and increases cardiac work load. *Hyperkalemia* (potassium excess) precipitates cardiac arrhythmias. Calcium imbalances may lead to muscle weakness or tetany because of a change in cell-membrane permeability. The regulation of anions is not as critical for specific body functions as that of the cations, but a correct ratio between positive and negative ions needs to be established in order to maintain acid-base balance. Regulation of this homeostatic mechanism is discussed later in this chapter.

Sodium

Sodium is the major component of extracellular fluid. Sodium and chlorine combine in water to form a saline solution that acts as a basis for the body fluids. Sodium does not easily penetrate most cell membranes. An increase in the concentration of sodium will cause an increase in total fluid volume because water tends to follow sodium passively.

Because of its vital role in body homeostasis, it is not surprising that the body very efficiently maintains sodium levels at approximately 142 mEq/liter in extracellular fluid. The sodium is selectively reabsorbed in the tubules of the nephron. The amount of reabsorption is regulated by the concentration of *aldosterone* in the body fluids. If large amounts of sodium are excreted, correspondingly large amounts of water will be lost. If sodium is retained, so is water.

Aldosterone is a hormone secreted by the adrenal cortex. The hormone increases the rate of sodium reabsorption in all segments of the tubular system, and the amount of sodium reabsorbed is a direct function of the amount of aldosterone present. In the absence of aldosterone the two kidneys will lose one-sixth to one-tenth of the total body sodiium chloride each day. Aldosterone secretion is increased by one or more of the following conditions: (1) a decrease in extracellular fluid sodium concentration; (2) a high extracellular potassium concentration; (3) a decrease in total blood volume or reduced cardiac output, and (4) conditions of physical stress precipitated by trauma, extreme exercise, burns, or other circumstances.

The mechanism of aldosterone secretion is hypothetical at this point. One of the more popular theories is that reduced renal blood flow or reduced sodium concentration in the extracellular fluid increases the secretion of *renin* from the *juxtaglomerular cells* of the kidney. Renin reacts with blood plasma to form *angiotensin*. The angiotensin increases aldosterone secretion, causing sodium conservation until serum levels of the electrolyte can return to normal. When renin secretion is inhibited by high sodium concentrations, angiotensin and aldosterone are not produced, causing increased excretion of sodium and water.

In addition to regulating total water balance, sodium also plays an important role in the conduction of nervous impulses. The nerve cell in its resting state has a positive charge outside and a negative charge inside. A large number of sodium ions are on the outside, with a smaller number of potassium ions on the inside of the cell. When the nerve cell is stimulated, membrane permeability changes, allowing sodium to enter the cell and potassium ions to exit. The sodium-potassium pump uses active transport to restore the previous ion balance. This electrolyte change is ultimately responsible for muscle contraction. It is obvious that any disturbance in sodium balance will be reflected by a change in neuromuscular function.

Hypernatremia

An excess in serum sodium concentration is referred to as *hypernatremia*. The cause of hypernatremia is either dehydration, resulting in an increase in the concentration of sodium rather than an increase in amount of total sodium, or conditions such as *Cushing's syndrome* in which large amounts of aldosterone are secreted. The main result of such an imbalance is water retention with a potential for fluid overload and, if prolonged, congestive heart failure. Signs and symptoms are compatible with those of fluid overload. These include *pitting edema,* excessive weight gain, elevated blood pressure, and as the system approaches congestive failure, rales, rhonchi, and dyspnea. If the excess is due to dehydration, the patient will have dry mucus membranes, flushed skin, thirst, oliguria, and *pyrexia.* The patient becomes agitated, at times to the point of mania or seizure activity. Laboratory findings will reveal an increased sodium level, if the cause is related to dehydration. If dehydration is not present, the sodium level will remain unchanged but total serum osmolarity may be lowered. Treatment of saline excess is directed toward the specific cause. If the patient is not dehydrated, the physician will order diuretics with the concurrent restriction of salt and fluids. The patient is usually limited to 1,500–1,700 ml of fluid per day, however, the restriction may be as severe as a 1,000–1,200 ml/day limit. If an extracellular fluid deficit is the cause of the problem, intravenous replacement therapy is usually instituted with an isotonic or hypertonic saline solution.

Hyponatremia

Hyponatremia, or sodium deficit, results either from a loss of sodium without a water loss, as may occur with the administration of thiazide diuretics, or from gains in water without corresponding gains in sodium, as when an individual perspires heavily and drinks large amounts of water without replacing the sodium loss. Other causes that may precipitate hyponatremia include gastrointestinal losses (as from vomiting, diarrhea, or continuous suctioning), infusion of electrolyte solutions, adrenal insufficiencies, renal disease, and loss associated with trauma such as burns. The initial clinical findings are usually the patient's subjective feeling of anxiety and a diffuse feeling of impending doom. The patient's level of consciousness may deteriorate to the point of delirium. Oliguria, pyrexia, flushed skin, abdominal cramping, and convulsions frequently occur with a deficit. The patient's overall status may reach one of hypovolemic shock accompanied by vasomotor collapse, hypotension, tachycardia, and *cyanosis*. A specific sign is that of *fingerprinting*. If pressure is applied on the sternum with a fingertip, a visible fingerprint will be visible after the pressure is released. This phenomenon is due to an increased elasticity in the body tissues. The extracellular fluid is now hypotonic and is readily absorbed into the cells, resulting in an overall reduction in extracellular fluid volume. Laboratory findings may reveal a decrease in serum sodium, but only if there is not a corresponding fluid deficit. If the actual extracellular fluid sodium concentration is decreased, the urine specific gravity will be 1.01 or lower because of a sodium decrease in the urine. Treatment of hyponatremia centers around replenishing the sodium levels without causing excessive fluid retention. A hypertonic solution is administered if the fluid levels are normal. Such a solution replaces sodium in the least amount of water possible. If a fluid deficit exists, an isotonic saline solution will be administered.

Potassium

Potassium is the major intracellular electrolyte. It acts with sodium in the propagation of nerve impulses along nerve fibers. Potassium is also necessary for the chemical reactions that occur to form ATP from carbohydrates and to build proteins from amino acids. Skeletal muscles and muscles of the heart and intestines are dependent on potassium for function. The intracellular compartment contains about 98% of all the potassium in the body. The extracellular fluid level is reflected in a normal serum potassium level of 3.5–5.5 mEq/liter. The potassium content of urine varies with the intake, usually amounting to 40–50 mEq daily. Potassium is also excreted through body secretions such as sweat, saliva, gastric juices, and feces.

Potassium must be ingested daily, as the body has no effective way of storing it. 40 mEq daily will supply the body with the potassium necessary for function. The average balanced diet contains from 60 to 100 mEq/day.

Potassium is regulated in two different ways. The first involves an aldosterone feedback mechanism exactly opposite of that of sodium. When aldosterone stimulates the distal tubules to reabsorb sodium, the exchange of positive ions causes potassium to be passively secreted into the tubules and eliminated via the urine. A high serum potassium level increases the rate of aldosterone secretion, which increases sodium reabsorption and decreases the potassium back to normal. The second method of potassium regulation is its direct effect on the distal tubules collecting ducts to cause an increase in potassium secretion into the tubular fluid. The basic dissimilarity between potassium and sodium is that the body can vigorously conserve sodium but cannot store potassium efficiently, particularly in those patients under stress.

Hyperkalemia

An excess of potassium in the body is referred to as *hyperkalemia*. In most cases potassium excess is due to renal failure or leakage of potassium from the intercellular component to the extracellular fluid. Patients experiencing renal failure wil have hyperkalemia, particularly if the failure is associated with oliguria or anuria. The principle limiting factor in the excretion of potassium is a reduced glomerular filtration rate. The problem is compounded when the patient consumes a diet high in potassium. Mass movement of potassium from the cells to the extracellular fluid usually follows cell damage, or lysis. Any kind of trauma, burns, or other injury will cause the potassium shift. Dehydration or infusion of hypertonic intravenous fluids can stimulate potassium movement out of the cells into the plasma because of a concentration gradient between the two compartments. Metabolic *acidemia*, discussed later in this chapter, may also be associated with hyperkalemia.

Physiological signs and symptoms that accompany hyperkalemia include irritability, nausea, diarrhea, and intestinal colic. As the imbalance progresses, the patients condition will deteriorate with weakness, flaccid paralysis, difficulty with respiration, and oliguria. Electrocardiograph changes include peaked T waves, P wave disappearance, and the eventual fusion of the QRS complex, RS–T segment, and the T wave. Because nervous transmission through the heart is slowed, intraventricular conduction disturbances occur, which progress to ventricular fibrillation and cardiac arrest. Laboratory analysis reveals repeated plasma potassium levels greater than 5.6 mEq/liter.

In the presence of functioning kidneys, treatment usually centers on a reduction in the intake of potassium. When hyperkalemia occurs as a result of renal failure, the physician may order the administration of carbonic anhydrase inhibitors or ion exchange resins such as Kayexelate enemas. The physician may order rapid intravenous glucose with insulin. As glucose moves into the cell the potassium is passively transported with it. Potassium inside the cell is not toxic. If necrotic tissue is causing the potassium excess, surgical debridement may be necessary to remove the injured cells. Hemodialysis or peritoneal dialysis are often used to decrease the serum potassium level.

Hypokalemia

Excessive loss of potassium or inadequate potassium intake can result in a decreased serum potassium level, referred to as *hypokalemia*. The leading cause of potassium deficiency is the administration of diuretics, which act on the tubules to inhibit potassium reabsorption. Examples of such diuretics include the thiazides and furosemide. Any loss of potassium-rich fluids such as gastrointestinal digestive juices may also result in a decreased serum potassium. Prolonged gastrointestinal suction, abdominal surgery, excessive vomiting or diarrhea are all common precursors of hypokalemia. Other conditions that may precipitate potassium deficiency include *pyelonephritis, thyroid storm* (see next section), crushing injuries, and wound healing. Excessive *diaphoresis*, fever, and emotional upset also contribute to potassium loss.

The clinical symptomotology associated with hypokalemia is due to the role of potassium in body homeostasis. Early symptoms may mimic those of hyperkalemia, making diagnosis of the precise alteration difficult without laboratory data. Muscle weakness and malaise are usually the initial signs. Loss of reflexes, muscle flabbiness, and polyuria secondary to renal tubule damage may result. Heart block, atrial and ventricular arrhythmias, weak pulse, and falling blood pressure occur as the deficit progresses. Anorexia, vomiting and *paralytic ileus* may accompany gastrointestinal muscle weakness. The electrocardiogram reveals a flattened T wave, a depressed S–T segment, and a prominent U wave. Laboratory diagnosis will reveal a potassium level of less than 4 mEq/liter with a corresponding low serum chlorine level (below 98 mEq/liter).

Treatment centers on replacement therapy, either by oral or parenteral routes. Substances high in potassium include meat, bananas, orange juice, coffee, tea, cola beverages, and chocolate. Potassium supplements are frequently bad tasting and may stain the teeth. The administration of the solutions in cold grape juice taken with a straw may facilitate the patient's compliance with at-home drug therapy.

Calcium

The cation calcium is important in relation to neuromuscular irritability, formation of bones and teeth, and the clotting of blood. It is the most abundant electrolyte in the body (1,200 gm), with approximately 90% of it stored in the bones and teeth. Because of this storage of calcium, relatively little is circulating in the serum. The normal range of 8.5–10.5 mg% measures the ionized calcium in serum. This is approximately equal to 5 mEq/liter. Much of the remaining calcium in the serum is bound to albumin and is not available for physiological activity. Only the ionized calcium is measured in serum levels.

One of the primary functions of calcium in the body is its role in the initiation of muscular contraction. Calcium ions normally decrease the permeability of the membrane to sodium, thus regulating to a degree the membrane excitability of the nerve cell, prohibiting an overcharging of the cell membrane. Calcium, in combination with specific molecules, activates ATP inside the muscle fiber. The muscle remains contractual until the energy source is depleted or the calcium

combines with other substances in the fiber. Of course the most important muscle contraction regulated by this mechanism is the heart. Calcium ions play an important role in blood clotting. The ion does not enter into any of the blood-clotting mechanisms but acts as a cofactor to cause the reactions to take place. Specifically, calcium works with factor V and X to convert prothrombin to thrombin. An additional role of calcium is its function in the strengthening of the capillary membrane. Of course calcium also has a primary role in the formation of bones and teeth. The normal adult needs about 1 mg of calcium daily. Sufficient vitamin D and protein must also be present in the diet, as both are necessary for calcium absorption from the gastrointestinal tract.

The serum calcium ion concentration is controlled principally by the parathyroid and thyroid glands. Low serum calcium levels stimulate the parathyroid glands to release parathyroid hormone, which acts directly on the bone to increase the rate of reabsorption of bone salts, thus releasing large amounts of calcium and phosphorus into the serum. The kidney also plays a part in calcium regulation, excreting large amounts of the ion when serum levels are elevated and very small amounts when serum levels are decreased.

Hypercalcemia

Calcium excess (*hypercalcemia*) may be associated with overconsumption of the ion, hyperparathyroidism, parathyroid tumor, or excessive administration of Vitamin D (over 50,000 IU daily). Fractures, bone tumors, or prolonged immobilization may cause calcium excess because of movement of calcium from the bone into serum. Calcium excess in the serum is noted in the early stages of osteoporosis when calcium moves from the bones to the serum.

Clinical signs associated with hypercalcemia include neuromuscular relaxation, hypotonicity of the muscle, deep bone pain, pathological fractures, and renal *calculi*. Constipation may occur because of smooth-muscle relaxation. As the excess worsens, the nervous system becomes depressed, producing lethargy and coma. *Hypercalcemic crisis* may occur, which if left untreated will lead to cardiac arrest. Symptoms include severe nausea and vomiting, dehydration, stupor, and *azotemia*. Laboratory findings during calcium excess will show a plasma concentration above 5.8 mEq/liter. Roentgenograms may reveal generalized bone demineralization and renal calculi.

Treatment is usually directed at the cause of the excess. Mobilization or weight-bearing exercises will decrease bone demineralization. Steroids may be given to assist the body's stress response. Steroids also inhibit the absorption of calcium. The nurse should be aware that calcium enhances digitalis intoxication.

Hypocalcemia

When the calcium level in the serum falls below normal, the condition is referred to as *hypocalcemia*. A calcium deficit may arise from prolonged gastrointestinal excretion of calcium such as occurs during diarrhea. Calcium is mobilized to wound sites and is frequently lost in wound exudation such as occurs in burns. Pancreatic disease precipitates calcium withdrawal from the extracellular fluid and prevents absorption of calcium from the gastrointestinal tract, causing a calcium imbalance. Severe hypocalcemia may occur during renal failure because of the lack of calcium absorption from the gastrointestinal tract. Clients who are in the immediate postoperative stage following a thyroidectomy may experience *thyroid storm,* a condition that results from a severe calcium deficit caused by possible excision or manipulation of the parathyroid glands during the surgery.

As with the other electrolytes a deficit in calcium will cause clinical signs that result directly from the function of calcium in the body. As the calcium level falls, the nervous system becomes increasingly more irritable. Both the peripheral and central nervous system are involved, though symptoms appear peripherally first. The first signs may be circumoral and digital tingling followed by abdominal and skeletal muscle cramps. Tetany occurs when the nerve fibers become so excitable that they discharge spontaneously, initiating nerve impulses that cause the muscles to go into severe contraction. *Latent tetany,* the period immediately preceding full-blown tetany, can be detected by placing a tourniquet on the clinet's arm. This causes ischemia of the peripheral nerves and increases excitability, causing the muscles of the forearm and hand to go into spasm. *Chvostek's* sign is also useful in diagnosing a calcium deficit. This is elicited by tapping the client's face over a facial nerve such as in front of the temple. If the face twitches, the results are positive. Prolonged tetany can be fatal when it results in respiratory paralysis. Seizures and coma also accompany severe hypocalcemia. A decreased calcium level may cause a change in the client's ability to clot blood. It causes marked cardiac dilatation and a decrease in the force of contraction. An additional result of hypocalcemia is *osteoporosis*. When serum calcium decreases, calcium salts are lost from the bones or not replaced after being depleted. The bones become more porous, brittle and fragile. Pathological fractures may occur. Laboratory evaluation usually reveals a serum calcium level below 4.5 mEq/liter, or 8.5 mg percent. The EKG will show a prolonged Q–T interval characteristic of calcium deficiency.

Hypocalcemia is treated by the oral or intravenous replacement of calcium. An increase of vitamin D in the diet is advisable because of the vitamin's role in aiding calcium absorption in the gut. If osteoporosis is present, restoration of weight bearing will prevent further bone demineralization. For the client experiencing acute hypocalcemia from renal failure, calcium is administered orally.

Magnesium

Magnesium is the fourth most common cation in the body. The distribution of the cation is similar to that of potassium in that the major concentration of the ion is within the cell. One of magnesium's intracellular functions is its action as a catalyst during carbohydrate metabolism. Magnesium also activates the systems associated with potassium, calcium, and protein use. In healthy adults the serum magnesium level is approximately 3 mEq/liter. The intracellular concentration is almost 10 times greater.

Very little is understood about the regulation of magnesium balance in the body. It is known that the renal tubules reabsorb magnesium from the urine in response to a decreased extracellular concentration of the ion, the kidneys acting in much the same way as they do in potassium regulation.

Hypermagnesemia

Magnesium excess (*hypermagnesemia*) is rare, usually only occurring in uremia related to renal failure. Clinical signs include overall sedation, lethargy, depressed respiration, coma, and eventual death. Symptoms arise as the serum magnesium approaches 6 mEq/liter. As the other electrolytes are brought into line through such means as dialysis, the magnesium level also decreases. The sedative effects of hypermagnesemia can be blocked by the administration of calcium.

Hypomagnesemia

A decreased concentration of magnesium in the fluid is referred to as *hypomagnesemia*. Alcoholism tends to cause magnesium deficit. Any disease that causes sustained gastrointestinal secretion losses will precipitate a magnesium deficit. A client with a high intake of calcium may also have hypomagnesemia because the absorption of calcium is inversely proportional to magnesium absorption. Additional factors in magnesium deficiency include toxemia of pregnancy, renal failure, malabsorption syndromes, and liver disease.

Because of the similarity in intracellular functions between magnesium and potassium, many of the symptoms that occur with magnesium deficit are similar to those in hypokalemia: tremor, *athetoid movements*, tetany, a positive Chvostek's sign, muscular irritability, and eventually convulsions. Hallucinations and tachycardia frequently accompany the imbalance. Laboratory analysis reveals a magnesium level of less than 1.4 mEq/liter.

Treatment is by replacement therapy. A 1% solution of magnesium sulfate given by mouth will result in an immediate improvement in the client's clinical picture.

Chlorine

Chlorine is the major anion of the body systems. The combination of sodium and chlorine in water form the basis for the entire fluid base of the body. Chlorine functions along with sodium to maintain the osmotic pressure of the blood. The ion is also essential for the homeostatic maintenance of acid-base balance in the body. The normal chlorine level in the blood is 95–105 mEq/liter. The intracellular concentration of clorine is much less.

Chlorine is regulated by the kidneys secondarily to positive ion concentration. Because of this the same regulatory mechanisms that increase the reabsorption of positive ions also cause reabsorption of negative ions, primarily chlorine.

Chlorine and sodium vary proportionately to each other in plasma. Chlorine excess and deficit are frequently associated with sodium and fluid changes. When sodium and chlorine are both elevated, intracellular fluid deficit is usually present. A decrease in sodium and chlorine indicates possible intracellular fluid excess. Signs and treatment of the deficit or excess are the same as for fluid excess discussed earlier in this chapter.

When chlorine decreases independently of sodium, it is usually due to a metabolic alkalotic state. The specific recognition and treatment of acidemia and *alkalemia* are discussed later in this chapter.

RESPIRATORY PHYSIOLOGY

Respiration involves the transport of oxygen from the atmosphere to the cells and the removal of carbon dioxide (CO_2) from the cells to the atmosphere. Respiration can be subdivided into external and internal respiration. *External respiration* involves the mechanical movement of oxygen into the pulmonary tree, diffusion across the alveolar-capillary membrane, and the movement of oxygen to the cell. External respiration also involves the removal of CO_2 from the cells in a similar manner. *Internal respiration* refers to the cell's ability to use oxygen (Chap. 12). This discussion applies to the physiology of external respiration and its regulatory control on the body systems.

The respiratory system permits the exchange of gases in the blood through the rhythmic expansion and deflation of the lungs. The changes in thoracic volume that occur during inspiration and expiration allow the passive movement of air into and out of the bronchial tree. *Tidal volume* is the volume of air inspired and exhaled with each normal breath in the healthy man and is equal to approximately 500 cc. A woman has about 20–25% less capacity. The maximum amount of air that a person can expel from his or her lungs after filling them to the maximum and then expiring to the maximum extent is known as *vital capacity*. In the young man this volume is approximately equal to 4.6 liters; in the young woman the volume should approximate 3.1 liters. Another measurement of importance when discussing respiratory volumes is the *minute respiratory volume*

(MRV): the total amount of new air moved into the respiratory passages each minute. It is equal to the tidal volume multiplied by the respiratory rate. In the young adult male the MRV averages 6 liters/min. The MRV provides the clinician with a much more accurate picture of a client's ability to inspire air than does the respiratory rate.

The alveolus is the functional unit of the lung, the site where gas exchange takes place. The movement of oxygen into the red blood cells from the alveoli occurs through diffusion. The oxygen concentration in the blood is less than that in the alveoli. This "down-hill" gradient is reversed for CO_2 exchange. (See Figure 11-1).

When oxygen diffuses into the plasma from the alveoli, almost all of it (98.5%) combines with hemoglobin in the red blood cells. When fully saturated, a hemoglobin molecule can carry four molecules of oxygen; so 1 gm of fully saturated hemoglobin will carry 1.34 ml of oxygen. The normal hemoglobin concentration in the blood is 15 gm/100 ml; hence there are approximately 20 m of oxygen in 100 m of blood. Normal female hemoglobin value is approximately 12–15 gm/100 ml.

When discussing the concentration of oxygen in the blood, it is necessary to understand the concept of *partial pressure* (p) of respiratory gases. The *partial pressure* of any gas in a mixture is the pressure that it would exert if it alone were present. The partial pressure of a gas is equal to its concentration multiplied by the total pressure of the gas mixture. Using the concept of partial pressure when discussing gases is advantageous because gases always diffuse in the direction of lower partial pressure but not always in the direction of lower concentration. The partial pressures of various gases in the body are given in Figure 11-6.

When the pO_2 is low, the oxygen content of the hemoglobin will also be low, and conversely, when the pO_2 is high, the oxygen content of the hemoglobin will be high. The relationship of the partial pressure of oxygen to

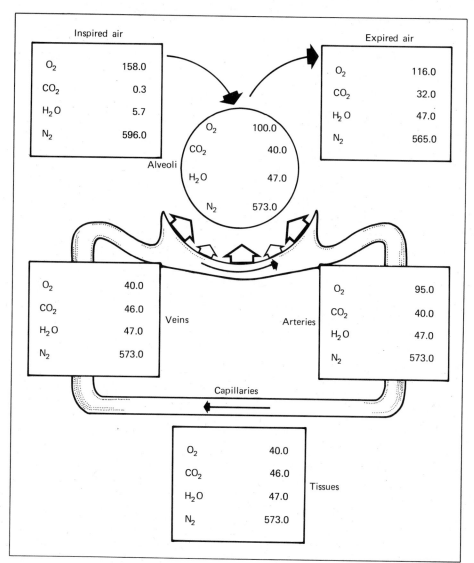

Figure 11-6. Partial pressures of gases in mm of Mercury.

the saturation of hemoglobin is shown in Figure 11-7. The relationship is not purely linear. When the pO_2 is very high, changes in the pO_2 have very little effect on hemoglobin concentration. However, when the pO_2 falls below 40 mmHg, very minute changes will cause large differences in the saturation of hemoglobin.

Respiration is regulated by several body systems. Centers in the brain and brain stem receive information from all parts of the body concerning their needs for oxygen, and these

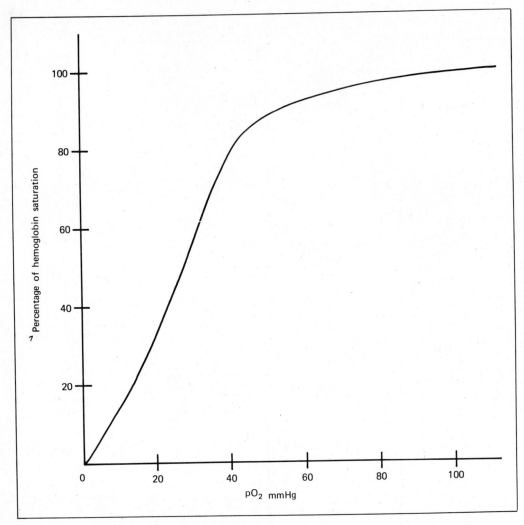

Figure 11-7. Oxyhemoglobin dissociation curve.

centers respond by increasing or decreasing respiratory rate. Two sets of *chemoreceptors,* the *aortic bodies* (located in the aortic arch) and the *carotid bodies* (located at the bifurcation of the common carotid arteries), respond to a decreased pO_2 and an elevated CO_2 in the blood to stimulate or inhibit respiration. An increase of CO_2 is the primary chemical stimulus of the respiratory neurons.

ACID-BASE BALANCE

Fundamental to the understanding of the acid-base balance in the body is an understanding of hydrogen-ion concentration, what an acid is, what makes a substance basic, and what the body buffer systems are.

When dissolved in water, many substances will dissociate to form positively charged ions and negatively charged ions. Electrolytes, discussed previously in this chapter, are examples of such substances. An *acid* is any substance that liberates hydrogen ions when placed in an aqueous solution. A common example of an acid found in the body is hydrochloric acid (HCL). When placed into solution, the substance dissociates into hydrogen ions and chlorine ions. This reaction is shown below:

$$HCl \rightleftarrows H^+ + Cl^-$$

The reaction may proceed in either direction, as shown by the double arrows.

Similarly, a *base* is a substance that will accept or bind with hydrogen ions in an aqueous solution. An example of a base is ammonia, which forms an ammonium ion in solution:

$$NH_3 + H^+ \rightleftarrows NH_4^+$$

The higher the concentration of acid in a solution, the more acidic it is. The higher the concentration of base, the more alkaline the solution is.

Because acids release hydrogen ions and bases accept them, the acidity or alkalinity of a solution can be shown by the concentration of hydrogen ions in the solution. The term *pH* represents a scale that measures the degree of acidity or alkalinity of fluids. If a solution has a low pH it is said to be acid, therefore containing a large number of hydrogen ions. If a solution has a high pH it is said to be alkaline and contains few hydrogen ions. To clarify, pH and hydrogen ion concentration ($[H^+]$) are inversely related. Water is a neutral substance and has a pH of 7. Those solutions with a pH below 7 are considered acidic; those with a pH greater than 7 are basic. The normal pH of blood is 7.43–7.45, very slightly alkaline. Intracellular fluid is slightly more acidic, with a pH of 6.8.

Cells depend on the correct body pH for optimum functioning. An abnormally low or high hydrogen ion concentration interferes with enzyme function during cellular metabolism and can result in cell death. Regulation of hydrogen ion concentration in body fluids is performed by means of chemical substances in the blood referred to as *chemical buffers*. pH can also be maintained by the respiratory and renal systems.

About 300 liters of carbon dioxide are formed each day by the metabolic processes of the normal adult. When dissolved in water, carbon dioxide produces an acid, carbonic acid. The acid dissociates thus forming about 13,000 mEq of hydrogen ions. Normally the lungs blow off carbon dioxide as fast as it is produced. Carbonic acid is not allowed to accumulate, and arterial pH thus remains constant.

Body Buffers

An acid-base buffer is a solution of two or more chemical compounds that prevent drastic changes in hydrogen ion concentration when either an acid or a base is added to the solution. Each buffer system for controlling hydrogen ion concentration consists of a solution of a weak acid and one of its salts, formed by neutralizing the acid with a strong base.

The largest and most important body buffer system is the carbonic acid–bicarbonate system. When a base is added such as NaOH, the following reaction occurs:

$$NaOH + H_2CO_3 \rightarrow NaHCO_3 + H_2O,$$

thus reducing the alkaline effect on the serum pH. A similar reaction occurs when an acid is added, such as HCl in the following equation:

$$HCl + NaHCO_3 \rightarrow H_2CO_3 + NaCl$$

The importance of the carbonic acid–bicarbonate buffer system is due to the fact that excess CO_2 can be blown off by the lungs and the bicarbonate ion can be conserved or excreted by the kidneys.

The phosphate buffer system acts in a similar manner but is composed of $Na_2H_2PO_4$ and NaH_2PO_4. When an acid such as hydrochloric acid is added to the solution, the following reaction occurs:

$$HCl + Na_2HPO_4 \rightarrow NaH_2PO_4 + NaCl$$

The phosphate buffer reacts with a base as:

$$NaOH + NaH_2PO_4 \rightarrow Na_2HPO_4 + H_2O$$

In this situation, a strong base, NaOH, is exchanged for a weak base, Na_2HPO_4, thus decreasing the overall alkaline effect on serum.

The most plentiful buffer in the body is the protein buffer system. It is known that at least 75% of all the chemical buffering power of the body fluids is inside the cell and results from the intracellular proteins. Some of the amino acids have free radicals that react as NH_3^+ and OH^-, thus operating in both acidic and basic solutions as powerful buffers.

A relatively weak buffer system is the oxyhemoglobin–hydrogenated hemoglobin system. Here again, the system takes up free hydrogen ions, thus reducing the acidity of the solution.

It must be remembered that all of the buffer systems coexist in the body fluids, working simultaneously to maintain body pH.

Respiratory Regulation of Acid-Base Balance

To understand the role of respiration in the maintenance of body pH, students must first understand the effect of carbon dioxide on pH. An increase in carbon dioxide concentration will cause a decrease in body pH; that is, it will shift the equilibrium to be more acidic. The following equation demonstrates the formation of carbonic acid from carbon dioxide:

$$CO_2 + H_2O \underset{dehydration}{\overset{hydration}{\rightleftharpoons}} H_2CO_3 \underset{association}{\overset{dissociation}{\rightleftharpoons}} H^+ + HCO_3^-$$

A decrease in pCO_2 will result in a decreased number of hydrogen ions and in a raised pH. Such a situation occurs when respiration is stimulated so that more CO_2 is expired than is produced, as in hyperventilation. An alkaline pH will result.

Alveolar ventilation normally is maintained at a level that does not cause changes from normal pH. Respiration not only affects hydrogen ion concentration but is regulated in response to it. Hydrogen ions directly affect the respiratory center in the medulla oblongata to increase or decrease ventilation. For example, when the body has an excess of hydrogen ions, which occurs in acidosis, respirations become deeper in order to allow time for the body to blow off the excess CO_2 via the respiratory system. Respiratory activity responds rapidly to acid-base stresses and shifts blood pH toward normal in a matter of minutes.

Renal Regulation of Acid-Base Balance

The kidneys regulate body pH by either (1) increasing the urinary excretion of hydrogen ions when the blood is too acid or (2) increasing the urinary excretion of bicarbonate when the blood pH is too high. In contrast to the rapidity of respiratory regulation, the renal system may take as long as 20 hours to return the pH to normal. The mechanism of reabsorption of bicarbonate is the most important in renal acid-base regulation.

A second important mechanism in the regulation of acid-base balance by the kidneys is the formation of titratable acid. The end product of this mechanism is an equivalent quantity of sodium bicarbonate added to the blood for each hydrogen ion combined with a buffer to form an acid.

The third mechanism in renal acid-base control is the excretion of ammonia. Ammonia is a weak base produced locally in the kidney from amino acids. Ammonia diffuses into the urine, where it combines with hydrogen ions to form ammonium ions. As the ammonia is excreted, so is the hydrogen ion. For each hydrogen ion excreted, an equal quantity of sodium bicarbonate is added to the blood.

Alterations in Acid-Base Homeostasis

Alterations in acid-base balance may arise from respiratory or metabolic causes. The change in homeostasis is reflected by a change in serum pH. When the pH drops below 7.35, this condition is referred to as *acidemia*. The lowered pH reflects a greater number of circulating hydrogen ions in the blood. *Alkalemia* is the condition in which the pH is above 7.45. When the body is in alkalemia, the total concentration of buffer base is greater than normal, with a relative decrease in the hydrogen ion concentration. Respiratory acid-base imbalances are caused by primary defects in the function of the lungs or changes in normal respiratory patterns. Metabolic alterations may be due to changes in the metabolism and use of particular nutrients.

Metabolic Acidemia

Metabolic acidemia is a result of losing bases and retaining too many acids. The carbonic acid–bicarbonate buffer system is altered by a decreased ratio between the two. Metabolic acidemia is probably the most frequently encountered acid-base disturbance. One of the most common causes is uncontrolled diabetes mellitus. In this alteration, insufficient insulin results in increased fat metabolism, which causes an excess accumulation of ketones and other acids in the blood. The same alteration occurs when a person has not eaten for a period of time or is suffering from undernutrition, only the accumulation of acids is much slower. Another cause of metabolic acidemia is renal insufficiency. In this alteration, waste products of protein metabolism (many of which are acidic) are retained. Another cause is muscle deprivation of oxygen, which causes carbohydrates to be incompletely metabolized, with lactic acid resulting as a

by-product. Excessive exercise or prolonged *hypoxia* can cause excessive lactic acid secretion. Severe diarrhea may cause acidemia because of the loss of normally alkaline intestinal and pancreatic secretions. Metabolic acidemia may also be caused by any over-ingestion of acids, as in salicylate intoxication or with a high-fat diet containing many acid-producing substances.

Signs of metabolic acidemia include the classic *Kussmaul's respirations*. This hyperventilation may be accompanied by a characteristic fruity odor. The body attempts to blow off extra carbon dioxide and counteracts the metabolic acidemia by producing respiratory alkalemia. Other clinical findings include headache, drowsiness, nausea, vomiting, diarrhea, stupor, coma, and convulsions. Dehydration may occur as a result of the nausea and vomiting. Laboratory data reveals a pH of less than 7.35. The serum bicarbonate reading will be below 22 mEq/liter. The serum potassium level is usually increased with acidemia caused by a change in cell-membrane permeability.

Treatment of metabolic acidemia is directed at the underlying cause of the condition. If the acidemia is severe, an intravenous solution of bicarbonate is administered.

Metabolic Alkalemia

Metabolic alkalemia may result from a malfunction of metabolism that yields either an increase in the amount of basic solutions in the blood or a reduction of available acids in the serum. There is a primary increase in plasma bicarbonate, a rise in pH, and usually an increase in pCO_2 because of respiratory compensation. Hypokalemia usually accompanies alkalemia. A primary cause of metabolic alkalemia is the loss of gastrointestinal fluid from vomiting or gastric lavage. The loss of upper gastrointestinal secretions that contain large amounts o hydrochloric acid and potassium results in a decrease in the number of hydrogen ions in the serum. Potassium-depleting diuretics can also precipitate al-

TABLE 11-5. Alterations in Acid-Base Homeostasis

	Acidemia		Alkalemia	
	Metabolic	Respiratory	Metabolic	Respiratory
Cause	Ketoacidosis, renal failure, lactic acidemia, diarrhea	Hypoventilation, COPD, sedation, pneumonia, atelectasis	Upper GI losses via vomiting, lavage; diuretic therapy	Hyperventilation
Clinical signs	Headache, nausea, vomiting, diarrhea, sensorium changes	Low ventilation, sensorium changes, coma, arrhythmia, tachycardia	Nausea, vomiting, diarrhea, sensorium changes, tremors, seizures	Tachypnea, numbness, tingling of hands and face, syncope
Laboratory data	pH less than 7.35; HCO_3 less than 22 mEq/liter; pCO_2 less than 35 mmHg; high K	pH less than 7.35; HCO_3^- greater than 28 mEq/liter; pCO_2 greater than 45 mmHg; high K	pH greater than 7.45; HCO_3 greater than 28 mEq/liter; pO_2 normal; pCO_2 greater than 45 mmHg; low K; low serum Cl	pH greater than 7.45; HCO_3^- less than 22 mEq/liter; pO_2 normal; pCO_2 less than 35 mEq/liter; low K
Treatment	Treat underlying cause; administer O_2, $NaHCO_3$ IV	Treat cause, IPPB, pulmonary toilet, ventilator, $NaHCO_3$ IV	Replace fluid loss with K and Cl added, ammonium Cl	Sedation

kalemia, as will an overingestion of bicarbonate.

The clinical signs of metabolic alkalemia are difficult to differentiate from those of hypokalemia and hypochloremia. The major signs include nausea, vomiting, diarrhea, apathy, mental confusion, shallow breathing, tetany, and spastic muscles. The EKG shows a low T wave merging with the P wave. Sinus tachycardia may be present. Laboratory data reveals a pH above 7.45 and a serum CO_2 level above 45 mmHg. The serum chlorine reading will decrease disproportionately to a decreased serum sodium reading. In other imbalances, sodium and chlorine decrease proportionately.

Treatment of metabolic alkalemia centers on treating the causes of the alteration. Many times, prevention of alkalemia is much easier than waiting until the alteration develops and treating it. If treatment is necessary, potassium and chlorine replacement should be initiated. Acidifying solutions such as ammonium chloride may be administered orally or intravenously.

Respiratory Acidemia

Respiratory acidemia results from a failure of the body to ventilate adequately and remove carbon dioxide from the body. In acidemia of this type the level of carbon dioxide and carbonic acid in the serum is increased and the ratio of carbonic acid to bicarbonate is increased. An increased hydrogen ion concentration in the blood results. Respiratory acidemia occurs in conditions in which there is an inadequate exchange of gases in the blood. Specific alterations that may precipitate acidemia include emphysema, asthma, bronchitis, pulmonary edema, pneumonia, sedation, *atelectasis,* or trauma to the medulla oblongata.

Clinical signs of respiratory acidemia include decreased ventilation, drowsiness, and decreased *sensorium.* Hypoxia becomes more advanced; diaphoresis, cyanosis, irregular tachycardia, and restlessness occur. Labora-

tory evaluation reveals a pH below 7.35. The arterial pCO_2 will be over 45 mmHg with a normal or slightly decreased pO_2. If the kidneys have had time to compensate, the serum bicarbonate will be above 28mEq/liter.

Treatment centers on improved ventilation. Intermittent positive pressure breathing, antibiotics, postural drainage, or assisted ventilation may be employed.

Respiratory Alkalemia

Respiratory alkalemia results from hyperventilation. Increased respiration causes excessive loss of carbon dioxide. A decrease in CO_2 will lead to a fall in plasma ion concentration and plasma bicarbonate. This type of alkalemia results from voluntary hyperventilation or overbreathing associated with anxiety, fear, meningitis or salicylate intoxication.

Clinical findings include an increase in the rate or depth of ventilation; dizziness; *paresthesias,* particularly circumoral; tetany; and eventual *syncope.* These symptoms are due to a decrease in cerebral blood flow because of a decreased CO_2. Laboratory analysis reveals a pH above 7.45, normal pO_2 and a pCO_2 below 40 mmHg. Hypokalemia may eventually occur.

Treatment involves sedation and reassurance, a rebreathing mask, or addition of dead space to the T tube set up if one is being used.

Table 11-5 summarized causes and effects of the states of acidemia and alkalemia.

BIBLIOGRAPHY

Arlin, M. J. *The Science of Nutrition.* 2nd Ed. New York: Macmillan, Inc., 1977.

Beland, I. L. *Clinical Nursing, Pathophysiological and Psychosocial Approaches.* 3rd Ed. New York: Macmillan, Inc., 1976.

Cohen, S. Blood-gas and acid-base concepts in respiratory care. *Am. J. Nurs.* 76:6, 1976.

Ganong, W. F. *Review of Medical Physiology.* 8th Ed. Los Altos, Calif.: Lange Medical Publications, 1977.

Guthrie, H. A. *Introductory Nutrition*. 4th Ed. St. Louis: The C. V. Mosby Co., 1979.

Guyton, A. C. *Textbook of Medical Physiology*. 4th Ed. Philadelphia: W. B. Saunders Co., 1971.

———. *Basic Human Physiology: Normal Functions and Mechanisms of Disease*. 2nd Ed. Philadelphia: W. B. Saunders Co., 1977.

Hines, B. Vitamins: Absorption and malabsorption. *Ann. Intern. Med.* 138:619, 1978.

Metheny, N. M., and Snevely, W. D. *Nurses' Handbook of Fluid Balance*. 2nd Ed. Philadelphia: J. B. Lippincott Co., 1974.

Passmore, R. Stores in the human body. In J. Borzek, Ed., *Human Body Composition*. Oxford: Pergamon Press Ltd., 1965.

Pflanzer, R. G. The blood. In E. Selkurt, Ed., *Basic Physiology for the Health Sciences*. Boston: Little, Brown & Co., 1975.

Pike, R. L., and Brown, M. L. *Nutrition: An Integrated Approach*. 2nd Ed. New York: John Wiley & Sons, Inc., Pubs., 1975.

Reed, G., and Sheppard, V. *Regulation of Fluid and Electrolyte Balance: A Programmed Instruction in Clinical Physiology*. Philadelphia: W. B. Saunders Co., 1977.

Selkurt, E. E., Ed. *Basic Physiology for the Health Sciences*. Boston: Little, Brown & Co., 1975.

Stroot, V. R., Lee, C., and Schaper, A. *Fluids and Electrolytes: A Practical Approach*. 2nd Ed. Philadelphia: F. A. Davis Co., 1977.

Vander, A. J., Sherman, J. H., and Luciano, D. S. *Human Physiology*. New York: McGraw-Hill Book Co., 1970.

Williams, S. R. *Nutrition and Diet Therapy*. 3rd Ed. St. Louis: The C. V. Mosby Co., 1977.

Wilson, E. D., Fisher, K. H., and Garcia, P. A. *Principles of Nutrition*. 4th Ed. New York: John Wiley & Sons, Inc., Pubs., 1979.

Worthington, B. S. Effect of nutritional status on immune phenomena. *J. Am. Diet. Assoc.* 65:123, 1974.

—Alex, te dejas engañar por las apariencias —le dije—. No se trata de que, de pronto, haya cambiado San Francisco, mi casa victoriana y todo aquello por este lugar. No he cambiado los libros para niñas por Tinseltown, en absoluto, no se trata de eso. He regresado para hacer algo que no debí dejar de hacer la primera vez que estuve aquí. Lo cual tampoco tiene mucho que ver con Hollywood. En realidad tiene que ver con el tiempo, con lo que tienes delante a través de los años y cómo lo ves o cómo lo utilizas. Y ésa es la razón por la que me encuentro perfectamente bien.

—Bueno, ahora empiezas a hablar como el Jeremy que conozco. Debo admitirlo. Ponle un poco de verdad a todo eso en mi honor y me convencerás.

Me dio una palmadita en el hombro y salió otra vez al jardín, donde estaba G.G. con las chicas, junto a la piscina. Los periodistas ya se habían ido. Belinda se estaba quitando los tejanos y la camisa para quedarse con el minúsculo biquini brasileño puesto. Acto seguido dirigió su cuerpecito arrebatador con las manos por delante hacia la piscina y se lanzó.

De nuevo estábamos Faye y yo solos. Perfecto. Te quiero, Faye.

Levanté la vista para mirarla, mi mente se llenó otra vez de cuadros nuevos que haría pronto. Estarían llenos de una luz poderosa y de oscuros degradados. Serían estudios luminosos de Alex, Blair, G.G. y Belinda, sí, sobre todo de Belinda, ella sería el centro de un nuevo concepto, de una nueva aventura más allá de lo que había hecho hasta ahora.

El contorno deslumbrante, sí, quería captarlo, y también quería descubrir las sombras que los focos habían difuminado hasta ahora e incluso el color y la textura de California. Tenía que hacerlo.

Pero estas relucientes imágenes no eran más que

una parte de lo que me esperaba. En efecto, ahora mi mundo estaba lleno con miles de seres de todas las edades, formas y actitudes, con imágenes del pasado, presente y futuro que nunca había observado ni visto antes. Por primera vez en mi vida podía pintar lo que quisiera.

Gracias a Belinda había salido del mundo de los sueños y había entrado en el mundo luminoso de la vida misma.

ÍNDICE

CHAPTER 12

Cellular Metabolism

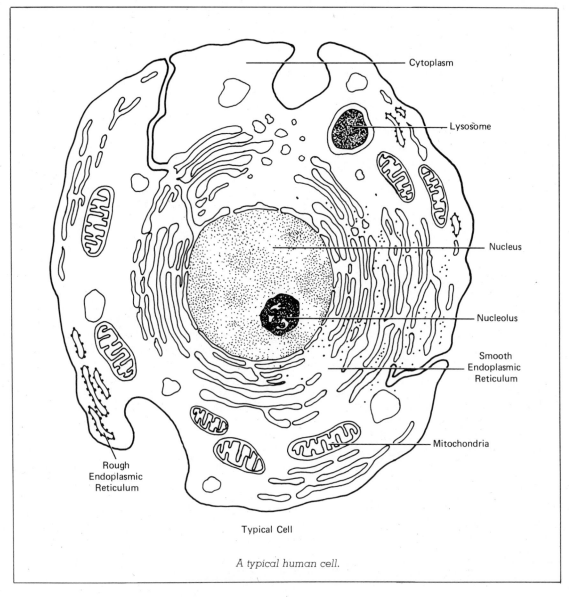

A typical human cell.

Two types of metabolic processes are operating simultaneously within the body: *Anabolism,* the synthesis or manufacture of new substances from simpler ones, and *catabolism,* the breakdown of complex substances into simpler ones, as in the degrading of food fats to glycerol and fatty acids. Anabolism and catabolism occur simultaneously, and together they are called *metabolism.* All metabolism takes place at the cellular level.

An understanding of cellular metabolism requires knowledge of the structure and functions of the components of the cell, which is the first topic in the chapter. The next is the production of energy, the major function of each living organism. Then the major anabolic and catabolic processes of carbohydrate, protein, and fat metabolism are presented, followed by a discussion of the role of the endocrine system in regulating metabolism and a brief introduction to specialized cells, tissues, and body systems.

CELLULAR PHYSIOLOGY

A cell is the smallest structural and functional unit of a living organism. It is capable of acquiring nutrients for its use (i.e., metabolism) and of eliminating its wastes. It is also capable of the physiological activities of adaptation, irritability, movement, and reproduction, activities it carries out to ensure its survival. The cell depends, however, on a supply of nutrients as its source of energy and for the synthesis of new substances. Proper nutrition is therefore the prerequisite for the existence of the cell; without suitable nutrients it fails to exist.

There is another way to consider the importance of nutrition to cellular physiology. Human life begins in a moment in time from the union of a male and female cell. This cell multiplies many times as the fetus continues to grow and develop. Nutrients from the mother's womb are provided to nourish the fetus from the moment of conception. One of the primary requirements for life is proper nutrition. Nutrition itself begins at the cellular level and continues there throughout the life of the organism. The use of all nutrients occurs within the cell for catabolism or anabolism.

The human body consists of around 100 trillion cells. To discuss cellular physiology the physiologist describes the structure and functioning of a typical cell. The multicellular organism shows cellular specialization with a division of labor among the cells. Nevertheless all cells do contain basic structures that allow them to carry out their functions. The cell is a marvelously efficient unit. It appears to be a very simple system composed of an outer plasma membrane, a nucleus located near the center, and several structures outside the nucleus. Yet close examination with the electron microscope reveals the high degree of complexity of these structures.

In transporting nutrients to the cell, the blood vessels end in a network of extensively branched capillaries. The final distance to the cell is bridged by the interstitial fluid. The tissue fluid brings to the cell nutrients and oxygen, which are received through the plasma membrane. The membrane is believed to be composed of a bilayer of lipids and proteins (see Fig. 12-1). The passage of nutrients through the plasma membrane by the transport methods was discussed in Chapter 11. The nutrients may diffuse through the pores in the membrane, be transported across by carriers, or be pumped across by active transport mechanisms. The factors regulating the composition of the substances inside and outside the cell are presented later in this chapter.

Cytoplasm

All of the different materials that compose the living substances of the cell are known collectively as *protoplasm. Protoplasm* is a viscid,

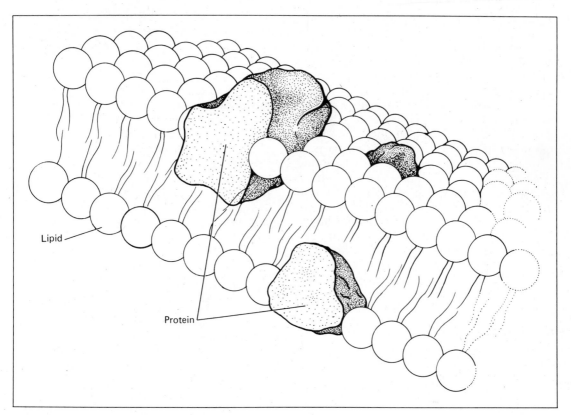

Figure 12-1. Structure of the cell membrane.

translucent colloid material with water as its continuous phase. It is composed of carbohydrates, proteins, lipids, electrolytes, and water. Stated another way, protoplasm is composed of nutrients. The substances outside the nucleus, but inside the plasma membrane, are collectively known as the *cytoplasm.* The cytoplasm is the true internal environment of the cell. It contains specialized structures called *organelles,* which carry out specific metabolic activities. Some of these organelles are the *endoplasmic reticulum,* the *mitochondria,* the *Golgi complex,* and the *lysosomes.* Each of these organelles and the cytoplasm itself perform both anabolic and catabolic functions.

The cytoplasm is composed of various proteins, water, ions, and soluble nutrients. There are also stores of glycogen and lipids. The cytoplasm is involved in part of the reactions that break down glucose (*glycolysis*). The reverse of these same reactions occurs for the synthesis of glucose (*glycogenesis*). The synthesis of some fatty acids also occurs in the cytoplasm.

Mitochondria

The mitochondrion has been described as the powerhouse of the cell because most of the energy required by the cell is produced in it.

It is a rod-shaped structure that contains large quantities of enzymes needed for extracting energy from the nutrients. Energy is produced from the oxidation of amino acids, fatty acids, and the continued oxidation of glucose. All three of the energy nutrients enter a common pathway for energy production called the *tricarboxylic acid cycle*. The individual reactions that occur in this cycle are discussed in the next section. The energy released from the oxidation of the energy nutrients is used to synthesize the high-energy compound ATP, which is then transported out of the mitochondrion throughout the rest of the cell to provide energy wherever it is needed for cellular functions. Other anabolic reactions also occur in the mitochondrion. This organelle is involved in the synthesis of fatty acids and the synthesis of nonessential amino acids as well as the synthesis of the heme portion of the hemoglobin molecule.

Endoplasmic Reticulum

The *endoplasmic reticulum* is a network of tubular structure flowing throughout all areas of the cytoplasm. Substances are synthesized within this organelle and then transported through the tubular network to another part of the cell or to the outside of the cell. The endoplasmic reticulum is mainly involved in anabolic activities. Part of the endoplasmic reticulum is referred to as the *granular,* or rough, endoplasmic reticulum; and part as the *agranular,* or smooth, endoplasmic reticulum. The granular designation refers to the presence of small granular substances called *ribosomes* on the surface of the endoplasmic reticulum. It is on these ribosomes that protein synthesis occurs. This synthesis of protein is under the direction of the nucleus. The agranular, or smooth, endoplasmic reticulum is involved in the synthesis of lipids and the storage of glycogen.

Golgi Complex

The endoplasmic reticulum is continuous with another organelle, the *Golgi complex.*

These two organelles function together in the manufacture and release of substances into the cytoplasm. The Golgi complex is involved with combining the previously synthesized carbohydrates, proteins, and fats into such substances as glycoproteins, glycolipids, and mucopolysaccharides, which are essential substances needed by every cell. For example, the mucopolysaccharides are important parts of mucus and of the cementing substance of the interstitial spaces and of cartilage and bone. Also many enzymes and hormones that have been synthesized by the ribosomes are concentrated and stored in the Golgi complex and prepared for final secretions. This organelle is also involved with the formation of the lysosomes.

Lysosomes

The lysosomes are the digestive system for each cell; they are analogous to bags containing digestive enzymes. Lysosomes allow the cell to digest and remove unwanted substances. They are involved strictly in catabolic activities. The enzymes present in the lysosomes may cause further digestion of proteins, glycogen, nucleic acids, and mucopolysaccharides into the end products of amino acids, glucose, phosphates, and so forth, which can then diffuse into the cytoplasm and be either reused by the cell as needed or excreted.

Nucleus

The nucleus is the central control for all the reactions occurring within the cell and for reproduction of the cell itself. Its major function is the synthesis of protein from a template, or "protein recipe." The nucleus contains large quantities of DNA. On the DNA strand are genes that contain the code for protein synthesis. A copy of the protein recipe is stored by the RNA, which is present in the *nucleolus* of the nucleus. During protein synthesis the RNA migrates to the cytoplasm and provides the information for the manufacturing of protein by the ribosomes on the endoplasmic reticulum. The actual sequence of events that occurs during protein synthesis is considered later in this chapter.

Specialized Cells

In the human organism the "typical" cell does not exist because of a high degree of specialization among the cells. All cells contain the basic organelles previously described, but the specialized cells contain a higher proportion of one or more of the organelles, depending on their specialized functions. Some of these specialized cells are liver cells, red blood cells, muscle cells, bone cells, nerve cells, adipose cells, and intestinal cells. The specialized function of the liver is metabolic, so liver cells contain high proportions of mitochondria. There are approximately 1,000 mitochondria present in each liver cell, but only 100 for each adipose-tissue cell. The endoplasmic reticulum and the Golgi complex are prominent in secretory cells such as the pancreas and intestine. Additional mitochondria are also present in the intestinal cell because of the production and release of energy to transport the nutrients into the intestinal mucosa. The mammary glands contain an extensive endoplasmic reticulum and Golgi complex for the synthesis and secretion of milk during lactation. Because the adipose tissue is mainly for storage, adipose cells contain only small amounts of mitochondria, endoplasmic reticulum, and Golgi complex. Lysosomes are the most prevelant in liver, white blood cells, and kidney cells, where the majority of detoxification reactions occur.

PRODUCTION OF ENERGY

Because the production of energy is the most important function of the living organism and because there is a final common pathway for the production of energy from carbohydrate, proteins, and fat, this important topic merits separate discussion here.

Regulators

The rate of chemical reactions within the cell is regulated by enzymes, cofactors, and hormones. To function, many enzymes require the presence of specific minerals or some vitamins. A number of hormones control the rate at which carbohydrate, protein, and fat are metabolized.

Enzymes

Enzymes are protein substances that are produced by the cell. They function as a catalyst to speed up the rate of a chemical reaction. Without enzymes some of the reactions necessary to obtain energy from the food eaten might take several months or years. Every cell manufactures thousands of enzymes for its use. Such a large number of enzymes are needed because of the high degree of specificity of enzymes; each is so constructed as to act only on one particular substances or substrate. The reader will already have seen how specific enzymes are produced during digestion that act only on certain classifications of carbohydrates, proteins, and fats. Enzymes are either *endoenzymes* produced for use within the cell or *exoenzymes* released by the cell and used elsewhere, as in the case of the digestive enzymes. Enzymes are used to speed up the chemical reactions, but they are not themselves changed in the process, and they can be reused many times.

The ultimate control of the functioning enzymes present within a cell lies in the genetic makeup. A genetic deficiency or the lack of an enzyme will result in a disorder of metabolism. Examples include a deficiency of the enzyme lactose results in a condition known as *lactose intolerance*. A lack of the enzyme galactose-1-phosphate uridyl transferase results in the disease *galactosemia*. The interested student is referred to the medical textbook *Duncan's Diseases of Metabolism* by G. G. Duncan (1974) for a complete discussion of metabolic disorders caused by enzyme deficiencies. Enzymes are classified by the names of the substances on which they act or by the type of chemical reaction they promote.

Cofactors and Coenzymes

Some enzymes require a specific factor to initiate the action of the enzyme necessary for its complete action. It is either a *coenzyme*, which is composed of one of the water-soluble vitamins, or a *cofactor*, which is a specific mineral. The vitamins that function as coenzymes are thiamine, riboflavin, niacin, pantothenic acid, pyridoxine, cobalamin, folic acid, and biotin. These serve to regulate both catabolism and anabolism of the energy nutrients. Some of the minerals such as potassium, manganese, magnesium, calcium, and zinc are required as cofactors for the reactions that release energy from the nutrients. Because these cofactors are not changed in the reactions, they can be used and reused many times. The daily requirement for vitamins and minerals is very small because of the body's continual conservation and reuse. A summary of the major cofactors and coenzymes in metabolism is presented in Table 12-1.

Hormones

Hormones are chemicals generally produced by the endocrine glands and transported by the blood to the various cells. Hormones serve to initiate or control the action of the enzymes. The effect of hormonal regulation of the digestive enzymes was discussed in the previous chapter. Some hormones are protein in nature, such as insulin and thyroxine, but others such as sex hormones are steroids, classified as derivatives of fat. Hormones regulate the metabolism of carbohydrate, protein, and fat and therefore the release of energy or the synthesis of new substances.

Common Metabolic Pathway

The common metabolic pathway for the release of energy from carbohydrate, protein, and fat is the Krebs cycle, or the tricarboxylic acid cycle (the TCA cycle). Another name for

TABLE 12-1. Common Coenzymes and Cofactors in Metabolism

Coenzymes	Vitamin
TPP (thiamine pyrophosphate)	Thiamine
NAD, NADH, NADP, AND NADPH (nicotine adenine dinucleotides)	Niacin
FAD and $FADH_2$, (flavin adenine dinucleotides)	Riboflavin
FMN (flavin mononucleotide)	Riboflavin
CoA (coenzyme A)	Pantothenic acid
Lipoic acid	Lipoic acid
Biotin	Biotin
Pyridoxal Phosphate	Vitamin B_6
Tetrahydrofolate	Folic acid
Vitamin B_{12}	Vitamin B_{12}
Vitamin C	Vitamin C
Vitamin K	Vitamin K
Vitamin A	Vitamin A

Cofactors	Mineral
Mg^{+2}	Magnesium
Fe^{+2}, Fe^{+3}	Iron
PO_4^{-3}	Phosphorus
Zn^{+2}	Zinc
Cu^+, Cu^{+2}	Copper
Mo^{+2}	Molybdenum
Co^{+2}	Cobalt
Mn^{+2}	Manganese

this cycle is the *citric acid cycle*. The end products from the digestion of carbohydrate, protein, and fat enter this common pathway as either pyruvic acid or acetyl-CoA. This cycle occurs within the mitochondria of the cell in the presence of oxygen. It is therefore an *aerobic process*. (Before entering this cycle the three energy nutrients have already been separately metabolized. These catabolic reactions are discussed in detail in the next section; this section deals just with the events from the entrance of pyruvic acid and acetyl-CoA into the Krebs cycle to the final yielding of energy.) See Figure 12-2 for the major events occurring in this cycle within the mitochondria.

The initial step in the Krebs cycle involves *pyruvic acid*, which is a three-carbon acid that results from the breakdown of some of the amino acids, lactic acid from muscle, glycerol, or glucose. The first reaction involves the *decarboxylation* (removal of CO_2) of the pyruvic acid and the activation of acetate. Pyruvic acid combines with coenzyme A to form acetyl-CoA (active acetate), releasing carbon dioxide and hydrogen. Five vitamins perform as coenzymes for this reaction to occur: thiamine as thiamine pyrophosphate, riboflavin as flavin adenine dinucleotide, niacin as nicotine adenine dinucleotide, lipoic acid, and pantothenic acid as part of coenzyme A. In the next step the activated acetyl-CoA combines with oxalacetic acid to form citric acid. The coenzyme A portion is separated and can be reused many times for the formation of additional acetyl-CoA from pyruvic acid. In the formation of acetyl-CoA, oxalacetate acts like a catalyst. Oxalacetate is the necessary fuel to keep the Krebs cycle going because it is the beginning and the ending point of the cycle. The TCA cycle always proceeds in a clockwise manner, and it is a repetitive process. The reactions proceed in the following order: pyruvic acid, acetyl-CoA, citric acid, α-ketoglutaoric acid, succinyl CoA, and oxalacetate, which recombines with more acetyl-CoA for a continuation of the cycle. The enzymes in the Krebs cycle are either *decarboxylases* that remove carbon dioxide or *dehydrogenases* that remove hydrogen. From the perspective of nutrition it is important to notice the cofactors required for each reaction, for this reveals the roles the vitamins and minerals play in specific metabolic reactions (see Fig. 12-2). It has already been pointed out that several of the B-complex vitamins were required as coenzymes in the conversion of pyruvate to acetyl-CoA; magnesium was also required as a cofactor in this reaction.

Oxidative Phosphorylation
Another very important role of the coenzyme forms of niacin and riboflavin occurs at many steps of the Krebs cycle. Several of the steps in this cycle involve *dehydrogenation,* or the removal of hydrogen. Were these hydrogens combined directly with oxygen, much of the energy would be wasted as heat. As nature's better alternative the vitamins niacin—as the coenzyme NAD—and riboflavin—as FAD—capture the released hydrogen atoms. These coenzymes are hydrogen acceptors, and they carry these hydrogens through a final cycle in which substantial energy is produced in the form of ATP. The name of this process is *oxidative phosphorylation,* and it is a process that includes a series of steps called the *electron transport chain.*

Up to this point very small amounts of ATP (energy) have been produced despite all the complex reactions that have occurred. The major portion (about 90%) of the ATP formation will occur from the further oxidation of the hydrogen atoms that were captured by the riboflavin and niacin coenzymes. Each turn of the TCA cycle has yielded four pairs of hydrogens and electrons. The hydrogens are transported to the nearby cytochrome system on the inner surfaces of the mitochondria.

The *cytochromes* are a group of iron-containing enzymes that readily accept hydrogens and transfer them along. Energy is released at each step and is captured and stored as ATP (see Fig. 12-2). The oxidation of hydrogen and the phosphorylation to form ATP are coupled and occur together. Tremendous amounts of ATP are formed during this process. For example, the oxidation of one molecule of glucose releases only 2 ATP molecules during the citric acid cycle, but 34 ATPs are released during the oxidative phosphorylation process.

THE ENERGY NUTRIENTS

The human body is composed of approximately 62% water. Protein composition is 17% and fat about 14%. The entire mineral portion of the body makes up only 6% of the

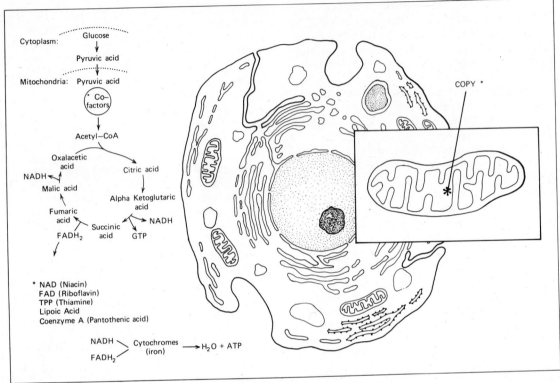

Figure 12-2. Entry of glucose and pyruvic acid into the citric acid cycle.

total weight, and the remaining 1.5 percentage is carbohydrate. Note that vitamins do not compose any of the structural parts of the body. They are required in only very minute amounts, and their main function is to regulate the metabolism of carbohydrate, protein, and fat. The anabolic and catabolic metabolic reactions are primarily those reactions involving the energy nutrients. In the next three major sections the major anabolic and catabolic reactions of carbohydrate, protein, and fat will be examined.

Carbohydrate

The major function of carbohydrate is to supply energy. This energy is available to every cell of the body in the form of glucose.

(With the exception of the cells of the central nervous system, most cells of the body can also use fatty acids for energy.) Following digestion the three monosaccharides that are absorbed are glucose, fructose, and galactose. They enter the portal circulation and travel to the liver. Before entering the bloodstream for transport the cells galactose and fructose are converted to glucose. Thus the metabolism of carbohydrates is really the metabolism of glucose.

Anabolism
There are two major anabolic reactions involving glucose. When surplus glucose is available it can be converted to a storage form called *glycogen* and stored in the liver. This process is known as *glycogenesis*. Another

anabolic process involving the formation of glucose is called *gluconeogenesis*. This process is the formation of glucose from noncarbohydrate sources such as some of the amino acids, the glycerol portion of fat, and lactate from muscle metabolism.

The regulation of carbohydrate metabolism is one of the major functions of the liver. The blood level of glucose is maintained within a specific range (60–120 mg/100 ml) in the healthy person. The liver makes available additional glucose by converting glycogen, the storage from of glucose, into glucose for transport into the bloodstream. The liver also removes excess glucose from the blood and converts the excess to glycogen. The blood levels of glucose are regulated by hormones through the actions of a widely distributed substance called *cyclic AMP* (adenosine monophosphate).

GLYCOGENESIS. The major anabolic process of carbohydrate metabolism is *glycogenesis,* or the formation of glycogen. All cells of the body are capable of converting glucose to glycogen, and all cells contain a small storage reserve of glycogen. The muscle and the liver manufacture the largest amounts of glycogen. The muscle tissue of the body stores about 240 gm of glycogen and the liver only about 100 gm. This represents a total of about 340 gm of glycogen, or the equivalent of about 1,360 Calories. If no food is consumed at all, this storage of glycogen will last a 70-kg (154-lb) man for about 13 hours of moderate activity. During fasting the body's glycogen stores are completely depleted within 24 hours, and the adipose tissue will have to be used to supply energy needs. There is a major difference, however, between the storage of glycogen in the muscle and that in the liver. The glycogen stored in the muscle is used as a source for muscular exertion when the level of blood glucose is low. Muscle glycogen can only be used within the muscle during muscular exertion; it cannot be used to replenish blood levels of glucose. The glycogen in the liver, however, can be reconverted to glucose and be used to replenish glucose levels in the blood.

The initial step in the metabolism of glucose involves its phosphorylation. This involves the addition of inorganic phosphorus to *adenosine diphosphate* (ADP) to yield ATP. The source of this phosphorus comes from foods in the diet. This reaction requires use of ATP, the enzyme *glucokinase,* and the presence of magnesium. In most tissues this reaction is irreversible. This process of phosphorylation captures the glucose within the cell and prevents its diffusion back out of the cell. Specific phosphatase enzymes are available within the liver, the kidney tubules, and the intestinal epithelial cells where reversal of this reaction does occur. The liver must be able to reconvert glycogen all the way back to glucose so it can be used to replenish the blood levels. One of the functions of the kidney is reabsorption of valuable nutrients and their return to the bloodstream. Glucose is reabsorbed in the renal tubules, and if necessary the phosphatase enzyme that is present can be used to convert any phosphorylated glucose back into pure glucose to be returned to the blood. Once glucose has been phosphorylated to *glucose-6-phosphate*, it may either be converted by a series of reactions to glycogen or further oxidized for energy.

Next a *mutase enzyme* assists in changing the location of phosphate. Glucose-6-phosphate is converted to glucose-1-phosphate. The building of glycogen requires the input of energy in the form of UTP (*uridine triphosphate*), a high-energy compound similar to ATP, which was used to form the UTP. Glucose-1-phosphate must react with UTP to form an active form of glucose called *uridine diphosphoglucose* (UDPG). As a bond is formed between the incoming glucose molecule and the already existing glycogen residue, the UDP is split off and returns to activate another glucose molecule.

Glycogen is a large molecule that consists of from 6,000 to 30,000 glucose units. The glucose molecules are arranged in straight chains (amylose portion) and branched chains (amylopectin portion). The glycogen is synthesized one glucose molecule at a time by the action of the enzyme *glycogen synthetase*. When the chain has been lengthened to between 6 and 11 glucose residues, a branching enzyme acts on the molecule to form a bond at a different location of the molecule, thus creating a branching point. The size of the glycogen molecule constantly changes as part is reconverted to glucose or used within the cell for energy or as additional glucose units are added. Glycogen can be seen as solid granules within the cell.

Potassium is required for the conversion of glucose to glycogen. Some potassium is bound to the phosphate required for glycogenesis. The potassium is stored with the glycogen and released when the glycogen is broken down. Disease states that deplete the glycogen stores also deplete the body of some of its potassium.

Insulin is the one hormone that stimulates glycogenesis. The main action of insulin is to lower blood glucose, and one way it does this is by promoting the conversion of glucose to glycogen. Most of the other hormones have the opposite action. Their basic action is to raise blood sugar and therefore foster the breakdown of glycogen.

GLUCONEOGENESIS. Glucose can also be formed from noncarbohydrate sources in a process called *gluconeogenesis,* literally, the formation of glucose from new sources. A portion of each of the energy nutrients is capable of forming glucose and thus assisting in maintaining blood glucose levels within a normal range. Approximately 60% of the amino acids can be converted to glucose, but only about 10% of the fat—the glycerol portion—can be converted to glucose. Protein is converted to glucose only when the glycogen reserves are depleted as in fasting, strenuous exercise, or diabetes mellitus. This is another example of the protein-

sparing effect of carbohydrate. The actual reactions involve all of the metabolic pathways.

SYNTHESIS OF CARBOHYDRATE COMPOUNDS. Although carbohydrate composes only a very small portion of the body's weight, the monosaccharides are synthesized into important compounds that regulate metabolism. Only the names and general functions of some of these compounds, not their actual synthesis, are within scope of this book. Two carbohydrates derived from the metabolism of glucose, *ribose* and *deoxyribose,* are constituents of RNA and DNA. *Glucuronic acid* acts as a detoxifying agent in the liver, and it is also a component of many mucopolysaccharides. *Hyaluronic acid* is part of the structure of connective tissue. *Chondroitin sulfate* is found in skin, tendons, cartilage, and bone. There are immunopolysaccharides that help the body resist infection. A classification of carbohydrates called *galactolipids* are part of nerve tissue. Carbohydrate compounds called *glycosides* are part of the steroid and adrenal hormones.

The monosaccharide galactose is required for the synthesis of lactose, the carbohydrate component of breast milk during lactation. Lactose is a disaccharide composed of glucose and galactose. The conversion of these two monosaccharides into lactose is a fairly simple reaction that takes place in the liver. Some of the galactose present in the liver is diverted into the production of lactose instead of being converted to glucose. These two monosaccharides are linked together with the aid of lactose synthetase to form lactose. The formation of lactose is very similar to that of glycogen, although the process is much shorter because only two monosaccharides must be linked together.

Catabolism
The two catabolic reactions involving carbohydrates are *glycogenolysis* and *glycolysis.* *Glycogenolysis* is the breakdown of glycogen to

glucose. *Glycolysis* is the breakdown of glucose to release energy. Glycolysis is divided into an anaerobic (without oxygen) and an aerobic (with oxygen) phase. Not only are these major pathways important for the breakdown of glucose and glycogen; but they provide points of entry for amino acids, glycerol, and fatty acids into the general metabolism. Additional interrelationships and interconversions of all the nutrients will be discovered as the metabolism of each energy nutrient is studied.

GLYCOGENOLYSIS. Glycogenolysis is not simply the reversal of glycogenesis. The end results appear to be the same, but different enzymes are involved. In the liver, kidney, and intestinal cell, glycogen is converted all the way back to free glucose because these cells contain the specific phosphatase enzyme for this task. This free glucose can then enter directly into the bloodstream. The other cells of the body, including the muscle, lack the phosophatase enzyme and convert the glycogen only back as far as glucose-6-phosphate, which can be used for energy only within the cell.

In recent years a mechanism has been discovered that more clearly explains hormonal regulation of metabolism at the cellular level. The substance involved is *cyclic AMP,* a nucleotide with only one phosphate attached. It is directly related to the other nucleotides, ADP and ATP, all of which exist with magnesium within the body.

Adenyl cyclase, an enzyme present within the plasma membrane, forms cyclic AMP from ATP. When the body is in need of glucose, the adenyl cylase is stimulated by epinephrine, *glucagon,* and *ACTH.* This enzyme stimulates the production of cyclic AMP, which in turn inhibits the synthesis of glycogen. The phosphorylase enzyme is activated by the presence of cyclic AMP, and glycogen breakdown begins. The enzyme phosphorylase removes one glucose molecule at a time; when a branched link is reached, a debranching enzyme removes this glucose molecule. In the muscle

the reaction proceeds only as far as glucose-6-phosphate. In the liver and kidney, however, the specific enzyme glucose-6-phosphatase converts the glucose-6-phosphate into free glucose. This final step in glycogenolysis is reflected by a rise in blood levels of glucose.

ANAEROBIC GLYCOLYSIS. The anaerobic stage of glycolysis occurs in the cytoplasm of the cell. It converts glucose into two molecules of pyruvic acid through a series of 10 reactions. If sufficient oxygen is available the pyruvic acid moves on into the mitochondria, where there is further oxidation and release of energy through the TCA cycle. This pathway of reactions is sometimes known as the *Embden-Meyerhof pathway* or simply as glycolysis.

The entrance of glucose into the cell is facilitated by insulin, in the process, lowering blood glucose levels. Once within the cell, the first reaction requires ATP, a *kinase enzyme,* and magnesium. Insulin is also thought to be involved in this phosphorylation of glucose. As stated previously this enzyme is found only in the liver, kidney tubules, and intestinal epithelial cell.

Once glucose is within the cell it undergoes a series of some 10 chemical reactions to split the six-carbon glucose molecule into two molecules each containing three carbons. Glucose is first phosphorylated and rearranged to form a fructose derivative. This compound is split in the next reaction to either two molecules of *glyceraldehyde-3-phosphate* or one molecule of *dihydroxyacetone phosphate* and one molecule of glyceraldehyde-3-phosphate. This is a significant reaction because the six-carbon monosaccharide is split into three carbon molecules. This reaction is also important because the main compound, glyceraldehyde-3-phosphate, can be further changed eventually to yield energy. The secondary compound, dihydroxyacetone phosphate, may be converted to fat and used for the synthesis of fat from excess dietary carbohydrate.

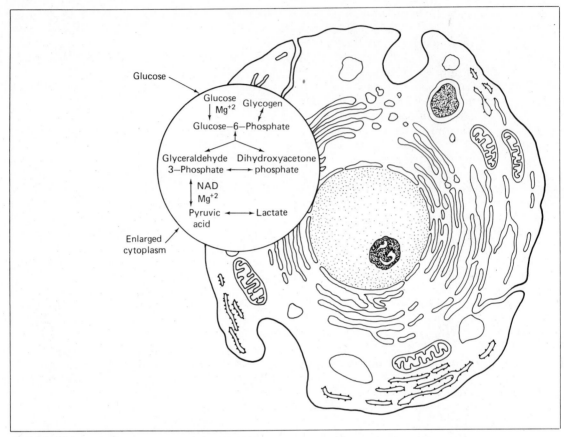

Glucose

Glucose   Glycogen
Mg^{+2}

Glucose–6–Phosphate

Glyceraldehyde   Dihydroxyacetone
3–Phosphate   phosphate

NAD
Mg^{+2}

Pyruvic   Lactate
acid

Enlarged
cytoplasm

Figure 12-3. Anaerobic glycolysis (Embden-Meyerhof pathway)

See Figure 12-3 for a summary of these reactions.

The purpose here, however, is to follow the reactions of the glyceraldehyde-3-phosphate. In the first reaction the niacin-containing coenzyme NAD is required. In the second of five reactions the first mole of ATP is formed. Magnesium is required as a cofactor in this reaction and one other. Finally, in the last reaction *phosphoenolpyruvic acid* is converted to pyruvic acid, and second mole of ATP is formed. At this stage if there is sufficient oxygen available, the pyruvic acid will enter the TCA cycle for a more efficient production of energy within the mitochondria. If, however, sufficient oxygen is not present, anaerobic glycoysis can occur within the cytoplasma.

When insufficient oxygen is available, as during intense muscular exercise or a temporary cessation of oxygen supply such as choking, the production of energy and therefore life itself does not end immediately. The body has a back-up system whereby energy production can continue without oxygen (anaerobic metabolism). In this case the pyruvic acid will be converted to lactic acid with the aid of the enzyme lactic dehydrogenase. This conversion of pyruvic to lactic acid requires the coenzyme NADH and in the process re-supplies NAD, which is needed for the continued breakdown of glucose and for ATP production. The lactic acid that accumulates leaks out of the muscle cell into the blood. It travels to the liver, where it is converted to pyruvic acid and then to glucose. The glucose leaves the liver and travels by the blood back to the muscle, where it continues to supply energy for muscular exertion. When a person "catches his breath," oxygen is once again supplied and aerobic metabolism once again resumes. This lactic acid cycle involving the liver, blood, and muscle is known as the *Cori cycle*, shown in Figure 12-4. The heart muscle can also use lactic acid as a temporary source of energy during an emergency.

AEROBIC GLYCOLYSIS. The *pentose phosphate shunt*, or the *hexose monophosphate shunt*, is a series of side reactions of the anaerobic Embden-Meyerhof pathway. At first glance it does not seem to have much nutritional significance, but on closer examination its importance becomes obvious. This pathway is a series of complex reactions, of which only those of most obvious nutritional significance are presented here.

The shunt begins with glucose-6-phosphate; and after a series of reactions that alter the number of carbon atoms, it ends up with glyceraldehyde-3-phosphate. During these reactions several interesting events have occurred. First of all these reactions do not require ATP. During the reactions another

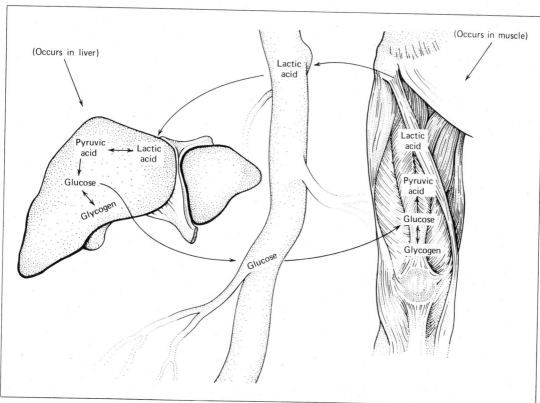

Figure 12-4. Lactic acid cycle.

niacin-containing enzyme, NADPH, is formed. This coenzyme is particularly needed for the synthesis of fatty acids and the use of lactic acid during muscular work. One of these reactions of the pentose phosphate shunt results in the formation of ribose, the five-carbon sugar necessary for the synthesis of the nucleic acids, RNA and DNA. Several of the reactions also require the thiamine coenzyme, TPP, and magnesium. This pathway is very active in the mammary gland, testis, leukocyte, and adrenal cortex. About 30% of the metabolism of glucose in the liver accurs by this pathway.

The final major aerobic pathway for the release of energy from glucose begins when pyruvic acid is converted to acetyl-CoA and enters the TCA cycle, the details of which have already been presented as the means by which 90% of the energy production occurs from carbohydrate, protein, and fat.

Fat

The two major locations of fat metabolism in the body are the liver and the adipose tissue. It is probably no surprise that the liver is involved in fat metabolism, but the adipose tissue is often thought to be just a storage reservoir of fat. Quite on the contrary, fat is constantly recycled out of the adipose tissue; and there is a complete turnover every two to three weeks. Both the liver and the adipose tissue are involved in anabolic and catabolic reactions involving fat. The major difference between the two is that the adipose tissue stores fat, but the liver does not. Storage of fat by the liver is an abnormal condition the body seeks to avoid. More details about the roles of the adipose tissue and liver in fat metabolism are presented in Figure 12-5.

Catabolism

The breakdown of fat is called *lipolysis,* a term that refers both to the process by which fat is split into fatty acids and glycerol in the liver and to the breakdown of fatty acids into acetyl-CoA.

LIPOLYSIS.   Dietary fat that has been digested and absorbed is transported in the blood as triglycerides in the form of a water-soluble lipoprotein complex called a *chylomicron.* These chylomicrons give the serum a milky appearance following a meal. The adipose tissue as well as the liver and other tissues contain the enzyme *lipoprotein lipase.* This enzyme is also known as the *cleaning factor* because it removes the chylomicrons from the serum. This removal involves the hydrolysis of the triglycerides from the chylomicrons into fatty acids and glycerol. The fatty acids can now gain entrance into the adipose cell to be used for energy or resynthesized into triglycerides for storage. The glycerol diffuses back into the plasma, where it will be used for energy by either the kidney or the liver cell.

Adipose tissue lipolysis results in the release of nonesterified fatty acids that travel in the blood bound to serum albumin. These fatty acids are the most metabolically active of the blood lipids. They are rapidly taken up by tissues in the body for further oxidation as a source of energy.

Most of the cells of the body are capable of using fatty acids for energy. Fats as a source of energy are equally as important as carbohydrates. From 30 to 50% of the carbohydrate eaten at a meal is converted to triglycerides and stored for later use for energy. From two-thirds to three-quarters of cellular energy is supplied by the fatty acids of triglycerides instead of by carbohydrates. This serves to emphasize that the major source of energy is not carbohydrate but actually fat.

The breakdown of fatty acids occurs only within the mitochondria of the cell. The fatty acids diffuse from the blood into the cytoplasm of the cell, but the mitochondrial membrane is not permeable to fatty acids. How then does the fatty acid gain entrance into the mitochondrion where it can be broken down

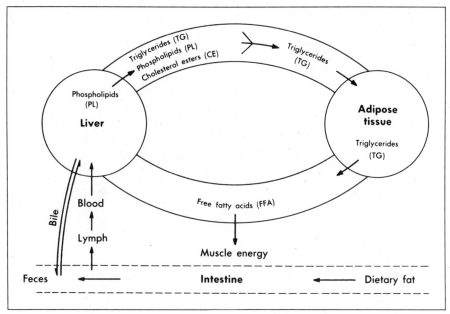

Figure 12-5. Liver–adipose tissue fat exchange. (Reprinted with permission from Sue Rodwell Williams, *Nutrition and Diet Therapy*, 3rd Ed. St. Louis; The C. V. Mosby Co., 1977)

for energy? A compound called *carnitine* acts as a carrier substance to transport the fatty acid into the mitochondrion. It also serves to transport the end product of fatty acid oxidation, acetyl-CoA, out into the cytoplasm.

The first actual step in fatty acid oxidation is its activation through a reaction with ATP and in the presence of CoA and an enzyme called *thiokinase*. This enzyme is found both inside and outside the mitochondria. This reaction forms an activated fatty acid or what is called the *acyl-CoA derivative*. Now the fatty acid can be oxidized in a stepwise series of reactions called *β-oxidation*. Each time a series of five reactions occurs, the fatty acid is two carbons shorter, and a molecule of acetyl-CoA has been formed. The acetyl-CoA enters the TCA cycle for further release of energy. One of the five reactions requires FAD, and another one requires NAD. The hydrogens that

are produced are used to produce ATP. Most of the common fatty acids have even-numbered carbon chains, and they yield only acetyl-CoA. Fatty acids with an odd number of carbon atoms are metabolized the same way, except the last compound formed is *propionyl CoA*, which contains three carbons. It can, however, be converted to succinyl CoA, which is a component of the TCA cycle. Two reactions are required for the conversion of propionyl CoA to succinyl CoA, one of which requires biotin and the other, vitamin B$_{12}$ as cofactors. Figure 12-6 summarizes the major steps in fatty acid oxidation.

The energy yield from the oxidation of one fatty acid is quite high. Energy is released when the acetyl-CoA molecules are formed and also when the acetyl-CoA molecules are oxidized by the TCA cycle. *Palmitic acid* is a common saturated fatty acid that is 16 car-

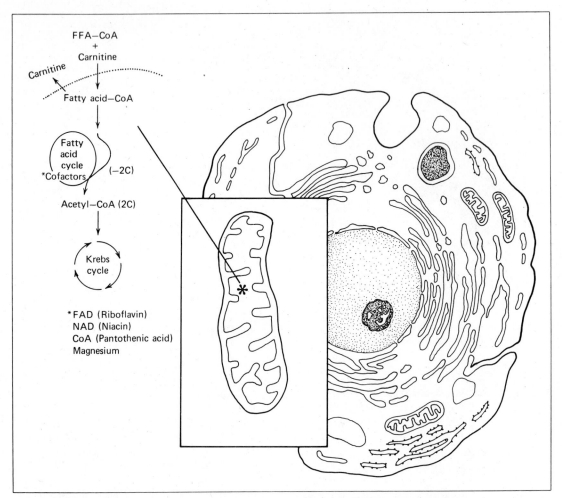

Figure 12-6. Fatty acid oxidation. Each turn of the fatty acid cycle results in the removal of 2 carbons and the formation of acetyl CoA.

bons in length. Eight molecules of acetyl-CoA are formed yielding 35 ATP molecules. An additional 96 are formed during the TCA cycle. One ATP molecule was used initially to activate the fatty acid, so there is a net production of 130 ATP molecules.

KETOGENESIS. Fatty acid oxidation usually does not result in the accumulation of the intermediary *metabolites,* a group of three com-

pounds called *ketones.* The muscle and other body cells can use ketones for energy, but the liver does not possess the enzymes for their further oxidation. When these ketones accumulate in small amounts, the liver can detoxify them, and they are simply excreted in the urine. In some conditions, however, these ketones accumulate in large amounts and cause a disturbance in the acid-base balance of the body. An inadequate amount of carbohydrate in the diet or a decreased availability of carbohydrate to the cells (as in diabetes mellitus) leads to an increased amount of acetyl-CoA being formed from the breakdown of fat. Because there is little or no carbohydrate to be used for energy, the body turns to fat as its source. Fat is broken down at an abnormally rapid rate in an attempt to meet the energy needs of the body (see Figure 12-7). Because there is a reduction of carbohydrate metabolism, there is less oxalacetic acid to combine with the acetyl-CoA in the

TCA cycle. Also, additional amounts of acetyl-CoA are combined to form one of the ketones, *acetoacetic acid*. This acid then gives rise to the formation of the other two ketones, *β-hydroxybutyric acid* and *acetone*. Because the liver cannot oxidize the ketones, they diffuse out of the liver cell into the blood. These ketones rise in the blood (*ketonemia*) and may even spill over into the urine (*ketonuria*). The ketones are fairly strong acids, and they combine with an available base such as sodium and cause a disturbance in the acid-base bal-

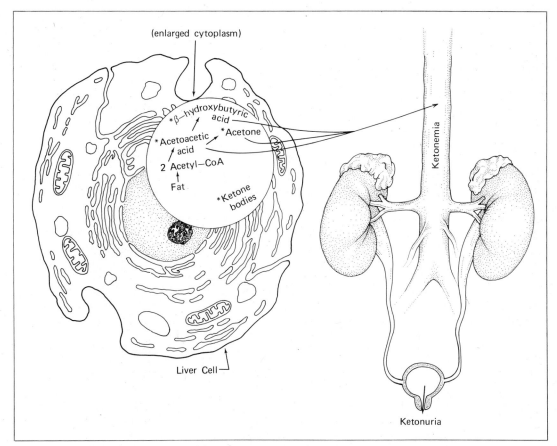

Figure 12-7. Ketogenesis is the formation of ketone bodies. When there is decreased glucose available, fatty acid oxidation is increased and ketones accumulate in the blood and urine.

ance of the body. The manifestation of clinical symptoms depends on the blood levels of ketones and on the client's individual tolerance for them. If *ketoacidosis* is allowed to proceed it may lead to coma and possible death.

FATE OF GLYCEROL.   The glycerol portion of the triglyceride molecule is metabolized through glycolysis (Embden-Meyerhof pathway) and either on through the TCA cycle or as a potential source of glycogen. It will be recalled that when fructose 1,6 diphosphate splits it forms glyceraldehyde-3-phosphate, dihydroxyacetone phosphate or both. This latter compound can then form glycerol. This is the point, then, where glycerol from fat metabolism enters the glycolytic pathway. Glycerol may also be used to form the backbone of another triglyceride molecule. Glycerol is first converted to *α-glycerophosphate* by the enzyme *glycerokinase*. This enzyme is present mainly in the liver, which is the major site of glycerol metabolism.

Anabolism

The synthesis of fat is known as *lipogenesis.* Lipogenesis includes the formation of fatty acids, triglycerides, and fat-related compounds primarily by the liver, adipose tissue, and intestinal mucosa. Other tissues such as kidney, brain, lung, and mammary gland participate to a limited extent in fatty acid synthesis.

The two major locations of fat synthesis are the adipose tissue and the liver. The adipose tissue is mainly involved with the synthesis, storage, and release of triglycerides. The functions of the liver are more complex than those of the adipose tissue. The liver synthesizes fatty acids and triglycerides. It also is involved with the conversion of fatty acids to triglycerides and phospholipids as well as the synthesis of lipoproteins and cholesterol. The liver functions in the synthesis and release of fat, but it does not store fat. To prevent the accumulation of fat in the liver, substances called *lipotropic factors* are present. These fac-

tors are protein in nature, and they serve to mobile the fat out of the liver by forming lipoproteins. Some of the common lipotropic agents are *choline, betaine, inositol, serine, lecithin,* and *methionine.* All of these factors are related either directly or indirectly to the amino acids. Methionine is an essential amino acid; serine is a nonessential amino acid; and lecithin contains choline. Choline and betaine are both derived from the simplest amino acid, *glycine.*

When the content of any one of the energy nutrients is high in the diet, the synthesis of fatty acids and triglycerides is stimulated. An excess of dietary carbohydrate stimulates the synthesis of fatty acids by the liver. These fatty acids eventually stimulate the synthesis of triglycerides by either the liver or the adipose tissue. These triglycerides are then stored as adipose tissue. An excess of protein in the diet will result in a conversion of the excess amino acids into either glucose or fatty acids with the eventual conversion into triglycerides for storage. Eating excess dietary protein is an expensive way of simply adding to one's fat stores. When the caloric intake from the energy nutrients is less than the energy requirements, the triglycerides in the adipose tissue will be broken down to fatty acids and released to supply energy. The same thing occurs during fasting or starvation. The synthesis or breakdown of fat, then, is directly related not only to the amount of dietary carbohydrate but to the energy balance of the body.

FATTY ACID SYNTHESIS. New fatty acids within the body originate from either excess carbohydrate or protein in the diet. Excess glucose and some of the amino acids are converted to a acetyl-CoA, which is the "building block" of fatty acid synthesis. The acetyl-CoA is available within the mitochondria because this was the site of lipolysis and the oxidation of pyruvate from glucose. Because the mitochondrial membrane is not permeable to acetyl-CoA, it needs a carrier to assist its movement into the cytoplasm, where fatty acid synthesis can occur. Carnitine is probably the carrier that transports the acetyl-CoA into the cytoplasm; it was the carrier that transported the fatty acid into the mitochondria so that lipolysis could occur.

Fatty acid synthesis in the mitochondria consists of a series of stepwise reactions in which acetyl-CoA is added to lengthen the fatty acid chain by two carbons (Fig. 12-8). Fatty acids may also be synthesized in the cytoplasm from citric acid by the addition of

two carbons each time until the desired length of the fatty acid is achieved.

The synthesis of fatty acids in the cytoplasm is referred to as de-novo synthesis. The first step involves the moving of the citric acid of the TCA cycle from the mitochondria out into the cytoplasm and its conversion to acetyl-CoA. The next step is the fixation of carbon dioxide into acetyl-CoA. This reaction requires energy (ATP) and the B-complex vitamin biotin. The resulting compound is *malonyl CoA,* which is a three-carbon com-

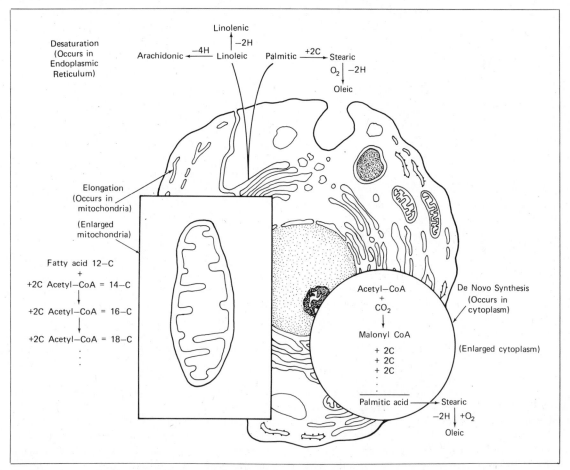

Figure 12-8. Lipogenesis occurs in the mitochondria, endoplasmic reticulum, and the cytoplasm.

pound. The next step uses the niacin-containing coenzyme NADPH to add hydrogen to the compound. The next reaction removes the double bond through the use of NADPH and the addition of hydrogen. The NADPH required for fatty acid synthesis is conveniently a product of the hexose monophosphate shunt, which also occurs in the cytoplasm. Thus a supply of NADPH, which is essential for fatty acid synthesis, is readily available in the cytoplasm. The addition of hydrogen to the carbons on either side of the double bond is referred to as *saturation*. This saturation of the carbons with hydrogen removes the double bond. These reactions are repeated until the fatty acid is the desired length. Each two-carbon unit added to the fatty acid is supplied by malonyl CoA, and carbon dioxide is liberated. Malonyl CoA is readily synthesized each time from acetyl-CoA in the presence of ATP and biotin.

The incorporation of double bonds into exisiting fatty acids is another method of fatty acid synthesis. *Oleic acid,* which contains one double bond, can be formed from *stearic acid,* a saturated fatty acid. *Linoleic acid* has the same chain length as oleic acid, except linoleic acid contains two double bonds. The human body, however, is not capable of adding this second double bond to oleic acid. Three polyunsaturated fatty acids—linoleic acid (C18:2), *linolenic acid* (C18:3), and *arachidonic acid* (C20:4)—are classified as essential because the body cannot synthesize them and a deficiency results in a clinical symptom. A dietary deficiency of the essential fatty acids produces a characteristic type of eczema in infants. Current research indicates that only the addition of linoleic acid to the diet has any positive effect on relieving the leision. Arachidonic acid can be synthesized from linoleic acid. Linoleic acid cannot be manufactured within the body so it must be obtained from the diet. It may be that linoleic acid is the only true essential fatty acid. This synthesis of unsaturated fatty acids or the lengthening of existing fatty acid chains is ac-

complished within the mitochondria instead of in the cytoplasm.

TRIGLYCERIDE SYNTHESIS.   Triglycerides are the storage form of lipid in the adipose tissue. This form of fat is also known as *depot fat.* Following a meal, excess quantities of the energy nutrients travel to the liver, where they are converted to fatty acids. The excess fatty acids are then transported to the adipose tissue via the serum lipoproteins. These lipoproteins are composes of varying quantities of triglycerides, phospholipids, and cholesterol mixed with protein. Fatty acids are then converted to triglycerides within the adipose tissue. Triglycerides may also be synthesized within the liver or intestinal mucosa.

The synthesis of a triglyceride requires that three fatty acids be incorporated into a glycerol molecule. Both the glycerol and the fatty acids must be in an activated state before this formation can occur. Glycerol is supplied from either the breakdown of fat or the oxidation of glucose by the Embden-Meyerhof pathway. In the liver the activation of glycerol to α-glycerophosphate takes place with the use of ATP and the enzyme *glycerokinase.* Adipose tissue lacks this enzyme, so the major source of α-glycerophosphate in this tissue comes from the oxidation of glucose. Dihydroxyacetone phosphate can be converted to α-glycerophosphate with the niacincontaining coenzyme NADH.

The fatty acids to be incorporated into the triglyceride molecule are supplied either by the hydrolysis of fats or from the supply of fatty acids synthesized by the liver. The fatty acids are activated to an acyl-CoA derivative using ATP and CoA. Two molecules of the activated fatty acid are added to the activated glycerol molecule with the aid of *phosphatidic acid.* The phosphate group of the phosphatidic acid is removed, and diglyceride is the result. A *diglyceride* is a fat compound that contains two fatty acids. One final activated fatty acid (acyl-CoA) is added, and coenzyme A is removed. This final step results in the desired result, the formation of a new triglyceride.

PHOSPHOLIPID SYNTHESIS. Phospholipids are part of all cells of the body and are especially important components of brain and nerve cells. The three major types of phospholipids are the *lecithins,* the *cephalins,* and the *sphingomyelins.* The liver is the major site for the synthesis of phospholipids. Phospholipids are classified as a *compound lipid;* that is, they are a derivative of a triglyceride. Phospholipids have a phosphoric acid component and a nitrogenous compound that replaces one of the fatty acids. The synthesis of phospholipids begins with α-glycerophosphate, like the initial step in triglyceride synthesis. The details of the synthesis of phospholipids is beyond this text, but the student should remember that the synthesis of these compounds is closely related to triglyceride synthesis.

CHOLESTEROL SYNTHESIS. Cholesterol has a complex structure, and therefore all but a few of the important details about its synthesis, production, and degradation are beyond the scope of this text. *Cholesterol* is the chief *sterol* of the body, and it is classified as a *derived lipid.* This means that cholesterol is derived, or formed, when dietary fats are broken down within the body. Cholesterol is available from both an exogenous source (the diet) and an endogenous source (internal synthesis). Cholesterol is synthesized by the intestinal mucosa and skin as well as by the liver.

Cholesterol is a complex structure consisting of five cyclic structures plus other portions. The primary compound involved in the synthesis of cholesterol is acetyl-CoA. This central metabolic compound is the source of all the carbon atoms of cholesterol. Any nutrient that can form acetyl-CoA is a potential precursor of cholesterol; therefore fatty acids, glucose, and some amino acids are potential sources for its synthesis. The coenzyme NADPH is required at several steps.

The liver synthesizes about 1,000–15,000 mg of cholesterol daily, independent of the daily diet, which contains about 500–800 mg. The cholesterol manufactured by the liver is used for the formation of certain hormones and of bile acids, which are a component of bile salts. About 80% of the cholesterol synthesized by the body is excreted as bile salts. Research indicates that diets high in saturated fat and cholesterol may have the effect of elevating serum cholesterol inasmuch as a reduction in dietary intake of cholesterol often leads to a reduction of blood levels. A diet high in polyunsaturated fats has the effect of lowering serum cholesterol, probably by enhancing its excretion as bile acids.

Protein

Protein is the structural component of every cell of the body; therefore the major function of protein is to build and maintain body cells. Because protein is a necessary component of body secretions, enzymes, hormones, and antibodies, it also has the function of regulating numerous body processes. The major metabolic activity of protein is synthesis (anabolism). The body seeks to protect and preserve the anabolic function at all costs by sparing and conserving not only the protein ingested from food but the protein in the body tissues and fluids.

Anabolism

One-half of the dry weight of the human body is protein. It is contained in the muscle, bone, skin, and body fluids. Protein is also a part of enzymes, some hormones, and antibodies. The terms *gene, DNA,* and *RNA* bring to mind the transmission of hereditary characteristics to a fertilized ovum for the reproduction of a new human being. Yet the body uses DNA and RNA as tools for the minute-by-minute construction of complex body proteins. The synthesis of glycogen and triglycerides were somewhat complex, but the synthesis of body protein is even more so. The topic of protein synthesis provides a fascinating and exciting glimpse into how complex and yet at the same time how specific and ordered the human body is.

PROTEIN SYNTHESIS. Each cell of the body is capable of synthesizing protein for its own functioning. The events of protein synthesis begin in the nucleus of the cell. The nucleus contains a set of 23 pairs of chromosomes, and on each chromosome are approximately 3,000 genes. There is a specific gene for every protein that needs to be synthesized by the cell. The genes are composed of DNA, and they contain the information needed for protein synthesis. When a given protein needs to be synthesized by the cell, the first step is the transfer of this information to *RNA*.

Before proceeding with a discussion of the events of protein synthesis, the composition and structure of DNA and RNA need to be explained. DNA and RNA are classified chemically as *nucleic acids,* which are composed of many smaller units called *nucleotides.* RNA and DNA both consist of four nucleotides. A nucleotide is composed of a pentose sugar (ribose or deoxyribose), a base (a *purine* or a *pyrimidine*), and a molecule of phosphoric acid. DNA is composed of the five-carbon sugar deoxyribose, phosphoric acid, and either a purine or pyrimidine base. Each of the four nucleotides which compose DNA contains a different base. The two purines are *adenine* and *guanine,* and the two pyrimidines are *thymine* and *cytosine.* The purines and pyrimidines are classified as nitrogenous bases because they contain nitrogen. The basic structure of RNA is similar except that the five-carbon sugar is ribose. The one other difference is that RNA contains the pyrimidine base *uracil* in place of thymine. This substitution is very important in determining the code for each amino acid, which is explained later.

The exciting sequence of events in protein synthesis (see Fig. 12-9) begins in the nucleus with DNA. DNA is actually part of the gene,

and it must remain in the nucleus. The DNA, however, contains the specific arrangement of amino acids for the synthesis of a given protein. Because the actual synthesis of the protein will occur on the ribosomes of the endoplasmic reticulum in the cytoplasm, the information on the DNA molecule must somehow be transferred into the cytoplasm. The pattern for protein synthesis is imprinted onto the nucleic acid RNA directly from the DNA. This form of RNA is known as *messenger RNA* because it travels from the nucleus into the cytoplasm, where it attaches itself to the ribosomes. The ribosomes contain another type of RNA, *transfer-RNA.* It exists in short chain sections in the cytoplasm. The purpose of the transfer RNA is to bring specific amino acids to the ribosome so that the amino acid can be lined up along the messenger RNA in the sequence specified there.

The specific way in which the two types of RNA direct the proper sequencing of the amino acids to form a protein is a fascinating subject that reveals much about the nature of proteins. As the discovery of the structure of the atom opened wide the field of inorganic chemistry, so the discovery of the molecular structure of DNA by J. D. Watson and F. H. C. Crick in 1962 unraveled the mysteries of protein synthesis of biochemistry. Once the structure of DNA was unveiled, the genetic code for each amino acid was broken, and protein synthesis was no longer a complete mystery. Watson and Crick described DNA as a double-coiled chain consisting of two intertwined strands. The pentose (deoxyribose) and the phosphate alternate to form both sides of the chain. The deoxyribose portions of each chain are each bonded to a base. The two bases are bonded to each other in the center by hydrogen bonding. The pairing of the bases is very important. A specific purine base always pairs up with a specific pyrimidine base. In DNA adenine always pairs up with thymine, and guanine always pairs up with cytosine. Each of these bases is represented by a letter in Figure 12-9.

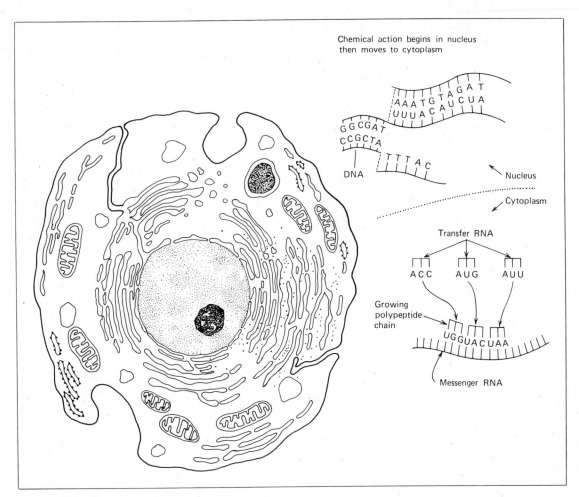

Figure 12-9. Protein synthesis.

The sequence in which these bases occur contains the code for the arrangement of specific amino acids to form a given protein. It is now known that a sequence of three base "pairs" is the code for an amino acid. This *triplet code* for each amino acid must be transferred from the DNA molecule to RNA for protein synthesis to proceed on the ribosomes in the cytoplasm.

The structures of DNA and RNA are similar except that RNA contains ribose and the base uracil is substituted for the thymine of DNA. There are three types of RNA. Messenger RNA in the nucleus is imprinted with the code for protein synthesis directly by DNA. Transfer RNA is present in the cytoplasm and serves to direct the specific amino acids to the exact location on the ribosomes for the synthesis of a given protein. *Ribosomal RNA* is manufactured in the nucleus from the small amount of RNA that occurs there. The RNA is complexed with some proteins to form the ribosomes, which then move out of the nucleus into the cytoplasm and attach themselves to the endoplasmic reticulum. The rough, or granular, endoplasmic reticulum, which contains ribosomes, is responsible for protein synthesis. The smooth, or agranular, endoplasmic reticulum participates in lipid synthesis and glycogen resorption.

The messenger RNA moves out of the nucleus into the cytoplasm and attaches itself to the ribosomes. Messenger RNA is a long single strand that contains the specific sequence for the amino acids. It therefore serves as a template, or pattern, for the attachment of the amino acids. The transfer RNA present in the cytoplasm is composed of short chains that contain only three bases at one end. These three bases are the code for one of the amino acids. The function of the transfer RNA is to gather the individual amino acids and carry them to the corresponding site on the messenger RNA. There is a specific transfer RNA for each amino acid.

Very important here is the concept of the all-or-none law of protein synthesis. All of the amino acids required for the synthesis of a given protein must be present simultaneously and in the proper amounts for a given protein to be synthesized. This is analogous to the manufacture of a radio on an assembly line. If one of the electronic components is missing, the radio cannot be completed. In the same way, if one of the amino acids is missing in the cytoplasm, the synthesis of a given protein will not occur. The body can manufacture any of the nonessential amino acids, but the nine essential amino acids must be included in the diet.

The all-or-none law is a good reason to include some complete protein or complementary combinations of vegetable proteins in every meal. An example, though oversimplified, may serve to illustrate this principle. A busy student only had time to eat a bag of potato chips and drink a cola beverage before rushing to a 10:00 AM class. Later in the afternoon this person cut her finger in chemistry

lab. After the bleeding stopped, the cells around the cut tried to synthesize some collagen (a protein) to repair the damaged tissue; but because all of the essential amino acids were not present, the collagen could not be synthesized at that time. To repeat, all of the amino acids must be present simultaneously and in the proper amounts for protein synthesis to occur. The only source of the nine essential amino acids is from a complete protein in the diet or a complementary combination of proteins.

Now, to continue with the synthesis of a protein on the ribosomes, the transfer RNA in the cytoplasm finds the corresponding amino acid as specified by the combination of the three bases on the end of the transfer-RNA molecule. Transfer RNA acts as a carrier to transport the amino acid to the ribosome. As the messenger RNA moves along the ribosome, the three bases attract the corresponding transfer-RNA and amino acid complex. Recall that the bases always match up in pairs. The three bases contained in the messenger RNA determine the amino acid. The transfer RNA has the bases that correspond to the bases of the messenger RNA. The bases of messenger and transfer RNA are loosely bonded to each other by hydrogen bonding. As each successive amino acid is added in the proper sequence to form a polypeptide chain and eventually a specific protein, it is linked to the preceding amino acid by the peptide linkage that bonds the peptide end of one amino acid to the carboxyl (acid) end of another. Once the peptide linkage has been formed, the transfer RNA separates from the amino acid and returns to the cytoplasm to transport more of the same amino acids.

This process of protein synthesis occurs continuously and rather rapidly within the cell. Many proteins contain 150–200 amino acids, but they are synthesized in approximately one minute. Each cell of the body synthesizes proteins continuously to meet the everyday demands for maintenance and repair. One can readily see the increased demands for protein synthesis imposed on the body during physiological growth and injury to body tissue (surgery, wounds, burns). These periods of physiological stress have the natural effect of increasing the dietary requirement for protein.

SYNTHESIS OF NONESSENTIAL AMINO ACIDS. The nonessential amino acids are classified as such because they can be synthesized within the body from the essential amino acids. The eight amino acids known to be essential in humans are *threonine, valine, lysine, leucine, isoleucine, phenylalanine, tryptophan,* and *methionine. Histidine* is an amino acid that is essential for infants; recent work suggests that it may also be essential for adults. As long as there are adequate quantities of complete protein in the diet, there will be adequate quantities of essential amino acids in the body. Some nonessential amino acids are formed directly from the essential amino acids:

Methonine→Cysteine

Phenylalanine→Tyrosine

One of the simplest ways nonessential amino acids are formed within the body is through a reaction called *transamination.* This reaction uses two of the alpha keto acids from carbohydrate metabolism, pyruvic acid and α-ketoglutaric acid. The amino group (—NH₂) is simply transferred from one compound to another, forming a new amino acid and a new acid. The overall reaction may be summarized as:

(Amino acid)$_A$ + (Keto acid)$_B$ ⇌ (Amino acid)$_B$
    + (Keto acid)$_A$

The coenzyme *pyridoxal phosphate,* a form of vitamin B₆, is required for all transamination reactions. All of the nonessential amino acids can participate in transamination reactions except *proline, hydroxyproline,* threonine, and lysine (see Figure 12-10).

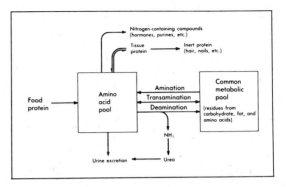

Figure 12-10. Interrelationships between the amino acid pool and the common metabolic pool of residues from carbohydrates, fats, and amino acids. (Reprinted with permission from Sue Rodwell Williams, *Nutrition and Diet Therapy,* 3rd Ed. St. Louis; C. V. Mosby Co., 1977)

All of the amino acids have specific functions in the body, but some act as precursors of important body compounds. Tryptophan is a precursor of the B-complex vitamin niacin. Tryptophan is also a precursor of *serotonin,* a powerful vasoconstrictor that participates in brain and nerve function and in gastrointestinal secretions and peristalsis. Phenylalanine, through its conversion to tyrosine, serves as precursor of the melanin pigment in hair and skin. Phenylalanine and tyrosine together participate in the formation of the hormones thyroxine and epinephrine. *Glycine,* the simplest of all the amino acids, participates in the synthesis of such important compounds as purines, the porphyrin ring of hemoglobin, and conjugated bile salts. Glycine is also very useful in its role as a detoxifying agent. It combines with toxic substances and converts them to harmless forms that can be excreted in the urine. Pantothenic acid, one of the B-complex vitamins, is partially formed from the amino acid *alanine.*

Catabolism

Although amino acids are used primarily for protein synthesis within the body, there are

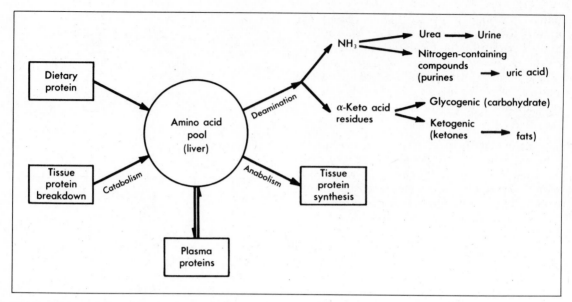

Figure 12-11. Balance between protein compartments and amino acid pool. (Reprinted with permission from Sue Rodwell Williams, *Nutrition and Diet Therapy*, 3rd Ed. St. Louis; The C. V. Mosby Co., 1977)

several circumstances in which they must be degraded to form either carbohydrate or fat. About 60% of the amino acids in protein can be converted to glucose and used for energy. If inadequate Calories are available in the diet from carbohydrate and fat, the body is forced to use a large proportion of the amino acids for energy instead of for protein synthesis. When inadequate quantities of essential amino acids are consumed, either because of poor food selection or inadequate quantities of protein, there are insufficient quantities of essential amino acids available for protein synthesis to occur. In this case the amino acid will have its amino group removed and be metabolized as either fat or carbohydrate. Amino acid catabolism involves the removal of the amino (—NH_2) group, leaving a compound called a *keto acid*. The major events are the fate of the ammonia (NH_3) that results from the removal of the amino group (*deami-*

nation) and the fate of the keto acid (see Fig. 12-11).

DEAMINATION. The first step in the catabolism of any amino acid is the removal of its amino group. This is accomplished by either of two processes. One of these is the process of transamination, already described. This reaction may be thought of as both anabolic and catabolic, anabolic in the sense that a different amino acid has been synthesized, catabolic because the original amino acid has lost its amino group. This is a good example of the difficulty in making a clear-cut distinction between anabolic and catabolic reactions in metabolism.

Another way the amino group of an amino acid may be removed is through the process of *deamination*. This process simply converts the amino acid to its corresponding keto acid through the removal of the amino group.

This reaction requires either a riboflavin coenzyme (FMN or FAD) or the niacin coenzyme (NAD). The splitting off of the NH_2 groups involves hydrolysis, with the resulting formation of ammonia (NH_3). This ammonia may be used in the formation of other nitrogen-containing compounds such as purines or *pyrimidines* or used in the synthesis of other amino acids. If it is not used in either of these ways, it must be detoxified either through the synthesis of urea or the formation of *glutamine*. It should be noted that once the essential amino acids are deaminated they cannot be reformed because the reaction only proceeds in one direction.

Glutamic acid, one of the nonessential amino acids, is capable of picking up free ammonia in the cell. The resulting compound is called *glutamine,* the amine form of glutamic acid. This is a safety mechanism to guard against the accumulation of ammonia within the cell. The glutamine can transfer the ammonia to other compounds or release it into the distal tubules of the kidney for excretion. The glutamic acid is now free to pick up and transport another molecule of ammonia.

The ammonia from deamination is removed from the blood and transported to the liver, where it is converted into urea. The overall reaction is:

$$NH_3 \; + \; CO_2 \; \rightleftarrows \; NH_2CONH_2 \; + \; H_2O$$
(Ammonia)   (Carbon dioxide)   (Urea)   (Water)

Notice that urea is actually composed of two molecules of ammonia bonded together by a carbon atom. The overall process of urea synthesis is actually a cyclic process that involves several steps.

The liver is the only organ capable of synthesizing urea and thereby detoxifying ammonia. The cycle involves three other nonessential amino acids, *ornithine, arginine,* and *citrulline.* The cycle requires energy in the form of ATP. The first step is the combining of ammonia with carbon dioxide and ATP to form a compound called *carbamoyl phosphate.*

Note the combining of two waste products of metabolism, ammonia and carbon dioxide, in this reaction. Next, this compound combines with the first amino acid, ornithine, to initiate the cycle and form citrulline. Then citrulline reacts with *aspartic acid,* which has contributed another molecule of ammonia, to form arginine. Now, in the presence of a specific enzyme and the mineral magnesium, arginine is converted to one molecule of urea and one of ornithine. One turn of the cycle has yielded one molecule of urea, and ornithine has been resynthesized so that the cycle can be perpetuated and repeated. In summary, carbon dioxide and ammonia entered as carbomoyl phosphate and exited as urea. The urea diffuses out of the liver and is excreted by the kidney. The urea cycle is summarized in Figure 12-12.

FATE OF KETO ACID.   After the removal of the amino group from an amino acid, the carbon skeleton that remains is referred to as a *keto acid.* These keto acids enter the common pathway of energy metabolism at several different points. Amino acids enter general metabolism as different metabolic end products. Those that enter as acetyl-CoA or one of the ketone bodies will be metabolized like fat. Those whose metabolic end products are pyruvic acid or any member of the TCA cycle will be metabolized like carbohydrate. Amino acids may be classified as either *ketogenic* (forming fat) or *glucogenic* (forming glucose). Most of the amino acids are glucogenic, and only a few are ketogenic. This distinction between the two types of amino acids is somewhat arbitrary. For example those amino acids that are converted to pyruvic acid (a glucogenic compound) may be further converted to acetyl-CoA (a ketogenic compound). A summary of the pathways by which the amino acids enter the general pathway of metabolism is found in Figure 12-13. The important fact to remember is that amino acids are capable of forming either carbohydrate or fat. Actually almost all the amino acids are

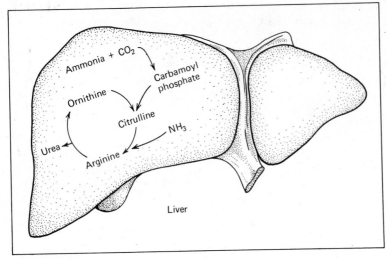

Figure 12-12. Urea cycle in the liver.

potentially ketogenic because they may be first converted to carbohydrate, which in turn can be converted to fat.

Almost all the amino acids are potentially glucogenic, but the nonessential amino acid alanine is especially so. A cycle that involves alanine operates between the muscle and liver via the bloodstream in cooperation with the previously discussed Cori cycle. Some of the pyruvate in the muscle is easily transaminated to form alanine. The alanine travels through the bloodstream to the liver, where it releases its amino group for subsequent conversion to urea. This deamination of alanine results in reconversion to pyruvate, which is a potential source of glucose. The glucose travels via the bloodstream, back to the muscle, where it is used as a source of muscular energy. It is then converted to pyruvate, and the cycle is repeated. This cycle serves two major purposes. First, it provides a means of removing nitrogen from muscle and transporting it to the liver without the formation of ammonia. Second, the alanine serves as a source of glucose for muscular work during periods of low supply.

Nitrogen Balance

The metabolic processes of anabolism and catabolism of protein occur continuously and simultaneously within every cell. The concern of medical personnel is the net effect of these reactions on a client. Is there a higher proportion of anabolic reactions occurring, for a building-up effect; or are there more catabolic reactions occurring, which have a breaking-down effect?

There is a method for measuring the degree of protein anabolism and catabolism within the body. This method is based on the fact that all protein contains 16% nitrogen. Studies of nitrogen balance measure the amount of nitrogen consumed in the diet from protein and the amount of nitrogen excreted in the urine. This method, although quite useful for determining minimum protein requirements for individual subjects, is not practical for the usual hospital setting. The studies require precise control of dietary intake and collections of urine and feces for a period of several weeks. The technique is quite precise, expensive, and time consuming. The overall concept of nitrogen balance does however have merit and application in the hospital setting. Common laboratory tests of the blood and urine yield a reasonable picture of protein metabolism.

Nitrogen balance may be defined as a measurement of the state of nitrogen equilibrium in the body; that is, anabolism and catabolism are equal. Nitrogen equilibrium can be established in an adult at any level of protein intake that exceeds the minimum requirement. In this case nitrogen intake from the diet exactly equals nitrogen excretion through the

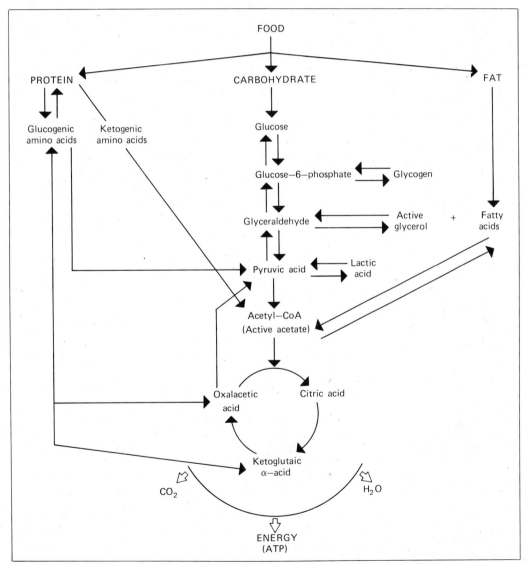

Figure 12-13. Summary of metabolism.

urine, feces, and skin. When this balance is altered in either direction, however, the result is either positive or negative nitrogen balance, indicating that either anabolism or catabolism of protein is predominating. Several laboratory tests can be used to assess the state of protein metabolism and give an indication of the relative state of positive or negative nitrogen balance. The tests include blood levels of protein fractions and the nonprotein constituents of nonprotein nitrogen, urea nitrogen, creatinine, and uric acid. The nitrogenous constituents in the urine can also be used as an indication of protein catabolism.

Positive nitrogen balance exists whenever the intake of nitrogen exceeds its excretion. This occurs during periods of anabolism or growth of body tissue. There is a slightly higher protein requirement during periods of physiological growth. The body uses the protein for building new tissues, as in growing children and during pregnancy. Positive nitrogen balance is also evidenced during lactation because of the manufacture of the breast milk. If negative nitrogen balance is evident during any of these stages, then it is quite likely that the protein intake of the diet is inadequate or that some disease or condition of the body is interfering with the use of the protein. Positive nitrogen balance is also evident whenever damage or depleted tissues are being replenished following surgery or injury. Note that positve nitrogen balance occurs only when the healing process has begun. Athletes in training are also in an anabolic state because new muscle tissue is being developed. (See Fig. 12-14.)

Negative nitrogen balance occurs whenever the excretion of nitrogen is greater than the intake. This excretion of nitrogen represents the catabolism, or breakdown, of body tissue (protein). Negative nitrogen balance usually exists for several days following surgery, injury, or burns. This is an undesirable physiological state because the body is breaking down its own tissues to meet its increased needs for protein, Calories, or both; and measures should be employed immediately to correct it. Other conditions that lead to negative nitrogen balance are inadequate Calorie content of the diet, inadequate protein, or poor quality of protein. All three of these conditions cause the body to catabolize its own tissue in an attempt to meet the protein and energy needs. (See Fig. 12-14.)

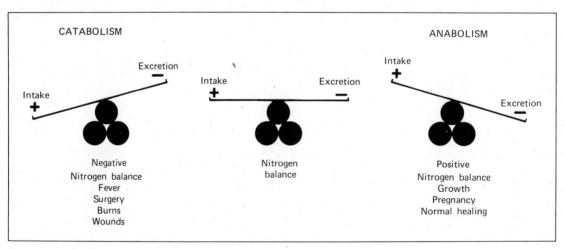

Figure 12-14. Nitrogen balance.

It must be remembered that the anabolic and catabolic reactions of carbohydrate, protein, and fat do not occur in isolation. Metabolism of the energy nutrients involves continual interdependency among the nutrients.

A summary of the major interrelationships in metabolism is in Figure 12-13. A summary of cellular metabolism and the role of ATP in metabolism is presented here as a review for the student (Tables 12-2 and 12-3).

TABLE 12-2. Summary of Cellular Metabolism

Region of Cell	Major Functions	Nutrients Required
Plasma membrane	Surrounds the cell; provides for selective permeability.	Lipid ——— Structure of Protein membrane
Protoplasm	Provides optimum environment for life.	All nutrients.
Nucleus	Replication of DNA by formation of messenger RNA; DNA contains hereditary information.	DNA contains a sugar (deoxyribose), a phosphate, and a nitrogen base; RNA contains the sugar ribose.
Endoplasmic reticulum	Transports biological materials through the cell via membranes.	
Smooth (agranular)	Synthesizes phospholipids, triglycerides, cholesterol, mucopolysaccharides, and glycogen.	Carbohydrates, proteins, and fats.
Rough (granular)	Synthesizes protein.	All essential amino acids; nonessential amino acids.
Golgi complex	Packages and stores cellular secretions such as digestive enzymes.	Amino acids. Zinc
Lysosome	Serves as digestive system of the cell; stores hydrolytic enzymes for use as required to destroy foreign substances or degrade worn out cellular components.	Amino acids for synthesis of enzymes; vitamins A and E to maintain and stabilize lysosome membrane.
Cytoplasm	Site of cellular secretion and absorption.	
	Glycolysis.	Glucose, magnesium, phosphorus, oxygen, and niacin (NAD).
	Glycogenesis.	Glucose.
	Fatty acid synthesis.	Glucose, biotin, niacin (NADPH).
	Hexose monophosphate shunt.	Ribose, glucose, thiamine.
	Activates amino acids prior to protein synthesis.	
Mitochondria	Oxidizes end products of glycolysis in citric acid cycle.	Niacin (NAD), thiamine (TPP), riboflavin (FAD), pantothenic acid (CoA), magnesium, and sulfur.
	Oxidizes fatty acids.	Riboflavin (FAD), niacin (NAD), pantothenic acid (CoA), and magnesium.
	Forms high-energy bonds (oxidative phosphorylation) in the electron transport system.	Iron, copper, niacin (NAD), riboflavin (FAD), and phosphorus.
	Degrades amino acids for energy (deamination) and for synthesis of nonessential amino acids (transamination).	Vitamin B_6 (pyridoxine).
	Synthesizes fatty acid.	Niacin (NADPH)

TABLE 12-3. Summary of the Role of ATP in Metabolism

	Catabolic Reactions (Release ATP)	Anabolic Reactions (Use ATP)
Carbohydrate	Glycolysis Oxidative phosphorylation	Glycogenesis Gluconeogenesis
Protein	Deamination Fate of keto acid	Cell maintenance Protein synthesis
Fat	Lipolysis Fatty acid oxidation	Lipogenesis

ENDOCRINE REGULATION OF METABOLISM

The endocrine system consists of hormones that act as blood-borne messengers that regulate cell function. Hormones serve to control and integrate many bodily functions including reproduction, organic metabolism, energy balance, and mineral metabolism.

Insulin

Insulin is a polypeptide protein hormone secreted by the B cells of the pancreas. The hormone acts directly or indirectly on most tissues of the body except for brain tissues. The most important effect of insulin is the stimulation of glucose entry into cells by increasing cell permeability. An increase in glucose uptake in turn stimulates glycogen synthesis and inhibits enzymes that cause glycogen breakdown. Insulin also stimulates an increase in membrane permeability to amino acids and potassium. This mechanism leads to increased protein synthesis and increased enzyme activity in the glucose metabolic pathway. In addition, the increased entry of glucose into adipose tissue facilitates fatty acid synthesis and, subsequently, triglyceride synthesis. When the insulin level in the blood is decreased, the above reactions reverse.

The regulation of insulin release is very complex, involving, as it does, several separate mechanisms. Some of the factors believed to increase the release of insulin include (1) a rise in blood glucose level; (2) the release of a substnace similar to pancreatic glucagon in the jejunum when glucose is present; (3) stimulation of the vagus nerve; (4) glucagon; and (5) amino acids. Insulin secretion is inhibited by epinephrine and norepinephrine.

The effect of insulin lack on carbohydrate metabolism is illustrated in Figure 12-15. With the *hyperglycemia* that accompanies an insulin deficit, severe *glycosuria* may result. The *osmotic diuresis* that occurs depletes the body of water and electrolytes. Dehydration eventually occurs, with a resultant decrease in total blood volume and blood pressure. As circulation fails, *anoxia* occurs, causing a shift to anaerobic metabolism. An elevation of hydrogen ions in the cells appears, resulting in a falling pH. Death from heart failure occurs unless supplemental oxygen is administered.

Fat metabolism is equally affected by insulin lack. Figure 12-16 illustrates the alterations in fat metabolism brought about by insulin lack. When glucose cannot be metabolized, large amounts of fat are released from fat stores and are excreted into the blood in the form of fatty acids. The fatty acids are incompletely metabolized, resulting in accumulation of acids in the blood and metabolic acidemia. The loss of keto acids in the urine precipitates the passive loss of sodium, potassium, and water. Blood volume drops, and circulatory failure ensues.

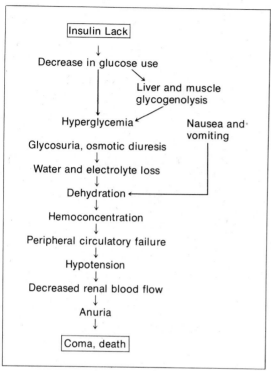

Figure 12-15. Effect of insulin lack on carbohydrate metabolism. (Reproduced with permission from J. Tepperman, *Metabolic and Endocrine Physiology*, 3rd Ed. Copyright © 1973 by Year Book Medical Publishers, Inc., Chicago.)

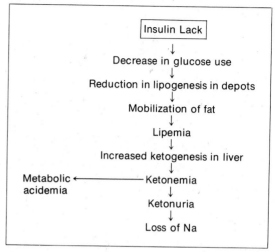

Figure 12-16. Effect of insulin lack on fat metabolism. (Reproduced with permission from J. Tepperman, *Metabolic and Endocrine Physiology*, 3rd Ed. Copyright © 1973 by Year Book Medical Publishers, Inc., Chicago.)

Protein synthesis is reduced in the presence of an insulin deficit. Protein catabolism begins to exceed protein anabolism, resulting in an increase in circulating amino acids. Nitrogen and potassium are lost from the body. *Hypovolemia* and its associated effects then occur. Figure 12-17 summarizes altered protein metabolism from insulin lack.

Obviously, insulin has a profound effect on total metabolism. Adequate insulin supplies facilitate glucose use as well as fat and protein synthesis. If insulin is not present in sufficient amounts, cell nutrition is reduced; water and electrolytes are lost; and circulation to the tissues is threatened.

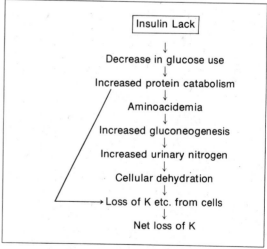

Figure 12-17. Effect of insulin lack on protein metabolism. (Reproduced with permission from J. Tepperman, *Metabolic and Endocrine Physiology*, 3rd Ed. Copyright © 1973 by Year Book Medical Publishers, Inc., Chicago.)

Glucagon

Glucagon is a hormone produced by the nine cells of the pancreas. Many of the functions of glucagon are in direct opposition to insulin. When blood glucose levels are below normal, glucagon is secreted into the portal circulation and inhibits glycogen synthesis in the liver. Glycogenolysis occurs, resulting in an increase in blood glucose level. Glucagon also exerts a direct effect on adipose tissue, which increases the release of free fatty acids and glycerol. Many of the body cells are able to use fatty acids partially in their individual metabolism, thus sparing glucose for use by those tissues for which glucose is the sole means of metabolism. Excessive glucagon release can create a condition similar in effect to diabetes mellitus. Glucagon deficit can result in an abnormally low serum glucose level.

Epinephrine

Any stimulus to the sympathetic nervous system will initiate the release of *epinephrine* or the neurotransmitter *norepinephrine*. The bulk of epinephrine is produced in the adrenal medulla; norepinephrine is produced at the sympathetic postganglionic terminals. Epinephrine and norepinephrine are released when the body undergoes any kind of stress. A low plasma glucose level also stimulates epinephrine release. The cardiovascular system responds through vasoconstriction to increase the blood flow to the vital organs. Blood pressure rises. Gastrointestinal smooth-muscle activity and mobility decrease during the stressful period.

Epinephrine and norepinephrine have a marked effect on tissue metabolism. The hormone increases the activity of the enzymes that catalyze the breakdown of glycogen. An abrupt increase occurs in blood glucose and lactic acid levels. Blood glucose levels slowly decline as the glucose is used by the tissues.

Epinephrine also has an effect on lipid metabolism. An increase in circulating free fatty acids and glycerol occurs. The fatty acids are metabolized to CO_2 and water by way of the citric acid cycle or to ketone bodies by the liver. Glycerol is metabolized and enters the glycolytic pathway. It is apparant that the metabolic effects of epinephrine oppose those of insulin.

Cortisol

Cortisol is secreted subsequent to stimulation of the adrenal cortex by *ACTH* from the anterior pituitary. Stressful stimuli tend to increase the amount of cortisol production. Cortisol itself causes an elevation in blood glucose level and is a powerful inhibiter of glucose uptake by many of the tissues. The action of epinephrine is enhanced when steroids are present.

Protein breakdown is stimulated in all tissues except the liver, where reverse glycolysis is stimulated. This mechanism assures a constant supply of glucose in the blood, though it occurs at the expense of body protein.

Thyroid Hormones

Two of the hormones released by the thyroid, *thyroxine* (T_4) and *triiodothyronine* (T_3) function to increase the rate of metabolism of all cells. A general increase in calorogenic activity is noted, correlating with an increase in the rate of oxidation in body cells. Growth, maturation, and tissue differentiation results. In addition to increasing the overall metabolic rate in the body, T_4 and T_3 stimulate an increase in quantity and activity of enzymes; glucose absorption and use; and an increased demand for vitamins, which function as coenzymes during the metabolic processes.

Both synthesis and breakdown of carbohydrate, lipid, and protein are increased. Because of the general increase in glucose use, gluconeogenesis and glycogen breakdown are also increased. Because amino acids play an important role in gluconeogenesis, protein breakdown also increases. Fat metabolism is enhanced in order to spare glucose for use by the nervous tissue. Thyroid hormone is important for the ill patient in that it promotes healing and regeneration of injured body tissues.

Growth Hormone

Growth hormone is secreted by the anterior pituitary. It is responsible for normal growth in children and maintenance of normal carbohydrate, lipid, and protein metabolism. The general affect of growth hormone is the anabolism of protein. The hormone increases lipid breakdown in adipose tissue, freeing fatty acids for use as metabolic fuel. The hormone tends to have an effect opposite of insulin, thus increasing blood glucose level. As long as sufficient amounts of glucose and fatty acids are available for metabolism, gluconeogenesis is decreased, inhibiting protein breakdown. In general, the presence of growth hormone inhibits cellular glucose uptake to slow glucose use in those tissues that can burn fatty acids.

SPECIALIZED CELLS

To this point, this chapter has been concerned with the activities of the "typical cell," including energy production and the anabolic and catabolic processes of carbohydrate, protein, and fat metabolism. There is, however, no such entity as a typical cell. Each cell of the body is adapted to its particular function. Some of the body cells are modified to perform specialized functions that make life possible.

A human being develops from one cell, a fertilized ovum, into an adult with 10^{14} cells (100,000,000,000,000) (Pike and Brown, 1975). During the development of a human being, differentiation and specialization of the cells occur. These changes are accompanied by morphological and physiological changes that result in specialization of the cell's func-

tions. As a result of this specialization certain cells have specific nutrients needs. Some of the specialized cells in the human body are cells of the liver, the bone, the muscle, and the nerves. Red blood cells and adipose cells are two other specialized cells.

Some of the specialized cells are adapted to perform a special function such as the nerve cell with its long axon to conduct and transmit nerve impulses; the muscle cell with its ability to adjust its length; or the bone cell, which is specially adapted to attract calcium and other minerals to produce a skeleton with rigidity and strength (Fig. 12-18). The lifespan of cells differs greatly, from those that have an existence of only a few days (such as the skin cells and the red blood cell) to those that last a lifetime (such as the nerve cell). Some cells, such as the nerve cell, cannot be replaced; whereas other cells, such as those of the liver and skin, rapidly regenerate if they are diseased or injured.

Table 12-4 is a summary of the functions of the specialized cells. The liver cell (*hepatocyte*) is involved with the metabolism and storage

TABLE 12-4. Selected Functions of Specialized Cells

Specialized Cell	Function
Liver cell (hepatocyte)	Regulation of blood glucose level; gluconogenesis, formation of acetyl-CoA and ketone bodies, plasma protein synthesis, creatine and urea synthesis, plasma lipid synthesis, cholesterol synthesis and degradation, bile acid synthesis, and bile pigment formation
Red blood cell (erythrocyte)	Hemoglobin synthesis, iron delivery, and globin synthesis
Bone cell (Osteocyte)	Collagen synthesis, mucopolysaccharide synthesis, and mineral deposition and resorption
Muscle cell (myofibril)	Muscle contraction and relaxation
Nerve cell (neuron)	Transmission of nerve impulses

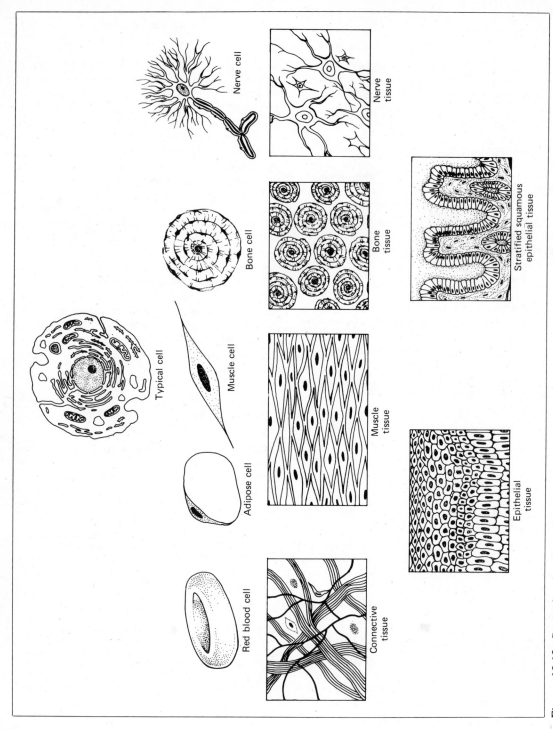

Figure 12-18. Specialized cells and tissues.

Nerve cell

Nerve tissue

Bone cell

Bone tissue

Stratified squamous epithelial tissue

Typical cell

Muscle cell

Muscle tissue

Adipose cell

Epithelial tissue

Red blood cell

Connective tissue

of nutrients. It may also be thought of as a transfer, or nutrient redistribution, center. The liver cell receives nutrients from the small intestine following absorption and also from the blood for further metabolism or redistribution. The function of the red blood cell is to transport oxygen and carbon dioxide to and from all the other cells of the body. The bone cell (*osteocyte*) is involved with the deposition of calcium and other minerals in the bony skeleton. Muscle cells are specialized for the process of contraction and relaxation that result in body movement. The nerve cells (neurons) transmit messages to and from muscles and sense organs to the brain. The adipose, or fat, cell has the primary function of synthesizing, storing, and releasing fat.

BODY TISSUES

Groups of cells all having a similar structure and function are called *tissues*. There are four basic types of tissues in the body, each having specific functions: *epithelial, connective, muscle,* and *nerve tissue.*

Epithelial Tissue

Epithelial tissue forms glands, covers body surfaces, and lines body cavities. These tissues function in protection, absorption, secretion, and excretion. The epithelial tissues lack blood vessels. Nutrient supply and waste removal are provided by the underlying connective tissue.

Connective Tissue

Connective tissue binds the cells of the body together. There are several types of connective tissue, each composed of a specific proportion of collagen, *elastin,* or reticular fibers embedded in a matrix called *ground substance*. The connective-tissue fibers are composed of protein. The ground substance is composed primarily of mucopolysaccharides. Some examples of specialized connective tissues are cartilage and bone. Although they are more

fluid in their composition, blood and lymph are also considered to be connective tissue.

Muscle and Nerve Tissue

Muscle tissue is composed mainly of protein. The proteins of muscle tissue are very elastic and have much contractile power (Harper et al., 1979). Nerve tissue is composed of complex lipids and protein. The lipids in nerve tissue are phospholipids (lecithins, cephalins, and sphingomyelins); cholesterol *cerebrosides,* or galactolipins; sulfur-containing lipids, and some aminolipids.

Body tissues with similar functions are grouped together to form body organs such as the heart, lungs, liver, stomach, and skin. The system forms the basic structural plan of the body. The major systems of the body are:

- Skeletal system
- Muscular system
- Nervous system
- Integumentary system
- Circulatory system
- Respiratory system
- Digestive system
- Urinary system
- Endocrine system
- Reproductive system

By using the nutritive process as the organizational framework for this unit, some of these

TABLE 12-5. Role of Body Systems in the Nutritive Process

Nutritive Approach	Body System
Digestion and absorption	Digestive
Transport	Circulatory
	Respiratory
Metabolism	Skeletal
	Muscular
	Nervous
	Integumentary
	Endocrine
Excretion	Digestive
	Urinary

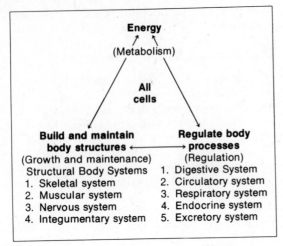

Figure 12-19. Summary of nutrient functions as they relate to body systems.

systems have already been discussed. Table 12-5 shows the relation of the body systems to the nutritive process. Figure 12-19 summarizes the three major nutrient functions as they relate to all the body systems.

BIBLIOGRAPHY

Duncan, G. G. *Duncan's Diseases of Metabolism.* 7th Ed. Philadelphia: W. B. Saunders Co., 1974.

Guthrie, H. A. *Introductory Nutrition.* 4th Ed. St. Louis: The C. V. Mosby Co., 1979.

Guyton, A. C. *Basic Human Physiology: Normal Functions and Mechanisms of Disease.* 2nd Ed. Philadelphia: W. B. Saunders Co., 1977.

Harper, H. A., Rodwell, V. W., and Mayes, P. A. *Review of Physiological Chemistry.* 17th Ed. Los Altos, Calif.: Lange Medical Publications, 1979.

Krause, M. V., and Mahan, L. K. *Food, Nutrition, and Diet Therapy.* 6th Ed. Philadelphia: W. B. Saunders Co., 1979.

Nat's Dairy Council. The role of lactose in the diet. *Dairy Council Digest* 45(5):25, 1974.

_____. Interrelationships of diet, gut microflora nutrition, and health. *Dairy Council Digest* 47 (4):19, 1976.

_____. Gut ecology and health implications. *Dairy Council Digest* 50(3):13, 1979.

Pike, R. L., and Brown, M. L. *Nutrition: An Integrated Approach.* 2nd Ed. New York: John Wiley & Sons, Inc., Pubs., 1975.

Robinson, C. H., and Lawler, M. R. *Normal and Therapeutic Nutrition.* 15th Ed. New York: Macmillan, Inc., 1977.

Routh, J. I. *Introduction to Biochemistry.* 2nd Ed. Philadelphia: W. B. Saunders Co., 1978.

Speck, M. L., and Reynolds, W. M. Contributions of microorganisms to foods and nutrition. *Nutrition News* 38(4):13, 1975.

Williams, S. R. *Nutrition and Diet Therapy.* 3rd Ed. St. Louis: The C. V. Mosby Co., 1977.

Wilson, E. D., Fisher, K. H., and Garcia, P. A. *Principles of Nutrition.* 4th Ed. New York: John Wiley & Sons, Inc., Pubs., 1979.

CHAPTER 13

Metabolism of Structural Body Systems

Cora Kurtz

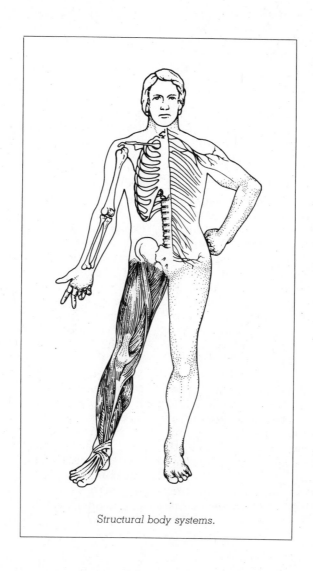

Structural body systems.

Development and maturation of structural body systems described in this chapter refer to a single, continuous growth process that begins at conception and proceeds through numerous stages characteristic of childhood, adolescence, adulthood, and old age, finally culminating in death. Development encompasses a series of highly regulated events. Once fertilization has occurred, cell proliferation results in growing cells, tissues, organs, and body systems that take on increased complexity of function. Maturity marks the attainment and maintenance of body size, conformation, and capabilities common to humans. Growth is most rapid during the early years. Rate of change slows in the adult and may be further retarded in old age.

Hormonal, genetic, and environmental factors influence individual rates of development. The nutrients in the food eaten and the nutritive process of metabolism regulate the supply of nourishment to the body systems. The setting for optimal development and maturation is one in which a person can reach his full genetic potential not only in terms of physical size, strength, and endurance but in behavioral and intellectual capacities as well.

Nutrients function within the entire body in an interrelated pattern to produce a synchronized, harmonious organism. Although the total body is growing at an observable rate, different structures within it are at various phases of growth at any given time. Nutrient concentrations within one system will affect related systems. For example, a constant and normal concentration of ionized calcium in extracellular fluid is of great importance in muscular contraction, neural and neuromuscular transmission, and activity of several enzymes. If ionized calcium is low, tetanic spasms, convulsions, or even death may occur. If plasma calcium is above normal, cardiac function is disturbed, and calcium is excessively deposited in the kidney or other tissues (Bell et al., 1976). The following discussions of nutrient roles and functions are based on normal nutrient concentrations throughout the body.

SKELETAL SYSTEM

Bones

The skeletal system is the body's basic structure. Its framework is composed of over 200 bones with their joints. Joints, in response to muscular action, enable the bones to perform a great variety and range of motion. Connective tissue bands, called *ligaments,* hold the bones together. Ligaments are found in relation to all the freely movable joints and many of the less movable ones. The slightly movable and immobile joints form continuous structures in which either cartilage or fibrous connective tissue fills the space between the bones. These soft tissue areas are largest in the child, become smaller in the adult, and may become completely filled by bone in old age.

Functions

In addition to being a sturdy and resilient framework with movable levers for the entire body, bones serve as protection for such delicate organs as the brain and spinal cord. Bones are also necessary for the production of blood cells and for the storage of calcium, which may be removed when an inadequate supply is available (Memmler and Wood, 1977).

Development

Bones have their own blood system, lymphatic vessels, and nerves. In the embryonic stage of organic bone development, long bones appear in the fetus as cartilaginous models that are later replaced by bone. Others, such as the flat skull bones, are formed directly into bone within the connective tissue membranes without an intermediate cartilage stage (Bell et al., 1976).

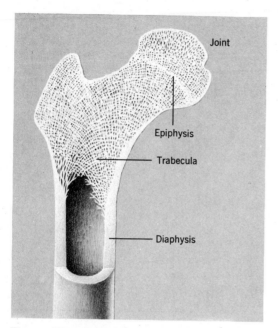

Figure 13-1. Schematic drawing of trabecula in bone. (From E. D. Wilson, K. H. Fisher, and M. E. Fuqua, *Principles of Nutrition*, 3rd Ed. Copyright © 1975 by John Wiley & Sons, Inc. Reprinted by permission of John Wiley & Sons, Inc.)

Deposition of calcium compounds, or inorganic bone development, begins in in the fetus as early as the second and third months of prenatal life. The process of depositing these crystalline salts continues throughout life, more rapidly at certain stages in the life cycle than at others. Figure 13-1 illustrates the major components of bone. The *diaphyseal* (shaft) of the long bones calcifies to become rigid and strong, capable of supporting the upright weight of the body, as early as eight months after birth, before the infant begins to walk (Guthrie, 1979).

Long bones continue to grow in length during early and middle childhood. *Epiphyseal cartilage,* in which cells are arranged in regular longitudinal columns, is produced by repeated cell division. Each row of cells, enclosed in a tunnel of cartilage, has thin partitions between the cells. As the cells approach the diaphyseal side of the *epiphyseal plate* (the end of long bones), they enlarge, and the cartilage around them calcifies. The cells next to the marrow cavity die, and thin transverse partitions of cartilage disappear, leaving tunnels that are invaded by capillaries and *osteoblasts* (cellular components for bone formation). Osteoblasts form a layer of bone on the tunnel's inner walls, and this process is repeated. During these developmental periods of the life-span, the interstitial growth of epiphyseal cartilage is always present as a thin and regular zone. Cartilage is not transformed into bone; it is replaced by it (Bell et al., 1976).

Practically every skeletal dimension in the body takes part in the growth spurt of puberty and early adolescence. Even the diameter of the head shows a small growth increase in most people. Although growth essentially ceases in late adolescence, minimal growth can continue into early adulthood. The epiphyses of the long bones, though not all fusing at the same time, cannot once fused be stimulated to grow again, as seen in Figure 13-2 (Guthrie, 1979). The maturing of bone (*ossification*) can be observed by increasing numbers of dark areas on x-ray film as calcium is deposited in the cartilage and the bone grows. This process of cartilage degeneration and bone replacement is completed by approximately 25 years of age, or adulthood. The processes of bone maintenance, the deposition and resorption of calcium salts, however, continue throughout adulthood, decreasing somewhat with old age.

Bones that grow by surface deposition may continue to grow in response to stimulation at any stage of the life cycle. Physical stress stimulates formation of new bone material; thus, athletes often have bones of higher density. In contrast, the weightless astronaut or the immobile invalid may lose large amounts of bone calcium unless exercised (Arlin, 1977;

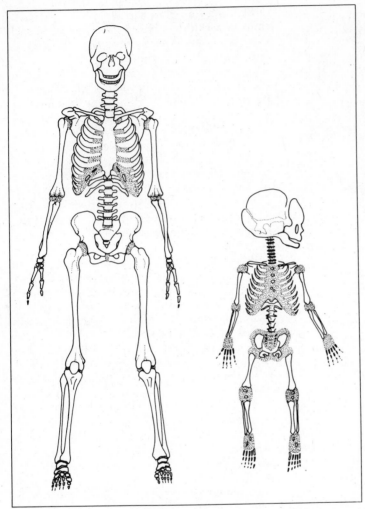

Figure 13-2. Closure of epiphyses of bones in the adult.

Timiras, 1972). The jaw and bones of the face will respond to abnormally increased levels of growth hormone; this is seen in *acromegaly*, a condition accompanied by a tumor and hyperfunctioning of the anterior pituitary.

Between the third and fifth decades of life, a general phenomenon of bone loss occurs, progressing twice as fast in postmenopausal women as in men. Certain factors, such as small stature, hasten bone loss whereas less bone loss occurs in taller people (Pike and Brown, 1975).

Composition
Bone is cellular and well vasculated, with a collagenous protein matrix that has been im-

pregnated with mineral salts, especially phosphates of calcium.

Osteoblasts are the bone-forming cells that secrete collagen. Collagen polymerizes rapidly to form collagen fibers. The resulting tissue becomes *osteoid*, a cartilage like material that differs from cartilage in that calcium salts are precipated in it. As the osteoid is being formed, some osteoblasts become entrapped in the osteoid and are then called *osteocytes*. Osteocytes initiate processes in the *canaliculi* (channels) that dispurse throughout the bone and are capable of considerable bone resorption. *Osteoclasts* are multinuclear cells that erode and resorb previously formed bone. All types of bone cells arise from a common *stem cell*. Transformation from one cell to the other is frequent. Osteoblasts or osteocytes are both formed from the same root cell. Either cell has potential for being formed, depending on the role the cell is needed to play. These interchangeable activities of the cells enable a fractured bone to heal and remodel in accordance with the applied stresses (Ganong, 1977; Guyton, 1977; Zuidema, 1977).

Bones of small children are relatively pliable because they contain a larger proportion of cartilage and a smaller amount of the firm calcium salts than those of adults. In old age, by contrast, there is less of the softer tissues such as cartilage and a much higher proportion of calcium salts. Thus, bones of the elderly are brittle. Bone fractures in the elderly heal with difficulty, mainly because of their relatively high proportion of inert material and the small amount of vascular softer tissues.

Long bone shafts are made of a hollow cylinder of hard, compact bone containing marrow. Compact bone is nearly as strong as cast iron but much more flexible. In adults the marrow is primarily fatty with a small amount of hematopoietic marrow at the shaft ends of long bone. The formed elements of blood—red cells, white cells, and platelets—originate in the bone marrow cavity (Bett et al., 1976; Zuidema, 1977).

Nutrition

Calcium and phosphorus are the primary crystalline salts deposited in the organic matrix of bone. These inorganic salts consist of small crystals of calcium phosphate in the form of *hydroxyapatite* and of noncrystalline, or amorphous, *tricalcium phosphate*. Small amounts of magnesium, sodium, carbonate, citrate, chlorine, and fluorine are also present (Bell et al., 1976; Mitchell et al., 1976).

Initiation of calcification involves fixation of phosphorus to the matrix of bone. Failure of calcification to occur can result from lack of either calcium or phosphorus. Calcification of cartilage is defective in vitamin D deficiency, so that the epiphyseal cartilage is much wider than normal. Vitamin A is required for the deposition of cartilage at the growing ends of bones.

The calcium of bone is of two types: a readily exchangeable reservoir and a larger pool of only slowly exchangeable, stable calcium. Plasma calcium is in equilibrium with the readily exchangeable bone calcium (Ganong, 1977). Figure 13-3 illustrates calcium turnover in a healthy person. Urinary and fecal excretion equal calcium intake from dietary sources while bone resorption and accretion are equal. The parathyroid hormone controls the resorption of calcium from bone; *thyrocalcitonin*, a thyroid hormone, inhibits calcium withdrawal from bone (Bell et al., 1976).

Differing nutritional conditions cause the relative ratio of calcium to vary greatly in the body. On a weight basis, the calcium to phosphorus ratio varies between 1.3 and 2.0 (Guyton, 1977). Rate of skeletal development determines bone calcium needs. Children tend to store calcium at an accelerated rate during the year or so that precedes the periods of rapid gains in height. Children and pregnant women maintain a calcium to phosphorus ratio of approximately 1.0 (Williams,

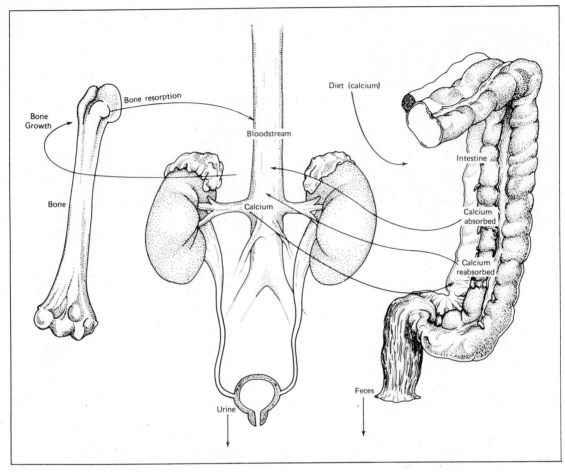

Figure 13-3. Calcium turnover in the healthy person.

1977). Adults have a calcium ratio of approximately 1.5 (Bell, et al., 1976). Throughout life, mineral in the skeleton is being actively turned over, and bone is continuously being remodeled and maintained. Calcium in bone turns over at a rate of 100% a year in infants and 18% a year in adults (Ganong, 1977).

Bone matrix, composed primarily of collagen, is also composed of *glucosaminoglycans,* glycoproteins, lipids, and peptides. Collagen contains a unique amino acid, *hydroxyproline,* whose formation requires the presence of as-

corbic acid. Bone mineral can be added or removed from the matrix, depending on the body's need for calcium.

Nutritional Imbalance

Bone mineralization is impaired when vitamin D is deficient. The deformed bones symptomatic of *rickets* indicate abnormal calcium metabolism and incorporation into the bones. As illustrated in Figure 13-4, rickets is a deficiency disease characterized by pliable, malformed, and distorted bones. The result-

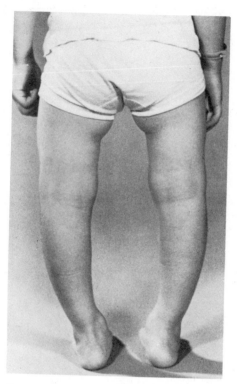

Figure 13-4. Infant with bowed legs of rickets. (Photo courtesy of Upjohn Co.)

ing enlargement or beading of the ribs (frequently called the *rachitic rosary*), enlarged wrists and ankles, bowed legs, or knock knees appear when the bones are too soft to support the child learning to walk. Early symptoms of rickets in infants are profuse sweating and restlessness.

Calcium, phosphorus, and vitamin D are the major nutrients involved in the prevention of rickets. In geographical regions where exposure to sunshine is limited, a vitamin D supplement or cod liver oil is recommended for infants who are breastfed. Commercial formulas in the United States contain vitamin D supplements.

Between the third and fifth decades of life, bone resorption exceeds bone accretion, and there is a slow but progressive loss of bone (Bell et al., 1976; Pike and Brown, 1975). This resulting condition of bone becoming more porous is called *osteoporosis*. Surveys indicate that 15–50% of elderly people over the age of 65 in the United States suffer from osteoporosis. The incidence is shown to be four-to-six times greater in women than in men. Approximately 14 million women suffer from various forms of the disease (Arlin, 1977). At present, no satisfactory evidence indicates that bone loss is due to low calcium intakes or that protection is afforded by high intakes. Epidemiological observations suggest that fluorine plays a significant role in this relationship. Experimental studies indicate simultaneously increased consumption of fluorine and calcium results in harder bones, because of the incorporation of fluorine with calcium into newly formed hydroxyapatite crystals. Fluorine increases bone crystallinity and decreases bone mobility (Wei, 1974).

A constant and normal concentration of ionized calcium in the extracellular fluid is of great importance in the activity of several enzymes (Bell et al., 1976). For example, the stability of collagen in connective tissue and bone also depends on cross linkages that require oxidative deamination steps involving oxidases. Lack of these enzymes and ascorbic acid oxidase, another copper-containing metalloenzyme, are thought to contribute to the pathogenesis of skeletal lesions characterized by a copper-deficient state (Hambidge, 1977).

Retarded growth in preschool children is consistent with zinc deficiency. Severe depletion of chromium, a cofactor for insulin, may cause impaired growth. Magnesium deficiency can explain extensive skeletal abnormalities associated with impaired activity of the epiphyseal cartilage plate (Hambidge, 1977).

Lead and some toxic elements are taken up and released by bone in a manner similar to calcium turn over. Because it serves to remove them from the body fluids, the rapid bone uptake of these elements is sometimes called a *detoxifying mechanism.* The radioactive elements radium, plutonium, and strontium are also taken up by bone, however, which is a harmful situation because radiation from these elements may cause malignant degeneration of bone cells and the formation of osteogenic sarcomas (Ganong, 1977).

Teeth

Nutrition plays a significant role in the formation and development of the teeth; conversely, the teeth exert considerable influence on the nutritional status of their owners. They determine the capacity to consume an adequate diet. Painful or loose teeth, missing teeth, and poorly fitting bridges and dentures all interfere with normal chewing and ingestion of certain foods so that the diet frequently has to be limited to a few foods that can be eaten without discomfort (Arlin, 1977).

The major functional parts of the masticatory apparatus are the teeth and the *periodontium.* The major parts of the teeth are *enamel, dentin, cementum,* and *pulp.* The tooth can also be divided into the *crown* (the portion that protrudes out of the gum into the mouth) and the root (the portion that protrudes into the bony socket of the jaw). The collar between the crown and the root, where the tooth is surrounded by gum, is the *neck* (Guyton, 1976). The tissues that surround and support the tooth are known as the *periodontium.* Anatomically, the periodontal structures are described as the *gingiva,* the *periodontal ligament,* the *alveolar bone,* and the cementum. See Figure 13-5 for an illustration of the parts of a tooth.

Functions
The purpose of the teeth is to cut, grind, and mix food. To perform these functions, the jaws have powerful muscles capable of a maximal occlusive force of 50–100 lb between the front teeth and 150–200 lb between the jaw teeth. Lower and upper teeth are provided

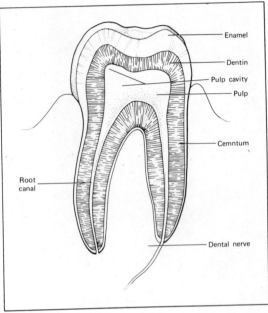

Figure 13-5. Functional parts of a tooth. (Redrawn by permission from *Textbook of Medical Physiology,* 5th Ed., by A. C. Guyton. Philadelphia: W. B. Saunders Co., 1976.)

with projections and facets that interdigitate to allow each set of teeth to fit with the other. Occlusion, or fitting, allows even small particles of food to be caught and ground between the teeth surfaces (Guyton, 1976).

Development
The earliest teeth are called the *deciduous,* or *milk,* teeth. These 20 teeth begin to calcify in the fetus around the twentieth week of prenatal life (Mitchell, et al., 1976). They erupt in the mouth between the seventh month after birth and the second year of life. They remain until the sixth through the thirteenth year. After each deciduous tooth is lost, a permanent tooth replaces it. An additional 8–12 teeth also erupt. The permanent teeth number 28 to 32, depending on whether the four *wisdom teeth* appear. Not all four wisdom teeth erupt in everyone. Calcification of the

permanent teeth begins at birth (with the first permanent molar, or 6-year-old molar) and ends around the age of 16 years (with the wisdom teeth) (Mitchell et al., 1976).

Teeth erupt by protruding upward from the jaw bone through the oral epithelium into the mouth. The cause of eruption is currently unknown, though several theories exist. Teething is often a time when gum discomfort causes a child to become irritable, especially at feeding time.

Teeth structures, particularly dentin and enamel, are metabolically more stable than bone. Once teeth are completely matured there is not a continuous state of mineral salt resorption and deposition as in bone. Pregnant women whose diets are inadequate in calcium were once thought to calcify the fetal skeleton by calcium lost from their teeth. The old adage A Tooth for Every Child has since been disproven. In such circumstances an expectant mother might lose calcium from her bones, including her jaw bone, but it is less probable that she derives calcium from her teeth (Arlin, 1977).

Teeth become more firmly seated in the jaws as one reaches adulthood and older. This results from the cumulatively applied pressure and strain on the teeth from chewing and grinding, which cause the layer of cementum to become thicker and stronger (Guyton, 1976).

Composition

The outer surface of the tooth is covered prior to its eruption by a layer of enamel that is formed by special epithelial cells, called *ameoblasts*. Once erupted, no more enamel is formed on the tooth. Enamel is composed of small hydroxyapatite crystals with adsorbed carbonate, magnesium, sodium, potassium, and other ions embedded in a fine meshwork of very strong and almost completely insoluble protein fibers similar to (but not identical with) the *keratin* of hair. The small size of the crystalline salt structure makes the enamel extremely hard, much harder than dentin. The

special protein-fiber meshwork makes enamel very resistant to acids, enzymes, and other corrosive agents. The calcium salts in dentin make it extremely resistant to compressional forces, while the collagen fibers make it tough and resistant to tensions that result from solid objects striking the teeth.

Cementum, a bony substance secreted by cells of the periodontal membrane, lines the anatomic roots of the teeth. Bundles of continuous, intermingling collagen fibers, which are produced by fibroblasts with the periodontal membrane, form periodontal ligaments that run from the tooth root to the alveolar bone proper. By being embedded into the alveolar bone and the cementum, these fibers serve as the primary attachment of the tooth in the bony socket.

Pulp, the inside portion of each tooth, is composed of connective tissue with an abundant supply of nerves, blood vessels, and *lymphatics*. The cells lining the surface of the pulp cavity are called *odontoblasts*. The odontoblasts remain viable throughout life and send projections into small dentinal tubules that penetrate all the way through the dentin. These tubules provide an important pathway for nutrition (Guyton, 1976).

Nutrition

Few adults in Western countries are free of tooth decay. Studies estimate that only about 2% of the US population have no dental cavities. *Dental caries* is a microbial disease of childhood that causes loss of tooth substance, mainly in the pit and fissure and on the interproximal surfaces of the crown and less frequently on the back surfaces. Dental caries has no single cause; it is instead a disease in which environmental factors play a decisive role. The ecological triad for dental caries includes the presence of specific cariogenic microorganisms, a susceptible tooth, and dietary factors.

Poor tooth structure, reflected by increased susceptibility to dental caries, may be the result of inadequate calcium during the periods of teeth formation (Mitchell et al., 1976). *Nursing bottle syndrome*, a condition resulting from excessively prolonged sucking on the bottle during the tooth-erupting stage, induces an irregular shape and decay of the teeth (Wei, 1974). Although the nutritional environment exerts little influence on the structure of mature adult teeth, it profoundly influences their development in the prenatal stage and is important in encouraging and sustaining bacterial colonies on the teeth surfaces in subsequent years (Arlin, 1977).

Heredity, combined with nutrition during tooth development, affects resistance to decay at a later date (Mitchell et al., 1976). Probably the most important factor in caries prevention is the acid-resistant enamel that results when fluoridated water is consumed from infancy until the last tooth has erupted (Arlin, 1977). Water sources that do not provide adequate amounts of fluoride, that is, well or spring water, can be standardized to a concentration of 1 m/liter of water. Public health authorities, in areas where the drinking water is low in fluoride content advocate the fluoridation of public drinking water in the amount of 1 ppm (Mitchell et al., 1976).

Dental plaque is an assemblage of microorganisms that adheres directly to the tooth surface. Organisms within dental plaque do not require dietary foodstuffs for survival and growth. Diet composition, especially its sucrose content, will, however, affect the metabolism and pathogenic potential of dental plaque, particularly with regard to dental caries. A diet with a high sucrose content, especially of a sticky consistency, will aid in plaque adhesion and selectively influence retention of nutrients and metabolic products within plaque. Frequent ingestion of carbohydrate, especially sucrose, will affect the composition of the oral microbiota by promoting the growth of acidogenic and aciduric types of organisms and preventing the survival and growth of acid-sensitive types.

Physical consistency of food will also affect microbial retention and growth at various sites in the oral cavity. Salivary gland function is selectively influenced by diet consistency and taste. Liquid diets have been shown to cause a significant reduction in the principal salivary buffer, bicarbonate. Hard or fibrous foods have the opposite effect (Morhart and Fitzgerald, 1976).

Thus, good oral hygiene and less frequent consumption of sweets will help reduce the incidence of dental caries. Foods that adhere to the teeth, like caramels, pastries, chocolates, and candied apples, are especially damaging. Soft drinks, sweetened juices, and hard candies can also be harmful. Carrot sticks, apples, and "roughage foods" have a protective influence on dental health (Mitchell et al., 1976).

Nutritional Imbalance

Calcium, phosphorous, and vitamin D deficiencies during and preceding eruption of teeth account for some of the faulty tooth structure. The teeth, once developed, are less apt to be influenced by diet. Inadequate vitamin A produces faulty enamel-forming epithelial cells, thus impairing the soundness of the tooth structure. Vitamin C deficiency affects the collagen framework of dentin (Arlin, 1977).

Calcification of the teeth may be influenced by various genetic, nutritional, and hormonal factors as well as by the use of certain medications during developmental stages. As a somewhat permanent health record, the teeth show manifestations of past diseases by changes in structural form and color (Timiras, 1972). An increased consumption of selenium during tooth development, for example, has been associated with a high incidence of dental caries (Hambidge, 1977).

Excess fluoride is recognized in some geographical areas as the cause of mottled enamel in the permanent teeth. This condition, endemic in a few areas such as the Texas panhandle, is commonly known as *dental fluorosis*. Very mild or mild mottling can occur when fluoride in the drinking water ranges between 2 and 5 ppm. Moderate or severe mottling can occur when fluoride in drinking water is above 5 ppm (Menaker, 1980; Morhart, 1979).

Table 13-1 illustrates the interdependency of nutrients in the development and maturation of bones and teeth. A deficiency of any nutrient results in a physiological change within the system. Onset of a deficiency disease is subject to the amount and duration of the deficient nutrients. Excessive or antagonistic trace metals compete for ionized substances to which they can attach themselves. This interference results in an inability of the system to develop and function normally.

MUSCULAR SYSTEM

The major skeletal or longitudinal growth of the body is a result of bone development, but growth of the muscular system accounts for a considerable portion of the increase in body weight. Muscles constitute approximately 43% of adult body weight, contain more than one-third of all the body proteins, and contribute about one-half of the metabolic activity of the resting body.

Both the skeletal and muscular systems are fundamental to the development and maintenance of the body's shape, posture, and locomotion. Influenced by the center of gravity located near the spine, changes that take place in the skeleton and muscles during infancy are consolidated in the erect posture attained in early childhood.

The structural units of muscle consist of thousands of fibers or cells. The three broad classes of muscle differ in structure (histologically), location (anatomically), function (physiologically), and in their manner of innervation (neurologically) (Schottelius and Schottelius, 1978; Timiras, 1972).

Functions

Despite the various functions and characteristic differences of muscles, they possess in common the property of contractility. Muscles are essentially machines for converting chemical energy into mechanical work. They allow purposeful movement of the whole body from one point to another or movement of a limited body part in respect to the whole body or the environment. Posture is maintained against the effects of gravity. Vital processes, such as contraction of the heart, con-

TABLE 13-1. Nutrients and the Skeletal System

Normal Structural Component	Nutrients or Nutrient Compounds	Abnormal State of Nutrient Imbalance
Bones Joints Ligaments Cartilage Collagen Teeth Enamel Dentin Cementum Pulp	*Major* Calcium, phosphorus, vitamin D *Auxiliary* Magnesium, sodium, potassium, carbonate, citrate, chlorine, fluorine, copper, chromium, zinc, vitamins A and C, glucosaminoglycans, glucoproteins, lipids, peptides, hydroxyproline *Antagonists* Lead, selenium, radium, plutonium, strontium	*Deficiencies* Rickets, osteoporosis, skeletal lesions, retarded growth, faulty tooth structure, faulty enamel formation, dental caries, skeletal lesions *Excesses* Malignant degeneration of bone cells; osteogenic sarcomas; dental caries, fluorosis

NOTE: See Chapters 19 and 24 for further information on clinical signs of nutritional deficiencies.

striction of blood vessels, breathing, and peristalsis all depend on muscular activity (Schottelius and Schottelius, 1978).

Both muscles and liver store glycogen. Approximately 340 gm of glycogen can be stored by a man, 240 gm in the muscles and 100 gm in the liver. Liver glycogen, however, is more quickly available for replenishing blood sugar. Muscle glycogen is used primarily as fuel for the muscles (Mitchell et al., 1976).

The prevention or recovery from objective fatigue, as opposed to subjective fatigue caused by boredom, is a matter of disposal of waste products and the supplying of oxygen and nutrients. Lactic acid and pyruvic acid, intermediate waste products are either oxidized further into carbon dioxide and water or, by the expenditure of energy, are built up into higher compounds, such as glycogen. Lactic acid formed in skeletal muscle may be removed by the circulating blood and carried to the heart, there to be used as such in the production of energy for cardiac activity.

To prevent fatigue, oxygen and nutrients must also be brought to the muscles from the "supply organs." These activities all depend on blood circulation and on respiration. Onset of fatigue is hastened by any interference with the blood supply, as is seen in the contracted position of leg muscles during motionless standing. Capillaries and small veins are compressed because of the high degree of tension in the tonically contracting muscles, and circulation is made difficult. Hence, this form of work, as distinct from rhythmic muscular activity (e.g., walking), fatigues a person rapidly (Schottelius and Schottelius, 1978).

Development

Muscles are generally divided into three types: smooth, cardiac, and skeletal. Refer to Figure 13-6. *Smooth* (also called unstriated, visceral, or involuntary) muscles possess a single, centrally located nucleus and are devoid of cross striations, although they exhibit faint longitudinal striations. The fibers, found in the walls of internal or visceral organs (generally hollow organs), are usually not subject to conscious control and receive their innervation through the autonomic nervous system. *Cardiac* (heart) muscle fibers possess cells that show both longitudinal and imperfect cross striations and have a single nucleus. Cardiac muscle is innervated by the autonomic nervous system. *Skeletal* (striated or voluntary) muscle fibers are multinucleated and display longitudinal and cross striations. In nearly all instances these muscles are attached to bones. To a large extent their innervation is under voluntary control (Schottelius and Schottelius, 1978).

The number of fibers in a muscle increase considerably with maturation. The thickness of muscle fiber increases dramatically between the first and seventh year of life, changes very little in the preadolescent period, undergoes accelerated growth at approximately 14 years of age, and continues to grow up to and beyond the twenty-fifth year of life. There seems to be no built-in limit to the potential thickness of a muscle. It is known to decrease in old age when general atrophy occurs. Physical activity and gymnastics at any age are capable of exerting considerable influence on muscle fiber thickness, especially during adolescence but also to some extent in adult life. Adult muscle growth consequent to strenuous exercise is believed to be due to an increase in diameter of individual fibers rather than an increase in cell number. Excess body weight from the accumulation of fat lessens muscle efficiency (Schottelius and Schottelius, 1978).

Muscle tissue, once injured, repairs itself only with difficulty or not at all. Injured tissues are frequently replaced with scar (connective) tissue.

Composition

The structural single unit of a muscle is the fiber. A muscle fiber is composed of a number

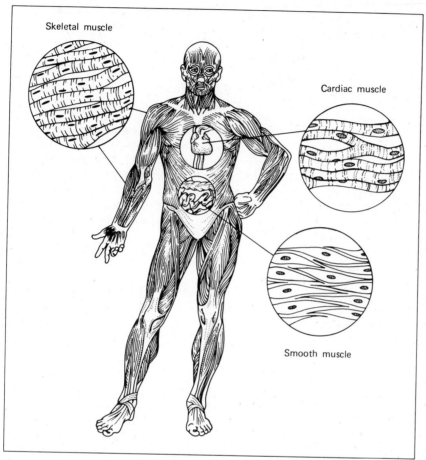

Skeletal muscle

Cardiac muscle

Smooth muscle

Figure 13-6. Muscles of the human body and the three major types of muscles. (Redrawn with permission from R. L. Memmler and D. L. Wood, *The Human Body in Health and Disease*, 4th Ed. Philadelphia: J. B. Lippincott Co., 1977.)

of delicate *fibrils* (one of the fine threads into which a striated muscle can be longitudinally split) surrounded by a semifluid *sarcoplasm* (muscle-fiber protoplasm). A respiratory pigment, *myoglobin* (muscle hemoglobin), that functions in the transport of oxygen from the capillaries to the oxidation sites (the mitochondria) is also present in the sarcoplasm. Some fibers contain more myoglobin than others and are called red muscles. This red-pigmented protein resembles red blood cell hemoglobin, which contains iron, and gives the fiber a red appearance. Fibers deficient in myoglobin are pale or white. Most muscles contain both kinds of fibers. Muscle fibers rich in myoglobin have a high capacity for oxidative metabolism and electron transport enzymes. A high rate of anaerobic glycolysis with intense activity of glycolytic enzymes and phosphorylase are characteristic of white muscle fibers.

Red fibers, considerably slower in their contractile action, undergo fatigue less rapidly than white fibers. Thus red fibers are well adapted for static or postural contractions. Body posture is largely achieved by muscles well supplied with red fibers. Changes in body or limb position, on the other hand, are brought about by the more rapidly acting white fibers predominat in flexor muscles.

Many of the nonprotein constituents of muscle are soluble in water (75% of muscle composition is water) and are usually spoken of as extractives. These substances include components of the glycolytic cycle: creatine, creatine phosphate, ATP, ADP, amino acids, and lactic acid. One of the most important substances in muscle cells is ATP. An energy-rich bond links the terminal phosphate group of this compound to the structure. Rupturing of this bond produces inorganic phosphate and ADP, with the simultaneous release of a large amount of energy.

$$ATP \rightarrow ADP + H_3PO_4 + Energy$$

The breakdown of ATP releases energy used in the performance of work.

Carbohydrate in muscle is present mostly as glycogen. Lipids constitute about 2% of muscle weight, and salts about 1%. The principal salt ion is potassium. Only small amounts of sodium, calcium, chlorine, and magnesium are present.

The enzyme components of muscle that catalyze the steps in glycolysis (the breakdown of glycogen to CO_2 and H_2O) are proteins. Other muscle proteins include different enzymes and the structural proteins. Greater than one-half of the total protein in skeletal muscle is made up of structural proteins: *actin, myosin, tropomyosin,* and *troponin* (Schottelius and Schottelius, 1978).

Nutrition

Muscle function requires sources of energy for regeneration of ATP. Both fatty acids and glucose, derived principally from glycogen, are used, the proportion varying relative to the kind of work being done. Fatty acids provide most of the energy for resting muscle and light-to-moderate physical activity. Glucose, a more rapidly mobilized fuel, will furnish energy in the absence of oxygen. It is called on to generate a quick burst of energy or to supplement the oxygen-requiring fatty acids during extended periods of vigorous exercise. The capacity to meet demands required of marathon or skiing races often depends on the extent of glycogen reserves available in liver and muscle tissues (Arlin, 1977).

Myoglobin, related to blood hemoglobin in both structure and function, is found only in muscle tissue. Small but essential amounts of iron, found in myoglobin, are capable of supplying oxygen to the muscles (Mitchell et al., 1976).

The contracting unit of muscle, the *myofibril*, contains filaments of actin and myosin, two proteins found only in muscle. Approximately 2,500 of these filaments, bundled into each myofibril, are arranged in alternate layers. On receipt of a nerve impulse, the filaments of actin and myosin slide along each other and shorten the muscle fiber. They resume their original positions during relaxation, and the fiber lengthens. A delicate balance of calcium, sodium, and potassium ions govern the transmission of nerve impulses to the muscle fiber. Calcium and magnesium ions are involved in the reactions that cause filaments of actin and myosin to move across each other (Arlin, 1977). Sodium ions, which play a large part in transmitting electrochemical impulses along nerve and muscle membranes, maintain normal muscle irritability and excitability. Sodium and potassium ions regulate the nerve response to stimulation, the transport of nerve impulses to muscles, and the resulting contraction of the muscle fibers. Ionized potassium is a significant component in the activity of striated (skeletal and cardiac) muscle. Ionized chlorine provides the main balancing anion in the extracellular fluid.

Storage of nitrogen as muscle protein requires potassium. When muscle tissue is broken down, potassium together with nitrogen is lost in muscle protein (Williams, 1977).

Nutritional Imbalance

In some body structures, nutrition and the ability for continued muscle functioning depend to a certain extent on their own activity. This phenomenon is especially true for skeletal muscles, in which nutrition and function are inseparable. No matter how well supplied with blood and food, an inactive muscle undergoes atrophy (progressive wasting) (Schottelius and Schottelius, 1978). The body will support the maintenance of muscle tissue only when there is a demonstrated need. Unused muscles degenerate rapidly and often are replaced with fatty tissue. Consuming large amounts of protein without additional exercise will support not muscle development but fat production (Arlin, 1977).

Abnormal serum levels of sodium may adversely affect the function of muscles such as the cardiac muscle. Studies suggest that hypertension is most common among population groups who consume an excessive salt intake and least common in groups who consume very little salt (Christakis, 1974; Wilson et al., 1979).

Marked loss of potassium from muscle tissue in malnutrition can be measured by decreased hand-grip strength. A plasma potassium level less than 3.5 mEq/liber is often accompanied by a disorder of smooth-muscle function. Muscle weakness and cardiac arrhythmias may occur. Occasionally ascending skeletal-muscle paralysis and interference in

the muscle functions of respiration and swallowing lead to a serious and sometimes fatal event (Goodhart and Shils, 1973).

Decreased ionized serum calcium causes tetany, a state of severe, intermittent spastic contractions of the muscle and muscular pain. Tetanylike responses may be caused by an increase in the serum phosphorus fraction in the ratio of calcium to phosphorus. "Milk tetany" is a condition that has been reported in newborns fed undiluted cow's milk. The calcium to phosphorus ratio in cow's milk is greater than in human milk. Because the kidneys of these infants could not clear the phosphorus load, elevated serum phosphorus levels caused a compensatory serum calcium decrease and in turn caused tetanic muscular spasms (Williams, 1977). Tetany can occur at serum calcium levels below 30% of normal (Arlin, 1977). Magnesium deficiency is also characterized by twitching, tremors, irregular pulse, muscle weakness, jerkiness, leg and foot cramps, and shaking hands (Wilson et al., 1979).

Selenium has a sparing effect on vitamin E. Although the mechanism and significance of its effect on human muscle are not known at this time, it has been shown to be beneficial in certain experimental animals with muscle disorders (Arlin, 1977). Selenium supplements have been known to prevent muscular dystrophy in vitamin E deficient lambs (Hambidge, 1977).

As depicted in Table 13-2, muscles are dependent on their nutritional supply both for growth and performance. In the absence of adequate protein and exercise their structural fibers become wasted. These conditions occur when the diet provides an inadequate supply of Calories or protein, as in famine, poverty, postsurgical mismanagement of diet, and the inability of some elderly to provide adequately for themselves. In disease conditions when there is an imbalance of ions or energy sources, normal work performance is diminished and fibers atrophy. Normal devel-

TABLE 13-2. Nutrients and the Muscular System

Normal Structural Component	Nutrients or Nutrient Compounds	Abnormal State of Nutrient Imbalance
Muscle fiber Myoglobin Myofibril	*Major* Water, glucose, glycogen, lipids, proteins, i.e., actin, myosin, tropomyosin, troponin, iron *Auxiliary* Lactic acid, amino acids, creatine, creatine phosphate, ATP, ADP, potassium, sodium, calcium, chlorine, magnesium, nitrogen *Antagonists* Phosphorus	*Deficiencies* Muscular atrophy, muscle weakness, cardiac arrhythmias, tetany, twitching, jerking, leg and foot cramps, irregular pulse *Excesses* "Milk tetany" of newborn

NOTE: See Chapters 19 and 24 for further information on clinical signs of nutritional deficiencies.

opment and maturation depends on adequate Calorie and protein sources acting together in an environment where exercise (voluntary or involuntary muscle use) stimulates hormonal release and resulting nutrient compounds.

NERVOUS SYSTEM

The nervous system is the main coordinator of the body's activities. The central processing unit, as well as the memory, is located in the brain. Each body system is in direct communication with the brain by means of its own computer cables called *nerves*. The nerves from even the most remote parts of the body come together and form the lead cable called the *spinal cord,* which in turn enters the main terminal, or the brain. Messages come in and are processed, and relayed responses are emitted 24 hours a day. This entire communication network including the brain is made up of nerve tissue. Sometimes these processes rise to conscious levels, but frequently activities of the body are regulated without conscious awareness.

Functions

The primary role of the nervous system is to regulate the numerous activities of the body by delegating assignments or appropriating functions to the body's respective systems or organs. It receives cues from the external environment and internal mechanisms. In addition, such components as the brain support a very high level of intellectual and metabolic activity.

The nervous system can be divided into central and peripheral portions. The brain and spinal cord constitute the central nervous system CNS. Outside the CNS 43 pairs of nerves leave the cerebrospinal axis and pass to the various organs of the body. These peripheral nerves contain *afferent,* or sensory, fibers carrying nerve impulses *from* the periphery *to* the CNS and *efferent,* or motor fibers, carrying impulses *from* the CNS *to* muscles, glands, and other organs (Bell et al., 1976) (see Fig. 13-7).

Nerve cells, or neurons, have a specialized capacity to conduct and to connect with other nerve cells or with *receptors* or *effectors* (Timiras, 1972). Points of junction for trans-

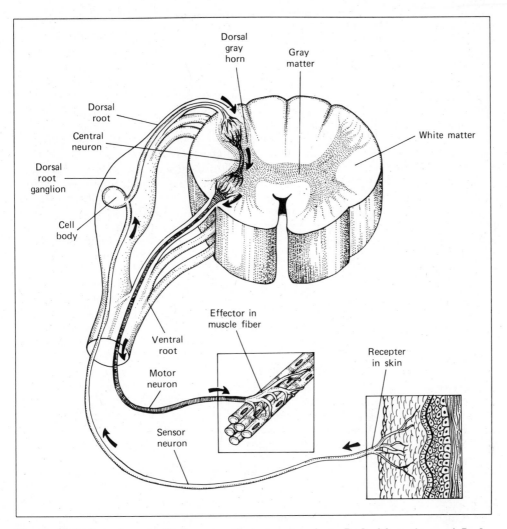

Figure 13-7. Spinal cord. (Redrawn with permission from R. L. Memmler and D. L. Wood, *The Human Body in Health and Disease*, 4th Ed. Philadelphia: J. B. Lippincott Co., 1977.)

mission of nerve impulses are called *synapses,* from the Greek word meaning "to clasp."

The afferent nerves bring information to the CNS about the external world from receptors that are sensitive to light, sound, temperature, or pressure stimuli and also information about the internal state of the body, for example, about muscle tension. Arrival of these impulses produces impulses that the CNS sends along the efferent nerves to induce appropriate movements of muscles or secretion of glands. Although the pathways taken by impulses once they arrive at the CNS are very complex, the basic principle is that impulses are handed on from nerve cell to nerve cell until finally they emerge in an efferent nerve to produce a response in an effector organ such as a muscle or a gland (Bell et al., 1976).

As cable wires are insulated to keep them from short-circuiting, so are nerve fibers, which transmit a current similar to electricity. Insulating material of nerve fiber is called *myelin*. Myelin lowers the nerve-fiber threshold and increases both conduction velocity and the ability to carry repetitive impulses (Timiras, 1972). Groups of these fibers are called *white matter* because of their appearance. Not all nerves have myelin. Nerves that control action of the glands, the smooth muscles and the heart do not. The cell bodies of all nerve cells also are not covered with myelin. Nerve cells to begin with are all gray. Because a large collection of cell bodies are found in the brain, the great mass of brain tissue is termed *gray matter*.

The function of the autonomic nervous system is to regulate actions of glands, the smooth muscles, and the heart. Whenever a change calling for a regulatory adjustment occurs, it is automatic without any conscious awareness.

The sympathetic nervous system acts largely as an accelerator, especially under stress conditions. Once the crisis has passed, the parasympathetic part of the autonomic system acts as a balance for the sympathetic system.

Cerebrospinal fluid (CSF) acts as a cushion between the brain's soft and delicate substance and the rigid skull. In addition to supporting the weight of the brain, it distributes the force of blows on the head. CSF also acts as a "valve" in that high concentrations of solutes in the extracellular fluid of the brain diffuse into the CSF and are carried into the blood (Bell et al., 1976).

Development

Although development of the neurological system begins early in embryonic life, nervous structures develop at differing rates and are not completed until after puberty. Periods of active growth and differentiation of the CNS are referred to as *critical periods* in its development. The plasticity of the neurological system, that is, its capacity to be molded by social, cultural, and nutritional influences, is most dramatically demonstrated by its greater susceptibility during these significant developmental stages. The function of the adult neurological system, therefore, can only be considered an outcome of genetic, biological, and environmental factors (Timiras, 1972).

Throughout the fetal period the human brain is relatively large. During postnatal years, however, the spinal cord increases from .9 to 2% of the brain weight. The spinal cord is considered to be the most organized part of the CNS. Although secondary form changes occur, the spinal cord preserves its early embryonic tubelike shape throughout life. A column of central gray matter is divided into two principal regions: dorsal, which is chiefly sensory, and ventral, which is predominantly motor. By the fourth fetal month, the gray substance is arranged into essentially the adult form.

Development of myelin around many fibers in the marginal layer of the spinal cord is responsible for the appearance of a peripheral layer of white substance arranged in tracts, which attains maturity in the middle of the prenatal period. Continued myelin deposition in the cervical cord and extending progressively to lower levels accounts for the thickening of the white substance until adolescence. Ventral root fibers acquire myelin before the dorsal roots. Last in the spinal cord to develop are certain descending motor tracts which myelinate during the first and second years of life.

Beginning with the second fetal month, the relatively simple spinal cord structure is gradually superseded by a more complex secondary system. Thus, during fetal development the once independent and autonomous spinal cord is placed under the control of higher centers in the brain (Timiras, 1972).

The active period of brain and spinal cord cell multiplication begins in early fetal life and proceeds through two peaks of cell division or deoxyribonucleic acid (DNA) synthesis. The first stage marks the development of neurons, or basic nerve cells. All 10,000 million neurons are formed by the sixth month of prenatal life. The second stage is *glial-cell* development. Each neuron is surrounded by about 10 glial cells. Glial cells multiply rapidly, especially in the last few months of prenatal life and the first 18 postnatal months (Bell et al., 1976; Christakis et al.). Neurons generally do not undergo further division after differentiation, whereas glial cells continue to proliferate throughout life. Although numbers of neurons in CNS structures remain constant, neuronal volume increases during early stages of maturation. Number, and perhaps volume, of the glial cells increases with maturation of the CNS. The constancy in the number of neurons is perhaps significant in the role they play in the memory processes: the storage and availability of experiences throughout life. Glial-cell function includes response to injury by foreign agents; regulation of neuronal metabolism; and the contribution of electrical activity to the retina, brain, and spinal cord. Glial cells participate in development, degeneration, regeneration, myelination, demyelination, and allergic responses of the brain. They are also thought to play a role in the process of transmitting impulses across the synapse and to serve for storage and retrieval of innate and learned behavioral responses (Timiras, 1972).

Myelin formation reaches its peak of development between the ages of 1 and 2 years and continues into the fourth year (Christakis, et al., in press). The slow but final stage of myelin maturation is reached between 13 and 25 years of age (Timiras, 1972).

The critical periods of CNS growth occur between the sixth prenatal month natally and the eighteenth postnatal month, which coincide with the maximum DNA-synthesis and myelin-formation rates. All brain regions and cell types are most susceptible to insult during these periods of rapid growth (Christakis, et al.).

The progressively slowing responses of the CNS with aging have not been fully understood. Theories exist but are still inconclusive. Obvious changes can be observed, however, in motor function with advancing age. There are varying degrees of loss of fine motor coordination and rapid initiation of movement in older people. Such physiological changes can be observed in the absence of disease, although associated diseases hasten the onset of numerous neurological responses (Timiras, 1972).

Composition

A neuron is the basic structural unit of nerve tissue. It consists of a nerve cell body plus small branches called *fibers*. Neurons can be tremendously long. Neurons are not only distinguished by specific physiological properties but also by differences in their biochemical makeup. Figure 13-8 illustrates the structure of a motor neuron.

The water-soluble proteins of brain tissue are similar to those of other tissues and have a comparable rate of turnover. Lipoproteins of the myelin sheath contain protein with such a low turnover rate that they are almost metabolically inert.

The concentration of free amino acids in brain tissue is eight times higher than in blood plasma. An adequate blood supply to the brain is of utmost importance. More than five seconds' arrest of cerebral circulation is followed by unconsciousness. An arrest of longer than three minutes causes irreparable damage to the gray matter and other brain cells (Bell et al., 1976).

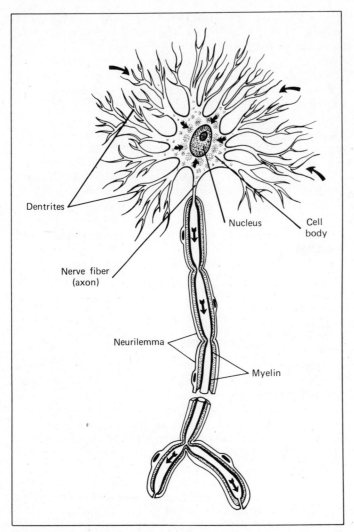

Figure 13-8. Motor neuron. (Redrawn with permission from R. L. Memmler and D. L. Wood, *The Human Body in Health and Disease*, 4th Ed. Philadelphia: J. B. Lippincott Co., 1977.)

Neuroglial cells constitute from one-fourth to one-half of brain-tissue volume. Glial cells are rich in glycogen, contain about one-tenth of the RNA of the neurons, and have more lipid and very much more carbonic anhydrase than neurons. The membrane potential of glial cells is due to the difference in potassium concentration between the interior of the cell and narrow clefts between cells.

Nerve tissue, or clusters of neurons, is supported by connective tissue except in the brain. All peripheral nerves have a thin coating known as *neurilemma*. As part of the repair mechanism, neurilemma aids in the repair of damaged peripheral nerves. On the other hand, the brain and spinal cord have no neurilemma; if injured, their injury is permanent.

A lipid membrane, known as the *blood-brain barrier,* separates the blood from the CSF and the extracellular fluid of the brain. This means that drugs and other lipophobic substances cannot pass directly into the brain; whereas oxygen, carbon dioxide, alcohol, barbituates, glucose, and lipophilic substances pass quickly into the brain from the blood (Bell et al., 1976).

Nutrition

Brain tissue uses glucose almost excusively as its source of energy. This dependence on glucose makes it very sensitive to hypoglycemia. Because the brain stores only about 0.1% glycogen, it does not constitute a significant energy source. In the absence of glucose, for example in fasting and diabetic states, the brain can use small quantities of two ketone bodies, 3-hydroxybutyrate and acetoacetate (Bell et al., 1976).

The CNS is especially rich in lipids, which are primarily associated with membranes such as myelin. Cholesterol, certain phospholipids (and other lipids during brain development) provide, in varying amounts and composition, membranes that serve as a barrier for the diffusion of undesirable substances (Goodhart and Shils, 1973; Timiras, 1972).

Brain and spinal cord development is accompanied by an increase in protein content. At birth, approximately 2% of the body consists of nitrogen. This is contrasted with only slightly over 3% nitrogen in the adult. Most of the nitrogen increase occurs during the first year of life. Considering the role of protein synthesis in cellular development and growth, it is not surprising to find that the periods of greatest nitrogen increase coincide with the critical periods of CNS development. In addition to being constituents of protein, certain amino acids, or neurotransmitters, are thought to have an influential effect on behavior (Christakis et al.; Pike and Brown, 1975; Timiras, 1972). Recent evidence suggests that nutrition-induced changes in the CNS of the elderly may accelerate or retard geriatric changes by influencing brain neurotransmission. The ability of CNS cells to communicate with one another via the release of neurotransmitter compounds may be more insidious and commonplace in the elderly than was previously thought (Lytle and Altar, 1979).

Water and electrolytes play an important role in the physiology and biochemistry of nerve tissue. Magnesium and calcium influence nerve-membrane permeability. Levels of sodium and potassium ions inside and outside the nerve cell facilitate transmission of nerve impulses. The stimulants in such beverages as coffee, tea, and cocoa influence excitability of nerve tissue by increasing the ease of impulse transmission (Arlin, 1977).

The composition of CSF and fluid of the extracellular space of brain is to some extent independent of blood plasma composition. Compared with plasma, CSF contains a higher concentration of sodium and chlorine, making it slightly hypertonic. Both sodium and magnesium seem to be actively transported from the blood to CSF. Glucose content is lower in CSF, and ionized calcium is similar in plasma and CSF (Bell et al., 1976). Normal hydration and electrolyte balance is essential to maintaining a fine-tuned, responsive neurological system.

Because zinc is involved in protein synthesis, it is essential to brain growth in fetal development (Guthrie, 1979; Pike and Brown, 1975). *Carbonic anhydrase,* an enzyme important to respiration, is a protein that contains an atom of zinc in each molecule (Ganong, 1977).

Nutritional Imbalance

Severe protein malnutrition called *kwashiorkor* and protein and Calorie malnutrition known as *marasumus* are conditions that not only predispose children to high morbidity and death rates but subject those who survive to suboptimal neurological development. Extended periods of kwashiorkor or marasumus during the critical periods of CNS growth induce irreversible damage to the neurological system. Protein and Calorie deprivation during other developmental periods may not cause permanent damage, but the effects could be detrimental to overall CNS and behavioral development if rehabilitation does nòt occur early (Adolph, 1972; Mitchell et al., 1976; Christakis et al.).

Beriberi and pellagra, vitamin deficiency diseases, are characterized by symptoms involving degenerative changes in the neurological system. Beriberi, the classical disease of thiamine deficiency, is marked by peripheral nervous disorders and eventual paralysis. Because thiamine is a necessary component of carbohydrate metabolism, early symptoms of thiamine deficiency include impaired neuronal activity, diminished alertness and reflex responses, general apathy, and fatigue.

Pellagra, the deficiency disease caused primarily by lack of niacin, is marked by deterioration of the neurological system resulting in irritability, in signs of emotional instability, and eventually in extreme mental aberration. Tryptophan, as a niacin precursor, is also an important nutrient in preventing pellagra.

Neurological damage associated with vitamin B_{12} deficiency appears to be related to increased levels of branched-chain fatty acids such as methylmalonic acid and its precursor proprionic acid as well as of odd-numbered fatty acids. Patients receiving anticonvulsant therapy have lower CSF levels of folic acid. Administration of folic acid to these patients causes the drug serum level to fall but does not increase the folate level of CSF.

Deficiencies or excesses of trace metals have been shown to effect CNS development and function. One of the chemical transmitters of nerve impulses is acetylcholine. It is released when the nerve cell is stimulated if adequate amounts of calcium ions are present. When blood calcium falls below normal, the characteristic neuromuscular hyperirritability of tetany occurs (Mitchell et al., 1976).

Severe copper deficiency occurs as Menkes's steely-hair syndrome. The hair in this syndrome resembles the steely wool hair seen in copper-deficient sheep. Other features include striking abnormalities of the blood vessels and hypothermia. The progressive neurological degeneration of this disease begins in early infancy, with onset of convulsions at approximately three months of age and death in later infancy or childhood (Hambidge, 1977).

Lead is an example of a metal ingested in excess. Children between the ages of one and six years are sometimes the victims of lead poisoning from ingestion of flaking paint from old dilapidated cribs or houses. Of children who survive lead poisoning, some have permanent neurological damage and others are mentally retarded (Mitchell et al., 1976).

Development of all body tissues, including the brain, depends on normal metabolism of various chemical compounds. Any disturbance in the orderly sequence of maturational events during prenatal life may result in "errors" of metabolism. Many inborn errors of metabolism have been ascribed to genetic factors; the etiology of others is still unknown. Several of these biochemical abnormalities are accompanied by mental retardation. Other chemical dysfunctions are categorized by nutritional classifications, such as carbohydrate (galactosemia, fructosemia), lipids (sphingolipidosis), or amino acids (phenylketonuria) dysfunctions (Timiras, 1972). A description of these diseases and their relationships to CNS development is not within the scope of this unit. For a more extensive description of these inborn errors of metabolism refer to Chapter 27.

To carry out its mission as a central processing, storing, and communications unit, the neurological system depends on a delicately balanced array of nutrients and nutrient compounds. Table 13-3 summarizes some of the major, auxilliary, and antagonistic nutrients involved in the well-being of the human neurological system.

Vision

Vision, as a special sense, is considered part of the nervous system because its "interpretation" is controlled by a specialized area of the cerebral cortex in the brain. Sense impulses arise from receptors designed to report changes that occur either within or outside the body.

Visual sense from the eye is one of the special senses, which also include hearing, taste, smell, and equilibrium. Other senses are hunger, thirst, and touch, which are influenced by sensory mechanisms from muscles, joints, and various internal parts of the body.

Functions
The eyes, within their protective casing, have a layer of receptors, a lens system for focusing light on the receptors, and a system of nerves for conducting impulses from the receptors to the brain. Light rays striking the retina initiate impulses that, when conducted to the brain, produce the sensation of vision. The retina allows the eye to adapt to light or dark environments. The eyes adapt to increased illumination within about five minutes upon passing suddenly from a dim to a brightly lighted environment.

Visual acuity, or 20/20 vision as measured by the Snellen letter charts, is the degree to which details and contours of objects are perceived. Color vision allows for varieties of sensations in hue, intensity, and saturation of nonwhite objects. Range of vision is directed by specialized eye muscles (Ganong, 1977).

Development
The sensory epithelium of the eye, like that of the nervous sytem, begins its development as a neural plate composed of undifferentiated, proliferative epithelial cells. Further development progresses similarly to the CNS system development (Timiras, 1972).

As illustrated in Figure 13-9, the outer layer, or white of the eye, is called the *sclera*. It

TABLE 13-3. Nutrients and the Neurological System

Normal Structural Components	Nutrients or Nutrient Compounds	Abnormal State of Nutrient Imbalance

Brain
Nerve tissue
Sensory receptors and effectors
Synapse
Myelin
Neuron
Glial cell
Cerebral spinal fluid
Spinal cord
Eye
	Major
	  DNA, lipoproteins, amino acids, glycogen, lipid, glucose, protein, thiamine, niacin, vitamin A
	Auxiliary
	  Potassium, cholesterol, phospholipids, nitrogen, water, magnesium, calcium, sodium, chlorine, zinc, copper, vitamin B_{12}, folic acid, riboflavin, vitamin C
	Antagonists
	  Lead
		Deficiencies
		  Kwashiorkor, marasmus, beriberi, pellagra, convulsions, corneal vascularization, night blindness, xerosis
		Excesses
		  Neurological changes and mental retardation

NOTE: See Chapters 19 and 24 for further information on clinical signs of nutritional deficiencies.

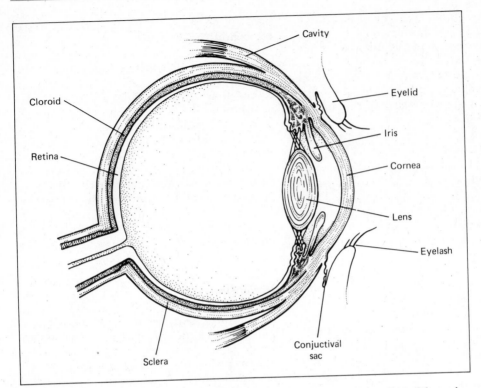

Figure 13-9. Major parts of the eye. (Redrawn with permission from R. L. Memmler and D. L. Wood, *The Human Body in Health and Disease,* 4th Ed. Philadelphia: J. B. Lippincott Co., 1977.)

is made of firm, tough connective tissue. Sclera is modified anteriorly to form the transparent *cornea,* through which light rays enter the eye. A name frequently used for the cornea is "window" of the eye. The *choroid,* or second coating of the eyeball, is a pigmented layer that contains many of the blood vessels that nourish the structures of the eyeball. The inner coat, or *retina,* includes approximately 10 different layers of nerve cells, including the receptors cells known as *rods* and *cones.* These end receptors generate the sense of vision.

The eye is well protected by a strong bony orbit (cavity) and by eyelids, which are lined by *conjunctiva* on their inner surfaces. A number of sensitive hairs (eyelashes) project from the lid. The cornea is kept clear and moistened by tears, which wash away foreign objects that may enter the lid area. Separating the front of the eye from the eyeball proper is a sac lined with an epithelial membrane. This sac aids in the destruction of some pathogenic bacteria that may enter the eye from the outside (Bell et al., 1976; Ganong, 1977).

The *iris,* or colored, pigmented part of the eye, regulates the amount of light entering the eye. The pupil changes size according to the distance of the viewed object. This process of contraction and dilation is controlled by intrinsic muscles.

The optic cup, destined to become the retina, begins forming during the fourth week of prenatal life. Binocular vision is achieved between the third prenatal month and birth. In fetuses of six months all layers of the adult retina can be recognized, including the rods and cones. The eye is sensitive to light by the seventh fetal month. Form perception is acquired in the first year of postnatal life, and color vision in the second year (Timiras, 1972).

Changes in eye function with aging show great individual variation and do not come on suddenly at any age. Ocular age changes do not necessarily mirror changes in other body systems consistent with a given chronological age. Certain physiological changes however do occur with progressive aging. Examples of these include gradual loss of accommodation, drying of the lens, depigmentation of the iris, and loss of retinal reflexes. With aging, eyelids and surrounding skin become thinner, wrinkled, and more pigmented.

Other conditions that occur with aging but are believed to be associated with diseases rather than physiological changes include glaucoma, lens opacities, high myopias, vascular changes, and progressive forms of muscular disease (Timiras, 1972).

Composition

Corneal epithelium is the eye's primary barrier to infections. As with epithelial tissue elsewhere in the body, vitamin A has a vital role in the formation and maintenance of these mucous membranes that line the ocular cavity (Goodhart and Shils, 1973; Williams, 1977).

The presence of a light-sensitive pigment, *rhodopsin* (commonly known as *visual purple*), in the rods of the retina allows the eye to adapt to changes in light. Rods are sensitive to light of low intensity and function in dim light. Cones are sensitive to high-intensity light and function in bright light and color vision. *Iodopsin* (commonly known as *visual violet*), the main pigment in cones, contains vitamin A. The same vitamin A fraction, retinal, is present in all visual pigments but in combination with different proteins.

Light hitting the retina causes rhodopsin to split into two parts and is referred to as *bleaching*. When healthy people are stimulated with constant light, an equilibrium occurs in which rate of rhodopsin bleaching and rate of regeneration are equal. This process of retinal bleaching and regeneration in respose to light is a photochemical event that makes vision possible.

Nutrition

Vitamin A in the epithelial tissues of the eye prevents keratinization. Keratin is a protein that forms scalelike, dry tissue such as hair and nails. Vitamin A aids in giving the skin turgor and keeping tear ducts moist and lubricated. Without vitamin A, epithelial cells would lack luster and lose their elasticity. Although vitamin A is a required component in visual pigment, there is no evidence that it can cure color blindness (Goodhart and Shils, 1973; Williams, 1977).

The crystalline lens of the eye is devoid of nerves and vascular supply. It is freely suspended in an aqueous humor on which it depends for its nutrition. The function of vitamin C in the lens and surrounding fluid seems to be to act with glutathoine and cystine in the mediation of oxygen uptake of the lens (Goodhart and Shils, 1973).

Nutritional Imbalance

The first symptoms of vitamin A deficiency are deterioration of dark adaptation and night blindness (see Fig. 13-10). The deficiency results in destruction or dysfunction of nervous elements and prevents the rods, cones, or both from participating to their full capacity in the visual process. Changes in the color sensitivity of the retina also accompany deterioration of dark adaptation.

Further deprivation of vitamin A results in a condition called *xerosis*. Xerosis is found most frequently in undernourished infants who have been weaned to an inadequate diet. Loss of elasticity in the conjunctiva causes

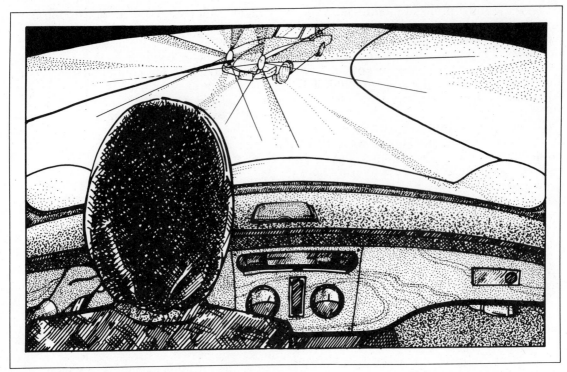

Figure 13-10. Left: Night blindness may be a symptom of vitamin A deficiency. The headlights of an oncoming car cause unusual discomfort for the driver. The driver may be blinded temporarily and have difficulty seeing.

wrinkling. If the process advances further, the cornea becomes dull and finally perforates.

Corneal vascularization is probably the first sign of riboflavin deficiency. As the deficiency progresses, symptoms include itching and burning, roughness of the eye, photophobia, and impairment of visual acuity. A similar type of corneal vascularity occurs in rats on diets deficient in protein or any of the essential amino acids. A similar type of vascularization has also been demonstrated experimentally in zinc deficiency, sodium deficiency, and thallium poisoning. It has been suggested as a result of research that riboflavin has a special function during twilight, transforming light of short wave frequency to a frequency for which the eye has a greater sensitivity (Goodhart and Shils, 1973).

INTEGUMENTARY SYSTEM

The integumentary system derives its name from the word *integument,* meaning "covering." It is composed of skin, oil and sweat glands, hair, toenails, and fingernails. The skin is an enveloping membrane that contains epithelial, connective, and nerve tissue. It can also be subdivided into several strata, or layers, as seen in Figure 13-11.

The outer layer, or *epidermis,* is made entirely of epithelial cells with no blood vessels. The "true skin," or *dermis,* has a framework of

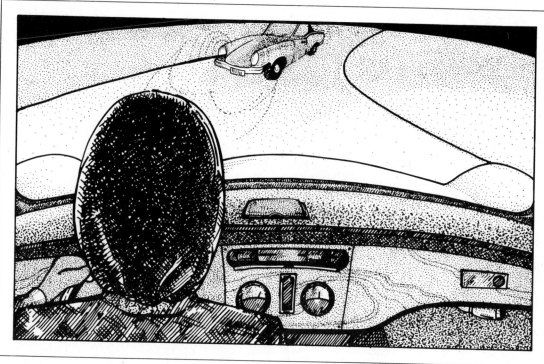

Figure 13-10. (*Continued*) Right: An adequate dietary intake of vitamin A helps prevent or correct this symptom.

connective tissue and contains many blood vessels, nerve endings, and glands. The third, or "under-the-skin" layer is the *subcutaneous layer.* It is a combination of elastic and fibrous tissue and deposits of adipose tissue. This layer is a means of connecting the skin to the surface muscles. Adipose tissue serves as insulation as well as an energy reserve.

Epithelial tissues cover both the exterior surface of the body and the interior, or major cavities, and line all the tubular structures. The external surface provides a resilient, protective covering. Internal tissue is a secretory mucous membrane.

Skin and appearance offer clues to a person's emotions as well as to his general health. Color of skin depends not only on the amount of pigment in the epidermis but on the quantity of blood circulating in surface blood vessels. Concentration of hemoglobin, presence or absence of oxygen, and existence of such substances as bile, silver compounds, or other chemicals in blood serve the skilled clinician as an index of health. Skin reflects such emotions as fear, embarrassment, anger, anxiety, and joy. People are also identified by characteristic skin markings, such as fingerprints or moles (Goodhart and Shils, 1973).

Functions

The primary function of epithelial tissues is protection of vital organs and other body tissues from drying and invasion by pathogenic

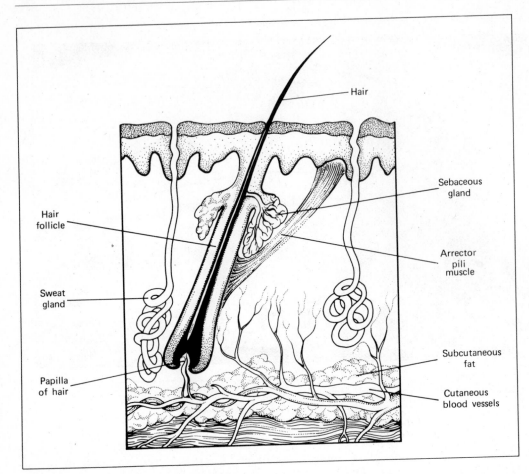

Figure 13-11. Structure of the skin.

organisms or their toxins. Skin regulates body temperature by dissipating heat to the surrounding air. It also obtains information from the environment via nerve endings profusely distributed throughout it.

In addition to its physiological roles, the integumentary system receives much attention as an element of personal appearance (Arlin, 1977). The care with which and the manner in which a person arranges the hair, manicures the nails, and hygienically grooms the skin speaks vividly of cultural conditioning and personality characteristics.

Development

Increase in cellular epidermal thickness and epidermal keritinization begin early in fetal life (Timiras, 1972). Thickness of epidermis and dermis varies. Some areas, such as the soles of the feet and the palms of the hands, are covered with very thick layers of skin. Skin of the eyelids is very thin and delicate.

Outer cells of epidermis are horny and flat. These cells are pushed outward from deeper layers in the epidermis. The specialized protein keratin forms the outer layer of skin. Two forms of keratin exist. Hard keratin is relatively inert and occurs in durable structures such as nails. Soft keratin is capable of sloughing and appears in softer skin tissue. A strand of hair is composed of an inner core of soft keratin surrounded by an outer shaft of hard keratin. Large amounts of the sulfur-containing amino acids, cystine and methionine are found in keratin and account for the characteristic odor of singed hair (Arlin, 1977).

There are two kinds of skin appendages derived from the epidermis: glands (sweat and oil) and keritinized structures (hair follicles, hair, and nails) (Goodhart and Shils, 1973). Most of the skin appendages extend into the dermis and often deeper into the subcutaneous layer. Before an infant is born, *sebaceous,* or oil, *glands* produce a substance like cream cheese, called vernix caseosa, which covers the infant's body.

The skin's outer surface continually sloughs away throughout life. Usually scaling is unnoticed. This constant turnover of cells is due to cells proliferating in the lower epidermal layer, gradually working their way to the surface, and scaling off.

Melanin, one of several pigment granules, is found in the germinating part of the epidermis. Positioned between each cell nucleus and the outer skin surface, melanin protects the chromosomes from damage by ultraviolet irradiation. When the skin is exposed to the sun's ultraviolet rays, as in suntanning, melanin is increased to protect the nuclei, and the result is a general darkening of the skin (Arlin, 1977).

The dermis, or *corium,* has a framework of elastic connective tissue and is well supplied with blood vessels and nerves. Because of the many nerve endings (receptors) for pain, touch, pressure, and temperature, the skin is regarded as one of the chief sensory organs of the body. Many reflexes originate in the dermis, which make it possible for a person to adapt to the environment. A child, because of having a relatively greater skin surface per kilogram than the adult body, loses heat faster than the adult. The elderly also do not produce heat as efficiently as the young. It is therefore important to protect the very young and very old from undue exposure to extreme cold.

The subcutaneous layer of skin provides support for most of the skin appendages, is a good heat insulator, and is an excellent shock absorber (Goodhart and Shils, 1973). A mixture of fatty substances empties through the subaceous glands into hair follicles. This oily material gives luster to the hair and softens the layers of skin by preventing water loss (Arlin, 1977).

Structural and functional changes that affect the skin of the elderly,—that is, atrophy, dryness, roughness, loss of elasticity, partial disappearance of capillaries, and decreased ability of vessels to dilate—occur in the connective tissue and elastin of skin. Investigators currently hold controversial views concerning reasons for their occurrence (Timiras, 1972).

Composition

Epidermis is composed of four or five layers of cells. The only actively growing layer after birth is the layer adjacent to the blood supply. These cells continuously divide, multiply, and migrate outward to form surface layers. As they progress to the outer layer, they gradually lose their nuclei and cellular constituents and are almost entirely protein in the form of keratin.

Melanin is formed from tyrosine, an amino acid. Absence of melanin results in blond hair. Varying shades of hair coloring ranging from brown to black reflect (in true hair coloring) the amount of pigment present. It is theorized that graying of hair results from an inability to convert tyrosine to melanin, possibly as a result of diminished hormone activity.

The dermis layer is composed of fat, protein, connective tissue, nerve endings, and blood capillaries. Dermis also contains involuntary muscle fibers, particularly where there are hairs. This skin layer is also a large potential storehouse for water, blood, and electrolytes. Exposure to sunlight enables ultraviolet radiation to change the cholesterol-like precursor in the dermal layer to vitamin D (Arlin, 1977). Although the exact role of vitamin A in epithelial tissues is not known, it is believed to be necessary to the mucus-secreting cells.

The highly vascularized dermal layer gives a pinkish appearance to skin and nails. Blood, near the surface in the lips because the layering of skin is so thin, imparts a red coloring to their appearance (Arlin, 1977).

Subcutaneous tissue is a storehouse of Calories in the form of fat. Because of their thick subcutaneous layers of fat, obese people tend to become overheated easily and sweat more profusely.

Nutrition

Zinc, because of its role in protein synthesis, is a necessary component in the epidermis layer of skin, including the keratin of hair and nails. Zinc is present in greater amounts in skin with greater pigmentation (Guthrie, 1979).

Linoleic acid, an essential fatty acid, is important for strengthening capillary and cell-membrane structure. It helps prevent an increase in skin permeability. Essential fatty acids also combine with cholesterol to form cholesterol esters.

Vitamin A is essential in the formation and maintenance of healthy epithelial tissue. Vitamin A appears to contribute to soft tissue growth and mucous membranes through an effect on protein synthesis, mitosis, or stability of cell membranes. Exact mechanisms have not been clearly elucidated.

Vitamin C plays a role in tyrosine metabolism and collagen formation. It is necessary for healthy gums and wound healing (Williams, 1977).

Sulfur also appears to be necessary for collagen synthesis and formation. Sulfur found in keratin-containing tissues—that is, hair, skin, and nails—is in combination with the sulfur-containing amino acids cystine and methionine (Guthrie, 1979).

Nutritional Imbalance

Plasma proteins, especially albumin, exert an essential osmotic influence in preventing water loss from the vascular system. People suffering from kwashiorkor, a protein deficiency disease, exhibit a characteristic edema and skin lesions. Low-protein diets of long exposure result in skin changes characterized by dryness; scaliness; inelasticity; and a gray, pallid appearance. A brownish pigmentation with a blotchy, dirty appearance may appear anywhere on the body but is most often seen on the face (Goodhart and Shils, 1973). Skin lesions are characteristic of the rare zinc-deficiency disease *acrodermatitis enteropathica* (Hambidge, 1977).

Changes in color and texture of skin and hair are also associated with deficiencies in iron or folic acid (anemia), niacin (pellagra), vitamin A, riboflavin, and pyridoxine. The latter three nutrient deficiencies may be accompanied by a greasy dermatitis affecting specific body areas. Copper deficiency is associated with decreased pigmentation of the skin and hair (Hambidge, 1977). Essential fatty acid deficiency produces a characteristic eczema of the skin (Arlin, 1977).

Scurvy, the classical vitamin C deficiency, presents symptoms of a horny growth in the hair follicles (*follicular keratosis*) that occur on the legs, buttocks, arms, and back. These symptoms are followed by hemorrhages around the hair follicles and scorbutic changes in the gums. Gums appear red and swollen and bleed easily (Wilson et al., 1979).

Although vitamin A deficiency causes a dermatitis similar to acnelike pustules, there seems to be no relationship between the two conditions (Arlin, 1977). Oral vitamin A has been used extensively in acne therapy for its theoretical inhibition of keratinization. It has, however, been found ineffective unless used in potentially toxic doses. Topical vitamin A acid, when initiated conservatively, seems to have beneficial effects on the skin of patients with acne (Gellis and Kagan, 1978).

Perspiration lost through the sweat glands is a means of regulating body temperature. Insensible perspiration (perspiration without strenuous exertion) through the skin averages a loss of 400–600 ml(12–18 oz)/day. Perspiration lost during strenuous exercise may amount to several liters a day (Goodhart and Shils, 1973). When sweating is particularly heavy, water and sodium chloride are lost and should be replaced. Commercial sweetened drinks that contain electrolytes, glucose, and lactic acid are unnecessary but probably harmless (Hodges, 1980). Beverages that promote "balanced electrolyte replacement" have no particular merit in that salts of minerals other than sodium chloride are not lost in significant amounts unless profuse sweating of long duration occurs. Salt dissolved in water, although not always palatable, replaces the necessary nutrients lost through perspiration. Salt tablets along with a liberal intake of water may be advised for conditions where copious sweating occurs (Arlin, 1977).

People who live in environments where they are not exposed to adequate sunlight need supplemental vitamin D. Atmospheric smoke, fog, window glass, and clothing protect from ultraviolet light and inhibit the activation of provitamin 7 dehydrocholesterol in the skin (Wilson et al., 1979).

There appears to be no valid rationale for the popular belief that gelatin strengthens fingernails. Nails contain a high proportion of sulfur. Gelatin is an incomplete protein and is itself deficient in one of the sulfur containing essential amino acids found in nails. The amino acid glycine found in gelatin supports collagen formation. Because nails consist of keratin and not collagen, there appears to be little justification for this stated relationship (Arlin, 1977).

The healthy glow radiating from shiny hair, ruddy complexion, and clear skin is characteristic of well-nourished people. As shown in Table 13-4, the interrelationships of a variety of nutrient compounds account for this appearance.

NUTRITIONAL REQUIREMENTS

This chapter has considered the nutritional needs of the various structural body systems for their development and maintenance. These nutritional needs were discussed in terms of the specific roles of individual nutrients in the structural body system and the results of nutrient imbalance. Human nutritional requirements are based on the nutrient needs of the body at various stages of the life cycle. These requirements are not easily arrived at because the specific nutritional requirements of the body systems are not known and also because human nutritional requirements are vary among individuals at each stage of the life cycle. A general discussion here of aspects of nutrient needs throughout the life cycle both summarizes the nutrient needs of structural body systems and introduces the nutritional requirements of the separate stages of the life cycle, the topic of Unit III.

The effort in establishing nutritional recommendations is to promote a level of dietary intake that will maintain the majority of the population in a state of "good nutrition" ultimately resulting in "good health." Differences in standards between countries and within a country reflect the inevitable variations of recommendations among population groups as well as differences of opinion in the interpretation of nutritional studies. Although specific levels of nutrient recommendations

TABLE 13-4. Nutrients and the Integumentary System

Normal Structural Component	Nutrients or Nutrient Compounds	Abnormal State of Nutrient Imbalance
Skin	*Major*	Deficiencies
Oil and sweat glands	Protein, i.e., collagen and keratin; fatty acids; lipids;	Dry, scaly skin; edema and skin lesions;
Hair	vitamins A and D	acrodermatitis enteropathica;
Toe and finger nails	*Auxiliary*	pallor; greasy dermatitis;
Adipose tissue	Tyrosine, cystine, methionine, albumin, linoleic acid,	decreased skin and hair pigment; Eczemalike rash;
Gums of teeth	cholesterol, sulfur, zinc, copper,	follicular keratosis;
Mucous membranes	vitamin C, iron, folic acid, niacin, riboflavin, pyridoxine	bleeding gums; scurvy; pellagra;
		Excesses
		Obesity, excess vitamin A (yellow-orange color)

NOTE: See Chapters 19 and 24 for further information on clinical signs of nutritional deficiencies.

can be debated, general trends in the nutritional needs of each age group are observable.

Nutritional needs differ between late prenatal life and early infancy. Glucose use prevails in the fetal period; fatty acids are also being synthesized. In infancy, glucose is in short supply, and fatty acids are used to a greater extent. A high-fat diet is desirable during this developmental stage. After weaning, metabolic processes adapt to the prevailing meal pattern common to each culture (Hahn, 1972).

Significant improvements in the health of the populations of the United States and other industrialized nations have been attributed to decreased intakes of fat, sugar, and salt. Although epidemiological studies indicate a relationship between diet and early onset of chronic disease, the mechanisms of modified dietary regimens that influence survival are not clear. Animal studies indicate that the higher the total intake of food, the shorter the life-span. In humans a diet that appears to promote optimal health and longevity is one in which caloric intake does not contribute to obesity. Recommended

levels of essential macro- and micronutrients that would be most conducive to long life, based on normal developmental changes associated with aging, have not been defined. Note that no age-specific nutrient recommendations are made beyond age 51 in the RDA (see back cover). The major physiological change occurring in old age is a decrease in the number of functioning cells that result in a slowing down of metabolic processes. Organ systems decrease in function (up to 60%). Cell death is the major phenomenon associated with the aging process. Although the total organism is aging at an observable rate, different systems within that organism are at various phases of aging at different times.

Nutrient requirements do not appear to change markedly with advancing age. Changes, however, such as lifestyle, socioeconomic status, psychological climate, and the presence of chronic disease alter nutrient intake in the elderly. In general, health in later life depends on the attitudes, health, and nutritional practices established during earlier years (Kent, 1978; Ross, 1977; Todhunter and Darby, 1978; Young, 1978).

Nutrient Effects on Total Body Composition

Body composition represents a balanced state of equilibrium between each nutrient and component body part. Both constancy and change in composition imply a continuous turnover process of its constituents. No nutrient remains in body tissue indefinitely throughout life. Whether it be inorganic ion or protein enzyme, some component is lost and replaced daily from infancy through old age.

Increase in body weight is most rapid during the early months of life. Infants double their birth weight by approximately five to six months of age. Poolsize of nutrients in the infant is much larger per unit mass than at any other time in the life cycle. Infants retain metabolic excesses that adults would excrete. For some of the nutrients this pool size can be explained by the relatively large extracellular fluid volume in infants (Adolph, 1972; Mitchell et al., 1976). Because of the intense metabolic demands during this rapid developmental stage, a change in the quantity or quality of diet and fluid intake may have far-reaching consequences more pronounced than those resulting from a change in adult diets.

At birth, girls have a greater skeletal maturity (by about one month) than boys. From one month of age through adolescence, 62% of boys' body weight is water and 55% of girls' (Cheek et al., 1969). Muscles are poorly developed at birth. The amount of subcutaneous fat is limited but will increase during the first year of life. When the toddler begins to walk, baby fat disappears, muscles increase in size, and bones begin to harden.

The head of the infant is large in proportion to the entire body. During rapid brain and nervous system development, the head continues to grow rapidly. In childhood, body proportions become more like the adult form as limbs lengthen at a rapid rate and head growth decelerates (Mitchell et al., 1976).

The period of adolescence is one of dramatic development. During the growth spurt, girls grow approximately 3 in (7.5 cm)/year, and boys may grow as much as 4 in (10 cm)/year. Under the influence of steroid hormones, changes in body size, amount and proportion of various tissues, and energy metabolism begin to take place. Bones grow in length and width; muscles increase in mass; body fat is layed down in soft tissues; shoulders widen in boys; and hips broaden in girls. There is accelerated growth of reproductive organs in both sexes. Corresponding to the peak of adolescence, caloric, protein, and mineral requirements exceed comparable needs both previously and subsequently in life (Garn and Wagner, 1969).

Linear growth is virtually complete by 21 years of age in men and by 17 in women. In the United States the average person tends to continue to gain in weight until approximately 60 years of age. Lateral growth, or lean muscle mass, may continue during the third decade, especially in people undergoing rigorous physical training.

Aging is associated with a loss of *parenchymal cells*. Histologists can distinguish old from young tissues in the heart, skeletal muscle, brain, cartilage, and kidney. These tissues have no capacity for regeneration. The number of nonglial cells per unit of cerebral cortex decreases with advancing age. The greatest slope occurs between the ages of 45 and 55 years. Linear reduction in discrete renal function occurs between 30 and 90 years of age, as indicated by a loss of functioning nephrons. Age-wise decrements in body water occur without a decrease in oxygen consumption. This suggests that functioning cells are lost, but those that remain have normal oxygen uptake. Loss of lean body muscle with increasing age has been measured by total body potassium. Height and weight decrease with advancing years. Postponement of biological aging has been the subject of much research and controversy. Although numerous theories exist, a clear definition of biological aging remains elusive (Masoro, 1976). Further studies are needed to define the unique role nutrition plays in senescense and quality of life in the elderly.

BIBLIOGRAPHY

Adolph, E. F. Development of physiological regulations. In M. Winick, Ed., *Nutrition and Development,* pp. 1–25. New York: John Wiley & Sons, Inc., Pubs., 1972.

Arlin, M. J. *The Science of Nutrition.* 2nd Ed. New York: Macmillan, Inc., 1977.

Bell, G. H., Emslie-Smith, D., and Paterson, C. R. *Textbook of Physiology and Biochemistry.* 9th Ed. New York: Longman, Inc., Churchill Livingstone, 1976.

Cheek, D. B., Graystone, J. and Reba, R. Human growth and body composition. In F. P. Heald, Ed., *Adolescent Nutrition and Growth.* New York: Appleton-Century-Crofts, 1969.

Christakis, G. *Salt and Hypertension: The Enigmas Remain.* Essays on Hypertension, No. 2. Nutley, New Jersey: Hoffman La Roche, Inc., 1974.

Christakis, G., Fordyce, M., LaRocco, A., and Kurtz, C. *Nutrition and Social Deviancy: A New Hypothesis.* Ford Foundation Monograph. New York, prepared for publication.

Food and Nutrition Board, Nat'l Research Council. *Recommended Dietary Allowances.* 9th Ed. Washington, D.C.: Nat'l Acad. of Sciences, 1980.

Garn, S. M., and Wagner, B. The adolescent growth of the skeletal mass and its implications to mineral requirements. In F. P. Heald, Ed., *Adolescent Nutrition and Growth.* New York: Appleton-Century-Crofts, 1969.

Gellis, S. S., and Kagan, B. M. *Current Pediatric Therapy,* pp. 506–508. Philadelphia: W. B. Saunders Co., 1978.

Goodhart, R. S., and Shils, M. E., Eds. *Modern Nutrition in Health and Disease.* 5th Ed. Philadelphia: Lea & Febiger, 1973.

Government releases guide for nutrition. *The Nation's Health,* pp. 1, 4. Washington, D.C.: Amer. Pub. Health Assoc. ISSN: 0028-0496, March 1980.

Guthrie, H. A., *Introductory Nutrition.* 4th Ed. St. Louis: The C. V. Mosby Co., 1979.

Guyton, A. C. *Textbook of Medical Physiology.* 5th Ed. Philadelphia: W. B. Saunders Co., 1976.

———. *Basic Human Physiology: Normal Functions and*

Mechanisms of Disease. 2nd Ed. Philadelphia: W. B. Saunders Co., 1977.

Hahn, P. Lipid metabolism and nutrition in the prenatal and postnatal period. In M. Winick, Ed., *Nutrition and Development,* pp. 129–130. New York: John Wiley & Sons, Inc., Pubs., 1972.

Hambidge, K. M. Trace elements in pediatric nutrition. In L. A. Barness, Ed., *Advances in Pediatrics* 24:191, Chicago: Year Book Medical Pubs., Inc., 1977.

Herbert, V. Facts and fictions about megavitamins therapy. *Resident and Staff Physician* 24:43, 1978.

Hodges, R. E. *Nutrition in Medical Practice.* Philadelphia: W. B. Saunders Co., 1980.

Kent, S. Can dietary manipulation prolong life? *Geriatrics* 33(4):102, 1978.

Lytle, L. D., and Altar, A. Diet, central nervous system, and aging. *Fed. Proc.* 38:2017, 1979.

Masoro, E. J. Physiological changes with aging. In M. Winick, Ed., *Nutrition and Aging.* New York: John Wiley & Sons, Inc., Pubs., 1976.

Memmler, R. L., and Wood, D. L. *The Human Body in Health and Disease.* 4th Ed. Philadelphia: J. B. Lippincott Co., 1977.

Menaker, L., *The Biology of Dental Caries.* New York: Harper & Row, Pubs., Inc., 1980.

Mitchell, H. S., Rynbergen, H. J., Anderson, L., and Dibble, M. V. *Nutrition in Health and Disease.* 16th Ed. Philadelphia: J. B. Lippincott Co., 1976.

Morhart, R. E. Dental research, personal communication, Dec. 1979.

Morhart, R. E., and Fitzgerald, R. J. Nutritional determinants of the ecology of the oral flora. *Dent. Clin. North Am.* 20:473, 1976.

Nutrition Education in Medical Schools. Hearings before the Subcommittee on Nutrition of the Committee on Agriculture, Nutrition, and Forestry, United States Senate, Ninety-Sixth Congress, Part II. Washington: U.S. Gov. Printing Office, 1979.

Pike, R. L., and Brown, M. L. *Nutrition: An Integrated Approach.* 2nd Ed. New York: John Wiley & Sons, Inc., Pubs., 1975.

Ross, M. H. Dietary behavior and longevity. *Nutr. Rev.* 35:257, 1977.

Schottelius, B. A., and Schottelius, D. D. *Textbook of Physiology.* 18th Ed. St. Louis: The C. V. Mosby Co., 1978.

Thomas, B. A., Ed. *Scope Manual on Nutrition.* Kalamazoo, Mich.: W. E. Upjohn, 1975.

Timiras, P. S. *Developmental Physiology and Aging.* New York: Macmillan, Inc., 1972.

Todhunter, E. N., and Darby, W. J. Guidelines for maintaining adequate nutrition in old age. *Geriatrics* 33(6):49, 1978.

Wei, S. H. Y. Nutritional aspects of dental caries. In S. I. Fomon, Ed., *Infant Nutrition*. 2nd Ed., pp. 338–358. Philadelphia: W. B. Saunders Co., 1974.

Williams, S. R. *Nutrition and Diet Therapy*. 3rd Ed. St. Louis: The C. V. Mosby Co., 1977.

Wilson, E. D., Fisher, K. H., and Garcia, P. A. *Principles of Nutrition*. 4th Ed. New York: John Wiley & Sons, Inc., Pubs., 1979.

Young, V. R. Nutrition and aging. *Advances in Experimental Med. Biology* 97:85, 1978.

Zuidema, G. D., Ed. *The Johns Hopkins Atlas of Human Functional Anatomy*. Baltimore, Md.: The John Hopkins Univ. Press, 1977.

CHAPTER 14

Excretion of Nutritive Wastes

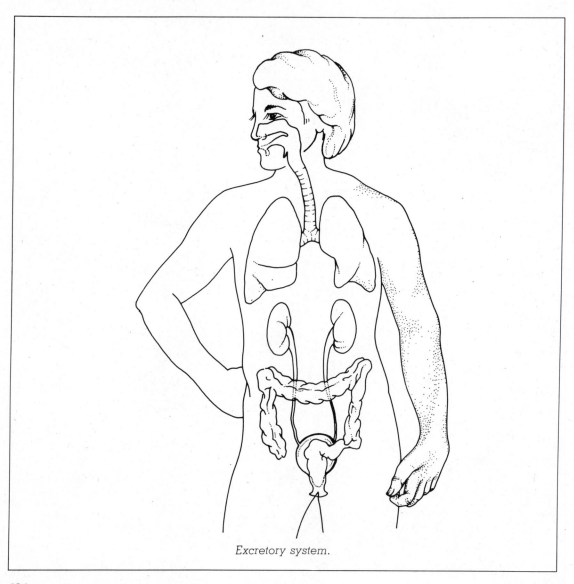

Excretory system.

The nutrition process as discussed thus far has involved the ingestion, absorption, transport, and use of nutrients from food for the purpose of growth, maintenance, energy, and regulation. The ingestion of food and the use of nutrients produce metabolic waste products and excess nutrients that must be excreted. Metabolism of the energy nutrients produces carbon dioxide, nitrogenous products, heat, and excess water as waste products. Other waste products include materials that were not digested nor absorbed, such as cellulose and fiber; some nutrients that may have been absorbed but could not be used; and nutrients consumed in excess of the body's need or storage capacity. Excretion rids the body of excesses of some nutrients and final products of metabolism that if left to accumulate in the body would be toxic. The excretion of nutritive wastes involves four systems of the body: the urinary, digestive, respiratory, and integumentary systems. The organs of excretion are the kidney, colon, lungs, and skin. Excretion through these organs helps to maintain the normal composition of the components of the internal environment, such as the blood and the tissue fluids.

KIDNEY

The nutritional significance of the kidney lies in its role in maintaining the nutrient composition of the blood. The elimination of urine is only one function of the kidney. The kidney is also involved in regulating the composition of the internal environment, that is, the fluid and electrolyte balance and the acid-base balance.

Every four to five minutes the entire blood supply circulates through the kidney. This constitutes 20% of the cardiac output or 1,200 ml (41 oz) of blood being delivered to the kidneys each minute. Out of this amount, 120 ml (4 oz) of filtrate is formed each minute, but from this amount only 1–2 ml (.03–.06 oz) of urine is formed per minute for excretion. Over an entire 24-hour period the kidney concentrates 180 liters (191 qt) of fluid into only 1–2 liters (2–4 pt) for elimination from the body. Obviously, something happens to the large quantities of fluid that pass through the kidneys. The kidney filters, reabsorbs, and secretes some substances in the preparation of the urine for excretion, but these functions are also vitally important in regulating the acid-base balance and fluid and electrolyte balance of the body.

Formation of Urine

The functional unit of the kidney is called the *nephron. Nephrons* are microscopic units within the kidney that carry out the functions of filtration, reabsorption, and secretion. It has been estimated that there are approximately 1 million of these units in each kidney. The nephron consists of a bed of capillaries called a *glomerulus* and a proximal and a distal convoluted tubule, which are connected by the *loop of Henle.* The parts of the nephron are shown in Figure 14-1. If the tubules of the nephrons were uncoiled and laid end to end, they would stretch 75 miles.

The formation of urine is a series of complex events involving complicated physiological mechanisms. The details of these events are left to the study of physiology. The intention here is to present a basic explanation of the events that are of nutritional significance.

The first step in the formation of urine is filtration of the blood through the glomerulus of the nephron. The blood enters Bowman's capsule, which surrounds the glomerulus. The semipermeable membrane of the glomerulus acts somewhat like a sieve that strains out large molecules, such as proteins, fats, and blood cells, retaining them in the bloodstream. The smaller molecules such as salts, glucose, amino acids, and vitamins become part of the glomerular filtrate. The rate at which blood filters through the glomerulus is referred to as the *glomerular filtration rate*

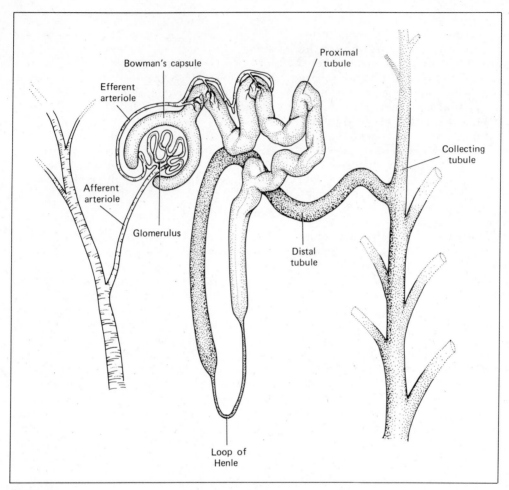

Figure 14-1. A nephron, the functional unit of the kidney.

(GFR). This rate of flow is 125 ml (4 oz) of blood per minute in people with normally functioning kidneys. This glomerular filtrate has essentially the same composition as the blood except that it is protein free.

At this point the glomerular filtrate enters the tubules of the nephron. In a sense the essential nutrients are on their way out of the body, but during the brief time in the tubule most of them are selectively reabsorbed and returned to the blood. It is by this mechanism

of reabsorption that the kidney has final control over maintaining the composition of the internal environment. The process of secretion also helps to maintain nutritive balance within the body.

The tubules of the nephron participate in selective reabsorption and secretion. The first section of the tubule is called the *proximal convoluted tubule*. It is within this section of the tubule that major nutrient reabsorption occurs. About 80–90% of these useful nutrients are reabsorbed into the blood. Among those actively transported are glucose, amino acids, vitamin C, calcium, sodium, and potassium (Crouch and McClintic, 1976). Because the reabsorption of these nutrients involves active transport, this process requires energy. Fatty acids are the primary source of energy if the reaction occurs in the cortex portion of the kidney, but glucose and fructose can also be used. If the reaction occurs in the medulla of the kidney, glucose is the primary source of energy (Robinson and Lawler, 1977). About 80% of the water is also reabsorbed here. The epithelium of the proximal convoluted tubule is not permeable to some of the waste products such as urea, so these substances pass on through the tubule.

As the filtrate reaches the loop of Henle, water passes into the surrounding fluid, and the relative concentration of sodium is increased in the ascending limb of the tubule. Energy is required for the operation of the sodium pumps, but the net effect is the conservation of water and the concentrating effect on the urine.

There are two hormonal mechanisms that control water and electrolyte balance: the secretion of the antidiuretic hormone (ADH) and aldosterone. ADH is secreted by the posterior lobe of the pituitary gland. It stimulates the reabsorption of water in the distal convoluted tubule. It is secreted in response to osmoreceptors located in the hypothalmus that are sensitive to changes in osmotic pressure. The purpose of ADH secretion is the conservation of body water.

The aldosterone mechanism regulates the renal control of electrolyte and water balance. It is primarily involved in the conservation of sodium, but it has a secondary effect on the conservation of water. This mechanism involves a chain of events that begins with the secretion of the enzyme renin by the renal cortex into the blood. The secretion of this enzyme is initiated in response to a decrease in sodium intake, a loss of body sodium, or a decrease in total body fluid volume. In the blood, renin acts on a substance manufactured by the liver called *angiotensinogen* to form *angiotensin I,* which then forms *angiotensin II.* This compound stimulates secretion of aldosterone by the adrenal cortex. Aldosterone increases the reabsorption of sodium and also of water (see Fig. 14-2).

A final function of the kidney involves the secretion of certain substances to control the resulting acidity or alkalinity of the urine. This secretion occurs primarily in the distal convoluted tubule. The secretion may be of potassium, ammonium, or hydrogen ions. These substances are secreted from the blood into the fluid in the renal tubule to combine with the substances there to form a more acidic or alkaline urine. The metabolic end products of foods and their effect on the urine are often the opposite of what might be expected. For example, most fruits and vegetables yield alkaline end products. Meats and breads and cereals, on the other hand, leave acidic end products in the urine. There are a few foods, such as cranberry juice, that contain a high proportion of organic acids that are not changed during metabolism. Drinking large amounts of cranberry juice is thought to have the effect of acidifying the urine. Because an equal proportion of acid- and alkaline-yielding foods is usually consumed, there is little concern over the acidic and alkaline components of the diet.

Micturation

After passing through the collecting tubules, the tubular fluid, which has traveled through the nephron, is now called *urine.* The urine travels from each kidney through a muscular tube called the *ureter* into the urinary bladder. The *urinary bladder* is a hollow organ that serves as a temporary storage for urine. When 200–300 ml (7–10 oz) of urine have accumulated, there is a desire to urinate. The filling of the bladder stretches its walls and stimulates nerves in the pelvis that send the impulse through the spinal cord to the brain for pro-

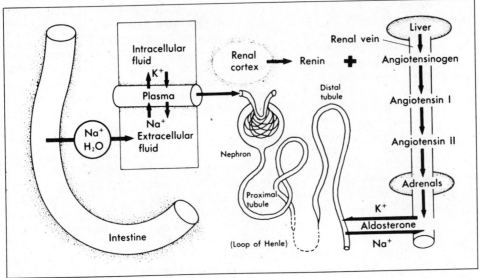

Figure 14-2. The aldosterone mechanism, which conserves sodium in exchange for potassium and causes increased reabsorption of water. (Reprinted with permission from Sue Rodwell Williams, *Nutrition and Diet Therapy,* 3rd Ed. St. Louis: The C. V. Mosby Co., 1977)

cessing. Motor neurons travel back to the bladder and bring about relaxation of the internal sphincter of the bladder so that urine is emptied into the urethra and out of the body.

Composition of Urine

Urine is composed mainly of water, electrolytes, and the end products of metabolism. The concentrations of various substances in the urine are presented in Table 14-1.

About 50–100 mOsm more acid than alkali are found by the urine each day. To maintain a blood pH of 7.35–7.45, the kidneys must continually remove the excess acid. This causes the pH of the urine to be about 6.0.

One of the most important urinary measurements is the volume of urine formed each day. In renal failure the volume is usually reduced. Urine output less than 500–800 ml (17–27 oz) per 24 hours is usually indicative of inadequate fluid intake or renal insufficiency. Normal output is 600–1,000 ml (20–34 oz) a day.

The ability of the kidneys to concentrate urine may be measured by taking the specific gravity of the urine. The specific gravity, normally 1.015–1.035, varys considerably with the amount of fluid ingested.

Urinary Nutrient Excretion

From both a nutritional and a clinical perspective it is important to understand the normal routes of excretion of the various nutrients. The presence of abnormal constituents in the urine and feces leads to the diagnosis of specific medical conditions. The condition may result from a disorder of the organ of excretion itself, such as the kidney or colon, or from a disorder of metabolism that leads to the excretion of abnormal metabolites into the urine or feces.

TABLE 14-1. Concentrations of Substances in the Urine

Normal Urine Characteristics	
Color	Straw, amber, transparent
pH	4.5–7.5
Specific gravity	1.010–1.025
Amount	1,200–1,500 ml a day
Odor	Specific aromatic

Substance	Concentration	
Sodium (Na^+)	128	mEq/liter
Potassium (K^+)	60	mEq/liter
Calcium (Ca^{+2})	4.8	mEq/liter
Magnesium (Mg^{+2})	15	mEq/liter
Chlorine (Cl^-)	134	mEq/liter
Bicarbonate (HCO_3^-)	14	mEq/liter
Glucose	0	mg
Urea	1,820	mg
Uric acid	42	mg
Creatinine	196	mg

The major solid component of the urine is the excretion of nitrogenous wastes, the end products of protein metabolism. Urea is the major waste product of protein metabolism, and it is present in the urine in the highest concentration. The excretion of urea is directly related to the protein intake. The higher the protein intake, the higher the amount of urea excreted. Urea excretion is increased whenever catabolism of body protein is increased, as in fever, infection, or burns. The liver usually takes the ammonia produced from protein metabolism and converts it to urea for excretion by the kidney. In liver disease this detoxification of ammonia to urea does not occur, and the ammonia gains entrance into the general circulation. In kidney disease where there is a decreased urinary output because of impaired filtration, the urea is returned to the blood, where it increases the level of blood urea nitrogen to toxic levels. Other end products of protein metabolism excreted in the urine are creatinine and creatine, some ammonia, uric acid, and small quantities of amino acids.

Excess quantities of water-soluble vitamins and electrolytes that have been absorbed but that cannot be used by the body are removed from the bloodstream by the kidney, filtered through the nephron, and excreted in the urine. The minerals generally excreted by way of the urine are excess sodium, potassium, chlorine, fluorine, iodine, sulfur, and phosphorus.

LARGE INTESTINE

The other major organ of excretion is the large intestine (the colon). It is the organ for the excretion of waste material from the gastrointestinal tract. About 12–72 hours after food is eaten, it enters the large intestine. It remains here for about 18 hours or longer. The length of time varies with the kind of food eaten and the characteristics of the person who has consumed the food.

About 500 ml (17 oz) of chyme gains entrance into the colon from the small intestine through the ileocecal valve. There are two major structural differences between the large intestine and the small intestine that are related to the function of the large intestine. The large intestine does not secrete any digestive enzymes, for all digestion was completed in the small intestine. The large intestine secretes instead large quantities of alkaline mucus. This mucus helps to neutralize the irritating acids formed by the intestinal bacteria. It also aids in the passage of the feces out of the body by serving as a lubricant. Movements in the large intestine are not the same as in the rest of the gastrointestinal tract. The movements are more limited and are generally back-and-forth movements. Instead of the peristaltic waves in the small intestine, special mass movements are initiated three or four times a day to move the fecal mass toward the anus.

Formation of Feces

The formation of feces is a relatively simple process involving the reabsorption of water and the action of intestinal bacteria. The mass of undigested food remains in the colon for a longer period of time than in all of the other digestive organs combined. The purpose is to allow maximum absorption of water and electrolytes to occur. Water is continually reabsorbed throughout the colon. After entrance from the ileocecal valve, the fecal mass changes from a fluid to a semifluid, a mush, a semimush, and a solid state as it approaches the rectum. If motility through the colon is too slow, the result will be the formation of small, hard fecal particles that are often difficult to evacuate. By contrast, if motility is too rapid, the result will be the passage of semiliquid material commonly known as diarrhea. This general knowledge of fecal consistency is important for the nurse assisting clients with colostomy care. A colostomy is the formation of an artifical opening from the colon to the outside of the body for the elimination of fecal waste. Knowing the region of the colon surgery for the formation of the colostomy will give a clue to the general consistency of the drainage from this opening.

Certain strains of bacteria are normal inhabitants of the gastrointestinal tract. In the upper part of the small intestine the predominant types of bacteria are streptococci, staphylococci, lactobacilli, and fungi. In the lower part of the small intestine and the colon, the predominant bacteria are the anaerobes, bacteroids, and lifidobacteria (Bell et al., 1976). These bacteria will attack any food that has not been absorbed, resulting in the production of gas. The presence of intestinal gas is uncomfortable and may cause cramping pains and diarrhea. The gases released are ammonia, methane, carbon dioxide, and hydrogen. Certain indigestible carbohydrates such as those found in baked beans or other legumes may result in the production of intestinal gas. Milk may be a source of excess gas in people with a lactose intolerance. The enzyme lactase is missing or present in such small quantities that the lactose passes into the colon undigested and is attacked by the intestinal bacteria. A portion of the intestinal gas is absorbed in the colon, and part is excreted by the lungs; but the remainder (about 500 ml) passes out of the rectum each day (Bell et al., 1976). Although some foods are considered to be gas formers and certain foods seem to be greater offenders than others, there are no foods known to produce gas in everyone. Gas formation is an individual matter and depends on the completeness of digestion and the composition of each person's intestinal bacterial flora. The composition of the diet seems to influence the action of certain types of bacteria. A high carbohydrate intake favors the fermentative bacteria; a high protein intake favors the putrefactive bacteria (Robinson and Lawler, 1977).

The intestinal bacteria are also involved in the synthesis of some vitamins, particularly those of the B-complex group. The B vitamins that are manufactured by the intestinal bacteria are vitamin B_{12}, thiamine, and riboflavin (Guyton, 1977). The colon bacteria are also involved with the synthesis of biotin, folic acid, and vitamin K (Williams, 1977). With the exception of vitamin K, the intestinal synthesis of the B-complex vitamins is minimal and the significance of this synthesis is uncertain.

It will be remembered that there is no recommended dietary allowance for vitamin K because it is plentiful in a wide variety of foods and because the intestinal bacteria synthesize adequate quantities. When medical conditions interfere with the intestinal synthesis of vitamin K, a supplement is advisable. Prolonged antibiotic therapy destroys the normal bacterial flora so that adequate vitamin K cannot be synthesized. Intestinal diseases that cause a rapid passage of the intestinal contents in the form of diarrhea may also interfere with adequate synthesis of vitamin K. A supplement of this vitamin may need to be administered either orally or intravaneously.

Defecation

The fecal contents move somewhat slowly toward the anus. The colon acts as a storage for fecal material until enough accumulates to move the fecal material into the rectum and initiate defecation. *Defecation* is the passage of feces through the anal opening to the outside of the body.

Normally the rectum is empty. When food enters the stomach it may initiate the gastrocolic reflex, which may bring about a mass movement within the colon. This may cause fecal material to move into the rectum, thus initiating the desire to defecate. This often occurs following the first meal of the day. The defecation reflex involves contraction of the muscles around the rectum and relaxation of the anal sphincters, which allow the passage of the feces to the outside of the body. A high-fiber diet usually will result in the production of a softer stool that is easier to eliminate. A low-fiber diet may lead to the formation of a smaller and harder stool, which may lead to straining.

Aids to normal elimination include a diet of moderate fiber content, the ingestion of at least six to eight glasses of water daily, sufficient rest, and regular exercise. It is also help-ful to establish a daily routine that allows for regular elimination at approximately the same time each day, for example, after breakfast. A daily bowel movement is not necessary for all people.

Composition of the Feces

Table 14-2 describes the composition of feces. The brown color of feces is caused by derivatives of *bilirubin*. The odor is caused principally by the products of bacterial action and vary from person to person. Most water is reabsorbed by the time defecation occurs. Only about 100 cc of fluid is excreted in the feces.

Fecal Nutrient Excretion

The feces consist primarily of nutrients that were undigested or unabsorbed. The major solid component of the feces is due to the presence of indigestible carbohydrates. The greater the fiber content of the diet, the larger the bulk of feces produced. This is evidenced by a comparison of the diets of African natives and inhabitants of Western countries. Burkitt and Meisner (1979) reported that Africans who consumed a diet containing over

TABLE 14-2. Composition of Feces

Normal Stool Characteristics	
Color	Brown (influenced by foods and meals)
Form	Cylindrical
Consistency	Soft
Odor	Varies with diet, meals, person
pH	6.8–7.3
Amount	Approximately 150 gm (5 oz) a day
Frequency	3 times a day to biweekly
Water	75%
Solid matter	25%
Dead bacteria	30%
Fat	10–20%
Inorganic matter	10–20%
Protein	2–3%
Roughage and digestive juices	30%

20 gm of crude fiber a day had an average daily stool output of 300–500 mg (10.5–17.5 oz). The ingested food passed through the alimentary canal from mouth to anus in 30–35 hours. This is referred to as intestinal transit time. In contrast, the average stool weight of inhabitants of Western countries was only slightly over 100 gm (3.5 oz), and the intestinal transit time was about three days in healthy young adults and up to two weeks in the elderly. The significance of a high-fiber diet decreasing the intestinal transit time and increasing the bulk of the stool is being intensely studied by researchers.

Small amounts of undigested protein and fat are also found in the stool. The feces is also the major route for excretion of the unabsorbed mineral content of the diet. The regulation of mineral absorption occurs in the small intestine. The quantity of minerals required by the body tissues is absorbed from the chyme by the small intestine. The remainder passes into the large intestine unabsorbed. The minerals that are predominantly excreted with the feces are calcium, iron, zinc, copper, manganese, and magnesium. Beyer and Flynn (1978) compared the effects of consuming high- and low-fiber diets on human fecal output. It is found that the losses of carbohydrate, protein, fat, and ash (minerals) were over twice as much on the high-fiber diet than on the low-fiber one.

TABLE 14-3. Routes of Excretion of Water and Electrolytes

Substance	Organ of Excretion
Water	Skin
	Kidney
	Lung
	Intestine
Sodium	Kidney
	Skin
Potassium	Kidney
Calcium	Intestine
	Kidney
Magnesium	Intestine
	Kidney
Chlorine	Kidney
	Skin
Bicarbonate	Lung
Phosphate	Kidney
	Possibly gastrointestinal tract

place the amount lost through perspiration. The water lost by excessive sweating should be replaced by drinking fluids. The dangers of dehydration were discussed in Chapter 11.

The waste products excreted by the lungs are water vapor and carbon dioxide in the form of bicarbonate. The functioning of the respiratory system was discussed in Chapter 11. Table 14-3 summarizes the principal routes of excretion for water and electrolytes and lists some usual amounts.

SKIN AND LUNGS

The skin and lungs are the other two organs that excrete nutrient wastes. The skin excretes primarily excess water and salts in the form of perspiration. The salts are primarily sodium, chloride, and small amounts of potassium. Strenuous exercise or prolonged exposure to a hot, humid environment may call for the inclusion of additional salt to re-

BIBLIOGRAPHY

Arlin, M. J. *The Science of Nutrition.* 2nd Ed. New York: Macmillan, Inc., 1977.

Bell, G. H., Emslie-Smith, D., and Paterson, C. R. *Textbook of Physiology and Biochemistry.* 9th Ed. New York: Longman, Inc., Churchill Livingstone, 1976.

Beyer, P. L., and Flynn, M. A. Effects of high and low-fiber diets on human feces. *J. Am. Diet. Assoc.* 72:271, 1978.

Burkitt, D. P., and Meisner, P. How to manage constipation with a high fiber diet. *Geriatrics* 33(2), 1979.

Crouch, J. E., and McClintic, J. K. *Human Anatomy and Physiology.* 2nd Ed. New York: John Wiley & Sons, Inc., Pubs., 1976.

Guyton, A. C. *Basic Human Physiology: Normal Functions and Mechanisms of Disease.* 2nd Ed. Philadelphia: W. B. Saunders Co., 1977.

Robinson, C. H., and Lawler, M. R. *Normal and Therapeutic Nutrition.* 15th Ed. New York: Macmillan, Inc., 1977.

Williams, S. R. *Nutrition and Diet Therapy.* 3rd Ed. St. Louis: The C. V. Mosby Co., 1977.

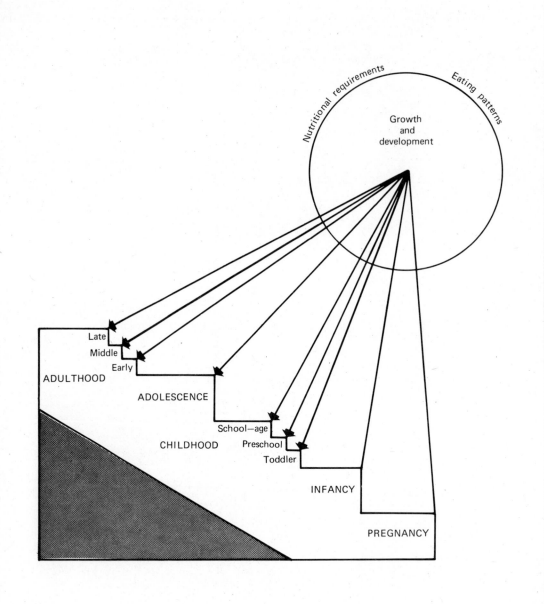

Conceptual model for Unit III.

NUTRITION THROUGHOUT THE LIFE CYCLE

In Unit III the life cycle provides the framework for the discussion of nutritional requirements. Alterations in requirements that occur during pregnancy and lactation are discussed in Chapter 15. The physiological changes that occur during these periods are discussed in relation to their effect on nutrient intake. Chapter 16 reviews the nutrient needs of children from infancy to adolescence. In addition to RDA requirements, feeding patterns are discussed.

The unit concludes with Chapter 17, in which the particular needs of adult clients in relation to maintenance and repair are summarized. Common alterations that affect nutritional requirements are outlined, including medications, exercise, and general lifestyle. The special nutritional needs of older adults are explained, and programs aimed at prevention of malnutrition in the elderly are summarized briefly.

BEHAVIORAL OBJECTIVES

After completing this unit, the student will be able to:

1. Discuss the nutrients required during each phase of the life cycle.
2. Identify methods of intervention that can be used to meet altered nutritional demands during the life cycle.
3. Discuss changes in eating habits that occur throughout the life cycle.

CHAPTER 15

Nutrition During Pregnancy and Lactation

Judith Bonner

Optimal growth, development, and health of the infant depend on the nutritional status of the mother before conception and on the quality of the diet she consumes while she is pregnant (Fig. 15-1). Routine prenatal care should include (1) an assessment of nutritional status that is specifically designed to identify women at nutritional risk, (2) the provision of adequate dietary advice consistent with the nutritional assessment, and (3) follow-up care designed to monitor changes in nutritional status.

The nine-month antepartum period can be divided into three stages. The first stage, frequently referred to as the *germinal period*, begins at conception when fertilization of the egg occurs. This stage continues for two weeks, during which time the single cell begins the complex process of cell division and also begins the journey through the fallopian tubes to the uterus, where implantation normally occurs in the uterine wall.

The second stage of pregnancy extends from the second to the eighth week. This stage is called the *embryonic period* and is characterized by the differentiation of tissues, organs, and body parts. By the end of the eighth week the new life only weighs about 1 oz but can be recognized as a human fetus with a head, face, arms, legs, fingers, toes, and with internal organs including a heart that beats.

The third and final stage of pregnancy, which is the *fetal period,* begins at the beginning of the ninth week and ends with birth.

During this period the organs and structures continue to develop and to assume their specialized functions, but the dramatic change that occurs during this period is growth. At no other time during the life cycle will the developing human grow as fast and in such a brief period of time.

Because of the physiological changes that occur during pregnancy it is readily apparent that the nutritional status of the woman before conception is important. Most women are unaware that they are carrying an unborn child until most of its body parts have been formed. During the first eight weeks the nutritional requirements for fetal development can probably be met without change in maternal diet, providing the woman enters pregnancy in good nutritional status. The nutritional requirements of the woman do not increase greatly until the third stage of pregnancy, when the period of rapid growth of the fetus occurs.

NUTRITIONAL REQUIREMENTS DURING PREGNANCY

Food Energy, Weight, and Weight Gain

During pregnancy a woman requires additional food energy to support the growth of the fetal and maternal tissue, to provide for the increase in resting metabolic rate, and to provide for the increased cost of activity that

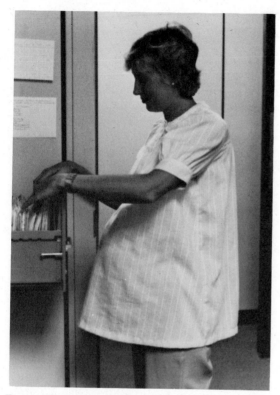

Figure 15-1. The nutritional needs of the pregnant woman require special attention.

growth of the baby and for the changes in the mother necessary to support and protect the baby. Maternal changes include enlargement of breast tissue, uterus, amniotic fluid, blood, and extracellular fluid. The pattern and composition of weight gain is as important as the total amount gained during the nine-month period. During the first trimester 1–2 kg (2–4 lb) should be gained. Subsequently, the weight gain should average 0.4 kg (0.9 lb)/week. Weight gain should represent growth in fetal or maternal tissue rather than fluid retention. A physical examination, together with careful weighing and dietary evaluation, help to distinguish the type of weight gain. Women who enter pregnancy underweight and women who are having their first child generally gain slightly more weight; women who enter pregnancy obese or who are having a second or subsequent child generally gain slightly less weight.

Women who enter pregnancy underweight (10% or more under ideal weight for height) or who have a monthly weight gain of less than 1 kg during the second and third trimesters of pregnancy have an increased risk of delivering low-birth-weight or premature babies. The reason for the inadequate weight gain should be determined so that appropriate measures can be taken.

A common reason weight gain may be inadequate during pregnancy is fear of obesity. Some women enter pregnancy obese; others fear they will become obese. These women may try to lose weight or to limit their weight gain either at the advice of their physicians or because of their own desire. These women and their physicians should be counseled that weight reduction during pregnancy is a questionable practice that is not in the best interest of the mother or the child. Women who gain less than 8 kg (17.6 lb) during their pregnancy must to some extent catabolize their own tissue in order to provide for the growth of the baby, placenta, amniotic fluid, and other necessary maternal tissues. Also, diets that are restricted in Calories may provide in-

results from her larger body size. Providing her activity level remains the same the pregnant woman requires an additional 300 Calories/day. This represents 60 Calories/kg of pregnant body weight for the 11- to 14-year-old, 45 Calories/kg for the 15- to 18-year-old, and 40 Calories/kg for the woman older than 18 years. Women who are more active and women who enter pregnancy underweight may need additional food energy to ensure an appropriate weight gain.

The most useful parameter to use in assessing whether or not the diet of a pregnant woman contains sufficient food energy is her weight. Women should gain from 10 to 13 kg (22 to 28 lb) during pregnancy. This amount of weight is necessary to account for the adequate amounts of other nutrients. Obese women should be counseled that the appropriate time to begin a weight reduction regimen is before conception, after the delivery of the baby, or after they no longer desire to breast-feed.

On the other end of the spectrum, women who gain 3 kg (6.6 lb) or more per month are gaining too much weight. It is important to determine whether the excessive weight gain is secondary to excessive caloric intake resulting in the deposition of extra fat or to fluid retention. Excessive weight gain from overeating predisposes the woman to postpartum obesity. After the twentieth week of pregnancy, however a sudden weight gain may be due to edema and should alert the nurse to the possibility of fluid retention and of the complications associated with toxemia of pregnancy.

If weight is to be used successfully as a tool to monitor adequacy of caloric intake, care must be taken to obtain accurate measurements. Scales should be checked routinely. Women should be weighed wearing only preweighed gowns. Inaccurate measurements are virtually meaningless.

Nutrient Increases Needed

Protein

Protein requirements increase during pregnancy to provide the amino acids and nitrogen necessary for the growth of the fetus and the accessory maternal tissue. An additional 30 gm of protein per day is recommended for the pregnant woman. This represents 1.7 gm of protein per kilogram of pregnant body weight for 11- to 14-year-olds, 1.5 gm/kg for 15- to 18-year-olds, and 1.3 gm/kg for women older than 18 years. Use of protein for anabolic purposes requires that adequate food energy also be provided. Reasons for increased protein requirements include rapid fetal growth; placental growth and development; increased maternal tissue growth, particularly of the breasts and uterus; and an increased maternal circulating blood volume. In addition, protein stores are increased to prepare for the demands of labor, delivery, and lactation.

Calcium and Vitamin D

At birth, the healthy, full-term baby contains between 25 and 30 gm of calcium. Fetal deposition of calcium occurs primarily during the last trimester. For the calcium required by the fetus to be provided without mobilizing maternal skeletal reserves, 1,200 mg calcium per day is recommended, which represents a 50% increase over that required for the nonpregnant state. Proper use of calcium requires vitamin D. The amount of vitamin D recommended for the pregnant woman is double the 5 μg recommended for the nonpregnant woman.

Although there are numerous methods of providing the increased requirement for most nutrients, it is virtually impossible to provide the amount of calcium recommended for pregnant women without using dairy products. For instance, 1 qt of milk provides not only the allowance for calcium but the allowance for vitamin D and is an excellent source of protein of high biological value and also of other nutrients. Other foods that can contribute substantially to the calcium content of the diet include cheese (1½ oz of cheese = 8 oz of milk) and products such as cream soups and puddings that have nonfat dry milk solids added.

It has been suggested that leg cramps during pregnancy were caused by a decrease in serum calcium and an increase in serum phosphorus. It was further suggested that eliminating milk from the diet because of its high phosphorus content and administering aluminum hydroxide, which binds dietary phosphate, and thus preventing its absorption would aleviate the leg cramps. To date there is no research to justify this practice. Nevertheless, some physicians continue to recommend the routine elimination of milk and dairy products during pregnancy.

Iron

Iron requirements are increased during pregnancy primarily because maternal blood volume increases in order to provide for placental circulation and because the fetus receives iron stores that should last for the first three to six months of postnatal life. These iron stores are deposited during the final two months of pregnancy.

The average American diet contains 6 mg of iron per 1,000 Calories. Even with the increased caloric requirement it is difficult for the pregnant woman to obtain adequate quantities of iron from diet alone. Therefore, during pregnancy women should receive a supplement of 30–60 mg of elemental iron. They should be counseled that iron will cause their stools to be black and may cause either constipation or diarrhea. Gastrointestinal upset can be avoided by administering medicinal iron with meals. Absorption of iron can be improved by the concomitant administration of foods high in ascorbic acid, such as citrus fruit.

Anemia is a common problem during pregnancy, and 90% of the anemia encountered results from iron deficiency. Women at risk of iron-deficiency anemia include adolescents; women who have had several children, particularly when there have been short intervals between pregnancies; and women who have habitually consumed diets low in iron.

Hemoglobin and hematocrit are routinely used as parameters to screen for iron deficiency, but are not sensitive indicators. Iron stores are depleted before decreases in hemoglobin and hematocrit will occur. Adequate assessment of iron status requires determination of more sensitive indicators of iron status. Two tests commonly performed include serum iron (normal: greater than 42 mg%) and percentage saturation (normal: greater than 16%).

Folacin

During pregnancy the recommended intake for folacin is 800 μg, which represents a 100% increase over nonpregnant requirements. Folacin is necessary for DNA synthesis and thus for growth. Folacin deficiency has been shown to result in fetal damage. It is therefore imperative that the folacin intake during pregnancy be adequate. A medicinal supplement may be required to obtain adequate quantities of this nutrient. A supplement that provides 200–400 μg of folacin throughout the last half of pregnancy should sufficiently augment dietary intake and protect most pregnant women from folacin deficiency anemia.

Iodine

Iodine needs are increased from 150 μg to 175 μg. Pregnancy causes an increased BMR and a subsequent increase in thyroxine production. The requirements of iodine can usually be met by using iodized salt during food preparation.

Magnesium

Magnesium is a coenzyme in energy and protein metabolism and thus is necessary for tissue growth and muscle action. Magnesium requirements are increased from 300 mg to 450 mg during pregnancy. Magnesium-rich foods include nuts, soybeans, cocoa, seafood, and dried beans.

Vitamin A

Vitamin A requirements are increased from 800 μg Retinol Equivalents to 1,000 μg Retinol Equivalents. Essential for cell development and fetal tooth bud formation, vitamin A can usually be obtained in sufficient quantities from foods. Green and yellow vegetables and fortified margarine are good sources.

Vitamin E

Vitamin E, necessary for tissue growth and cell-wall integrity, can be found in leafy vegetables, cereals, meats, eggs, and milk. Vitamin E requirements during pregnancy are 10 mg α-tocopherol Equivalents, compared to

8 mg α-tocopheral Equivalents for nonpregnant adult women.

Vitamin C

Vitamin C requirements are also increased by one-third during pregnancy. Vitamin C is vital to tissue formation and integrity. Well-known sources such as citrus fruits; strawberries; cantaloupes; tomatoes; and green, leafy vegetables are incorporated into the diet. The pregnant woman requires 80 mg of vitamin C daily, compared to 60 mg for the nonpregnant woman.

B Vitamins

Vitamins B_6 and B_{12} are both coenzymes in protein metabolism. Because of maternal and fetal growth additional amounts of both vitamins are required. The vitamin B_6 requirement is raised from 2.0 mg for the nonpregnant woman to 2.6 mg for the pregnant one. 4 μg of Vitamin B_{12} is required, compared to 3 μg for the nonpregnant woman.

Sodium

In the past it has been a routine practice to restrict dietary sodium during pregnancy. It now appears that this dictum is not only unfounded but potentially dangerous. There appears to be an increased requirement during pregnancy to maintain normal sodium levels in the plasma and various tissues. Imposing a dietary sodium restriction can result in a deficit, and because the glomerular filtration rate increases by 50% early in pregnancy, the kidneys are more efficient in handling sodium.

Vitamin and Mineral Supplementation

Despite the increased requirement for every vitamin and mineral during pregnancy, if the diet contains a wide variety of foods from all of the food groups and is adequate in food energy, protein, and calcium, and if a folacin and iron supplement is used, further supplementation is unnecessary. The use of a vitamin pill may provide a false sense of security for both the expectant mother and the nurse and doctor who care for her. The method of choice for ensuring nutritional adequacy is through the selection of a balanced diet. Efforts to improve the dietary habits of pregnant women will affect not only their health and the health of their unborn but the health of the rest of the family.

DIET-RELATED PROBLEMS OF PREGNANCY

Understanding the physiological basis for the physical discomfort some women experience during pregnancy should enable the nurse to be of greater assistance to her clients. Heartburn is a common problem, particularly during the latter part of pregnancy. It occurs because the cardiac sphincter becomes relaxed in pregnancy, allowing the contents of the stomach to empty back into the esophagus. Smaller, more frequent meals may ease the back pressure and decrease heartburn for some women. An even simpler solution is to remain sitting for at least one hour after food is eaten. Reflux into the esophagus is much more common in the recumbent position than while sitting or standing. Dietary modifications would include the avoidance of spicy and highly acidic foods such as tomatoes.

Constipation may also be a problem for the expectant woman. Constipation may result from the relaxation of the smooth muscles in the gastrointestinal tract, from the pressure exerted on the digestive tract by the growing fetus, or from the medicinal iron the woman is taking. A diet high in fiber and foods with a laxative effect together with an increased intake of fluids should provide some relief for the constipation.

Vomiting may present problems during the first trimester. Dehydration may result from excessive vomiting. It may be caused by the decreased gastric emptying time of the stomach resulting from decreased gastric acid and pepsin concentrations. Restricting the fat in the diet and eliminating fluids with meals during this period may reduce or eliminate the vomiting. If the vomiting persists past the twelfth week or results in an inappropriate weight gain or loss, medical attention should be sought.

There has been increasing concern over the risks associated with alcohol consumption during pregnancy. Recently, the Department of Health, Education, and Welfare's National Institute of Alcohol Abuse and Alcoholism advised women that as little as two drinks of hard liquor consumed daily on a regular basis can cause fetal defects. The risk rate ranges from 10% for women consuming 2–4 oz of hard liquor a day to 74% for heavier drinkers. Babies born to mothers who consumed alcohol during their pregnancies have a variety of congenital defects including eye, ear, or heart defects, disturbed sleep patterns, seizure disorders, mental retardation, and facial abnormalities.

NUTRITIONAL REQUIREMENTS DURING LACTATION

Women who choose to breast-feed their babies should receive appropriate information about their nutritional needs, which are even greater during lactation than during pregnancy. If women gain weight normally during pregnancy, they store from 2 to 4 kg (4.4–8.8 lb) of fat, which can offset the energy cost of lactation. In this case, approximately 500 Calories in addition to normal needs are required to support lactation during the first three months after the baby's birth. If lactation continues beyond 3 months, however, or if substantial weight loss occurs, caloric intake will need to be increased. If caloric requirements are not met, the quantity of milk produced may be affected.

Caloric requirements should be supplied by a well-balanced diet that contains more protein, vitamins, and minerals than the woman normally requires. The iron supplement recommended during pregnancy should be continued for at least the first three months of lactation to replenish maternal iron stores. In addition to eating a well-balanced diet (Fig. 15-2), the lactating woman should drink plenty of fluids (six to eight glasses a day). If the fluid intake is inadequate, the mother may become dehydrated, and the quantity of milk she produces may be decreased.

Circumstances other than diet can influence the mother's milk supply, and so to avoid problems anticipatory guidance should be provided in appropriate breast-feeding technique. Practices in the hospital should be structured to support a successful lactating experience. Unless it is otherwise contraindicated, the baby should be put to its mother's breast in the delivery room. Furthermore, the mother should be allowed to have her baby in

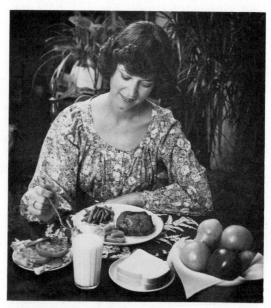

Figure 15-2. Nutritional needs are increased during lactation. (Courtesy Ross Laboratories)

her room with her so that she can feed on demand and can put the baby to her breast more frequently than generally occurs when a baby is kept in the nursery (Fig. 15-3).

When the infant begins to suck, a message is carried to the mother's hypothalamus via the nervous system to signal the anterior pituitary gland to release *prolactin* and to signal the posterior pituitary gland to release *oxytocin.* Prolactin is necessary for the synthesis of the protein, carbohydrate, and fat necessary for milk production. Oxytocin causes the cells to contract so that milk can be released from the breast, a process called *milk letdown.* A mother can usually feel a tingling sensation that accompanies milk letdown some 30–60 seconds after sucking begins.

Although there may be advantages to feeding on demand, mothers still need some guidelines as to how often and for how long their babies need to be fed. The medical literature reports far too many cases of the breast-fed baby who was simply "too good." These babies did not cry very often and thus were not fed enough by the usually best-intending mothers. Mothers should understand that initially the capacity of their babies' stomachs is only an ounce or two. In addition, human milk is easily digested. Thus a baby may need to be put to the breast every two hours for 5 to

10 minutes. As the baby grows and the stomach capacity increases, the interval between feeding will increase, as will the length of feedings. By one month of age most babies will nurse every three to four hours for 15 to 20 minutes. It is also preferable to feed from both breasts during a feeding period. Using only one breast during a feeding reduces the stimulation for milk production, and most of the milk can be emptied from a breast in the first 10 minutes of active sucking. To continue sucking on the same breast provides more oral satisfaction than actual nourishment.

Having the baby suck at the breast provides the necessary stimulus for production of an adequate supply of milk. The nurse can tell if the milk supply is adequate by evaluating how well the baby is growing (discussed in the next chapter) and by the number of wet diapers. If there are no other sources of fluid, the breast-fed baby will have at least six to eight wet diapers a day.

Common practices that make it difficult for a nursing mother to establish an adequate milk supply include giving commercial formula during the first few days of life "until the milk comes in." Although the *colostrum* produced by the mother is thin and watery in appearance, it contains the nutrients and other properties needed by the baby. Putting the baby to the breast as soon after delivery as possible and then every two to three hours will not only make the milk "come in" sooner but provide health benefits to the baby that can be obtained from no other source.

If for any reason the mother must feed her infant from a bottle during the first four to eight weeks, she should be encouraged to express the milk from her breasts manually. This practice will not only continue the stimulation necessary for milk production but prevent the discomfort for the mother from breasts being too full.

Other factors that may interfere with the mother's ability to produce sufficient milk are her mental and physical state. Mothers who are too tired or who are upset or anxious may not have an appropriate letdown reflex.

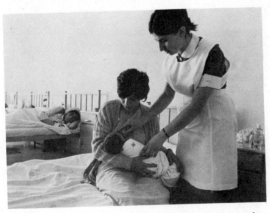

Figure 15-3. The nurse shows this new mother how to breast feed her infant. (WHO photo by J. Mohr)

Stress can inhibit the release of oxytocin and hence of milk letdown. Stress can establish a vicious cycle. The baby becomes frustrated because sucking does not produce the desired result. As the baby gets more hungry and more irritable, the environment for the mother becomes more stressful. Without proper support from her family and from the nurse, lactation failure can follow. While a woman is breast-feeding she should be encouraged to take care of herself as well as her baby and to get plenty of rest.

Excessive amounts of coffee or soft drinks high in caffeine, smoking, and some drugs can interfere with the letdown reflex or with milk production. Drugs should be taken only with a physician's approval.

NUTRITIONAL REQUIREMENTS AND ORAL CONTRACEPTIVES

Approximately 10 million American women take oral contraceptives as a means of birth control. Oral contraceptives have been on the market for almost 30 years. With the experience obtained during this interval has come the realization that nutrient use may be adversely affected by the prolonged use of oral contraceptives. Nutritional aberrations attributed to oral contraceptives include decreased blood levels of folacin, vitamin B_{12}, riboflavin, ascorbic acid, zinc, and vitamin B_6. Although rare, the lowered blood levels have been followed by clinical evidence of a nutritional deficiency for all the nutrients except ascorbic acid and zinc. It is not currently known whether the nutritional status of women before using oral contraceptives contributed to the deficiencies observed.

The currently recognized nutritional problems associated with using oral contraceptives are not sufficient to warrant discontinuing their use but are sufficient to warrant the routine assessment of the nutritional status of women on these medications. If diets are found to be inadequate in any nutrient, appropriate dietary counseling should be provided to improve the quality of the diet. In addition, a biochemical and clinical evaluation should be preformed to rule out a frank deficiency state.

The issue of whether women taking oral contraceptives should also take a multivitamin and mineral preparation is currently unresolved. If dietary intake is marginal the risk of developing a nutritional deficiency is probably greater. These women would probably benefit from taking a multivitamin preparation as a prophylactic measure. As in pregnancy, however, this practice should not be substituted for appropriate dietary advice and proper eating habits.

BIBLIOGRAPHY

Committee on Maternal Nutrition. *Maternal Nutrition and the Course of Pregnancy.* Washington, D.C.: Nat'l Acad. of Sciences, 1970.

Committee on Nutrition. *Nutrition in Maternal Health Care.* Washington, D.C.: Nat'l Acad. of Sciences, 1974.

Committee on Nutrition of the Mother and Preschool Child. *Laboratory Indices of Nutritional Status in Pregnancy.* Washington, D.C.: Nat'l Acad. of Sciences, 1978.

Food and Nutrition Board, Nat'l Research Council. *Recommended Dietary Allowances.* 9th Ed. Washington, D.C.: Nat'l Acad. of Sciences, 1980.

Hibbard, B. M. The role of folic acid in pregnancy with particular reference to anemia, abruption and abortion. *J. Obstet. Gynaecol. Br. Commonw.* 71:529, 1964.

Higgins, A. C. Nutritional status and the outcome of pregnancy. *J. Am. Diet. Assoc.* 37:17, 1976.

Hytten, F. E., and Leitch, I. *The Physiology of Human Pregnancy.* 2nd Ed. Oxford: Blackwell Scientific Publications Ltd., 1971.

Jacobson, H. N. Weight and weight gain in pregnancy. *Clin. Perinatol.* 2:233, 1975.

Kitay, K. Z., and Harbort, R. A. Iron and folic acid deficiency in pregnancy. *Clin. Perinatol.* 2:255, 1975.

Pike, R. Further evidence of deleterious effects produced by sodium restriction during pregnancy. *Am. J. Clin. Nutr.* 23:883, 1970.

Pike, R. and Smiciklas, H. A reappraisal of sodium restriction during pregnancy. *Int. J. Gynaecol. Obstet.* 10:1, 1972.

CHAPTER 16

Nutrition During the Growing Years

Judith Bonner

GROWTH

The way children grow is the single most useful indicator of their nutritional status. Moreover, it is impossible to evaluate the adequacy of children's diets without also evaluating how well they are growing. Growth is the most highly sensitive indicator of nutrient intake. Each child's growth potential is determined by his genetic endowment. Proper evaluation of growth must take into consideration the size of the parents and the size and growth rate of the siblings. Many things can influence whether or not a child achieves his growth potential, including state of health, home environment, and nutrition.

Growth occurs in an orderly fashion, although the rate at which children grow varies considerably between children and at different ages. The following landmarks may be useful in putting into perspective the average size of children at various ages. The average birth weight for children born in the United States is 3.4 kg (7.5 lb) (range: 2.5–4.6 kg, or 5.5–10 lb). During the first four to six months of life, infants gain an average of 20 gm/day. By four to six months most have doubled their birth weight. During the second six months infants gain an average of 15 gm/day. By the first birthday infants have tripled their birth weight. Around this time the rate of growth begins to slow down. Yearly gains average 2.5 kg (5–6 lb) until the adolescent growth spurt begins. For girls this may be as

early as age 10 or as late as age 14, whereas for boys the age range is 12–16 years.

The average birth length is 50 cm (20 in) (range: 45–55 cm, or 18–22 in). Infants increase their length by 50% in the first year. By four to six months the average length is 66 cm (26 in), and by one year it is 75 cm (30 in). During the second year of life most toddlers grow another 10–12 cm (5 in). From then on, yearly increases in length average 5–7 cm (2–3 in), until the pubertal growth spurt.

Head circumference is a useful measure of nutritional status for the first two years of life. At birth the circumference of the average infant's head is 34–35 cm (14 in). By four to six months the head is 44 cm (18 in); by one year, 47 cm (19 in); and by two years, 49 cm (20 in).

For growth rate to be a clinically useful tool, weighing and measuring must be done with great precision, and the measurements obtained must be plotted on appropriate growth charts. Beam scales with nondetachable weights should be used to weigh infants and children. Scales should receive proper maintenance, including calibration, at routine intervals. For accuracy, infants should be unclothed and children should wear lightweight underclothes or a preweighed hospital gown. Whenever possible, weights should be obtained at approximately the same time of day and under the same conditions.

Until the infant is 3 years old, recumbent length should be recorded. This measurement requires the assistance of two examiners. The child lies on a firm table to which a measuring stick has been permanently attached. One examiner holds the child's feet against a foot board. The other examiner places a headboard at right angles to the child's head and the tape measure. Preferably, the examiners then exchange positions, and a second measurement is taken. If a discrepancy between the measurements occurs, the reason is determined and the measurement is corrected.

For children over 3 years old, a measuring stick is permanently attached to the wall so that standing height can be accurately recorded. It is too easy to make errors when using the measuring stick attached to most platform scales. The child should be instructed to stand so that his heels, buttocks, shoulders, and head are flat against the measuring stick. Again, a headboard is brought down so that it is at right angles to the top of the child's head and the measuring stick, and the measurement is read and recorded.

A nonflexible tape measure is used to measure head circumference. The tape should be placed firmly around the head so that the maximum circumference is obtained.

The next step in evaluating the way in which a child is growing is to plot the measurements obtained on the appropriate growth chart. The most recent growth charts were constructed by the National Center for Health Statistics and are reproduced free of charge by several infant formula manufacturers for use in hospitals and health clinics. There are four separate charts for infant boys and girls from birth to 36 months and for boys and girls from 2 to 18 years.

Growth charts are divided into percentiles. The measurements of a large statistical sample of children have been ranked in size from the smallest to the largest and have been assigned percentiles that correspond to their positions in the rank order. The middle measurement, or the median, is called the fiftieth

percentile. Approximately half of the children of the same sex and age are smaller and half are larger than a child whose measurements fall at the fiftieth percentile. A percentile of 90 indicates a measurement that is as great or greater than that of 90% of the children in the sample. Half of the children can be expected to fall between the twenty-fifth and the seventy-fifth percentiles; 80% of the children can be expected to fall between the tenth and ninetieth percentiles. Any percentile from 1 to 99 can be determined, although growth charts have specific percentiles, called *percentile levels,* marked with black lines to show the extent to which measurements deviate from the median. The major percentile levels are the fifth, tenth, twenty-fifth, fiftieth, seventy-fifth, ninetieth, and ninety-fifth.

It is an all-too-common mistake to have the fiftieth percentile as a goal for growth. If this were realistic, all children of the same age and sex would be identical in size. A single plot on a growth chart merely tells how big a child is in relation to other healthy children of the same age and sex. Several plots over time are necessary to indicate how well a child is growing. By the time a child is 2 or 3 years of age, growth will begin to follow in the same track or channel. It is then easy to detect early signs of obesity or malnutrition, provided accurate measurements are taken and plotted and the genetic potential of the child is considered. Changes in weight reflect recent changes in diet, whereas changes in height measurements reflect the long-term effects of diet.

Children whose weight plots above the ninety-fifth percentile or whose weight or height plots below the fifth percentile deserve a more detailed assessment of their nutrition and health status as described in chapter 19. Although 10% of all healthy, well-nourished children will exceed these limits, the limits are useful in detecting the child with nutritional problems. One should in fact begin to look more closely at the children who plot above the seventy-fifth or below the twenty-fifth percentile. If their genetics does not indicate a predisposition for the current size, nutritional assessment and counseling, will be most effective if done immediately, while the problem can still be prevented, rather than later, when treatment is required. Other times the growth chart should signal concern include:

1. *When there are 2 percentile levels difference between the weight and the height.* For example, if height is at the twenty-fifth percentile and weight is at the seventy-fifth, the child is probably overweight. Or, if the child's height is at the fiftieth percentile and weight is at the fifth, the child may be underweight. In this case, if the child's weight has been following the fifth percentile for a number of years or if the child's family are lean in build, there may be no reason for concern. If, however, the child's weight has followed along the fiftieth percentile for a number of years and has suddenly dropped to the fifth percentile, the nurse should look for a nutritional problem or another health concern for which the child needs help.

2. *When there is a sudden change in percentile levels so that the child's measurements cross 2 percentile levels.* For example, if a 7-year-old child who has been growing steadily at the twenty-fifth percentiles for weight and height for several years suddenly jumps to the seventy-fifth percentile for weight and height, his dietary intake should be evaluated to make certain the child's diet is not excessive. Frequently, overweight children grow taller faster. If this trend is not picked up and help provided, in a few years their weight will markedly exceed the ninety-fifth percentile. At that point successful therapy is frequently not possible.

It is important to weigh, measure, and plot growth each time a child comes for health care. The growth chart should moreover be explained to the mother and, when appropriate, to the child, to let them know how the child is doing and to serve as a motivating aid in counseling.

NUTRITIONAL REQUIREMENTS

Nutrient requirements vary considerably during the pediatric period. Requirements reflect the child's needs for growth and maintenance.

Fluid

The body of a newborn contains proportionally more water than that of an adult. The adult value of 60–65% is reached by 1 year of age.

Water is required for growth, to replace the losses that occur through the gastrointestinal tract, urinary tract, respiratory tract, and skin. Factors that increase fluid requirements include a diet containing a high renal-solute load, fever, diarrhea, vomiting, and hot weather. Approximate daily fluid requirements of healthy children under normal conditions are:

Age	ml/kg of Body Weight
Birth to 2 weeks	60–100
2 weeks to 1 year	125–150
1–3 years	125
4–6 years	100
7–12 years	75
Over 13 years	50

It is particularly important to assess the fluid needs of infants, for they cannot make their feelings of thirst known.

Food Energy

The pediatric age group require food energy to cover the cost of basal metabolism, specific dynamic action, maintenance, activity, and growth. Caloric requirements for growth are greatest during growth spurts. Activity varies considerably among children. Differences in growth rate and in activity pattern explain most of the variability in caloric requirements. Dramatic differences can even be seen during infancy. Infants who sleep a lot and rarely cry need fewer Calories than infants who are awake most of the day (and sometimes night!) and who cry a lot. Assessment of how well a child is growing is necessary to determine whether caloric intake needs to be adjusted upward or downward. Table 16-1 lists the RDAs of certain nutrients for infants and children.

Protein

Infants require over twice as much protein per unit of body weight as adults do. The amount of protein needed gradually decreases as the rate of growth decreases. Although protein is essential for the promotion of growth and health, the average US diet provides ample protein. Surveys designed to evaluate the nutritional status of population groups in the United States have revealed that protein deficiency is not a serious problem for children who do not suffer from a chronic illness. If caloric needs are met using a wide variety of foods and all four food groups, protein needs will probably also be met. Children at risk of a protein deficiency are those who simply do not get enough food or those whose parents follow a fad diet such as the Zen macrobiotic diet, a diet that ultimately restricts everything in the diet except brown rice.

Minerals

Recommendations for calcium and phosphorus are high during the growing years but can easily be met if milk and dairy products are included in the diet. It is recommended that by 6 months of age a daily intake of 15 mg of iron be included in the diet. The difficulties of getting adequate iron (18 mg) in the diets of adult women are well known. It is difficult to meet an infant's iron requirement unless an iron-fortified formula is fed. Infant cereal also contributes significantly to the iron content of the diet. Although breast milk contains very little iron, the amount pre-

sent is readily absorbed. Authorities continue to debate whether the breast-fed baby needs supplemental iron. The best way to ensure that the iron needs of children are being met is to assess iron status on a routine basis by determining the hemoglobin, hematocrit, serum iron, percentage of saturation, and total iron-binding capacity.

Flouride

Fluoride has been shown to be effective in reducing the incidence of dental disease. When fluoride is not included in the water supply, a supplement is indicated. The nurse can check with the local water system to determine the fluoride content of the water supply. Do not assume that because a city does not have a fluoridation program that there is inadequate fluoride in the water. Fluoride is naturally occurring in many water supplies. If a family uses water for which the fluoride content is unknown, collect a sample and have it analyzed. The state Department of Health can usually advise where to send the water for analysis. Mottling of the teeth can occur when too much fluoride is ingested.

The amount of fluoride recommended varies with the age of the child and the concentration of fluoride in the water. If the water contains more than 0.7 ppm, a fluoride supplement is not needed; if the fluoride concentration is less than 0.3 ppm, children less than 2 years old need 0.25 mg; those from 2 to 3 years, 0.50 mg; and those from 3 to 14 years, 1.0 mg. If the concentration of fluoride is between these two levels, children less than 2 years of age do not need additional fluoride; those from 2 to 3 years need 0.24 mg; and those from 3 to 14 years need 0.5 mg.

Vitamins

Infant formula and cow's milk to which vitamin D has been added are the only significant dietary sources of vitamins in milk. The breast-fed baby should receive a supplement

TABLE 16.1 Recommended Daily Dietary Allowances of Selected Nutrients

Age (yr)	Weight (kg)	Height (cm)	Food Energy (Calories)	Protein (g)	Vitamin A (µg RE)	Vitamin D (µg)	Vitamin E (mgαTE)	Vitamin C (mg)	Calcium (mg)	Phosphorus (mg)	Magnesium (mg)	Iron (mg)
0–0.5	6	60	kg × 95–145	kg × 2.2	420	10	3	35	360	240	50	10
0.5–1.0	9	71	kg × 80–135	kg × 2.0	400	10	4	35	540	360	70	15
1–3	13	90	900–1,800	23	400	10	5	45	800	800	150	15
4–6	20	112	1,300–2,300	30	500	10	6	45	800	800	200	10
7–10	28	132	1,650–3,300	34	700	10	7	45	800	800	250	10
Boys 11–14	45	157	2,000–3,700	45	1,000	10	8	50	1,200	1,200	350	18
Girls 11–14	46	157	1,500–3,000	46	800	10	8	50	1,200	1,200	300	18
Boys 15–18	66	176	2,100–3,900	56	1,000	10	10	60	1,200	1,200	400	18
Girls 15–18	55	163	1,200–3,000	46	800	10	8	60	1,200	1,200	300	18

SOURCE: Adapted from *Recommended Dietary Allowances*, 9th Ed. (1980), with the permission of the Nat'l Acad. of Sciences. Washington, D.C.

of vitamin D even though rickets is rarely observed in breast-fed babies.

A varied diet containing all four food groups and meeting caloric requirements will probably supply the vitamins needed by the pediatric population. Care should be taken to include citrus fruit for vitamin C and a dark-yellow or dark-green vegetable for vitamin A. The B-complex vitamins will be supplied in adequate amounts if good-quality protein foods, breads, and cereals are included in the diet.

Many parents worry about whether to give their children multivitamins. Although probably unnecessary, one multivitamin a day will do no harm. It cannot, however, take the place of a balanced diet.

FEEDING PRACTICES IN INFANCY

During the first year of life the newborn undergoes an intense period of growth, development, and maturation. Nutritional requirements are greater per unit of body weight than they ever will be again. Although meeting nutritional needs will not guarantee a healthy and happy baby, a loving and stimulating environment is incomplete without a good diet.

Human Milk

Milk is an infant's most important food. There are many forms of milk available for mothers to choose from. Nurses must be knowledgeable about these alternatives to assist mothers in making a wise choice.

The American Academy of Pediatrics has recently reaffirmed their position of encouraging the use of human milk as the sole source of nutrition for the first six months of life and as a major source of nutrition during the second six months. The advantages of breast-feeding are many and include benefits for both the mother and the infant. In addition to the maternal bonding that occurs, the mother may derive benefit from an earlier involution of her uterus and from mobilization of fat deposited during pregnancy for lactation. The infant also benefits from the close physical contact with the mother. In addition, human milk is unquestionably superior in quality to commercial milk. Human milk contains a number of ingredients that may offer protection against infections. These factors include *secretory IgA, Lactobacillus bifidus, lysozyme, lactoferrin,* and *lactoperoxidase.* Intake of human milk may reduce the incidence of allergies. In cases where there is a strong family history of allergy, the mother is generally encouraged to consider breast-feeding.

The percentage of Calories from carbohydrate, protein, and fat appears optimal in human milk. Interestingly, the concentration of fat in the milk changes during a single feeding period. The milk initially produced (*foremilk*) contains 2% fat. As the baby nurses, the concentration of fat increases until the milk produced at the end of the feeding (*hindmilk*) contains 7% fat. It has been suggested that the higher fat content of the hindmilk may be involved in appetite regulation. Many references give the fat content of human milk as 3.2%; this figure is an average value. Table 16-2 compares the food energy and distribution of Calories from protein, fat, and carbohydrate in various forms of milk.

The concentration of protein is low, as is the concentration of electrolytes such as sodium, potassium, and chlorine. Protein (nitrogen) and minerals consumed in excess must be excreted in the urine, thus presenting the kidney with a high *renal-solute load.* Because the kidneys of newborns may not be as efficient at concentrating the urine, the low renal-solute load of human milk may be advantageous. Table 16-3 compares the renal-solute load of various forms of milk.

Human milk is also easier to digest. Digestibility is influenced by the proportion of milk protein that is casein or whey. In human milk 40% of the protein is casein, and 60% is whey; in cow's milk, 82% of the protein is

TABLE 16-2. A Comparison of Food Energy and Nutrient Content of Various Forms of Milk

| | Food Energy (Calories/oz) | Distribution of Calories from: | | |
		Protein (%)	Fat (%)	Carbohydrate (%)
Recommended range	—	7–16	30–55	35–65
Human milk	20	7	55	38
Milk-based formula	20	9	48–50	41–43
Soy-based formula	20	9	48	43
Cow's milk				
Whole	20	22	49	29
2%	18	28	35	37
Skim	10	40	2	58

casein, and 18% is whey. Lactose is the primary carbohydrate in human milk as well as in cow's milk, but the concentration of lactose is greater in human milk. Human milk is a rich source of cholesterol and polyunsaturated fats, particularly linoleic acid, the essential fatty acid. The fat is more easily digested than the fat in cow's milk. Table 16-4 gives the fat, cholesterol, and linoleic acid content of various forms of milk.

Commercial Milk Formulas

An iron-fortified commercial formula is an acceptable alternative for the woman who chooses not to breast-feed her baby. As with human milk, formula should be the sole source of nutrition for the first four to six months of life and a major source of nutrition during the second six months of life (see Fig. 16-1). Nutrient composition of standard milk-based formulas (Similac, Enfamil, and

SMA) is as similar to the nutrient composition of human milk as the manufacturing process permits. It is obviously impossible to duplicate the milk synthesized by the mammary glands, but women who choose to use a commercial formula should be assured that the nutritional needs of their infants can be met.

Standard milk-based formulas can be purchased ready to feed with or without iron; Mothers may be instructed to use the iron-fortified ones. Formulas can be purchased ready to feed (already in the bottle with the nipple attached); in 32- or 8-oz ready-to-pour cans with formula in the correct concentration; in 13-oz cans of concentrated formula that must be diluted with an equal volume of water; and powdered in cans. Serious consequences can result if ready-to-feed formula is diluted with an equal quantity of water or if concentrated formula is fed straight from the can. Thus, mothers need to be instructed about the use of the various types.

TABLE 16-3. Renal-solute Load of Various Forms of Milk

	Renal-solute Load (mOsm/liter)	Protein (gm/liter)	Sodium (mEq/liter)	Potassium (mEq/liter)	Chloride (mEq/liter)
Human milk	79	12	7	13	11
Milk-based formulas	99	14	8–10	12–20	10–15
Soy-based formulas	140	24	12–20	18–20	12–15
Cow's milk, whole	221	33	25	35	29

TABLE 16-4. Fat, Cholesterol, and Linoleic Acid Content of Various Forms of Milk

	Total Fat (gm/liter)	Cholesterol (mg/liter)	Linoleic Acid (% Calories)	Polyunsaturated to Saturated Ratio
Human milk	43	130–360	3.8	0.2 : 1
Milk-based formulas	36	12	20	1.8 : 1
Soy-based formulas	32	0	23	3.8 : 1
Cow's milk, whole	35	140	1.1	0.08 : 1

A wide variety of soy-based formulas are available for the infant who shows symptoms of allergy or intolerance to the milk-based formulas. These formulas are made from protein isolated from soy and are fortified with various minerals. Soy-based formulas are also lactose free. The carbohydrate used is generally sucrose, corn syrup or a mixture of the two. All soy-based formulas contain iron or are fortified with it. They are usually available in the same dilutions as the standard milk-based formulas.

Although cow's milk makes an important contribution to the nutritional quality of the diets of toddlers, children, teens, and adults, it is not recommended during the first year of life. Cow's milk is not a good source of iron, for it only provides 0.5 mg/liter (or quart). Feeding cow's milk during the first couple of months of life is associated with gastrointestinal bleeding. Both the low concentration of iron in the milk and the blood loss may contribute to the iron deficiency seen in infants fed cow milk. Also, cow's milk is deficient in vitamin C and contains excessive protein, minerals, and renal-solute load.

The problems associated with whole cow's milk are also associated with 2% and skim milk. In addition, skim milk is deficient in linoleic acid, the essential fatty acid, and in Calories. Although babies fed skim milk grow, they grow more slowly than babies fed human milk or commercial formula, and part of the growth apparently occurs at the expense of depositing fat that provides the needed reserve in case of illness.

The first birthday is the age at which it is appropriate to introduce whole or 2% milk. By this age most children have developed adequately and are eating a sufficient variety and quantity of other foods from all the food groups to make the concerns about feeding cow's milk no longer relevant.

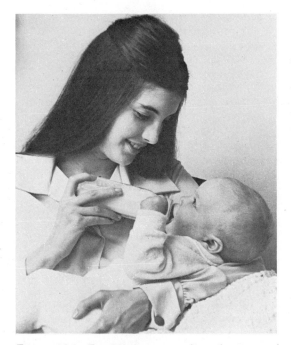

Figure 16-1. Feeding time can be relaxing and pleasurable for both mother and baby. (Courtesy Ross Laboratories)

Solid Foods

The current recommendation concerning solid foods is to delay their introduction until the infant is at least four months and preferably six months old (see Fig. 16-2). Nutritionally speaking, there is no need to introduce them sooner. Human milk or commercial formula alone provides all the nourishment required during this period. Introducing solid foods earlier may lead to an excessive caloric intake, which leads to an excessive rate of weight gain, which in turn leads to infantile obesity. Because infancy is a time when weight reduction is not advocated, it is imperative to initiate practices that establish good eating habits.

Solid foods, particularly strained meats and vegetables, increase the renal-solute load. A high solute load without additional fluid may impose an undue burden on immature kidneys. It particularly puts the infant at risk of dehydration if the high renal-solute load is superimposed on an illness that includes fever, vomiting, or diarrhea. All the enzymes needed for the digestion and subsequent absorption of foods are not present. This is particularly true of pancreatic amylase, which hydrolyzes starch. Activity of pancreatic

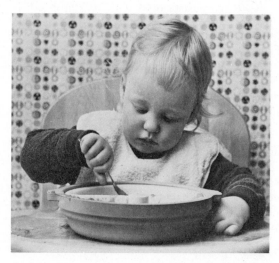

Figure 16-2. Eating solid foods presents a new challenge to the baby. (Courtesy Ross Laboratories)

amylase increases around the third month of life. Nor is the baby developmentally ready to take food from a spoon until three to four months. The presence of rooting, suckswallow, and extrusion reflexes make spoon feeding more difficult, as does poor head control and inability to sit.

The order in which solid foods are introduced is, by and large, a matter of individual preference rather than scientific reasoning. One method is to introduce cereals first, followed by vegetables, fruits, meats, and then eggs. Each time a new food is introduced it is wise to allow a few days before another new food is introduced to see if any symptoms of allergy or intolerance appear. For this same reason it is always preferable to introduce each ingredient separately before giving mixtures. For example, if the first cereal introduced is mixed cereal and the child breaks out in a rash, it will not be clear which ingredient is causing the problem.

Today, more and more mothers are interested in making their own strained food rather than purchasing commercial products. If wise shopping habits are used, preparing one's own baby foods can be more economical. Mothers who make their own baby food should, however, be counseled to prepare it without adding extra salt, butter, sugar, or cream sauces. Most commercial manufacturers have reduced or eliminated the sugar and salt and have eliminated the additives in their products.

Commercial manufacturers produce a wide range of infant desserts. A quick glance at the label will show that the primary difference between a fruit and a dessert made from that fruit, such as applesauce versus apple Betty or peaches versus peach cobbler, is the fact that sugar is added to the desserts. There are sufficient numbers of fruits, vegetables, breads, cereals, meats, and dairy products available to choose from without ever offering the products in the dessert line. Many people wonder at what age people establish a "sweet tooth." Research has established that babies come into this world with a preference for the sweet taste.

By the time babies are seven to nine months of age, they should have foods with different textures. One method of achieving this is to offer table foods that are soft enough for the baby to manage, for example, scrambled eggs, mashed potatoes, macaroni and cheese, or mashed vegetables. If foods with different textures are not offered during this sensitive period of development, babies may not readily accept them later.

When babies can sit alone, have developed eye-hand coordination and the *pincer grasp* (can pick up objects with the thumb and pointing finger), and can transfer objects from hand to hand, they are ready to begin finger foods. This generally occurs between 9 and 12 months of age. Green beans, slices of banana, peaches, hot dog, pieces of toast, or other similar foods can be managed independently. Hard pieces of food such as peanuts, popcorn, hard candy, or berries may cause choking. At this same time babies can hold their own bottles or begin to drink from a training cup.

Babies should be taken off the bottle when they are developmentally ready to drink from a cup. This means that they not only have mastered the ability to finger feed but have lip control. Although the cup should be introduced sooner, most babies will not master cup feeding until 1 to 1½ years of age. After a baby has teeth, however, it is important not to put the baby to bed with milk or any sweetened liquid. Some liquid usually remains in the mouth after the infant goes to sleep and continually bathes the teeth, promoting tooth decay.

Also around 1 year of age children will begin to play with the spoon. Although most are not yet developmentally ready to master spoon feeding, it is important to allow them to try. Even though spills will inevitably occur, the youngsters will in time learn to feed themselves.

The rapid rate of growth that occurred during the first year begins to slow down. At this time many mothers become concerned that their children's appetites have decreased. Both diet and growth should be evaluated to make certain there are no problems. Then mothers should be reassured that this is one of nature's ways of protecting against obesity. Children require and demand more food when growth rate increases than during periods of quiescence.

FEEDING PRACTICES FROM TODDLER TO TEEN

The variety of foods necessary to meet the nutritional needs of healthy, active children throughout the period of growth are the same as for adults. Their diets are also built around the basic four food groups, but the amounts of these foods needed to supply Calories and nutrients vary with age.

Preschool Children

Many preschool children prefer simply prepared foods; appreciation of gourmet cooking occurs at a later age. Initially, toddlers prefer plain foods served individually rather than in mixtures. Serving foods individually gives young children the assurance that they are getting what they are expecting. It also provides an opportunity for them to explore differences in color, shape, and texture.

Toddlers fed a wide variety of foods as infants are more likely to accept a wide variety of foods (Fig. 16-3). When new foods are introduced, young children should be allowed to learn to accept them at their own rate. They are great imitators; if parents or older siblings refuse certain foods, chances are greater that preschoolers will too. Nurses should counsel mothers never to use force to get children to eat. It rarely works. More often than not both the mother and the child turn out to be the loser.

By 3 or 4 years of age, children begin food jags. These jags usually do not last long. They

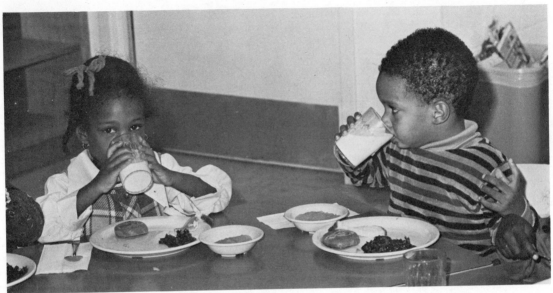

Figure 16-3. Well-balanced meals give preschoolers the nutrients needed for growth. (USDA photo by Jack Schneider)

are one of the few ways in which a child this young can exert his independence. Unless the food jag is for food that provides mainly Calories with little or no other nutritional value, little harm results from catering to the child's wishes. The less that is said about the food jag, the less likely that problems will occur.

Appetites and food intake fluctuate considerably from day to day. Foods children eat with relish one day will be refused the next. This is typical eating behavior for children in this age group. Mothers soon learn when the loss of appetite reflects impending illness. A careful evaluation of the child's growth should reassure the mother that no harm is resulting from either the food jags or the daily variations in appetite, providing sweet drinks and candy between meals are not causing a mealtime loss of appetite.

Snacks for children are as much a part of life's routine as coffee breaks are for adults. Snack time should provide a nutritious rounding out of the child's diet. Foods to

choose from include juice, milk, fruit, raw vegetables, cheese, crackers, and peanut butter.

One of the most common problems mothers and health professionals alike have in evaluating the diets of preschoolers is in estimating portion size. A rule of thumb is to provide 1 T for each year of life. For example, a serving of green beans for a 2-year-old would be 2 T. Frequently parents become concerned that their children are not eating enough when their expectations may be the only problem. Children with small appetites generally respond better to smaller portions.

Another common feeding problem is the use of food as a reward or punishment. When parents use this approach they lose sight of the true purpose of food. Children should not be given ice cream for being good or refused juice for misbehaving.

Diets of preschoolers are most often low in calcium, vitamin A, and iron. The milk intake, and therefore the calcium intake, decreases with weaning. Children this age should continue to drink 16–24 oz (.5–.7 liters) of milk or to substitute other dairy products. Unless children are offered a wide variety of vegetables earlier in life, their acceptance may be low, resulting in low levels of vitamin A in the diet. Most milks have vitamin A added, however, which is another reason for encouraging milk intake. It is simply impossible to provide the recommended intake of 15 mg of iron when caloric needs only average 1,300, unless liver and foods that have iron added to them are used frequently. The only other alternative is to provide an iron supplement. Iron deficiency continues to be a problem for this age group.

A common problem that begins during the preschool years and continues for many people until old age is tooth decay. Approximately one-quarter of the 2-year-olds and two-thirds of the 3-year-olds in the world have at least one decayed tooth. (Arlin, 1977). The incidence for the United States may be even higher. After eating, plaque forms around teeth. If the plaque is not removed by brushing, it forms organic acids from sugars in the mouth. The enamel of the tooth is the target of the acids. Foods high in sugars that are sticky and adhere to the teeth contribute to the formation of decay. Such foods include carbonated beverages, caramels, other candies, jams, jellies, honey, chewing gum, cake, and cookies. On the other hand, crisp foods such as apples, carrots, and celery partially prevent other foods from adhering to the surface of the teeth and thus may help retard cavities. Fluoride, as has already been discussed, is also important in preventing decay. The best dental insurance policy is the establishment of good dietary and hygienic practices.

School-age Children

When children begin school their families lose control to a certain extent over their eating behavior. Suddenly their teachers and the school feeding programs begin to influence their habits. Even more important, their peers begin to exert pressure. Children must become independent and decide whether to follow the crowd or the advice of their families (see Fig. 16-4).

The appetites of most elementary school children are good, although many children may need to be coaxed into eating breakfast. Adhering more rigidly to a bedtime schedule and being more creative in planning breakfast may help improve its acceptance. Children are not likely to accept breakfast if the rest of the family do not join them.

By the time children begin the first grade, portion sizes of the foods commonly served should be average servings as recommended in the basic four plan.

Adolescents

As children approach adolescence the complexity of their lives and their problems increases. Eating a balanced diet is frequently not a high priority for them. As a group their diets have been frequently lacking in calcium, iron, ascorbic acid, and vitamin A. Their intakes of sugar, saturated fat, and salt are fre-

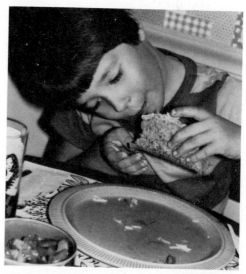

Figure 16-4. Finger foods such as tacos are a favorite of school-age children.

quently excessive. This results, in part, from frequent meals or snacks at fast-food chains.

During this period young men may get more interested in diet as they begin to show some promise as athletes. Most aspiring athletes will try anything in hopes of obtaining some competitive advantage. In general the only difference between the diets of athletes and nonathletes should be in the number of Calories consumed. During periods of active training, athletes may require from 500 Calories to 3,500 Calories more. The additional Calories should be from a nutritionally balanced diet supplying approximately 15% protein, 30–35% fat, and 50–55% carbohydrate.

On the day of an athletic performance, foods containing protein or fat should be eaten at least three or four hours ahead of the event because protein and fat slow gastric emptying. Strenuous exercise on a full stomach not only can cause discomfort but can impair performance. Carbohydrates can be taken up to 30 minutes before the event because they are more rapidly digested and absorbed into the bloodstream. Liquids can also be taken up to 30 minutes before the event. Dehydration is a common problem of athletes. Care should be taken to ensure proper hydration. During the event, blood glucose levels and state of hydration should be maintained. If physical exertion exceeds an hour in duration, replacement of glucose, water, and electrolytes becomes necessary.

There continues to be considerable interest in carbohydrate loading before athletic events that require endurance (more than 30 minutes of strenuous activity). The carbohydrate molecule contains more oxygen than does a fat molecule. This makes carbohydrate a preferable energy source because it requires less oxygen to produce the same amount of energy than does fat. Also, the length of time a person can perform hard work is directly proportional to the amount of muscle glycogen, which is a form of carbohydrate. Carbohydrate loading is designed to increase muscle glycogen content. One method of carbohydrate loading frequently used is first to deplete the muscles of glycogen through stenuous exercise beginning one week before the event. This is followed by three days of a diet high in protein and fat designed to continue to deplete any muscle glycogen reserves. Next, extremely high levels of carbohydrate are added to the high protein and fat diet for the remaining days before the event. Muscle biopsies have shown the method to be useful in increasing glycogen stores. More than 700 gm of glycogen can be stored in the muscles, which results in 2,800 Calories of available energy.

Young adolescent women are frequently preoccupied with fashion, figure, and dates. For a few, and the incidence appears to be on the rise, there may be an extremely abnormal desire to be thin. Young people affected with this suffer from a disease called *anorexia nervosa*. Victims are usually adolescent or preadolescent girls from middle-class or upper-middle-class families who have been "model" children. The victims are frequently striving to achieve an unattainable goal. They relentlessly pursue excessive weight loss despite severe hunger. They have an exaggerated fear of gaining weight. If anorexia nervosa is not detected and treated successfully, the consequences can be fatal. Although the disease results in malnutrition, diet is only a minor portion of the therapy. The thrust of the treatment program must revolve around resolving the psychological and social problems that these youths face.

A common problem for both sexes in adolescence is *acne*. Acne usually begins at puberty. The pathogenesis is due to the androgenic stimulation of the sebaceous glands and to defective keratinization, which ultimately results in the formation of *comedones* (blackheads and whiteheads). Although many physicians impose various dietary restrictions on their acne patients, carefully controlled studies refute any benefit derived from such restrictions. Nevertheless, some patients believe that eliminating certain items from their diets improves their skin condition. Foods frequently eliminated include soft drinks, fried foods, and chocolate. Vitamin A acid has been shown to be effective in the treatment of acne when used as a topical agent. This preparation causes irritation and peeling, thereby sloughing off and expelling the whiteheads.

BIBLIOGRAPHY

Arlin, M. J. *The Science of Nutrition.* 2nd ed. New York: Macmillan, Inc., 1977.

Babson, F. E. and Benda, G. I. Growth graphs for the clinical assessment of infants of varying gestational age. *J. Pediatr.* 89:814, 1976.

Cheek, D. B., and Hill, D. Changes in somatic growth after placental insufficiency and maternal protein depri-vation. In D. B. Cheek, Ed., *Fetal and Postnatal Growth: Hormones and Nutrition.* New York: John Wiley & Sons, Inc., Pubs., 1975.

Children's Bureau. *Infant Care.* Washington, D.C.: U.S. Dept. of Health, Education, and Welfare, 1973.

Foman, S. J. *Infant Nutrition.* 2nd Ed. Philadelphia: W. B. Saunders Company, 1974.

Food & Agriculture Org. of the United Nations. *Energy and Protein Requirements.* FAO Nutrition Meetings Rep. Series 52 and WHO Tech. Rep. Series 522. Rome, 1973.

Fryer, B. A., Lamkin, G. H., Vivian, V. M., Eppright, E. S., and Fox, H. M. Growth and preschool children in the North Central Region. *J. Am. Diet Assoc.* 60:30, 1972.

Kallen, D. J., Ed. *Nutrition, Development and Social Behavior.* DHEW Publ. No. (NIH) 73-242. Washington, D.C.: Dept. of Health, Education, and Welfare, 1973.

U.S. Dept. of Health, Education, and Welfare. *Preliminary Findings of the First Health and Nutrition Examination Survey, United States, 1971–1972.* DHEW Publ. No. (HRA) 75-1229, Washington, D.C., 1975.

CHAPTER 17

Nutrition During the Adult Years

Catherine Justice

This chapter is about nutrition and the adult, those from ages 23 to 50 and those over 50 years old, the differences between nutrient needs for growth and development and for maintenance of the mature adult, the nutrition-related problems common among adults, and the programs and guidelines needed to add life to one's years. The influence of nutrition on performance, body structure, and life expectancy is cumulative. The effects of maternal diet on the outcome of pregnancy depend on the adequacy of the mother's diet during her own growing years as well as on her nutritional status at the time of conception and the foods that she consumes during the pregnancy. Nutrition does influence the growth and development of a child, but once youth is past a person cannot grow taller by changing diet habits (although he may grow fatter or leaner). Deficiency states do not develop as a result of eating poorly for one day or even one month unless one has been eating a marginal diet for a long time. For example, in the 1930s a young, well-nourished physician put himself on a vitamin C–deficient diet to learn more about scurvy (Crandon et al., 1940). Six months were required before any symptoms of scurvy were apparent. On the other hand, English sailors in the 1700s commonly developed scurvy within 30 days of going on sea rations. Their voyages usually began in the early spring, and winter diets in the northern European countries at that time supplied very little vitamin C.

Diseases are not cured by following a special diet, but a modified diet may be critical in the control of a disease such as diabetes mellitus or *phenylketonuria*. Diet may, however, be extremely important in the prevention of disease and the maintenance of body function. Overeating causes obesity, and obesity is associated with an increased incidence of cardiac failure, diabetes, and hypertension. Underweight patients usually have less ability to respond to treatment and to recover from surgery. The association of critical body weights with the initiation of the growth spurt, the attainment of maximum growth rate, and the menarche during adolesence suggest the influence of nutrition on body function (Firsch and Revelle, 1970). Both early- and late-maturing girls generally experience their first menstrual period when they reach a body weight of around 105.2 lb (47 kg). Extremely undernourished women often stop menstruating. A critical fat to lean ratio seems necessary to maintain regular ovulatory cycles ("Radcliffe Athletes Participate . . . ," 1980). Frisch has said: "When women lose between 10 to 15 percent of their total body weight, they also lose about one-third of their body fat. The result is that the menstrual cycle 'turns off'. We believe that this change in ratio of lean mass to body fat may be a crucial factor in the cessation of cycles" (p. 398). Such secondary *amenorrhea* has caused considerable anxiety among women athletes, ballet dancers, high-fashion models, dieters, and women who wish to conceive and bear children.

State of health at any age is influenced by what is eaten—not just one day but all of the days before. One cannot have the best of health unless one eats wisely. Nutrition makes a difference in the way people feel, act, and resist disease. Sometimes providing a good diet is the only treatment available for an illness. Then, good patient care requires careful attention to what the patient eats and what he reports he does *not* eat of what he is served.

Maintenance and repair is the theme for nutrition and the adult. Neglect of maintenance and repair can lead to irreparable damage. The adult who seeks optimal health must practice good nutrition. Life expectancy has increased because more of the population survive the perils of infancy and childhood today. The number of people in our population over 75 years old makes this our most rapidly growing population age group. Good nutrition can improve the quality of life for all age groups if started in time and practiced continuously.

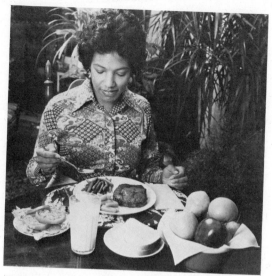

Figure 17-1. Adults have varied nutritional needs depending on lifestyle, culture, and food preferences. (Courtesy Ross Laboratories)

AGING AND CHANGING

Whereas a child grows taller as he matures, adults lose stature. They continue to have changes in body composition; and as the years pass, functional capacities show a tendency to diminish as well. Disease, medication, and death are more common among the mature population. Illness makes it difficult to distinguish between the effects of aging and the effects of disease. The cumulative effects of maturation, disease, medication, and previous health practices influence the nutrient needs of adults; but the variability introduced by lengthening individual histories complicates the formulation of recommended dietary allowances (Fig. 17-1). The RDAs are formulated to provide enough of the nutrients to meet the needs of practically all healthy, normal people (Food and Nutrition Board, 1974). To meet the needs of "practically all," the allowances must overstate the need of most people and yet underestimate the nutrient needs of a few who have unusual needs associated with disease and medication.

Physiological Changes

Most gerontologists believe that the mechanism of aging is a decline in the number of cells along with changes within the cells that damage the cellular organelles and changes in the basic genetic material that affect cell replication. In addition, a gradual decrease in the levels of certain hormones probably reduces integration among the body systems.

Shock (1970) studied many people of different ages and concluded that loss of function with increasing age does not occur at the same rate in all organs and systems. Comparing the average for people 75 years old and 30 years old, he noted the following differences:

- Brain weight was almost unchanged (93%).
- Basal metabolism declined to 84%.

• Filtration rate of the kidneys was only 69%.
• Maximum breathing capacity was only 43%.

This loss of function is probably the result of a loss of cells from individual organs. Nevertheless, most adults manage quite well despite these reductions in function. The differences between younger and older people become more apparent when a body system is challenged by disease or injury. The return to equilibrium is slower in the older person.

The changes in body composition considered characteristic of aging could also be the result of a loss of cells. With age, the percentage of water decreases, and the percentage of the body that is fat increases. The proportion of collagen also increases. There is more water in muscle and visceral cells and less water in fat cells. Collagen is a tough, insoluble protein that is important in body structure, but increasing amounts of it make the skin and vascular system less elastic and the connective tissue stiff. Losses of bone account for the lower bone densities observed in the aged. Rossman (1971) has suggested that the loss of height observed in aging is caused by the collapse of the spine, which results from these lower bone densities. Trotter and Gleser (1971) have noted an average decrement of height of 1.2 cm (0.5 in) each 20 years of adult life. Rossman (1971) generalizes that people experience a 2-in (5 cm) loss of height in the 50 years between ages 20 and 70.

The changes in posture produced by the collapse of some of the vertebrae are perhaps somewhat less universal than the redistribution of fat that accompanies aging. Even elderly in good nutritional condition tend to experience an atrophy of fat depots on the arms and breasts. There may be a loss of fat from the face also at the same time fat is being deposited on the abdomen and hips.

Disease, Medication, and Death

A mortality equation formulated in the early nineteenth century states that the likelihood of death doubles every eight years of adult life (Strehler, 1971). Disease, surgery, and accidents of minor nature for young adults can be life-threatening for aged people. Reserve physiological capacities seem to diminish, and the aged recover less quickly than the young faced with the same challenges to health and strength.

Health among older adults can hardly be defined as freedom from disease. Practically every old person has something wrong with him (Public Health Serv., 1970). It has been said that 86% of those over 65 have at least one chronic condition. Despite their chronic illnesses more than half of the over-65 population continue to carry out normal roles and responsibilities in the community. Only 1 in 20 of the aged lives in an institution. More than two-thirds live in their own homes (Public Health Serv., 1970). If health is defined as the ability to function and live outside an institution, the aged are quite healthy and usually maintain this state of health almost until the end of life.

The control of chronic conditions with medication and diet is a concern for many adults. The interactions between prescribed medications and between certain medications and nutrients needs to be examined when establishing health care plans for adults (Roe, 1976). Some common nutrient-drug relationships are:

1. People required to take isonicotinic acid hydrazide (INH) and several other antitubercular drugs usually need a supplement of vitamin B₆ in therapeutic amounts.

2. People taking tetracycline should not consume milk or milk products within one hour before or two hours after taking this medication.

3. People taking an anticoagulant should avoid foods that contain large amounts of vitamin K in one serving. Turnip greens and spinach should be eliminated from their diets.

4. People on tranquillizers of the monoamine oxidase (MAO) inhibitor type must avoid fermented foods such as aged cheeses and Chianti wine.

Pharmacists are helping identify possible drug-nutrient interactions and providing label information to help patients avoid these kinds of problems.

The need to modify diets to control disease is recognized but often not acted on. A study of community needs for nursing service showed that the need to modify food habits outranked all other categories of potential health problems (Mikey, 1963). Another study stated that the need for help with modified diets ranked third among community health needs.

Public health goals emphasize the achievement of healthier and longer lives. Between the ages of 15 and 24, 50% of all deaths are caused by accidents; but the major causes of death among people over 65 years old—diseases of the heart, cancer, and stroke—are the leading causes of death for the population as a whole. Although the role of diet as a cause of these diseases is not entirely understood, estimates from a joint task force representing the State Agricultural Experiment Stations and the USDA suggested that 20–25% of the cardiovascular disease and 20% of the malignancies could be prevented if we simply practiced what we now know about good nutrition (Weir and the Agricultural Policy Advisory Comm., 1971). The Weir report also stated that probably 50% of the cases of diabetes mellitus and other carbohydrate disorders could be avoided or improved if better diets were consumed. The task force also predicted that improvements in mental health and work efficiency would correlate with improvements in dietary habits. The report stated: "Most all of the health problems underlying the leading causes of death in the United States would be modified by improvements in dietary habits" (p. 2).

The Surgeon General's Report on Health Promotion and Disease Prevention continued the emphasis on better diet as a means of attaining public health goals (Public Health Service, 1979). The report identified five health goals for the United States for the next decade. Two of the five goals seek better and longer life for adults:

• To cut by 25% the death rate of those from age 25 to 65
• To lower by 20% the average days those over 65 spend in hospitals

The report states that a better diet would cut the death rate and reduce the incidence of disease and disability.

RECOMMENDED DIETARY ALLOWANCES

Growth and development are the chief determinants of nutrient needs before maturity. Adults need nutrients to maintain and repair their tissues and systems. Foods should be selected to provide the building materials needed to replace those lost in the dynamic equilibrium constantly occurring in the living organism. The total nutrients needed for replacement and repair of the mature adult are more than the total nutrient needs of children except for calcium, phosphorus, and vitamin D. With the exception of periods of pregnancy and lactation, the current RDAs for adults are stated for only two age groups: 23–50 years and 51 years and over (Food and Nutrition Board, 1980).

Experiments to determine the nutrient needs of adults have generally used college students as subjects. The balance studies to measure nutrient needs have been conducted on only a limited number of people over 30 years of age. The findings of nutrient needs of mature adults are confusing because they are often contradictory. Allowances for people 51 years of age and over are the same as the allowances for other mature adults except for a reduction in the iron allowance for women past the childbearing years and a reduction in the suggested caloric intake. Because the recommended allowances include margins of safety to allow for variation between individuals, allowances established on the basis of studies in healthy young adults are probably ample for older adults as well if they are in good health.

Caloric Needs

The reduction in basal metabolism observed as a change accompanying aging and a reduction in activity explain the reduction in the suggested caloric intake. Durnin and Passmore (1967) estimate a decline in basal metabolism of about 2% per decade starting at age 21, but they emphasize that declines in activity are not so universal. Some older homemakers whose energy expenditures Durnin and Passmore measured were actually using more Calories than younger women of the same size.

Changes in body composition characteristic of aging may explain the decline of basal metabolism. Although fat as well as lean tissue carries on metabolic activities, the fat tissue seems to have a lower metabolic rate. As the proportion of body fat increases, the caloric cost of basal metabolism declines. The caloric cost of basal metabolism at age 70 is at least 10% less than at age 21—a reduction of 120–200 Calories/day for most people.

Although basal metabolism accounts for the largest part of the total caloric need for most people, differences in activity must be considered in estimating a person's total caloric need. Most nursing-home residents are less active than the "average" person recognized in the RDA tables. The RDA "average person" engages in standing and walking only two hours a day and is otherwise sedentary. The 1979 RDA suggest a caloric range of 1,600–2,400 Calories for women 23–50 years of age, 1,400 to 2,200 Calories for

women 51–75, and 1,200 to 2,000 Calories for women over 75. For men, the suggested caloric ranges are 2,300 to 3,100, 2,000 to 2,800, and 1,650 to 2,450, respectively.

Nutrient density is a more critical problem for the adult than for the adolescent. The USDA studies of food consumption reveal that men and women over 65 years of age more often fail to consume recommended allowances of minerals and vitamins than do adolescents (USDA, 1968). Adolescents tend to consume so many kilocalories that mineral and vitamin intakes accumulate to equal or exceed the RDA even when some food choices are relatively "empty Calories." Adults generally need fewer Calories with each passing decade. The nutrient density of their Calories must increase with age if allowances are to be attained in the face of decreased total caloric need. Food selection requires greater care if minerals, vitamins, and protein allowances are to be achieved from foods providing fewer Calories.

Protein Allowances

It is possible that the protein needs of older adults could be lower than the 0.8 gm of protein per kilogram of body weight recommended for all adults (Young et al., 1976). Possibly the essential amino acid requirements are different for older and younger adults. Most nutritionists favor planning for at least 1 gm of protein per kilogram per day for institutionalized adults. Total protein intake for adults should probably average between 45 and 90 gm/day. A well-selected diet will include milk, grain products, and vegetables as well as meat as sources of protein. The nonmeat items will supply between one-third and one-half of the protein allowance for the day, so 4–6 oz of cooked lean meat is enough to provide the rest of the dietary protein. Legumes and cheese should be used occasionally as meat substitutes. Peanut butter is also acceptable as a meat substitute once in a while.

Calcium Allowances

The calcium allowance for a child under 10 years of age is the same as the calcium allowance for adults (800 mg). Long-term calcium deficiencies deplete the calcium stores of the bone to maintain the calcium level of the blood. Whether or not enough calcium is absorbed from the diet depends, however, not only on how much calcium is in the diet but on whether the body can provide the active form of vitamin D, which causes the gut to synthesize the calcium-carrying protein that moves calcium from the gut into the bloodstream.

B Vitamins

There are National Research Council recommended allowances for only six of the eight B vitamins, but the 1979 RDA do include estimated safe and adequate daily dietary intakes for the other two, biotin and pantothenic acid. These two vitamins are so common in foods that they become nutritional concerns only when long-term intravenous feeding replaces food or when enough raw egg whites are consumed for a protein in the egg white to combine with dietary biotin so that the vitamin cannot be absorbed from the gut.

Surveys of food consumption have not provided much information about how much folacin, vitamin B_{12} and vitamin B_6 various population groups are consuming because only limited food-composition data has been available for these three vitamins. The 1979 RDAs for folacin and vitamin B_{12} are the same for adolescents, for adults 23–50, and for people over 50 years of age: folacin, 400 μg; vitamin B_{12}, 3 μg. The vitamin B_6 1979 RDA increases slightly through the growing period, reaching a maximim of 2.0 mg/day for women 15 and older and of 2.2 mg/day for men 19 and older.

Vitamin B_6 deficiencies in adults have developed as a consequence of taking antitubercular medications. A supplement of vitamin B_6 should be prescribed along with those drugs identified as antagonists to vitamin B_6. The RDA is not an appropriate guide for B_6 requirements for people on medications that act to deter the metabolic functions of the vitamin; 50 mg/day is usually given to adults on the antitubercular drug INH (Roe, 1976).

Measures of vitamin B_6-dependent enzyme activity in the blood have suggested that older people on the same diet do not have as much vitamin B_6 in their blood as younger adults, but recognizable clinical symptoms of deficiency—neurological impairment and skin oiliness—have been observed in adults only when given an antagonist of this vitamin.

Adult women taking oral contraceptives probably need more vitamin B_6 than their diets provide. Tests for vitamin B_6-dependent enzyme activity indicate an abnormal metabolic pattern in women on the pill. Researchers are currently attempting to determine the supplement that these women need to maintain normal B_6 blood levels ("Inhibition of the Hemopoietic Activity. . .," 1979).

Folacin and vitamin B_{12} are both necessary for the maturation of normal blood cells. A deficiency of either or both of these vitamins causes a *macrocytic anemia:* immature blood cells appear in the peripheral circulation, and the number of red blood cells is low. Treating a folacin-deficiency anemia with vitamin B_{12} allows the anemia to become worse. Treating a B_{12} deficiency with folacin will improve the blood picture but permits the neurological degeneration caused by the vitamin B_{12} deficiency to advance to a point that is usually beyond repair.

A diet low in vitamin C is apt to be low in folacin also. There seems to be some risk of folacin deficiency among older adults (Girdwood, 1969) and hospital patients as well as among pregnant women. Folacin deficiencies seem to develop as a result of the failure to eat raw vegetables and fruits frequently. Like vitamin C, folacin is easily destroyed by cooking, and folacin may even require vitamin C to prevent its destruction in the gut. It has been suggested that excessive intake of alcohol blocks the hemopoietic activity of folacin ("Inhibition of the Hemopoietic Activity. . . ," 1979).

Pernicious anemia is the result of a deficiency in vitamin B_{12}. This anemia is pernicious because, if not treated soon enough, the neural system suffers permanent damage. Oral supplements will not be effective because the missing link is not inadequate consumption of the vitamin but rather the inability to absorb dietary vitamin B_{12}. The vitamin requires a carrier to move it from the lumen of the gut into the bloodstream. The carrier, called *intrinsic factor,* is secreted by the stomach. Middleaged and older adults sometimes lose the ability to secrete intrinsic factor. Adults who have had most of the stomach surgically removed or a resection of the lower part of the small intestine (the absorption site for vitamin B_{12}) also risk B_{12} deficiency. The treatment is regular injections of vitamin B_{12} to bypass the problems of absorption of the vitamin. Pernicious anemia can be controlled successfully if infections of B_{12} are initiated in time and continued for the rest of the patient's life.

Fairly complete food-composition data is available for the other three B vitamins: thiamine, riboflavin, and niacin. There is, however, a problem in interpreting niacin consumption. The tabled values for niacin do not include the niacin available from the essential amino acid tryptophan. A diet adequate in protein is practically certain to be adequate in niacin even if the total of preformed niacin is less than the RDA. To calculate the total niacin available from the diet, it is necessary to add 1 mg of niacin for every 60 mg of tryptophan in the diet. It is usually estimated that 1% of the dietary protein is tryptophan.

Dietary thiamine is often less than the RDA even though enriched breads and cereals contain as much thiamine as the whole grain product. Thiamine intakes less than the allowances are almost inevitable if a person avoids starchy foods such as enriched or whole grain breads and cereals, legumes, and pork. Adults on low-carbohydrate diets and alcoholics frequently consume insufficient amounts of thiamine.

Riboflavin is supplied abundantly by meat as well as by milk products. Although many adults do not drink enough milk, the high consumption of meat in the United States tends to provide enough riboflavin. If both milk and meat are omitted, only the consumption of larger amounts of grain products can supply enough riboflavin. Enriched breads and cereals contain more riboflavin than whole grain products. Fruits and vegetables are poor sources of riboflavin.

The RDAs of thiamine, riboflavin, and niacin have been correlated with the suggested caloric allowances so that the recommended allowances are higher for adolescents than for adults and higher for men than for women and sometimes higher for adults 23–50 than for adults over 51 years of age. Current thiamine allowances are from 1.0 to 1.4 mg for adults. Riboflavin allowances range from 1.2 to 1.6 mg. Recommended allowances for total niacin for adults are from 13 to 18 mg/day. About 9 mg of niacin per day are necessary to prevent the development of pellagra, the deficiency disease caused by a lack of niacin. Thiamine intakes should never be less than 1 mg/day.

Ascorbic Acid

The current RDA for vitamin C is 60 mg/day for both men and women over 15 years of age. Consumption of 60 mg can hardly be attained unless one selects a vitamin C–rich food such as oranges, grapefruit, strawberries, or cantaloupe or has two foods as high in vitamin C as baked potatoes, tomatoes, cabbage, broccoli, or spinach.

Tissue saturation with vitamin C can be maintained on intakes of 70–100 mg/day. Intakes of vitamin C and serum levels of the vitamin correlate remarkably well until saturation is attained. Excessive intakes of the vitamin are excreted in the urine. Excretion of a test dose is used to determine whether or not tissue saturation has been achieved. When the tissues are saturated, the test dose is quickly excreted. Assays of serum for vitamin C have indicated that some older adults fail to consume enough vitamin C–containing foods. They regard these foods as too costly or too acidic, failing to recognize the essential role of fruits and vegetables in the diet.

Fat-soluble Vitamins

Although many adults in the United States consume less than the 800–1,000 Retinol Equivalents of vitamin A recommended in the RDA, low blood levels of vitamin A are found less often in adults than in children and adolescents. Probably the ability of the body to store appreciable amounts of the fat-soluble vitamins provides adults some reserve against inadequate daily intakes. There are RDAs for only three of the four fat-soluble vitamins, and only vitamin A intakes can be calculated because food composition values for vitamins D, E, and K are not readily available.

Foods contain no significant amounts of vitamin D unless they are fortified with vitamin D; but a precurser of vitamin D in the skin is converted to vitamin D when skin is exposed to sunlight. Adults whose work or disability keeps them out of the sun should have vitamin D supplements of about 200 IU/day. This is the amount of vitamin D an adult will get when by drinking 2 cups of vitamin D–fortified milk. The milk purchased for residents of extended care facilities should always be vitamin D fortified.

Dietary vitamin K is a concern only for those adults who may need to limit their intake because they are required to take an anticoagulant. Physicians should standardize the dosage of the anticoagulant while the patient is consuming a normal diet because avoiding vitamin K-containing foods completely is neither practical nor desirable. An estimated safe and adequate daily dietary intake of vitamin K is 70 to 140 μg, which is present in most diets. Most of the foods providing significant amounts of vitamin A also supply vitamin K.

The RDA for vitamin A is 800 Retinol Equivalents for all females over 10 years of age and 1,000 Retinol Equivalents for all males over 10. The 1979 RDA for vitamin E has been reduced to 8 Tocopherol Equivalents for all females over 10 and to 10 Tocopherol Equivalents for all males over 15. Allowances expressed in equivalents are expressions of biological activity rather than of weight. Retinol Equivalents and Tocopherol Equivalents represent entirely different weights. A Retinol Equivalent represents the vitamin A activity of 1 μg of preformed vitamin A. A Tocopherol Equivalent has the vitamin E activity of about 1 mg of the most active form of vitamin E. Equivalents rather than weights are used because there are several forms of vitamin E, each with a different biological activity, and because the carotenoids in foods as well as the preformed vitamin A can help meet the body's need for vitamin A.

Food-composition data for vitamin E is so confusing that it is virtually impossible to calculate the vitamin E activity of a diet. Researchers, however, can destroy the vitamin E activity of a diet, using rigorous laboratory procedures not ordinarily experienced in food preparation. Adults participating in long-term studies and consuming only diets from which vitamin E activity had been stripped developed low serum levels of vitamin E. Surveys of other populations consuming many different diets reveal almost no low serum levels of vitamin E (Horwitt, 1976). On these bases we assume that diets generally provide adequate amounts of vitamin E.

Studies of food consumption conducted by the USDA do calculate the vitamin A activity of the foods consumed. Consumption of less than the recommended amounts seems to be fairly common among both children and adults, but low serum levels seldom occur among adults. Autopsy data, however, suggest that many "healthy" adults lack liver stores of vitamin A, probably because they do not select enough vitamin A-containing foods. Unless the diet includes, at least four times a week, servings of dark-green, leafy vegetables, such as greens or broccoli, or deep-yellow foods, such as carrots, winter squash, sweet potatoes, apricots, or cantaloupe, or a 2-oz serving of cooked liver, the diet will probably not provide the recommended allowance for vitamin A. Head lettuce, green beans, peas, and corn do not contain significant amounts of vitamin A.

Trace Minerals

The quantities of trace minerals needed in the diet are similar to the quantities of vitamins recommended, but tables of food composition provide much more information about the vitamin content of foods than about trace minerals. There are RDAs for three trace minerals—iron, zinc, and iodine—and the 1979 Committee on Recommended Allowances has published estimates of safe and adequate daily dietary intakes for six other trace minerals: copper, manganese, fluorine, chromium, selenium, and molybdenum. One-a-day supplements advertised to "ensure" adequate nutrition include most vitamins but only rarely include any minerals, either trace or major, except iron. Trace minerals are required as they occur in foods—in trace amounts, the same as vitamins. Too much of any trace mineral can be toxic. Supplements of one mineral may increase the need for another, and these relationships are still not well defined. The percentage of absorption of a trace mineral seems to vary according to need, the presence of dietary fiber, and in the case of iron, for example, whether or not vitamin C is present and whether the iron is heme iron or nonheme iron (Cook and Monsen, 1977).

The best advice at present to insure adequate intakes of the trace minerals is to eat a variety of foods from all four of the basic four food groups in sufficient amounts to meet protein, calcium, vitamin, and energy needs. This dietary pattern will probably ensure sufficient amounts of the trace minerals except for iodine and fluorine. To be sure that iodine is supplied, use iodized salt. To be sure that fluorine is supplied, drink water whose fluorine content is regulated to provide 1 to 2 ppm of fluoride.

Iron

The RDAs for iron assume that only 10% of the iron in the diet will be absorbed. The RDA for iron is 18 mg for women during the childbearing years and 10 mg for all other adults. The iron in vegetables and egg yolk is poorly absorbed; that found in meat is absorbed much better. The actual percentages absorbed depend on a person's need for iron and on the presence of vitamin C in the gut. Few diets, even well-selected ones, will contain 18 mg of iron, but supplements should not be taken unless laboratory tests confirm that a person has an iron deficiency.

Zinc

In the 1960s zinc deficiency was identified in young men whose growth and sexual development were arrested. Zinc supplements caused a growth spurt and sexual maturation. The roles of zinc in wound healing and taste acuity seem to indicate the importance of dietary zinc for adults as well as young people. Zinc supplements do not necessarily improve taste acuity, however. In 1974 the first RDA for zinc was set at 15 mg for all people over 10 years of age. This estimate has been repeated in the 1979 RDA.

Major Minerals

The major minerals are needed in larger amounts than the vitamins and trace minerals. The RDAs for three of the major minerals are in hundreds of milligrams but still less than the quantities of carbohydrate, protein, and fat needed:

- Calcium: 800 mg for all adults
- Phosphorus: 800 mg for all adults
- Magnesium: 350 mg for adult men; 300 mg for adult women

All but a small part of the calcium and phosphorus are in the bones and teeth. Part of the magnesium is also found in the hard tissues of the body, but these three minerals as well as sodium, potassium, and chlorine are also important electrolytes in body fluids. Safe and adequate adult dietary intakes of these three additional major minerals are estimated in the 1979 RDA:

- Sodium: 1,100–3,300 mg
- Potassium: 1,875–5,625 mg
- Chloride: 1,700–5,100 mg

Phosphorus and potassium occur so plentifully in food that eating almost insures getting these amounts. Calcium is the nutrient most often low in the diets of adults in the United States. Unless one uses daily products equivalent to 2 cups of milk daily, it is almost impossible to get recommended amounts of calcium from food. Much of the calcium in vegetables, grains, and legumes is not absorbed from the gastrointestinal tract, and there is almost no calcium in meat.

Some have associated lifelong low intakes of calcium with the development of osteoporosis. Osteoporosis is the most common form of disability among the aged. Both the mineral matter and the protein framework of the bone are lost. The thinned bone fractures easily and is usually the cause of the hip fractures and the spontaneous vertebral collapse so common among the elderly. There is still no agreement about the cause of this severe loss of bone. Probably there are multiple causes. Possibly inadequate calcium, vitamin D, and fluorine as well as the hormonal changes of aging and still other factors are implicated.

Not all of the sodium in the diet comes from table salt (sodium chloride), but most of it does. Most of us consume far more than 1,100–3,300 mg of sodium daily. Many adults have to restrict their sodium intakes to help control high blood pressure. Animal foods must be limited for these adults because they contain sodium even if prepared without added salt. Grains and vegetables contain little sodium but are usually salted in cooking. Fruits, however, contain almost no sodium and are the only food group not restricted on strict sodium diets. Sodium intakes are seldom limited to less than 1,000 mg per day, but no added salt at all is permitted if only 1 gm (1,000 mg) of sodium is allowed. Limited amounts of salt are allowed a person on a 2–3 gm sodium diet; 1 t of salt adds 2,000 mg of sodium. Salt substitutes are potassium chloride. Some people may be restricted in potassium as well as sodium, so salt substitutes should be used only if the physician approves.

The weakness experienced by some hospital patients and people on certain potassium-wasting diuretics for hypertension or cardiac insufficiency may be a potassium deficiency. When one eats very little, one gets very little potassium. Potassium medications are bitter and often irritating to the stomach. One banana or one tall glass of orange juice provides more than 500 mg of potassium. Baked potatoes, melons, and avocados, if not salted, are also useful sources of potassium for the person who needs to avoid sodium but push potassium.

Magnesium is not concentrated in any single food but requires a varied diet including whole grain cereals and legumes. Chlorine, too, is a dietary essential. Table salt is sodium chloride, and 1 t provides about 3,000 mg of chlorine as well as 2,000 mg of sodium.

COMMON NUTRITIONAL PROBLEMS AMONG ADULTS

Adults in underdeveloped areas of the world often exhibit the effects of childhood nutritional deficiencies such as kwashiorkor, xeropthalmia, beriberi, and pellagra. Adults in the United States are more apt to show health problems that stem from overconsumption and the failure to select foods wisely. Vitamin and mineral and protein deficiency diseases are rare in the United States, but adults might be healthier if they followed better dietary patterns. Hospital patients would respond to medical care better if their nutritional status were maintained more effectively. Hospitals provide plenty of good food, but patients sometimes cannot or will not eat. Some lifestyles block the attainment of optimal health.

Dangerous Lifestyles

The Canadian Department of Health and Welfare designated the La Londe Committee to examine the causes of disease and disability (La Londe, 1976). The committee drew up a list of eight dangerous lifestyles. While acknowledging that disease has environmental and genetic causes, the committee elected to focus attention on lifestyles that cause disease and disability. A person has limited control over environmental causes of disease and even less control over his genetic makeup, but he makes the choices that determine his lifestyle. The committee predicted that, in general, a man of 45 who would avoid these eight dangerous lifestyles would live at least 11 years longer than the average life-span.

Four of the eight dangerous lifestyles are related to eating and drinking:

1. Obesity
2. Gluttony
3. Skipping breakfast
4. Alcoholism

The other four are:

5. Lack of sleep
6. Lack of exercise
7. Smoking
8. Accidents

Although gluttony usually results in obesity, the committee seems to have listed gluttony separately to point out the dangers of consuming too large a portion of ones total Calories as fat, or sugar, or meat. Obesity has been identified as a concurrent problem in several of the degenerative diseases. Weight reduction has been associated with reduction of blood pressure in people with hypertension and with relief of clinical symptoms in people with mature-onset diabetes.

Skipping meals seems to promote obesity. At least people who skip meals are more often obese than people who eat at least three meals a day. A study of breakfast habits demonstrated that going without breakfast did not promote weight reduction (Cereal Instit., 1976). The Iowa Breakfast Studies also showed that skipping breakfast resulted in decreased efficiency and ability to do work in the late-morning hours. The Iowa group suggested that breakfast should provide one-fourth of the day's Calories and one-fourth of the day's protein. Some of the subjects in this study benefited from a midmorning snack, but less than 50% of those in the Iowa study performed as well with a midmorning snack as with a light or moderate breakfast. A heavy breakfast actually seemed less helpful than a moderate breakfast of cereal or an egg, toast, fruit, and milk. Breakfast does not have to be based on cereal or an egg, however. An equally good breakfast might include a hamburger or cottage cheese, but some significant source of protein is needed to keep up one's efficiency as noon approaches.

The *Indiana Diet Manual* (Indiana Diet Manual Comm., 1974) published some useful criteria from the Wisconsin State Board of Health for good distribution of food consumption. These guidelines require that health care institutions serve as follows:

1. Serve at least three meals a day; a bedtime nourishment should also be served.
2. No more than 50% of the total Calories for the day should be served in any five-hour period.

3. No more than 14 hours should elapse between the evening meal and breakfast.

4. Two meals per day and three nourishments may not provide the appropriate distribution of Calories and nutrients.

The checklist from the Indiana State Board of Health (1974) requires affirmative answers to the following questions before approving the food service in a health care institution:

1. Is there meat or another protein food in each dinner and supper?

2. Is there at least one serving of a fruit and/or vegetable in each meal?

All of these criteria developed to evaluate food service in health care institutions are equally appropriate guidelines for individuals managing their own lives.

Alcoholics often eat poorly; but the liver damage usually found in alcoholics cannot be avoided by good eating habits or by the consumption of mineral, vitamin, and protein supplements. The liver damage sustained by alcoholics is proportional to the amount of alcohol consumed (Shaw and Lieber, 1978).

Nutrient Intakes and Nutritional Status in the United States

Evaluations of nutrient intakes are calculations of nutrients in the foods consumed followed by comparisons of the calculated consumption with the recommended allowances for those nutrients. Because allowances include margins of safety, some people consuming less than the allowances are getting enough but others are certainly consuming less than they need of the nutrient. Studies of nutritional status attempt to identify people who are actually getting less of a nutrient than they require by examining blood, urine, and tissue samples and by taking anthropometric measures. Three nationwide surveys discussed in Chapter 7 provide some current information about nutrient intake and nutritional status.

The USDA Survey of Food Consumption evaluted nutrient intake, not nutritional status. As of 1965, calcium, vitamin A, and iron were the nutrients most often consumed in less than the recommended amounts (USDA, 1968). Fluctuations in the RDA for vitamin C moved this nutrient from the list of those most often consumed in less than the recommended amounts to the list of those whose intakes were generally adequate. The RDA for vitamin C for adults has fluctuated from about 60 mg/day in the 1968 RDA to 45 mg in the 1974 RDA and back to 60 mg in the 1979 RDA. Using the lower standard there is almost no reason to suggest that people in the United States have low intakes of vitamin C. It is well to keep in mind that evaluations of nutrient intake are calculations, not examinations of the physiological state of an individual.

The Ten-State Nutrition Survey teams collected information about foods consumed as well as laboratory studies of the blood and urine samples obtained from a subsample of their subjects, who also had physical examinations. The sample population in the Ten-State Nutrition Survey was selected to represent low-income people. Obesity and iron deficiency anemia were the two major nutritional problems identified (Public Health Serv., 1972). The findings in the survey suggest that nutritional problems of middle-income people are probably similar to the problems of low-income groups.

The Health and Nutrition Examination Survey, also known as HANES, (U.S. Dept. of Health, Education, and Welfare, 1975) employed sampling techniques designed to make the sample representative of all income groups. Again, obesity was identified as a major problem. No significant number of those examined showed evidence of nutritional deficiencies by the methods used. The people examined in the both Ten-State Survey and the HANES, however, represent a population well enough to get to the laboratory site to have blood and urine samples taken and to be examined. Institutionalized people were not included.

Dietary Guides

The RDAs state the amount of each nutrient that most nutrition scientists think is enough for practically everyone. The RDAs do not tell us what foods to eat, although nutrition authorities agree that it is better to get our nutrients from food than to depend on supplements in pills and capsules. The basic four concept was developed to help people select foods to provide the nutrients needed, but it says nothing about saturated or polyunsaturated fats, cholesterol, salt, and sugar.

Since the early 1960s the American Heart Association has been urging people to reduce their consumption of cholesterol and fats and to alter their selection of fats so that the amount of saturated fat does not exceed the amount of polyunsaturated fat. Not all nutrition scientists endorse these recommendations for the general public, but both the American Medical Association and the National Academy of Sciences (Food and Nutrition Board and Council on Foods and Nutrition, 1972) think that people identified as being at risk of cardiovascular accidents should be taught to modify their diets along the lines advocated by the American Heart Association, but specifically to fit individual needs.

The McGovern committee's *Dietary Goals for the United States* (included and discussed in Chap. 7) incorporate and extend the dietary recommendations of the American Heart Association. Nutritionists working with the public generally believe these goals will help improve the quality of diets in the United States, although some nutrition scientists are extremely critical of them. Scientists who endorse the goals point out that these specifics must be subject to revision as more knowledge becomes available but consider it helpful to tell people how much salt, sugar, fat, complex carbohydrates, and so on they should have in their diet. Some people think the goals should also call for a decreased consumption of alcohol inasmuch as it accounts for about 12% of all the Calories consumed in the United States. Although the goals themselves do not make any promises, the rationale behind them and the suggested changes in food selection and preparation is to reduce the incidence of the "killer diseases." No one can promise that those who select food and prepare it as the goals suggest will never have a heart attack, a stroke, a malignancy, or diabetes, but epidemiological evidence suggests that they are less apt to be so afflicted.

Probably the leading journal publishing human nutritional research in the United States is the *American Journal of Clinical Nutrition*. In May 1979 the American Society of Clinical Nutrition assembled a panel of research people. This panel endorsed no goals nor guidelines but reported a "strong association" between:

- Sugar and dental caries
- Salt and hypertension
- Cholesterol and saturated fat and coronary artery disease (King, 1979)

In July 1979 *The Surgeon General's Report on Health Promotion and Disease* (Public Health Serv., 1979) included dietary guidelines for better health. Although less specific than the Dietary Goals, the surgeon general's guidelines are quite similar.

Dietary Goals for the United States

The original set of goals was revised before the end of 1977 to emphasize the importance of avoiding being overweight and to clarify the goal for reduced salt intake. The revised goals and the changes necessary in food selection and preparation to implement them were previously discussed in Chapter 7. The changes required to achieve the goals of limiting fat and cholesterol have already been initiated by many people, but cholesterol cannot be kept below 300 mg/day if one selects an egg for breakfast; and almost any 3-oz serving of meat, even if lean, will provide 75 mg of cholesterol. Organ meats such as liver, heart, and brain are so high in cholesterol that they would have to be eliminated from the diet to achieve the Dietary Goal limiting cholesterol to 300 mg/day.

The proportion of dietary fat provided by polyunsaturated fat has been increasing but, on the average, people in the United States consume fats far in excess of 30% of their total caloric intake. To reduce total fat intake would generally mean selecting only lean cuts of meat, trimming off all visible fat, discarding meat drippings, and avoiding practically all fried foods. To be sure that one-third of the fat is polyunsaturated would mean avoiding lard, butter, and animal fats, for these fats are largely saturated. Vegetable oils and soft margarines would replace these animal products.

The part of the Dietary Goals most people find hardest to accept is the large amount of plant foods and the small amount of animal foods suggested. Most adults in the United States are very critical of diets high in starchy foods, and consumption trends for foods providing "natural" sugars such as milk, fruits, and vegetables have been declining. Dietary patterns consistent with the goals depend on starchy foods to supply about 45% of the protein in the diet. These patterns are not vegetarian diets; milk and meat are included. The meat, however, is used more like a seasoning than like a main dish. The total amount of protein provided would exceed the RDA, but the amounts of meat suggested for people on 1,800–2,400 Calories are less than the 4–5 oz required in the basic four pattern of food selection. The amounts of meat allowed in the Dietary Goals would be consistent with the basic four for adults whose caloric needs reach 2,700 Calories ("Dietary Goals for the United States," 1979).

Patterns of daily food selection consistent with the Dietary Goals can be planned to meet different caloric needs. The patterns can be expressed in diabetic exchanges, with sugar listed as a separate item, as the goals would permit sugar up to 10% of the total Calories. People with diabetes normally have not been allowed to use table sugar. In household measures an 1,800-Calorie pattern would include:

2 cups skim milk

2 oz cooked, lean meat

11 t fat (vegetable oil and margarine) or fat exchanges for other-than-lean meats)

3 T sugar

4 small servings of fruit or 1 cup fruit juice and 1 large fruit

(Sugar listed might be used to sweeten these)

1½ cup low-Calorie vegetables

1 medium potato

1 cup starchy vegetable like peas or limas

1 large serving of breakfast cereal

4 slices whole grain bread

The 5 gm of salt (1 t) permitted in the revised goals applies only to salt added in processing and preparation of food and that added at the table. The goal limits salt because, although salt is the major source of dietary sodium, it is not the only source of sodium in the diet; a well-balanced diet, prepared and eaten without any added salt, will provide about 1,200 mg of sodium or as much sodium as 3 gm of salt. The goal would permit a total of 3,200 mg of sodium per day. The teaspoon of salt provides 2,000 mg sodium.

The McGovern committee drew up these goals in the belief that they were dealing with the nutritional problems common among adults in the United States. The National Academy of Sciences continues to make recommendations in terms of allowances for specific nutrients for various age-sex groups and has not endorsed the stringent dietary restrictions embodied by the Dietary Goals for the general population. Many health care professionals, however, believe that the restrictions proposed by the committee are needed to help prevent the most common "killer" diseases among adults.

Healthy People

The surgeon general (Public Health Serv., 1979) has stated:

Given what is already known or strongly suspected about the relationship between diet and disease, Americans would probably be healthier, as a whole, if they consumed:

- only sufficient Calories to meet body needs and maintain desirable weight (fewer Calories if overweight);
- less saturated fat and cholesterol;
- less salt
- less sugar
- relatively more complex carbohydrates such as whole grains, cereals, fruits and vegetables; and
- relatively more fish, poultry, legumes (e.g. beans, peas, peanuts), and less red meat.

Adequate, balanced nutrition can be obtained by eating—in quantities sufficient to maintain desirable weight—a wide variety of foods each day, including meat or meat alternates, fruits and vegetables, cereal and bread-type products, and dairy products.

The surgeon general's report recognizes that there are variations in people's nutritional requirements and even those of the same person at different stages of the life-span.

TECHNIQUES AND PROGRAMS TO HELP ADULTS AT NUTRITIONAL RISK

Recognizing "Risk"

Data from the USDA Household Food Consumption Surveys have shown the diets of a significant proportion of adults to be "poor" when the nutrient composition is compared to the RDAs. That is, the diet is "poor" if it fails to provide at least two-thirds of the recommended allowance of one or more of the seven key nutrients calculated in the survey: protein, calcium, iron, vitamin A, thiamine, riboflavin, and ascorbic acid. A diet providing

more than enough Calories is not classified as "poor" in these surveys, but diets deficient in Calories are almost inevitably deficient in one of the calculated nutrients as well. Nevertheless, both caloric excess and caloric deficit are forms of malnutrition.

While obesity is a common nutritional problem among middle-aged adults, many older adults are painfully thin. Lack of ability to shop and to prepare food, as well as poverty and loneliness, promote undernutrition. Underweight people are less able to recover from surgery, to resist infection, and to respond to treatments such as chemotherapy and radiation. Bedfast patients who are undernourished are more apt to develop decubitus ulcers. Maintaining a desirable weight is important at all ages, but being underweight may be more critical to the maintenance of life itself than obesity.

Adults should keep a record of their body weights. Once a week is often enough to weigh, but differences because of clothing need to be avoided by weighing in the nude or in the same clothing each time. If one weighs at the same point in one's daily schedule each week, for instance, before breakfast on Wednesday mornings, many fluctuations caused by food and drink and excretory functions can be eliminated. Daily fluctuations of plus or minus 2 lb (1 kg) are usually caused by food intake and kidney and bowel function. Women should also anticipate some fluid retention before the beginnning of each menstrual period. Regular weighing helps one recognize the beginnings of obesity. It is easier to lose 5 lb than to lose 10. Weight records are also useful in identifying early stages of disease. Adults who lose 10 lb (4.5 kg) without trying should seek a physician's advice. One of the early signs of malignancies and one of the symptoms of untreated insulin-lack diabetes is an unexplained weight loss.

Skin-fold thickness is a better measure of body fat than body weight, for about one-half of the fat in the body is just under the skin.

Tables of standards for skin-fold thickness are based on younger adults, however, and may not be valid for the aged who have undergone the characteristic redistribution of body fat. Serial readings of skin-fold thickness on the same adult, however, could provide a useful guide to increasing or decreasing fat stores over a period of chronic illness. Skin-fold measures can also be combined with estimates of muscle circumference to assess loss of body protein resulting from illness and malnutrition.

People responsible for long-term care should be sure that weights or skin-fold thickness and muscle circumference are charted on a regular basis. Caloric excess or caloric deficit are the most easily identifiable forms of malnutrition. Assessing the fat deposits and muscle wasting in people who are chronically ill provides a convenient index to their nutritional status. It is inexcusable that records of weight or skin-fold thickness are often neglected.

Feeding Techniques to Help the Weak and the Handicapped

Patients who must be fed or handicapped people who feed themselves require longer mealtimes. The food needed to maintain an adult represents about 2,000 spoonfuls a day. Volunteers can often help patients who need to be fed, but nursing should allow extra time in staffing to assist the handicapped and those who feed them. It is not unusual for such patients to need an hour to get enough to eat.

Patients who must be fed are apt to leave considerable amounts of food on their trays because they tire easily and because they think they are taking too much of the feeder's time. It may be useful to put priorities on the foods. For some patients fluids are of primary importance; but for many, milk, eggs, meat, and cheese are more important than gelatin, applesauce, and lettuce, for example. Make a meal a social occasion. Feeders should talk to patients even if they cannot respond and try to find some way to communicate if only by signals. People generally eat better when social contacts are provided along with the food.

Almost inevitably the patient who must be fed is the patient who does not get enough to eat. Feeding a person who cannot feed himself requires special empathy. He should be helped to help himself, and the goal should be maximizing his limited abilities to do so. The person being fed should be encouraged to hold his napkin and, if possible, his bread and butter and to bring these to his mouth as often as he wishes. Frequent sips of milk, water, or coffee may help him swallow, and he may be able to sip from a bent straw better than from a cup or glass.

Handicapped people can often feed themselves if someone supplies special eating aids:

- A slippery glass may have a stretch-cloth slipcover.
- A plate may have a bumper added.
- Forks and spoons with bent handles, elongated handles, or even swivel handles can be made at home or purchased.
- A rocker knife requires only one hand to cut up food.

The physical therapist is often especially resourceful in helping handicapped people feed themselves. Blind people need to know how their dishes will be arranged on the tray and how the food will be arranged on their plate.

Foods may have to be altered or selected to help those with chewing and swallowing problems. These patients are often afraid of choking. Not all foods have to be cooked to be soft: ripe bananas and melons are soft fruits. Many meats may have to be ground or chopped for certain patients, but fish that has been steamed or baked is usually soft enough without further treatment. If a patient cannot chew certain foods such as meat, they may be chopped into bite-size pieces; if chopping is not enough, they may be ground; if grinding is not enough, as a last resort they may be blended. Remember that an adequate diet must include bread and cereals as well as meat, milk, and fruits and vegetables. It may be necessary to put the bread into the blender as well as the meat, vegetables, and fruits. Foods other than bread or milk should not be blended with other food. The meat, the vegetable, and the fruit should be kept as identifiable products. The patient should be told that this is pureed roast beef or apricot nectar. All of his food should not be mixed in one bowl. Pureeing, grinding, and chopping should be done as little as possible but should not fail to be done if the patient's handicaps make it impossible for him to swallow otherwise.

More aged than younger adults require dietary restrictions to control disease, but these restrictions should be handled on an individual basis. Food for the elderly should be seasoned with the same care appropriate for younger people. One of the changes characteristic of aging seems to be a decrease in the number of taste buds. Unless a person is on a sodium restriction so strict that he needs to use "salt-free" bread, his food should be cooked with salt. Sweet, sour, and bitter, as well as salt, are needed to provide a variety of flavors. Current diet theory advises ulcer patients to avoid pepper and caffeine, but such restrictions are not appropriate for the elderly as a group.

Many but not all elderly people have difficulties in chewing and swallowing, sometimes need help in eating, or require a modified diet. Nevertheless, the idea that the elderly should be fed a thin gruel concocted in a blender to compensate for dentures and diminished powers of digestion is as wrong as the idea that vitamin and mineral supplements can replace food. Food supplies more than nutrition. The taste, color, form, and texture of foods contribute to the joy of eating. No food should be provided or denied simply because a person is old. Favorite foods shared with family and friends are among the pleasures of life that should be provided both old and young.

Community Programs to Provide Meals for Shut-ins

During the past 25 years over 1,000 communities in the United States have started programs to deliver meals to the aged and the sick who are physically well enough to remain in their own homes but unable to prepare their own meals. Money to provide both the payments for those accepted into the program but without funds to pay for their meals and the funds to hire a part-time director for the program are provided by community chests or local service clubs. These community-based programs are known as Meals on Wheels. Volunteers deliver the meals and collect the payments. A local hospital or other health care facility usually provides the meals and charges only enough to recover food costs.

Usually a physician's referral and diet order is required before one is eligible for the service. Some of the people referred to Meals on Wheels have special diet prescriptions. A dietitian must work with the program if modified diets are to be provided. Most programs can serve only 25 to 30 recipients and have more requests for service than they can meet. There is no age restriction for those receiving the meals, and the criterion for acceptance into the program is the need for the service. Community support makes it possible for Meals on Wheels to keep costs low and to serve many who are not able to pay. The needs of participants are reviewed frequently to encourage those who can go out for meals and prepare their own meals to do so. This means that Meals on Wheels is meant to be a temporary service that contributes to the return of shut-ins to society and to independent living.

Recently, federal funding has become available to expand delivery of meals to aged who are homebound. In some communities

Meals on Wheels have been contracted for this service, but Home-Bound Meals are part of the Congregate Feeding Program initiated by Title VII in 1972. Meals on Wheels is a nonprofit, volunteer service, locally funded and usually limited to urban areas.

Government Programs to Improve the Nutritional Status of Adults

Federally funded programs to improve the nutritional status of people in the United States started with the School Lunch Act in 1945. Federal funding of the school lunch programs encouraged school corporations to provide a hot meal at noon at nominal cost to students. Surplus foods were used in the school lunch programs, and these foods were also distributed to needy families. Surplus and commodity foods have been replaced by food stamps for individuals and families. The Expanded Foods and Nutrition Education Program (EFNEP) directed by the Cooperative Extension Service of the USDA is an educational program to help low-income families use their food resources wisely. Originally the aides employed by EFNEP tried to help homemakers use the commodity and surplus foods. Now the EFNEP aides help homemakers learn to shop wisely using their limited resources, which may include food stamps, to obtain maximum nutritional benefits and to prepare good, low-cost meals and snacks. Whereas the school lunch program provides direct benefits to school children, and food stamps and assistance from EFNEP focus on households, the newest federal nutrition program is for the aged. The initial legislation for congregate meal programs for the aged was passed in 1972. Child nutrition programs continue to expand, but adult programs are also developing.

Expanded Foods and Nutrition Education Program

EFNEP does not distribute foods, nor does it give out food stamps or money for food. Originally funded in 1968 with a $10 million grant from the Cooperative Extension Service and budgeted currently at just over $50 million annually, EFNEP is the outgrowth of a series of pilot projects in nutritional education. In its first 10 years of operation on a national basis, the program has enrolled more than 1.5 million families, including more than 6 million individuals. The Cooperative Extension Service continues to supervise both the family and the youth programs.

EFNEP is distinguished by its efforts to provide accurate nutritional information in a form that can be understood and applied. Areas in which the program is funded have a supervising home economist selected and employed by the Cooperative Extension Service. This professional works with state and national specialists in foods and nutrition and is responsible for the activities of a group of local paraprofessionals called *program aides.* The pilot programs demonstrated the effectiveness of employing and training paraprofessionals who lived in the community to work with their neighbors. The aides take training in the basics of food and nutrition, completing an initial series of 15 hours before contacting any homemaker, and receiving continuing education as long as they stay on the job. Educational materials distributed and explained by the aides are prepared or approved by state and national extension specialists. In 1978 there were more than 5,000 people employed as nutrition aides (Science and Education Admin., 1979).

Although the aides do reinforce their teaching with printed information, they work primarily with homemakers individually in the home of the program family. Aides help the homemaker improve her skills in food preparation, grocery shopping, and menu planning. Sometimes they help families start gardens. Aides emphasize the importance of handling food to keep it safe as well as nutritious. State programs have purchased an audiovisual tool called the *Phonoviewer* for the aides to use with families. The Phonoviewer is like a portable television except that it plays only a filmstrip and a record. The Phonoviewer tapes are about topics such as food safety, diet in pregnancy, feeding the young child, food for the elderly, and other nutritional concerns.

Obviously not all the low-income families in the United States can be enrolled in EFNEP at the same time. One aide can work with 20 to 50 families, depending on how much assistance each family requires. Because they usually live in or near the area where they work, aides are able to select families most in need and most receptive to educational efforts. If a family agrees to accept help, the aide begins calling on a scheduled basis. Each call is an informal lesson selected according to the observed needs of the family. Families are expected to remain in EFNEP about two years and then be graduated so that the aide can enroll another family. Over 300,000 low-income families were enrolled in 1977/1978.

A major effort of EFNEP is to "increase the homemakers ability to manage resources that relate to food" (Science and Education Admin., 1979). The effectiveness of this effort is measured by changes in the homemaker's diet over the two-year period during which the family is in the program. Both a *minimum diet* and an *adequate diet* are defined in terms of the basic four. A minimum diet must include foods from all four food groups, whereas an adequate diet includes at least two servings of milk, two servings of meat or meat substitutes, four servings of fruits or vegetables, and four servings of breads or cereals. About one-half of the homemakers have had minimum diets when they entered the program. After two years, about three-fourths of the homemakers have achieved at least minimum diets, and the number achieving adequate diets has increased four times.

Adults and youths of all ages can participate in the educatinal programs traditionally carried out through the Cooperative Extension Service. The home economics divisions of the Extension Service have a long history of providing reliable information for the homemaker. The traditional programs in Foods and Nutrition Extension continue to reach chiefly middle- and upper-income families; but since 1968, the nutritional education program known as EFNEP has expanded its audience to include a significant fraction of the low-income families in the United States.

Food Stamps

Not all low-income families in the United States are issued food stamps. In fact, only about one-half of the families enrolled in EFNEP are using food stamps, although the stamps are regarded as part of the food resources available to low-income families. A person or family must contact the food stamp office in his county of residence and complete a 5-page questionnaire to determine eligibility and the money value of the food stamps available to that person or family. Families are not required to participate in EFNEP to be eligible to receive food stamps. The food stamp application includes questions about income, assets, utility bills, rent or mortgage payments, and debts to help the eligible workers determine how much of their cash resources the family or person can reasonably be expected to use to purchase food. Food stamps are issued in the amount of the difference between the money reasonably available for food and the money required to purchase an adequate diet based on the current cost of the *thrifty diet* as defined by the USDA. The USDA has drawn up lists of the foods people might ordinarily select to provide an adequate diet at three cost levels: low, moderate, and liberal. The grocery store prices of the foods on each list are collected quarterly, and the information is published, providing the costs for individuals of various age-sex groups and for typical family groupings. The cost of a thrifty diet is estimated at one-fourth less than that of the *low-cost diet*. If price data indicate that a young couple could purchase a low-cost diet for $32, the cost of a thrifty diet would be $24. If the couple had no income they would qualify for $24/week in food stamps. If the couple could reasonably be expected to have $12 available from their own resources for food, they would receive an additional $12 in food stamps. Every six months, current food prices replace earlier prices in the formula used to estimate the total cost of a thrifty diet for food stamp recipients. Only families with no income can receive enough food stamps to equal the total cost of the thrifty diet. Other recipients are expected to use the food stamps as supplements to their own cash for food.

Food stamps may be used in many groceries and supermarkets the same as money except that they purchase only food and not nonfood items such as soap, paper goods, pet foods, alcoholic beverages, tobacco or cigarettes, or vitamins and medicines (Food and Nutrition Serv., 1979).

Food stamps do not ensure an adequate diet. Purchasing an adequate diet at the thrifty cost level requires more knowledge about foods and nutrition than most people have achieved. Traditional patterns of eating must be altered if a balanced diet is to be obtained at such a low cost: Less meat and more meat substitutes must be used. Grain foods must be used in larger quantities than most people find acceptable. Instant nonfat dry milk should be substituted for fresh milk, and most homemakers will need to spend more time in grocery shopping and food preparation than is customary.

The Food Stamp Program has replaced the distribution of surplus foods and commodity foods. Commodity foods were added to surplus foods to attempt to insure needy families of enough of the right foods to avoid nutritional deficiencies, but many of these "right" foods were wasted. Food stamps allow the participant to purchase the foods he thinks he will use.

Nutrition Programs for the Aged

During the late 1960s the Administration on Aging identified poor nutrition and isolation as the two critical problems among the aged. Participants in research and in demonstration nutrition programs initiated in 1968 stated that the social benefits of these programs were as important as the food. Evaluation of these pilot projects led to the selection of group meals in a community setting as the vehicle to deliver various health and social services to the aged. In 1972 Congress passed amendments to the Older Americans Act, under Title VII, to start meal service and related services for people over age 60 and their spouses. Funds were allocated to the various states to establish congregate meal sites and such related services as transportation, outreach, information, referral, escort, health and welfare counseling, recreation and shopping assistance, and nutritional education.

A strong emphasis on the congregate aspect of the program originally restricted home-delivered meals to 10% of the meals served. Home-delivered meals are less effective in relieving loneliness than meals eaten with other people at the nutrition site. It has proved difficult to limit the number of home-delivered or homebound meals. A program worker must assess and reassess the need for meals delivered to the home, but without this meal service many people living independently would have to be institutionalized. By 1979 some programs were delivering 40–50% of their meals to homebound aged. Late in 1979 steps were initiated to reduce this percentage to about 30% of the total meals.

Meals are seldom prepared on the site or even in a central project kitchen. Contract meals are common. Some contract meals are for profit; some are nonprofit; and occasionally the meals are purchased from a school. Pans of food are delivered to the meal sites ready to serve, and individual meals are delivered hot to homebound participants living near the meal sites. Meals for people in rural areas are frozen and delivered as packages to provide meals for several days. A 1973 survey revealed that meal costs were high: from $0.59 to $3.99 per meal. The average cost in

1979 was $2.72 per meal, but this includes the cost of supportive services and delivery of homebound meals.

The meals must provide no less than one-third of the RDAs for eight key nutrients—protein, calcium, iron, vitamin A, thiamine, riboflavin, niacin, and ascorbic acid—and one-third of the suggested Calorie intake. Most meals provide considerably more than one-third of the caloric needs of most older people and more than one-third of the protein allowance; but it is believed that many participants eat little the rest of the day, and not much food is returned or wasted.

Although congregate meals for the aged were originally called "Title VII" Meals, they have subsequently been funded under Title III and have also contracted for Title XX funds, which can be used only to help low-income people. Most communities seem to refer to their nutrition programs for the aged as simply "The Nutrition Program." Although these programs generally provide five hot meals a week at noon, like the School Lunch Program does, there are several differences:

• The participants in nutrition programs for the aged are asked to pay what they feel they can afford. The money is put into a contribution box or envelope. There is no fixed charge for the meal whether it be congregate or homebound.

• The pattern for the meal includes a simple dessert. Both coffee and milk are offered.

• Meals for the aged are rarely served in schools, although it has been proposed that school lunch facilities might be appropriate. Churches and community centers often provide the meal site.

• Meals are served year-round, not just during the school year.

Each state governor has designated an agency to distribute the funds allocated to his state for nutrition services to the aged. Usually the agency selected is the state commission on ag-

ing. The state agency tries to distribute these funds on the basis of the needs of the aged living in the various areas of the state. Each area in turn develops projects that organize the individual meal sites. During the first seven years of the program, 1,200 nutrition projects were organized. Each of these projects operates about 15 meal sites. In 1979, meals, either congregate or homebound, were distributed daily to more than .5 million older people.

BIBLIOGRAPHY

Cereal Instit., Inc. *A Complete Summary of the Iowa Breakfast Studies.* Chicago, 1976.

Cook, J. D., and Monsen, E. R. Vitamin C, the common cold, and iron absorption. *Am. J. Clin. Nutr.* 30:235, 1977.

Crandon, J. H., Lund, C. C., and Dill, D. B. Experimental human scurvy. *N. Engl. J. Med.* 223:353, 1940.

Dietary goals for the United States. 2nd Ed. and Addendum. *J. Am. Diet. Assoc.* 74:529, 1979.

Durnin, J. V. G. A. and Passmore, R. *Energy, Work, and Leisure.* London: Heinemann Ed. Book, Ltd., 1967.

Food and Nutrition Board, Nat'l Research Council. *Recommended Dietary Allowances.* 8th Ed. Publ. No. 2216. Washington, D.C.: Nat'l Acad. of Sciences, 1974.

_____. *Recommended Dietary Allowances.* 9th Ed. Washington, D.C.: Nat'l Acad. of Sciences, in press.

Food and Nutrition Board, Nat'l Research Council, Nat'l Acad. of Sciences, and the Council on Foods and Nutrition, Am. Med. Assoc. (Joint statement). Diet and coronary heart disease. *Nutr. Rev.* 30:223, 1972.

Food and Nutrition Serv. *How to Apply for and Use Food Stamps.* Program Aid No. 1226. Washington, D.C.: U.S. Dept. of Agriculture, 1979.

Frisch, R. E., and Revelle, R. Height and weight at menarche and a hypothesis of critical body weights and adolescent events. *Science* 169:397, 1970.

Girdwood, R. H. Folate depletion in old age. *Am. J. Clin. Nutr.* 22:234, 1969.

Horwitt, M. K. Vitamin E—a reexamination. *Am. J. Clin. Nutr.* 29:569, 1976.

Indiana Diet Manual Comm. *Indiana Diet Manual.* Indianapolis, 1974.

Indiana State Board of Health. *Menu planning check list.* State Board Health Publ. No. 25-007. Indianapolis, 1974.

Inhibition of the hemopoietic activity of folic acid by ethanol. *Nutr. Rev.* 37:254, 1979.

King, S. S. New U.S. dietary guide may be hard to swallow. From *The New York Times* News Service. *Chicago Tribune*, Nov. 8, 1979.

La Londe, M. *A New Perspective on the Health of Canadians.* Ottawa: Minister of National Health and Welfare, 1976.

Mikey, J. B. Findings of study of extra-hospital nursing needs. *Am. J. Public Health* 53:1047, 1963.

Public Health Serv. *Working with Older People.* Publ. No. 1459, Vol. 1, p. 63. Washington, D.C.: U.S. Dept. of Health, Education, and Welfare, 1970.

———. *Ten-State Survey in the United States, 1968–1970.* Washington, D.C.: U.S. Dept. of Health, Education, and Welfare, 1972.

———. *Healthy People: The Surgeon General's Report on Health Promotion and Disease Prevention.* Publ. No. 79-55071. Washington, D.C.: U.S. Dept. of Health, Education, and Welfare, 1979.

Radcliffe athletes participate in study on effect of athletics on menstruation. (Radcliffe) *Centennial News.*, p. 16, Jan. 1980.

Roe, D. *Drug-induced Nutritional Deficiencies.* Westport, Conn.: AVI Pub. Co., 1976.

Rossman, I. The anatomy of aging. In I. Rossman, Ed., *Clinical Geriatrics.* Philadelphia: J. B. Lippincott Co., 1971.

Science and Education Admin. *The Expanded Food and Nutrition Education Program—Historical and Statistical Profile.* Washington, D.C.: U.S. Dept. of Agriculture, 1979.

Shaw, S., and Lieber, C. S. Nutrition and alcoholic liver disease. *Nutrition in Disease.* Columbus, Ohio,: Ross Laboratories, 1978.

Shock, N. W. Physiologic aspects of aging. *J. Am. Diet. Assoc.* 56:491, 1970.

Strehler, B. L. Aging at the cellular level. In I. Rossman, Ed., *Clinical Geriatrics.* Philadelphia: J. B. Lippincott Co., 1971.

Trotter, M., and Gleser, G. The effect of aging on stature. *Am. J. Phys. Anthrop.* 15:171, quoted in I. Rossman, Ed., *Clinical Geriatrics,* Philadelphia: J. B. Lippincott Co., 1971.

U.S. Dept. of Agriculture. *Food Consumption of Households in the United States.* USDA Household Food Consumption Survey, 1955–1965, Reps. 1–4. Washington, D.C., 1967.

———. *Food Intake and Nutritive Value of Diets of Men, Women, and Children in the United States, Spring 1965.* USDA ARS 61-18. Washington, D.C., 1968.

U.S. Dept. of Health, Education, and Welfare. *Preliminary Findings of the First Health and Nutrition Examination Survey, United States, 1971–1972.* DHEW Publ. No. (HRA) 75-1229, Washington, D.C., 1975.

Weir, C. E., and the Agricultural Research Policy Advisory Comm. *Benefits from Human Nutrition Research.* Washington, D.C.: U.S. Dept. of Agriculture, 1971.

Young, V. R., Perera, W. D., Winterer, J. C., and Scrimshaw, N. Protein and amino acid requirements of the elderly. In M. Winick, Ed., *Nutrition and Aging.* New York: John Wiley & Sons, Inc., Pubs., 1976.

THE APPLICATION OF NUTRITION TO NURSING PRACTICE

Part II is intended to help nursing students apply principles of nutrition to the delivery of nursing care. It is divided into two units. Unit IV introduces the nursing process and applies it to nutritional care of the client. Assessment, the first step in the nursing process and an important part of clinical nutrition as well, has two chapters devoted to it. Next, a series of nursing diagnoses based on assessment of the nutritive process is presented to help students understand the importance of nutrition to the delivery of effective client-centered nursing care. Specific nursing interventions in the nutritional support of selected medical interventions are discussed in a separate chapter. The nursing diagnoses in Unit IV provide the framework for the discussion of dietary interventions in Unit V.

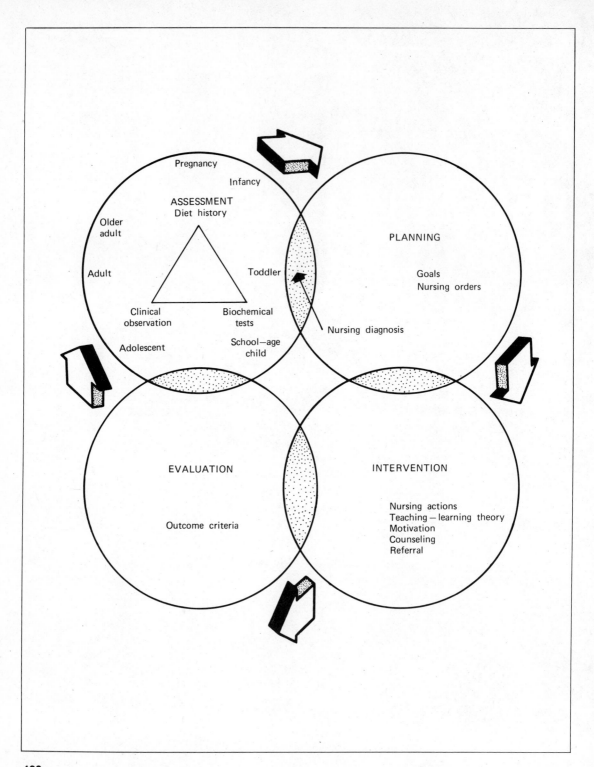

THE NURSING PROCESS IN NUTRITIONAL CARE

In Unit IV the nursing process is used as an overall framework for delivering nutrition-centered nursing care. Chapter 18 presents an overview of the nursing process as a problem-solving model. The components of assessment, planning, intervention, and evaluation are introduced and explained. Chapter 19 discusses the components of nutritional assessment in depth. Dietary intake surveys, clinical and anthropometric data, and laboratory analysis are the tools explained as a basis for an in-depth nutritional assessment. Hospital-acquired malnutrition is discussed to emphasize the relevance of nursing assessment. Chapter 20 explains how the basic nutritional assessment is altered for each stage of the life cycle. Emphasis is placed here on individual rather than group or community assessment.

Chapter 21 introduces the concept of nursing diagnosis in relation to nutritional problems of clients. Diagnoses centering on interferences with each step of the nutritive process—ingestion, digestion, absorption, nutrient transport, metabolism, and excretion—are categorized and discussed as they are manifested in the client.

Chapter 22 covers general nutritional care of the client and incorporates the planning, intervention, and evaluation steps in the problem-solving process. The concepts of patient teaching, hospital-based food source, comfort measures, and goal setting are applied to clients without severe alterations in nutritional states. Evaluation of client learning and nursing care are also discussed. *Audit, peer evaluation,* and *self-study* are examples of the evaluation methodologies discussed.

Finally, Chapter 23 describes dependent nursing functions related to nutritional care. Test diets, drug-diet interactions, intravenous therapy, total parenteral nutrition, and tube feedings are all discussed in detail.

BEHAVIORAL OBJECTIVES

After completing this unit, the student will be able to:

1. Apply the nursing process as a problem-solving model to nutritional situations.
2. Assess the nutritional status of a client or group of clients by using biochemical, clinical, and dietary data.
3. Establish nursing diagnoses specific to a client's needs.
4. Delineate specific nursing orders that will help meet a client's nutritional needs.
5. Use outcome criteria to evaluate nursing care.

CHAPTER 18

The Nursing Process as a Problem-solving Model

The nurse is constantly confronted with myriad problems to solve requiring a complex array of resources and thinking processes. Approached systematically, many problems that initially appear overwhelming and insolvable evolve into manageable details. Such a system, when applied to nursing, is called the *nursing process*. This chapter provides a theoretical basis for the nursing-process concept.

PROBLEM SOLVING

Most people have been solving problems throughout their lives. By the time they are students in nursing school, they have probably become fairly proficient at problem solving. To illustrate the sequence of problem solving, take the familiar example of weight control:

The first thing that must occur is the *recognition that a problem exists*. This usually occurs by *collecting* various bits of *information*. For example, one notices clothes are becoming a little "snug" or that one has to buy a size larger blue jeans. In addition, a "significant other" may ask if one is gaining a little weight. To add insult to injury one also can "feel" a few extra inches around the middle. If one is perceptive enough to pick up on these signs, one automatically goes to the next step of problem solving: *comparing the information* gathered with *standards*. The standards, influenced by both culture and values, may include: (1) no flab around the middle, (2) no increase in clothing size, and (3) a nor-

mal weight plus or minus 5 lb for height. For example, assume normal weight is 135 lb. At this point one is ready to *define the problem*. One labels one's problem as extra weight, chubbiness, or an acute case of shrinking clothes. One may notice that at this point more information is needed to identify, validate, and confirm the problem precisely. For example, one could weigh oneself and measure the waist line. Such observations will validate the problem and may possibly lead to a more accurate label for the problem.

Now that the problem is tentatively defined, one needs to decide what to do about it. A long-term goal may be to lose 15 lb. A short-term goal may be to lose 5 lb. One may make additional objectives centering on reducing one's waist measurement or dress size. These goals consciously or unconsciously provide direction for actions that follow. *Plans* are based on goals. If a goal is to lose 5 lb, one may plan to: (1) eat a 1,200-Calorie diet, (2) exercise 30 minutes/day, or (3) fast for three days. Before these plans are implemented one determines which of the alternatives are most likely to solve the problem and which may only create new difficulties. At this point one also must consider concurrent problems and conditions that may be influenced by actions. For example, exercising for 30 minutes a day is a reasonable solution; yet one may not be able to make such a time commitment. One may decide that the best plan is to follow a 1,200-Calorie diet.

The next step involves the actual "doing." One follows the diet outlined according to plan. After this step one would determine if what was done about the problem helped to solve it. The most accurate way to do this is to see if the *goal was met.* Have 5 pounds been lost? Other data related to satisfaction with the diet and rate of weight loss might be gathered in evaluating the success of action. The entire process is a circular one, with the final step providing information that may be helpful in redefining the problem.

The process as illustrated may appear rather tedious; but when it is used with more complex problems and carried out systematically, a reasonable outcome may be assured.

NURSING PROCESS

This problem-solving process applied to nursing care is the *nursing process.* It involves a pattern of observation and logical thinking that provides the basis for nursing care. The process has been broken down into four basic steps: assessment, planning, intervention, and evaluation. This series of actions have one purpose: maintaining a client's optimal level of wellness. They are analogous to the steps used in any problem-solving situation.

Using the example of weight gain, *assess-*

ment occurred when (1) there was recognition that a problem existed, (2) information was collected, (3) information was compared with standards, (4) the problem was defined. *Planning* involved: (1) determining what needed to be accomplished (establishing objectives), (2) listing several ways in which the objective might be accomplished, and (3) selecting the appropriate or most important possible solutions. The *intervention* phase is the action step. At this time the plans decided on are carried out. In the example, this involved following a 1,200-Calorie diet. The *evaluation* phase consists of: (1) gathering data to determine if the objectives have been met and (2) providing information to help recognize further problems. Figure 18-1 outlines the problem-solving aspect of the nursing process.

The nursing process, if used consistently and systematically, will guide the nurse in providing comprehensive nursing care. There are many reasons for this. The first is the fact that the nursing process provides the nurse with a useful tool to focus attention on being goal directed rather than task oriented. For example, instead of seeing each client as a series of diets to plan, the nurse will direct her

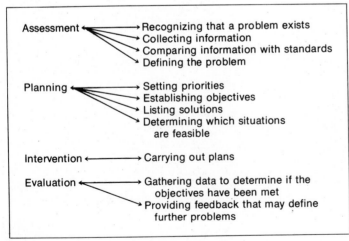

Figure 18-1. The nursing process as problem solving.

activites toward identifying the specific nutritional needs of each client and finding ways to fulfill those needs. Because of this the nursing care given is client centered; that is, it focuses on the client and his needs.

When using the nursing-process model to direct thinking, the nurse is provided with a method of organizing seemingly involved thoughts, concepts, and ideas from the physiological, social, and psychological sciences and the arts. In addition, intellectual, interpersonal, and technical skills the nurse has developed are integrated into a meaningful care plan. For example, to assess and meet a toddler's nutritional needs the nurse would apply principles of growth and development, biochemistry, communication theories, psychology, and family interaction theories.

Finally, the cyclic characteristic of the nursing process assures that the client will be quickly and purposefully assisted in meeting his needs. There is constant feedback in and among the four components of assessment, planning, intervention, and evaluation. For example, when caring for a toddler the nurse may assess a need for additional finger foods to increase his caloric intake. Planning may include the addition of hot dogs to his meal plan. During intervention, the nurse may note that the toddler will eat only if his mother is with him. Thus, more information is sent back to the assessment phase, which may identify another problem. When evaluating the intervention, the nurse notes that the child has increased his caloric intake but eats hot dogs only with catsup. This information again provides a basis for reassessment. The interrelatedness of the nursing process is illustrated in Figure 18-2. The nursing process is a systematic way of assisting a client toward high-level wellness through the process identification of problems or potential problems.

Assessment

The initial phase of the nursing process is *assessment*. The purpose of assessment is to iden-

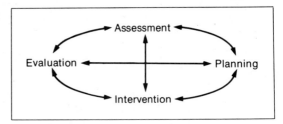

Figure 18-2. The interrelatedness of the phases of the nursing process.

tify, collect, and interpret data about the client that will enable the nurse to make a statement about actual or potential health problems the client may have that the nurse can do something about. The end product of assessment is a statement that describes these problems. As noted in the previous discussion of problem solving, a problem must be accurately identified before it can be solved. It would be very difficult to assist a client with his diet if the nurse did not know that the client is a vegetarian. This statement of patient problems is commonly labeled *nursing diagnosis*.

Assessment begins with data gathering. Sources from which data may be gathered include client, family, significant others, health record (chart), literature, and other members of the health care team through systematic observation and interaction. When beginning to assess a client to determine the presence or absence of problems, the nurse must use every source available to make the most accurate diagnosis possible.

A major part of assessment involves interaction between nurse, family, and client, which makes communication skills essential. Data gathered through the use of communication techniques is referred to as *subjective data*. In collecting such data the nurse must use a deliberative approach, taking care to structure the questions purposefully. Open-ended questions will usually provide more accurate information than direct yes-no questions. For example, asking a client to describe what he had for breakfast and lunch yesterday will provide much more useful information than asking if he eats a good breakfast.

Data may also be obtained by using all of the senses a nurse has. Data can be gathered through touch, smell, hearing, and sight. Such information, observed directly by the nurse, is *objective data.* Examples of such data include blood pressure, heart rate, intake and output records, or the noting of edema (Table 18-1).

There are specific techniques the nurse can develop to collect objective data (Table 18-2). The most used and probably most important is observation. The use of this skill will validate much of the subjective data obtained by interview. For example, if the client enters the hospital and states, "I eat like a bird," the nurse would particularly note how much and what kind of food the client actually eats.

Palpation is the use of touch to examine the body. For example, by lightly but firmly touching the abdomen and ankles, the nurse is able to gather such information the presence and degree of ankle edema, any abdominal tenderness and masses, and the presence or absence of a fecal impaction.

Percussion is a similar skill, which when used accurately can provide a great deal of information the nurse can use as a basis for diagnosis. The technique involves thumping of body surface to produce sounds. To execute the technique, the nurse places one or two fingers on the body surface to be percussed

TABLE 18-1. Comparison of Objective and Subjective Data

Type of Data	Definition	Examples
Objective	Information directly perceived by the person collecting the data	Blood pressure, Calorie count, noting edema
Subjective	Information gathered through the use of communication techniques	Chart, diet, history

TABLE 18-2. Objective Assessment Techniques

Technique	Observation
Observation	Atrophy, pallor
Palpation	Edema, masses, tenderness
Auscultation	Blood pressure, heart sounds
Percussion	Flatus, fluid in lungs

and taps them gently with the forefinger of the opposite hand. Usually this technique is employed to determine the presence or absence of fluid or flatus.

Auscultation involves listening to sounds produced by the body, usually with a stethoscope. Active bowel sounds can be observed in this way.

Objective data can also be gathered through the use of various devices that yield data about a client. Examples of such information gathering include taking a temperature with a thermometer, taking blood pressure with a sphygmomanometer, recording the electrical activity of the heart with an electrocardiograph, or taking a weight with a scale.

It is important that all of the data needed be collected. To accomplish this, data collection needs to be done in a systematic, purposeful manner. It is helpful to use an assessment tool such as those presented in Chapters 19 and 20 as a guide for data collection. With any guide, however, the questions and areas presented cannot be inclusive or appropriate in all nursing situations. It is imperative that the nurse listen actively to a client's verbal and nonverbal responses to all areas of inquiry. The information the nurse receives should provide direction for the next area of assessment. Any tool used must be adapted to the client, family, and setting in which the nurse is involved.

The task of data collection is not all there is to assessment. The information gathered is meaningless unless the nurse is cognizant of how that information compares to what is considered normal for a person of a specific age and developmental level. For example, the nurse weighs a 3-year-old child and finds that the child weighs 20 lb (9 kg). It is also necessary to know that normal weight for a 3-year-old child should fall between 28 and 38 lb (12.5 and 17 kg).

After the data gathered is compared to the population standard, it is necessary to compare the data to what is normal for the person you are assessing. Many times what is normal for an individual is quite different from the population standards. An example of this would be an athlete whose heart rate may be 40 beats/minute. The population standard is 60–100 beats/minute; yet if the athelete's heart was beating consistently at 90 beats/minute, it would be abnormal for him.

It is obvious why the nurse should be aware of both the individual norm and the population standard. If, for example, the nurse is going to teach a client about a proper diet, she might assume that he will be able to eat all four basic food groups. Yet he may be a vegetarian, of a different cultural background in which certain foods are not eaten, or may not have the financial means to buy a meat everyday. The time spent teaching would leave both client and nurse frustrated because the nurse did not explore the client's normal eating patterns before teaching. In summary, a *population standard* is an average of what is normal for all people. A *person's norm* is what is normal for that person.

After the data is collected and the norms and standards are explored, the nurse will sort, compare, analyze, and synthesize the information. At this point a judgment is made regarding whether a problem exists or if there is the potential for a problem to develop. Once this step is completed, the nurse has a label for a problem or a potential problem. The statement that evolves from the thinking process described above is the *nursing diagnosis,* the last phase of assessment. It is a brief description of actual or potential problems nurses are capable of treating and

licensed to treat. Unless a nursing diagnosis is made, the entire nursing process is useless. A problem cannot be solved, prevented, or helped unless it is first precisely identified.

In general, nursing diagnoses describe health problems that are potential or actual blocks to need fulfillment. When making a nursing diagnosis, the nurse needs to consider the three major components of a diagnostic statement: (1) the health problem, (2) the known or suspected etiology, and (3) the signs that lead to the diagnosis. It helps to write the diagnosis in the form of the *problem related to its possible etiology.* An example of a nursing diagnosis in this form is "chewing difficulty related to poorly fitting dentures" or "obesity related to lack of responsibility for eating habits."

Nursing diagnosis is the one aspect of the nursing process that documents what nursing does and is. It can be used to validate nursing as a profession that contributes a unique and necessary component to total health care delivery. The most critical aspect of making a nursing diagnosis is the thinking and judgment involved. The nurse needs to make certain that the signs, symptoms, and reasons for the diagnosis are carefully documented. Documentation is best done in a standardized manner, frequently using an assessment sheet, a nursing history form, a problem list, or nursing notes.

It must always be kept in mind that assessment is a continuous process in itself (Fig. 18-3). It must be done before and simultaneously with the other parts of the process. The nurse's senses must be constantly in tune and aware of what is taking place within the client's internal and external environment. These observations must also include what the client is perceiving as happening. Assessment involves subjective and objective data collection, comparing data with the client's norms and the population standards, and concluding with a precise and accurate statement of the patient's potential and actual problems.

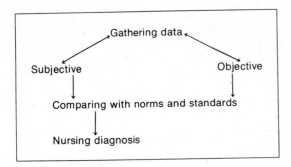

Figure 18-3. Assessment.

Planning

Once the problem is identified the next logical step is determining possible ways to solve the problem. The *planning* of nursing care depends on and arises from the nursing diagnosis. Trying to establish a plan of action without accurately identifying the problem is fruitless.

What occurs during the planning step is: (1) a determination of the relative importance of the problems identified, that is, establishing a priority list of the problems; (2) the establishment with the client, family, and other members of the health care team of mutual goals that describe the anticipated resolution of the problems; (3) the delineation of specific actions to help solve the problem and move the client toward the goals identified; and (4) the communication of the planned goals and actions to other health team members to assure continuity of care.

Setting Priority

The first consideration in the planning step is assigning priority to the problems identified. In the real world, nurses do not have an unlimited amount of time to spend with each client; the time they do have must be spent in solving the most important problems identified. Often it is obvious what is most important, such as when a client has an insulin reaction. At other times the priority is not so clear.

When assigning priority to problems it is helpful to keep in mind a hierarchy, such as Maslow's (1962) hierarchy of needs (Fig. 18-4). When making a priority judgment, it is important to consider the importance the client has placed on the identified problem. For example, the nurse might not consider the change in body image caused by an appendectomy scar important, whereas a very body-conscious adolescent might.

HUMAN NEED THEORY.   *Human need theory* provides a theoretical basis for giving nursing care. The client can be viewed as an integrated, organized whole motivated toward fulfilling his basic human needs. Through the recognition that all people are moving toward the fulfillment of these needs, the nurse is able to provide meaningful nursing care.

A *need* may be defined as a biopsychosocial force that initiates behavior to maintain or improve a sense of adequacy and well-being or to relieve distress. Many areas and levels of needs are present in every person. Maslow (1962) established his hierarchy of needs by delineating those more crucial for existence than others. He believed that a person faced with a lack of one or more needs is motivated to meet those needs on which survival most directly depends. An example of this would

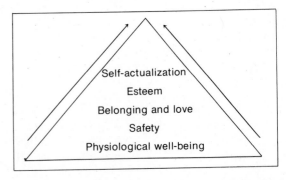

Figure 18-4. Maslow's hierarchy of needs. (From A. H. Maslow, *Toward a Psychology of Being.* Princeton, N. J.: Van Nostrand Reinhold Co., 1962.)

be a person lacking both food and air. Air is more critical to survival than food. The person would first try to meet his need for air. Only after this need was met would he attempt to find food.

Maslow's hierarchy consists of five basic needs: physiological needs, safety needs, belonging and love needs, esteem needs, and the need to be self-actualized. Thinking of needs in a hierarchy makes it is easy to see that each need must be met before the next higher need can build upon it. Although each level of need may never be completely satisfied, it will be met to the extent possible. Because of this, every person may have unsatisfied needs at many levels simultaneously.

The most important needs are the physiological needs: air exchange, food and fluid, elimination, activity and rest, and sexuality. Even within this category of needs some have a higher priority than others.

The next category of needs, which emerge only when the phsyiological needs are reasonably well satisfied, are the safety needs. *Safety* means the absence of threat or danger perceived in the internal or external environment. Safety and security needs are present when threats occur from such stimuli as war, illness, social upheaval, hospitalization, or separation. People generally need an established routine to be free from fear and anxiety.

After physiological and safety needs are met, a person is able to move away from himself and begin to test out relationships with other people. From this emerges the next level of need fulfillment, that of belonging and love needs. These are evident in a person's relationships with parents, family, colleagues, peers, spouse, children, and acquaintances. In meeting these needs, people may explore where they belong in society and the characteristics of their cultural heritage.

The next level on the hierarchy is need for esteem. When a person is satisfied that he can love and is loved, he attempts to discover his own attributes. Self-evaluation occurs, and self-respect is initiated. A person tends to use these ideas as a basis for evaluation of others. If esteem needs are unmet, a person may feel inferior, weak, and helpless. The nurse should carefully consider the effect of discontinuing, because of hospitalization and illness, those activities that have provided for self-esteem in the past.

Maslow's highest category of need is self-actualization. This includes the desire to be fulfilled, that is, to make actual all the potentials of self. The behavior that meets this need is unique to each person. It may be possible to be self-actualized in one area of life and not in all of them.

Setting Objectives

The second aspect of the planning phase centers on the development of goals or objectives that express the intended outcome of nursing care. The primary purpose of setting objectives is to provide direction for the remainder of the nursing process. These objectives, often termed *expected outcomes,* will provide criteria for determining how effective the nursing care is in meeting the patient's needs. All objectives need to be established with the client, family, and other care team members. For the client to participate actively in health care, it is imperative that he know what will be done and the reasoning behind the activities. The more specific the expected outcome statement is, the more direction it will provide. An example of such a statement is: "By the end of Mr. Jones's first week in the hospital, he will be able to plan a one-day, 1,800-Calorie diabetic diet using the American Dietetic Association's exchange lists." The objective provides precise direction. The time involved, the exact behavior expected, and how the behavior is to be accomplished is outlined. The usefulness of a well-constructed objective is evident when it is compared to one not so precise; the statement, "Mr. Jones will eat correctly," is vague and provides little precise direction.

Nursing Orders

After the nurse has developed the objectives—the "blueprints for action"—that specify direction, it becomes necessary to determine how to meet those objectives. To do this the nurse constructs a series of actions that are aimed at achieving the objectives. These actions, often termed *nursing strategies, nursing orders,* or *nursing measures,* are supported by scientific and behavioral facts shown to be effective in similar situations in the past. All nursing orders must be clear, precise, and specific to the individual receiving care. The way the nurse approaches each client's problems must be tempered by her knowledge of the uniqueness of that person. There are no "cookbook" lists of nursing orders that will meet the same objective in separate situations. This interaction between the planning and assessment phases of the nursing process is typical of the dynamic nature of the process.

Following are three examples of nursing orders that are exact and specific to each client:

1. Offer 100 ml of water and/or grape juice every 1 hr to encourage fluid intake.
2. Encourage Mrs. Smith's choice of her own menu selection by reading the menu aloud to her before lunch.
3. Stay with Mr. Doe while he eats to encourage socialization.

Each nursing order is based on a sound scientific rationale. Frequently, documenting the rationale for each order will strengthen the student nurse's problem-solving skills, for by so doing the student becomes increasingly adept at making plans that are apt to meet the stated objective.

Communicating Plans

The final aspect of the planning process is probably the most important and the least likely to be carried out. It is simply communicating plans to other health team members. The same nurse will probably not be with a client during his entire hospital stay. To provide for continuity of care all plans and any results of those plans need to be communicated to all the health team members. It is obvious how much time would be wasted if every nurse the client saw had to devise her own care plan for that client without the benefit of knowing what the previous nurse had discovered. For example, a nurse determines that 6-year-old Johnnie loves to take his medicine with grape juice but will spit it out if he takes it with anything else. Once this fact is discovered, it will save Johnnie, his parents, and the next nurse a great deal of frustration if his likes are communicated. The nursing Kardex or unit care plan is a reliable means of communicating the nursing orders to other health team members.

Intervention

The third step of the nursing process is *intervention.* During this phase, planned, purposeful interaction occurs with the client and health team members. The nursing orders are carried out. Because of the work done during the planning phase, the nurse is goal directed and not task oriented. It is during the intervention phase that the nurse must use management skills. The nurse coordinates the care to be given, carries out the actions, makes referrals as necessary, and records what is done.

Charting

The *chart* is written record of what happens to a client while he is in the health care delivery system. The chart serves many purposes, one of the most important of which is communication. In a busy health care delivery system it is virtually impossible for all the health team members involved with a specific client to sit down together and discuss the status of his health care intervention. If the necessary information is kept in a permanent written record, all health team members will be able to keep informed on the client's progress toward the established goals. It is necessary to record all phases of the process, particularly diagnosis, plans, interventions, and evaluation statements.

A second purpose served by the chart is substantiation of the interventions carried out. For example, when record keeping is complete, a survey of the effectiveness of using demonstrations as a teaching method would be possible.

The fact that the chart is a legal document cannot be overlooked. As such, it is used to investigate the commission or omission of care given by a health team member as well as to evaluate an entire institution's quality of care.

Charting needs to be concise yet complete. It must be given priority in health care delivery in order to assure quality care. All nursing actions carried out during the implementation phase need to be documented. As with all the steps of the nursing process, assessment will occur continuously during intervention. For example, a nurse discovers while assisting Mr. Johnson with his lunch that he has difficulty chewing nonground meat. New data is collected, a new nursing diagnosis is made, and new plans evolve.

Evaluation

The final step of the nursing process is *evaluation*. It is the phase in which the nurse decides if the nursing actions taken actually met the client's needs. The objectives specified in the planning step serve as guidelines for evaluation. When objectives are well constructed it will be obvious if the client has been able to demonstrate the behavior cited. The nurse must also consider the degree to which the behavior is demonstrated. For example, if the objective concerned menu planning on an 1,800-Calorie diet, does the client plan the menu independently or is some assistance required? Of course any judgment about the effectiveness of the nursing actions must include the client. If he does not feel confident planning his diet, the future compliance with the regimen may be low.

The conclusions reached in the evaluation phase should indicate whether the nurse needs to reassess, replan, and implement new intervention strategies or to continue with the present course of action. If the expected outcomes are not fully achieved, the nurse has not necessarily failed; rather, the client has been assured of optimal care by the checks and balances built into the nursing process.

In summary, during evaluation the nurse determines the effectiveness of the nursing actions. Objectives set during the planning phase serve as a guide for comparing the client's current status with that before intervention. New data will emerge from evaluation that will indicate if a reassessment should be made.

CASE STUDY: How the Nursing Process Can Be Applied to a Patient with a Nutritional Problem

Mrs. L. is a 40-year-old school teacher admitted to the hospital for treatment of low back pain and to rule out a herniated lumbar disc. Even though her primary medical diagnosis is not nutritionally based, she does have some nutritional concerns. Several weeks before admission Mrs. L. had discussed with her physician the influence of excess weight on her low back pain. At that time they agreed to work toward a slow weight loss to be accomplished by Mrs. L.'s adherence to a 1,200-Calorie diet. Mrs. L. was familiar with the diabetic exchange system and chose this method for her diet therapy.

ASSESSMENT

A. *Dietary habits:* Mrs. L. is trying to lose weight. She is quite knowledgeable about various diets and has placed herself on a 1,200-Calorie diabetic diet. She is familiar with the diabetic exchange system. During her three-week adherence to the diet she has lost a total of 7 lb (4.2 kg). She wishes to continue the diet during her stay in the hospital. Her physician has complied with this request.

B. *General appearance:* Mrs. L. appears well developed, not obese. She has pink skin tones, fine hair, and intact skin.

C. *Attitudes toward eating:* Mrs. L. states that she enjoys eating. She and her husband review the day's activities during the dinner hour. She enjoys cooking, particularly using foods that she has canned or preserved from her summer garden.

D. *Factors influencing food ingestion:* Mrs. L. denies any nausea or vomiting. She reports that she has had some difficulty with constipation because she has become less active as a result of her back pain. She denies any difficulty with ingestion of food.

E. *Additional data:*
Weight, 150 lb (68.2 kg)
Height, 66 in (167.6 cm)
Triceps skin fold, 19.3 mm

INITIAL NURSING DIAGNOSES

From the above data, preliminary diagnoses can be made, including:

1. Potential difficulty with appropriate selection of food related to lack of information concerning a 1200 Calorie diabetic diet

2. Constipation related to decreased activity

3. Excess weight related to chronic over ingestion of nutrients (Calories) and lack of exercise

Of course additional diagnoses could be made as more data is gathered.

PLANNING

For each diagnosis, goals and nursing orders would be documented. Following is an example for the first diagnosis:

Diagnosis

Potential difficulty with appropriate food selection related to lack of information concerning the 1,200-Calorie diabetic diet.

Goals

Mrs. L. will be able to choose food within the 1,200-Calorie diet that meets her nutritional requirements and is satisfying to her.

Nursing Orders

---

1. Coordinate activities between patient and dietitian regarding education about 1,200-Calorie diet.
2. Reinforce dietitian's teaching, reviewing Mrs. L.'s food selections with her at each meal.

INTERVENTION

Dietitian, nurse, and patient began review of 1,200-Calorie diet. Mrs. L. is practicing choosing foods from the hospital menu that fit into her 1,200-Calorie diet. In addition, she has been reading the literature the dietitian gave her on the diabetic exchange system.

EVALUATION

Evaluation is based on the goals set during planning. An example of an evaluative statement would be: "Mrs. L. has a beginning understanding of the exchange system as evidenced by her ability to plan a menu from a list of foods."

QUESTIONS

1. What additional data should be collected to further clarify or expand the nursing diagnoses?

2. Which data given in the assessment would be categorized as being subjective (S)? Objective (O)?

3. What would be the goals and nursing orders for the other two nursing diagnoses identified in the case?

4. What data would be used to evaluate whether or not the goals were accomplished?

Assessment Chart

Data Gathering	Data Gathered	Patient Norm	Population Standard	Nursing Diagnosis
I. Assessment Tool	(Indicate if data is (S) subjective or (O) objective)	(Before illness or hospitalization)		Potential difficulty c appropriate selection of food related to 1,200-Calorie diet.
Food and fluids:				
1. Dietary habits Is trying to lose weight. Has placed herself on 1,200 Calorie ADA diet c recommendation of physician. Knows exchange system. Has been on diet × 3 weeks. Has lost 7 lb. (S)		1,200 Calories for past 3 wks.	4 basic groups.	
2. General appearance Well-developed, not obese. (O)			Well-developed.	
3. Attitudes toward eating Enjoys eating (S)				
4. Factors influencing food ingestion No nausea, vomiting, or diarrhea. (O)				
5. Lab values	Na, Cl, K, CO_2. (O)		Na = 135–145 Cl = 90–100 K = 3.0 CO_2 = 4.5	
II. Additional Data-gathering Techniques				
Food and fluids:				
1. Weigh patient.				
2. Keep I&O.	Weight 150 lb (68.18 kg)			
3. Keep diet record.	Intake = 3500 cc			
4. Check skin turgor.	Output = 3120 cc			
5. Auscultate for bowel sounds.	Active, all four quadrants			

Evaluation Chart

Goal	Planning	Intervention	Evaluation
Selection of food	Obj: Pt will be able to choose food within the 1,200-Calorie diet that is nutritious and satisfying. 1. Refer to dietitian for patient teaching regarding 1,200-Calorie ADA diet. 2. Reinforce dietitian's teaching, reviewing number of exchanges with each meal.	Dietitian, nurse, and patient began study of 1,200-Calorie diet. Mrs. L. is practicing choosing foods from the hospital menu that fit into her 1,200-Calorie diet.	Mrs. L. has a beginning understanding of the basic four and 1,200-Calorie diet.

BIBLIOGRAPHY

Carlson, S. A practical approach to the nursing process. *Am. J. Nurs.* 72:1589, 1972.

DuGas, B. W. *Introduction to Patient Care.* 3rd Ed. Philadelphia: W. B. Saunders Co., 1977.

Gebbie, K., and Lavin, M. A. Classifying nursing diagnosis. *Am. J. Nurs.* 74:250, 1974.

Gordon, M. Nursing diagnosis and the diagnostic process. *Am. J. Nurs.* 76:1298, 1976.

Jones, D. A., Dunbar, C. L., and Gurobec, M. M. *Medical-Surgical Nursing, a Conceptual Approach.* New York: McGraw-Hill Book Co., 1978.

Lewis, L. This I believe . . . about the nursing process—key to care. *Nurs. Outlook* 16:26, 1968.

Little, D. E., and Carnevali, D. L. *Nursing Care Planning.* 2nd Ed. Philadelphia: J. B. Lippincott Co., 1976.

Maslow, A. H. *Toward a Psychology of Being.* New York: Van Nostrand Reinhold Co., 1962.

Mason, M., Wenberg, B. J., and Welsch, P. K. *The Dynamics of Clinical Dietetics.* New York: John Wiley & Sons, Inc., Pubs., 1977.

McCain, R. S. Nursing by assessment—not intention. *Am. J. Nurs.* 65:82, 1965.

Mitchell, P. H. *Concepts Basic to Nursing.* 2nd Ed. New York: McGraw-Hill Book Co., 1977.

Walter, J. B., Pardee, G. P., and Noble, D. M. *Dynamics of Problem-oriented Approaches: Patient Care and Documentation.* Philadelphia: J. B. Lippincott Co., 1976.

Yura, H., and Walsh, M. B. *The Nursing Process.* 3rd Ed. New York: Appleton-Century-Crofts, 1978.

CHAPTER 19

The Framework
of Nutritional Assessment

Assessment, the first phase of the nursing process, involves the collection and organization of data in such a way that a judgment can be made about the status of a client's needs. This interpretation of data into a nursing diagnosis provides the nurse with a list of potential and actual problems that can be treated.

The level of wellness a person will be able to achieve depends largely on nutritional status, so the nurse must be able to assess a client's level of nutritional function accurately and completely. This chapter discusses the components of nutritional assessment and provides suggestions for carrying out the investigation.

The integration of nutritional status into a client's level of wellness is illustrated by the following definition: *nutritional status* may be viewed as the "health condition of an individual influenced by his intake and utilization of nutrients, determined from the correlation of information obtained from physical, biochemical, clinical, and dietary studies (Christakis, 1973, p. 3). The nurse is in an excellent position to make clinical assessments because of the client-nurse relationship, the diagnostic skills of the nurse, and the close proximity of the nurse to the client and the client's environment.

There are three kinds of data that can be gathered to provide a basis for making a nursing diagnosis. The first is dietary data that describes the client's actual food intake, environmental conditions that may be a factor in decisions about food, and behaviors that may affect food intake or selection. The second is data on the basic physiological status of the client, including various anthropometric measurements as well as specific clinical findings. The final kind of data is biochemical data such as analysis of serum and urine metabolic constituents, chemical data, and information on certain nutrient-dependent metabolic processes. Figure 19-1 illustrates these components.

To insure that all available data is gathered for each of the three components of nutritional assessment, it is often helpful to use a guide that will cue the nurse to gather the specific information. Such a tool is to be used as a *guide* and not as a verbatim questionnaire (Harry, 1978). Each nurse should integrate her own personality, therapeutic communication techniques, active listening, and a sound knowledge of nutritional standards with the assessment tool to gather an accurate picture of a client's nutritional status. Figure 19-2 illustrates an assessment tool that could be used for data gathering.

Sources of information that may aid the nurse in the assessment of a community's nutrition include general agricultural data that provide information on availability of food supplies to a population; socioeconomic data that demonstrate the distribution and use of food supplies; dietary surveys that yield data on the rate of food consumption; biological studies that indicate the nutrient value of various foods; vital statistics that indicate risk-prone population groups; environmental data that may provide information on the acquisition and preparation of food; and general health practices of a population, which yield data on the possible interrelationship be-

477

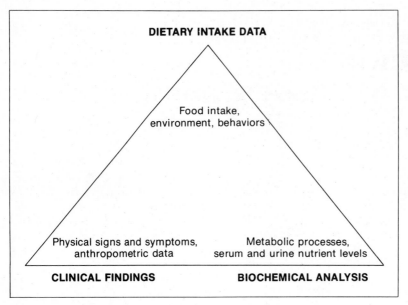

Figure 19-1. Components of nutritional assessment.

tween nutrition and disease (World Health Org., 1963).

It must always be remembered that determination of nutritional status depends on an assessment of the whole person as a unique being with a variety of interrelated needs and characteristics. In addition, the nurse needs to investigate the community of the client in order to establish a complete data base from which judgments and decisions can be made.

DIETARY INTAKE DATA

The collection of information about the food consumption of a community, family, or person will, in many instances, be the nurse's starting point when initiating a nutritional assessment. The information gathered will quite often be largely subjective, requiring the use of sophisticated communication techniques by the nurse. It is of primary importance that the nurse be aware of the prejudices, values, assumptions, and perceptions

she may have that could influence the nurse-client interaction.

Communication Skills

The purpose of communication among the health care team is to exchange information that will serve to promote coordination and continuity of care. Communication with a client should be purposeful and client centered. The accuracy of the diet history will depend on the communication techniques used by the interviewer.

The two broad categories of communication are verbal and nonverbal. *Verbal communication* involves the use of spoken or written words. *Nonverbal communication* is the exchange of messages without the use of words, for example, by crying, touching, moving closer to a person, or using symbols or signals.

For effective and meaningful communication to occur, five essential components of the communication process must be met: (1) A message must be *delivered*. (2) The receiver's *attention* must be directed to the message sender. (3) The receiver must *perceive* and *interpret* the message. (4) The language or symbols used must have a *common meaning* to both the sender and the receiver. (5) *Validation* must occur between the sender and the receiver, confirming that the message was delivered and understood. Figure 19-3 illustrates the interaction of the essential components in the process.

Several elements may affect the communication process. One of the most obvious is the possibility of difficulty with language. Common examples are the overuse of medical

---

I. Initial Data Gathering

Name _____   Age _____

Hospital admission date _____

Occupation _____   Estimated daily energy expenditure: Low

Medium

High

Avocation (hobbies) _____

Reason for admission to hospital or clinic _____

Past medical history (include diseases, illnesses, and previous hospitalizations) _____

Briefly relate what has occurred since admission (include lab work, tests, surgical procedures, etc.) _____

Past hospitalizations _____

Client's perception of intervention (it's helping, frustrating, etc.) _____

Activity level: Medications client is currently taking:

Allergies:

Social and cultural background:

A. Marital status _____

B. Significant others who provide a support system _____

C. Children _____

D. Education _____

E. Religious affiliation _____

Figure 19-2. Guide for nutritional assessment.

II. Food Intake Data

A. *24-hour recall:*

	Today		Yesterday	
	Food	*Amount*	*Food*	*Amount*
Breakfast				
Lunch				
Dinner				
Between-meal intake				

B. *Estimate of usual weekly intake:*

Food	Daily Guide	Amount Consumed	Method of Cooking
Milk	1 pt		
Cheese			
Milk desserts			
Citrus fruit	1 daily		
Other fruits	1/day		
Leafy green vegetables	1 serving		
Other green vegetables	1 serving		
Yellow vegetable	1 serving		
Potato or rice	1 serving		
Lean meat, fish, or fowl	4 oz		
Eggs			
Nuts			
Peanut butter			
Legumes			
Bread and cereals	4 servings		
Fats	3 T		
Candy			
Carbonated beverages			
Cake, cookies, pies			
Alcoholic beverages			
Coffee, tea			
Other:			
party foods			

Figure 19-2. (*Continued*)

Is this diet typical?

C. *Actual dietary intake:*

Date	Meal	Food	Amount (Weighed)	Calculations
				Total Calories _____
				Total Protein _____ gm
				Fat _____ gm
				Carbohydrates _____ gm
				H_2O _____ cc

D. *General information regarding intake:*
   1. Person responsible for food preparation _____
   2. Outstanding characteristics of past eating habits (food fads, special diets, IV therapy, NPO for diagnostic tests, etc.) _____
   _____
   3. Foods liked best _____
   4. Foods disliked and/or avoided _____
   _____
   5. More than half of meals eaten away from home? _____
   6. Evidence that income and/or meals may not be adequate for needs _____
   _____

III. **Clinical Assessment**
   A. *Anthropomorphic data:*
   Weight _____ kg   If infant,

   Height _____ cm   Head circumference _____ cm

   Triceps skin fold _____   Growth percentile _____

   Midarm circumference _____

   B. *Objective assessment data:*
   Area to be assessed   Findings
      1. Hair
      2. Eyes:
         Conjunctiva
         Bitot's spots?
         Presence of lesions?

Figure 19-2. (Continued)

481

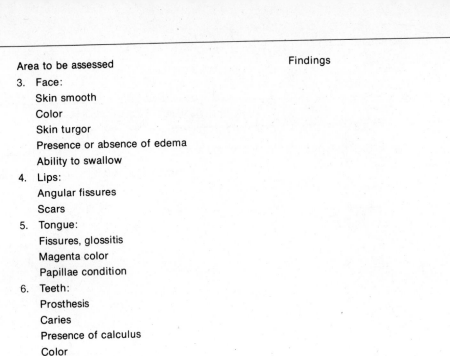

Area to be assessed   Findings

3. Face:
   Skin smooth
   Color
   Skin turgor
   Presence or absence of edema
   Ability to swallow

4. Lips:
   Angular fissures
   Scars

5. Tongue:
   Fissures, glossitis
   Magenta color
   Papillae condition

6. Teeth:
   Prosthesis
   Caries
   Presence of calculus
   Color

7. Gums:
   Inflammation
   Bleeding

8. Thyroid:
   Enlargement?

9. Skin:
   Lesions
   Pigmentation
   Turgor
   Petechiae
   Subcutaneous tissue
   Dry, moist?

10. Nails:
    Color
    Shape
    Brittleness

11. Muscles:
    Tone
    Tenderness
    Weakness
    Spasticity

Figure 19-2. (Continued)

	Area to be assessed	Findings
	12. Extremities:	
	Sensation	
	Pulses present	
	Vibratory sense	
	13. General appearance	
	14. Mentation	
	15. Orientation	
IV.	**Laboratory Assessment**	
	RBC	_____
	Hemoglobin	_____
	Hematocrit	_____
	Creatinine-height index (% of standard)	_____
	Total lymphocyte count	_____
	Serum levels:	
	Ascorbic acid	_____
	Folacin	_____
	Albumin	_____
	Creatinine	_____
	B_{12}	_____
	Vitamin A	_____
	Vitamin E	_____
	BUN	_____
	Urine levels:	
	Thiamine	_____
	Riboflavin	_____
	Pyridoxine	_____
	Creatinine	_____
	Urea	_____

Figure 19-2. (*Continued*)

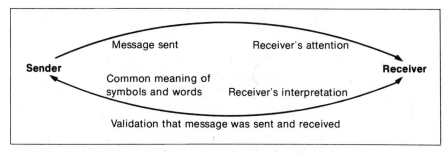

Figure 19-3. Essential components of the communication process.

terminology with clients and the differences in meaning of similar terms, which may vary with location. The physical or mental status of the client can also influence his ability to perceive messages or direct attention toward the message sender. A client who is in pain, for example, may not be able to provide accurate answers to questions about eating patterns. Another influence is the client's and the nurse's value systems. If for example a client is in the hospital for ketoacidosis resulting from eating a large amount of sweets, the nurse may unconsciously exhibit signs of disapproval because the client did not follow the prescribed diet regimen. In this case the nurse values compliance and becomes disturbed when dealing with a person who does not comply. Another influence is degree of familiarity between participants involved in the communication process. Quite frequently, if the nurse has dealt with a client previously, message validation may occur more readily.

The nurse as a health professional has several tasks to carry out during the nurse-client interaction process. The first is to *establish trust*. Although there is no prescription for the establishment of trust, it often occurs if the nurse is honest, open, and truly interested in helping the client achieve the highest level of wellness possible. The nurse should *support the client's abilities*. This includes discovering and using the unique contributions each person is able to make to his own care. One of the most important tasks the nurse has is to fulfill the role of a *client advocate*, noting deficiencies and inequities in the health care delivery system and following through with change strategies. To carry out these basic tasks, the nurse needs to understand the concept of the *therapeutic use of self*, that is, helping through the way she is rather than through the use of external tools such as a physician's medications or diagnostic procedures.

Therapeutic communication techniques also encourage client verbalization. Examples of therapeutic communication techniques likely to promote a positive nurse-client relationship faster are illustrated in Table 19-1. Through the use of these techniques the nurse allows the client to take the lead in an exchange, providing for an accepting and open atmosphere in which the client feels free to discuss his concerns. In communicating with clients, three general principles need to be remembered. The first is that the client should do most of the talking. The nurse's verbal response should be minimal—confined to comments that will aid the client in expression of needs. The second principle is that, on the whole, the more direct the questions asked, the less reliable the information gathered. When asked a direct question, most people will respond with what they think the interviewer wants to hear or will fabricate a response to avoid embarrassment. If the nurse allows the client to take the lead by using broad opening statements, the client will volunteer only the information that is emotionally safe for him. An example of this approach would be to state, "I'd like for you to tell me about your eating patterns and concerns about food," rather than "Can you tell me what you had for lunch yesterday?" The latter statement could be perceived as threatening and, if used in the early phases of the interview, might block effective communication between nurse and client. Examples of other blocks are given in Table 19-2. The third principle is that, if the nurse has a caring and open attitude and is aware of her own values and feelings that could influence communication, effective communication will be more likely to occur.

Interview

In general, the interview is a more structured interaction than most nurse-client exchanges. Within the interview structure, nurses and clients develop a trusting, nonjudgmental relationship in which reliable data is collected.

TABLE 19-1. Therapeutic Communication Techniques

Technique	Purpose	Example
Making broad opening statements	Allows client to take the lead and talk about his concerns.	Is there something bothering you? Tell me about your concerns regarding food.
Giving general leads	Encourages the client to continue.	Yes? Oh? Go on.
Reflecting	Prompts client to continue; allows client to hear, consider, and expand what was said (may be obvious if overused).	Repeat or rephrase what the client said.
Selective reflecting	Prompts the client to expand on what was previously stated.	Repeat or rephrase part of what was said, usually what the nurse considers to be the main idea, e.g., *Client:* I've been so rushed, I haven't eaten a thing for two days. *Nurse:* You haven't eaten for two days?
Sharing observations	Focuses on the client, conveys interest and concern.	*Nurse:* "You're trembling"; "You seem upset."
Acknowledging the client's feelings	Lets the client know his feelings are understood and accepted.	*Nurse:* "I can see how that would be frustrating."
Verbalizing implied thoughts and feelings	Validates the nurse's impressions.	*Client:* "It's a waste of time to study these food exchanges." *Nurse:* "You feel they aren't benefiting you?"
Being silent	Slows pace, provides time for the client to think.	No verbal response; nonverbal response is important, needs to convey acceptance and interest.
Clarifying	Clarifies meaning of client's statement or behavior.	*Nurse:* "I'm not sure I understand what you mean"; "Are you saying . . .?"
Validating	Confirms something	*Nurse:* "Are you feeling better now?"

TABLE 19-2. Blocks to Communication

Block	Possible Results	Example
Using reassuring cliches	Conveys that the nurse is not interested or does not with to discuss.	"Everything will be all right"; "Don't worry about it."
Giving advice	Implies that the nurse imposes own opinions, values, etc. Client may resent nurse.	"What you should do is. . . ,"
Giving approval	Implies nurse's concepts of right and wrong are used in judging client's behavior.	"That's the right attitude."
Requesting an explanation	Makes client feel uneasy; quite often puts the client on the defensive. Usually asks "why."	"Why didn't you follow your diet?" "Why are you upset?"
Expressing disapproval	Intimidates or angers client; the interaction is based on the nurses values.	"You shouldn't eat that."
Belittling client's feeling	Denies the importance and uniqueness of client's feelings.	"I know just how you feel"; "Everyone feels that way sometime."
Defending	Communicates nonacceptance of client's feelings.	"This hospital is an excellent one"; "She's an excellent nurse."
Using stereotyped comments	Communicates on a superficial level.	"Isn't it a beautiful day?" "How are you?" (with no follow-up).

The nurse needs to structure the interview, providing always a warm, open climate. The following guidelines will assist the nurse in carrying out the interview.

1. Prepare for the interview. Remember that each client is unique; therefore obtain basic information about the client and his environment. Use an assessment tool similar to the one illustrated in Figure 19-3 to aid in data gathering. Do not follow forms too routinely, however. Active listening must still be the fundamental component of the interview.

2. State the purpose or dominant theme of the interview. Use a broad opening statement such as "I'd like to discuss your eating patterns" to promote the development of a purpose.

3. Use open-ended questions because they will allow the client to express concerns, feelings, and specific information. The therapeutic techniques previously discussed will help in data gathering. The techniques should be integrated *into* the interviewer's personality. The use of therapeutic techniques may at first seem uncomfortable or foreign—as with the use of any new tool (recall how strange it was to use a sphygmomanometer or stethescope for the first time). With practice, the techniques will become useful additions to the repertoire of therapeutic actions.

4. Observe the client for signs of anxiety that indicate the interview may be inhibiting expression of feelings or getting close to some threatening or uncomfortable information. Reflect on interviewing behavior and assess the possible overuse of confrontation or requests for explanation.

5. Encourage spontaneity and the expression of feeling. Honest, open expression will many times provide useful information that will later aid in planning nursing care.

6. Listen to what is *not* said, as well as what *is* said. Active listening requires observation and participation in the interview by the nurse.

7. At the conclusion of the interview, summarize what has occurred, validate impressions, and set the time and purpose of future interviews.

It is often easier to determine what should be avoided when carrying out an interview than to follow a precise list of directions that may not be adaptable to all situations. Examples of pitfalls to avoid follow.

1. If possible, avoid creating a negative impression. Long waits in clinic offices, crowded conditions, lack of privacy during the interview, or any other uncomfortable environmental condition may delay or prohibit effective information exchange between nurse and client. If the nurse is frequently interrupted during the interview, the client may perceive her as too busy to talk.

2. Avoid getting off to a poor start. A yes-no question at the start of the interview will inhibit further open expression. Construct the first question carefully, in an open-ended form.

3. Avoid letting personal biases interfere with the interview. People are drawn toward people who are like themselves, and withdraw from those who are different. Nurses need to be wary of associating a client's appearance and mannerisms with those of prior acquaintances and thus having them influence perception of the client.

4. Avoid misinterpreting nonverbal messages. A common example is assuming a client is bored because he yawns, when in fact, the schedule of the interview may interfere with the normal sleeping pattern of the client.

5. Avoid failing to probe the client's interpretation. For example, a client may state, "I eat like a bird." Clarify statements to obtain specific information. Follow such a statement with, "Tell me what you eat during a typical day."

6. Avoid rushing the interview. Allow the client to respond adequately to questions. To

conclude the interview use a statement such as "We have just five minutes left; is there anything else you'd like to discuss before we close?" (Kessler, 1977).

The structure and style of the interview will affect the amount and accuracy of information obtained during a nurse-client interaction.

Data-gathering Methods

The *dietary history* is a tool used to evaluate someone's dietary intake. Determining the food that a client does or does not consume provides a starting point for a total nutritional assessment. Food intake data may be recorded by a variety of methods, most of which involve subjective collection. The nurse wishes to determine what foods are being eaten in what quantities. The level of physical activity and conditions surrounding food consumption and preparation also need to be assessed.

All the methods have limitations and advantages. The choice of method should depend on the intent of the survey and on the client involved. Any method is limited by the skill of the history taker and the degree of cooperation and memory of the client. The use of skilled communication techniques will increase the reliability of the data gathered. A second limitation is that data from short-term studies will probably not accurately reflect total nutrient intake over long periods of time. A third and uncontrollable limitation is the wide individual variability in nutritive needs that results from differences in people's ability to ingest, absorb, and use nutrients. In addition, our knowledge of absolute nutritional requirements is still evolving.

24-hour Recall

The major function of the *24-hour recall* method is to provide a means of obtaining an accurate estimate of the quantity of all foods eaten during the 24 hours preceding the interview. The interviewer asks the client to recall the kinds and amounts of food consumed. The client is often shown models of food and measuring cups to aid in the estimation of quantities. The interviewer may prompt the client to include data on gravies, dressings, sauces, margarines, and beverages. One advantage of the 24-hour recall is that dietary intake can be gathered in 20–30 minutes. The 24-hour recall will, however, yield primarily qualitative rather than quantitative data. Most people are unaware of the true amount of food consumed. Information obtained by this method may not represent the person's usual intake. Repeating the 24-hour recall randomly over a period of time will increase the accuracy of the sample. The accuracy of the recall at any time depends on the ability of the client to remember what has been eaten and his willingness to share the information truthfully. Unlike other studies, the 24-hour recall is not announced in advance. Otherwise the client might change his behavior because of increased awareness of what is eaten. An additional advantage of this method is that the recall does not require the client to be literate. By asking carefully constructed questions, the nurse is able to elicit otherwise unobtainable information. If a more general picture of a client's food consumption is desired, the nurse may question the client about his usual intake. Such a method used in conjunction with the 24-hour recall is more likely to yield meaningful data.

Food Diary

The *food diary* is a written record of food intake for a specified period of time, usually three to seven days. The length of recording depends on the purpose of the record, the nutrients being assessed, and the interest level of the client. A common medical problem that demands this kind of assessment is the determination of foods to which a client may have allergies.

Consideration must be given to the days chosen to observe intake. Food consumption on weekends is usually different from weekday food intake. The combination of week-days and weekends in the record will reflect a more accurate picture of intake.

Instructions given to the client must be clear. For each day the food diary is kept, the client records the names of foods eaten, the way the food was prepared, and, if needed for the purpose of the assessment, the time and place the food was eaten.

An obvious limitation of this method is that the client may change eating patterns for the time of the recording. The food diary will yield qualitative rather than quantitative data.

Weighed Intake Record

When a very accurate record of food consumption is required, the *weighed intake record* provides the best means of obtaining it. The client is taught to weigh all food consumed during a given period of time. A correction must be made for *plate waste* (food served but not eaten). Because this method is very tedious the client must be well motivated for accurate results to be obtained. Frequently the client will try to find shortcuts in preparation to make the weighing less time consuming. There remains the possibility that the client's eating patterns may change during the time of the recording. The weighed intake method is the one used most frequently in controlled laboratory studies.

Food Inventory

Used mainly when studying food consumption by family groups, the *food inventory* reflects total food consumption during a specified period of time. The food inventory may be carried out in two ways, depending on the purpose of the study. The first, called the *food record*, is the most time consuming. It involves making a record of (1) all foods available in the household at the beginning of the assessment, (2) all food brought into the home during the length of the study (usually two to six weeks), and (3) the food remaining at the study's end. An estimate of waste that occurred during the study must be made.

Food eaten in restaurants or in other settings must also be noted. The weight of the food is frequently taken into account. The second method, referred to as a *food account,* consists of a record of all food brought into the household during a specified length of time. No record is made of food available before or after the study. If the family relies on a large storage of food, such as in a freezer, the food account would not accurately assess their intake. Because of this potential for inaccuracy the food account is used primarily in groups whose diet is not too complex. With both methods the nurse must determine the number of people consuming the food.

Food List

The *food list* is a recall method in which the person responsible for food preparation is asked to estimate the quantity of food consumed for a specified period, usually a week. The food list is used by the USDA as a basis for calculating per capita food consumption. When used in an individual clinical setting, the food list yields qualitative data. The client tends to omit some food items and to estimate incorrectly the amount of food consumed.

Food-frequency Record

The *food-frequency form* is used to determine the number of times per day, week, month, or year a client consumes a specific food or category of food. The data is obtained in an interview situation by a trained interviewer. This data then is analyzed by a computer so that the data is translated into an average daily nutritional intake. The data can then be compared with the RDA to check the nutritional adequacy. Because this method of taking a diet history is more time consuming and requires a trained interviewer and a computer analysis, it is used most frequently for research studies.

Analysis of Dietary Data

After the data is collected it must be interpreted before a judgment about the adequacy of nutrient intake can be made. The first step in dietary analysis is to convert the food recorded as being eaten into nutrient quantities or food groups. The simplest analysis of food consumption is a comparison of the data gathered with the recommended amount of the basic food groups. Table 19-3 illustrates one such method of calculating intake. Such a daily food guide can be used quickly and easily. The nurse must remember that individual differences must be taken into account. Food consumption data may also be calculated by hand, using food composition data for specific nutrients. The standard reference for food composition is the USDA Handbook Number 8, which takes into account method of preparation, influences of climate, and degree of maturity. As always when applying the nursing process, the nurse needs to be aware of how population standards compare

TABLE 19-3. A Daily Food Guide

MILK GROUP: two or more servings
Count as a serving 1 cup of milk.
Cheese can be used in place of milk part of the time:
  1 oz of Cheddar-type process cheese = $\frac{2}{3}$ cup milk
  1 oz of American-type pasteurized process cheese
    food or spread = $\frac{1}{2}$ cup milk
Count milk you drink and milk in food you eat:
  $\frac{1}{2}$ cup cottage cheese = $\frac{1}{3}$ cup milk
  $\frac{1}{2}$ cup ice cream = $\frac{1}{3}$ cup milk
Guide for number of servings each day:
  Two to three servings for children under 9 years
  Three or more servings for children 9–12 years
  Four or more servings for teenagers
  Two or more servings for adults
  Three or more servings for pregnant women
  Four or more servings for nursing mothers

VEGETABLE-FRUIT GROUP: four or more servings
Count as a serving $\frac{1}{2}$ cup or 1 portion (serving sizes may be smaller for young children).
A serving may be:
  $\frac{1}{2}$ cup cooked or raw fruit or vegetable
  1 portion, as 1 banana, 1 potato, or $\frac{1}{2}$ grapefruit
Choose citrus fruits, tomatoes, and green peppers as good sources of vitamin C. Also select dark-green, deep-yellow, and other fruits and vegetables as sources of vitamin A. Choose a vitamin C source daily, and a source of vitamin A at least every other day.

TABLE 19-3. (Continued)

MEAT GROUP: two or more servings
Count as a serving 2 oz of cooked lean meat, poultry, or fish (serving sizes may be smaller for young children.)
A serving may be:
  2 large chicken wings
  A hamburger patty
  A piece of fish
In place of $\frac{1}{2}$ serving meat, you may use:
  $\frac{1}{2}$ cup dry beans or peas (cooked)
  2 T peanut butter
  1 egg
  1 oz hard cheese, as natural or process Cheddar
    or Swiss (when used in place of meat, cheese
    may not be used in place of milk)

BREAD-CEREAL GROUP (whole grain or enriched): four or more servings
Count as a serving:

1 slice bread	1 biscuit or muffin
1 cup puffed or flaked cereal	$\frac{1}{4}$ cup granola
$\frac{1}{2}$ cup bran-type cereals	$\frac{1}{2}$–$\frac{3}{4}$ cup cooked cereal
$\frac{1}{2}$–$\frac{3}{4}$ cup cooked macaroni, spaghetti, rice, cornmeal, or grits	

If cereal is not included in the four servings, an additional serving from this group should be selected.

Choose extra servings from the four food groups and, as needed, other foods such as butter or margarine, salad dressings and oils, and jams and jellies to round out meals.

SOURCE: Food and Nutrition Ser., Agricultural Research Ser., *A Daily Food Guide*, rev., FNS-13. USDA, 1975.

with the data obtained from a specific client. Standards for nutrient intake are given in Table 19-4.

In calculating dietary data, the nurse can encounter several problems. One of the most common is inaccuracies in converting household portion size to a weighed amount. A second mistake can occur when the nutrient tables used do not reflect nutrient variations, storage differences, or differences in preparation methods.

Nutrient calculations become difficult when processed foods are used in large quantities. The current nutritional labeling requirements on all processed foods are an excellent resource for the nurse in nutrient calculation.

TABLE 19-4. Guide to Interpretation of Nutrient Intake Data

Kcal Standards

Age	kcal/kg Body Weight
0—1 month	120
2–5 months	110
6–11 months	100
12–23 months	90
24–47 months	86
48–71 months	82
6–7 years	82
8–9 years	82
10–12 years	
Male	68
Female	64
13–16 years	
Male	60
Female	48
17–19 years	
Male	44
Female	35
20–29 years	
Male	40
Female	35
30–39 years	
Male	38
Female	33
40–49 years	
Male	37
Female	31
50–59 years	
Male	36
Female	30
60–69 years	
Male	34
Female	29
over 70 years	
Male	34
Female	29

For second and third trimesters of pregnancy, increase basic standard 200 kcal.
For lactating women, increase basic standard 1,000 kcal.

Protein Standards

Age	gm Protein/kg Body Weight
0–11 months	2.2
12–23 months	1.9
24–47 months	1.7
48–71 months	1.5

Kcal Standards

Age	kcal/kg Body Weight
6–9 years	1.3
10–16 years	1.2
17–19 years	1.1
20 years and over	1.0

For second and third trimesters of pregnancy, increase basic standard 20 gm.
For lactating women, increase basic standard 25 gm.

Calcium Standards

Age	mg/day
0–11 months	550
12–71 months	450
6–9 years	450
10–12 years	650
13–16 years	650
17–19 years	550
Adults	400

For third trimester of pregnancy, increase standard 400 mg.
For lactating women increase standard 500 mg.

Iron Standards

Age	mg/day
0–11 months	10
12–47 months	15
48–71 months	10
6–9 years	10
10–12 years	
Male	10
Female	18
13–19 years	
Male	18
Female	18
20 years and over	
Male	10
Female (to 55)	18
Female (55 on)	10

Vitamin A Standards

Age	IU
0–1 month	1,500
2–5 months	1,500
6–11 months	1,500

TABLE 19.4 *(Continued)*

Kcal Standards

Age	kcal/kg Body Weight
12–23 months	2,000
24–47 months	2,000
48–71 months	2,000
6–7 years	2,500
8–9 years	2,500
10–12 years	2,500
over 12 years	3,500

For lactating women increase standard 1000 IU.

Vitamin B Standards

Age	Thiamine	Riboflavin	Niacin
For all age groups including adult	0.4 mg/ 1000 kcal	0.55 mg/ 1000 kcal	6.6 mg/ 1000 kcal

Vitamin C Standards (Ascorbic Acid)

All age groups	45–60 mg/day

SOURCE: US Dept. of Health, Education, and Welfare Publ. No. (HSM) 72-8133, n.d.

Any food to which a nutrient is added or any food for which a nutrition claim is made must carry a nutrition statement. In addition to usual information, such as name, net weight, and ingredients, the label will provide amounts of Calories, protein, carbohydrate, fat, vitamin A, vitamin C, thiamine, riboflavin, niacin, calcium, and iron (Food and Drug Admin., 1974). Figure 19-4 is an example of the minimum requirements for labels. Figure 19-5 is an example of such a label with added information on cholesterol, fats, and sodium. All nutrition information is per serving.

The nutritional standards used in the United States are the RDA prepared by the Food and Nutrition Board of the National Research Council. The purpose and use of these allowances has been discussed in Chapters 2 and 6. It is important to consider differences in individual norms when using population standards as a basis for nursing diagnosis. Failure to meet RDA standards does not necessarily mean that malnutrition exists, for with the exception of Calories, the RDAs are calculated above average physiological requirements for each nutrient (Christakis, 1973). On the other hand, an apparently adequate diet may be consumed by a client with deficiency symptoms. These deficiency symptoms may be the result of inadequate absorption or use of the nutrients. When determining if nutrient quantities are important, the nurse needs to consider (1) human individuality, (2) the number of repetitive food intake assessments carried out, and (3) the reliability of the food intake data.

Assessing Environmental Determinants of Food Intake

Many variables influence the way a client perceives his nutritional needs and preferences. Food habits have been described as "the characteristic and repetitive acts that [the client] performs under the impetus of the need to provide himself with nourishment

NUTRITION INFORMATION
(per Serving)
Serving Size = 1 oz
Servings per Container = 12

Calories	110
Protein	2 gm
Carbohydrate	24 gm
Fat	0 gm

PERCENTAGE OF US RECOMMENDED DAILY ALLOWANCES (US = RDA)[a]

Protein	2
Thiamine	8
Niacin	2

[a] Contains less than 2% of US-RDA for vitamin A, vitamin C, riboflavin, calcium, and iron.

Figure 19-4. Nutrition information contained on most food labels.

NUTRITION INFORMATION
(per serving)
Serving size = 8 oz
Servings per Container = 1

Calories	560	Fat (percent-	
Protein	23 gm	age of Cal-	
Carbohydrate	43 gm	ories 53%)	33 gm
		Polyun-	
		saturated	2 gm
		Saturated	9 gm
		Cholesterol[a]	
		(20 mg/100	
		gm)	40 mg
		Sodium	
		(365 mg/100	
		gm)	830 mg

PERCENTAGE OF US RECOMMENDED DAILY ALLOWANCES (US RDA)

Protein	35	Riboflavin	15
Vitamin A	35	Niacin	25
Vitamin C		Calcium	2
(ascorbic acid)	10	Iron	25
Thiamine			
(vitamin B₁)	15		

[a] Information on fat and cholesterol content is provided for individuals who, on the advice of a physician, are modifying their total dietary intake of fat and cholesterol.

Figure 19-5. Labeling information including optional listings for cholesterol, fats, and sodium.

and simultaneously to meet an assortment of social and emotional goals" (MacBryde, 1970). Food habits are difficult to assess, although certain determinants of food behavior that can be investigated are listed below (Mason et al., 1977). The generalizations usually made from such factors must be validated for each individual client. It should not be assumed that a specific environmental characteristic will have a predicted effect on a client's eating behavior.

FAMILY STATUS

• The family structure will influence the eating patterns of the family members. The number and ages of dependents influence the cost of maintaining the family. The composition of the family will also determine who is responsible for food preparation and the time available to prepare a nutritionally balanced diet. These principles were discussed in Chapter 1.

OCCUPATION

• The level of income will affect the kind, type, and amount of food available, as well as such resources as transportation and freezers (see Chap. 8). Occupations can provide a clue to stress-related diseases such as cardiovascular diseases or serve as determinants of self-esteem.

EDUCATION

• Educational level will provide clues to the use of resources by a client and, to some degree, to the level of nutritional education to which the client may have been exposed. It will also give a clue to what teaching strategies may be successful with the client.

ETHNICITY

• Cultural background will have an influence on the type, kind, and preparation of food. Chapter 1 described many of the cultural determinants of eating.

RELIGION

• Awareness of the client's religion may provide the nurse with clues regarding dietary laws and regulations that may influence his eating patterns. If a trusting relationship is established, the client should be able to express his degree of compliance with any dietary restrictions his religious beliefs may impose.

LEISURE ACTIVITIES

• The kind and amount of leisure activities a client participates in will give a clue to caloric consumption, time allocation, and to a degree, coping behaviors. For example, the young executive who regularly jogs long distances will require more Calories than his sedentary peer. Likewise the young college student who spends her leisure time reading will require fewer Calories than average.

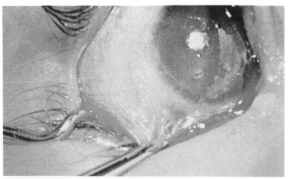

Plate 1.
Xerosis. Cause: lack of vitamin A.

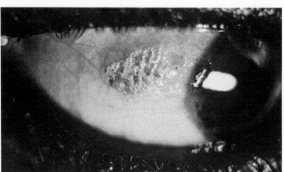

Plate 2.
Bitot's spots. Cause: lack of vitamin A.

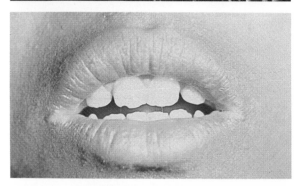

Plate 3.
Cheilosis and angular fissures.
Cheilosis. Cause: lack of niacin and/
or riboflavin. Angular fissures.
Cause: lack of niacin, riboflavin, iron,
or vitamin B$_6$.

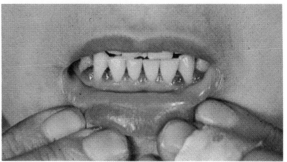

Plate 4.
Scorbutic gums. Cause: lack of
vitamin C.

Plates courtesy of *Nutrition Today*.

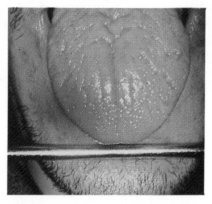

Plate 5.
Glossitis. Cause: lack of folic acid, niacin, riboflavin, vitamin B_{12}, vitamin B_6, tryptophan, or iron.

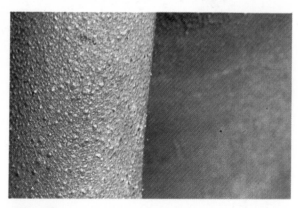

Plate 6.
Follicular hyperkeratosis. Cause: lack of vitamin A or insufficient unsaturated fatty acids.

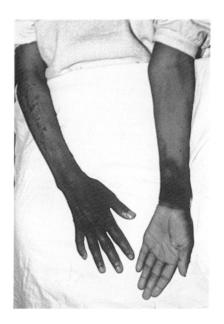

Plate 7.
Hyperpigmentation. Cause: chronic niacin lack, lack of vitamin B_{12} or folic acid.

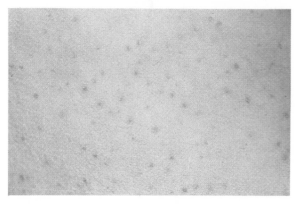

Plate 8.
Perifollicular petechiae. Cause: lack of vitamin C or vitamin K.

Plates courtesy of *Nutrition Today.*

MOTIVATIONAL DATA

• Examining what motivates the client will give a clue to what values, attitudes, and beliefs stimulate his eating patterns. Such data are not easily assessed by direct means but may be determined through careful observation of the client's lifestyle and behaviors. If, for example, the client is motivated to succeed by peer pressure, he may learn more in a group situation than from individual teaching.

CLINICAL ASSESSMENT OF NUTRITIONAL STATUS

Clinical evaluation as a fundamental component of nutritional assessment will provide the nurse with clues to overt nutritional deficiencies or potential difficulties with ingestion, absorption, digestion, or excretion of nutrients. Clinical assessment consists of two phases: *use of anthropometric findings* and *direct objective assessment.*

It must be emphasized that signs of malnutrition are often nonspecific. Frequently, there may be more than one cause of a specific clinical finding. Dry skin, for example, may be caused by sun exposure or by vitamin A deficiency. Because of this fact, clinical findings may not correlate well with biochemical or dietary findings. Frequently, clinical findings will reflect a combination of nutritional deficiencies.

The nurse must remember that the clinical examination reflects the results of long-term nutritional status. The variations among clinicians' assessment techniques must be considered when comparing physical findings made by several clinicians over a period of time. Because of the possible misinterpretation of clinical data by different clinicians, it is of utmost importance that all data observed be recorded as accurately as possible. The signs should be described in precise terms, using actual sizes of lesions, not vague terminology such as "large" or "small." The terms "poor," "fair,"

and "good" should be avoided, as should the often charted "ate well."

Direct Objective Assessment

Direct physical examination of clients was the earliest means of evaluating nutritional status. Only a few signs of nutritional deficiency result from the lack of a specific nutrient. Further, it must be remembered that the signs of progressed malnutrition are multiple and rarely localized. Any physical finding suggestive of a nutritional abnormality should be considered a clue to be pursued further. Such signs could also give clues to metabolism-related diseases such as diabetes mellitus and hyperthyroidism. In general, if a client manifests one or more of the following signs, he may be said to be suffering from malnutrition: edema, dyspigmentation of the hair, easy pluckability of the hair, muscle atrophy, moon face, flaky-paint rash, and dermatosis (Christakis, 1973).

The parts of the body that most commonly exhibit abnormalities consistent with malnutrition include the skin, eyes, mouth, skeleton, and nervous system. The specific clinical signs and possible causes of nutritional deficiency are amplified in Table 19-5. Table 19-6 lists specific signs of macromineral deficiency and excess as well as the serum levels that may be expected when symptoms occur.

General clinical symptoms of malnutrition may begin in a client with a subjective feeling of vague ill health. Later, lack of energy and general malaise may be present. The most common nutritional defect is thinness with failure to gain weight or caloric balance with weight loss. The next most frequent disturbance is dehydration, usually secondary to diarrhea, vomiting, or polyuria. The most common of all chronic deficiencies is that of iron, producing iron-deficiency anemia (MacBryde, 1970).

In children, failure to grow is the most common manifestation of malnutrition. The possible underlying causes are numerous,

TABLE 19-5. Clinical Signs of Nutritional Disorders

Affected Body Area	General Population Standard	Signs of Nutritional Disorders	Possible Nutrition-related Causes
Hair	Shiny, firm, not easily plucked.	Lack of natural shine; dryness, dullness. Ease of plucking. Thinness, sparseness. Changed color (flag sign).	Protein-Calorie deficiency.
Face	Skin smooth, with color uniform, according to cultural heritage. No edema.	Loss of skin color; dark skin over cheeks and under eyes; scaling of skin around nostrils; edematous face (moon face).	Iron deficiency; inadequate caloric intake; lack of B-complex vitamins; protein deficiency.
Eyes	Bright, clear, shiny, with pink, moist membranes. No lesions or tissue mounds.	Pale conjunctiva.	Iron deficiency.
		Dull cornea; soft cornea; Bitot's spots (Color Plate 2).	Vitamin A deficiency.
		Redness and fissuring of eyelid corners.	Riboflavin, niacin, pyridoxine deficiency.
Lips	Smooth; no edema; no lesions.	Redness and edema of mouth and lips, angular fissures (Color Plate 3).	Niacin, riboflavin deficiency.
Tongue	Deep pink; no edema. Papillae visible.	Edema; redness, rawness; fissures (Color Plate 5).	Folic acid, niacin, vitamin B_{12}, pyridoxine deficiency.
		Magenta color.	Riboflavin deficiency.
		Pale color.	Iron deficiency.
		Atrophy of papillae.	Niacin, folic acid, vitamin B_{12}, iron deficiency.
Teeth	White; free of pain and caries.	Mottled enamel, occasionally with brown spots.	Excess fluoride during development.
		Caries.	Poor dental hygiene; excess sugar.
Gums	Deep pink, do not bleed easily, no edema.	Sponginess; proneness to bleed easily; receding (Color Plate 4).	Ascorbic acid deficiency.

494

Glands	No edema or tenderness.	Thyroid edema.	Iodine deficiency.
		Parotid enlargement.	General malnutrition; protein deficiency.
Skin	No lesions, dark or light spots. No rashes.	Dryness, sandpaper feel of skin (follicular hyperkeratosis) (Color Plate 6).	Vitamin A deficiency; deficiency in unsaturated and essential fatty acids.
		Red, swollen pigmentation of exposed areas (pellagrous dermatosis).	Niacin or tryptophan deficiency.
		Petechiae (Color Plate 8). Hyperpigmentation (Color Plate 7).	Ascorbic acid deficiency. Vitamin B_{12}, folic acid, niacin deficiency.
		Lack of subcutaneous tissue.	Prolonged-Calorie deficiency.
Nails	Firm, with pink nail beds; not brittle.	Spoon-shaped nails that are brittle and ridged.	Iron deficiency.
Musculoskeletal system	Pain-free during the usual activities of daily living.	Muscle atrophy, dependent edema.	Protein-Calorie deficiency.
		Thin, soft frontal and parietal bones; soft, thin infant skull bones; epiphiseal swelling; knock-knees; bowlegs.	Vitamin D deficiency.
		Small bumps on both sides of chest wall (beading on ribs).	Vitamin D and calcium deficiency.
Neurological system	Intact muscle innervation and tactile senses.	Burning-foot syndrome.	Pantothenic acid deficiency.
		Tetany; neuromuscular irritability.	Magnesium deficiency.
		Mental confusion, irritability.	Thiamine, niacin deficiency.
		Sensory loss; loss of vibratory sensation, particularly in feet and ankles; calf tenderness.	Thiamine deficiency.

TABLE 19-6. Signs of Deficiency and Excess of the Macrominerals

Mineral	Signs of Deficiency	Deficiency Level	Signs of Excess	Excess Level
Calcium	Probably rickets, tetany, seizures, abnormal clotting times, leg cramps, tingling at ends of fingers.	<4.5 meq/liter	Hypotonicity of muscles, renal calculi, deep bone pain.	>5.8 meq/liter
Phosphorus	Muscle weakness.	<3 mg/100 ml	Tetany (usually from low calcium to phosphorus ratio).	>6 mg/100 ml
Sodium	Apprehension; abdominal cramps; cyanosis; cold, clammy skin; rapid, thready pulse; hypotension; oliguria.	<137 meq/liter	Dry, sticky mucous membranes; flushed skin; thirst; high temperature; rough, dry tongue.	>147 meq/liter
Potassium	Flaccid paralysis, malaise, weak pulse, faint heart sounds, anorexia, vomiting, paralytic ileus, heart block.	<3.5 meq/liter	Mild excess: irritability, nausea, diarrhea. Severe excess: weakness, flaccid paralysis, difficulty in phonation and respiration, cardiac arrhythmia and standstill. EKG: elevated T wave, depressed ST segment.	>5.6 meq/liter
Magnesium	Twitching, tremors, irregular pulse, tachycardia insomnia, muscle weakness, leg cramps, hand tremors, high startle response.	<1.4 meq/liter	Lethargy, coma, impaired respiration.	>2.3 meq/liter

ranging from physical and psychological neglect to any of a number of malabsorption syndromes or nutritional deficiencies.

Fatigue and weakness are often the only signs in mild cases of malnutrition. A diet inadequate in Calories may bring about an impairment of physical efficiency within a matter of days. In prolonged semistarvation, muscle strength is diminished greatly, and muscle endurance is strikingly decreased. Starvation can produce a neurotic state characterized by irritability, depression, and a decrease in self-initiated activity. Paradoxically, anorexia usually accompanies malnutrition. This may be caused by ketosis, which develops secondarily to using lipid stores as caloric sources.

Skin Lesions
Skin lesions are usually the result of mixed nutritional deficiencies. Vitamin deficiencies manifest themselves in varying degrees of dermatitis. Healthy skin results from adequate nutrition, protection from trauma, and cleanliness. People who are poorly nourished tend to have skin that is not resistant to blunt trauma. Because of this lack of resistance, the skin tends to have a variety of abnormalities that do not fit into any one category. It should not be forgotten that single nutrient deficiencies rarely occur in clinical situations. Skin lesions on areas of skin exposed to the sun are caused by niacin deficiency. Fragility in the capillary wall as evidenced by petechiae is frequently a sign of ascorbic acid deficiency, particularly in infants.

Ocular Lesions
Vitamin A deficiency is one of the major causes of blindness in the world (Sandstead and Pearson, 1973). When vitamin A deficiency is severe, the epithelium of the conjunctiva becomes dull with a wrinkled appearance. *Bitot's spots* may also appear in the cornea at this time. They appear as foamy spots in the cornea; the next stage is opacity of the cornea.

Oral Lesions
The lips, tongue, and membranes of the mouth mirror the adverse effects of nutrient deficiencies on the entire gastrointestinal tract. Cracks at the corners of the mouth, referred to as *angular stomatitis*, and vertical cracks followed by redness, swelling, and ulceration in other areas of the lips are characteristic of a riboflavin deficiency.

The nurse should observe the teeth during the nutritional assessment. The dental examination may generally reflect flouride intake and the general effect of diet on the formation of dental caries. The nurse should look for (1) obvious dental caries, (2) periodontal disease, and (3) calculus deposit.

Glandular Lesions
One of the first known nutritionally associated clinical signs was the enlargement of the thyroid gland associated with a lack of iodine intake. The World Health Organization has recommended a system for thyroid gland assessment (Table 19-7). Even such grading is subject of course to various clinicians' interpretations.

Neurological, Skeletal, and Extremity Signs
Signs associated with the neurological and skeletal systems and the extremities reflect a variety of deficiencies including vitamin B_{12} and thiamine. In the United States, neurolog-

TABLE 19-7. The World Health Organization Recommendations for Assessment of Iodine-deficient Goiter

Grade	Physical Findings
Normal	One lobe of the thyroid is the size of the first phalanx of the client's thumb.
1	One lobe is greater than the size of the first phalanx of the client's thumb.
2	Gland is visible with neck extended.
3	Gland is visible with neck in normal position.
4	Gland is visible across the room.

ical abnormalities associated with nutritional deficiencies are most frequently found in alcoholics, in clients with alterations in the gastrointestinal tract secondary to surgery or malabsorption, and in those people with chronic pernicious anemia. Edema of the legs in the absence of underlying cardiovascular or renal disease is usually indicative of severe protein deprivation. One difficulty in determining the etiology of extremity edema is that many clients subject to protein deficiency have many underlying pathophysiological disorders.

Anthropometric Measurements

Assessment of growth in relation to age and sex provides important clues to a person's nutritional status. Retardation of growth is one of the nonspecific hallmarks of nutritional deficiencies. On the whole, anthropometric evaluations are useful for indirectly determining fat deposition, protein catabolism, and height-weight correlations. They may be particularly useful when used longitudinally to evaluate clients' nutritional status. Anthropometric measurements are designed to provide the most meaningful data possible, using the least amount of staff, equipment, and complicated techniques. The most frequently used anthropometric measurements are height, weight, and skin-fold thickness.

Weight and Height

Weight should be recorded using a beam balance. If successive weights are going to be kept for longitudinal evaluation, the weight should be taken at the same time of the day and under the same conditions. Most accurate are before breakfast weights taken with the client wearing similar amounts of clothing, such as a hospital gown. Height should be measured without shoes, with the head in a level position.

In the client with concurrent disease, weight may be an unreliable index of protein depletion or Calorie deficiency. Any disease

process that has fluid retention as a side effect will cause weight gain.

Weight loss is an important index of change in nutritional status, for it usually reflects caloric inadequacy in the diet (Schneider et al., 1977). The following formulas provide data on the significance of a client's weight loss (Blackburn et al., 1977). The client's percentage of ideal body weight is calculated as follows:

$$\text{Percentage of ideal body weight} = \frac{\text{Actual weight}}{\text{Ideal body weight}} \times 100$$

(Refer to Appendices E and F for desirable body weights of men and women.) The percentage of body weight change may be similarly calculated:

$$\text{Percentage of weight change} = \frac{\text{Usual weight} - \text{actual weight}}{\text{Usual weight}} \times 100$$

Many tables giving "ideal" body weights use three classifications of body build—small, medium, and large—on which to base weights. These charts generally reflect more accurate ideal body weights than similar data based on ages, but they entail the difficulty caused by lack of standardization of the determinants of each body build.

Growth charts are used extensively for evaluating the growth of children. Such charts, as illustrated in Figures 19-6 through 19-9, plot a child's growth in relation to the average by placing the child in a certain percentile. The value of such a record is that, first, it provides the nurse with an accurate comparison of a child's growth with that of the entire population; and second, the child's progress over time can be easily monitored. Trends toward either upper or lower percentiles can be early indicators of childhood obesity or failure to thrive.

Table 19-8 illustrates an accurate alternative method of assessing acceptable childhood growth. The method, espoused by Garn (1965), recognizes the role of heredity factors

TABLE 19-8. Parental Midpoint Scale for Evaluating Growth of Children[a]

| | Midparent Stature[b] | | | | | |
| | 64.0 in | | 66.5 in | | 69.0 in | |
Age	Boys	Girls	Boys	Girls	Boys	Girls
1	29.0	29.0	29.5	29.0	30.5	29.5
2	33.6	33.0	34.5	33.5	35.0	34.5
3	36.5	35.5	37.5	37.0	39.0	38.0
4	39.0	38.0	40.5	41.0	42.0	41.0
5	41.5	40.5	43.5	43.0	44.5	43.5
6	43.5	43.5	45.5	45.5	47.0	46.0
7	45.7	46.0	48.0	47.5	49.0	49.0
8	48.0	48.0	50.0	49.5	51.5	51.0
9	50.0	50.5	52.0	52.0	53.5	54.0
10	52.0	53.0	54.0	54.0	55.5	56.5
11	54.5	55.5	56.0	56.5	58.0	59.0
12	57.0	58.0	58.5	59.0	60.0	61.5
13	59.5	60.5	61.0	62.0	63.0	63.5
14	62.5	62.5	63.5	63.0	66.0	65.5
15	65.5	63.0	66.0	64.0	69.0	66.5
16	66.5	63.0	68.0	64.0	69.5	67.0
17	67.5	63.5	69.0	64.5	70.0	67.5

SOURCE: S. M. Garn, "The Applicability of North American Growth Standards in Developing Countries." Originally published in *Canadian Medical Association Journal* 93:914, October 23, 1965.)

[a] Age-size tables for Ohio white children whose midparent stature (or parental midpoint) is the average of the stature of the two parents. All values rounded off to the nearest half inch.

[b] Average of maternal and paternal statures.

in childhood development. Standards have been developed for height based on the average height of both parents.

Skin-fold Measurements

Fatness is an indirect indicator of previous caloric intake. An accurate assessment of body fatness is made by determining body density. This is done by measuring body specific gravity. This may be more easily assessed by measuring triceps skin-fold thickness. The special calipers used to measure skin-fold thickness exert a specific pressure on a specific area of skin fold (see Fig. 19-10). The thickness of a skinfold in various parts of the body is measured as an indication of the amount of subcutaneous fat. The deltoid and triceps sites are usually used, although chance of error in measurement increases with obesity. The lower thoracic site is the best location for measurement of all people; but this site is not always easily acceptable. The standards for triceps skin fold are given in Tables 19-9 through 19-12.

Midarm circumference, a measurement of the arm half way between shoulder and elbows, reflects body fat and muscle mass. *Midarm muscle circumference*, a more direct calculation of protein stores, can be calculated using the midarm circumference and the triceps skin-fold measurement:

Midarm muscle circumference
= Midarm circumference
+ [3.14 × Triceps skin fold] (in cm)

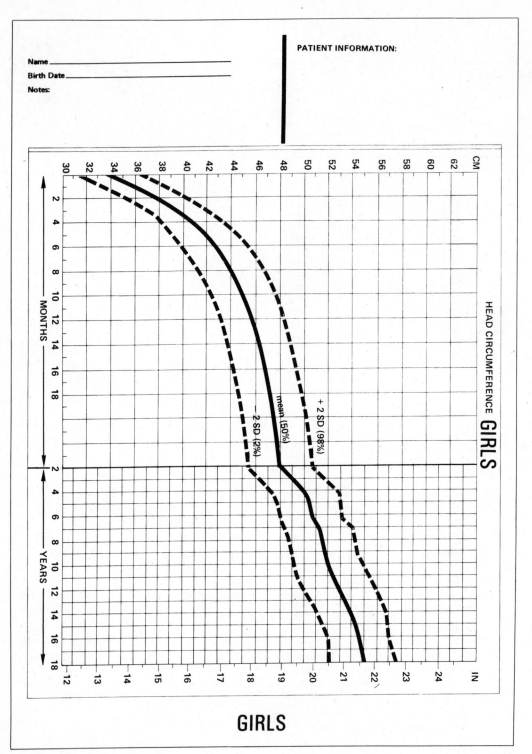

Figure 19-6. Growth chart for evaluating girls' head growth. (Courtesy Mead Johnson Laboratories)

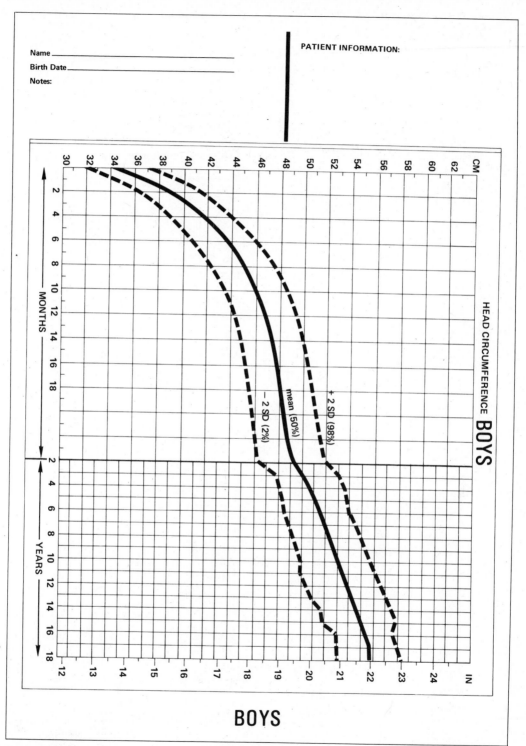

Figure 19-7. Growth chart for evaluating boys' head growth. (Courtesy Mead Johnson Laboratories)

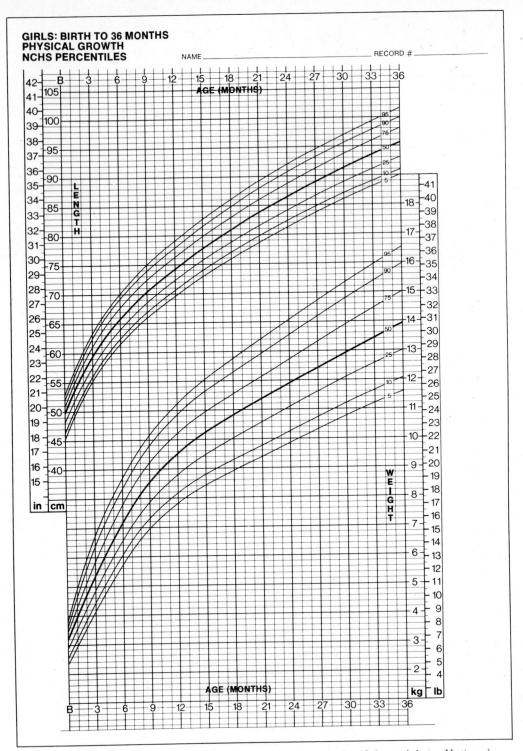

Figure 19-8. Growth chart for evaluating girls' body growth. (Adapted from National Center for Health Statistics, "NCHS Growth Charts, 1976." *Monthly Vital Statistics Report.* Vol. 25, No. 3, Suppl. (HRA) 76-1120. Health Resources Administration, Rockville, Md., June 1976. Data from The Fels Research Institute, Columbus, Ohio. © 1976 Ross Laboratories.)

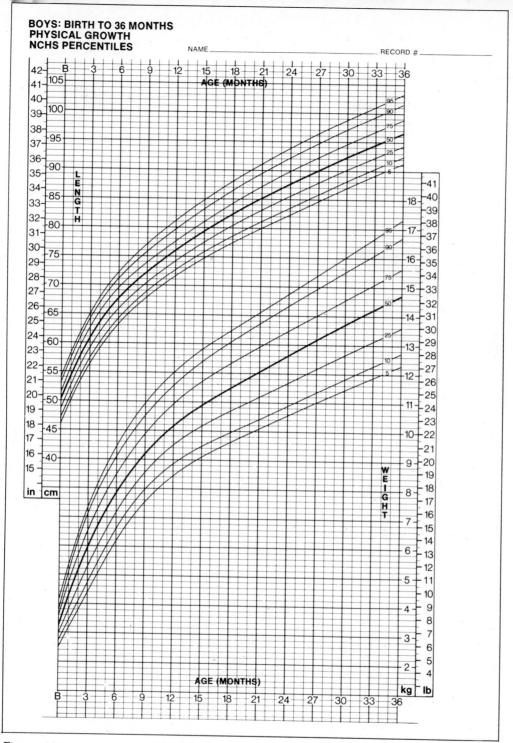

Figure 19-9. Growth chart for evaluating boys' body growth. (Adapted from National Center for Health statistics, "NCHS Growth Charts, 1976." *Monthly Vital Statistics Report* Vol. 25, No. 3, Suppl. (HRA) 76-1120. Health Resources Administration, Rockville, Md., June 1976. Data from The Fels Research Institute, Columbus, Ohio. © 1976 Ross Laboratories.)

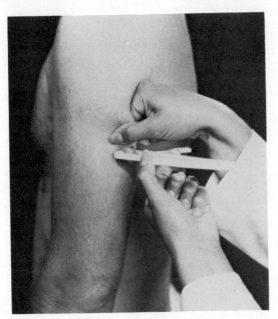

Figure 19-10. The triceps skin-fold measurement helps to assess body fat stores.

This measurement is of particular importance in evaluating the relative contribution of muscle and visceral protein to catabolism (Schneider et al., 1977) and is most useful when taken regularly over a long period of time.

LABORATORY ASSESSMENT

Laboratory evaluation is the third component of a total nutritional assessment. It is a precise approach to determining levels of nutrients in blood or urine or to evaluating certain biochemical functions that depend on an adequate supply of specific nutrients. Precision depends on accuracy of the sample obtained. In general, urinary excretion levels fluctuate more than serum levels and reflect recent rather than usual intake. Values from a single determination may be misleading.

The purpose of biochemical assessment is to detect subclinical deficiencies before the onset of overt clinical signs. In many instances the body's homeostatic mechanisms mask changes that would otherwise reflect nutritional status. Biochemical evaluation enhances clinical and dietary assessment by confirming suspected deficiencies or pointing out possible causes.

Classifications of blood constituents may be evaluated. The first of these is *nutritional substances*. Nutrients absorbed from the gastrointestinal tract or products for cellular use are in this category, for example, glucose, amino acids, minerals, vitamins, lipids, pyruvic acid, lactic acid, creatinine, and circulating hormones. The second classification is *excretory*

TABLE 19-9. Standards of Triceps Skin Fold, Birth to 60 Months, Sexes Separate

Age (Months)	Triceps Skin Fold (mm)									
	Standard		90% of Standard		80% of Standard		70% of Standard		60% of Standard	
	M	F	M	F	M	F	M	F	M	F
Birth	6.0	6.5	5.4	5.9	4.8	5.2	4.2	4.6	3.6	3.9
6	10.0	10.0	9.0	9.0	8.0	8.0	7.0	7.0	6.0	6.0
12	10.3	10.2	9.3	9.2	8.2	8.2	7.2	7.1	6.2	6.1
18	10.3	10.2	9.3	9.2	8.2	8.2	7.2	7.1	6.0	6.1
24	10.0	10.1	9.0	9.1	8.0	8.1	7.0	7.1	5.6	5.8
36	9.3	9.7	8.4	8.7	7.5	7.8	6.5	6.8	5.6	6.1
48	9.3	10.2	8.4	9.2	7.5	8.2	6.5	7.2	5.5	5.7
60	9.1	9.4	8.2	8.5	7.3	7.5	6.4	6.6		

SOURCE: Adapted from Hammond, 1955.

TABLE 19-10. Standards of Triceps Skin Fold, 5–15 Years, Sexes Separate

	Triceps Skin Fold (mm)									
	Standard		90% of Standard		80% of Standard		70% of Standard		60% of Standard	
Age (Years)	M	F	M	F	M	F	M	F	M	F
5	9.1	9.4	8.2	8.5	7.3	7.5	6.4	6.6	5.5	5.7
6	8.2	9.6	7.4	8.6	6.6	7.7	5.8	6.7	4.9	5.8
7	7.9	9.4	7.1	8.5	6.3	7.5	5.5	6.6	4.7	5.7
8	7.6	10.1	6.8	9.1	6.1	8.1	5.3	7.1	4.5	6.1
9	8.2	10.3	7.4	9.2	6.6	8.2	5.8	7.2	4.9	6.2
10	8.2	10.4	7.4	9.3	6.6	8.3	5.7	7.3	4.9	6.2
11	8.9	10.6	8.1	9.6	7.2	8.5	6.3	7.5	5.4	6.4
12	8.5	10.1	7.6	9.1	6.8	8.1	5.9	7.0	5.1	6.0
13	8.1	10.4	7.3	9.4	6.5	8.3	5.7	7.3	4.9	6.2
14	7.9	11.3	7.1	10.1	6.3	9.0	5.5	7.9	4.8	6.8
15	6.3	11.4	5.7	10.2	5.0	9.1	4.4	8.0	3.8	6.8

Adapted from Hammond, 1955.

substances, which are substances enroute to elimination by the kidneys, lungs, or liver. Examples include carbon dioxide, creatinine, urea, bilirubin, amylase, and phosphatase. The final classification is those intrinsic *functional substances* that are fundamental blood components: hemoglobin, glutathione, plasma proteins, fibrinogen, and electrolytes. These functional substances usually exist in a narrow range of normal concentration.

Table 19-13 summarizes specific vitamin substances to be assessed biochemically, levels of deficiency, possible results from the deficiency, and precautions to be taken when interpreting the data. The nurse should note that the fat-soluble vitamins A, D, E, and K are best absorbed in the presence of fat in the diet. Thus, diseases that interfere with fat absorption may precipitate certain fat-soluble vitamin deficiencies.

The minerals most frequently assessed biochemically are iron, calcium, and iodine. A deficiency of iron usually results in anemia. The most accurate reflection of iron intake is the measurement of hemoglobin and hematocrit levels; Table 19-14 provides standards. Serum levels of calcium are essentially constant over a wide range of intakes. Fluctuations that do occur are most frequently caused by pathophysiological processes in the body or by the increased demand for calcium during pregnancy. Iodine intake is most frequently evaluated by clinical assessment of the presence or absence of goiter.

Because of the epidemic of coronary artery disease in the United States, measurements of

TABLE 19-11. Standards of Triceps Skin Fold, Adults, Sexes Separate

	Triceps skin-fold (mm)				
Sex	Standard	90% of Standard	80% of Standard	70% of Standard	60% of Standard
Male	12.5	11.3	10.0	8.8	7.5
Female	16.5	14.9	13.2	11.6	9.9

TABLE 19-12. Obesity Standards for Caucasian Americans (Minimum Triceps Skin-fold Thickness in Millimeters Indicating Obesity)

Age (Years)	Skinfold Measurement	
	Male	Female
5	12	14
6	12	15
7	13	16
8	14	17
9	15	18
10	16	20
11	17	21
12	18	22
13	18	23
14	17	23
15	16	24
16	15	25
17	14	26
18	15	27
19	15	27
20	16	28
21	17	28
22	18	28
23	18	28
24	19	28
25	20	29
26	20	29
27	21	29
28	22	29
29	23	29
30–50	23	30

SOURCE: Adapted from C. C. Seltzer and J. Mayer, "A simple criterion of obesity." *Postgraduate Medicine* 38:A101–107, 1965. NOTE: Figures represent the logarithmic means of the frequency distributions plus 1 SD.

serum lipid levels have become common. Elevated serum cholesterol levels are viewed by many as a risk factor in the development of coronary artery disease. Elevated serum cholesterol level is discussed further in Chapter 26.

Biochemical evaluation of protein status is difficult. It is generally assumed that protein deficiencies are uncommon in the United States. Yet because of the possible catabolic state that may exist in hospitalized patients, a measure of protein status is advisable. Measurement of creatinine will give an indirect indication of protein supply. The amount of creatinine in the urine is a direct reflection of a person's muscle mass and has been assumed to be constant (Hills, 1971). The excretion of creatinine may be higher with an increased intake of lean meat. The results of the evaluation are expressed as milligrams of creatinine excretion in 24 hours/cm of body height. Table 19-15 provides the ideal values for the *creatinine-height index* for both men and women. The percentage of ideal lean body mass may be calculated using the formula:

$$\text{Creatinine-height index} = \frac{\text{Actual urinary creatinine}}{\text{Ideal urinary creatinine}} \times 100$$

An additional laboratory test that provides evidence of a client's nutritional status involves the performance of *skin tests* that reflect a client's *immune status*. Protein-Calorie malnutrition has a profound impact on immune function. In fact, the most common form of acquired immunodeficiency is malnutrition (Bistrian, 1977). An easy method to test immune function is to use skin tests of various organisms to which most of the US population have become immune. These include mumps virus, Candida, and streptokinase-streptodornase (SKSD). The skin tests are administrered intradermally (see Figure 19-11) and read 48 hours later. Positive results in two of the three tests indicate that a client's immune system is not dangerously suppressed (Madura, 1979). A negative reaction will provide data that, used in combination with other laboratory and anthropometric data, will lead to a conclusion of malnutrition.

In total, laboratory abnormalities become evident sometime before physical signs are seen. Laboratory data reflects more immediate intake than physical findings and, therefore, correlates better with dietary evaluation than with clinical examination.

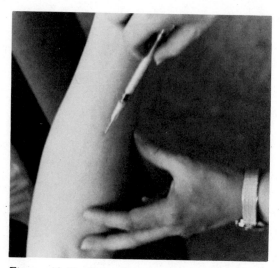

Figure 19-11. Skin testing is one method of biochemical evaluation.

RACIAL DIFFERENCES AND NUTRITIONAL ASSESSMENT

It is important to consider racial differences when conducting the physical exam, collecting anthropometric data, or using biochemical analysis of serum and urine samples. The Afro-American population differs from Anglo Saxon norms largely in anthropometric data. It is known that black infants are smaller than white infants at birth. Part of this difference is due to socioeconomic factors, but the dimensional differences remain even after family incomes are matched. By adolescence, however, black children stand taller than white children of the same age. This rapid increase in size over white children of the same age slows after puberty, resulting in no significant height differences between black and white adults. Black children obtain a greater portion of their adult stature earlier. Because of these differences, black children cannot accurately be evaluated against norms that have been developed from white population standards. To do so would be to place some proportion of black children who are

actually at nutritional risk within normal range.

People of largely African ancestry also have a greater skeletal mass, a larger mineral mass, and a higher whole-bone density than their white counterparts. Because one of the clinical manifestations of protein-Calorie malnutrition is the loss of mineral mass, black people are less likely to be diagnosed during the early phases of the depletion than are white people.

This difference in norms between the white and black population extends also to biochemical data. Black hemoglobin ranges average 1.0 gm/100 ml lower than whites; hematocrit levels average 3% percent lower. These differences exist from birth throughout life and have been shown to be unrelated to socioeconomic status.

RELEVANCE OF NUTRITIONAL ASSESSMENT OF HOSPITALIZED CLIENTS

The relevance of a strong emphasis on nutritional assessment may not be easily recognized for the nurse working in an institutional system where physicians, nutritionists, and other health professionals abound. Butterworth and Blackburn (1975) give three reasons for a thorough, fundamental assessment. The first is that many hospitalized patients are malnourished and may suffer a combination of nutritional deficiencies. Second, people who are nutritionally healthy will have a greater resistance to infection and will have an increased capacity for wound healing. Third, many new techniques and products have been developed that can meet a variety of nutritional needs. Further, Butterworth (1974) states that the largest population of unrecognized malnutrition cases in the United States and Canada occurs not in slums or ghettos but in hospitals.

Protein-Calorie malnutrition, is a state that develops in the hospital in one-fourth to

TABLE 19-13. Biochemical Evaluation of Vitamin Deficiency

Substance	Age	Deficient Level	Acceptable Level	Possible Results of Deficiency	Precautions in Interpretation
Ascorbic acid (vitamin C) (mg/100 ml)	All	over 0.1	0.2+	Scurvy.	Depends on intake immediately preceding the test.
Thiamine (in urine) (μg/g creatinine)	1–3	over 120	175+	Morbidity in alcoholics; beriberi.	Spot samples may not be an accurate indication of nutritional statistics.
	4–5	over 85	120+		
	6–9	over 70	180+		
	10–15	over 55	150+		
	16+	over 27	65+		
	Pregnant	over 21	50+		
Riboflavin (in urine) (μg/g creatinine)	1–3	over 150	500+	Scaly skin, weight loss, weakness, skin lesions.	Variability of riboflavin excretion is high.
	4–5	over 100	300+		
	6–9	over 85	270+		
	10–16	over 70	200+		
	16+	over 27	80+		
	Pregnant	over 30	90+		
N-1-methyl-nicotinamide (in creatinine); reflects niacin intake	All	over 0.2	0.6+	Pellagra, dermatitis, diarrhea.	Urinary excretion may not be constant.
	Pregnant	over 0.8	2.5+		
Folacin (in serum) (mg/ml)	All	over 2.0	6.0+	Anemia; occurs first in pregnant women or those on oral contraceptives.	Standards for interpreting data are controversial.

Nutrient	Age			Deficient signs	Comments
Pyridoxine (vitamin B₆) (in urine) (µg/g creatinine)	1–3	over 90	90+	Anemia, seizures, peripheral neuropathy.	Values may be greatly increased in pregnancy or in women taking oral contraceptives.
	4–6	over 80	80+		
	7–9	over 60	60+		
	10–12	over 40	40+		
	13–15	over 30	30+		
	16+	over 20	20+		
Vitamin B₁₂ (in serum) (µg/ml)	All	over 100	100+	Anemia.	
Vitamin A (in serum) (µg/100 ml)	All	over 10	20+	Dry skin, night blindness, follicular hyperkeratosis.	
Vitamin D	All			Rickets in children; osteomalacia in adults.	Elevated serum alkaline phosphatase was once used. Currently no accurate way to determine levels.
Vitamin E (in serum) (mg/100 ml)	All	over 0.2	0.6+	Uncertain; possible red blood cell fragility.	High unsaturated fat consumption increases need for vitamin E.

SOURCE: Values taken from C. E. Butterworth and G. L. Blackburn, "Hospital Malnutrition." *Nutrition Today* 10:8–18, 1975. Derived from "Table of Current Guidelines for Criteria of Nutritional Status for Laboratory Evaluation," in G. Christakis, Ed. "Nutritional assessment in health programs." *American Journal of Public Health* (Supple.), 63:34, 1973.

TABLE 19-14. Standards for Hemoglobin, Hematocrit, and Serum Iron Levels by Age

Age	Standard	
	Hemotocrit (Percentage)	Hemoglobin (gm/100 ml)
6–23 months	31	10.0
2–5 years	34	11.0
6–12 years	36	11.5
13–16 years, male	40	13.0
13–16 years, female	36	11.5
Over 16 years, male	44	14.0
Over 16 years, female	38	12.0
Pregnant, second trimester	35	11.0
Pregnant, third trimester	33	10.5

	Serum Iron (gm/100 ml)
6–23 months	30
2–5 years	40
6–12 years	50
Over 12 years, male	60
Over 12 years, female	40

one-half of all medical-surgical patients hospitalized for two weeks or more, can be divided into three separate categories. The first is the adult kwashiorkorlike state caused by a diet deficient in protein. The syndrome is characterized by *unchanged* anthropometric data despite severe depression of serum proteins, tranferrin, and albumin. The second type, adult marasmus, is characterized by decreased anthropometric measurements with normal serum albumin. The syndrome is one of prolonged gradual muscle mass atrophy and subcutaneous wasting. The third and most serious state is the marasmic-kwashiorkorlike state. The life threatening characteristics include atrophy, decreased serum albumin, edema, and depressed immunological competence. Protein-Calorie malnutrition is hypothesized to result from several undesirable yet common hospital practices including: (1) failure to record height and weight, (2) frequent staff rotation, particularly between separate units, (3) diffusion of responsibility for patient care, (4) prolonged intravenous feedings of saline solution or glucose, (5) failure to note a client's actual food intake, (6) meals withheld because of diagnostic tests, (7) tube feedings of inexact amounts and uncertain composition, (8) lack of knowledge about vitamin mixtures and other nutritional products, (9) failure to recognize increased nutritional needs resulting from the stress of injury or illness, and (10) lack of communication between all health team members.

Nurses must take responsibility for the deplorable state of their clients' nutrition. Nutritional assessment will provide a base line of information with which to compare later findings and will point out potential nutritional deficiencies before severe physiological alterations occur.

TABLE 19-15. Urinary Creatinine per Centimeter of Body Height for Men and Women of Ideal Weight for Their Height

Height		Medium Frame, Ideal Weight		Total mg Creatinine/ 24 Hr	mg Creatinine/cm Body Height/ 24 Hr
Ft and In	cm	lb	kg		
Men: Creatinine Coefficient—23 mg/kg/Body Weight					
5' 2"	157.5	124	56.0	1,288	8.17
5' 3"	160.0	127	57.6	1,325	8.28
5' 4"	162.6	130	59.1	1,359	8.36
5' 5"	165.1	133	60.3	1,386	8.40
5' 6"	167.6	137	62.0	1,426	8.51
5' 7"	170.2	141	63.8	1,467	8.62
5' 8"	172.7	145	65.8	1,513	8.76
5' 9"	175.3	149	67.6	1,555	8.86
5'10"	177.8	153	69.4	1,596	8.98
5'11"	180.3	158	71.4	1,642	9.11
6' 0"	182.9	162	73.5	1,691	9.24
6' 1"	185.4	167	75.6	1,739	9.38
6' 2"	188.0	171	77.6	1,785	9.49
6' 3"	190.5	176	79.6	1,831	9.61
6' 4"	193.0	181	82.2	1,891	9.80
Women: Creatinine Coefficient—18 mg/kg/Body Weight					
4'10"	147.3	101.5	46.1	830	5.63
4'11"	149.9	104.0	47.3	851	5.68
5' 0"	152.4	107.0	48.6	875	5.74
5' 1"	154.9	110.0	50.0	900	5.81
5' 2"	157.5	113.0	51.4	925	5.87
5' 3"	160.0	116.0	52.7	949	5.93
5' 4"	162.6	119.5	54.3	977	6.01
5' 5"	165.1	123.0	55.9	1,006	6.09
5' 6"	167.6	127.5	58.0	1,044	6.23
5' 7"	170.2	131.5	59.8	1,076	6.32
5' 8"	172.7	135.5	61.6	1,109	6.42
5' 9"	175.3	139.5	63.4	1,141	6.51
5'10"	177.8	143.5	65.2	1,174	6.60
5'11"	180.3	147.5	67.0	1,206	6.69
6' 0"	182.9	151.5	68.9	1,240	6.78

SOURCE: Reproduced with permission of *Nutrition Today* magazine, 703 Giddings Avenue, Annapolis, Maryland, 21404. © March/April, 1975.

BIBLIOGRAPHY

Anderson, L., Dibble, M., Mitchell, H., and Rynbergen, H. *Nutrition in Nursing.* Philadelphia: J. B. Lippincott Co., 1972.

Bistrian, B. Interaction of nutrition and infection in the hospital setting. *Am. J. Clin. Nutr.* 30:1228, 1977.

Blackburn G. L., Bestrian B. R., Marni, B. S., Baltey, S., Schlamna, H. T., and Smith, M. F. Nutritional and metabolic assessment of the hospitalized patient. *J. Parenteral Enteral Nutr.* 1:11, 1977.

Boykin, L. S. *Nutrition in Nursing.* Flushing, N.Y.: Medical Examination Pub. Co., Inc., 1975.

Brown, M. L., Myrtle, L., and Pike, R. *Nutrition: An Inte-*

grated Approach. 2nd Ed. New York: John Wiley & Sons, Inc., Pubs., 1975.

Butterworth, C. E. Iatrogenic Malnutrition: The Skeleton in the Hospital Closet. *Nutrition Today* 9:4, 1974.

Butterworth, C. E., and Blackburn, G. L. Hospital malnutrition. *Nutrition Today* 10(2):8, 1975.

Christakis, G. Nutritional assessment in health programs. *Am. J. Public Health.* 63 (Supple.), 1973.

Food and Drug Admin. *Nutrition Labels on Food.* DHEW Publ. No. (FDS) 74-2039. Rockville, Md.: U.S. Dept. of Health, Education, and Welfare, 1974.

Futrell, M. F., Windham, F., and Kilgore, L. T. Hydroxyproline Index: An indicator of nutritional status. *J. Am. Diet. Assoc.* 65:125, 1975.

Garn, S. M. The applicability of North American growth standards in developing countries. *Can. Med. Assoc. J.* 93:914, October 23, 1965.

Gifft, H. H., Washbon, M. B., and Harrison, G. G. *Nutrition, Behavior and Change.* Englewood Cliffs, N.J.: Prentice-Hall, Inc., 1972.

Guthrie, H. *Introductory Nutrition,* 4th Ed. St. Louis: The C.V. Mosby Co., 1979.

Harry J. *The Nursing Process: An Approach to Problem Solving.* Indianapolis: Indiana University School of Nursing, 1978.

Howard, R. B., and Herbold, N. H. *Nutrition in Clinical Care.* New York: McGraw-Hill Book Co., 1978.

Kessler, A. Pitfalls to avoid in interviewing outpatients. *Nursing 77* 7(9):70, September, 1977.

MacBryde, C. and Blacklow, R. *Signs and Symptoms,* ed 5. Philadelphia: J. B. Lippincott Co., 1970.

Madura, J. Nutritional assessment. Lecture, Indiana University School of Medicine, June 1977.

Mason, M., Wenburg, B., and Welsch, P. K. *The Dynamics of Clinical Dietetics.* New York: John Wiley & Sons, Inc., Pubs., 1977.

Meiling, R. L. The institutional system. *Nutrition Today* 9(4):34, 1974.

Overton, M. H., and Lukert, B. P. *Clinical Nutrition: A Physiological Approach.* Chicago: Year Book Medical Pubs., Inc., 1977.

Sandstead, H., and Pearson, W. N. Clinical evaluation of nutritional status. In R. S. Goodhart and M. E. Shils, Eds., *Modern Nutrition in Health and Disease,* 5th Ed. Philadphia: Lea & Febiger, 1973.

Schneider, H. A., Anderson, C. E., and Coursin, D. B., Eds. *Nutritional Support in Medical Practice.* New York: Harper & Row, Pubs., Inc., 1977.

Thiele, V. F. *Clinical Nutrition.* St. Louis: The C. V. Mosby Co., 1976.

Univ. of Alabama Hospitals. *Assessment of Nutritional Status.* Unpublished checklist. Birmingham, Ala., n.d.

Watt, B. K. and Merrill, A. C. United States Department of Agriculture, Agricultural Research Service. *Agricultural Handbook #8 Composition of Foods, Raw, Processed and Prepared.* Washington D.C., 1963.

Wellman, N. S. The evaluation of nutritional status. In R. B. Howard and N. H. Herbold, Eds., *Nutrition in Clinical Care.* New York: McGraw-Hill Book Co., 1978.

World Health Organization. *WHO Report of Expert Committee on Medical Assessment of Nutritional Status.* World Health Organization Technical Report Series 258, 1963a.

CHAPTER 20

Nutritional Assessment Throughout the Life Cycle

The nurse conducts a nutritional assessment to detect overt and potential cases of malnutrition and overnutrition. People's nutrient requirements vary because of differences in age, sex, body size, physiological state, activity, and environment. From this assessment, problems may be identified that can be treated by nursing interventions. As people develop, their nutritional needs change, thereby changing the focus of the assessment. The purpose of this chapter is to explore some aspects of nutritional assessment at each phase of the life cycle. Case studies and assessment tools illustrate the suggested methods. These assessment tools are to be used as *guides* to assist the nurse in data collection and interpretation. The nurse must always adapt her assessment techniques to each client and avoid collecting meaningless information by following a form too routinely. The depth of nutritional assessments will vary with the nurse's purpose, time, and expertise.

PREGNANCY

Pregnancy has at long last come to be viewed as a normal physiological process. Yet, because of the additional physiological demands placed on a woman during the development of the fetus, her nutritional status may change dramatically throughout the course of her pregnancy. The outcome of the pregnancy will be affected by both short- and long-term nutritional patterns and illnesses. Several purposes are fulfilled by a nutritional assessment during pregnancy, including the iden-

tification of risk factors that may influence fetal or maternal health, the opportunity to reinforce healthy nutritional patterns, and the collection of information as a basis for planning nutritional education to promote the well-being of both the mother and baby. Pregnant women, because of increased medical contact, are usually more available for an individualized teaching program. As in every nurse-client interaction, of course, the health professional must not stereotype the client. Active listening to each person is the only way to validate any nutritional concerns present. Nutritional assessment and intervention during the prenatal phase of human development may have the rewarding effect of a cycle of poor nutritional habits passed down through generations. The nurse's interventions can have a great impact on the quality of life of future generations.

Certain groups of women may be at a greater risk for developing complications related to alterations in nutritional status and must, therefore, be assessed even more thoroughly than usual. Some of these people include: adolescents, particularly if obesity or malnutrition is present; women who have had more than three pregnancies; women who are self-supporting, have a low income, or must supply food for a large number of dependents; women who have borne low-birth-weight infants or postmature infants; women who have any complicating medical-surgical problem or who are depressed; women who use drugs such as alcohol or nicotine; and women who are not familiar with nutritional concerns or who participate in fad diets (Christakis, 1973).

The assessment of the expectant mother involves the three major components of nutritional assessment discussed in Chapter 19—dietary history, clinical exam and history, and laboratory assessment. The collection of sophisticated data on these components is expensive in both practitioner and laboratory time, but much of the assessment data can be gathered effectively from the client by health professionals during routine visits during and after pregnancy. Figure 20-1 is a typical assessment tool that can be used for maternal nutritional assessment.

Dietary History

The expectant mother is often uncertain about the physiological changes she is experiencing. She may be extremely vulnerable to familial, cultural, and traditional influences on food choices. Good communication techniques and skills are required of the interviewer to determine what foods the client is eating and what she is avoiding. Nutritional status before pregnancy needs to be assessed for potential problems as well.

Cultural norms play a large role in a pregnant person's choice of a diet pattern. In urban regions eating bacon, ham, and beans may be discouraged during pregnancy. It is not unusual to hear a client state that she cannot eat green vegetables during pregnancy. *Pica* (abnormal cravings) is generally associated with various ethnic and geographical groups. The nurse should ask the client if she

Name ______________________________

Age ______________

Cultural background ____________________

Pregravid weight ____________________ Current weight

Height ____________

Dietary History:

24-hr recall:

Breakfast	
Lunch	
Dinner	
Snacks	

Allergies:
Food preferences:
Food restrictions:

Economic status: ____________________

Understanding of nutritional concepts ____________________

Medications:

Presence of:	Yes	No
Nausea		
Vomiting		
Constipation		
Indigestion		
Alcohol intake		
Tobacco habit		

Figure 20-1. Nutritional assessment tool for the pregnant woman.

Physical Assessment:

Weight _____   Prenatal _____

Height _____

Physical Exam:

	Date								
	Weight								
	Fundal height								
	Fetal heart tones								
	Fetal position								
	Urine Glucose/Protein								
	Weeks of gestation								

HEENT:
Chest:

Heart:

Abdomen:
Extremities:
Neurological:

History:

OB & Gyn _____   Para _____   Gravida _____   Abort _____

Age of menarche: _____

Average duration of menses: _____

Birth weights of children: _____
Medical:

Immunizations _____

Diseases, illnesses _____

Laboratory Evaluation:

Hb/Hct. _____   Urine glucose/albumin _____

Blood type _____

VDRL _____

Serum folate _____

Figure 20-1. (*Continued*)

is eating clay, cornstarch, flour, or dirt. The approach used in presenting such questions is crucial. An explanation that the consumption of such substances is not unusual may help to elicit meaningful information. Above all, an open, caring attitude will do much to elicit complete and reliable answers. Religious restrictions as well as personal dietary preferences must be assessed to provide for sup-

plements where needed. The portion of the diet consisting of iron-containing foods is particularly important to validate. If the nurse shares the reasons why particular food groups need to be included in the diet, the client is more likely to participate in and comply with a prescribed diet regimen.

In addition to assessing the actual food consumed and the specific foods not eaten, the nurse must note the medications the client is receiving. If the client was taking oral contraceptives at the time she became pregnant, deficiencies of vitamins C, B_6, B_{12} and folacin may be present.

The nurse must advise expectant mothers that vitamin supplements are not replacements for food. Frequently the physician prescribes a multivitamin-and-iron supplement. The nurse has the responsibility of teaching the client the purpose, content, and correct administration of any supplements given. Within the past few years, research has shown that the pregnant woman should take no medications (including alcohol, nicotine, or aspirin) unless prescribed by her physician. The nurse can reinforce this warning at the same time vitamin and mineral supplements are discussed.

Allergies and milk intolerance must be considered in the diet history. Cravings for particular foods are usually psychologically initiated and need to be considered for their potential contribution to or interference with a client's diet regimen.

Special concerns unique to pregnancy may interfere with the expectant mother's nutrition. Nausea and vomiting, perhaps caused by endocrine or psychological alterations, usually pass by the sixth month of pregnancy. *Hyperemesis* that results in severe electrolyte losses, ketosis, or fluid imbalance may require hospitalization with replacement therapy. Nausea and vomiting, if they occur, need to be dealt with as valid concerns. Antiemetic drugs may be necessary. Home remedies such as small carbohydrate meals are occasionally successful.

Slowed gastrointestinal motility and pressure from the fetus may cause constipation in the latter months of pregnancy. Hemorrhoids secondary to the pressure of the fetus may further impair elimination. Increasing dietary fiber and fluids may provide relief. Such common-sense nursing strategies as encouraging a regular bowel routine, moderate exercise, time for relaxation, and

privacy will also assist the client. "Indigestion" and gas are frequent occurrences as the baby grows and applies pressure on the mother's upper gastrointestinal system; small, frequent meals supplemented by milk may help. Antacids or baking soda should be discouraged because of the potential for developing alkalemia from the bicarbonate or anemia as a result of the antacid combining with iron. Any acute illness in which nutritional intake is hindered may be followed by a negative nitrogen balance that could jeopardize both the mother and the fetus.

Weight losses from a self-prescribed diet may be a precursor to maternal malnutrition. Macrobiotic, vegetarian, and "natural" diets, if strictly followed, need to be carefully assessed. Self-medication with large doses of the fat-soluble vitamins can lead to toxicity with severe results for the mother and fetus. Alcoholism, drug abuse, and smoking may impair fetal growth or interfere with nutrient uptake by the mother. Again, effective communication skills are necessary to gather accurate data in these sensitive areas.

Socioeconomic concerns are usually addressed during the diet history, because the mother's socioeconomic status will affect her dietary habits. Where economic resources are limited, protein-rich foods tend to be replaced by high-Calorie carbohydrates or fats. (See Chap. 1 for a full explanation of influences on food habits.)

Physical Assessment

Chapter 15 noted the effects of maternal health and nutrition on fetal development. A child's normal growth may be severely retarded because of maternal malnourishment. Compared to a normal infant, an underdeveloped newborn will be more likely to become ill, have slowed central nervous system development, and experience difficulty in adapting to a stressful environment.

Two of the most important predictors of the potential for a low-birth-weight baby are the mother's prepregnancy weight and her weight gain or loss during pregnancy. Prepregnancy weight is a result of the expectant mother's genetic inheritance, sociocultural and economic heritage, and previous nutrient consumption. The expectant mother should be considered at nutritional risk if her weight is 10% or more below ideal or 20% or more above the norm for her height and age grouping (see Appendices E and F for correct weights according to height). Figure 20-2 illustrates the approximate weight gain considered normal for each week of pregnancy, but individual variations need to be considered when assessing an expectant mother's total weight gain.

When conducting the physical examination, the nurse must be careful not to confuse alterations present with those normally occurring from pregnancy. For example, *gingival hyperplasia* often occurs normally during pregnancy, but it may also represent a vitamin C deficiency. Increased cheek pigmentation may either be a sign of niacin deficiency or occur as a result of normal alterations in body chemistry. Ankle edema may be a sign of fluid imbalance but more frequently occurs from a decreased venous return caused by fetal pressure on the veins of the legs.

The classic clinical signs that manifest themselves during longstanding malnutrition are rarely observed in the United States. It is important, however, that the health professional use the clinic visits to assess the typical findings that could predict latent malnutrition or deficiency. Assessment should include a dental examination and an inspection of the skin, mucous membranes, eyes, tongue, and hair. Careful record keeping by the same practitioner will facilitate the discovery of any potential nutritional deficits.

Historical Data

Past medical and health histories provide the nurse with clues to potential physical, phychosocial, and nutritional problems an expectant mother may encounter. Factors such as environmental conditions, socioeconomic status, and available support systems may play a great part in the mother's ability to accept and comply with a prescribed nutritional or medical regimen. Age is an important factor. Adolescents and older women have an increased risk of developing complications during pregnancy. Frequently women in these categories have low-birth-weight babies.

Gynecological History
Age of menarche is significant because of its relationship to nutritional status. Menarche is usually delayed when under- or overnutrition exists. Average age at menarche in the United States today is 12.5 years. Constantly improving national nutrition accounts for the steady decline in the age of onset of menstruation. Likewise, *amenorrhea* or a scanty menstrual flow may be associated with nutritional deficiency.

Pelvimetry should be conducted to determine the potential for natural birth. Deviations from normal may have resulted from rickets or calcium deficiency during the woman's developmental years. Pelvic measurements provide advance warning of the potential necessity for Cesarean section. Such advance notice would provide time to build up the mother's nutritional reserves.

Obstetrical History
The total number of previous pregnancies and their outcome needs to be determined. If the client is multiparous with intereonceptional periods of less than a year, there is a greatly increased chance that her nutritional reserves may be severely depleted. A past history of having had a premature infant, a stillborn infant, an abortion, or a low-birth-weight infant may provide clues to overall nutritional status. A history of having given birth to a low-birth-weight infant may suggest past nutritional problems.

Any complications after birth that were experienced by either mother or infant need to

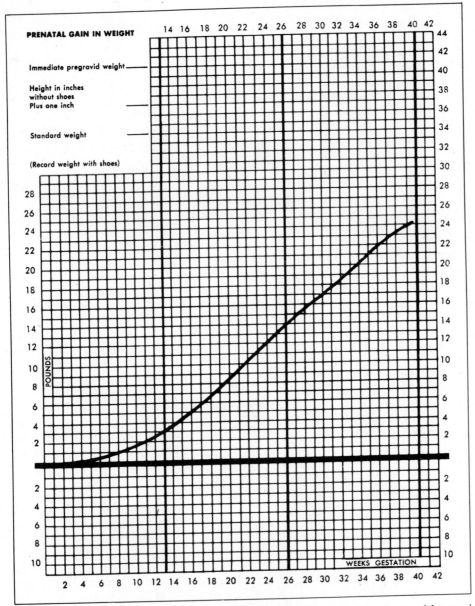

PRENATAL GAIN IN WEIGHT

Immediate pregravid weight

Height in inches
without shoes
Plus one inch

Standard weight

(Record weight *with* shoes)

POUNDS

WEEKS GESTATION

Figure 20-2. Pattern of normal prenatal weight gain. (From Committee on Maternal Nutrition, Food and Nutrition Board, National Research Council, National Academy of Sciences: *Maternal Nutrition and the Course of Pregnancy*. Washington, D. C.: Government Printing Office, 1970.)

518

be documented. For example, a child with a birth weight of 10 lb (4.5 kg) or more may signal the presence of latent diabetes in the mother. Neonatal hypocalcemia in the infant may point to maternal hyperparathyroidism or a decreased calcium intake.

Any previous complications of pregnancy such as excessive vomiting, *preeclampsia*, toxemia, anemia, or postpartum infection need to be noted. Frequently, complications occur after poor prenatal care or because of lack of compliance with prescribed regimens. Nutritional imbalances have long been postulated to be a significant factor in the development of prenatal problems.

Medical History

Family and personal history of disease should be evaluated for potential relationships to nutritional concerns. Diabetes, cardiovascular disease, and infectious illnesses are among those conditions that seriously alter nutritional requirements during pregnancy.

Drug use and abuse need to be documented. Alcoholism, frequently difficult to detect, interferes with nutrient ingestion and may be a precursor of nutritional deficiencies. If an expectant mother smokes, the length of time she has smoked and the number of cigarettes smoked per day are significant. Women who smoke give birth to a disproportionate number of low-birth-weight infants.

Laboratory Assessment

Laboratory evaluation of nutritional status may reveal more short-term nutritional problems or ones of recent onset. The interpretation of laboratory results should be made with knowledge of how pregnancy alters many values.

Hemoglobin and hematocrit values can point out potential or overt anemia in the expectant mother. Deficiencies in the ingestion of protein, folacin, vitamin B_{12}, and iron may be reflected in a lowered hemoglobin

level. If the hemoglobin level falls below 11 mg/100 ml of serum, anemia is overt and needs medical treatment. Frequently the cause of anemia in pregnancy is the dilutional effects of the fetal circulation on maternal blood volume. Documentation of iron-deficiency anemia can be made by determining serum iron level and total iron-binding capacity level. Serum iron levels below 50 mg/100 ml in pregnancy indicate possible iron deficiency. Levels of less than 15% iron saturation indicate iron-deficiency anemia.

Folacin deficiency, estimated to occur in 50–60% of all pregnant women, is best reflected by the measurement of serum folate levels.

A serological test for syphilis is frequently required by law. Results may reveal a latent disease process that can have severe adverse developmental effects on both fetus and mother.

Urine is frequently tested for glucose and protein (albumin), which can signal diabetes, preeclampsia, or renal disease. Urinalysis obtained by clean catch midstream can identify a urinary tract infection. Norms for pregnancy have not generally been established for the more sophisticated laboratory tests. If a specific nutritional deficiency is suspected, supplemental therapy should be instituted immediately.

CASE STUDY: Pregnant Woman

As Jane P., a pregnant 24-year-old, enters the obstetrics clinic for her monthly checkup, the nurse observes that Jane appears to be comfortable and well-groomed. The nurse begins to make a complete assessment of Jane to obtain information that will be helpful in meeting her needs throughout her pregnancy. The physician has notified Jane that her pregnancy test is positive and that her anticipated delivery date is in 32 weeks. Jane states that she is married and that both she and her husband are eagerly anticipating their first child, indicating that the pregnancy is planned. The nurse questions Jane about her lifestyle. Jane relates that she and her husband live in a one-story ranch house in one of the developments near the city. Neither she nor her husband has relatives nearby, but they are in close touch with several other young couples in their neighborhood. Jane volunteers that her job as a secretary keeps her busy but prevents active exercise. When asked about her diet history, Jane states that since the onset of her pregnancy she has been extremely fatigued. The nurse notes that Jane is rather pale and that her laboratory studies indicate a mild anemia. The physician has prescribed an iron supplement for Jane. A detailed 24-hour recall of what Jane ate is listed below. She confirms that this is a typical diet pattern for her during the week.

7 AM Breakfast:
1 piece toast (whole wheat) with butter
1 T jelly
8 oz milk
6 oz coffee with cream

10 AM Coffee Break
1 milk chocolate candy bar
6 oz coffee with cream

12 Noon Lunch
¼ lb hamburger on bun
4 oz French fries
16 oz cola

2 PM Coffee Break
8 oz cola

6 PM Dinner
1 cup spaghetti
½ cup meat sauce
4 slices French bread
½ cup green salad
2 T salad dressing
1 glass wine

11 PM Snack
1 apple

QUESTIONS

1. What additional data is needed to make a nursing diagnosis?
2. What nursing orders should be implemented in regard to the physician's order for iron supplements?
3. What approach should be used to teach Jane about the importance of nutrition to a normal pregnancy?

INFANCY AND CHILDHOOD

At no other time in the life cycle is adequate nutrition so important to normal growth and development as during infancy and childhood. Such conditions as obesity, atherosclerosis, and perhaps hypertension may have their roots in childhood malnutrition or overnutrition. See Chapter 15 for the basic requirements for infants and children.

The goal of nutritional assessment during infancy and childhood is the detection of potential and overt undernutrition and overnutrition. The detection of a problem in infancy or childhood frequently points to additional problems occurring with other members of the family group. Simply by measuring body weight and height serially in grade school, gross estimates of the adequacy of nutrition in families can be made.

Gross nutritional deficiencies are rare in the United States; yet more subtle subclinical problems exist including caloric under- and overnutrition, dental caries, iron-deficiency anemia, hypercholesterolemia, and trace mineral deficiencies. The Ten-State Nutrition Survey showed that certain nutritional problems could be predicted by general family characteristics. Among the findings were: The incidence of malnutrition increased as the income level of the family decreased; the higher the educational level of the family member who was responsible for buying the food, the better the nutritional status of those family members under 17 years of age; and poor dental health was positively associated with the increased consumption of candy, soda pop, and pastries. Further, undernutrition is more common in families with a large number of children. Environmental concerns such as poverty, food-faddist parents, or a family history positive for diabetes or obesity necessitate even more careful nutritional assessment by the health professional.

Dietary History

Dietary histories are generally gathered from a child's parents or guardian. Usually the person responsible for food preparation will be able to provide a fairly accurate history. In today's society, frequently the child's baby sitter or day care center may have to be consulted to obtain full intake data.

School-age children who attend school where nutritious lunches are served usually have the opportunity to consume at least one-third of the RDAs for the major nutrients. The Type A lunch includes: 2 oz of meat or meat substitute; ¾ cup total of at least two fruits or vegetables; 1 slice of whole grain or enriched bread; 1 t of butter or margarine; and ½ pt of milk. Of course merely providing the nutrients does not guarantee that they will be consumed. It has been shown that children obtained a significantly higher level of nutrients from school lunches than from bag lunches (Head and Werks, 1975). Total Calories obtained are usually fairly equivalent; but lunches brought to school by students frequently contain lower food value.

To obtain an accurate record of nutrient intake the dietary history should be based on actual food eaten, with plate waste subtracted. Frequently, the most satisfactory way of obtaining a dietary history in childhood is to have the parents keep a thorough daily food diary and occasionally to request 24-hour recalls during clinic visits.

In one study (Head, 1975) based on short-term food diaries and diet histories, the investigator found that the protein intake of children tends to be one and one-half to two times greater than the RDA. Vitamin A intake was supplemented by daily vitamin therapy in nearly 40% of preschool children. About one-third of lower-income children reported ascorbic acid intakes below 20 mg. Similarly, iron intake was inadequate for 20–30% of the children in the study, with the highest deficiencies occurring in the lower socioeconomic groups.

In general, three basic concepts need to be considered when assessing the nutritional status of a child. First, the health professional needs to remember that the energy requirement per unit of weight is higher in the infant and child than in the adult. Second, the child needs a higher proportion of tissue-building foods for growth and development than the adult. Finally, variety is limited because the child's digestive ability is immature.

The diets of children at various ages are now described.

The Infant Diet

The major item on the young infants diet is, of course, the formula, or "mothers milk" if breast fed (Fig. 20-3). Most infants require about 5 oz of fluid per kg of body weight per day. This includes the allotment for water and juice. Some doctors recommend 1.5 to 2 oz of formula per pound (never to exceed an 8-oz feeding); thus a 7 lb baby might receive 10 to 14 oz of formula per day. The breast-fed baby may need Vitamin D to supplement his formula. A comparison of human and cow's milk is given in Chapter 16.

CALORIES.   The growth spurt in infancy is greater than at any other time in life, and the baby needs Calories to meet these growth needs. A newborn requires 110 to 150 Calories/kg; from age 2 to 12 months about

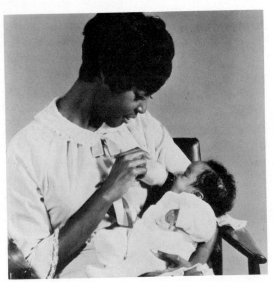

Figure 20-3. The infant's feeding patterns are learned quickly by his mother. (Courtesy Ross Laboratories)

100 to 110 Calories/kg are required. If it is considered that the adult usually needs less than 40 Calories/kg, it can be recognized at once that a major dietary difference owing to energy needs and growth is present. Frequent crying may indicate that the baby may need more calories. If the baby receives sufficient food and love, he will usually not cry or be restless after feeding and will double his birth weight at 4 to 5 months and triple it at 1 year.

PROTEIN.   The infant needs 2.5 to 3.5 gm of protein per kg per day; this need gradually drops to 2 gm/kg by the age of 1 year. This still exceeds the 0.8 gm/kg requirement for adults. Breast milk provides 2 to 2.5 gm of protein per day, while cow's milk provides 3 to 4 gm.

FATS.   Some fats are needed in infancy and are supplied adequately by milk. Breast milk has more linoleic acid than cow's milk. Infants with a deficiency of the essential fatty acid and linoleic acid have more eczema than normal infants.

SUPPLEMENTARY FOODS.   An infant cannot thrive on milk alone beyond early infancy. Particularly, the infant will need additional Vitamin C and iron. The fetal store of iron is usually depleted at 3 to 5 months of age, and milk is a poor source of iron and Vitamin C. Foman (1974) states that there appears to be no advantage in introducing supplementary foods prior to 6 months of age.

The age at which supplements begin varies widely; there is difference of opinion among pediatricians regarding the development of increased digestive ability. Most foods are added one at a time to test tolerance. Cereal is often the first supplement. Since rice is usually not allergenic, it is often the first cereal and may be introduced in small amounts as early as 2 weeks or as late as 6 months. Patience is needed, since the infant will experience some difficulty at first with the consistency of the food and the tongue thrust used in sucking. The early introduction of foods other than milk or formula tends to occur as a result of social custom rather than nutritional need. Other than the increased cost of supplemental foods, the only problem arising from early supplemental feedings is the possibility of overfeeding and the development of childhood obesity (Foman, 1974).

Fruit may be introduced with cereal or shortly thereafter. Vegetables are introduced when the infant is about 4 months and meats and soups at 5–6 months. Most infants have been introduced to all the pureed supplements by the end of the sixth month. Chopped foods begin at 9 to 12 months. Finger foods such as zwieback are often introduced with teething. By 10 months a baby can feed himself a cracker with fair skill.

WEANING.   At 4 to 6 months of age most babies show a readiness to take *small* amounts from a cup. Mothers may then give orange juice or water by cup. Serious weaning usually begins at 7 to 10 months and varies with the readiness of the individual child and mother. Breast-fed babies may begin weaning a little earlier than bottle-fed; 7 to 8 months is common for beginning and 9 to 10 months for completion. The bottle-fed baby is usually weaned by 1 year, though the early morning or bedtime bottle may be continued a while longer. Weaning should be gradual (Fig. 20-4).

SCHEDULE. Most babies will establish an eating pattern if the mother allows flexibility early and responds to the infant's indication of need. A more flexible approach is usually rewarded with a minimum of feeding problems later.

Childhood Diet

ONE YEAR. The 1-year-old generally eats three meals a day containing a variety of simple foods and some mashed table foods, with a juice or cracker snack and about a pint of milk. Finger foods are very popular. The child may want to hold a spoon of his own

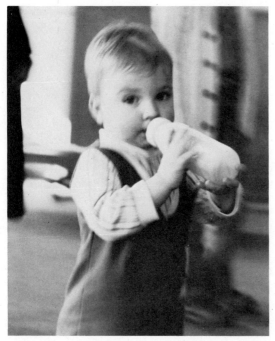

Figure 20-4. The toddler may still enjoy a bottle during the day.

while being fed. At about 15 months the child is able to feed himself, though with much spilling.

TWO YEARS. The child now enjoys chopped foods, whole grain and enriched cereals and breads, and green and yellow vegetables. He does well with one egg every other day and enjoys fruit (pulp only) and fruit juices. Toast and simple desserts are very popular.

THREE TO FIVE YEARS. The child in this age group eats from the family table and begins to enjoy whole fruits and vegetables. He still likes basic, bland foods and rejects casseroles or mixtures. Between 2 and 4 years a child may appear to "lose his appetite" or become "finicky" at meals. Actually, his growth rate slows down and he needs less food. The child also may enjoy a "refusal" at times as he tests a new-found sense of independence. Eating and attitudes are very closely related. If mealtime is a happy time, if food is attractive, and if there is minimal stress on how much one must eat, there will usually be few problems. A healthy child will not starve and will tend to select healthful foods. Small servings look much more "possible" to the young child.

SIX TO TWELVE YEARS. The child in this age group is not fussy about food selection. He likes variety but is developing definite food habits during these years. There should be evidence of great improvement in table manners if example and guidance have been available. The school lunch program makes a significant contribution to the child's daily nutritional intake (Fig. 20-5). A good breakfast is also an important consideration for the school-age child (see Fig. 20-6).

Clinical Assessment

A background medical history is helpful when assessing the clinical status of children. The birth weight, the prenatal course, and the occurrence of acute or chronic illnesses are sig-

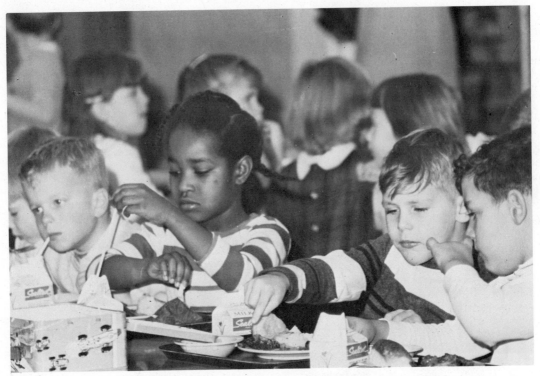

Figure 20-5. Elementary schools provide children with a hot lunch at noon. (USDA photo by Jack Schneider)

nificant. The health professional must remember that physical examination alone is not a reliable indicator of nutritional status because visible signs occur only after prolonged periods of malnutrition.

The general appearance is observed for obesity or emaciation. Color, pallor, and turgor of the skin are noted. The hair is observed for texture, shine, and the presence or absence of lice. Teeth are inspected for visible caries.

Anthropometry compares the relationships of height, weight, specific body parts, and subcutaneous fat. Longitudinal records of anthropometric data reveal trends in nutritional status. The nurse in an outpatient setting has the opportunity to initiate and keep such records. Chapter 19 contains examples of growth charts that could be used for longitudinal assessment. Length from heel to head, weight, and head circumference should be recorded. Length generally correlates better with socioeconomic status than weight and therefore should be carefully monitored. Children over 2 should be weighed and measured on a balanced-beam scale. Table 20-1 provides standards for children's anthropometry.

Interpretations of a child's nutritional status should never be made without serial observations of growth. Children under 2 years are usually observed at three-month intervals; six-month to yearly assessments are appropriate for older children. The rationale for such observations is that a child's vulnerability to malnutrition and its developmental

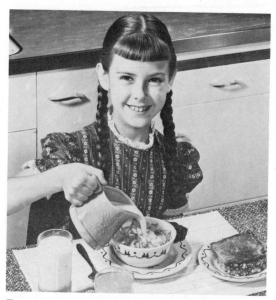

Figure 20-6. This school-age girl begins the day with a good breakfast (USDA photograph)

considerations occurs during rapid growth stages. Undernutrition affects such central nervous system functions as perception, attention, learning, and language development. Generally, undernutrition should be suspected in children who are classified below the tenth percentile.

Determination of skin-fold thickness provides an independent measurement of body fat and may be useful in evaluating childhood overnutrition. Childhood obesity in the United States is present in at least 10% of the population. The use of calipers will accurately provide information on total adipose content, whereas weight-to-height charts fail to distinguish between muscle and soft-tissue bulk. Arm circumference measurement in children is taken halfway between shoulder and elbow on the left arm, which should hang loosely by the side at the time of measuring. The tape must be applied to the skin surface around the whole arm but not so tight as to cause an indentation. (See Chap. 19 for details on anthropometric measurement.)

Laboratory Assessment

Laboratory assessment of children is usually carried out only when undernutrition is suspected. Abnormal hemoglobin, protein, cholesterol, and vitamin A levels reflect long-term dietary inadequacy. The clinician must note that many disease processes may also alter the biochemical levels of the child. Frequently malnutrition in American children is the result of such alteration.

Serum transferrin saturation greater than 15% indicates an iron level capable of producing hemoglobin. A hemoglobin level of 10.5 gm/100 ml is the lower limit of normal for children aged 1 to 6 years.

Plasma ascorbic acid levels reflect the level of intake up to an adequate level. The normal range of plasma ascorbic acid values is between 0.1 and 3.1 mg/100 ml. Generally, plasma vitamin levels are not necessary as long as vitamin supplements are being administered to the child.

Other nutritionally related tests that are important include sickle cell detection, serum lead levels, and blood urea nitrogen levels. The necessity for such detection usually arises out of a pathophysiological process suspected in the child.

Figure 20-7 is a typical assessment tool useful for longitudinal monitoring of the nutritional status of a child.

CASE STUDY: An Infant's Routine Checkup

Mrs. G. has just brought her 3-month-old daughter, Angela, into the clinic for a routine checkup and immunizations. Mrs. G. explains that she is returning to work full time next week. Until now, she has been breast-feeding Angela.

Angela appears normal for her age. She weighs 10 lb (4.54 kg), a weight gain of 4 lb (1.8 kg) from her birth weight. She is alert and responds obviously to her mother's voice.

It is apparent that Mrs. G. is quite concerned about the transition to the bottle formula the doctor has prescribed for Angela.

QUESTIONS

1. What additional data needs to be collected to arrive at an accurate nursing diagnosis of Angela's nutritional status?

2. What resources would be helpful in teaching Mrs. G. about formula preparation and feeding?

3. What specific teaching guidelines could be used to help Mrs. G. with the transition to formula?

CASE STUDY: A Toddler's Finicky Eating

Mr. S. has asked for some advice about his 3-year-old son, Alan. Mr. S. explains that Alan refuses to eat practically anything except peanut butter and jelly sandwiches. Obviously an attentive father, Mr. S. is quite concerned about Alan's behavior. He states that he has never had difficulty getting Alan to eat a wide variety of foods before and, in fact, has made certain that Alan not overeat.

QUESTIONS

1. What questions should Mr. S. be asked about Alan's eating patterns?

2. Given that Alan's growth and development are normal for his age, what information should Mr. S. be given about Alan's eating patterns?

CASE STUDY: A School-age Child Admitted for Tonsillectomy and Adenoidectomy

Jonathan W. is a 10-year-old child admitted to the hospital for evaluation and removal of his tonsils and adenoids. Before admission he had several serious infec-

tions that were treated with antibiotics in home therapy. Jonathan's 2-day hospital course has been uneventful, and he is to be discharged to his home this afternoon. Jon's mother works part time as a teacher's aide in the school that Jonathan and his only sibling, an older brother, attend. Jon's intake since yesterday's surgery has been minimal, consisting mainly of liquids including jello, pudding, and ice cream. He has experienced two episodes of post-operative nausea and vomiting, with a total emesis output of 200 cc.

Jon's mother reports that he enjoys eating meats and desserts but ignores most vegetables. He usually eats dry cereal for breakfast, the school lunch, and a moderate-size dinner consisting of meat—usually hamburger, fish, or chicken—potatoes, and a green vegetable. He and his brother have an afternoon snack of an apple, cookies, or milk.

Jon's admitting weight and height were 63 lb (28.6 kg), 54 in (137.1 cm).

QUESTIONS

1. What information is most important for Jon and his mother to have before discharge from the hospital?

2. What problems might occur after Jon's discharge? What nursing interventions could prevent or lessen them?

3. What diet might be suggested to Jon's mother for the first few days after Jon's discharge?

ADOLESCENCE

Adolescence is second only to infancy in the nutritional requirements necessary for normal growth and development. During adolescence, a substantial amount of new tissue is built. Girls may double their body weight between the ages of 8 and 14; boys will do so between 10 and 17 years of age. During this period there is an increase in the apparent

TABLE 20-1. Anthropometry of Children, Aged 12–71 Months

Age (Months)	Height (cm)	Weight (kg)	Head Circumference (cm)	Thorasic Fat Fold (mm)
		Boys		
12–17	78.0	10.6	47.0	4.6
18–23	84.0	12.0	48.0	4.3
24–29	89.0	12.8	49.0	4.2
30–35	93.0	14.1	50.0	4.0
36–41	97.0	14.5	50.0	4.2
42–47	101.0	15.8	50.0	4.1
48–53	103.5	16.6	50.0	4.0
54–59	107.0	17.5	51.0	4.0
60–65	110.0	19.0	51.0	4.2
66–71	114.0	20.0	51.0	4.2
		Girls		
12–17	76.0	10.2	46.0	4.6
18–23	83.0	11.2	47.0	4.4
24–29	88.0	12.2	48.0	4.4
30–35	91.0	13.5	48.5	4.6
36–41	96.0	14.5	49.0	4.3
42–47	100.0	15.2	49.0	4.6
48–53	103.0	16.2	50.0	4.2
54–59	107.0	17.4	50.0	4.2
60–65	109.0	18.1	50.0	4.6
66–71	113.0	20.0	50.0	4.8

SOURCE: Public Health Service, *Preschool Nutrition Survey*, PHS Publ. No. 2158. DHEW, 1971.

basal metabolic requirement. There is also an increased demand for Calories and nitrogen. Both are correlated with physiological events: menarche in girls, and the adolescent growth spurt in boys.

Certain trends are evident in the nutrition of children in the United States population. Age-adjusted height and weight of children is greater today than in past generations. Improved nutritional status, absence of chronic disease, and urban living are postulated to have influenced earlier maturation.

Adolescent obesity, particularly in girls, may precipitate malnutrition from fad dieting. Because of the adolescent's increasing body awareness, self-consciousness may result when the real self does not compare favorably to the self idealized from advertisements and models. Failure to meet the additional requirement for protein at this stage of devel-opment may cause a decrease in resistance to infection.

Nutrient requirements during adolescence are altered by increased growth and the metabolism that accompanies it. Caloric requirements are increased, often resulting in between-meal snacks. Calcium and iron requirements are also increased by bone growth, increase in muscle mass, and the onset of menarche in girls. A tool for assessing adolescent nutritional status is Figure 20-8.

Dietary History

The evaluation of dietary intake of an adolescent can prove to be very difficult because of the frequency of between-meal snacks. Qualitative and quantitative data are useful when nutritional alterations are suspected. The most accurate method of collecting data is

	Name									
	Date of birth									
	Birth weight									
	Date									

Anthropometric Data	Height									
	Weight									
	Percentile									
	Head circumference									
	Skin fold									
	Significant clinical findings									
Dietary History	Foods eaten and amount									
Laboratory Values	Serum: Hemoglobin									
	Proteins									
	Vitamin A									
	Cholesterol									
	Other:									

Figure 20-7. Nutritional assessment tool for the child.

probably a food diary kept concurrently with intake. The 24-hour recall will provide data on the type of food consumed at meals, but it may omit the food taken on-the-run, between meals, or at social gatherings. Data on eating patterns, cultural influences, food preferences and dislikes, and client's knowledge of good nutrition need to be assessed during the interview.

Clinical Assessment

The client's age, position in the family, and medical history, such as his immunization record, may reveal important information that will suggest a potential problem. The teenager's experiences with childhood diseases should be noted. Current health status history should include information on social habits

Name _____ Age _____

Medications _____

Medical History:
Diseases:

Childhood illnesses:

Medications:

Dietary History:

24-Hour Recall	
Breakfast:	Snacks:
Lunch:	
Dinner:	

Clinical Evaluation:

Date								
Weight								
Height								
Triceps								

Immunizations:

Laboratory Evaluation:

Hb _____
Hc+ _____
UA _____ Glucose _____
Protein _____

Albumin _____

Iron _____

Transferrin _____
Creatinine _____

Figure 20-8. Nutritional assessment tool for the adolescent.

such as smoking and drinking. The clinician must use care and discretion in gathering such data and explain why the information is needed. The adolescent should be interviewed in privacy so that accurate data can be collected. Allergies need to be documented, along with a summary of the family medical history. The disease history of client and family is necessary for determining how nutrient intake or disease processes have affected growth and development.

The physical examination should include a brief review of systems, with particular attention to those areas most prone to nutritional deficiency, such as skin, eyes, mouth and pharynx, and growth.

Anthropometric data is most meaningful when gathered serially at specified intervals. Height and weight should be taken because longitudinal growth is one of the best indexes of nutritional status over time. When obesity is suspected, measuring skin-fold thickness is a method of assessing adequate nutritional consumption. If severe malnutrition is suspected, roentgenograms of the wrist will provide data on bone density and epiphyseal closure.

Laboratory Assessment

Minimal laboratory evaluation should include hemoglobin and hematocrit levels and urinalysis for glucose and protein levels. A more in-depth evaluation should include plasma levels of albumin, iron, and total iron-binding capacity; blood urea nitrogen levels; and vitamin and trace-mineral assays. Urine may be tested for creatinine, nitrogen, zinc, and thiamine levels. Many of the tests are expensive and should be conducted only when overt disease is suspected.

CASE STUDY: An Adolescent Having a Physical Examination

Susan O. is a 16-year-old who arrives in the physician's office for a precamp physical examination. She explains that she plans to be at camp for three weeks. She is obviously obese, weighing 160 lb (72.7 kg) for her 60 inches (152.4 cm). Susan states that she has never been hospitalized nor had any serious illnesses. She is a junior in high school and participates in the music program. Susan comments that she takes physical education in school but prefers studying or reading to more active pastimes. Previous medical records reveal that Susan was 20% above her ideal weight when examined three years ago.

Susan seldom eats breakfast, preferring to eat a lunch consisting of a hamburger, French fries, and a candy bar. She usually eats dinner with her family. Dinners consist mainly of a meat, vegetable, and salad. She admits that she frequently snacks while studying or when spending evenings with her friends. Her snacks consist of a variety of foods ranging from fruit to potato chips and pizza.

The clinical evaluation reveals no abnormalities or specific alterations. The triceps skin fold is 30 mm (1.2 in).

QUESTIONS

1. Given the above data, what nursing diagnosis would be made?
2. What approach might one use in setting goals with Susan?
3. To what community resources might Susan be referred in her efforts to lose weight?
4. What mechanism for follow-up could a nurse establish with Susan?

ADULTHOOD

Frequently, the adult client is seen by a nurse only when a disease alteration is present. Although there is an increasing move toward preventive health care through community health services, most adults do not seek regular follow-up unless they think some need is not being met. Because of this, the nurse needs to conduct some kind of nutritional assessment on every patient given treatment.

It is at the adult stage of development that many of the long-term nutritional deficiencies or alterations first manifest themselves as disease. The most common disorder in the United States is heart disease resulting from atherosclerosis from a diet high in saturated fat and cholesterol. Early identification of alterations in eating patterns allow diet and activity modification to occur at a time when the body can return to a more healthy state.

The role of nutrition in the development of such diseases as cancer, diabetes mellitus, gout, hyperlipidemias, cerebrovascular accidents, and skin lesions is incompletely understood. Most experienced clinicians will testify to the apparent role of good nutrition in rehabilitation and client recovery from disease or injury. Most adults assessed will fall into one of four major categories of nutritional diagnosis. The first category is those adults who require no intervention for health maintenance. These clients are usually living in the community and entering the health care system for preventive intervention only. The second category is clients with excessive intake of various nutrients. In the United States the excess foods are usually carbohydrates, fats, or those foods containing excess sodium. Occasionally, however, because of food fads, excesses of other nutrients may occur. The client with deficiencies in specific nutrients or Calories is in the third major category of nutritional diagnosis. Most nutritional intervention is directed toward these clients.

The fourth category are those adults with problems that are not directly related to nutritional concerns but that affect nutritional intake or requirements. Examples of such clients include those undergoing surgery or radiation therapy or those who have such diseases as ulcerative colitis or alcoholism. It is this group of patients whose nutritional concerns are most often left unmet by health professionals. The nutritional concerns, although not primary, frequently have a significant bearing on how the disease or therapy progresses. The potential problems associated with nutritional status are those that can be prevented if only they are recognized early.

Nutritional assessment of the adult involves all three components of the nutritional assessment. The depth to which each component is carried out depends on the client's problems and the nurse's purpose in intervening.

Dietary History

The diet history yields most meaningful data if two or more methods are utilized. Commonly, information regarding a client's "usual" intake coupled with a 24-hour recall will provide a firm basis for continued investigation. The nurse must be especially alert for clues to present food habits, ethnic influences, meal patterns, any trend toward "empty-Calorie" consumption, and the use of dietary supplements or substitutes (Fig. 20-9). If no quantitative data are necessary, an in-depth dietary history, a household survey, or a three- to seven-day diary may yield substantive data.

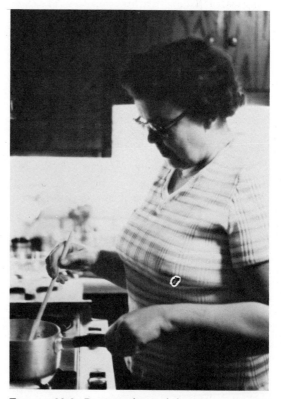

Figure 20-9. During the adult years nutrient needs stabilize but caloric requirements decrease with each decade.

Clinical Assessment

General medical history should include information regarding socioeconomic level; family size and structure; past health problems and concerns; and a brief review of body systems in relation to any problems experienced. The family's history of disease, particularly that of a chronic nature, needs to be investigated. An estimate of physical activity levels and energy expenditure patterns is useful in determining necessary daily requirements for the client.

The physical examination should provide data about all the systems. The nurse should pay particular attention to the hair, skin, eyes, nose, oral cavity, and mucous membranes. Goiter and deep tendon reflexes are also evaluated. Vital signs including blood pressure are important indexes of physiological status that need to be evaluated.

Anthropometric data should include height and weight, triceps skin-fold thickness, and arm circumference. Such techniques are easy to carry out accurately and yield meaningful data rapidly.

Laboratory Assessment

Laboratory data should include hemoglobin and hematocrit values, urine glucose and ketone levels, and a white cell differential. Skin tests for common antigens such as mumps will aid in the detection of those adults with visceral protein depletion. Albumin and transferrin levels are also important to evaluate available serum protein levels. More sophisticated tests involving concentrations of various nutrients are called for in the client with suspected nutritional deficiency.

After the data is gathered, it needs to be evaluated for validity and reliability. Just as a nurse with keen assessment skills notes a patient's pending anoxia, so the same nurse may detect a patient's pending protein-Calorie malnutrition. The nurse should use all the resources of the entire health care team when attempting to meet the needs of the adult client.

It is important that the nurse, as a professional clinician, be dedicated to nutritional assessment as one phase of total patient assessment. Only through the nurse's ability to view the patient continuously can a total nutritional program be initiated. Figure 20-2 is an appropriate assessment tool for use with adults.

CASE STUDY: A Middle-aged Adult Admitted for a General Work-up

Martha C. is a 59-year-old former legal secretary admitted to the hospital for evaluation of chronic obstructive lung disease (emphysema type) and a weight loss of 38 lb (17.3 kg) over the past five years. Her current weight is 88 lb (40 kg). She has smoked for 40 years, averaging two packs of cigarettes a day. Her doctor first diagnosed her emphysema two years ago. Since that time she has decreased her smoking to about four cigarettes a day. In addition to her weight loss, Martha has become increasingly exhausted and short of breath with exertion. She becomes short of breath when making a bed or when eating. Her symptoms are worse in the morning, with her ability to tolerate activity progressively increasing throughout the day. The physician has diagnosed Martha as having "pink puffer" emphysema. After extensive diagnostic tests he attributes her weight loss to lack of ingestion of food and the increased work of breathing she experiences whenever she eats.

QUESTIONS

1. Given that Martha must cook her own meals, what resources might make this chore less difficult?

2. How could Martha conserve her energy level during and after eating?

3. What mechanism should be used to gather dietary intake data on Martha?

4. What types of goals would be realistic for Martha? What would be a specific example of such a goal?

OLDER ADULTHOOD

The older adult has special needs and concerns, both physiological and psychological, that must be met for continued well-being. It is well known that certain physiological alterations occur normally with aging. These include a decreased cardiac output, decreased elasticity of the skin, slowed gastrointestinal mobility, decreased renal perfusion, slowed nerve conduction, lessened olfactory and gustatory senses, and a decreased vital capacity. Although many of these changes occur in most people, the degree to which and the speed with which they occur vary significantly among people.

The changes that occur in aging are related to a general loss of cells by organ systems or to the reduction in the cellular metabolism of tissues with age. Because of the individual rate at which people age, the nutritional needs and requirements also vary uniquely. The special nutritional concerns of aging arise from medical, psychological, social, and economic conditions that create a person's internal and external environment. Good nutrition for the aged must take these concerns into account in addition to the basic nutritional requirements. The role of adequate nutrition in aging is not completely understood, although case studies seem to indicate that good nutrition from conception through late maturity may mean the difference between a continued active life and disability. Good nutrition is known to affect development during youth and middle age so as to prevent disease and disability that ultimately manifest themselves as serious alterations in the older adult.

The nutritional requirements of older adults differ from those of younger people, with the required Calorie intake proportional to energy expenditure. In general, necessary Calorie intake will decrease after age 55. Because of the relatively high incidence of atherosclerosis in the aging, the older adult usually should adhere to a diet moderate in total fat with a high percentage of the fat in the form of unsaturated oil. Despite strong circumstantial evidence in favor of restricting total fat and of substituting unsaturated for saturated fats, the American Medical Association has cautioned that no direct causal relationship between dietary or serum lipids concentrations and atherosclerosis has been proved. It should be remembered in any event that the prevention or treatment of atherosclerosis is not the prevention of aging. Atherosclerosis is a disease; aging is a normal process. Finally, carbohydrate requirements are not effectively altered by aging. The major problem with the aging adult's diet is obtaining sufficient nutrient concentrations for health maintenance in a diet of limited Calories.

Socioeconomic conditions frequently have the greatest effect on the nutritional status of the older adult. The decline of the extended family and the increased mobility of families in American society decrease the available support systems for the elderly. Housing, transportation, and socialization become frequent problems for the aged. It is obvious how such concerns interfere with the ingestion of a balanced diet. The isolated elderly often become victims of fads that substitute low-nutrient foods for a balanced diet. Such dietary patterns tax an already limited budget. The Meals on Wheels program meets the nutritional needs of its clients as well as assisting with their socialization. Many have no visitors other than the Meals on Wheels volunteers, who may come daily or five days a week. The volunteer server often becomes a good friend of the client. Over one-third of the aged in the United States live below poverty level. Because of fixed incomes, the diets of the aged may consist of cheaper, low-protein foods.

The clinician's creativity is taxed when teaching the elderly person to buy and prepare nutritious foods he can afford and eat. Many large stores provide a discount on selected food items for those over 65 years of age. The client's ability to prepare nutritious meals and the facilities available for preparation must be considered in the nutritional assessment of the aged person. Finally, it must be determined if the client is able to get to the grocery or market to buy food. Those people living in widely scattered rural areas may need to be encouraged to keep a few weeks' supply of food on hand in case inclement weather should occur. Figure 20-10 is an assessment tool for use with the older adult. In conducting any evaluation of an older adult, the nurse must be aware that the person's attitudes, beliefs, and habits are a result of a lifetime of experience. Change, if it occurs at all, will occur slowly and only when the client perceives and believes that a change will be valuable to him.

Dietary History

Minimal dietary information should include the number of meals eaten per day and the regularity of them. The average one- or two-day meal plan is evaluated for the inclusion of the four food groups. In addition, the usual dietary intake should be evaluated against the essential nutrients. The amount of empty food sources such as alcohol or candy should also be noted. The client's likes and dislikes should be noted. Any supplemental vitamins or protein concentrates taken regularly need to be included in background data. It is help-

Name _____

Age _____   Cultural background _____

Dietary History:

Number of meals eaten per day _____   Times _____

Snacks _____
Medications, vitamin supplements:
_____

Usual Intake/24-Hour Recall		
Time	Amount	Food Consumed

Transportation _____
Facilities available for food preparation

Family member responsible for food

preparation _____
Income range _____
Sources of income _____

Medical History:
Past hospitalizations:

Date	Occurrence

Presence of fainting _____, dyspnea _____,

memory loss _____, pain _____, altered

sight _____, loss of hearing _____, urinary

frequency _____, usual bowel pattern _____.

Clinical Evaluation:

Height _____   Weight _____   Skin fold _____

Figure 20-10. Nutritional assessment tool for the older adult.

Review of systems:
    Head, Ears, Eyes, Nose, Throat:

    Skin:

    Neck:

    Chest:

    Heart:

    Back:

    Abdomen:

    Rectum:

    Extremities:

    Neurology:

Laboratory Data:

Hemoglobin ―――――   Serum albumin ―――――   Other: ―――――――――

Hematocrit ―――――   BUN ――――――――――   ――――――――――――

Serum iron ―――――   Glucose ――――――――

Figure 20-10. (*Continued*)

ful to evaluate the client's general knowledge of nutrition and what constitutes a balanced diet. Knowledge of facilities available for transportation and for meal preparation and eating, including the presence or absence of a companion, and of the approximate income level of the client will assist the nurse in developing a meal plan for client and family.

If a detailed dietary intake history is desired, 24-hour recalls are taken at intervals. If the client is hospitalized, Calorie counts are helpful in pointing out problems in consumption.

Clinical Assessment

A detailed medical history is important for gathering information on chronic or acute illnesses that can alter nutritional requirements or ingestion patterns. The medications the client is taking must be considered to prevent potential food-drug interactions. A family history including the spouse's health status is important in estimating physiological and psychological stress. The client's symptoms such as fainting, dizziness, pain, altered sight or hearing, the presence or absence of dentures, and any altered bowel or bladder habits, should be noted. A brief review of symptoms will provide information on the general health and nutritional requirements of the client. If possible, increased communication can be prompted by evaluation of the client's attitudes, fears, and values. Of course, such history taking requires a great deal of interviewing skill. Data gathering may be better accomplished by a series of interviews rather than one long one.

Anthropometric data should include height and weight measurements. Height and weight of people over 60 years of age may not be accurate indication of body composition and nutritional status because of osteoporotic changes. Skin-fold measurements provide some data on fat composition.

The physical examination must be a thorough evaluation of the client's current condition. Overt *cachexia* or obesity should be noted. The mouth should be inspected for dentures, caries, and general oral hygiene. Cardiovascular status needs to be evaluated via blood pressure; peripheral pulse rates; and inspection, auscultation, and percussion of the chest. An EKG will be of some benefit in pointing out overt abnormalities. The client's abdomen should be evaluated for masses, tenderness, and hypo- or hyperactive bowel sounds. The integrity of the skin should be observed carefully, particularly over bony prominences. A gross neurological examination of both motor and sensory status can be easily and quickly carried out on the cooperative client. Included in the examination should also be a gross evaluation of the client's visual and auditory senses.

Laboratory Assessment

Laboratory data that will provide information on which to base a nutritional diagnosis includes hemoglobin and hematocrit values, urinalysis, serum iron level and iron-binding capacity, serum albumin level, blood urea nitrogin level, glucose tolerance, vitamin assays. Specific tests such as barium roentgenography, and lower gastrointestinal evaluation may be done as well.

It is important to remember that renal function decreases normally with aging; therefore, creatinine and blood urea nitrogen levels may be slightly elevated in comparison with those of younger people. Vitamin levels are most frequently altered in older adults with malabsorptive syndrome or in whom ingestion occurs unpredictably.

CASE STUDY: An Older Adult Living in a Nursing Home

Alma R., 80 years old, has been a resident of the county nursing home for eight years. Alma was admitted after surgery for a broken hip. She remains alert and oriented, although she wears glasses and uses a hearing aid. Alma's general mobility is limited; she can walk only with assistance or a walker. Alma's general physical status remains stable. She has documented congestive heart failure controlled by digitalis and furosemide. She generally has pitting edema in her ankles, relieved by elevation. Her gastrointestinal system is normal, but she has occasional bouts of diarrhea. She eats a soft diet because of poor-fitting dentures, and she enjoys peppermint sticks between meals. Alma is 5 ft (152.4 cm) tall and weighs 96 lb (43.6 kg). Her primary social activities are occupational therapy, group singing, and knitting. Alma enjoys going to church on Sunday mornings in the recreation room of the nursing home.

Alma's food intake is limited by the menu at the home. She usually has mashed potatoes, ground meat, a green vegetable, and fruit or ice cream for both lunch and dinner. Breakfast consists of hot cereal, scrambled eggs, and milk. Between-meal candy and other sweets are occasionally provided by volunteers from various community agencies.

QUESTIONS

1. What would be the nutritional nursing diagnoses for Alma?
2. What type of dietary intake data would help establish this diagnosis?
3. What specific effect does Alma's nutritional status have on her total health status?

4. How might an extended care facility make mealtimes more enjoyable for patients?

BIBLIOGRAPHY

Caly, J. C. Assessing adults nutrition. *Am. J. Nurs.* 77:1605, 1977.

Christakis, G. Nutritional assessment in health programs. *Am. J. Public Health* 63 (Supple.), 1973.

Dansky, K. Assessing children's nutrition. *Am. J. Nurs.* 77:1610, 1977.

Fisher, S., Hendricks, D., and Mahoney, A. W. Nutritional assessment of senior rural adults by biochemical and physical measurements. *Am. J. Clin. Nutr.* 3:667, 1978.

Foman, S. J. *Infant Nutrition.* 2nd Ed. Philadelphia: W. B. Saunders Co., 1974.

Gain, S., and Clark, D. C. Problems in the nutritional assessment of black individuals. *Am. J. Public Health* 66:262, 1976.

Hanson, R. G. Considering "social nutrition" in assessing geriatric nutrition. *Geriatrics.* 33(3):49, 1978.

Head, M., and Werks, R. Major nutrients in the type a lunch. *J. Am. Diet. Assoc.* 67:356, 1975.

Lechtig, A., Delgado, H., Yarbrough, C., Habint, J. P., Martouee, R., and Klein, R. A simple assessment of the risk of low birth weight to select women for nutritional intervention. *Am. J. Obstet. Gynecol.* 125:25, 1976.

Luke, B. A nutritional assessment of the expectant mother: How and why. *Keeping Abreast Journal* 2(4):280, 1977.

Markesbery, B., and Wong, W. Points for maternity patients. *Am. J. Nurs.* 77:1612, 1977.

Snyderman, S., and Holt, L. E. Nutrition in infancy and adolescence. In R. S. Goodhart and M. E. Shils, Ed., *Modern Nutrition in Health and Disease,* 5th Ed. Philadelphia: Lea & Lebiger, 1973.

Sun, U., Ghai, O. P., and Rangaswami, R. An evaluation of age: Independent anthropometric indices for the assessment of nutritional status in pre-school children. *Indian J. Med. Res.* 63:66, 1975.

Zerfas, A. F., Shorr, I. J., and Neumann, C. G. African assessment of nutritional status. *Pediatr. Clin. North Am.* 24:253, 1977.

CHAPTER 21

Nursing Diagnosis Based on Assessment of the Nutritive Process

For many years nurses have been formulating "problem lists," "statements of patient needs," "assessment lists," and other assorted lists that describe a client's condition so that nursing actions and interventions can be purposeful. More recently, the field of nursing has come to believe that nurses can state health problems intelligently based on a systematic evaluation of a client's biopsychosocial status. The end product of such directive investigation is aptly termed a *nursing diagnosis*. Because of the rather recent development of a scientific approach to in-depth nursing assessments, nursing diagnosis remains in its infancy. More often than not, nurses return to their more comfortable dependent role and use the medical diagnosis as a basis for intervention. In so doing, nurses once again fall into the trap of not acknowledging the difference between nursing and medicine and thereby negating the very real and unique contribution independent nursing activities can make to quality comprehensive client care. Nurses should begin to document their contribution to the client's care. If they ignore this challenge, they render nursing forever a dependent, task-oriented occupation rather than a true profession.

One of the most exciting ways of documenting what nursing does is by developing and using nursing diagnoses. The professional nurse possesses a selective body of knowledge derived from the biological, physical, and psychosocial sciences that enables her to make statements about the health status of a client. In addition, the nurse is uniquely able to identify those problems that are truly nursing concerns and that nurses are capable of treating and licensed to treat. When the nurse recognizes a health problem beyond the scope of independent nursing practice, she must work in conjunction with physicians, dietitians, and other health professionals.

In the not-too-distant future, particularly after the onset of third-party payment for nursing, nurses will be reimbursed for and evaluated on the accuracy and scope of their nursing diagnoses for a particular client or group. Diagnoses based on the areas of independent nursing function will document nursing's contribution to health care.

Because nursing diagnosis remains unfamiliar territory for many of the practitioners providing care today, guidelines have been developed that help to narrow a client's problem to the areas where specific nursing interventions can be implemented. The diagnostic statement is a culmination of the assessment process. Frequently the problem of the practitioner centers around narrowing all the data into groups of problems that can be assigned priorities and be addressed by specific actions.

Campbell (1978) has developed the following criteria that can be used to evaluate a statement to determine whether or not it is a nursing diagnosis:

1. The statement describes a human response or a limitation of resources.

2. The problem identified can be dealt with by the professional nurse independent of medical direction.

3. The diagnosis occurs repeatedly in a significant number of clients. Of course, the circumstances surrounding the problem create a unique situation for each client.

4. The problem is a consequence of, contributing factor to, or potential danger leading to illness, injury, disease, or health maintenance (p. 12).

The client or group of clients may have one or more needs that have bearing on the diagnosis. The nurse can use Maslow's (1962) hierarchy (see Chap. 18) to determine the relative importance of each need identified. The data that supports the diagnosis can be obtained through nursing assessment. Further, the analysis and judgments required to deduce the problem can be made by the professional nurse in the light of nursing knowledge and the growing body of nursing science. Finally, to assure that the nursing diagnosis is unique, the patient problem or alteration must not be identified as a disease in the standard medical classification systems.

The fact that medical diagnostic statements do not address the areas of hygiene, assistance, comfort, and prevention and safety confirms that these areas of health care are within the scope of nursing. Nurses are generally much more cognizant of the physician's role than physicians are of the nurse's. Because of this, the nurse's practice is saturated with medical terminology, making it difficult even to discuss nursing therapy without functioning within the scope of medicine. Such a problem is not easily overcome, nor should it be completely. The nurse must recognize that there are many areas of overlapping responsibility between the nurse, the physician, and other health professionals. Gray areas must be recognized and accepted, but a nurse should not focus her practice solely on these mutual domains.

The purpose of this chapter is to delineate specific nursing diagnoses that can be anticipated in nursing situations with clients having problems with ingestion, digestion, absorption, nutrient transport, metabolism, or excretion. The diagnoses identified are meant to include both potential and actual interferences with client needs. The specific setting and client will determine whether a problem is overt or covert.

The diagnoses discussed include a problem statement, the probable cause or causes, and the assessment data the nurse can anticipate finding. Interventions and methods of evaluation are discussed in Unit V. The problems are classified according to the general nutritional concern involved. The student is encouraged to use the remainder of this chapter as a reference tool when developing nutritionally related nursing diagnoses.

Campbell (1978) has developed an extensive listing of nursing diagnoses and appropriate nursing interventions. She has laid the groundwork for the development of a classification of nursing diagnosis centering on human need theory. Because the diagnoses presented in this chapter are nutritionally related, a classification system developed around the nutritive process and altered nutritional states is used. The diagnoses are classified by areas of potential alteration rather than by specific disorders, so that the student can develop pertinent nursing interventions for the problem identified. An example of such classification is the diagnosis "electrolyte imbalance related to calcium intake." This diagnosis is classified under "nutrient transport" rather than "ingestion" because the primary *effect* of the alteration is in the area of nutrient transport rather than ingestion. In other words, the underlying cause is actually a disorder or condition, but the nursing diagnosis describes the effect of the alteration on the client. The student should note that not all nursing diagnoses centering on nutritional status require dietary modifications. Those that do are discussed in Unit V.

OVERVIEW OF NUTRITIONAL NURSING DIAGNOSES

I. Interferences with ingestion
   A. Manifested by a lack of information
   B. Manifested by the inaccessibility of nutrients
   C. Manifested by a lack of desire to ingest food and fluids
   D. Manifested by the inability to ingest food and fluids
   E. Manifested by oral discomfort and/or obstruction
   F. Manifested by alterations in ingestion that have already occurred

II. Alterations in digestion and absorption
   A. Manifested by alterations in motility
   B. Manifested by alterations in secretions
   C. Manifested by alterations in absorptive surface

III. Alterations in nutrient transport
   A. Manifested by alterations in vascular physiology
   B. Manifested by blockage of nutrient transport
   C. Manifested by electrolyte imbalance
   D. Manifested by oxygen/carbon dioxide alterations
   E. Manifested by fluid volume alterations
   F. Manifested by changes in blood pH

IV. Alterations in metabolism
   A. Manifested by alterations in nutritional requirements
   B. Manifested by alterations in endocrine physiology
   C. Manifested by alterations in structure

V. Alterations in excretion
   A. Manifested by alterations in fluid output
   B. Manifested by alterations in solid waste output

DETAILED CLASSIFICATION OF NUTRITIONAL NURSING DIAGNOSES

I. Interferences with ingestion
   A. Manifested by a lack of information
      1. Dependence on communication assistance related to
         a. Impaired speech delivery
         b. Impaired writing ability
         c. Impaired reading ability
         d. Impaired hearing ability
         Assessment data may reveal:
         A subjective feeling of frustration, isolation, anxiety; objective observation of the inability to form words or make sounds, inability to recognize words, difficulty in speaking, inability to read or write, difficulty hearing or interpreting words.
      2. Inadequate information related to foreign-food hazards
         Assessment data may reveal:
         Client may be planning a trip to a foreign country. Client's lack of information about the specific foods to avoid in foreign countries, lack of information about how to request foods to be prepared.
      3. Inadequate information about food allergies related to
         a. Lack of instruction
         b. Lack of communication
         Assessment data may reveal:
         Client's lack of understanding of signs of allergy; client's lack of understanding of what an allergy is; client's lack of understanding of the causes of allergy. (Signs of allergic reaction may include: hives, rash, respiratory distress, pruritis, nasal congestion, oral edema, vomiting, diarrhea.)
      4. Lack of information about proper food intake related to
         a. Lack of instruction
         b. Adherence to cultural food patterns

Assessment data may reveal:
The presence or history of food faddism, ingestion of unbalanced diet, obesity, malnutrition, client's lack of understanding about proper food intake.

5. Dependence on instruction on prenatal nutrition related to
   a. Pregnancy
   b. Lack of information
   Assessment data may reveal:
   Reliance on nurse for guidance on weight control, nutrient intake, and exercise. Woman is pregnant.

6. Reliance on instruction on postnatal nutrition related to
   a. Pregnancy
   b. Lack of information
   Assessment data may reveal:
   Reliance on nurse for guidance on weight control, nutrient intake, and exercise. Woman has recently delivered.

7. Noncompliance with therapeutic regimen related to
   a. Lack of information
   b. Hostility
   c. Denial
   d. Dependency conflict
   e. Lifestyle
   Assessment data may reveal:
   Anger, anxiety, misperception of directions, multiple excuses for noncompliance. Client has not complied with diet or other therapeutic regimens.

B. Manifested by the inaccessibility of nutrients

1. Potential inadequate fluid intake related to
   a. Fluid inaccessibility
   b. Refusal to drink fluids
   c. Inability to drink fluids
   d. Fluid restriction
   Assessment data may reveal:
   Mouth tenderness, weakness, dysphagia, inability to ingest fluids without assistance, confusion, hostility, poor skin turgor.

2. Thirst discomfort related to
   a. Fluid restriction
   b. Increased sodium retention
   c. Excessive fluid loss
   d. Lack of fluid intake
   Assessment data may reveal:
   A subjective feeling of dry mouth, preoccupation with the attainment of fluids, poor skin turgor, dry mouth and mucous membranes; laboratory data showing an increased sodium level and an increased serum osmolality.

3. Inadequate nutrient intake related to
   a. Poor eating habits
   b. Lack of available foods
   c. Lack of knowledge about proper diet
   d. Difficulty with ingestion
   Assessment data may reveal:
   Weakness, hunger, nausea, fatigue, peripheral numbness and tingling, chronic weight loss to the point of being underweight, pallor, restlessness, pica.

C. Manifested by a lack of desire to ingest food and fluids

1. Anorexia related to
   a. Emotional stress
   b. Drug toxicity
   c. Nausea and/or vomiting
   d. Concurrent illness
   Assessment data may reveal:
   A lack of enthusiasm for food, preference not to eat, consumption of only small portions of foods, lack of ingestion of food.

2. Impaired ability to taste food related to
   a. Cranial nerve impairment
   b. Central nervous system lesion
   c. Nasal infection

d. Use of tobacco

e. Injury to olfactory end organs

Assessment data may reveal:
Reports of foods tasting flat or the same; inability to distinguish tastes such as bitter, sweet, sour, salty; decreased appetite.

3. Nausea related to

a. Reduced peristalsis

b. Acidosis

c. Impaired cardiac circulation

d. Gastric irritation

e. Infection

f. Decreased blood pressure

g. Adrenal insufficiency

h. Displaced stomach by mass or pregnant uterus

i. Altered hormonal levels

Assessment data may reveal:
A subjective feeling of uneasiness and queasy stomach, difficulty eating.

4. Intra-abdominal pressure discomfort related to

a. Diminished peristalsis

b. Surgery

Assessment data may reveal:
Abdominal tightness with severe pressure sensation, restlessness, abdominal distention, mild dyspnea, hypoactive bowel sounds.

5. Food selection dissatisfaction related to

a. Lack of food variety

b. Cultural food patterns

c. Need for increased attention

d. Need to maintain control over own environment

Assessment data may reveal:
Anger, withdrawal, frequent complaints about food preparation, irritability, refusal to eat available food.

6. Difficulty maintaining a religious diet related to

a. Dependence on diet preparation by others

b. Need for specific therapeutic diet

c. Hospitalization

d. Change in lifestyle

Assessment data may reveal:
Anxiety, guilt feelings, inability to use or avoid required or prohibited foods (see Table 21-1).

D. Manifested by the inability to ingest food and fluids

1. Inability to feed self related to

a. Muscle weakness

b. Limited range of motion

c. Immobility

d. Neuromuscular incoordination

Assessment data may reveal:
Client is unable to feed self. Client relies on nurse for positioning. Use of assistive devices, frequent spilling of foods, impaired visibility, temporary or permanent immobility.

2. Inadequate fluid intake related to

a. Fluid inaccessibility

b. Refusal to drink fluids

c. Inability to drink fluids

d. Fluid restriction

Assessment data may reveal:
thirst, decreased urine output, fluid intake less than 800 cc per 24 hours, dry skin, poor skin turgor, weight loss; laboratory data showing increased urine specific gravity, hematocrit, and red blood count. Client may have a limited range of motion that prohibits fluid ingestion.

3. Fatigue upon eating related to

a. Endocrine imbalance

b. Malnutrition

TABLE 21.1 Prohibited Foods and Food Combinations of Selected Religions

Faith	Foods and Food Combinations
Jewish (Kosher)	Pork and pork products; shellfish; fish without fins and scales; meat from animals who do not have cloven hooves and do not chew their cuds; birds of prey; meat from the hind quarters of the animal; meat and milk at the same meal; fish on the same plate as meat or dairy products
Seventh-Day Adventist	Coffee, tea, meat, alcohol, caffeinated beverages
Mormon	Coffee, tea, caffeinated beverages, alcohol

NOTE: There may be certain food practices (such as using separate plates, utensils, and cooking vessels for dairy and meat meals) that the practitioner should be aware of when working with a client.

c. Energy depletion from prolonged illness

Assessment data may reveal:
Dyspnea after eating, extreme fatigue, inability to eat more than one or two bites of food.

4. Difficulty feeding (in infants) related to

    a. Intolerance of formula

    b. Small stomach capacity

    c. Inadequate muscle development

Assessment data may reveal:
Generalized infant weakness, intake of only small amounts of food, intolerance to food (regurgitates food taken).

5. Diminished sucking ability (in infants) related to

    a. Immature nervous system development

    b. Weakness

    c. Gastrointestinal disturbance

Assessment data may reveal:
General weakness; lack of sucking reflex on stimulation.

6. Dependence on tube feeding management related to

    a. Inability to obtain adequate nutrition through oral ingestion

Assessment data may reveal:
Presence of gastrostomy, jejunostomy, or nasogastric tube. Client relies on nurse for administration of feeding and maintenance of tube.

7. Hiccough related to

    a. Contraction of diaphragm

    b. Irritation of phrenic nerve

Assessment data may reveal:
Fatigue, nausea, persistent hiccough spasm, emesis

8. Vomiting related to

    a. Increased intercranial pressure

    b. Intestinal infection

    c. Electrolyte imbalance

    d. Gastric irritation from foods or drugs

    e. Equilibrium imbalance

    f. Acidosis

    g. Impaired cardiac circulation

    h. Internal organ irritation or inflammation

Assessment data may reveal:
Weakness, bad taste in the mouth, regurgitation of stomach contents.

9. Hyperemesis related to

    a. Endocrine or metabolic imbalance

    b. Pregnancy

    c. CNS alteration

Assessment data may reveal:
Headaches, dizziness, weakness, prolonged vomiting, weight loss, tachycardia, signs of dehydration (poor skin turgor, decreased urine output, dry skin and mucous membranes). Client may be pregnant or have a history of toxemia, liver car-

cinoma, or glomerulonephritis. If related to pregnancy, hyperemesis occurs primarily in the morning hours.

10. Dependence on hyperalimentation management related to
    a. Lack of oral intake
    b. Malabsorption syndrome
    c. Increased nutritional requirements such as occur after surgery, burns, or wounds
    Assessment data may reveal: Client relies on the nurse for: hyperalimentation/intralipid administration, maintenance of sterile IV line and dressing, observation of potential complications of therapy.

E. Manifested by oral discomfort and/or obstruction
    1. Oral tenderness related to
       a. Chronic tissue irritation
       b. Cancer
       c. Surgery
       d. Trauma from chemical, thermal, or mechanical means
       e. Radiation therapy
       f. Drug effects
       Assessment data may reveal: Pain in mouth; edematous oral mucosa, tongue organs; oral ulceration.
    2. Oral-cavity bleeding related to
       a. Trauma
       b. Blood-clotting disorders
       c. Blood dyscrasias
       d. Radium therapy
       Assessment data may reveal: Bleeding in the mouth, blood clots in the mouth, oral petechiae; spitting up blood.
    3. Bleeding gums related to
       a. Blood dyscrasias
       b. Clotting disorders

       c. Infection
       d. Tartar accumulation on the teeth
       e. Poisonings: lead, arsenic, mercury
       Assessment data may reveal: Blood oozing from the gums, clot formation around the teeth, a history of poor dental hygiene.
    4. Sensitive teeth related to
       a. Loss of tooth enamel
       b. Gum disease
       c. Rapid ingestion of hot or cold substances
       Assessment data may reveal: Generalized pain in all the teeth stimulated by hot, cold, or very hard foods.
    5. Teething pain related to normal tooth development
       Assessment data may reveal: Pain in area of erupting tooth, irritability, anorexia, crying, drooling, appearance of teeth.
    6. Predisposition to tooth decay related to
       a. Poor dental hygiene
       b. Poor nutrition
       c. Position of teeth in mouth
       Assessment data may reveal: Infrequent tooth brushing, client residing in an area where water is not fluoridated; use of a nonfluoride toothpaste; overingestion of carbohydrates; crowded teeth; profuse salivation.
    7. Toothache related to
       a. Tooth decay
       b. Dental pulp inflammation
       Assessment data may reveal: Localized throbbing, continuous pain in areas surrounding the tooth, restlessness, inability to sleep, jaw swelling.

8. Oral discomfort related to poorly fitting dentures

   Assessment data may reveal:
   Oral pain, reddened gums, gum tenderness or swelling, loose-fitting dentures.

9. Throat soreness related to infection

   Assessment data may reveal:
   Localized, continuous throat pain, increased with swallowing; throat redness; edema; fever; lymph-node enlargement; throat exudate.

10. Difficulty chewing related to

    a. Loss of teeth

    b. Muscle weakness

    c. Nerve injury

    d. Inflamed oral mucous membrane

    e. Poorly fitting dentures

    Assessment data may reveal:
    Painful chewing, poor control of food when chewing, impaired jaw movement, inability to clench teeth.

11. Difficulty swallowing related to

    a. Edema of throat; obstruction, inflammation, or irritation

    b. Emotional stress

    Assessment data may reveal:
    Throat tightness, pain on swallowing, ability to swallow only small amounts of food, drooling.

F. Manifested by alterations in ingestion that have already occurred

   1. Obesity related to

      a. Overingestion of nutrients

      b. Endocrine imbalance

      c. CNS damage

      Assessment data may reveal:
      Chronic fatigue, weight 20% over ideal body weight, triceps skin-fold thickness greater than 20 mm, dyspnea on exertion.

   2. Excessive caffeine intake related to

      a. Habit

      b. Need for stimulation

      Assessment data may reveal:
      Consumption of five or more cups of coffee a day, irritability in absence of caffeine consumption, reliance on coffee to offset fatigue.

   3. Food poisoning related to

      a. Ingestion of staphylococci (2–4 hours onset)

      b. Ingestion of salmonellae (6–48 hours onset)

      c. Mushroom poisoning (15 hours)

      d. Botulism (18–48 hours onset)

      Assessment data may reveal:
      Cramping abdominal pain, nausea, chills, fever, diarrhea, vomiting. If botulism, client may also experience dizziness, blurred vision, muscle weakness, and respiratory rigidity.

   4. Excessive vitamin and mineral ingestion related to

      a. Lack of education

      b. Food faddism

      c. Overdosage

      Assessment data may reveal:
      Alopecia, bone and joint pain, dry skin, jaundice.

   5. Food allergies

      Assessment data may reveal:
      Itching, headache, gastrointestinal inflammation, and swelling.

   6. Excessive intake of alcohol related to

      a. Habit

      b. Need for social acceptance

      c. Addiction

II. Alterations in digestion and absorption

   A. Manifested by alterations in motility

      1. Biliary colic pain related to

         a. Bile-duct obstruction

         Assessment data may reveal:
         Localized and/or referred pain to

right upper quadrant and/or abdominal pain. Pain may radiate to right shoulder and back. Pain is acute, severe, and continuous. Client may experience excessive belching, yellow-green emesis, gurgling bowel sounds.

2. Gastrointestinal spasms related to

   a. Vagal-nerve stimulation

   b. Overwork

   c. Severe stress or excitement

   Assessment data may reveal:
   Intermittent, localized, abdominal pain; hyperperistalsis, alternating diarrhea and constipation.

3. Excessive regurgitation related to

   a. Stomach contents pressing against the cardiac sphincter.

   Assessment data may reveal:
   Regurgitation after meals, accompanied by a sour taste in the mouth.

4. Flatulence related to

   a. Swallowed air

   b. Rapid eating

   c. Ingestion of gas-forming foods

   Assessment data may reveal:
   A subjective feeling of fullness, gas pains, mild abdominal distention, abdominal tympany upon percussion, gurgling bowel sounds.

5. Indigestion related to

   a. Intolerance of food or drugs

   b. Decreased motility

   Assessment data may reveal:
   Nausea, abdominal cramps, abdominal distention, diarrhea, anorexia.

6. Potential impaired intestinal circulation related to

   a. Hernia

   Assessment data may reveal:
   Nausea, a visible abdominal hernia, a history of heavy lifting or recent surgery.

7. Pain in esophagus related to

   a. Inflammation of esophageal wall

   b. Burns

   c. Prolonged gastric intubation

   d. Ingestion of poisonous substances

   Assessment data may reveal:
   A history of ingestion of poisonous substances, prolonged nasogastric tube placement, heartburn, pain following ingestion of very hot or cold foods, dysphagia.

B. Manifested by alterations in secretions

   1. Gastrointestinal-cardiac pain related to

      a. Gall bladder pain

      b. Pancreatic enzyme action on cardiac muscles

      c. Peptic ulcer

      Assessment data may reveal:
      Vomiting, anorexia, normal cardiogram, normal cardiac enzymes, localized or referred pain. In gall bladder: radiation to substernal region, cramping pain. In pancreatic enzyme action: right epigastric, midepigastric, and left lower epigastric pain; radiation to sternum or scapula. In boring stomach ulceration: lower anterior bandlike pain, radiation to intrascapular area of right shoulder (aching, burning, gnawing pain).

   2. Potential development of stress ulcer related to

      a. Hyperacidity

      b. Steroid therapy

      c. Rapid protein loss

      d. Chronic stress

      Assessment data may reveal:
      A history of major infection, surgical procedures, burns, or serious gastric ulcer. Lifestyle may entail frequent stress.

   3. Potential gastric distress related to the ingestion of irritating foods or chemicals

Assessment data may reveal:
A history of ingestion of drugs known to be gastric irritants, of highly spiced foods, or of substances that have consistently caused gastric distress.

4. Heartburn related to
   a. Hiatal hernia
   b. Esophageal distention
   c. Reflex of stomach contents into esophagus
   d. Habitual air swallowing

   Assessment data may reveal:
   Burning, wavelike sensation issuing from the stomach; chest tightness; recent history of ingesting heavy, spicy foods. Client may receive relief by opening the mouth with occasional belching.

C. Manifested by alterations in absorptive surface
   1. Inadequate nutrient availability related to malabsorption

      Assessment data may reveal:
      Diarrhea, nausea, loss of weight, fatigue, weakness, skin lesions.

III. Alterations in nutrient transport

A. Manifested by alterations in vascular physiology
   1. Predisposition to cardiovascular disease related to
      a. Genetic predisposition (familial hypertension)
      b. Prolonged stress

      Assessment data may reveal:
      A subjective feeling of prolonged fatigue; smoking, lack of leisure time or activities, obesity; hypertension; diet high in saturated fats and salts; increased serum cholesterol levels, multiple jobs; lack of regular exercise.

   2. Lifestyle inappropriate to cardiac disease related to
      a. Lack of information about heart disease
      b. Stressful environment

      Assessment data may reveal:
      A subjective feeling of urgency, restlessness, little leisure time, frequent mobility in job and home, multiple jobs, lack of social or leisure activities, a history of myocardial infarction.

   3. Predisposition to hypertension related to
      a. Obesity
      b. Lifestyle
      c. Familial tendency
      d. Physical status

      Assessment data may reveal:
      Smoking, sedentary lifestyle, agressive behavior, obesity, high salt and fat intake, gradual increase in blood pressure, pregnancy, client black, family history of hypertensive disease.

   4. Dependence on nursing supervision of controlled hypertension related to
      a. Hypertension
      b. Antihypertensive therapy
      c. Lack of ability to monitor own blood pressure course

      Assessment data may reveal:
      Reliance on nurse for blood pressure monitoring, required observation of antihypertensive therapy and side effects, required observation of diet therapy, required observation for hypertensive complications.

   5. Increased arterial blood pressure related to
      a. Obesity
      b. Atherosclerosis
      c. Fluid overload
      d. Increased metabolic rate
      e. Drug side effects
      f. Increased arterial resistance (e.g., renal disease)

      Assessment data may reveal:
      Weakness; dizziness; fatigue; headache; flushed face; epistaxis; blood

pressure significantly higher than client's norm, usually greater than 140/90.

6. Decreased arterial blood pressure related to
   a. Decreased cardiac output
   b. Severe blood loss
   c. Anaphylactic shock
   d. Drug side effect
   e. Blood-flow obstruction

   Assessment data may reveal:
   A subjective feeling of weakness, anxiety, dizziness, or fatigue; a blood pressure significantly decreased from client's norm, usually below 90/60; tachycardia; weak, thready pulse.

B. Manifested by blockage of nutrient transport
   1. Impaired lymph circulation related to
      a. Obstructed lymph flow (e.g., after surgery)
      b. Bacterial infection
      c. Inflammation of subcutaneous lymph vessels

      Assessment data may reveal:
      Pain; nonpitting edema; a history of carcinoma, radical mastectomy, or filariasis.

   2. Potential airway obstruction related to
      a. Structural abnormality of respiratory organ
      b. Poor control over respiratory and swallowing reflex

      Assessment data may reveal:
      Dyspnea; alterations in consciousness; ENT surgery; nasal edema; thick airway secretions; rapid eating or drinking, laughing, or coughing when eating; eating while lying down.

   3. Potential peripheral anoxia related to
      a. Peripheral vascular disease
      b. Constrictive clothing

      Assessment data may reveal:
      Cold skin at peripheral extremities, peripheral cyanosis, pain at site, tingling of hands and feet, numbness of hands and feet, decreased mobility.

C. Manifested by electrolyte imbalance
   1. Potential electrolyte imbalance related to potassium infusion

      Assessment data may reveal:
      Client is receiving prolonged intravenous therapy with large doses of potassium.

   2. Potential electrolyte imbalance related to inadequate fluid intake

      Assessment data may reveal:
      Less than 1,500 cc daily fluid intake over a prolonged period of time.

   3. Potential electrolyte imbalance related to dextrose infusion

      Assessment data may reveal:
      Client is receiving intravenous therapy of electrolyte-free solutions.

   4. Potential electrolyte imbalance related to T-tube drainage (and subsequent loss of sodium and potassium)

      Assessment data may reveal:
      Presence of a T tube with profuse bile drainage.

   5. Potential electrolyte imbalance related to colostomy drainage (and subsequent loss of sodium and potassium)

      Assessment data may reveal:
      Excessive colostomy drainage without replacement of electrolytes.

   6. Potential electrolyte imbalance related to adrenal-steroid therapy (that raises the reabsorption of sodium)

      Assessment data may reveal:
      A history of prolonged steroid therapy.

   7. Potential electrolyte imbalance related to gastric suction

      Assessment data may reveal:

A prolonged period of gastric suction in which secretions are removed without peripheral replacement.

8. Potential electrolyte imbalance related to inadequate sodium intake

    Assessment data may reveal:
    A subjective feeling of weakness coinciding with prolonged low sodium intake.

9. Potential electrolyte imbalance related to excessive sodium intake

    Assessment data may reveal:
    Edema, overingestion of sodium, and chronic use of saline laxatives.

10. Electrolyte imbalance related to
    a. Prolonged emesis
    b. Prolonged diarrhea

    Assessment data may reveal:
    Weakness, apathy, confusion, headache, vertigo, fatigue, muscle cramps, decreased blood pressure, flabby muscles, poor skin turgor. Client will have a history of prolonged vomiting or diarrhea. Laboratory data will show decreased serum potassium and sodium levels.

11. Electrolyte imbalance related to fistula drainage (and subsequent loss of sodium)

    Assessment data may reveal:
    Abdominal and muscle cramping, fatique; headache; vertigo; decreased blood pressure; poor skin turgor; laboratory data showing a decreased serum sodium. A rectal, vaginal, or colonic fistula will be present.

12. Electrolyte imbalance related to diaphoresis

    Assessment data may reveal:
    Chilling, very wet skin, a decreased serum sodium. Client may be experiencing fever, shock, or hypoglycemia.

13. Electrolyte imbalance related to diuresis

    Assessment data may reveal:
    Weakness; apathy; soft, flabby muscles; cardiac arrhythmias; laboratory data showing a lowered serum potassium level. Client will have been taking potassium-depleting diuretics. Less than 30 mEq of potassium is being replaced daily.

14. Electrolyte imbalance related to malnutrition

    Assessment data may reveal:
    Weakness; apathy; confusion; soft, flabby muscles; laboratory data showing a decreased serum potassium. Client will have a history of inadequate dietary intake particularly of potassium-containing foods.

15. Electrolyte imbalance related to inadequate calcium intake

    Assessment data will reveal:
    A numbness and tingling of extremities, muscle twitching, muscle cramping, palpitations, irritability, laboratory data showing a decreased serum calcium with elevated serum phosphate. Client will have a history of inadequate calcium intake. If depletion is chronic, client will manifest rough, dry skin and sparse hair. Hypocalcemia may result from intensive blood transfusion therapy.

16. Electrolyte imbalance related to excessive calcium intake

    Assessment data may reveal:
    Muscle weakness, headache, polyuria, thirst, nausea, fatigue, anorexia, constipation, coma; laboratory data showing increased serum calcium and decreased serum phosphate. Client may have a history of excessive and prolonged milk, alkali, vitamin D, or calcium intake.

D. Manifested by oxygen/carbon dioxide alterations

    1. Oxygen toxicity related to prolonged high levels of oxygen inhalation

Assessment data may reveal:
Pink skin, depressed respirations, confusion, restlessness, increased arterial oxygen levels.

2. Oxygen insufficiency related to
   a. Impaired circulation
   b. Reduced hemoglobin
   c. Impaired respiration
   d. Lack of oxygen available
      Assessment data may reveal:
      Nausea, headache, anxiety, dyspnea, cyanosis, confusion, lethargy, restlessness, vomiting, decreased serum arterial oxygen levels.

3. Carbon dioxide insufficiency related to
   a. Respiratory center damage
   b. Drug depression
   c. Hyperventilation
      Assessment data may reveal:
      Numbness and tingling of nose, ears, toes; light-headedness; depressed respirations; muscle twitching; decreased arterial carbon dioxide levels.

4. Carbon dioxide toxicity related to
   a. Decreased alveolar ventilation
   b. Administration of concentrated oxygen
      Assessment data may reveal:
      Headache, drowsiness, coma, excessive yawning, muscle twitching, tachycardia, sweating, increased arterial carbon dioxide levels.

E. Manifested by fluid volume alterations
   1. Dependence on intravenous infusion management related to intravenous therapy
      Assessment data may reveal:
      Presence of an IV with the corresponding needs of infusion regulation, site maintenance, and medication administration.
   2. Emergency phase circulatory overload related to

a. Too rapid administration of intravenous fluids
b. Cardiac failure
   Assessment data may include:
   Dyspnea, anxiety, back pain, coughing, hemoptysis, tachycardia, neck-vein distention, cyanosis, central venous pressure above 10 cm of water, increased pulmonary-artery wedge pressure, laboratory data usually showing dilutional hyponatremia and a decreased urine specific gravity.

3. Potential cardiac overload related to
   a. Increased energy requirements and metabolic rate
   b. Excessive exercise
   c. Overeating
   d. Emotional exitement
   e. Rapid fluid replacement
      Assessment may reveal:
      Overexertion, emotional excitement, pregnancy, rapid fluid replacement.

4. Potential hemorrhage related to
   a. Blood dyscrasia
   b. Endocrine imbalance
   c. Malignant growth of cells applying pressure on arteries
   d. Interrupted integument
      Assessment data may reveal:
      Recent bleeding episode; easy bruising; bleeding gums; external wounds; laboratory data showing increased bleeding time, clotting time, plasma thromboplastin, partial thromboplastin time, or decreased Factor VIII levels, hemoglobin, and hemocrit.

5. Actual hemorrhage related to
   a. Blood vessel rupture
   b. Platelet deficiency
   c. Blood-clotting defect (e.g., Factor VIII deficiency, disseminated intravascular coagulopathy)

Assessment data may reveal:
Weakness, a subjective feeling of doom, blood pressure decrease, decreased pulse pressure.

6. Hemorrhage related to
    a. Spontaneous blood vessel rupture
    b. Blood-clotting defect
    c. Platelet deficiency
    d. Radiation or chemotherapy
    e. Hemouralysis
    f. Surgery

   Assessment data may reveal:
   Subjective anxiety, weakness, decreased blood pressure and pulse pressure, tachycardia, dyspnea, pallor, cold skin, cyanosis, coma, hematemesis, tarry stools, hemoptysis, hematuria, postpartum hemorrhage; a history of gastric or peptic ulcer, esophageal varices, hemophilia, carcinoma, trauma, or surgery.

7. Increased fluid requirements related to
    a. Excessive fluid loss
    b. Increased metabolism
       Assessment data may reveal:
       thirst, fever, diarrhea, vomiting, profuse diaphoresis, hemorrhage, infection, renal caliculi symptoms.

8. Potential fluid overload related to ascites and edema
       Assessment data may reveal:
       Jaundice, increased abdominal girth, respiratory girth, respiratory distress. Client may have a history of liver disease.

F. Manifested by changes in blood pH
    1. Acidemia requiring immediate intervention related to
       a. Kidney impairment
       b. Excessive ingestion of acid
       c. Profuse sweating
       d. Poor nutritional intake

Assessment data may reveal:
A feeling of weakness and malaise, nausea, abdominal pain, dehydration, Kussmauls, respirations, progression to shock. Laboratory data include a blood pH below 7.2 and increased blood carbon dioxide.

2. Acidemia requiring immediate intervention related to diabetes mellitus

   Assessment data may reveal:
   A subjective feeling of malaise, hunger, dizziness, nausea, thirst. Objective parameters include restlessness; Kussmaul's respirations with acetone breath; vomiting; dehydration; dry, flushed skin; polyuria. Related laboratory findings include glucosurea; a decreased blood sugar and arterial carbon dioxide levels; serum pH below 7.2.

3. Potential acidemia related to
    a. Excessive fat and protein catabolism
    b. Fever
    c. Poor nutritional intake
    d. Impaired carbohydrate metabolism

   Assessment data may reveal:
   Fever; prolonged low carbohydrate intake; prolonged intake of acidic drugs; impaired carbohydrate metabolism; laboratory data showing an increased serum carbon dioxide.

4. Potential alkalemia related to
    a. Excessive carbonic acid loss
    b. Excessive bicarbonate intake

   Assessment parameters may reveal:
   Prolonged vomiting; prolonged diarrhea; prolonged nasogastric suctioning; prolonged potassium depletion; hyperventilation; prolonged adrenocorticol steroid therapy; excessive intake of alkalis; laboratory data showing a decreased serum potassium and/or decreased arterial carbon dioxide level.

5. Alkalemia requiring immediate intervention related to
   a. Excessive sodium bicarbonate ingestion
   b. Potassium loss through diuresis
   c. Chlorine loss through hyperemesis
   Assessment data may reveal:
   Anxiety; lethargy; restlessness; tetany; tremor; convulsions; flaccid muscle weakness; cardiac arrhythmias; laboratory data showing elevated blood pH, normal or decreased serum chlorine, a decreased serum potassium.

IV. Alterations in metabolism
  A. Manifested by alterations in nutritional requirements
     1. Increased nutritional requirements

Related to	Assessment Data
Blood loss	Dyspnea; fatigue; palpitations; dizziness; pallor; tachycardia; no gastrointestinal bleeding; low blood hemoglobin level, red blood cell count, and iron.
Lactation	Mother is lactating in postpartum period.
Increased metabolic rate	Hunger, fatigue, fever, hyperactivity, elevated T_3 and thyroxine levels.
Smoking habituation (vitamin C and B depletion)	Fatigue, person smokes three or more cigarettes, cigars, or pipes per day.
Tissue healing	Presence of healing wound or infection.
Infection	Fatigue, symptoms of protein-Calorie malnutrition.
Fever	Infection, increased metabolic rate, impaired circulation.

2. Decreased protein requirement related to elevated levels of ammonia, blood urea nitrogen, nonprotein nitrogen
   Assessment may reveal:
   Confusion, disorientation, jaundice.

3. Alterations in nutritional requirements related to inborn errors of metabolism
   Assessment data may reveal:
   Mental retardation, eczema, hyperactivity, seizures, irritability.

B. Manifested by alterations in endocrine physiology
  1. Impending thyroid crisis related to
     a. Thyroid hypofunction
     b. Surgical removal of thyroid
     Assessment data may reveal:
     Weakness, fatigue, tachycardia (usually greater than 130/min), increased respirations, restlessness, irritability, elevated temperature. Condition occurs most frequently within 12 hours after surgery.
  2. Potential goiter related to lack of iodine in diet
     Assessment data may reveal:
     A feeling of throat fullness, use of noniodized salt, lack of ingestion of iodine-containing foods, thyroid enlargement upon palpation. Condition is seen most frequently in the Pacific Northwest and Great Lakes regions.
  3. Predisposition to diabetes related to
     a. Chronic excessive carbohydrate consumption
     b. Pregnancy
     c. Menopause
     d. Genetic determination

Assessment data may reveal:
Obesity, diet high in carbohydrates, multiparous women with neonatal birth weight of greater than 10 lb, a history of early myocardial infarction (before 40 in men, before menopause in women).

4. Insulin shock related to
   a. Lack of compliance with diet
   b. Overdosage of insulin
   c. Decreased activity level
   Assessment data may reveal:
   Generalized weakness, headache, nervousness, hunger, dizziness, pallor, tremors, restlessness, irritability, diaphoresis, confusion, laboratory data showing a decreased serum glucose level.

5. Lack of information about diabetes management related to lack of instruction and/or experience
   Assessment data may reveal:
   Client's confirmation of lack of understanding of the disease, its cause, complications, and management.

C. Manifested by alterations in structure
   1. Decubitus ulcer related to
      a. Immobility
      b. Malnutrition
      c. Chemical injury
      d. Circulatory impairment
      Assessment data may reveal:
      Pain at site, lesion of varied size and deepness, serosanguineous drainage present primarily on bony prominences.

   2. Skin discomfort related to
      a. Nutritional deficiency
      b. Allergic reactions to food
      Assessment data may reveal:
      Itching, burning, occasional tenderness of skin.

   3. Potential bone demineralization related to
      a. Immobility
      b. Failure of bone matrix to form
      c. Malnutrition
      Assessment data may reveal:
      Prolonged immobility; lack of weight bearing; lack of protein, vitamin D, and calcium intake.

   4. Pain in joints related to
      a. Gout
      b. Arthritis
      Assessment data may reveal: pain in joints, swollen, reddened joints, joints tender to touch.

   5. Muscular atrophy related to
      a. Immobility
      b. Aging
      c. Lack of exercise
      d. Malnutrition
      e. Inadequate protein intake
      Assessment data may reveal: abnormally low muscle mass, lack of weight bearing ability, decreased strength.

   6. Neuromuscular incoordination related to
      a. Deficiencies of B-complex vitamins
      b. Degenerative diseases of nervous system
      c. Degeneration of peripheral nerves
      d. Convulsions
      e. Seizures
      Assessment data may reveal: uncontrolled, involuntary muscle movements; lack of fine motor control, incontinence; in children, lack of normal motor development.

V. Alterations in excretion
   A. Manifested by alterations in fluid output
      1. Dependence on indwelling urinary catheter management related to

a. Urinary incontinence or retention

b. Inability to manage indwelling catheter

Assessment data may reveal:
Presence of or need for an indwelling catheter. Client is dependent on nurse for insertion, maintenance, and management of system.

2. Predisposition to development of renal caliculi related to

a. Prolonged immobility

b. Excessive calcium intake

c. Increased parathyroid activity (higher excretion of calcium and phosphorus)

Assessment data may reveal:
Decreased fluid intake, bed rest, ingestion of a high-calcium diet, a urine pH very acidic or very alkaline, a history of renal caliculi.

3. Inadequate urinary output related to urine retention

Assessment data may reveal:
Urinary frequency; dribbling of urine; difficulty urinating; lower abdominal pain, bladder distention; fluid upon percussion over bladder. If retention is prolonged (as in prostatic hypertrophy) blood urea nitrogen and creatinine levels may be elevated.

4. Inadequate urinary output related to inadequate fluid intake

Assessment data may reveal:
Thirst, urine output between 500 and 1,000 cc/day; fluid intake less than 1,200 cc/day; signs of dehydration.

5. Diuresis related to

a. Hypofunction of posterior lobe of pituitary gland

b. Infection

c. Renal failure

Assessment data may reveal:
Fatigue, urine output greater than 3,000 cc/day, urinary frequency, urine specific gravity less than 1.010, other symptoms of fluid depletion.

6. Painful urination related to

a. Infection of urinary tract

b. Inflammation of urinary tract

c. Low urine pH

Assessment data may reveal:
Localized pain during voiding, urinary retention, urinary frequency, difficulty in starting the stream.

B. Manifested by alterations in solid waste excretion

1. Painful defecation related to

a. Constipation

b. Lower bowel or rectal spasm

c. Obstruction

Assessment data may reveal:
Localized rectal or abdominal pain, acute onset during or immediately after elimination.

2. Fecal impaction related to

a. Decreased peristalsis

b. Excessive water reabsorption in colon

c. Prolonged constipation

Assessment data may reveal:
Abdominal and rectal discomfort: rectal distention; a hard fecal mass palpable on digital examination; oozing, liquid stool from the rectum.

3. Constipation related to

a. Lack of fluid intake

b. Decreased mobility

c. Ignoring defecation reflex

d. Antacid therapy

e. Emotional tension

Assessment data may reveal:
Headache; indigestion; abdominal fullness and/or tenderness; small, hard masses of stool; flatulence, dehydration.

4. Diarrhea related to

a. Mechanical, chemical, or bacterial irritation of the intestinal mucosa

b. Emotional stress

c. Increased peristalsis

Assessment data may reveal:
Gastrointestinal cramping, weakness, nausea, hyperactive bowel sounds, frequent unformed stools. Client may have a history of spastic colon, Crohn's disease, infectious process, colitis, diverticulitis, Addison's disease, tuberculosis, ciliac disease, Whipple's disease, Kwashiorkor, glomerular nephritis. Client may have been receiving tube feedings.

5. Dependence on nursing intervention for ostomy care related to presence of ostomy
   Assessment data may reveal:
   Presence of ostomy, inability of client to perform daily care of appliance, client asking questions about care of ostomy, or client appearing anxious while caring for ostomy.

In conclusion, The student is reminded that this listing is not meant to be comprehensive or inclusive. Rather, it is meant to provide a base line of nutritionally related nursing diagnoses on which to build a documented assessment of a client's nutritional status. The nursing implications arising from each nursing diagnosis must be individualized to the particular needs of the client.

BIBILIOGRAPHY

Campbell, C. *Nursing Diagnosis and Intervention.* New York: John Wiley & Sons, Inc., Pubs., 1978.

Maslow, A. H. *Toward a Psychology of Being.* New York: Van Nostrand Reinhold Co., 1962.

CHAPTER 22

Nutritional Care of the Hospitalized Client

The nutritional care of the hospitalized client is primarily the responsibility of three members of the health team, the doctor, the nurse, and the dietitian. They should coordinate their observation of the client and the plans for his care with each other and with the client. Because of the nurse's expertise in direct assessment and total time she spends with the client, primary responsibility for coordinating the health team rests with her. The student should remember that the client is the center of the health care team. Good rapport among client and doctor, nurse, and dietitian enables the members of the health team to individualize their aspects of care to the client.

The nursing process (described in Chap. 18) is the problem-solving model used by nurses to plan and implement nursing care. Dietitians have also begun recently to use this approach. It is described by Krause and Mahan (1979) as the "nutritional care process," and by Mason (1977) as a "systems approach to nutritional care." This process, similar to the problem-solving method used in scientific investigation, allows the members of the health team to proceed through a logical sequence of steps to plan and deliver nutritional care. This chapter shows how the four steps of the process—assessment, planning, intervention, and evaluation—are applied to therapeutic nutrition.

ASSESSMENT

The initial step in the nursing process is collecting from a variety of sources data about the client from which a determination can be made of the client's health and nutritional status. Nutritional status is influenced not only by the intake of nutrients but by the use of nutrients within the body. Specific nutritional needs are identified that will be the primary focus of planning and intervention.

The nurse takes all the data that has been gathered (using methods and tools discussed in Chaps. 19 and 20) and makes her assessment, culminating in the nursing diagnosis, which includes the statement of the client's specific nutritional needs. Each client has specific nutritional needs imposed on him not only by hospitalization and the disease process but by any dietary inadequacies or excesses prior to admission. The goal is identification of the client's nutritional needs early in hospitalization and immediate intervention to meet those needs. For example, if the nutritional assessment reveals low levels of hemoglobin, an iron supplement and a high-protein diet should be implemented if not contraindicated by concurrent disease processes. The earlier the intervention to correct nutritional deficits, the sooner the client's nutritional status will improve. In many cases, an improvement in nutritional status also means a detectable difference in total health status.

PLANNING

After assessment comes planning the client's nutritional care. The first step is to determine the type of diet best suited to meet the client's needs. Diets may be classified as preventive, corrective, supportive, or as the primary means of therapy. Many clients with a good nutritional status simply require a regular well-balanced diet to prevent any nutritional problems. Clients who have had prior nutritional deficiencies require a diet that will correct these deficiencies and restore the optimal nutritional status. Diet therapy may also be supportive of the medical treatment. For example, adherence to a low-sodium diet is quite beneficial in the treatment of hypertension. In certain metabolic diseases such as diabetes mellitus or some of the inborn errors of metabolism such as galactosemia or phenylketonuria, diet therapy is a major aspect of the medial treatment.

All therapeutic diets are planned as a modification of the regular hospital menu. The dietitian plans the daily hospital menu using the basic four food groups as a guide. Hospital meals contain at least the minimum number of servings from the basic four. Additional foods such as extra milk, fortified margarine or butter, desserts, and bread are added to increase the Calories and palatability of the diet. A sample hospital menu and the nutrients it contains is shown in Figure 22-1.

Therapeutic diets served in the hospital are modifications of this regular hospital menu. As such, they should be referred to as *therapeutic* or *modified diets;* the term *special diet* usually has a negative connotation to a client. Most people do not like to be told that they must eat special food. When a client is informed by physician, nurse, or dietitian that he has been placed on a special diet, his re-

sponse is often negative, for he feels different and separated from family and friends by the modifications in his eating habits. Reference to a "special" diet often has the same negative impact on the family, who feel they must greatly change their eating habits to accommodate the client's diet.

Reference to the diet as either a therapeutic or a modified diet is a more effective approach. Usually the diet is only a modification in one aspect and does not necessitate a complete change in eating habits. Reference to the diet as a therapeutic measure also has a positive effect. If the client understands that adhering to the diet as part of the medical treatment will speed recovery, help him live longer, or make him feel better, he is much more likely to follow its restrictions. When the diet is called by either of these names, the family members are also more likely to have a positive attitude. It is an important task of nurse and dietitian to explain to the client and the family how this modified diet can be incorporated into the regular family eating patterns with few or minimal changes. More about this aspect of dietary education is included in the next section.

Dietary Modifications

When contemplating what diet to order for a client, the physician must keep in mind that there are only a limited number of ways that food can be modified. Diets can be modified in texture, number of Calories, levels of specific nutrients, exclusion of certain foods or constituents in foods, and number of feedings. The texture of food can be modified to provide foods that are liquid or soft or foods that are high or low in fiber or residue. The caloric content of the diet can either be raised or lowered, as can the levels of specific nutrients or constituents. Certain foods may be excluded in the case of allergies. Sometimes foods that contain a specific constituent such as gluten or lactose may need to be eliminated.

INDIANA UNIVERSITY HOSPITALS GENERAL MENU	INDIANA UNIVERSITY HOSPITALS GENERAL MENU	INDIANA UNIVERSITY HOSPITALS GENERAL MENU

PATIENT NAME

WED 01/02/80   WED 01/02/80   WED 01/02/80

MORNING	NOON	NIGHT
===== FRESHLY SQUEEZED ORANGE JUICE	===== CANADIAN CHEESE SOUP WITH CRACKERS	===== EGGNOG WITH WHIPPED CREAM & NUTMEG
===== GRAPEFRUIT JUICE	===== CREAM OF TOMATO SOUP	===== STRAINED CREAM OF POTATO SOUP
=====	===== CLEAR BROTH	===== STRAINED JULIENNE BROTH
===== HOT OATMEAL	===== SKILLET CHILI WITH CRACKERS	===== FRIED BREAST OF CHICKEN
===== BRAN FLAKES	===== HOT ROAST PORK ON CRUSTY BUN	===== SKILLET GRAVY
===== SHREDDED WHEAT	===== (GROUND) PORK	===== BAKED BREAST OF CHICKEN
=====	=====	===== CHICKEN (GROUND)
===== SCRAMBLED EGGS	===== WHIPPED POTATOES	===== CORNED BEEF WITH POTATO
===== POACHED EGG	===== CRISPY CORN CHIPS	===== WHIPPED POTATOES
===== FRIED EGG SUNNY SIDE UP	===== BUTTERED SPEAR OF BROCCOLI	===== BUTTERED GREEN PEAS
===== FRIED EGG OVER LIGHT	===== BUTTERED FRESH JULIENNE CARROTS	===== BUTTERED BRUSSELS SPROUTS
===== FRIED EGG HARD	===== BUTTERED BLENDERIZED BROCCOLI	===== BUTTERED BLENDERIZED GREEN PEAS
===== SOFT COOKED EGG IN SHELL	===== LEAF LETTUCE SALAD	===== JELLIED CRANBERRY SAUCE
===== HARD COOKED EGG IN SHELL	===== HOT BACON DRESSING	===== CRISPY HEARTS OF LETTUCE
=====	=====	===== FRENCH DRESSING
===== FRESH SAUSAGE LINK	===== WARM KUMMELWECK ROLL WITH MARGARINE	===== WARM CRACKED WHEAT ROLL AND MARGARINE
===== TOASTED ENGLISH MUFFIN	===== WHITE BREAD OR TOAST WITH MARGARINE	===== WHITE BREAD OR TOAST WITH MARGARINE
===== WHOLE WHEAT TOAST WITH MARGARINE	=====	=====
===== WHITE TOAST WITH MARGARINE	===== TRIO OF SHERBET BALLS	===== WARM PUMPKIN PIE
===== WHITE BREAD WITH MARGARINE	===== WARM APPLE CRISP	===== CREME DE MENTHE ICE CREAM
===== MARGARINE	===== MARGARINE	===== MARGARINE
===== MILK	===== MILK	===== MILK
===== 2% MILK	===== 2% MILK	===== 2% MILK
===== SKIM MILK	===== SKIM MILK	===== SKIM MILK
===== BUTTERMILK	===== BUTTERMILK	===== BUTTERMILK
=====	===== COTTAGE CHEESE	===== COTTAGE CHEESE
=====	===== CRACKERS	===== CRACKERS
=====	===== CUSTARD	===== PUDDING
=====	===== VANILLA ICE CREAM	===== VANILLA ICE CREAM
===== JELLO ===== HOT TEA	===== JELLO ===== HOT TEA	===== JELLO ===== HOT TEA
===== BROTH ===== ICED TEA	===== ===== ICED TEA	===== ===== ICED TEA
===== JELLY ===== LEMON	===== JELLY ===== LEMON	===== JELLY ===== LEMON
===== CREAM ===== FRUIT DRINK	===== CREAM ===== FRUIT JUICE	===== CREAM ===== FRUIT JUICE
===== COFFEE =====	===== COFFEE ===== FRUIT DRINK	===== COFFEE ===== FRUIT DRINK
===== SANKA =====	===== SANKA ===== LEMONADE	===== SANKA ===== LEMONADE

Figure 22-1. The selective hospital menu. (Courtesy Indiana University Hospitals)

The number of feedings provided throughout the day may need to be modified. Many nursing homes and some hospitals have voluntarily changed to provide a four-, five-, or six-meal plan instead of the traditional three meals a day. For the infirm client with high caloric needs, it is easier to encourage consumption of additional Calories if a bedtime snack or snacks between each meal are offered. Some clients who simply cannot tolerate large quantities of food at one time do much better with three between-meal feedings or six small meals during the day. The provision of six small meals is common in the dietary management of clients with ulcers or after a partial or total gastrectomy. Three meals with three snacks or feedings between meals is common diet therapy for hypoglycemia or for any client with a need for additional protein and Calories. The client on a strict reducing diet may prefer to have the daily caloric allotment divided so as to provide at least one or two snacks during the day.

Fluid intake often needs to be modified with certain disease conditions. Ordinarily fluid balance is maintained through the normal physiological mechanism of thirst. The daily requirement for fluid amounts to about 1 ml/Calorie for the adult and 1.5 ml/Calorie for the infant. In some cases, as when a client has a urinary tract infection, the fluid intake is increased by the order "force fluids." In other cases, as when clients have congestive heart failure, renal failure, or increased intracranial pressure or when the excretion of fluids is impaired or dehydration is desired, the recommendation is for a "fluid restriction." These clients can be made more comfortable if the fluid intake is spaced throughout the day and partially filled by ice chips, Popsicles, or lemon-glycerin swabs.

Naming of Diets

The acceptable naming of diets is important as a means of communication among the members of the health team about the client's diet. A general recommendation is to specify the level of Calories or level of nutrients desired. Use of the general terms *high* and *low* only leaves room for various private interpretations.

A diet should not be named for the disease condition for which it is required nor for the person who developed it. For example, a client hospitalized for gall bladder surgery who receives a menu slip with each meal that has "gall bladder diet" after his name and room number is thereby unnecessarily and frequently reminded of his illness. This method of naming diets also reveals nothing about the actual dietary modification. Another example is Kempner's rice diet, which was used in the past for the treatment of hypertension. This diet is actually very low in sodium content; yet the name reveals nothing about the dietary modification.

Diet Order

The client's diet is ordered by the attending physician, who writes the diet order in the client's chart. This order is then transferred by the nursing staff or ward clerks from the client's chart to the nursing Kardex and to the dietary department. Writing a personalized diet order requires knowledge of the client's dietary history, his nutritional status, and the effects of the disease and treatment therapies on his nutritional status. Although in many cases the dietitian might be better equipped to prescribe the diet, it is still the physician and the nurse who are legally responsible for the client's nutrition. Most clinical dietitians do not assume full responsibility for prescribing diets, however they make recommendations to the physician concerning the diet order. With increasing emphasis on clinical specialties in dietetics and more emphasis on medical science courses at both the undergraduate and graduate levels, dietitians may eventually be given the responsibility for writing diet orders.

Because of the current procedure for ordering diets, there is often a need for interpretation and consultation. Ideally, the members of the health team would collaborate in planning a suitable diet with the client. Often this cooperative effort is not feasible, and consultation and recommendations are instead made after the diet has been ordered. The most frequently missing part of a diet order is the number of Calories it should contain. The normal or slightly modified hospital menu provides too many Calories for clients who are on bedrest. If all the food provided is consumed at each meal, some clients may actually gain weight during hospitalization. Some clients, however, have very high caloric requirements imposed by surgery, fever, or infection. The regular hospital menu may not provide enough Calories for these clients, and some may steadily lose weight during their hospital stay. Because the actual caloric requirements of diseased clients are not known and because the caloric levels are not usually specified in diet orders, a daily or at least a weekly assessment of weight should be recorded in a client's chart. Any significant changes should be brought to the attention of the physician so that needed adjustments can be made by the dietitian.

Krause and Mahan (1979) refer to the diet order as a "diet prescription," and they compare it to a drug prescription. The diet prescription specifies the type (what nutrients modified), amount (Calories), and route of food ingestion just as the drug prescription identifies the drug, dosage, frequency, and route of administration.

Diet Rationale and Objectives

Five major purposes of diet therapy are stated by Robinson and Lawler (1976): (1) to maintain good nutritional status, (2) to correct any deficiencies that may have occurred, (3) to afford rest to the whole body or to certain organs that may be affected, (4) to adjust the food intake to the body's ability to metabolize the nutrients, and (5) to bring about changes in body weight whenever necessary.

In addition to these general purposes of diet therapy, each modified diet has its own objectives and scientific rationale. Each therapeutic diet has a sound scientific rationale for its use with a specific disease condition. For example, the low-sodium diet is used in the treatment of edema because a reduction in sodium intake aids in the elimination of excess sodium and fluid and therefore reduces the edema. Objectives can be stated for each modified diet. They usually follow quite closely the objectives for medical and nursing care.

Diet Manual

The dietary department of each large hospital publishes its own diet manual, but the scientific rationale for all therapeutic diets in these manuals is the same, as are the general objectives for diet therapy. The difference lies in how the scientific rationale and objectives are interpreted into actual foods for the client. Different hospitals have slightly different ways in which they interpret the same diet order. The differences usually result in slightly different foods offered on individual diets. Small differences in interpretations such as these are actually policies of the hospital dietary department. Occasionally these differences cause the client some concern. A client originally instructed on a diet in one hospital may notice slight differences in another hospital. A brief explanation by the dietitian or the nurse of the reason for the slight difference will usually satisfy the client's questions.

The diet manual, then, is actually a means of communication among the members of the health team. The hospital dietary manual is written by members of the department of dietetics often in consultation with the major hospital physicians and representatives of the nursing staff. Copies are made available to each physician and nursing unit. The physician uses the diet manual as a guide for prescribing diets for his clients. The diet manual describes each of the diets offered by the dietary department. Nursing personnel use the diet manual as a reference source when they are asked a question about a specific diet by either the client or his family. It also provides a handy reference to the diets commonly ordered.

In addition to a description of each diet and the indications for use, the diet manual also contains the levels of nutrients commonly ordered. There are lists of foods allowed and foods to be avoided. Sample meal plans are usually provided for each diet. There are also numerous charts of nutritional requirements, height and weight tables, diets used for diagnostic tests, and food composition tables.

For the dietary department the diet manual serves as a policy and procedure manual. It is also used as a teaching tool for training new staff members. The diet instruction sheets used by the dietitian in instructing the client about his diet are patterned after the diets listed in the diet manual.

Principles of Planning Clinical Practice

After all the data is gathered and the diagnoses are made, the nurse usually has a plan for action. Many times a problem arises at this stage in the total coordination of the activities of all the people involved. Establishing goals and objectives toward which all intervention is aimed can prevent such problems.

A *goal* is the end toward which effort is directed. *Objectives,* on the other hand, are those observable, verifiable steps that are taken as practitioner and client move toward the attainment of goals. At this point in the nursing process, the nurse becomes a manager synthesizing resources and circumstances to optimize results. The creativity that is inherent at this point is what may determine the degree of success the client may realize in his effort to reach the established goals.

Setting goals requires a clear understanding of the mission and purpose of the framework within which the practitioner is working. For example, a goal that would be appropriate and attainable for one client may not be for another with a similar problem. To provide for continuity, it is important that the goal statements be documented.

After clear goals are established, the nurse must establish, with the client, objectives and their priority. The objectives should be stated in precise, measurable terms so that they may be used to provide direction for the client. An example of a goal statement and several objectives that might be helpful in reaching the goal might be:

GOAL

Mr. Jones will be able to manage his diabetes through dietary modification.

OBJECTIVES

1. Within one week Mr. Jones will be able to describe the diabetic exchange system.
2. Within one week Mr. Jones will be able to use the exchange lists to plan a meal.
3. Within two weeks Mr. Jones and his wife will be able to prepare a balanced diet for one week using the exchange lists and considering their own food preferences.
4. By the time of discharge, Mrs. Jones will be able to explain the exchange system to another client.

It is important for the client to sense success at goal achievement. The use of clear objectives can provide such success. It is vitally important that the client have a voice in setting his own objectives and in deciding how they may best be achieved. Setting priorities will aid in the accomplishment of objectives. The careful construction of meaningful objectives will often yield a logical sequence of actions to get to the goal.

INTERVENTION

Intervention, the next logical step in the problem-solving process in both nursing and nutritional care, means involvement, interaction, and the actual delivery of care with the client as the focus. In nutritional care, intervention is concerned with individualizing the diet to the client, serving meals in the hospital, and providing nutritional education for client and family.

Individualizing the Diet to the Client

A carefully planned diet is successful only when it is eaten. It is primarily the responsibility of the nurse and the dietitian to ensure that the client is provided with foods that are acceptable to him but still within the restrictions of the diet. Early in the client's hospitalization the nurse has obtained valuable information about the client's eating patterns and psychological, social, cultural, and economic influences on his eating habits. After the diet order has been received, the dietitian should visit the client as soon as possible, even before the first or second meal is served to him, to obtain information about his food preferences and food habits. Obtaining a list of the client's food preferences used to be quite important when hospital dietary departments served only one meal, with only slight modifications, to all clients. This procedure is still followed in many small hospitals. In recent years most larger hospitals have instituted selective menus that allow clients to make a selection among three or more food items within the broad categories of appetizer, entree, vegetable, salad, bread, dessert, and beverage.

The diet must be individualized to the client's eating habits and food preferences as much as possible for best acceptance in the hospital and better compliance after discharge. The meals served in a hospital cannot accommodate all the social and cultural variations in food habits. Most dietitians are quite willing to make as many substitutions as possible within the limits of the department. Most clients do not expect hospital food to be the same as the food they usually eat. A satisfac-

tory compromise can usually be worked out by client and dietitian to include some foods that are particularly important to the client. Suitable compromises with the vegetarian and the Jewish client can usually be reached fairly easily. Clients with distinct cultural food preferences are often the least satisfied with hospital food. Special permission may be granted for the client's family to supplement the food in the hospital with specific ethnic foods brought from home.

Many additional factors influence a client's attitude toward food during hospitalization. The client may be more concerned about his health status than about eating. Frequently he may be in pain. He often does not realize the role of good nutrition in recovery from disease. Numerous psychological, emotional, and economic worries, such as concern about his job and family, may decrease the client's interest in his diet. The hospital environment is strange and often frightening to clients of any age, especially children. The client must eat in bed, sometimes lying completely flat, often alone or surrounded by strangers. The mealtimes in the hospital often do not correspond to the client's schedule of eating.

Selective Menus

The first contact a client usually has with the dietary department is when the selective menu is presented. A menu for the current day or the next day is usually left by the client's bed. The selective menu allows the client to select foods for each meal from a sheet listing two or three choices for each major food category. Most hospitals have four or more slightly different sheets for the modified diets. These sheets are usually color coded with a certain category of diet. If the client selects any food from his selective menu, the selections will usually be within the restrictions of his diet. Dietitians or other members of the dietary staff check all client menu sheets before the meals are served and make minor changes when necessary.

Most clients can make their own selections by marking their own menus. Others may need some explanation about the menus before marking them. A few clients will be unable to mark their own menus because they are too ill, have difficulty seeing, or are in a physical position that makes writing impossible. The dietary and nursing staff should be alert for menus that have not been marked. Helping the client select his food for the next day by reading the menu to him is an effective means of interacting with and encouraging the client. The use of selective menus has improved food acceptance in most hospitals. They are also an effective method of teaching and evaluating. These two advantages are discussed further later in this chapter.

Hospital Food Service

The food service portion of the dietary department is managed in one of two ways. Under the first system the dietary department, and therefore food service to clients, is under the direct supervision of the hospital administration. All members of the dietary staff are employees of the hospital. The dietary staff is usually divided between the two major departments of food service and diet therapy. The director or administrator of dietetics is responsible for the operation of both departments and is directly responsible to hospital administration.

The other way of managing food service within a hospital is through a food service management or catering company. In this system the hospital contracts with an outside company to manage the dietary department. In some cases, all personnel in the dietary department are members of this management company, including the dietitians. In other cases, only the personnel directly responsible for food service are employees of the management company; the dietitians in charge of the nutritional care of clients are employed by the hospital. Either system, if properly managed, can provide quality food service to hospitalized clients.

The actual delivery of food to the client can also be accomplished in one of two ways. Food service delivery systems are referred to either as centralized or decentralized. In the *centralized system* all the food is prepared in one large food service area. The client's tray is made up assembly line fashion near the large food production area. The plates are peheated, and a stainless steel or plastic cover is placed over the hot food. It is then transported to the hospital ward or floor by a special preheated food cart, conveyor system, or dumb waiter. Most of these food carts have both a heated and a refrigerated side to keep both kinds of food at the proper serving temperature. On the floor the client's tray is checked by the nurse or dietitian before it is delivered by either the nurse or the dietary staff.

In *decentralized food service* all or most of the food is prepared in quantity in the large food production area. It is then transported in bulk to a kitchen on the floor or ward. The food is assembled onto clients' trays in this smaller kitchen and delivered to the bedsides after they are checked for correctness by the dietitian or nurse. Both systems require close cooperation and communication between the nursing and dietary staff regarding admissions, dismissals, and diet changes.

Mealtime

The time and effort expended by both dietary and nursing staff to make mealtime pleasant for the clients are well spent. Visiting hours, doctor's rounds, and laboratory tests should be arranged so as not to conflict with mealtimes. Hours should be flexible enough to allow for family socialization during mealtime if the client so desires. The nurse's role at mealtime is to prepare the client for eating and to provide assistance in feeding when necessary. The client may need help with mouth care and handwashing before eating. He should be positioned in the bed or in a chair so that he is ready to eat when the tray arrives. Some hospital units have pleasant client dining rooms where the ambulatory clients may eat. Clients should be encouraged to eat in the dining room whenever possible to maintain a more normal eating pattern.

The dietary department's responsibility is for the delivery of an attractive, orderly tray containing palatable food served at the proper temperature. The tray cover should be clean and neat, and the dishes and utensils should be immaculately clean. All the necessary utensils and condiments should be included. The food should be attractively arranged, and garnishes should be included where appropriate. The tray should be promptly delivered to the client following a quick final check by the nursing or dietary staff.

Some clients require only minimal assistance at the beginning of a meal, such as opening the milk carton or condiments, pouring coffee, buttering bread, or cutting meat. The person delivering the tray may have a few moments to do one or more of these tasks. If not, someone should be available to assist the client (see Fig. 22.2). If the client needs to be fed completely, someone should be available to begin feeding immediately. If someone is not immediately available to feed the client, the tray should be held in the heated food cart or unit kitchen until the client can be fed. A tray of cold food is not appetizing to anyone and especially not to a sick person. Many clients look forward to mealtime in the hospital, so staff should make every effort to make it pleasant. For the client who is not really interested in meals, extra effort should be made to serve hot, attractive, tasteful food according to personal food preferences. A pleasant atmosphere and an extra word of encouragement at mealtime may stimulate appetite.

Nutritional Counseling

Nutritional counseling is another important aspect of intervention in nutritional care. The specific principles of nutritional counseling in relation to the different therapeutic diets are

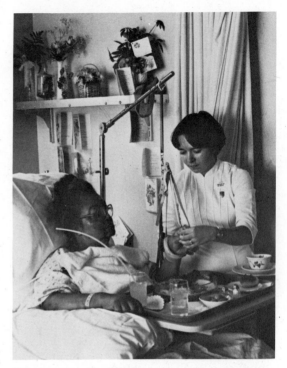

Figure 22-2. Assistive devices will often allow a client to regain relative independence at mealtime. Note the following devices in this picture: plate rim, hand brace, arm holder, and extra-long straw.

discussed in Chapters 24–28; some general methods of formal and informal counseling are mentioned here.

Both the nurse and the dietitian have responsibilities for nutritional education of their clients. The counseling process should begin early in a client's hospitalization. This is very important because the average hospital stay is only 11 days. Without early planning immediate after admission, many clients are released from the hospital before a diet instruction is given or else the dietitian rushes to the client's room to find him dressed, with suitcase packed, and ready to leave. The effectiveness of a diet instruction given under such conditions is questionable.

Informal counseling can be begun when the client is served his first meal. The selective menu is an excellent tool to use for informal counseling. After the client has checked those foods he would like to receive the next day, the nurse may look over the menu and comment briefly on his selection. For example, if no vegetables are selected, the reason may be investigated. A discussion could be initiated of the major nutrients and health benefits provided by vegetables. Helping the client select foods for his modified diet is also an opportunity for informal education about his diet.

Mealtime also provides an opportunity for informal nutritional counseling by the nurse or dietitian. A brief explanation about the role of certain nutrients in the recovery process is a useful nutritional education technique. Along with this, it can be explained why certain foods were provided on the tray, that is, what nutrients they contain. The pattern of the hospital menu can also lead to a natural discussion of the client's eating habits outside the hospital. Suggestions can be made about how to include certain foods in his daily eating habits. A client's eating habits should be viewed positively but with suggestions for improvement. Under no conditions should a client be told that his dietary habits are completely bad and that he must completely change them.

The major responsibility of the dietitian is dietary counseling and instruction of the client about his modified diet. The first step is to take a complete dietary history of the client. Next, the dietitian explains to the client the scientific rationale for the diet and the health benefits of following it. Next, she discusses the general principles of the diet and why certain foods are allowed and others not. After this she explains how the foods allowed on the diet can be incorporated into the client's own eating habits with a minimal amount of change. Suggestions for food purchasing and preparation are also included as well as suggestions and guidelines for eating

out in restaurants. From the amount and depth of material to be covered in a diet instruction, it should be evident that several 15- to 30-minute sessions are required for maximum understanding and compliance by the client. Many hospitals have initiated formal diet classes for some of the major modified diets such as the diabetic diet, the fat-controlled diet, and the low-sodium diet. These classes provide not only well-structured, consistent content but an opportunity for clients to interact and learn from each other.

Nurses provide valuable reinforcement to the dietitian's teaching about the modified diet. The nurse can answer most of the client's questions about the diet. She can reinforce its importance in relation to his health status. She can also offer practical suggestions about food purchasing and preparation to the client and the family. Providing client education about a therapeutic diet does not mean motivating a client to change his eating habits completely. Instead, it means instructing him in how his regular eating habits can be slightly modified to include in his meals those foods recommended on the diet.

Nutritional Education

Much of the nurse's efforts in nutritional care focus on education of the client to assure compliance and self-management. Learning is a process by which the behavior is modified by experience. Learning can therefore ultimately be measured as a change in behavior. When considering the definition of *learning*, it is important to realize that not all observed behavioral changes are attributable to learning. Other processes such as maturation and fatigue may also lead to changes in behavior. Learning, however, involves relatively permanent changes, whereas other processes may be transitory or independent of experience (Jung, 1968). For example, the nurse can determine that Mr. Jones has learned if he is able consistently to use the diabetic exchange lists to plan his meals.

After a plan for teaching has been developed by the nurse, dietitian, client, and other members of the health care team, the nurse is responsible for creating an environment in which the client can learn, can succeed, and can develop self-direction and motivation. *Teaching* is a system of actions intended to induce learning; that is, it is a deliberate, planned activity. Teaching is aimed at developing the potential of the learner while at the same time respecting his uniqueness. All too often nurses present information to a client and expect him to apply it immediately to his own experiences. Such activity usually ends in frustration for both client and nurse. The client is not certain what to do with the information, and the nurse has difficulty dealing with the client's needs if no learning has taken place. The nurse must remember that there is a difference between someone who has *learned* and someone who has been *informed*.

Domains of Learning

The client brings his whole being into the learning situation. Three major elements of the personality must be recognized. The first is the *cognitive domain*. This is the thought process itself, by which information is grasped. *Cognition* is the construction of concepts out of facts and principles. It can be summarized as "I know how to do it." It is to this element in the personality that most client teaching is directed.

The second element is the *emotion,* or *will,* usually referred to as the *affective domain*. In each person specific feelings and responses are associated with given items of knowledge in a given situation. It is in this domain that a client perceives a need to learn something. This element can be best summarized as "I want to do it." A client must be internally motivated to seek change and learning.

The third element is known as the *psychomotor domain*. In this domain are taught the basic skills for a client actually to do a task.

Usually, teaching in this domain centers on tasks a client can learn that require manipulation or dexterity. An example is teaching a client with rheumatoid arthritis to feed himself with assistive devices. The psychomotor domain can be summarized as "I can do it."

Types of Learning

In teaching a client the nurse deals with several types of learning. *Recall learning* is basically memory work. An example is memorizing the basic four food groups. Repetition is usually required for mastery. In adults, repetition by usage rather than rote repetition will aid in learning as well as increase motivation to learn. *Concept learning* involves the knowledge of basic content in a meaningful framework. Examples include learning the rationale behind a sodium-restricted diet to control hypertension or learning how to modify a diabetic diet to meet caloric demands based on activity level.

Before beginning to teach, it is necessary to determine if a client is truly ready to learn. Readiness involves both the physiological and psychological ability and desire to learn about a particular subject. A client must perceive a need and be willing to devote energy to meeting it. For example, a postoperative client who only two days ago had a colostomy for cancer may not perceive a need to learn about low-gas foods. He is still adjusting to the body image changes resulting from the colostomy, experiencing a moderate degree of pain, and attempting to deal with the fact of having cancer. In addition, he will probably still not be taking food orally. Nurses and dietitians need to address all the resulting needs before assuming the client is ready to discuss his diet.

The stage of illness a client is in will affect his learning needs and readiness to learn. During acute stages of illness, learning is unlikely to occur; pain, anxiety, fear, and exhaustion preclude it. Learning during the chronic stages of illness will be affected by the person's perception of the incapacitating effect of the illness, his dependency conflicts, his financial concerns, and the stage of grieving he is in.

Principles of Learning

Before setting out a specific teaching plan, the nurse must consider several principles of learning. Being familiar with these will assist in individualizing the care plan to the client and increase the probability of success.

1. *The learner must learn for himself according to his need, in his way, in his time, and for his purpose.* To teach, then, the teacher must discover who the learner is. By assessing the learner's past experiences, motivation, interests, and needs, the teacher can create a situation for him that is most likely to meet his individual needs. For example, if the nurse is teaching prenatal nutrition to a mother who has two children already, the nurse must investigate her previous experiences and current resources before making a teaching plan.

2. *The learner's interest and motivation increase when the learning experience has relevance.* Unless the learner is able to associate some payoff with learning the subject matter to be taught, he will probably never learn it. For example, unless a client feels a need to save money, he will probably not learn about economical ways to stretch the food budget, regardless of how innovative the nurse's teaching methods are.

3. *Positive reinforcement of a desired behavior increases the appearance of that behavior.* For example, if a child is praised every time he finishes the meal tray, the behavior is more likely to be repeated. The adolescent, however, may not value praise from an authority figure. It must be remembered that unless the client perceives the reinforcement as desirable, it will not influence the reoccurrence of the desired behavior.

4. *Rewards desired by the learner are more reinforcing than general or routine rewards.* To illustrate, the client who values independence will frequently learn the use of assistive devices more rapidly than the client who does not.

5. *Learning that proceeds from the simple to the complex aids understanding.* For example, it would not be helpful to attempt to teach a client about a Calorie-restricted diet without first defining what a Calorie is. Frequently health professionals start teaching from a level that is too complex for the client. The practitioner must include the "basics" in most teaching plans.

6. *Practice with feedback promotes improvement in performance.* Providing planned feedback during a teaching session not only reinforces correct behaviors but assures the learner that the teacher is involved and concerned with his progress. Any student can confirm that he will put forth greater effort if the teacher actively participates in the evaluation of the learning.

7. *The level of anxiety affects retention, attention, and the ability to learn.* Generally, the higher the anxiety level, the lower the ability to concentrate on what is being taught. The client who is anxious about impending surgery will probably not learn about his postoperative diet. Frequently, even when the client is interested in such information, it will be necessary to repeat the content more than once.

8. *Learning is more meaningful when the learner is actively involved in the learning activity.* For example, a client will retain more by choosing a diabetic diet with assistance than by listening to a lecture on the diabetic exchange system.

9. *The learning environment affects the rate, amount, and quality of learning.* The nurse who is constantly interrupted by the telephone or by other personnel will have a difficult time teaching the client anything. Likewise, the client will have difficulty concentrating on a subject if he is surrounded by visitors. The client's comfort must also be considered when preparing a learning environment. Proper lighting, temperature, and seating will enhance the learner's ability to concentrate on the subject matter. It is often helpful if the client can move to a place separate from his

room that is reserved just for learning, such as a classroom or a conference area.

10. *Finally, success in the achievement of goals leads to realistic goal setting and the tolerance of occasional failure.* For example, the client who is on a weight reduction diet may have set a goal of losing 20 lb (9 kg) at the rate of 2 lb (1 kg)/wk. Each week that 2 lb are lost will reinforce his desire to lose more weight.

Teacher Characteristics

Because learning is an active process involving both a teacher and learner, certain characteristics of the teacher will enhance the learning of the client. The key attribute of the teacher is *awareness*. Primary is the awareness of the client's uniqueness. The teacher must be sensitive to the client's cultural, social, psychological, and physiological needs and be willing to modify teaching strategies to fit the client. Second, the teacher must be aware of the dynamic nature of knowledge. The teacher should be continuously looking for new content, approaches, and methods. The teacher, building on a firm scientific data base, must be open minded to new advancements in subject matter. Research is continuously yielding new data in nutrition and nutritional care. Third, the teacher must be aware of the role her own feelings, personal experiences, and background can play in a teacher-client relationship. For example, if the teacher values physical fitness, she may have difficulty working with an overweight client. Many times such feelings can be handled if the teacher is aware of them. Finally, the teacher should be aware of the specific skills necessary for effective communication with others. Continuing to improve on communication skills will aid in diagnosing and meeting clients' needs.

Teaching Methods

A wide variety of teaching methods are available to the teacher, her choice depending on the type of information she wishes to teach and its purpose. The most effective teaching method is that of one-to-one interaction. The exchange occurs between teacher and client directly. The nurse is able to assess each client's needs, abilities, and resources independently and modify teaching strategies accordingly. If the client is not learning with the techniques used, the nurse can easily modify how the material is taught. Most short-term client teaching is probably carried out through this method at the client's bedside. Although one-to-one teaching is most effective, it is also the most expensive in time and duplication of effort.

A second teaching method effective for teaching nutritional content is using small discussion or sharing groups. Usually the members of the group have similar needs and goals. Many times the group members will learn vicariously from one another's experiences as well as gain a support system. An example of a successful group is Weight Watchers. The group support provides an additional incentive for reaching a goal. Group technique is more efficient than one-to-one teaching. The teacher should have some background in group process theory to make certain the group meets its goals.

The most efficient method of presenting information is through classes and group lectures. The same information can be given to a large group of people; yet it is difficult to determine just how much each person has learned.

Exhibits provide reminders of a message to a large number of people. The number of people who receive the information cannot be determined. Eye-catching phrases and colors will enhance the appeal of the information.

Books and pamphlets are a means of providing baseline data on a subject. A client can read at his own pace and have time to think about the material presented. Literature should always be followed up with a one-to-one discussion to allow opportunity for clarification and questions.

Teaching Strategies

In addition to the environmental strategies mentioned previously, many other strategies are available for the teacher to use to get the message across.

• *Expository strategies* are generally one-way messages to give clients information. Lecturing is the most common expository strategy. For it to be effective, close individual follow-up after the lecture is necessary to assess unmet client needs.

• *Discovery strategies* include discussion groups and question-asking sessions. The client must feel at ease and free to ask questions about the subject. Such sessions provide clues to the client's interests and level of knowledge about the subject.

• *Problem-solving strategies* include the use of case studies and situational questions. Such strategies are frequently used after a client has been given some baseline data. The use of such strategies provides feedback for client and nurse. An example of the use of such a strategy is having a client choose a prescribed diet from a list of foods.

Teaching Process

The process of effective teaching entails the same steps as the nursing process. Assessment must include all aspects of the client, identification of a need for learning, and identification of the resources available for learning. Planning must be thorough. The teacher must determine who, what, when, where, and how to teach. The expectations of the learner must be identified. The teaching style and strategies must be developed around the content. Included in planning must also be the method of feedback to be used.

Decisions to be made before intervention should include how the teaching setting will be analyzed; how the content, including termination of the session, will be paced; and what methods will be used to maintain a climate conducive to maximum learning. Eval-uation must be planned to include the method of feedback to be used, how the learning will be reinforced, and how the teaching methods will be evaluated.

Teaching Principles

When teaching any subject it is very important to be consistent, particularly when the client is unfamiliar with the subject matter. The most effective means of maintaining consistency is to have the same professional teach the client from start to finish. Such a process is made operational through the use of primary nursing as a method of nursing care delivery. Writing the lesson plan in the chart or Kardex provides another assurance of consistency.

A second principle of effective teaching is that the teacher's enthusiasm will promote learning. A teacher who is convinced that the subject matter is important and who conveys enthusiasm is more likely to convince a client that learning the subject is worthwhile.

Another fundamental principle is that, as a teacher, the practitioner must know the subject matter to be taught. Further, the teacher should organize and present the material so that the client believes the teacher knows what she is talking about.

The attitude of the teacher influences the amount of learning that occurs. This attitude will be reflected in the teacher's grooming, posture, and gestures and will either detract from or enhance learning. An essential aspect of an attitude that fosters learning is respect for the client as more important than a procedure, a disease, or a research project. The use of effective communication skills will create an attitude of acceptance and caring for the client.

Ideally, there should be no interruptions during a teaching session; realistically, this may not be possible. The nurse should plan for interruptions but attempt to keep them at a minimum. If the teacher is interrupted too frequently, the client may perceive that the nurse is too busy to take time out to teach and may avoid asking for clarification of points he does not understand.

Finally, the teacher must be realistic about teaching and learning. Both the client and the teacher will have good days and bad days. It is important not to overwhelm the client. It is not necessary to teach everything at once. The creative use of methods and strategies will assist the client with learning and subsequent movement toward health.

EVALUATION

Evaluation is the last and often most ignored phase of the nursing process. After intervention it is easy for the health practitioner to assume that the correct measures were taken and thus anticipate appropriate results. Validating that assumption is the essence of evaluation. Evaluation is a means of responding to the consumer's demand for accountability for health care provided by professionals.

When evaluating the health care given, the practitioner should focus on both the results and the quality of the care given. The results of the care given are reflected in measurable client behaviors. Examples are whether the client has gained an appropriate amount of weight or can prepare a meal within the limits of his diet. Measuring the quality of the care given involves a retrospective review of the correctness and appropriateness of the interventions carried out. For example, did the dietary teaching include periodic feedback from the client? Was proper technique used when administering a tube feeding?

Evaluating the Results of Nutritional Intervention

Evaluation of the results of nutritional interventions must be based on the client objectives set during the planning stage of the nursing process. It must be remembered that these objectives are examples of client behavior. To be effective, goals set should be specific to the client's needs. Following are examples of objectives specific to each nursing diagnosis category discussed in Chapter 21:

I. Interferences with ingestion
  A. Manifested by a lack of information
     Objectives: At the completion of the plan of care the client (or his family) will be able to
     1. Discuss the foods that he should eat to meet his nutritional requirements.
     2. Discuss alterations in the diet that may occur with changes in his nutritional requirements.
     3. Consume a diet that meets his nutritional needs.
  B. Manifested by the Inaccessibility of nutrients
     Objectives: Be able to
     1. Use community and personal resources necessary to obtain adequate nutrients.
     2. Discuss reasons for altered nutritional intake.
     3. Communicate increased satisfaction with nutrient intake.
  C. Manifested by a lack of desire to ingest food and fluids
     Objectives: Be able to
     1. Ingest food in the quantity and variety necessary to meet his nutritional requirements.
     2. Modify his intake to meet his nutritional requirements.
  D. Manifested by the inability to ingest food and fluids
     Objectives: Be able to
     1. Ingest nutrients in sufficient quantity and variety to meet his nutritional requirements, using available personal and community resources.
     2. Maintain a nourished state, using available resources.

3. Discuss the importance of nutritional care specific to his alteration, for example, hyperalimentation or tube feedings.

E. Manifested by oral discomfort and/or obstruction

Objectives: Be able to

1. Confirm his increased comfort.
2. Maintain appropriate ingestion patterns.

F. Manifested by alterations in ingestion that have already occurred

Objectives: Be able to

1. Confirm that an alteration in ingestion has occurred.
2. Seek medical intervention if ingestion is life threatening.
3. Discuss future behavior changes that may prevent future ingestion problems.

II. Alterations in digestion and absorption

A. Manifested by alterations in motility

Objectives: Be able to

1. Exhibit a return to normal motility.
2. Discuss measures that may prevent future problems with motility.
3. Confirm his increased comfort.

B. Manifested by alterations in secretions

Objectives: Be able to

1. Exhibit a return to normal secretory patterns.
2. Discuss behavior changes that may prevent future secretory problems.
3. Confirm his increased comfort.

C. Manifested by alterations in absorptive surface

Objectives: Be able to

1. Discuss altered intake patterns that provide necessary nutrients for normal growth, development, and maintenance.
2. Ingest a diet that provides necessary nutrients.
3. Maintain adequate nutrition.

III. Alterations in Nutrient Transport

A. Manifested by alterations in vascular physiology

Objectives: Be able to

1. Discuss altered ingestion patterns that may prevent vascular disease.
2. Plan a diet that provides for adequate nutrition, takes into account alterations necessary for vascular disease, and is satisfying.
3. Consume nutrients that are outlined in such a plan.

B. Manifested by blockage of nutrient transport

Objectives: Be able to

1. Discuss alterations in ingestion patterns that may be necessary to prevent further vascular blockage.
2. Consume a diet that will not contribute to further blockage.

C. Manifested by electrolyte imbalance

Objectives: Be able to

1. Follow a diet that provides for adequate nutrient intake and altered electrolyte status.
2. Discuss possible alterations in the diet that may occur with fluctuations in electrolyte status.
3. Plan a diet that meets necessary nutritional alterations and is satisfying.
4. Show a return to normal electrolyte patterns following ingestion of the prescribed diet.

D. Manifested by Oxygen/carbon dioxide alterations

Objectives: Be able to

1. Plan a diet that provides for adequate nutrient intake in the presence of altered oxygen/carbon dioxide status.
2. Consume a diet that meets his nutritional requirements.

E. Manifested by fluid volume alterations

Objectives: Be able to

1. State the purpose of various medical-nursing interventions aimed at reestablishing fluid volume homeostasis.
2. Plan a diet that takes altered fluid requirements into consideration.
3. Use nursing and medical resources to maintain adequate nutrition during emergency phase fluid alterations.

F. Manifested by changes in blood pH

Objectives: Be able to

1. Seek nursing and medical intervention to correct emergency phase serum pH alterations.
2. Discuss preventive measures that may maintain a normal blood pH.

IV. Alterations in metabolism

A. Manifested by alterations in nutritional requirements

Objectives: Be able to

1. Plan a diet that meets his altered nutritional requirements.
2. Consume a diet that meets his altered nutritional requirements.

B. Manifested by alterations in endocrine physiology

Objectives: Be able to

1. Plan a diet that meets his altered nutritional requirements.
2. Discuss a diet that may prevent endocrine imbalances.

C. Manifested by alterations in structure

Objectives: Be able to

1. Maintain (or regain) an intact integumentary system.
2. Ingest nutrients in a quantity and variety that will assist in maintaining skin and bone integrity.
3. Confirm his increased confort.
4. Follow a diet that is consistent with structural alterations.

V. Alterations in Excretion

A. Manifested by alterations in fluid output

Objectives: Be able to

1. Maintain an adequate urinary output.
2. Discuss the purpose of selected medical-nursing interventions.
3. Maintain a fluid intake consistent with his alteration.

B. Manifested by alterations in solid waste excretion

Objectives: Be able to

1. Maintain an adequate solid waste output.
2. Plan a diet that may help correct his alterations in solid waste output.

Achievement of the objectives can be confirmed only if the behaviors outlined during the planning phase of the nursing process are demonstrated by the client. Return demonstration of specific tasks is the most reliable way of determining success in teaching. A subjective affirmation from the client that he knows how to do something may not be a reliable indicator of true ability to perform. In most instances the period of performance evaluation will also serve as an assessment period to determine future needs.

If the objective is in the affective domain, determining whether it has been achieved is more difficult. Such an objective might be: The client will demonstrate a commitment to good nutritional habits by eating a well-balanced diet. The purpose of affective learning is to establish a new behavior or to increase, decrease, or extinguish an existing behavior. Confirmation of such behavior is difficult without continuous monitoring. Further, commitment to a pattern was opposed to simple compliance is extremely difficult to measure.

Any measure of motivation must reflect more than a single episode. Evaluation of motivation will probably require both the involvement of a trusted significant other selected by the client and the client's own self-reporting. The same data that was gathered in the assessment phase can be collected again.

In summary, the evaluation should focus on behavior changes in the client. The evaluation should look at both competence and motivation and should include a determination of the relevance to the client of performing the behavior. "Assurance that the client has, in fact, acquired or improved a desirable behavior, or eliminated a destructive one, is the first step in validating professional intervention" (Mason, 1977, p. 258).

Evaluating the Quality of Intervention

Evaluating the presence of desired behaviors in a client is only part of the evaluation that should occur at the conclusion of nutritional intervention. The appropriateness and accuracy of the intervention should also be evaluated. Such evaluation can be carried out on five levels. First, the client can be asked to evaluate the intervention. Frequently, affective data about how the client "felt" about the care giver will be gleaned from such an evaluation. In addition, important insights can be learned from the client's perceptions of what occurred during the time of intervention. Client-based evaluation is usually conducted

by a follow-up questionnaire after he is discharged from the care of the practitioner.

Peer evaluation is the second level of evaluation. Usually, peer evaluation will focus not on a single intervention or interchange but on total patterns of behavior. To be effective, peer evaluation should be self-initiated and carried out by a structured, nonthreatening method. Written evaluations followed by short discussions in the presence of a non-biased mediator can be such a method of evaluation. Such evaluation requires the establishment of trust, communication, and purposeful interchanges between health professionals.

Evaluation of the nurse by her supervisor is the third and most common level of evaluation. Such evaluations usually center on patterns of behavior rather than specific interventions. The superior may place the health professional's contributions in a larger context than that assumed by her colleagues. Evaluation by such a person not intimately caught up in a situation can provide meaningful insight into patterns of behavior.

A fourth and more formal level of evaluation involving many departments and professionals simultaneously is accomplished via an audit. A *patient care audit* is a means of professional self-regulation (Joint Commission for Accreditation of Hospitals, 1974). Systematic patient care evaluation can result in improved patient care, increased coordination of community resources by all members of the health care team, increased documentation of care performed, correction of deficiencies in agency-wide procedures, increased communication between departments and services, and increased research opportunities.

Two basic kinds of audit are common. One is an *outcome audit,* which focuses on client outcomes, that is, on what behaviors a client is demonstrating at the time of his discharge from an agency or department. The other audit is a *process audit,* which focuses on client management. An outcome audit identifies unacceptable client outcomes and, ideally, the inappropriate patterns of medical or nursing care that led to them. A process audit is intended as further exploration of a known or suspected problem in the process of care.

An example of how these two types of audit can be used is seen in a client on a diabetic diet. The nurse's notes show that the client had to be discharged to an extended care facility because he could not prepare a 1,500 Calorie diet. The client's behavior is reflected in the outcome audit. A process audit of the diabetic teaching program might reveal a deficiency in exploring the client's previous food patterns and cultural background. Process audit, then, functions as a management tool to determine whether specific nursing protocols are being followed, whether adequate assessment is occurring, and whether the nursing diagnoses documented have been well validated.

The audit, whether outcome or process, has three major components: identifying elements, setting standards, and specifying exceptions. *Element* refers to some aspect of the client's problem (such as a symptom), of the nurse's program of care (such as preventive measures), or of the client's clinical course (such as a desired outcome). Generally, audit criteria (the elements) are as specific and comprehensive as possible.

Standards are then assigned to the elements. Based on current knowledge, a standard can be specified by answering the question How often (in what percentage of cases) could it be expected that this element would occur or not occur or should this element be performed or not performed? An example of a standard for the element of a client being able to prepare his diabetic diet upon discharge is 100%. Usually, standards are written as 0% or 100%. Sometimes an all-or-none response is not possible. A common example is the discharge of a client free from pain. Generally, clients should not be having pain upon leaving the hospital or agency. But acceptable *exceptions* include clients with extensive car-

cinoma or who are discharged early on pain medication.

In a nursing process audit, two categories of elements are identified: those things nurses and health professionals should learn about patients and those things nurses should do to or for clients. Again, standards and exceptions are set for each element. Nursing audits represent a positive method for the profession to evaluate and critique itself systematically continuously.

Self-evaluation is the final level of evaluating client care. Self-evaluation should be conducted continuously to increase skill and consistency in performance. An honest appraisal of the client's behavior and how one responded to it is central to self-evaluation. Even more crucial is the health professional's ability first to determine when a different or better action could have been taken and then to act on that evaluation.

Evaluation at all levels looks at human, material, and environmental resources and how they contribute to the success of the total care plan. It requires a thorough comparison of the observed intervention with standards of competent professional practice.

BIBLIOGRAPHY

Bower, F. L., and Bevis, E. O. *Fundamentals of Nursing Practice.* St. Louis: The C. V. Mosby Co., 1979.

Hill, M. Helping the hypertensive patient control sodium intake. *Am. J. Nurs.* 79:906, 1979.

Joint Commission on Accreditation of Hospitals. *Accreditation Manual for Hospitals,* New York: JCAH, 1981.

Jung, J. *Verbal Learning.* New York: Holt, Rinehart & Winston, 1968.

Krause, M. V., and Mahan, L. K. *Food, Nutrition, and Diet Therapy.* 6th Ed. Philadelphia: W. B. Saunders Co., 1979.

Mason, M. *The Dynamics of Clinical Dietetics.* New York: John Wiley and Sons, Inc., Pubs., 1977.

Murray, R., and Zentner, J. Guidelines for more effective health teaching. *Nursing 76* 3:44, 1976.

Robinson, C. H., and Lawler, M. R. *Normal and Therapeutic Nutrition.* 15th Ed. New York: Macmillan Inc., 1977.

CHAPTER 23

Nutritional Support of Medical Intervention

One of the purposes of this book has been to focus on the independent functions of the nurse as a provider of nutritional care for the client. Through the use of the nursing process and a problem-solving method, the nurse is able to identify and correct potential or overt interferences with the client's health. Such independent activities contribute to the level of health a client is able to achieve.

Nursing does not exist in a vacuum; rather, it must be a part of the total care given by the health care team. A necessary part of the nurse's role as a health team member is to carry out those functions designated by the physician. Through knowledge of physiological and psychological norms, dexterity skills, assessment skills, and an ongoing relationship with the client, the nurse is able to assist the physician in the diagnosis and treatment of a specific illness. This chapter discusses several of the nurse's functions in relation to medical practice; specifically, nursing techniques used in intravenous fluid replacement, test diets, and diet-drug interactions, nasogastric feeding and total parenteral nutrition (hyperalimentation).

INTRAVENOUS THERAPY

Intravenous therapy is the infusion of water, electrolytes, glucose, nutrients, or combinations of these to prevent dehydration or electrolyte imbalance. IV therapy is initiated on the orders of a physician to (1) provide for daily fluid and electrolyte requirements, (2) replace losses of fluids and electrolytes that

are occurring, or (3) restore plasma volume after fluid and electrolyte losses have occurred. Generally, body reserves of protein and fat are sufficient to sustain most people for a week or more during inadequate nitrogen and caloric intakes without serious consequences. It has been shown, however (Randall, 1973), that even normal male volunteers who are immobilized will develop a small but significant negative nitrogen balance. The implications of a negative nitrogen status in regard to tissue repair and infection susceptibility will be discussed in Chapter 27.

The basic requirements for parenteral therapy can be categorized as (1) baseline requirements, (2) abnormal losses, and (3) fluid deficits or excesses.

Baseline Requirements

Daily baseline requirements are provided to minimize or prevent dehydration, starvation, and electrolyte imbalance that would occur during interruption of oral intake. Normal baseline water requirements vary from 1,250 to 3,000 ml/day depending on body cell mass, size, age, and sex. The following formula can be used to compute needed water in milliliters per day for relatively normal semistarving patients without massive trauma, dehydration, or prolonged illness. For all patients except infants who weigh less than 11 lb (5 kg), the patient's ideal body weight is used in the formula for the obese patient, and the actual body weight is used for others.

First 10 kg of body weight at 100 ml/kg/day
+ Second 10 kg of body weight at 50 ml/kg/day

+ All weight above 20 kg at 20 ml/kg/day if less than 50 years old

or at 15 ml/kg/day if greater than 50 years old

For example, a 45-year-old man weighing 85 kg should receive 2,800 ml of fluid volume per day to meet his basic metabolic requirements.

Daily body weight measurements are the single most important method of controlling water balance in the hospitalized patient. Rapid weight gain (more than 2 kg/day) usually indicates overhydration, whereas rapid weight loss usually indicates diuresis, dehydration, or both.

Baseline water requirements are increased by fever, sweating, and increased metabolism. A fever of 6.2 F (3.4 C), with its accompanying hyperventilation and increased water evaporation, will raise baseline water requirements by 500 ml/day. Similarly, an additional 500 ml of water will be required for every 5-degree rise in external temperature above 85 F (or for every 2.8-degree rise above 29 C), primarily because of losses from sweating.

Baseline water requirements are decreased during periods of lowered metabolism, as during hypothermia or a hypothyroid state. Clients experiencing congestive heart failure or acute renal failure with their concomitant fluid retention will also require less water intake.

Baseline electrolyte requirements are generally met by the administration of 500 cc of 5% dextrose and .9% sodium chloride solution (D_5NS). The solution provides 76 mEq of both sodium and chlorine. An addition of 40 mEq of potassium chloride will meet ongoing potassium requirements. Of course the electrolyte levels of all clients with severely altered ingestion patterns should be carefully monitored by regular serum samples.

Maintenance requirements of infants may be met by similar calculations. The formula just cited generally takes into account the decrease in metabolic rate per kilogram with increasing age. The very young infant (3 kg, or 6.5 lb, 1 month) should receive about 300–350 ml of water a day (approximately 100 ml/kg of body weight). Variations in the total requirements need to be made that take into consideration the infant's total body surface area and caloric expenditure. Because of the minute quantities required, the margin for error when dealing with infants is very small. The nurse must assume full responsibility for the prevention of accidental fluid overload or too little administration.

Abnormal Losses

Abnormal losses of fluid and electrolytes may be from the normal routes of excretion and secretion or from drains, fistulas, or wounds. The most common route of loss from the surgical patient is via the gastrointestinal tract and wounds.

The normal gastrointestinal tract secretes 8–10 liters of fluid per day. The components of this secretion include: saliva, 1–2 liters; gastric juice, 2,500 ml; bile, 500–750 ml; pancreatic juice, 1 liter; and upper small bowel juice, 2–3 liters. Usually all but 100–200 ml is reabsorbed by the lower small bowel and colon. Medical conditions in which a severe loss would occur include altered motility resulting in diarrhea or excessive vomiting; ileostomy or high colostomy; acute pancreatitis; and fistulas resulting from trauma, cancer, or another organic problem. All drainage should be carefully measured and recorded. The fluid volume lost is often replaced parenterally in amounts equal to that lost.

Deficits or Excesses

Fluid overload and dehydration were discussed in depth in Chapter 11. Decisions about replacement therapy are within the realm of medicine. The nurse must continually be alert for any signs of fluid or electrolyte imbalance and report them immediately to the physician.

Acute dehydration occurs with an almost total loss of extracellular fluid with the resultant shift of fluid out of the cell. A 2% loss of body weight secondary to fluid loss will produce thirst and some oliguria. A 4% loss of body weight will produce oliguria, tachycardia, and postural hypotension. At this point the client has lost 20% of his extracellular fluid. A 6% loss of body weight is life threatening. Hypotension and impending renal shutdown are imminent. Treatment with plasma expanders and fluid replacement should be instituted promptly at the first sign of severe dehydration.

The major reason for choosing the intravenous route for administering medication is to provide the medication rapidly and assure more accurate absorption. The exact rate and dose of medication can be accurately titrated to meet patient needs or provide for a therapeutic response. The very reasons for choosing IV therapy also point to many of its drawbacks. First of all, there is no room for error and frequently no time for an antidote or corrective therapy. In addition, the body perceives the IV catheter as a foreign body. As such, the catheter site is a potential site for sepsis, thrombus, or phlebitis formation. Infiltration of the intravenous medication can cause localized pain, swelling, and occasional extravasation of tissue.

Nursing Responsibilities in Intravenous Therapy

The nursing responsibilities associated with IV therapy can be discussed in terms of the nursing process. The scope of the responsibilities depends on the setting in which the nurse functions. In many settings the nurse is responsible for starting and maintaining the IV. In other settings a specially trained IV team starts and maintains the therapy. In still other settings the house interns and externs start the IV; then the nursing staff maintains the infusion and monitors the client for complications. IV therapy can be a major factor in the return of the client to normal functioning. Thus, the nurse should be actively involved in this aspect of medical care. Table 23-1 lists common IV solutions, their contents, and indications and contraindications.

Assessment
Assessment should include:

THE RATE. There are many factors that can affect the rate of flow of the solution, including the viscosity of the solution, the porosity of the final filters used, movement by the patient, height of the IV in relation to the heart and vein, medication additions, clot formations, and catheter size. The flow rate should be carefully calculated using the appropriate conversion factor for the infusion set used. To maintain precise infusion rates the nurse can use one of a variety of volumetric infusion pumps available. Whether a pump is used or not, the IV bottle or bag should be time-taped at the time it is hung to provide for ease in maintaining the rate throughout the infusion (see Fig. 23-1).

THE SITE. The IV site should be carefully observed for any signs of inflammation or infiltration (Fig. 23-2). Redness, pain, leaking around the site, edema, and lack of flow are all signs of impending phlebitis or infiltration. The nurse should use her judgment in deciding whether or not to discontinue an IV; of course infiltration necessitates immediate discontinuation.

THERAPEUTIC EFFECTS AND SIDE EFFECTS OF MEDICATION. The nurse must be aware of the reason intravenous therapy was initiated, the patient's electrolytes and other pertinent laboratory values, and the anticipated therapeutic effect of the drugs administered. The nurse should monitor the patient's fluid intake and output, daily weight, and vital signs. She should also be alert for the signs of electrolyte and fluid imbalance, as discussed in Chapter 11.

TABLE 23-1. Common Intravenous Solutions, Indications, and Contraindications

Solution	Contents	Indications	Contraindications
D₅W (5% dextrose in water)	Dextrose = 5 gm/100 ml	Need to prevent dehydration Need to supply water Need to promote sodium diuresis	Should not be given with blood Overhydration
D₅ ₁/₂ NS (5% dextrose in .45% sodium chloride)	Dextrose = 5 gm/100 ml	Fluid losses with sodium loss as from perspiration Need for hydrating solution to promote diuresis	Renal insufficiency Generalized edema as from cardial, hepatic, or renal disease
NS (.9% sodium chloride—normal saline)	Sodium = 14 mEq/liter Chloride = 154 mEq/liter	Alkalosis in the presence of fluid loss Diabetic acidosis	Elevated plasma electrolytes Edema
Ringers solution	Sodium = 14 mEq/liter Chloride = 155 mEq/liter Potassium = 4 mEq/liter Calcium = 4 mEq/liter	Dehydration from decreased water intake Water loss from vomiting, diarrhea	Severe deficiency of potassium or calcium Addison's disease
Lactated ringers	Sodium = 130 mEq/liter Potassium = 4 mEq/liter Calcium = 3 mEq/liter Chloride = 109 mEq/liter Lactate	Dehydration Need to restore fluid balance after fluid shift from extracellular fluid as from burns, infection Moderate metabolic acidosis	Liver disease Anoxic states Addison's disease
Sodium lactate	Sodium Lactate	Severe metabolic acidosis Need to reverse hyperkalemia	Liver disease Respiratory alkalosis when lactic acid levels are high
Normosol-MinD₃W	Dextrose = 5 gm/100 ml Nace = 234 mg/100 ml Potassium acetate = 125 mg/100 ml Magnesium acetate = 21 mg/100 ml Sodium bisulfate = 33 mg (3 mEq/liter) pH adjusted with HCl ≈ 1 mEq/liter	Need for maintenance solution Daily water and electrolyte losses Extracellular replacement Gastric replacement	Severe renal disease Severe liver disease
Normosol-R in D₅W	Dextrose = 5 gm/100 ml Sodium acetate = 222 mg/100 ml Sodium gluconate = 502 mg/100 ml Potassium chloride = 37 mg/100 ml Magnesium chloride = 15 mg/100 ml Sodium bisulfate = 33 mg (3 mEq/liter) pH adjusted with HCl ≈ 1 mEq/liter	Need for maintenance solution Daily water and electrolyte losses Extracellular replacement Gastric replacement	Severe renal disease Severe liver disease

Planning

The planning involved in IV therapy centers on maintaining patient comfort and safety. Because intravenous administration is largely a dependent function of the nurse, the nurse's main responsibility is the patient teaching about the need for treatment and explaining all procedures connected with IV therapy. Frequently all the patient needs is the assurance that the nurse sees him as a person instead of a task to be dealt with during the work shift.

Intervention

The methods of initiating, maintaining, and terminating IV therapy vary from setting to

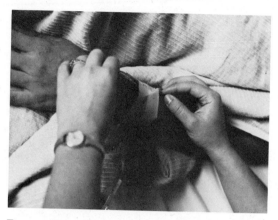

Figure 23-2. Checking the intravenous infusion site for signs of infiltration or phlebitis.

setting. Several policy and procedure books are available on this subject.

Several intravenous infusion pumps are available that control IV flow rates with great precision. Most pumps can be used with both bags and bottles, and many can be used for nasogastric as well as intravenous infusions.

Frequently, much of a nurse's time is spent attempting to maintain, correct, or troubleshoot intravenous therapy drip rates and infusions. Many times, experience provides the best teacher for dealing with the problems. Flow regulation can be achieved by careful monitoring, time taping the bottle, and dating the tubing. The careful use of padded armboards will prevent infiltration in many cases.

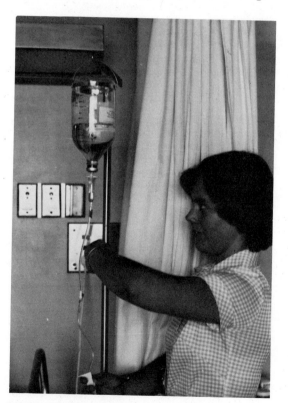

Figure 23-1. Setting the drip rate on an intravenous infusion.

Evaluation

Evaluation should focus on whether the nurse's responsibilities in IV therapy were carried out. Has the patient remained comfortable? Were all nursing measures taken that were necessary to ensure patient safety? Did the nurse use whatever technical skills were available to her to assist the physician in maintaining the IV site?

NUTRITIONAL PREPARATION FOR PATIENTS REQUIRING MEDICAL DIAGNOSTIC INTERVENTION

Frequently during the course of a client's hospitalization, the physician will order a series of radiological or diagnostic examinations. To achieve adequate visualization of the organ or system to be studied, the client may have to undergo a variety of preparations. Frequently alteration of the type or amount of a person's nutrient intake is required.

Each hospital has its own protocols and methods for preparing a patient for a particular study. There are some general guidelines and examples of nutritional variances that may occur in preparing patients for specific examinations:

• For a *barium enema*, obviously, the colon must be cleared of fecal material. To clear the bowel, a minimal-residue diet is provided for three days before the test. Table 23.2 lists foods acceptable on such a diet. The day before the examination the client receives only clear liquids to eat (Table 23-3). Clear liquids should be encouraged on the afternoon before the examination, with 8 oz of liquids given each hour between 11 AM and 10 PM. The client should receive nothing by mouth after 12 midnight. Usually cathartics and enemas are included in the preparation of the client. Other gastrointestinal examinations require similar preparation.

• A *cholecystogram* requires clearing of the intestinal tract of as much gas and fecal material as possible to achieve adequate visualization of the gall bladder. Enemas and mild cathartics are usually prescribed the day before the examination is scheduled. The evening meal the day before the test should consist only of dry toast, jelly, and a beverage. No milk, cream, butter, or fatty foods should be included. The patient should not take food by mouth after midnight. A commercial preparation of a fatty emulsion is given in the radiology department to stimulate gall bladder function.

• *Catecholamine levels* in urine are evaluated during endocrine evaluations and in those cases in which an adrenal tumor is suspected. The metabolites of the major catecholamines epinephrine and norepinephrine are excreted in the urine. One of these, vanillyomandelic acid (VMA), is used to reflect serum catecholamine levels. To obtain accu-

TABLE 23-2. Foods Allowed and not Allowed on a Minimal-residue Diet

Foods Allowed
Meat
Canned baby meats
Baked skinless fish
Finely chopped canned tuna
Cottage cheese, dry
Eggs
Cereal
Cream of Wheat
Farina
Fruit juices
Orange, grapefruit, pineapple
Apple, grape
Oil, butter, margarine
Clear broth or boullion
Beverages
Tea, coffee, decaffeinated coffee
Carbonated beverages
Sweets
Gelatin, sugar, strained honey
Marshmallows, vanilla wafers, sugar wafers
Seasonings
Foods not Allowed
Breads, fruits, vegetables, milk

TABLE 23-3. Clear-Liquid Diet

Food Group	Foods Included
Soups	Clear broth, consommé, and boullion
Beverages	Coffee, tea
	Synthetic beverages: lemonade, carbonated beverages
	Grape, apple, cherry, cranberry juice
Desserts	Gelatin
Sweets	Sugar, hard candy

rate results, any foods containing VMA must be omitted at least 48 hours before and during the urine collection. Foods that must be omitted include coffee, tea, cocoa, chocolate, cola beverages, bananas, vanilla, and nuts.

• *5-Hydroxyindole acetic acid* (5-H-IAA) is a test used to evaluate the presence of a *carcinogenic syndrome*. Tomatoes, bananas, avocados, vanilla, walnuts, and pineapple in any form should be omitted three days before the urine collection.

• A *meat-free test meal* is given to check for occult blood in feces. The test is rarely used except in cases of undetermined anemia. All meats, fish, and poultry are omitted from the diet for five to seven days.

• The *renin test diet* is used in the diagnosis of essential hypertension. A 500-mg sodium diet is recommended for at least three days before the test. A diet containing normal amounts of sodium will repress the plasma rennin level, giving inaccurate data.

• The *iodine radioisotope test diet* is given in preparation for thyroid function studies. The client is placed on a regular diet with the omission of all seafood products and iodized salt.

• The *100-gm fat test diet* is given to diagnose various malabsorption syndromes. The diet is usually followed for three to five days before the stool collection. Stool specimens are ana-lyzed for fecal fat, solids, and nitrogen content. Usually a level of 100 gm of fat is calculated into the diet by giving 1 egg (5 gm fat); 7 oz meat (35 gm); 2 cups whole milk (20 gm); and 8 pats of margarine, butter, cream, or salad dressing (40 gm).

• The *200-mg calcium test diet* is used when testing for hypercalciuria or in the treatment of acute hypercalcemia. When used for testing purposes the diet should be followed for three days before the test. All water used in the diet should be distilled. A sample menu for a 200-mg calcium diet is shown in Table 23-4.

• The *glucose tolerance test diet* is prescribed for the test to diagnose or confirm diabetes mellitus. The diet should contain a minimum of 300 gm of carbohydrate. Calories, protein, and fat are not limited. The diet should be eaten by the client for at least three days before the serum is drawn. The purpose of the regimen is to stimulate the pancreas before the test.

• The *restricted serotonin test diet* is prescribed when testing for urinary *indoles* and catecholamines. The test diet is given 72 hours before a 24-hour urine collection. Bananas, tomatoes, pineapples, shellfish, and mushrooms must be omitted on this diet, but Calorie, carbohydrate, protein, and fat content are normal.

TABLE 23-4. Sample Menu for the 200-mg Calcium Diet

Breakfast	*Lunch*	*Dinner*
Orange juice	Broiled halibut	Roast beef
Cream of rice	Buttered rice	Baked potato
Half-and-half	Buttered carrots	Buttered asparagus
Bacon	Lettuce wedge with French dressing	Grapefruit juice
Vienna toast	Vienna bread	Vienna bread
Margarine	Margarine	Margarine
Coffee made with distilled water	Jelly	Sugar cookies
Sugar	Salt	Salt
Salt	Gelatin	Coffee made with distilled water
Marmalade	Iced tea made with distilled water	
	Sugar	

DRUG-NUTRIENT INTERACTIONS

The maintenance or restoration of a person's health may require a number of medical and nursing interventions including nutritional, pharmacological, physical, and psychological support. Many of the nutrients and drugs prescribed can interact to create a completely different effect than originally intended. The nurse is in a unique position to know what medications and nutrients a client is receiving and therefore what possible interactions may occur.

Drugs can affect taste, appetite, intestinal motility, and absorption and metabolism of nutrients. Likewise certain foods or patterns of dietary consumption may alter drug absorption and response. Specifically, drugs can alter food intake by causing changes in appetite, taste, or smell. Nausea and vomiting are common side effects of many medications administered orally and parenterally. Absorption is changed through changes in gastrointestinal motility, changes in bile acid secretion, formation of drug-nutrient complexes, inactivation of enzyme systems, or changes in the mucosal cells lining the gastrointestinal tract. In addition, many drugs alter the normal metabolism and use of a specific nutrient or the rate and amount of nutrient excretion. These effects of a drug on nutrients are often due both to the intended therapeutic effect and to the incidental side effects of the drug.

Clinical deficiency states related to pharmacological therapy are usually the result of a combination of factors. Symptoms of nutrient depletion occur most frequently when a drug is used for an extended time, when the overall diet is inadequate or marginal, or when drugs alter widespread coenzyme functions, as with vitamin B_6. Consequently, effects of drugs on vitamins B_6, B_{12}, and folacin absorption account for the majority of drug-induced nutritional deficiencies.

The possible effects of nutrients on drug therapy are equally problematic. A food-drug interaction may occur in four ways. First, food may delay drug absorption, thus decreasing the blood level of the drug. When an antibiotic is administered, for instance, it is important to maintain a high blood level of the drug to treat an existing infection. Second, drug metabolism may be altered through enzyme induction or inhibition. Third, foods may alter the rate of drug excretion by changing the pH of the urine. Fourth, several common foods contain pharmacologically active substances that may alter the response of a drug administered simultaneously.

Determining diet composition while taking into consideration the potential nutrient-drug interactions is a difficult and complex task demanding the cooperation of the entire health team. The nurse is in a unique position to coordinate such efforts because of her increased exposure to client needs, habits, and long-term therapy. Oversights that occur in relation to drug-diet interaction are frequently due to a lack of knowledge about possible interactions, to the assumption that symptoms are due to disease rather than a nutritional deficiency, to an unrecognized existing problem such as alcoholism that places the client at risk, or to the concomitant administration of multiple drug therapies.

The nursing assessment must include clinical data; a listing of all drugs taken, including such home remedies as sodium bicarbonate; and a complete dietary history. Serum determinations of nutrient levels may aid the physician in making a diagnosis of an overt deficiency. Table 23-5 summarizes common drug-nutrient interactions; a more detailed explanation follows, as does a discussion of some of the more common problems associated with specific pharmacological agents.

Effects of Drugs on Ingestion

Drugs may affect nutrient ingestion by altering taste or appetite or by causing nausea with a resultant decrease in food intake.

Griseofulvin (an antifungal agent used to treat ringworm), penicillamine (used to chelate heavy metals), linomycin (an antibiotic), and 5-mercaptopyridoxal (an anticancer drug) all cause a decrease in taste acuity that could decrease intake.

Streptomycin (an antibiotic) frequently leaves a metallic taste in the mouth, even when administered intravenously. Likewise, potassium chloride (a potassium supplement), chloral hydrate and paraldehyde (both are hypnotics used to aid sleep), and vitamin B liquids have a bad taste and odor that are difficult to mask. The anticipation of the drug or concurrent administration with foods may decrease appetite and total caloric ingestion.

Drugs that decrease appetite include amphetamines (frequently given to induce weight loss), cholinergic agents (used for intestinal or urinary retention), glyceryl guaiacolate (an expectorant), and narcotic analgesics such as morphine or meperidine. High-fiber and bulk-forming medications such as methylcellulose, guar gum, and psyllium hydrophilic mucilloid tend to reduce appetite slightly by creating a feeling of fullness.

Gastrointestinal upset may be caused by phenformin (an oral hypoglycemic agent), cytotoxic drugs (cancer chemotherapeutic agents), and many antibiotics given by mouth.

Conversely, appetite may be increased by phenothiazine tranquilizers, antianxiety agents, tricyclic antidepressants, oral contraceptives, and glucocorticords, and when insulin-induced hypoglycemia is present. A small amount of alcohol taken before eating tends to increase appetite by stimulating taste and increasing saliva and gastric secretions.

Clients on restricted diets need to be monitored for the intake of drugs containing glucose, sodium, or other restricted nutrients. Cough syrups, expectorants, and elixers contain large amounts of glucose that need to be counted in the client's caloric intake. Many parenteral solutions and antibiotic tablets contain large amounts of sodium. For example, a 1-gm vial of naficillin contains 73 mg of sodium. The client on a severe sodium restriction to control fluid retention will need to be monitored carefully.

Drug-Nutrient Alterations in Absorption

One of the most frequently reported drug-diet interactions involves a change in the bioavailability of a drug because of concurrent food ingestion. Similarly, drugs may alter the absorption of various nutrients during the drug therapy. In fact, the majority of food-drug interactions seem to involve alterations in the absorptive process.

Absorption of drugs and absorption of nutrients occur by very different means. Absorption of most drugs is governed by lipid solubility, rate of dissociation, gastrointestinal pH, particle size, and physical form of the drug. Transport across gastric mucosa is primarily by passive diffusion. Nutrient absorption (discussed in Chap. 10) generally depends on gastrointestinal secretions, pH, and an intact enzyme system. The small intestine—the site of absorption for nutrients and most drugs—is also the major site of drug-nutrient interaction.

Drugs causing malabsorption induce diarrhea, steatorrhea, and weight loss. Flatulence, colic abdominal pain, and symptoms of specific nutrient deficiencies may occur.

Nutrient Effects on Drug Absorption

Food intake may alter the absorption amount and rate of a drug taken orally because drugs generally are absorbed more slowly when they are taken with food and because total absorption of the drug is often reduced. This effect is due to the delaying effect food has on gastric emptying. The decreased *rate* of absorption is more important when drugs are given as single doses in clinical situations requiring a rapid onset of drug activity. Analgesics, hypnotics, and antiasthmatics given as needed are examples of such drugs.

TABLE 23-5. Drug-Nutrient Interactions

Drug	Effect
Alcohol	Decreased absorption of thiamine, folic acid, vitamin B_{12}; increased urinary excretion of magnesium and zinc
Analgesics	
Aspirin (salicylates)	Decreased serum folate level; increased excretion of vitamin C
Colchicine	Decreased absorption of vitamin B_{12}, carotene, fat, lactose, sodium, potassium, protein, cholesterol
Amphetamines	Decreased appetite and caloric intake; possibly reduced growth
Antacids	
Aluminum hydroxide	Decreased absorption of phosphate
Other antacids	Decreased thiamine and fatty acid absorption
Anticonvulsants	
Barbituates	Decreased vitamin B_{12}, thiamine absorption; increased excretion of vitamin C; deficiency of folate and vitamin D
Hydantoins	Decreased serum folate, vitamin B_{12}, pyridoxine, calcium, and vitamin D levels; increased excretion of vitamin C
Antidepressants	Increased appetite; weight gain
Antimetabolites	General absorptive decrease secondary to intestinal-wall damage and oral mucus breakdown; specific malabsorption of B_{12}, folate, fat, and xylose
Antimicrobials	
Chloramphenicol	Increased riboflavin, pyridoxine, and B_{12} requirements
Neomycin	Decreased absorption of fat; carbohydrate; protein; vitamins A, B_{12}, D, and E; calcium; iron; sugar; potassium; sodium; nitrogen
Penicillin	Increased potassium excretion; inhibition of glutathione
Sulfonamides	Decreased synthesis of folic acid, vitamin K, and B vitamins
Tetracyclines	Decreased absorption of calcium, iron, magnesium, fat; increased excretion of vitamin C, riboflavin, nitrogen, folic acid, and niacin; decreased vitamin K synthesis
Cathartics	Decreased absorption of calcium, vitamin D, potassium, protein, glucose, fat
Chelating agents	Increased excretion of zinc, copper, pyridoxine; depression of appetite
Corticosteroids	Decreased absorption of calcium, phosphorus, iron; increased excretion of vitamin C, calcium, potassium, zinc, nitrogen; decreased tolerance of glucose; increased triglycerides and cholesterol absorption; increased vitamin D metabolism; increased appetite
Diuretics	
Furosemide	Increased excretion of calcium, magnesium, potassium
Mercurials	Increased excretion of thiamine, magnesium, calcium, potassium
Thiazides	Increased excretion of potassium, magnesium, zinc, and riboflavin
Triamterence	Decreased serum folate and vitamin B_{12} levels
Hypocholesterolemic agents	
Cholestyramine	Decreased absorption of cholesterol; potassium; vitamins A, D, K, and B_{12}; folate, fat, glucose, iron
Clofibrate	Decreased absorption of vitamin B_{12}, iron, glucose, potssium, sodium; decreased taste acuity, aftertaste
Hypotensive agents	Increased excretion of pyridoxine

TABLE 23-5. (*Continued*)

Drug	Effect
Laxatives	
Mineral oil	Decreased absorption of vitamins A, D, E, and K; calcium; phosphate
Phenolphthalein	Increased excretion of potassium
Levodopa	Decreased absorption of amino acids; increased use of ascorbic acid and pyridoxine; increased excretion of sodium and potassium
Oral contraceptives	Decreased serum levels of vitamin C, B_{12}, folate, pyridoxine, riboflavin, magnesium, zinc; increased absorption of iron; increased serum lipid levels; increased appetite
Potassium chloride	Decreased absorption of vitamin B_{12}
Sedatives	
Glutethimide	Increased metabolism of vitamin D
Sulfonamides	
Azulfidine	Decreased absorption of folate; decreased serum iron level
Other sulfonamides	Decreased synthesis of folate, vitamins B and K
Surfactants	Decreased absorption of fat
Tranquilizers	Increased appetite; weight gain

Food affects the *rate* of absorption of such drugs as aspirin but not the total amount absorbed. Such an interaction is not important if the aspirin is being taken continually for its antiinflammatory properties, as in the treatment of arthritis. If however the aspirin is being taken for a headache, serum titers may not rise to an effective level to combat pain. Another type of interaction is illustrated by tetracycline. Certain foods, such as milk or milk products, may affect the total *amount* of tetracycline absorbed but do not change the *rate* of absorption.

The type of food ingested may also have specific effects on drug absorption. An example of such an interaction is the dramatic slowing of gastric emptying following meals high in fat and low in fiber. Drugs absorbed from the upper small intestine will have a markedly delayed response time. Griseofulvin is an oral antifungal drug that is highly lipid soluble. The drug will reach different plasma concentrations depending on the amount of fat in a person's diet. Many beverages and juices, such as cola drinks, cranberry juice, and orange and grapefruit juices, are acidic and may affect acid-labile drugs such as ampicil-

lin, erythromycin, and penicillin G. Another food-drug interaction occurs when ferrous sulfate interferes with the absorption of tetracycline when given simultaneously. At least two hours should pass between iron and tetracycline administration.

Drug Effects on Nutrient Absorption

Drugs have two basic physiological effects that alter nutrient absorption: *luminal effects,* which change the intestinal environment, and *mucosal effects,* which change the ability of nutrients to be absorbed across the intestinal membrane.

One of the drug groups that most obviously affects the lumen is the cathartics. The intestinal transit time may be greatly reduced by those drugs, causing nutrients to pass through the small intestine too rapidly for absorption to occur. Other drugs bind with bile acids and thus impair the absorption of fat, fat-soluble vitamins, and cholesterol. Antacids change the pH of the stomach, causing a decrease in iron absorption because an acidic environment is needed to change iron from the ferric to the absorbable ferrous form.

Mucosal alterations that are caused by

drugs usually involve the destruction of the microvilli, interference with intestinal-wall regeneration and repair, or the inhibition of local enzyme activity. Effects observed depend on the physical and chemical properties of the drug as well as on drug dosage, general nutritional status, and the presence of concurrent disease.

Specific drugs that may cause malabsorption are:

- *Mineral oil,* which was the first drug discovered to cause malabsorption. The laxative interferes with absorption of carotene and vitamins A, D, E, and K, probably by creating a barrier at the mucosal surface. Phenolphthalein and bisacodyl can cause excessive diarrhea and the loss of nutrients, particularly calcium.

- *Broad-spectrum antibiotics* such as neomycin, which cause general malabsorption of fat, nitrogen, sodium, potassium, calcium, cholesterol, vitamin B_{12}, iron, lactose, and sucrose. These drugs may also cause a decrease in the synthesis of vitamin B_{12} by intestinal organisms. A vitamin K deficiency is possible if vitamin K intake is inadequate.

- *Hypocholesteremic agents,* which cause a decreased absorption of cholesterol, vitamin B_{12}, D-xylose, iron, and sugar. Many of the malabsorptive effects are due to changes in the intestinal mucosa.

- *Anti-inflammatory agents* such as colchicine (used to treat gout). Increased fecal excretion of sodium, potassium, fat, and nitrogen have been measured. Malabsorption of vitamin B_{12}, lactose, and cholesterol have also been reported.

- *Oral hypoglycemics* such as metformin and phenformin, which cause malabsorption of vitamin B_{12}.

- *Potassium chloride,* which taken orally causes a decrease in B_{12} absorption. Vitamin B_{12} absorption depends on an ileal pH above 5.5 and occurs best when the pH is above 6.6. Potassium chloride decreases the ileal pH.

Other examples of malabsorption of specific nutrients because of drug intake include a decrease in iron absorption because of aspirin; a decrease in folacin, vitamin B_{12}, and magnesium absorption because of alcohol; and a decrease in absorption of disaccharides, fat, folacin, xylose, and vitamin B_{12} because of cytotoxic agents.

Drug-Nutrient Alterations in Metabolism

Although the majority of drug-nutrient interactions occur during absorption, drugs and nutrients occasionally interfere with the way other drugs and nutrients are metabolized. Chemotherapeutic agents such as methotrexate and pyrimethamine interfere with the coenzyme action of a vitamin with its enzyme. Some drugs may interfere with a nutrient's metabolism by forming a complex with it and making it unavailable for use in the body; an example of such a combination is INH (an antitubercular drug). INH forms a complex with pyridoxine (B_6) and is excreted, making the B_6 unavailable for use. Drugs acting as antagonists may alter nutrient function by displacing the nutrient from a binding site. An example of a folacin antagonist is aminopterin, a drug used to treat leukemia.

Adrenocortical hormones cause breakdown of glycogen to glucose and of protein. Tissue wasting occurs, with mobility of fat to certain body areas, creating the characteristic "buffalo hump" and "moon face" common in long-time steroid users. Phenytoin, an anticonvulsant, causes enhanced metabolism of vitamin D resulting in deficiency. Chronic alcoholism will stimulate liver enzymes and increase the metabolism of other drugs such as warfarin. On the other hand, acute alcohol intake will decrease liver enzyme activity and slow drug metabolism.

Nutrients such as protein, carbohydrate, lipid, riboflavin, ascorbic acid, magnesium, and zinc affect drug metabolism by altering the hepatic system. Other influences on drug metabolism include the presence of other diseases, general nutritional status, liver function, and the concomitant administration of other drugs.

Nutrient-Drug Alterations in Excretion

Drugs affect nutrient excretion by altering reabsorption or transport. A drug may displace a vitamin from its binding site on a plasma protein and cause it to be excreted; an example being the effect of aspirin on folate. A drug may also alter the kidney's ability to concentrate or reabsorb a specific nutrient, a prime example being the effect that diuretic therapy has on calcium and potassium excretion.

Foods affect drug excretion by changing urine pH. The alkalinization of urine may increase the duration of such drugs as quinidene, imipramine, and amphetamines. Urinary pH also plays an important role in the precipitation of certain drugs, such as sulfonamides, in the urine.

Specific Drug-Nutrient Interactions

Anticonvulsants

The anticonvulsant drugs (diphenylhydantoin, phenobarbital, and primidone) can produce a clinical folate deficiency, a vitamin D deficiency, or both. Folate deficiency with resultant megaloblastic anemia might be a complication of long-term anticonvulsant therapy. The drugs appear to stimulate hepatic enzymes that metabolize folic acid. Folate deficiency can cause neurological alterations; yet large doses of folic acid may act as an anticonvulsant antagonist and increase seizure activity. Side effects attributed to anticonvulsant therapy that respond to folic acid administration include gingival hyperplasia, neurological impairment, and perhaps teratogenic tendencies.

A vitamin D deficiency leading to rickets can be seen in some clients receiving anticonvulsant therapy. Radiological examination of wrists, knees, and elbows shows morbidic changes in 15%–80% of all patients (Bowden, 1974). Such signs may include a low serum calcium level and an elevated serum alkaline phosphatase level. Whether a client will develop the rickets-like syndrome depends on: the dose of the anticonvulsant (the higher the dose, the greater the probability of bone changes); total vitamin D intake; sunlight exposure (the opportunity for vitamin D synthesis to occur in the skin); and skin color (darker skin allows less ultraviolet light absorption and thus less vitamin D synthesis). The ricketslike syndrome responds rapidly to vitamin D replacement.

Alcohol

Nutrient deficiencies that occur with alcoholism include those secondary to decreased absorption, increased need, increased excretion, of some combination of the three. The most common nutrients depleted include folacin, thiamine, riboflavin, niacin, ascorbic acid, vitamin B_6, vitamin B_{12}, magnesium, zinc, and protein. In addition to overt depletion alcohol also has a toxic effect on the pancreas that may cause acute pancreatitis. Contrary to popular belief a nutritious diet will not prevent the development of alcoholic liver disease. Rather, alcohol produces its nutritional effects not by causing a decreased intake but by acting directly on tissues and enzyme systems.

A deficiency of thiamine may lead to Wernicke's encephalopathy. The thiamine deficiency is accentuated if a magnesium deficiency is also present. Alterations in vitamin B_6 ingestion and use may lead to peripheral neuropathy, seizure activity, and anemia.

Alcohol increases magnesium excretion in the urine, resulting in a magnesium deficiency. Such a problem may lead to cardiomyopathy. Delirium tremors and seizures that occur during alcohol withdrawal may be secondary to decreased magnesium levels. Similarly, alcohol increases zinc excretion, which can lead to skin breakdown and poor wound healing.

Malnutrition occurring as a result of alcoholism is due to a combination of four major factors. Food intake may be sporadic and in decreased amounts. There are increased nutrient losses secondary to maldigestion resulting from pancreatitis and gastrointestinal malabsorption. Excretion is also altered by the toxic effect alcohol has on the renal system. The alcoholic's nutrient stores are decreased by hepatitis and cirrhosis. Finally, nutrient use is impaired by liver disease and ethanol toxicity.

Cancer Chemotherapeutic Agents
Chemotherapeutic agents interfere with cell replication or regeneration. Cancer cells are fast-growing immature cells susceptible to such interference. Unfortunately, the cells of the gastrointestinal mucosa are also rather fast growing and thus are also sensitive to chemotherapeutic agents. The most common nutritionally related side effects of the chemotherapeutic agents include stomatitis, nausea, vomiting, diarrhea, oral ulcerations, gingivitis, anorexia, alteration in taste, abdominal pain, glossitis, and anemias.

Generally, the client with cancer has a better chance of successful therapy if a balanced diet is eaten.

Antibiotic and Antimicrobial drugs
Tetracycline chelates when such minerals as calcium, magnesium, and iron are present. Both the absorption of tetracycline and the mineral are greatly reduced if administered together. At least two hours should pass after iron, calcium, milk, or antacid absorption before tetracycline is taken.

Neomycin causes malabsorption by damaging the intestinal mucosa and inhibiting gut enzymes. Vitamin B_{12}, carotene, iron, sodium, potassium, calcium, and nitrogen can be malabsorbed with this drug.

Salicylazosulfapyridine can cause folate malabsorption. Para-aminosalicylic acid (PAS) may interfere with folacin, vitamin B_{12}, iron, and cholesterol absorption and use.

Oral Contraceptives
Oral contraceptives have many effects on nutritional status. Generally, plasma levels of vitamins A and E are increased while levels of magnesium, zinc, riboflavin, vitamin C, folacin, and vitamins B_{12} and B_6 are decreased. In addition to altering nutrient use, oral contraceptives may also change actual requirements for specific nutrients.

Vitamin B_6 depletion is very common in oral contraceptive users. Depression and glucose intolerance may be related to the depletion. Folate levels are also decreased. The deficiency is particularly dangerous when it persists into pregnancy because folate deficiency may be associated with birth defects.

Oral contraceptive users have a decreased need for iron, probably because of decreased menstrual flow, and a decreased need for copper owing to increased absorption. Vitamin A levels increase during oral contraceptive use. There also seems to be a diminished requirement for vitamin K.

Antiparkinsonian Drugs
Parkinson's disease is an alteration that involves a dramatic decrease of the neurotransmitter dopamine in the brain, causing a loss of control over voluntary muscle movements. Dopamine cannot cross the bloodbrain barrier; so an amino acid, 3,4-dihydroxyphenylalanine (dopa), which is a precursor of dopamine is given orally and converted to dopamine in the brain. This conversion depends on the presence of pyridoxine (vitamin B_6). The presence of B_6 in the periphery, however, causes an increase in peripheral dopamine production, leaving less of the precursor available for dopamine formation in the brain. If pyridoxine and L-dopa are administered simultaneously, the antiparkinsonian effects of the drug are obliterated. A diet low in vitamin B_6 is not recommended during L-dopa therapy because

levodopa itself may induce a vitamin B_6 deficiency. Signs typical of vitamin B_6 deficiency include seborrheic dermatitis, hypochronic anemia, and peripheral neuropathy.

Cardiac Glycosides

The action of digitalis is modified by serum vitamin K and magnesium levels. For the therapeutic effects of digitalis to be exerted, a precise serum level of the drug must be maintained. The therapeutic dose is very close to toxic level, and therefore serum determinations must be made periodically. Digitalis has a much greater potential for toxicity in a magnesium-depleted client. Further, vitamin K depletion leads to increased ventricular irritability, which digitalis may accentuate. Frequently, magnesium-deficient clients also are vitamin K deficient. For the vitamin K deficiency to be corrected, the magnesium deficiency must also be corrected.

Corticosteroids

The administration of corticosteroids has many effects on a client's nutritional status. Calcium absorption is decreased; potassium and zinc are excreted in additional amounts. Vitamin D is metabolized more rapidly. There is also an increased need for vitamin B_6. There may be some relationship between the need for vitamin B_6 and a tendency for a client to become hyperglycemic and insulin resistant while on corticosteroid therapy.

Anesthetic Agents

The postsurgical effects of the anesthetic agent succinyl choline are modified by ascorbic acid. Oral vitamin C therapy before and after surgery appears to result in reduced muscle pain.

Antitubercular Drugs

Drugs used to treat tuberculosis include isoniazid (INH), PAS, and antibiotics such as streptomycin. INH is a vitamin B_6 antagonist that appears to inhibit various B_6-dependent enzyme systems. A niacin deficiency may also be present when vitamin B_6 levels are lowered, for pyridoxine is a necessary coenzyme in the formation of niacin in the body. In addition, the nurse should be on the alert for a vitamin B_{12} deficiency caused by PAS-induced malabsorption of the nutrient.

Pharmacologically Active Substances in Foods

Several foods contain substances that exert either an influence on drugs taken simultaneously or a pharmacological action of their own.

Tyramine

Probably the most well known drug-diet interaction is the one that occurs between monoamine oxidase (MAO) inhibitors and foods that contain tyramine. MAO inhibitors are used in the treatment of depressed clients to elevate their mental state. The drugs interact adversely with tyramine and amine derived from the amino acid tyrosine. MAO inhibitors block monoamine oxidase activity, and thus tyramine is allowed to reach the circulation rather than being neutralized in the liver. Tyramine causes the release of norepinephrine, which in turn induces a hypertensive crisis through sympathetic overstimulation. Symptoms include a marked rise in blood pressure, headache, and nosebleeds. Intracranial hemorrhage may occur, resulting in death. Foods containing tyramine include aged cheeses, dried fish, beer and ale, wines, vanilla, chocolate, yeast and yeast extract, soy sauce, yogurt, and spoiled meats. All foods containing tyramine must be avoided by clients receiving MAO inhibitors. Because of the difficulty of eliminating such foods for long periods of time, MAO inhibitors are not being used as frequently as they once were.

Licorice

Salt and water retention associated with hypokalemia has occurred in people who eat an excessive amount of licorice made with genuine flavorings (the root of the *Glycyr-rhiza*). (Licorice made in the United States is usually made with synthetic flavorings.) The active ingredient in genuine licorice is glycyrrhizic acid, a compound that acts as a mineral corticoid. Hypertension, myopathy, and myoglobinuria may also occur. Clients already receiving hypertensive therapy should be carefully monitored for excessive ingestion of the imported licorice.

Monosodium Glutamate

Monosodium glutamate is a flavor enhancer added to many processed foods. Chinese recipes, in particular, call for large amounts of it. Sensitive people may experience the Chinese restaurant syndrome with headache, burning sensations in the extremities, and facial pressure and chest pain mimicking angina. The syndrome is transient and appears to be dose related.

TUBE FEEDINGS AND NUTRITIONAL SUPPLEMENTS

Patricia A. Harvey

Malnutrition can be a serious consequence of severe illness and injury. It is very important to assess a client's nutritional status even if his outward appearance is that of a healthy human being. The normal daily nutritional requirement for hospitalized patients has been identified (Porter, 1978) as between 2,000 and 2,500 Calories and 70 gm of protein a day. Up to three to four times these amounts may be required to meet metabolic needs in the severely ill. When a need for additional nutritional support has been identified, there are two ways to meet the need: IV therapy (already discussed) and tube feedings.

A patient becomes a candidate for a tube feeding whenever he has lost the ability to take food orally but still retains adequate bowel function. The groups of patients for whom tube feeding may become necessary

have been identified by Walike (1975). The first group consists of those with physical impairments. This group includes patients with dental problems, facial fractures, head and neck surgery, burns, and upper-alimentary-tract surgery. The second group consists of those who have suffered neurological impairment. This group is composed of those with head injuries, paralysis, and loss of consciousness. The third group are those with mental disturbances. Clinically depressed and anorexic patients should be included in this group. According to Bennion (Bennion, 1979) 40% of tube feedings are used for patients who have had head and neck carcinoma and 32% for those with impairment of the CNS. Still another group is patients who are too weak to eat normally, such as premature infants with a decreased sucking reflex.

Tubes

When the decision to initiate tube feedings has been made by a physician, it is essential that the procedure be explained to the patient, when possible, and family. The insertion of the feeding tube may be unpleasant, and it is the nurse's responsibility to support the patient during this time.

There are various types of feeding tubes. Most are made of a synthetic material that is easily pliable. The length ranges from 15 in to 50 in; and the diameters vary. In choosing the tube size, both the patient and the feeding must be considered. The tube should be small enough that it can be inserted easily with the least amount of trauma to the patient but large enough so that the feeding chosen will pass easily through it.

Griggs and Hoppe (1979) identified through a study the advantages and disadvantages of four different tube types:

1. The *Keofeed tube* is made of silicone rubber with a column of mercury acting as a weight at its distal end. This tube is very soft and may be easily kinked, but most feedings will pass through easily.

2. The *Dobbhoff tube* is made of polyurethane and also has a mercury weight. It is passed to the distal duodenum or proximal jejunum.

3. The *Med Pro tube* is made of silicone rubber and enclosed in a stiff outer tube. The outer tube is removed when the tube is in place. This tube is smaller than the other tubes, and a pump is usually necessary for administration of the feedings.

4. The *Levin tube* is larger than the other tubes and causes more irritation during insertion. It also may cause irritation to the esophagus and make swallowing difficult.

After the feeding tube has been chosen, the patient should be prepared for its insertion. If possible, the client should sit at a 45-degree angle; this will aid insertion and lessen the chance of aspiration. If the patient is unable to sit, he should lie on his side. The tube may be placed in ice to stiffen it and ease passage. A topical anesthetic may also be applied to the throat to lessen the gag reflex. The tip of the catheter should be lubricated. Only a small amount should be used so the opening in the distal end of the tube does not become clogged. The nurse should offer an emesis basin if needed.

The patient should be asked if he has ever had a fractured nose or nasal defect, either of which could cause some difficulty in inserting the tube. The tube is placed in the nostril and gently pushed up and back until it reaches the back of the throat. The patient should then be instructed to swallow while the tube is being passed. If the patient has difficulty swallowing, he may drink sips of water while the tube is being inserted.

Placement of the tube should be checked immediately. If the client is unable to speak or if he experiences respiratory difficulty, the tube must be removed. If speech and respiration are functioning a syringe is used to aspirate contents from the stomach. A pH strip will show the contents to be acidic. Also, 5 cc of air are injected into the tube while listening with a stethoscope over the stomach. If the tube is properly placed, bubbling sounds can be heard.

In the past, tube placement has been checked by placing the end of the tube in a glass of water. It was assumed that, if the water bubbled, the tube was in the respiratory tract. There are several problems with this method of checking tube placement. The primary concern is the high potential for aspiration. If the patient inhales, water will be immediately sucked into the respiratory tract if the tube happens to be misplaced. *Aspiration pneumonia* could result. Another problem with using the water method for checking tube placement is that, frequently, flatus will rise out of the tube upon placement, causing air bubbles. Thus the tube may be placed correctly but still have air coming from it. If there is doubt, roentgenogram will show placement and location of the tube. When it has been ascertained that the tube is in place, it is taped securely to the patient's nose, but carefully so as not to cause trauma to the nasal mucosa. The first feeding should be delayed until the feeling of nausea has subsided.

Problems with Tubes

Serious problems associated with the anchored feeding tube can develop if proper care is not taken. The tube may cause *pressure necrosis,* which can result in hemorrhage and eventually in a tracheoesophageal fistula. This condition is characterized by gastric contents in tracheal excretions. The chance for this condition to occur is increased when the patient has both a tracheotomy and feeding tubes. If the feeding is to be given over a long time, pressure necrosis can be prevented by alternating the tube between nostrils every few days.

Because the tube is inserted into the nostril, the patient may breathe through his mouth, which may dry out the oral mucosa. Meticulous mouth care is thus essential. In addition, the tube often causes irritation and difficulty with swallowing. Any attempt to initiate foods orally may be met with resistance.

On some occasions a feeding tube through the nasal or oral passageway is not the recommended route for feeding. In these instances a tube may be surgically placed directly into the stomach or jejunum. Patients for whom this procedure would be beneficial have been identified by Wieman (1978). One such group of patients are those to whom tube feedings must be administered for an indefinite time. Placing the tube directly into the stomach greatly decreases the chances of aspiration and esophageal irritation. Another group are those with chronic respiratory disease. Breathing is compromised by the presence of the tube in the nasal passageway. The third group are those with basal skull fractures and CSF leaks, in whom the insertion of the nasogastric tube could cause further damage. The last group are those with a diseased oropharyx or esophagus. The presence of a tube could cause further irritation and damage.

Care must also be given to this tube when inserted. The skin around the tube should be kept clean and observed for signs of inflammation and breakdown. A small-gauze dressing may be kept around the tube to collect any drainage or gastric contents present on the skin. A baby nipple can be taped around the tube to provide support for the *gastrostomy tube.*

Kinds of Feedings

Various types of tube feedings are available, ranging from commercially prepared products complete in all nutrients to blenderized food made in the patient's home. Several points to consider in choosing the proper feeding have been identified (Gormican, 1975): cost of the supplement, packaging, shelf life, total nutrient content, nutritional precautions with use, osmolality, palatability, and nutrient omissions.

Hospital-formulated or blenderized diets are usually prepared ahead and require refrigeration. It has been recommended that they be prepared fresh each day (Kark, 1974). They can be placed in warm water after removal from the refrigerator, but this is not necessary. If allowed to become too warm, they are a good medium for bacterial growth. Warming the solution has also been found to break down water-soluble vitamins and cause the coagulation of proteins, which may clog the tube. If very cold fluids are given, however, they should be given slowly because of the possibility of cramping. Blenderized diets are often lacking in vitamins and minerals, so supplements of these should be given with feedings. Blenderized feedings are preferred for long-term therapy. These feedings are often milk based because milk is isotonic. Homogenized milk must be used because plain milk will turn to butter when blenderized. Feedings should also be strained several times to remove particles that might clog the tube.

Commercial feedings are available in liquid form in cans or in powder form in packages. They are convenient and contain all essential nutrients required. They are usually given at room temperature, but any remaining substance must be refrigerated.

Elemental diets provide nitrogen in the form of amino acids, fat in the form of triglycerides, and carbohydrate in the form of glucose. They have added vitamins and minerals. They require minimal digestion and are low in residue. The taste is usually unpleasant, however. See Table 23-6 for a comparison of common commercial tube feedings.

When choosing a feeding, Calories supplied, protein content, fluid and electrolytes supplied, and vitamin and mineral content should all be considered. Even though the commercial products are convenient, they may be costly and they must be used properly. Over- or underdilution and leaving unused portions of commercial feedings at room temperature can destroy their benefits.

TABLE 23-6. Common Tube Feedings

Feedings (1,000 cc)	How Supplied	Preparation	Uses	Calories	Carbohydrate (gm)	Protein (gm)	Fat (gm)	Sodium (mg)	Potassium (mg)	MOsm/kg	Points of Interest
Ensure	Canned	None	May also be given by mouth flavored.	1,060	144.5	37.1	37.10	740	1,270	450	Lactose free
Ensure Plus	Canned	None	May also be given by mouth flavored.	1,500	199.0	55.0	53.30	1,060	1,900	600	Lactose free
Nutri 1000	Canned	None	Also by mouth	1,060	101.0	40.0	55.00	520	1,458	400	Lactose free
Osmolite	Canned	None	Also by mouth	1,060	143.0	37.0	38.00	541	875	300	Lactose free, low residue
Sustacal	Canned and Powdered	1 pkt to 1 cup milk	Also by mouth	1,000	148.0	65.0	24.00	1,000	2,220	625	Lactose free, low residue
Citrotein	Powdered	¼ cup to ¼ cup water	Also by mouth	533	97.9	32.2	1.4	546	546	496	Lactose free, low residue
Flexical	Powdered	1½ cup to 3 cups water		1,000	152.5	22.5	0.34	350	1,250	805	Lactose free, low residue
Meritene	Powdered	4 T to 1 cup milk	Also by mouth	922	103.2	59.9	30.00	832	2,564	560	
Portagen	Powdered	1½ cups to 28 oz water	Also by mouth	1,000	112.0	34.0	46.00	400	100	354	Lactose free, midchain triglycerides
Precision LR	Powdered	1 pkt to 1 cup water	Also by mouth	1,080	215.0	21.0	0.70	600	1,500	600	Lactose free, low residue
Vipep	Powdered	1 pkt to 8½ oz water	Also by mouth	1,000	175.5	25.0	25.00	750	850	520	Lactose free, low residue
Vital	Powdered	1 pkt to 8½ oz water	Also by mouth	1,000	185.0	41.6	10.20	382	1,164	450	Lactose free, low residue
Vivonex	Powdered	1 pkt to 8½ oz water	Also by mouth flavored	1,000	225.0	20.4	13.00	860	1,170	550	Lactose free, low residue
Vivonex HN	Powdered	1 pkt to 8½ oz water	Also by mouth flavored	1,000	202.0	41.7	8.60	770	702	844	Lactose free, low residue

Administration

After the feeding regimen has been chosen, the type of administration needs to be decided. Many problems from tube feedings occur because too large a volume is given over a very short period of time. It is recommended that a patient receive 2 liters of fluid every 24 hours (Robinson, 1972). If the feeding is given by continuous drip, the amount should not exceed 250–350 cc over 20–30 minutes.

Various administration sets can be used for tube feedings, ranging from an enema bag cut off close to the bag and attached to IV tubing to manufactured gavage bags with suitable tubing and regulators already built in. Resterilized IV bottles are easy to use for more dilute feedings. Sterile irrigation sets can be hooked to IV tubing and used for this purpose. Also, if the amount of feeding is small, a large syringe can be used to administer the feeding by gravity.

According to two researchers (Griggs and Hoppe, 1979) the best method of administration is a continuous drip. When the feeding contains a high glucose concentration, this method is not always feasible. Griggs and Hoppe have set the following guidelines for continuous feedings: The feedings should be started at a slow rate (50 cc/hr), and the concentration should be only half of the prescribed feeding. If the patient has no symptoms of intolerance such as sugar in the urine or diarrhea for 24 hours, then the feeding may be raised to 75 cc/hr. The rate can then be increased 25 cc/hr each day until the prescribed rate is reached. After the rate is tolerated, concentration can be raised to full strength. For this type of feeding, the use of the resterilized IV bottle is ideal. To ensure that the accurate volume of feeding is given, the bottle can be timed as if it contained IV fluids. If a feeding gets behind, the bottle can be retimed. Giving the patient a bolus of feeding "to catch up" may be harmful.

There are several ways of regulating the fluid rate. When the patient is receiving a continuous feeding, it is advisable to use a food pump such as a Holter or IVAC pump to ensure accuracy of rate. A pump can be costly, however. The most commonly used method is a *gravity drip*. This method is less expensive for the patient but much harder to control. The gravity drip must be watched closely, and the nurse should monitor the patient closely while the feeding is being given. The last method is the use of a large syringe with the plunger removed. This must be given very slowly, and the nurse should remain with the patient. The feedings should never be given with force.

The patient's head should always be elevated at least 45 degrees for all feedings, and it should remain so for one-half hour after the feeding because of the chance of aspiration. If the feeding is continuous, the patient's head should remain elevated at all times. If the patient is to have some type of treatment that requires the head be lowered, the feeding should be stopped from one-half hour before treatment until one-half hour after it to decrease the chance of aspiration. The position of the tube should be checked before each feeding to make sure that it has not slipped out of the stomach. This should be done once each shift if the feeding is continuous. Suction equipment should always be kept ready at the bedside in case aspiration occurs.

Gastric contents should be aspirated before each feeding. If the amount of residual matter is more than 150 cc, the feeding should be withheld. This fluid should be given back to the patient to prevent the loss of electrolytes in the aspirate. When a continuous feeding is being prepared, the amount should be no more than will be infused within eight hours. Feedings may not be given at night so patients can maintain a sense of normalcy.

Patients will often be receiving medications along with the feedings. If the feedings are given intermittently, the medications can be added to the feedings. Pills and capsules should be crushed and dissolved in water.

Some medications are available in elixir form so they can easily be added to the nourishment. Often, antacids or cimetidine is added to the feeding to reduce regurgitation of the stomach contents and irritation of the esophagus by the tube.

After each feeding, the tubing should be rinsed with water to prevent old feeding from spoiling in the tubing. Administration sets should also be cleansed thoroughly. In the hospital setting, administration sets should be changed every 24 hours. It is helpful for the bag or bottle to be dated and timed so there is no question when the 24-hour period is over.

Problems with Feedings

Many of the problems encountered with tube feedings are due to the tube and its position, the liquid diet prescribed, and the rate and volume of the feedings. The most frequent complaint from patients receiving tube feedings is diarrhea. This condition can be caused by one or several of the following:

1. Bacterial contamination of the feeding from improper handling
2. Giving the feeding too quickly
3. Giving a feeding that is too cold
4. Allergic reaction of the client to any of the contents of the feeding
5. A high concentration of lactose found in most tube feedings
6. Improper placement of the feeding tube
7. High osmolarity of the feeding

If the reason for the diarrhea is found and it would be disadvantageous to correct the problem, antidiarrheal drugs may be given such as codeine, kaolin, morphine, or Lomotil.

Another common complaint is nausea, one major cause of which is delayed gastric emptying. This is why it is so important to check the residual matter before giving each feeding. If the feeding is not held, gastric distention may occur. This is characterized by left upper quadrant pain and an increase in the abdominal girth. Ambulation may help to decrease the distention if the patient can tolerate it.

The carbohydrate content should be monitored closely. If the concentration of carbohydrate is too great, the following symptoms may be seen: lethargy, thirst, glucosuria, and polyuria. The end result can be coma if steps for correction are not taken. For this reason it is important to check the *Clinitest* and *Acetest* of the urine every six hours. The Clinitest shows if the patient is spilling sugar in his urine. If so, a blood glucose level should be drawn, and insulin therapy may be initiated (Griggs and Hoppe, 1979). The Acetest indicates if ketones are being broken down and the patient's nutritional status is deficient in some area.

A high concentration of protein in the diet may also cause a set of problems designated the *tube-feeding syndrome* (Walike, 1975). It is characterized by confusion and decreased mental function. These symptoms are caused by dehydration, hypernatremia, hyperchloremia, and azotemia. Adequate protein is, however, needed for healthy tissue and for the prevention of decubitus ulcers.

The most serious complication of tube feedings is aspiration pneumonia. A healthy person has three defenses against aspiration according to Coyle and Arbet (1978): the gag and cough reflex, the cleansing ciliary action in the lining of the bronchi, and the automatic closing off by the glottis of the larynx during regurgitation or swallowing. A person with a nasogastric tube is therefore at risk.

Another complication is the patient's adjustment to this change in lifestyle. The normal process of food intake is changed. He may no longer be able to taste food. He no longer needs to chew and swallow. One researcher found that infants will tolerate feedings better if allowed to suck on a pacifier at meal time (Scipien et al., 1975). The family needs to be involved because they may be responsible for the preparation and administration of the feedings after discharge. Along with the tube feedings, the patient may also have to deal with a grave prognosis, radical surgery, loss of body image, and loss of identity as an active member of his family. The patient will require support and encouragement until he accepts the condition or until the need for the feedings no longer exists.

Despite all the potential problems, however, one study (Gormican, 1973) showed that a well-designed, standardized tube feeding containing the essential nutrients could provide adequate nourishment for an indefinite period of time if the caloric content was adequate and it was prepared properly and unless untoward symptoms appeared to decrease its beneficial effects.

TOTAL PARENTERAL NUTRITION

Total parenteral nutrition (TPN) is a technique of IV feeding designed to meet the nutritional requirements of patients when their own gastrointestinal tract cannot adequately provide these requirements. Blackburn (1975) has stated that more than 50% of hospital patients are malnourished. Frequently, patients are placed on nothing-by-mouth status and maintained for extended periods of time on IV solutions of 5% dextrose; 2 liters of D_5W supplies approximately 350 Calories/day for the body to use. Considering that the average basal Calorie requirement for an adult is 1,700 Calories/day, it is obvious why patients soon become nutritionally depleted. As discussed in Chapter 4, when starvation occurs, somatic and visceral protein is used for energy. The starved patient becomes more prone to sepsis and its complications because the immune system, dependent on visceral protein, is depleted. All patients who are not taking food orally for extended periods should be nutritionally assessed at regular intervals. (See Chap. 19 for a complete discussion of nutritional assessment.)

TPN should be used with four groups of patients. Those who are malnourished and must receive nutritional replacement before surgery compose the first group. Patients who have carcinoma of the colon, severe peptic ulcer disease, or esophageal stricture fall into this category. The second group of patients who are candidates for TPN are those with postoperative complications. Examples include patients with a prolonged ileus, fistula formation, or peritoneal sepsis. The third group of patients are those with inflammatory bowel disease that interfers with absorption. Colitis, regional enteritis, and gastroenteritis are conditions that may cause such an interference. Patients who have an inadequate oral intake compose the last group. These patients simply cannot ingest enough nutrients to meet their metabolic requirements. Examples include patients experiencing severe nausea as a side effect of chemotherapy, patients with a marked increase in metabolic rate such as occurs with severe burns, or those with short-bowel syndrome.

Catheter Placement

A central venous catheter is usually used to administer total parenteral nutrition because the high dextrose concentration tends to cause phlebitis and thrombosis in peripheral veins. In most cases the physician inserts the catheter with the nurse assisting. The insertion should be done in as clean an atmosphere as possible. Everyone in the room, including the patient, should be masked (Fig. 23-3). Once inserted, the tip of the catheter lies in the superior vena cava. The catheter is sutured in place. The nurse should watch the patient for any respiratory distress following the procedure. A *pneumothorax* may occur during the procedure if the pleura is punctured. A chest roentgenogram is usually taken in the patient's room after the procedure to rule out pneumothorax.

Catheter Care

Sepsis is the major complication of TPN. Diligent aseptic catheter care is necessary to pre-

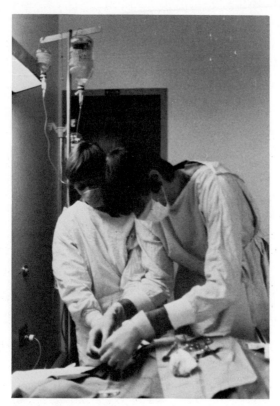

Figure 23-3. Establishing the central venous line for total parenteral nutrition.

vent this complication. The dressing should be occlusive and remain intact. Generally, the dirtier the environment is, the less often the dressing should be changed. Patients in an open-air intensive care unit, for example, should not have their dressing changed any more frequently than three times a week unless the dressing itself becomes contaminated. A general procedure used for changing the dressing follows:

1. Mask everyone in the room, including the patient.
2. Remove the old dressing, being careful not to pull on the catheter.
3. Check the catheter and site for any leaks, kinks, edema, or redness.

4. Clean the area with acetone swabs. This will remove dried blood, old Betadine, skin fats, and debris that can cause skin breakdown and proliferate bacterial growth.

5. Using sterile gloves, prepare the area with Betadine solution. Use at least four sponges, cleansing the area from the insertion site outward toward the periphery in a circular motion.

6. Apply Betadine ointment to the insertion site.

7. Cover the site completely, leaving the hub exposed. Occlusive tape should be used, and the dressing should be dated by the person changing the dressing.

The intravenous tubing should be changed every 24 hours to prevent the possible build-up of organisms along the inner lumen of the tubing. To prevent air embolis, the tubing should be changed rapidly while the patient is lying flat or in Trendelenburg position. If possible, the patient should be asked to hold his breath while the tubing is disconnected. The central venous catheter and tubing should never be used to draw blood nor to administer piggyback or other intravenous medications. A line that is used in such a way should be considered contaminated and no longer be used for *hyperalimentation*.

The TPN rate should be carefully monitored, preferably with an infusion pump. If the infusion rate is plus or minus 10% of what is ordered, the physician should be notified. No attempt to "catch up" should be made.

Determining the TPN Solution

The physician prescribes the quantity and contents of the TPN solution to be infused. Figure 23-4 is an example of an order form for a TPN solution. The nurse should be aware of how the physician determines the caloric content of the solution so that she can properly monitor the effect of the solution. The amount of glucose and amino acid to be given is calculated according to the stress the

9/79	HYPERALIMENTATION ORDER FORM	M 6405600	

DATE:
- ☐ CONTINUE OLD ORDERS UNTIL COMPLETED
- ☐ FORMULA CHANGE START AS SOON AS POSSBILE

I.V. NUTRITION PLAN_____Kcal/24hrs_____gm NITROGEN/24hrs
RATE OF ADMINISTRATION:_____

	BOTTLE # TIME DUE _____	BOTTLE # TIME DUE _____	BOTTLE # TIME DUE _____

Crystalline Amino Acids 8.5%
    10mEq Phosphate/500cc
    5mEq Sodium/500cc
    6.5gm Nitrogen equiv /500cc
	_____ cc _____%	_____cc _____%	_____ cc _____%

Dextrose 50% in Water 850 cal/500cc	_____ cc _____%	_____cc _____%	_____ cc _____%
Dextrose 70% in Water 1190 cal/500cc	_____ cc _____%	_____cc _____%	_____ cc _____%
Sodium Chloride 2.5mEq/cc	_____mEq _____cc	_____mEq _____cc	_____mEq _____cc
Sodium Lactate 5mEq/cc	_____mEq _____cc	_____mEq _____cc	_____mEq _____cc
Sodium Acetate 2mEq/cc	_____mEq _____cc	_____mEq _____cc	_____mEq _____cc

Sodium Phosphate
    4mEq Na+/cc
    3mM P/cc
	_____mEq _____cc	_____mEq _____cc	_____mEq _____cc

Potassium Chloride 2mEq/cc	_____mEq _____cc	_____mEq _____cc	_____mEq _____cc
Potassium Acetate 2mEq/cc	_____mEq _____cc	_____mEq _____cc	_____mEq _____cc

Potassium Phosphate
    4.4mEq K+/cc
    3mM P/cc
	_____mEq _____cc	_____mEq _____cc	_____mEq _____cc

Calcium Gluconate 10%
    90mg Ca++/10cc
    4.5mEq Ca++/10cc
	_____cc	_____cc	_____cc

Magnesium Sulfate 50%
    1Gm MgSO$_4$/2cc
    8.12mEq Mg++/2cc
	_____cc	_____cc	_____cc

MVI Concentrate (5cc)	_____cc	_____cc	_____cc
Solu-B-Forte (10cc)	_____cc	_____cc	_____cc
*Trace Metal Solution	_____cc	_____cc	_____cc
Zinc 2mg/5cc	_____cc	_____cc	_____cc
Copper 2mg/5cc	_____cc	_____cc	_____cc
Heparin 1,000units/cc	_____cc	_____cc	_____cc
Folic Acid 5mg/cc	_____cc	_____cc	_____cc
_____	_____	_____	_____
_____	_____	_____	_____
Sterile Water qsad	_____cc	_____cc	_____cc

*Usual adult dose: 2cc/day
    2cc provides: Zinc 2mg
             Copper 1mg
             Mn 0.4mg
             Cr 10mcg

Signed:_____ M.D.

MEDICAL RECORDS COPY	**PHYSICIAN'S ORDERS**						**T—6**		
B–CLIN. NOTES	E–LAB	G–X–RAY	K–DIAGNOSTIC	M–SURGERY	Q–THERAPY	T–ORDERS	W–NURSING	Y–MISC.	

Figure 23-4. A sample hyperalimentation order form. (Courtesy Indiana University Hospitals)

patient is experiencing. Table 23-7 gives the quantities of the base solution for different levels of stress. Stress level is determined by the entire clinical picture the patient presents. For example, a patient who has suffered extensive burns may be experiencing severe stress. An example of a patient under moderate stress is the fairly well-nourished patient experiencing a prolonged postoperative illness. Mild stress would be experienced by the normal patient undergoing a surgical procedure such as a cholecystectomy.

Excess Calories should be avoided because of the possibility of fatty liver development. The primary determinant of how much nutrient fluid to order initially rests on the patient's ability to handle a large glucose load. Glucose intolerance can be caused by diabetes mellitus, sepsis, hypokalemia, and high-dose steroids. The glucose concentration is usually increased gradually.

Minerals and electrolytes are added to the base solution. The requirements for these substances are generally the same as for those receiving standard intravenous therapy with the exceptions of potassium and phosphorus. More potassium than usual is needed because glucose, under the influence of insulin, moves intracellularly and is associated with the intracellular movement of amino acids and potassium. Increased potassium is needed to maintain normal extracellular and serum potassium values. Phosphate is added because patients receiving phosphate-free hypertonic dextrose–amino acid solutions may develop low serum phosphate levels in 7–10 days.

Other additives may include electrolytes, vitamins, heparin, trace metals, and intravenous fat emulsion. A trace-metal "cocktail" is frequently added to the TPN solution of patients on long-term therapy. Included are zinc

(necessary for enzyme function), copper, manganese, chromium, selenium, and cadmium. Essential fatty acids are supplied two to three times a week.

Intravenous Fat Emulsion

Derived from soybean triglycerides, intravenous fat emulsion (Intralipid 10% and Lyposyn) provides a caloric concentration (1.1 Calories/ml) substantially greater than amino acids or carbohydrates. Lipids, when added to the parenteral nutrition regimen, allow the patient to receive all the nutrients necessary for health parenterally. Use of lipid therapy is particularly beneficial when fluid volume, highly catabolic states, and essential fatty acid deficiencies complicate parenteral nutrition.

Intralipid is composed of 10% soybean oil, 1.2% egg yolk phosphatide, and 2.25% glycerol. The fatty acid content of Intralipid is: linoleic, 54%; oleic, 26%; palmitic, 9%; linolenic, 8%; and all others, 3%. The emulsified fat particles are less than 0.5 μm in diameter, which is similar in size to naturally occurring chylomicrons formed during absorption of fat from the diet (McNiff, 1977).

The use of fat emulsion is usually restricted to those patients who are expected to have a long-term requirement that cannot be met by alimentary tract feedings. In particular, lipids are used when a patient is maintained on long-term parenteral alimentation. Fatty acid deficiency tends to occur in these patients, and the addition of fat emulsion to the parenteral protocol will correct or prevent the deficiency. Fat emulsion therapy is contraindicated in patients with abnormal fat metabolism such as occurs in pathogenic hyperlipemia, lipid nephrosis, or acute pancreatitis. The emulsion should be used with extreme

TABLE 23-7.   Base-solution Requirements for Total Parenteral Nutrition

Solution	Mild Stress	Moderate Stress	Severe Stress
Glucose	25 Calories/kg/day	40 Calories/kg/day	60 Calories/kg/day
Amino acids	0.8 gm/kg/day	1.5 gm/kg/day	2–3 gm/kg/day

caution in patients with liver disease, pulmonary disorders, anemia, or coagulation disorders, or in any patients predisposed to fat emboli.

Hypersensitivity to the emulsion occasionally occurs. Early adverse reactions occur in less than 1% of patients. These reactions include dyspnea, cyanosis, allergic reactions, hypercoagulability, thrombophlebitis, hyperthermia, flushing, and acute thrombocytopenia. Delayed reactions include hepatomegaly, splenomegaly, thrombocytopenia, and leukopenia.

Ongoing laboratory evaluations are used to monitor fat emulsion therapy. Complete blood counts with liver function tests are done weekly. Serum triglycerides, cholesterol, and fatty acid levels are obtained biweekly. Nutritional assessment is done on a weekly basis, with weights being done every other day.

The normal adult dosage of intravenous fat emulsion is 2.5 gm/kg of body weight per day. The balance of Calories must be made up from carbohydrate and protein sources. The initial rate of infusion of soybean oil emulsion should not exceed 1 ml/min for the first 15–30 minutes. If tolerated with no signs of hypersensitivity, the infusion rate may be increased to provide 500 ml of fat emulsion in four hours. The fat emulsion should not be mixed with any other electrolyte solutions, and no drugs should be added to the emulsion in the infusion bottle. Usually, it is administered via a Y connection into the same catheter as the carbohydrate amino acid solution near the infusion site. The flow rates of both solutions should be controlled separately by infusion pumps. Filters should not be used with the emulsion. If any "oiling out" or discoloration of the fluid occurs, the solution should not be used.

Monitoring the TPN Solution

Strict aseptic technique is essential in preparing the TPN solution. Ideally, the solution should be prepared by an experienced technician in a Laminar Hood. The bottle should then be refrigerated and used within 24 hours. No bottle should be left hanging for longer than 12 hours.

Just as the patient cannot initially tolerate large amounts of glucose, neither can he tolerate abrupt cessation of the fluid. The physician will gradually titrate the glucose concentration until the pancreas is no longer producing large amounts of insulin. If the catheter is pulled or the solution is stopped before titration, the patient may go into insulin shock.

In addition to the temperature readings every four hours, daily weights, and routine vital signs, the patient should be monitored for glucose in the urine. Clinitests or *Diastix readings* should be taken every four hours or when the patient voids. Periodic electrolyte levels and weekly nitrogen balance determinations should also be done. A 24-hour urine collection is gathered to determine nitrogen balance. The urine urea nitrogen is then determined in the laboratory. Simply, the amount of nitrogen excreted by the patient is subtracted from the amount of nitrogen taken in. Nitrogen intake may be calculated as follows:

$$\text{Total nitrogen} = \frac{\text{Grams of amino acid taken in}}{6.25}$$

A positive nitrogen balance indicates that the patient is anabolizing more than he is catabolizing.

BIBLIOGRAPHY

Beaumont, E. The new IV infusion pumps. *Nursing 77* 31, 1977.

Bennion, M. Parenteral and tube feeding. In idem, *Clinical Nutrition*, New York: Harper & Row, Pubs., Inc., 1979.

Black, C. D., Popovich, N., and Black, M. Drug interactions in the GI tract. *Am. J. Nurs.* 77:1426, 1977.

Blackburn, G. L., Bestrian, B. R., Marni, B. S., Baltey, S., Schlamna, H. T., and Smith, M. F. Nutritional and metabolic assessment of the hospitalized patient. *J. Parenteral Enteral Nutr.* 1:11, 1977.

Bowden, A. M. Anticonvulsant and calcium metabolism. *Dev. Med. Child Neurol.* 16:214, 1974.

Buckley, J., Addicks, C., and Maniglia, J. Feeding patients with dysphagia. *Nurs. Forum* 15:69, 1976.

Carini, E., and Owens, G. Medical therapy. In *Neurological and Neurosurgical Nursing*, 6th Ed. St. Louis: The C. V. Mosby Co., 1974.

Coyle, N., and Arbet, E. How to protect your patients against aspiration pneumonia. *Nursing 78* 8:50, 1978.

Dicason, E. J., Schult, M., and Morris, E. M. *Maternal and Infant Drugs and Nursing Interventions.* New York: McGraw-Hill Book Co., 1978.

Dordoni, B. Reduction of absorption of paracetamol by activated charcoal and cholestramine: A possible therapeutic measure. *Br. Med. J.* 3:86, 1973.

Goldman, Guidelines for infection control in IV therapy. *Ann. Intern. Med.* 79:848, 1973.

Gormican, A. Tube feeding. *Dietet. Currents* 2(2):00 1975.

Gormican, A., Liddy E., and Thrush, B. Nutritional status of patients with extended tube feeding. *Research* 63:247, 1973.

Green, T. W. Pharmacology and clinical use of antacids. *Am. J. Hosp. Pharm.* 37:425, 1975.

Griggs, B., and Hoppe, M. Update: Nasogastric tube feedings. *Am. J. Nurs.* 79:481, 1979.

Hartshorn, E. A. Food and drug interactions. *J. Am. Diet. Assoc.* 70:15, 1977.

Hussar, D. Drug interactions: Good and bad. *Nursing 76* 61, 1976.

Kark, R. Liquid formula and chemically defined diets. *J. Am. Diet. Assoc.* 64:476, 1974.

Krause, M. V., and Mahan, L. K. *Food, Nutrition, and Diet Therapy.* 6th Ed. Philadelphia: W. B. Saunders, Co., 1979.

Kubo, W., Grant, M., Walike, B., Bugstrom, N., Wong, H., Hanson, R., and Padilla, G. Fluid and electrolyte problems of tube fed patients. *Am. J. Nurs.* 76:912, 76.

Kurdi, W. *Modern Intravenous Therapy Procedures.* Burbank, Calif.: Medical Education Consultants, 1976.

Lowenbraum, T. Infections from IV scalp-ven needles. *J. Am. Med. Assoc.* 212:451, 1970.

Manzi, C., and Masoorli, S. Troubles with IV's. *Nursing 78* 78, 1978.

McNiff, B. L. Clinical use of 10% soybean oil emulsion. *Am. J. Hosp. Pharm.* 34:1080, 1977.

Overton, M. H., and Lukert, B. P. *Clinical Nutrition: A Physiologic Approach.* Chicago: Year Book Medical Pubs., Inc., 1977.

Pennington, J. *Nutritional Diet Therapy.* Palo Alto, Calif.: Bull Pub. Co., 1978.

Porter, S. Feeding critically ill patients. *Nursing Times* 74:355, 1978.

Riella, M. C., Borviac, J. W., Wells, M., Essential fatty acid deficiency in human adults during total parenteral nutrition. *Ann. Int. Med.* 88:786, 1975.

Robinson, C. Nutrition in surgical conditions. In idem, *Normal and Therapeutic Nutrition*, 14th Ed. New York: The Macmillan Co., 1972.

Poe, D. *Drug-induced Nutritional Deficiencies.* Westport, Conn.: AVI Pub. Co., 1976.

Ryan, J. A. Catheter complications in TPN. *N. Engl. J. Med.* 290:757, 1974.

Scipien, G., Barnard, M., Chard, M., Howe, J., and Phillips, P. The gastrointestinal system. In *Comprehensive Pediatric Nursing.* New York: McGraw-Hill Book Co., 1975.

Scranton, P. E. *Practical Techniques in Venipuncture.* Baltimore: The Williams & Wilkins Co., 1977.

Sheinn, A., Collins, D., and Hoops, E. Drug interactions of common CCU medications. *Am. J. Nurs.* 74:1442, 1974.

Theuer, R. C., and Vitale, J. Drug and nutrient interactions. In H. Schneider, Ed., *Nutritional Support of Medical Practice.* New York: Harper & Row, Pubs., Inc., 1977.

Walike, B. Nasogastric tube feeding: The nursing perspective. *Dietet. Currents* (5):01 1975.

Wieman, J. Nutritional requirements of the trauma patient. *Heart Lung* 7:278, 1978.

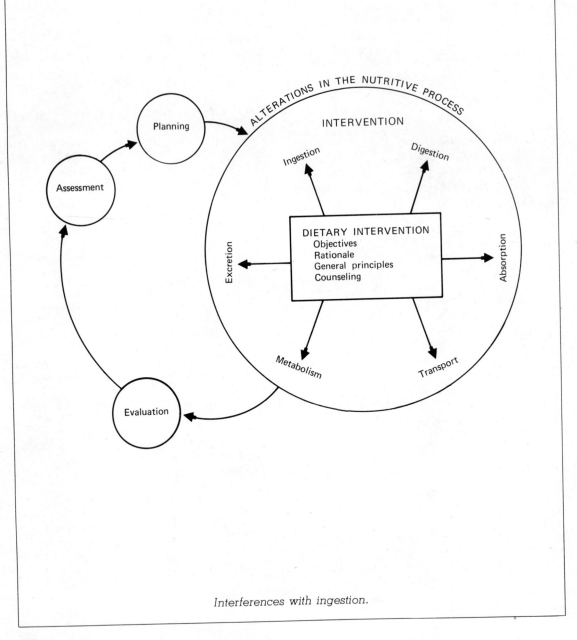

Interferences with ingestion.

V

DIETARY INTERVENTIONS FOR ALTERATIONS IN THE NUTRITIVE PROCESS

The purpose of this final unit is to demonstrate the use of the nursing diagnosis classification constructed around the nutritive process. Problems manifested by alterations in the nutritive process are discussed in terms of dietary interventions. Assessment data and possible causes of nutrition-related problems were presented in Chapter 21. This text does not emphasize specific diseases and their symptoms and management; rather, it discusses dietary interventions for many of the problems that interfere with the nutritive process. A client may evidence one or more of these problems, and a specific disease may affect one or more aspects of the nutritive process simultaneously. The approach here is intended to provide nursing students with a thorough understanding of the application of dietary management in total care of their clients.

The objectives and rationales of the dietary interventions for the individual nursing diagnoses are presented in this unit. Dietary principles are discussed in relation to the nutrients that are modified and the foods that are allowed and restricted. The discussion of dietary management emphasizes counseling clients about their diet. Client-centered objectives are provided for each nursing diagnosis. Practical aspects of the diet are also considered, such as suggestions for food purchasing and preparation.

As mentioned in Chapter 21 not all the nursing diagnoses that affect the nutritive process necessitate modifications in diet. Because this unit is concerned with dietary modifications, only those nursing diagnoses requiring specific changes in diet are discussed. Nursing diagnoses requiring medical intervention were discussed in Chapter 23.

BEHAVIORAL OBJECTIVES

After completing this unit, the student will be able to:

1. Explain the appropriate dietary intervention for a given nursing diagnosis.
2. State the general objectives of a given dietary modification as it relates to the nursing diagnosis.
3. Discuss the rationale for a given dietary intervention.
4. Describe the general principles of a given dietary modification, including the nutrient modifications and the foods allowed and not allowed.
5. Discuss practical considerations concerning food purchasing and food preparation for a selected diet.

CHAPTER 24

Interferences with Ingestion

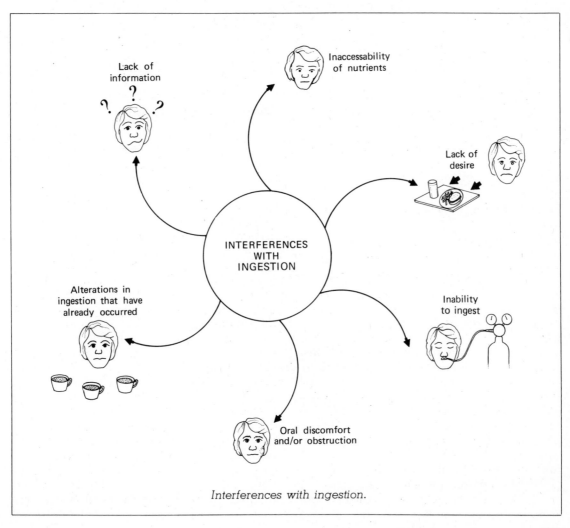

Interferences with ingestion.

The initial step in the nutritive process is the ingestion of food. A wide variety of factors can affect a client's ingestion, many of which were discussed in Chapter 1. This chapter is concerned with the six major categories of nursing diagnoses pertaining to ingestion that were listed in Chapter 21. The problems affecting the ingestion of nutrients from food are lack of information, inaccessibility of nutrients, lack of desire to ingest food, inability to ingest nutrients, oral discomfort and/or obstruction, and alterations in ingestion that have already occurred.

LACK OF INFORMATION

1. Dependence on communication assistance
2. Inadequate information related to foreign-food hazards
3. Inadequate information about food allergies
4. Lack of information about proper food intake
5. Dependence on instruction on prenatal nutrition
6. Reliance on instruction on postnatal nutrition
7. Noncompliance with therapeutic regimen

Hospital personnel frequently come into contact with people who have little or no knowledge about foods and nutrition or who have received inaccurate information. Some people eat primarily to stay alive; that is, they eat only to refuel their bodies. They give little or no thought to the kind or quality of food they consume. These people may subsist mainly on one food such as bread or beans or potatoes because of either personal taste preference or economic restrictions. In contrast, other clients have been influenced by food faddism to such an extent that a set regimen of food and supplements is consumed with almost a religious fervor. Whatever the reason for the inadequate nutrition informa-

tion, the nurse should be alert to the identification of this problem. If the client continues to practice current food habits, evidence of a nutritional deficiency or excess may appear.

Client Objectives

To be able to:

1. Discuss the foods that he should eat to meet his nutritional requirements.
2. Discuss alterations in the diet that may occur with changes in his nutritional requirements.
3. Consume a diet that meets his nutritional needs.

Dietary Interventions

The planning involved for the nutritional care and education of clients lacking information involves a careful consideration of each client's sociocultural, economic, and educational background. The major objective is to increase the client's awareness of the components of a nutritionally balanced diet and the accompanying health benefits. There is no specific dietary modification to be presented; the diet suggested to each client will be a modification of his existing or current diet.

Nursing intervention in any situation that involves inadequate or inaccurate nutritional information involves basic nutritional education. The nurse should take some of the responsibility for this teaching, since she is in close association with the client. The client's understanding of the importance of a balanced diet will be reinforced by nutritional education presented by both the dietitian and the physician. To be effective, a nurse must have a basic understanding of the components of a balanced diet (see Chap. 2), of the basic principles of normal nutrition, and of how the basic four food groups are modified to meet nutritional needs during different stages in the life cycle (Unit 3). The student is encouraged to review the basic four food groups as necessary.

The nurse should begin by informing the client of the health benefits that can be obtained from eating a well-balanced diet. She may then explain that food contains separate substances, known as nutrients, needed for the proper functioning of the body, and that three of these nutrients—carbohydrate, protein, and fat—are present in foods in varying amounts and contribute to the Calorie content of foods. She should emphasize that water is also an essential nutrient and that there are two other classes of nutrients— vitamins and minerals—that are required in only minute amounts though they have very important functions. As each food group of the basic four is explained, the major nutrients contributed by that food group can be named and their function explained. The number of servings required of each group and the amount considered to be a serving should also be explained.

After discussing the recommended servings from the basic four food groups, the nurse might plan an entire day's menu around the basic four. These menus should be planned using the client's usual eating habits. In this way the client can see the balanced diet as only a modification of his personal eating habits. The nurse may also include suggestions about economical and sensible food purchasing (presented in Chap. 8). The nurse may also review different methods of food preparation with the client as well as ways to prepare and store food for maximum retention of nutritive value (see Chap. 8). Finally, the nurse may mention agencies and organizations where the client can obtain more information about basic nutrition and foods.

Instructing the client about basic nutrition is generally most effective when there is discussion and interaction between client and nurse. To be effective the nurse should present the information at a level the client will understand, one geared to his sociocultural and educational background. The nurse

should be able to communicate with all levels of people from those who cannot read and write to those who have advanced college degrees.

Evaluation of the nutritional instruction could occur in a variety of ways. The nurse could ask the client to write some menus using the basic four food groups, which could be reviewed during the next visit. If the client is seen in a clinic, the nurse might ask the client to recall the food eaten during the past 24 hours and then review the list of food consumed with the client, using the basic four and making suggestions. Basic questions about food sources of common nutrients could be asked.

Dependence on Communication Assistance

When a client is hospitalized, the need for effective communication concerning food is crucial. Food preferences are a highly personal matter, involving each client's values, heritage, and desires. Frequently ingestion of food depends on how a client perceives its palatability. The method of preparation, texture, temperature, and mode of service all influence whether or not a food will be eaten. These preferences are usually made known through verbal communication.

The client who has lost the ability to communicate, either temporarily or permanently, becomes even more dependent on the nurse and on his significant others for food selection. Many times the person's only way of expressing disapproval of the loss of control is by refusing to eat. Nutritional depletion only serves to further compromise the physiological well-being of the client.

It is important to note that when there is impaired verbal communication there is frequently a concurrent physiological alteration that inhibits nutrient ingestion. A typical example is a cerebrovascular accident with resultant aphasia. Loss of control of one side of the mouth and *dysphagia* (difficulty swallowing) are also frequently seen. It is obvious that the nursing care of the client must be wholistic in approach and broad in scope.

The planning phase of the nursing process involves a comprehensive approach to the client with dependence on communication assistance. An awareness of the type of problem and its cause is necessary for carrying out effective nursing strategies. The causes of communication problems are many. Physiological alterations such as loss of hearing, loss of sight, removal of the pharynx, and mechanical interferences such as a tracheostomy or oral fixation, all may lead to a deficit in communication.

If the problem centers on the client not being able to read, the nurse should not give him pamphlets as a teaching device, although charts, pictures, and diagrams may be helpful. Such an undertaking demands creativity, knowledge, and patience from the nurse. The nurse must be careful not to talk down to the client. A person who cannot read because of loss of sight may be extremely articulate and able to learn quickly from conversations and group discussions. If the client has never had the opportunity to learn to read, he still retains a lifetime of experiences to build on in any kind of teaching program.

If the client cannot speak, erasable slates, alphabet boards, or a pad of paper and pencil may assist him in choosing what to eat. Such choices should be encouraged. Providing the client with real and valid choices enables him to exert some degree of control over his lifestyle and environment. Such active participation in care, though seemingly small, will encourage further participation. Such choices provide a firm basis on which to build a comprehensive rehabilitation program.

Hearing loss may prevent a client from understanding his or her environment completely. Many times, speech deficits are also present when the history of hearing loss goes back to infancy. Hearing aids, the use of sign language, or written communication may assist in planning the nutritional care of the client.

Similar difficulties arise when a client has no difficulty speaking or hearing but does not speak or understand English. Many hospitals have community interpreters available to them to assist in such cases. Small booklets can be made that use pictures instead of words to communicate client needs. With an effort and an attempt at understanding from both client and nurse, communication can usually occur.

The major intervention the nurse must use with the client with any kind of communication difficulty is *time*. Taking time to sit and attempting to understand a client's desires will go a long way in promoting further efforts at communication by both nurse and client. The attitude of caring that states, "You're worth my time; what you have to say is important; I want to understand your needs" is expressed almost subconsciously in the nurse's gestures, manners, approach, and appearance. If the client believes the nurse truly desires communication, he will continue to make every effort to communicate his needs. On the other hand, when a client senses a nurse is rushed and frustrated with his communication attempts, he is not likely to exert further effort to communicate, for to do so would bring further frustration, rejection, and dependence.

INACCESSIBILITY OF NUTRIENTS

1. Potential inadequate fluid intake
2. Thirst discomfort
3. Inadequate nutrient intake

This section focuses on problems of ingestion that occur because of inadequate quantities of nutrients available from food to maintain a person in an optimal nutritional status. Inadequate food or fluid intake can result in reduced amounts of nutrients available to the body cells. Inadequate fluid intake may occur during the summer, in the feeding of infants, or in the client who is on a restricted fluid intake and who experiences thirst discomfort. Inadequate food intake may be related to poor eating habits or to a lack of available food because of poverty or famine.

The clinical result of an inadequate intake of food over an extended period of time is a reduction in a person's nutritional status. This may first be manifested by weakness, malaise, apathy, loss of weight, and decreased resistance to infection. If this state of inadequate nutrition is left undetected, actual nutritional deficiency symptoms may develop. If the ingestion of food is not improved, the end result will be death. Recognition of the characteristic nutritional deficiency symptoms is an important skill for the nurse to have. Without adequate knowledge about nutritional deficiencies, some types of dermatitis, for example, might be dismissed as being due to poor hygiene or an allergy of some kind; whereas knowledge of nutritional deficiency symptoms can lead to identification of a nutrient deficiency. A detailed dietary history and the appropriate laboratory tests can confirm this diagnosis. Appropriate vitamin or mineral therapy can be initiated, and the disappearance of the symptoms occurs very rapidly.

It should be emphasized once again that, although there are classic nutritional deficiency diseases for the major nutrients, nutritional deficiencies of two or more nutrients often occur simultaneously in the same person. For example deficiencies of the B-complex vitamins thiamine, riboflavin, and niacin may all occur together. This phenomenon, however, should not necessarily interfere with diagnosis. Some of the deficiency symptoms are quite similar, but others are very specific to a certain nutrient. For example, in niacin deficiency a characteristic type of dermatitis occurs only on areas of the skin exposed to the sun.

Client's Objectives

To be able to:

1. Use community and personal resources.
2. Discuss reasons for altered nutritional intake.
3. Communicate increased satisfaction with nutrient intake.

Causes of Malnutrition

The causes of malnutrition are many and complex, but a basic knowledge of some of the interactions is quite helpful in understanding its development and treatment. Malnutrition in its broad sense was defined in Chapter 7. In this section the term *malnutrition* will be used to refer to undernutrition and, specifically, to nutritional deficiency diseases. Table 24-1 summarizes the major effects of the nutrient deficiencies on the body systems.

The emphasis in world nutrition has shifted away from the focus on the specific nutritional diseases to a concern for the general level of undernutrition, which is more evident. Previously, undernutrition in developing countries was accepted as a norm characteristic of these countries. However, the undernutrition present in these countries is no longer accepted and ignored. Efforts are being made to balance food supplies with the food needs of an expanding world population.

Malnutrition is caused by a complex interaction of many factors. It involves an inadequate intake of food by people living in a specific environment. The environment affects the supply of food and therefore the nutrient intake of the person. Some of the environmental factors that affect food availability are the soil, weather, and climate, as well as agricultural practices. Some countries export large amounts of high-protein foods to other countries because of the monetary gains to be realized. Some countries may also use their most productive soils to produce nonfood products such as coffee or tea for export. The rapidly increasing population of already crowded countries causes the short supply of food to be even more inadequate. Olness (1977) reported that cultural attitudes, beliefs, and taboos about food affect malnutrition. For example, in Laos it is believed that if the child eats eggs he will not have any teeth; in Kenya it is widely believed that children who eat eggs will have convulsions. In some

TABLE 24-1. Effects of Nutrient Deficiencies on Body Systems

Nutritional Deficiency	Integumentary System	Skeletal System	Muscular System	Nervous System (including Mental Attitude and Eyes)	Digestive System	Cardiovascular System
Protein	Flaky paint dermatosis; hair easily plucked		Mild wasting of fat and muscles	Mental changes (apathy)	Diarrhea	Edema; mild anemia
Protein and calories	Hair easily plucked		Severe wasting of fat and muscles	Impaired mental development	Diarrhea	Severe anemia
Vitamin A	Follicular hyperkeratosis, Xerosis (See Color Plates 1 and 6)			Eye Changes: Night blindness; dryness of the conjunctiva; photophobia; swelling and redness of the lids; Bitot's spots (See Color Plate 2); cornea becomes clouded and ulcers appear; keratomalacia; blindness		
Vitamin D		Failure of calcification; head appears enlarged and flattened; bowed legs; knock-knees; knobbing at wrists; bowing of arms; rachitic rosary	Decreased muscle tone; humpback (kyphosis); protuberance of abdomen			

Thiamine		Calf muscle tenderness; heaviness and weakness of legs; difficult walking; difficulty in rising from a squatting position	Malaise; tingling and numbness in legs; polyneuritis; Wernicke-Korsakoff syndrome; loss of immediate memory; disorientation; jerky movements of eyes; ataxia	Anorexia; vomiting; constipation	Increased pulse rate; palpitations; edema of legs, face, and trunk; high blood pressure; tachycardia; heart failure; dyspnea
Riboflavin	Cheilosis; angular fissures (See Color Plate 3); seborrheic dermatitis		Neuropathy; eye lesions may be present; photophobia; inflammation of cornea	Soreness of mouth and tongue; glossitis (See Color Plate 5); purple or magenta tongue; hypertrophy or atrophy of tongue papilla	Anemia
Niacin	Dermatitis on exposed area of the skin (See Color Plate 7)		Mental apathy; depression; anxiety; disorientation; confusion; dementia	Glossitis (See Color Plate 5)	Anorexia; indigestion; weight loss; diarrhea; stomatitis
Vitamin C	Skin is dry and rough; petechiae (See Color Plate 8); purpura; inadequate wound healing	Costochondral beading of ends of the ribs; Hemorrhages in muscles and joints; sunken chest		Gums swollen and bleed easily (See Color Plate 4)	Anemia

cultures the best food is saved for the fathers, or they are allowed to eat first. In Laos mothers prechew rice for their small infants. Young infants are breast-fed until the next baby arrives, at which time the older child is started on solid foods for the first time. This emotional trauma can lead to depression in these very young children and failure to eat even the food that is offered to them.

All these cultural and environmental factors have an effect on malnutrition, but the most dramatic precipitating factors are diarrhea and infectious diseases. Diarrhea may be precipitated by a contaminated water or food supply or by microbial and parasitic diseases. The malnourished child is more susceptible to infectious diseases, and the stress of these diseases increases the severity of the malnutrition. Thus a synergistic relationship is set up between malnutrition and infectious diseases (Gordon, 1976).

Synergism is the result of the interaction of two diseases that is more severe than the anticipated combined effect. The interaction involved can be understood better by examining the effect of each condition on the other. What are the effects of malnutrition on infection? A protein deficiency in humans can decrease antibody production, thus increasing the susceptibility to infection. Gordon (1976) reported that children with protein deficiency evidenced little or no leukocyte response to infection. The integrity of the skin, mucous membranes, and epithelial tissue acts as a protective barrier against infection, but deficiencies of vitamin A, ascorbic acid, niacin, or protein are likely to produce a lowered resistance. Wound healing, the closing of abscesses, and new collagen formation are all slowed by protein and ascorbic acid deficiencies. The infection itself also has an effect on nutritional status. One of the first manifestations of an infectious disease is loss of appetite and decreased tolerances for food. The infection and possible fever increase the metabolic rate and the actual nutrient requirements. At a time when the child requires more Calories

and nutrients, less is actually consumed. The protein requirement is higher because of the extra protein needed for repair. The low blood levels of vitamin A may be further reduced and xerophthalmia (vitamin A deficiency) may result. The end result of an untreated deficiency of vitamin A is permanent blindness. The following is an example of a child who develops malnutrition. The description should serve to illustrate many of the examples given in the previous paragraphs.

This child may be white or yellow or black or a combination of colors; he may be a boy or a girl; he may be handsome or ugly; born of average of or superior intelligence; and living on a farm or in a town. He is usually one of the older children in a family, probably the first or second. During the first year of his life he may do fairly well even though the family income may be insufficient to give him all the goodies which infants of upper classes receive in most countries. He takes his mother's milk until late in her second pregnancy and by that time he is likely to be about 18 months old. Toward the end of her second pregnancy he begins to have a premonition that things are changing for him. He gets less and less of his mother's milk and his mother seems less and less interested in allowing him to nurse her as if she is trying to create distance between them.

He feels very insecure because for 18 months he has stuck to her like a burr. If she has gone out to work on a shamba he has ridden on her back. If she has gone out to weed rice in paddies he has been comfortably tied to her back. So at the crucial age of 18 months, when separation anxiety is normally at its maximum, he is completely bewildered by the wrenching which he is undergoing. He is given food which he does not like because it is new and strange and he has never experienced solid food whether it is sticky rice or taro mush or cornmeal mush.

The new baby arrives and the separation is really complete. Now the intruder clings to the mother like a burr and there is no substitute mother for our tragic hero to clutch. If he had been a later sibling he might at least have had a comforting older sibling, but now he feels completely bereft. He sits in a corner and whines. He is acutely depressed and refuses food. He will not take even the carbohydrate-rich foods which are offered him and, of course, almost no animal proteins are offered. They are not for toddlers in his culture. Sometimes, in seeking comfort, he chews on sticks, stones or any chewable object. In the process he picks up intestinal parasites and bacteria and he almost always has diarrhea in the post-weaning period. His mother thinks of this as quite normal and ignores it unless it becomes terribly severe. But in 1976, this child may have had access to a clinic which has given immunizations. He may have been immunized against diptheria, whooping cough, tetanus, polio and measles—and even against tuberculosis. It is possible that his attacks of malaria are aborted by a medic or nurse in the vicinity who gives him the proper drug. Perhaps 50 years ago he would have died rather quickly during the period when he was so deprived of protein and so depressed. But, in 1976, life does not leave him and he survives the period of malnutrition. Not only does his system lack protein for full development of his brain (myelinization is essentially complete at age three) but he has missed the 12–18 months of exploring which is the right of every toddler. He has missed the very sensitive and crucial first impressions of the world about him as he huddled miserably in a corner or under a table with greenish stool spilling out under him. He has sat whining for months and his irritability has become an annoyance to other family members who begin to dislike him. They cannot sleep because he is miserable. If they recognize his malnutrition and tempt him with large amounts of special foods he may only develop a more severe diarrhea because protein deprivation also damages intestinal cells so that they can no longer accept nutrients in normal fashion.

He may get so ill that his feet become swollen, his skin looks burned; his parents begin to worry so much that they take him to a hospital. There he is treated with protein-rich foods and he improves in a month or two. Hospital staff may attempt to teach the mother about the cause of his illness and about its prevention. If she understands, this child may recover permanently in time for his brain to develop to capacity. But steaks and cream at age 4 and 5 may be

unable to reverse brain damage suffered before age 3. And also, some parents do not understand and take the child home to his former diet. He relapses and the final state is worse than the first.

If he lives through or squeaks through his period of protein deprivation, by age 5 or 6 he will be offered some proteins and he has teeth for chewing meat. Although he may be far below normal weight, ridden by parasites, and still not a very active or happy fellow, he goes on to maturity. He seems listless and apathetic much of the time. He missed the exciting period of exploration which every 2-year old needs and, at 7 or 8 or 10, he has no ability to learn what he should have learned as a toddler. If he was born with a superior mentality he may be of normal intelligence as an adult. If he began with normal intelligence he may mature with less than that. He can manage some types of thinking but his intellect has strange gaps. Abstractions are difficult for him and he does not know that there is a difference between himself and his schoolmates who were provided with proteins other than milk from early infancy on. He may feel cheated or left out and rightly so. Will he rear his children as he was reared? Animal nutrition studies show clearly that it takes more than one generation for well nourished offspring to regain normal intelligence when there has been a protein-deprived generation. Surely the world cannot afford more malnourished generations in its human population. [Olness, 1977, p. 283]

Protein-Calorie Malnutrition

The phrase *protein-Calorie malnutrition* covers a broad range of malnutrition disorders, including kwashiorkor at one extreme and marasmus at the other, with variations of each between. Kwashiorkor can be described as a deficiency of dietary protein, but caloric content of the diet is adequate or nearly adequate. Marasmus is chronic total undernutrition characterized by a diet not only inadequate in protein but also in total Calories and vitamins and minerals. These two conditions may be two manifestations of the same disease process, since no dietary differences have been found between children with kwashiorkor and marasmus (James, 1977). Marasmus may be an adaptation to chronic malnutrition, as evidenced by severe growth retardation, whereas kwashiorkor may be a dysadaptation to protein deficiency, as evidenced by edema and metabolic changes. Infectious diseases are usually the precipitating factor in kwashiorkor.

Kwashiorkor is an African word that means the sickness the older child gets when the next baby is born. It becomes evident in children ages 1–3 years who have been weaned from the mother's breast (Fig. 24-1). The child is given a diet consisting of a starchy cereal gruel, his first introduction to solid foods. Coupled with the traumatic experience of weaning and the nutritional inadequacies of the cereal gruel, the child's ingestion of nutrients is quite low. The child with kwashiorkor has severe edema that masks the muscle wasting (Fig. 24-2). The enlarged liver and the edema give the child the characteristic "pot belly" of kwashiorkor. To the nonmedical person, the child may appear to be healthy.

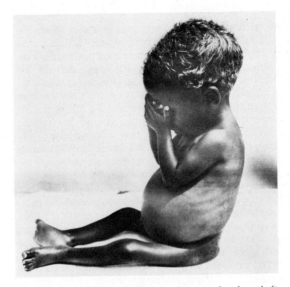

Figure 24-2. Kwashiorkor is the result of a deficiency of protein. The edema masks the muscular wasting. (WHO photo)

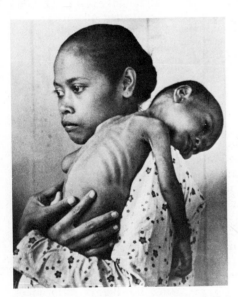

Figure 24-1. Malnutrition is a tragedy for millions of children and their families. (WHO photo)

Once treatment is begun the edema disappears, revealing the muscular wasting. The child is apathetic and irritable. He whimpers and moans but does not cry. He is very inactive and may even be unable to walk. A characteristic type of skin change, called "flaky paint" dermatosis, occurs. The patches of skin change in color from reddish to purple and finally dark brown. At this stage they become dry and peel off, leaving weeping areas. Some dyspigmentation of the hair occurs (grayish white, yellow, or reddish brown); the hair is sparse, finely textured, and easy to pluck out (DeMaeyer, 1976). The child's appetite is poor, and diarrhea is quite common. Laboratory values that are commonly low are serum potassium, serum albumin, and total serum protein. Very low serum levels of vitamin A are also present. Some of the symptoms of kwashiorkor resemble those of essential fatty acid deficiency. A deficiency of the essential fatty acid may be found to be a contributor to the disease (James, 1977).

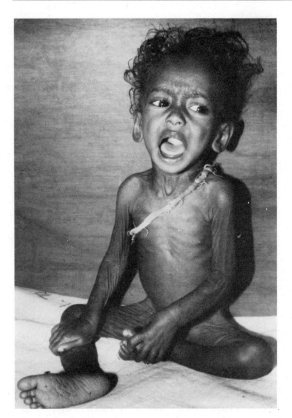

Figure 24-3. Marasmus is chronic total undernutrition. (Photo courtesy of T. Dallant)

Marasmus is chronic total undernutrition or severe starvation (Fig. 24-3). Both Calories and protein as well as other nutrients are very inadequate in the diet. The child with marasmus is usually younger than the child with kwashiorkor and has been exposed to an inadequate diet for a much longer period of time. Marasmus is often described as complete deprivation of food as well as physical and emotional care. The parents are either extremely poor, very uninformed about food values, may have severe mental or emotional problems, or various combinations of these problems (Williams, 1977). Marasmus is most common in infants between 6 and 18 months of age. In marasmus there is a very low body weight along with much muscular wasting and loss of subcutaneous fat tissue. The child is extremely emaciated and presents the appearance of a wizened old man. Many of the symptoms present in kwashiorkor are not present in marasmus, because the child has never had an adequate intake of food and physiological adaptation has occurred from the beginning of life. The child with marasmus usually is more alert and has a better appetite. There are usually no skin or hair changes in marasmus, and most of the laboratory values are within normal range.

Vitamin A Deficiency

A deficiency of vitamin A leads to changes in both the skin and the eyes. Since vitamin A can be stored in the liver, the time required for an adult to develop deficiency symptoms of this nutrient may be two years or more. A rapidly growing young child with minimal stores may show signs of corneal destruction of the eye within a few weeks on a diet deficient in vitamin A (Oomen, 1976).

With vitamin A deficiency the skin becomes dry and rough. One of these changes is known as follicular hyperkeratosis, or "goose flesh." (See Color Plate 6.) It gives the appearance of minute bumps evenly distributed over the skin. In this skin change the hair follicles have become blocked with keratin plugs from the epithelial lining (Krause and Mahan 1979). Xerosis, or drying of the skin, is manifested by the appearance of a powdery dandruff seen all over the skin, particularly on the legs. The advanced form of xerosis is called ichthyosis, or "fish scale" skin. All these skin changes are characterized by abnormal keratinization of the epithelium of the skin. Much care must be exercised, however, in the diagnosis of skin disorders due to a vitamin A deficiency. Deficiencies of other vitamins or of essential fatty acids may be the cause, or the client may have dry skin due to an allergy or sensitivity to some food or substance. Diagnosis of a vitamin A deficiency as evidenced by dry skin should always be further documented with a dietary history and laboratory tests supporting the diagnosis.

The deficiency disease associated with vitamin A deficiency is xerophthalmia. This condition is characterized by dryness of the cornea and conjunctiva of the eye, eventual softening of this cornea, and total blindness. Sommer (1976) states that it is thought to be the most important cause of blindness in children in many underdeveloped countries. It is often associated with kwashiorkor, or it occurs by itself as the result of a diet deficient in vitamin A. Newell (1978) reported that most cases of xerophthalmia occur in the rice-eating populations of Asia. It is estimated that 60,000–80,000 Indonesian children develop xerophthalmia each year and over half of these go blind. Twenty percent of these cases have corneal involvement and another fifty percent will develop the beginning stages of the disease before age 5. Xerophthalmia is probably the leading cause of blindness in the world today, and it is preventable.

There are several stages in the development of xerophthalmia. The first symptom may be night blindness, but this symptom is difficult to detect in infants and young children. For the purpose of describing the development of the disease, the primary signs can be divided into three stages (Oomen, 1976). The first stage involves conjunctival xerosis (dryness of the conjunctiva of the eye). The conjunctiva becomes dry, and there is a loss of transparency and an impaired ability to transmit light. There is also a thickening and wrinkling of the conjunctiva. The next step is the appearance of Bitot's spots. These are small, triangular, silvery gray patches that appear on the surface of the conjunctiva. (See Color Plate 2.) They represent degeneration of the epithelium. Some appear foamy, but they may also have a cheese- or grease-like surface according to Oomen (1976). The second stage involves dryness of the cornea. Stages 1 and 2 are reversible with vitamin A therapy. The final stage is irreversible. In this stage the cornea becomes clouded and ulcera-

tion usually occurs. The final events are softening of the cornea (keratomalacia), perforation, and total blindness.

Thiamine Deficiency

The specific deficiency disease caused by a deficiency of thiamine is *beriberi*. This disease was originally found in populations that consumed polished rice as a staple in their diet. The milling process of the rice had removed the thiamine, resulting in thiamine-deficient diets. This disease has largely been eradicated in countries where the rice is enriched, leaving the aleuron intact during milling, or by parboiling, which drives the thiamine into the endosperm portion of the rice.

Beriberi may occur as either wet or dry beriberi, depending on the presence or absence of edema. The symptoms involve the peripheral nerves and the related muscle functions in the autonomic, sensory, and motor systems. Symptoms common to both types are anorexia, malaise, heaviness and weakness of the legs, and tenderness of the calf muscle, which causes the client difficulty in rising from a squatting position. Early cardiac involvement is evident by palpitation upon exertion or from mental excitement. The polyneuropathy of dry beriberi involves both sensory and motor defects. These abnormalities begin distally and progress proximally. First, tingling and numbness appear in the calf muscles of the leg and later progress to the forearms, thighs, and the abdominal wall (Katsura and Oiso, 1976). Foot drop and wrist drop are evident in advanced polyneuropathy of dry beriberi. In wet beriberi edema is present in the face, legs, trunk, and around the heart. The pulse is rapid and the blood pressure is elevated. Death may result from sudden cardiac failure (Krause and Mahan, 1979). There are usually elevated levels of pyruvic acid and lactic acid in the blood, because thiamine is required in carbohydrate metabolism for the conversion of pyruvic acid to acetyl CoA.

Riboflavin Deficiency

Riboflavin deficiency is known as *arboflavinosis.* Because riboflavin is found in foods in combination with the other members of the vitamin B complex group, riboflavin deficiency often occurs along with thiamine or niacin deficiency. Milk and dairy products are especially high in riboflavin. If this one group of foods is avoided, it is possible for only a riboflavin deficiency to occur. Since riboflavin functions in protein metabolism, most of the characteristic symptoms of deficiency are evidenced by changes in the skin. The deficiency symptoms involving the tongue and the mouth are difficult to distinguish from deficiencies of other B complex vitamins. (See Color Plates 3 and 5.) There is a characteristic type of greasy dermatitis that may be seen in the folds around the nose, ears, and eyelids.

Niacin Deficiency

A disease of niacin deficiency, *pellagra,* often occurs along with a protein deficiency and other deficiencies of the B complex vitamins. The classic cases of pellagra occur in countries in which the diet consists mainly of corn (Fig. 24-4). Since corn is an incomplete protein and is particularly low in the essential amino acid tryptophan, a precursor of niacin, pellagra may develop. In the United States some cases of pellagra may still occur among the poor in the South who are forced, for economic reasons, to consume primarily cornmeal, salt pork, and molasses. The cornmeal is low in tryptophan, and the niacin it contains is present in a bound form that cannot be used by the body. In the preparation of tortillas in Central America the common practice of soaking the cornmeal in lye makes the niacin unavailable (Krause and Mahan, 1979). Since niacin is also involved with protein metabolism, some of the symptoms appear to resemble those of a riboflavin deficiency. (See Color Plates 3 and 5.) A distinguishing symptom of pellagra, however, is the characteristic type of

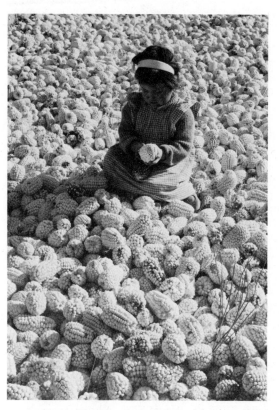

Figure 24-4. People in many countries suffer severely from malnutrition—even while there are surpluses of food on the market. A deficiency of niacin (pellagra) may occur from a diet that consists mainly of corn. (WHO photo by P. Almasy)

dermatitis that appears on exposed areas of the skin. This symptom frequently becomes evident in the spring and summer when more area of the skin is exposed to the sun. (See Color Plate 7.) The classic symptoms of pellagra are sometimes referred to as the 3 D's—dermatitis, diarrhea, and dementia. They therefore involve skin lesions, gastrointestinal disturbances, and mental changes (Barakat, 1976). The symptoms may also occur simultaneously with other deficiencies of the B complex group of vitamins.

Vitamin C

An inadequate quantity of vitamin C or ascorbic acid, in the diet may lead to the development of *scurvy*. Scurvy was more prevalent in the eighteenth and nineteenth centuries among sailors on long ocean voyages. When they began taking lemons along on the voyages, scurvy epidemics did not occur. Today it is recognized that lemons and other citrus fruits contain vitamin C, which prevents scurvy. Although scurvy is much less prvalent today, it still occurs. It may be the result of an increased requirement for or a decreased dietary intake of vitamin C. Such clinical conditions as fever, surgery, burns, infections, and physiological stress are known to increase the requirement for vitamin C (Williams, 1977).

The symptoms of scurvey are based on the role of vitamin C in the formation of hydroxyproline, a necessary constituent of collagen (Krause and Mahan, 1979). Collagen is the intracellular cement that binds the cells of bone, teeth, connective tissue, and capillaries together. The symptoms of ascorbic acid deficiency are related to changes within these specialized connective tissues and the capillaries (Woodruff, 1975). There may be changes within the skin, muscles, bones, joints, and gums. The skin shows evidence of follicular hyperkeratosis, which refers to bumps on the epidermis around the hair follicles. They resemble the goose flesh skin of a vitamin A deficiency. Small, pin-point hemorrhages called *petechiae* appear around these areas. (See Color Plate 8.) These hemorrhagic areas may spread into large, purplish spots called *purpura* or very large areas called *ecchymoses*. The gums are red, swollen, and bleed easily. (See Color Plate 4.) Hemorrhages may occur in the muscles of the thigh and leg. Hemorrhages in the joints lead to inflammation and painful swelling, especially around the knee joints (Goldsmith, 1977). The infant with scurvy lies in a position resembling a frog, with the knees slightly flexed and the thighs rotated to the outside (Woodruff, 1975). This position is the most comfort-

able for the infant with this condition because of the severe bone and joint pain. The infant will begin to cry if he has to move from this position. This position may remind the student nurse of the bowed legs characteristic of rickets, but these two symptoms should not be confused.

There are also disorders of the bone, especially if scurvy occurs during infancy or childhood. The growing ends of the long bones are affected in the region of the epiphyseal plate. Microscopic fractures and an accumulation of calcified cartilage lead to separation of the epiphyseal plate and malformation of the bone (Williams, 1977). Changes also occur at the costochondral junction of the ribs, the area where the ribs attach to the costal cartilage, which attaches to the sternum. Because of minute fractures and replacement of fibrous tissue at the growing ends of the ribs, these junctions are malformed. As the child breathes, the anterior chest wall is pulled toward the spine creating a sunken chest. The sharp projection of the ribs is called costochondral beading. It is quite similar to the beading of the ribs seen in rickets; however, with rickets the beading is more rounded (Woodruff, 1975).

Other body functions and processes are often affected in scurvy. Breathing may be more difficult because of internal hemorrhages in the intercostal muscles. Wounds may heal very slowly or fail to heal. Scars from previous wounds may separate, leaving an open sore. A client with a wound that does not heal within the usual length of time should be further examined concerning his nutritional status. It is quite likely that he may need additional vitamin C. Weight loss is common, and anemia may be present due to the hemorrhaging. The client's emotional state is one of depression, lack of motivation, and hypochondriasis (Hodges, 1976).

Vitamin D

Inadequate vitamin D leads to the development of the classic deficiency disease of *rickets*. It is a disease of the skeletal system in which calcification of the bones is incomplete. It usually becomes evident during infancy and early childhood, when the requirement for vitamin D is highest. The major clinical manifestations of rickets are the skeletal deformities. When the child begins to walk, the bones are soft and not strong enough to support the child's weight. The force of gravity exerted by standing and walking pulls the ends of the long bones out of position. This leads to the classic symptom of bowed legs and knock-knees. Ford (1974) states that the child may complain of painful knees. This symptom may be passed off simply as "growing pains" when a vitamin D supplement might alleviate the symptom. The wrists and ankles are also enlarged (Krause and Mahan, 1979) and there may be bowing of the arms. Another characteristic sign of rickets is the enlargement of the growing ends of the rib bones, which are attached to the sternum by costal cartilage. This bead-like effect is referred to as the "rachitic rosary." In severe rickets the costal cartilages may be pulled in, and the sternum protrudes producing a deformity known as "pigeon-breast" (Goldsmith, 1977). There may also be a general curving of the spine. Accompanying the sagging posture, there is usually a general sagging of the abdominal muscle and decreased muscle tone. Constipation is a common problem associated with rickets because of decreased intestinal muscle tone. Skeletal deformities of the head include the development of thickened areas of the skull causing it to appear larger. The top of the skull may appear flat and depressed toward the middle, and there may also be areas of softening of the cranial bones called *craniotabes* (Williams, 1977).

Osteomalacia is the adult form of rickets. It is extremely rare in the United States, but when it does occur it is usually associated with chronic malabsorption. The most frequent complaint is bone pain in the back and legs, especially when the client is walking or standing. Because minerals are not being deposited, there is a general softening of the bones. The bones are gradually losing the minerals.

Iodine

A deficiency of dietary iodine will lead to the condition of endemic *goiter*. Goiter is an enlargement of the thyroid gland. Iodine is an important component of the thyroid hormone thyroxine. When inadequate amounts of iodine are available in the diet, the thyroid gland enlarges in its attempt to produce adequate levels of the hormone (Fig. 24-5). Goiter is most prevalent in areas of the world where seafood is not available and where the iodine content of the soil is low. The midwestern region of the United States used to be known as the "goiter belt" because of the high incidence of goiter in the area. Since the advent of iodized salt, the incidence of goiter in the United States has greatly decreased. Endemic goiter is still a major health problem in certain areas of the world. It does not cause too many problems for the person with the condition; however, a long-term iodine deficiency passed onto succeeding generations does present problems. Severe iodine deficiency in the mother produces cretinism in the offspring. Cretinism is characterized by stunted growth and differing levels of mental retardation. Clements (1976) reported that the prevalence of cretinism, and other conditions such as deaf-mutism, correlates well with the prevalence rates and severity of goiter.

Dietary Interventions

Planning for nutritional care of the client who has been consuming inadequate quantities of nutrients should begin with an analysis of why there is an inadequate quantity of food or fluid consumed. Is the inadequate food intake from lack of knowledge about a balanced diet, poor eating habits, or an inadequate quantity of food available because of poverty? Or is the inadequate quantity of food consumed related to a difficulty with ingestion such as a decreased desire for food, pain experienced when eating, or difficulty swallowing? Once the reason for the ingestion of inadequate nutrients has been determined, a

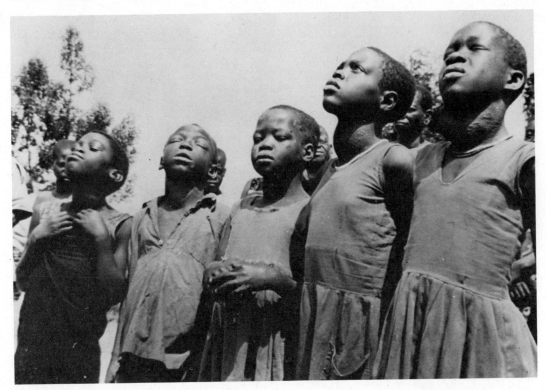

Figure 24-5. Goiter is the result of chronic iodine deficiency in the diet and drinking water. (WHO photo)

plan can be formulated. Planning for the nutritional care of clients who have been ingesting inadequate quantities of nutrients involves assisting the physician and dietitian in determining the methods of treating any specific nutritional deficiencies that may exist. Another important consideration is the social, cultural, psychological, and economic status of the client.

There are three general objectives to be achieved with the client who has been consuming inadequate quantities of nutrients from foods. The first objective is to treat any existing nutritional deficiencies. The second is to teach the client the principles and benefits of a nutritionally balanced diet. The third objective is to help the client plan and select a nutritionally balanced diet based on personal food preferences, food availability, and financial resources. The diet used in these instances is a nutritionally balanced diet. If a specific nutritional deficiency does exist, as evidenced by nutritional assessment, high doses of the deficient nutrient are administered, and in many cases additional vitamin or mineral supplements may be given.

In the first step, treating the deficiency disorder itself, the nurse should be involved with the physician and dietitian both in the planning and the implementing of the client's treatment. This involvement enables the nurse to have a better understanding of the nature of the client's disease. It also enables the nurse to be more supportive of the client during therapy. The nurse will also be able to monitor the laboratory values and the clinical signs more effectively if she has a broader knowledge of the nutritional deficiency disease.

The general treatment of a nutritional deficiency disease is the replacement of the deficient nutrient or nutrients in therapeutic doses. The diet served to the client also contains high amounts of the deficient nutrient. The nutrient supplements may be administered by injection, either intramuscularly, intravenously, or parenterally. Supplements are also given orally, either in liquid or capsule form. The specific doses depend on the age and body size of the client and on the severity of the deficiency disorder. For maximum use and tolerance by the client, doses of the nutrient supplement are administered throughout the day at regularly spaced intervals.

The initial treatment of protein-Calorie malnutrition, whether it is kwashiorkor or marasmus, involves first the correction of fluid and electrolyte inbalances. On the second or third day a dilute mixture of skimmed milk is begun. The caloric and protein levels are raised as quickly as possible by increasing the strength of the formula and the quantity (DeMaeyer, 1976). The provision of adequate Calories is essential to ensure that a large proportion of the protein will be used for the replenishment of body tissue. High levels of Calories are needed to meet the high energy demands of tissue replenishment and growth as well as the increased caloric demands imposed by possible fever, infection, and disease. Skimmed milk, weaning foods, or specially formulated foods such as Faffa or Incaparino, respectively, used in Ethiopia or Guatemala, are used (Kimm and Donoso, 1979). The client is also given a multivitamin and protein supplement to correct any subclinical deficiencies that might exist and an iron supplement during the first few weeks of treatment. The results of treatment are usually very dramatic.

Roberts (1978) reported on the treatment of four malnourished infants in Columbia, South America. The infants were severely malnourished and had the typical signs of marasmus. They were also suffering from external and internal parasites, abscesses and skin infections, respiratory infections, and anemia. The infants were admitted to an orphanage and given appropriate medical treatment including a high-protein diet. They received maximum care and stimulation by the nursery staff, who talked and sang to, cuddled, held, and rocked the infants. Visual and motor stimulation was provided by mobiles and manipulative toys placed in the cots. Music was also played during the day. The infants were observed to have ravenous appetites within a short period of time. They gained weight rapidly, although less than a normal child would gain in the same time. This maximum weight gain occurred during the first three to six months of treatment and then declined. This initial weight gain gave the children the appearance of being obese in contrast to their previous malnourished state. The condition, however, is self-limiting; by age 3, most of these children are of normal build.

In the treatment of vitamin deficiencies the amount of the vitamin administered as a supplement varies. For the fat-soluble vitamins A and D the amount given is approximately 6–10 times the RDA for children. The quantities of water-soluble vitamins administered is even higher because these vitamins cannot be stored. The levels range from 10 to 50 times the RDA. The doses of the water-soluble vitamins are also generally administered several times throughout the day. The usual procedure is to give injections of the vitamin for the first few days until the client is able to tolerate an oral dose. Oral doses are given either in a water-soluble preparation or in capsule form until all the symptoms of the deficiency disappear and usually for several additional weeks or months. If extensive amounts of diarrhea are present or if there is evidence of malabsorption, the fat-soluble vitamins should be administered intravenously or parenterally rather than orally.

In the second step, teaching the client or a family member the principles and benefits of a nutritionally balanced diet, the client must first be made to understand the cause of the nutritional deficiency disease. In the majority of cases the major contributing factor was probably an inadequate diet. Was the inadequate diet the result of inadequate knowledge, poor eating habits, or decreased availability of food? If the nutritional deficiency is due to inadequate knowledge or poor eating habits, the client must be made to understand the foods that were missing from the diet that led to the specific nutrient deficiency. He should be instructed in the principles and benefits of a nutritionally balanced diet. The foods that contain large amounts of the deficient nutrient should be discussed with the client. A determination may next be made as to which of the foods listed the client prefers and which could be realistically included in his diet. Even though orange juice is one of the common foods highest in vitamin C content, it will not benefit the client recovering from scurvy if he does not like the flavor of orange juice or if it is unavailable in the area.

Health workers working with clients in developing countries find that it is necessary to learn the cultural and social practices of the specific country before nutritional education can be of much benefit to the people. The most effective way to learn the culture of a country is actually to live among its people. Even then it may take several years before any noticeable improvement is seen in the overall nutritional status of an area or country. Patience, perseverance, and understanding seem to be very important keys to improving the nutritional status of a population. Copping (1968) relates some comments about an elderly African woman who criticized the Europeans for thinking that they had all the right answers: "You Europeans think you have everything to teach us. You tell us we eat the wrong food, treat our babies the wrong

way, give our sick people the wrong medicine; you are always telling us we are wrong. Yet if we had always done the wrong things, we should all be dead. And you see we are not" (p. 127). Undoubtedly the people of the developing countries become weary with the Americans and Europeans who tell them all the things they are doing wrong. A positive approach to nutritional education and integration of the basic principles into the culture of the country should have a more positive effect on the people.

In developing countries it is first necessary to determine which stages of the life cycle are at the greatest nutritional risk. In most countries, including the United States, these groups will be the infants and preschool children and the pregnant and lactating women. Another decision is where the nutritional education will actually take place. Copping (1968) suggests that nutritional education may take place in the home, community center, health center, hospital, youth club, or with a local community organization. Health workers have learned through experience that an important target group for nutritional education are the grandmothers, for it is they who often feed the young children. They are highly respected within the culture by the young mothers, and they have much influence over them. Two other groups who are receptive to nutritional education are (1) the young girls who remain at home to take care of the young children when the mothers go to work on the farm and (2) children in school. If children are given sound nutritional education in the schools, when they become adults they will have a better idea of the benefits of good nutrition.

The third step is to assist the client in planning and selecting a nutritionally balanced diet based on personal food preferences, food availability, and financial resources. Large-scale supplementary feeding programs or take-home feeding programs have been instituted in many countries for helping to adequately nourish infants, preschool children, and pregnant and lactating mothers. These are either on-the-spot feeding programs or take-home feeding programs. There are advantages and disadvantages to both, and neither has proved entirely satisfactory. In a take-home program a set quantity of food is distributed to be consumed in a specified amount of time by members of a family who are considered to be at high nutritional risk. The food is prepared and eaten at home. Once the food is in the home there may be extensive sharing of it among the family members. Most or all of it may be consumed by the adult males or older children and very little, if any, by the high-risk family members. The food may even be sold outside the family for money to buy some other product. The food may not be stored properly, and it may become infected or spoil. On-the-spot feeding may at first seem to have more advantages. At least the person who most needs to receive the food actually receives and eats the food at the feeding site. The distance to the feeding sites is often long, however, and the pregnant or lactating mother or the mother with the high-risk infant or child may only make the trip to the feeding site once or twice a week or less (Ramalingaswami and Tandon, 1979).

LACK OF DESIRE TO INGEST FOOD AND FLUIDS

1. Anorexia
2. Impaired ability to taste food
3. Nausea
4. Intra-abdominal pressure discomfort
5. Food selection dissatisfaction
6. Diffculty maintaining a religious diet

The ingestion of adequate quantities of food is important to the health of all people, but adequate food is even more important in the therapeutic treatment of the client who is ill. There are, however, many circumstances, both physiological and psychological, affecting the diseased client that may have a depressing effect on the desire to ingest food. The client may experience anorexia as a symptom of the diseased state, because of psychological stress, nausea and vomiting, or as a side effect of certain drugs (see Fig. 24-6). Anorexia may also be caused by specific metabolites produced in certain diseases. For example, the elevation of ammonia levels during cirrhosis and of the blood urea nitrogen in chronic renal failure both have a depressing effect on appetite.

A decreased desire to ingest food may also be caused by an impaired ability to taste food stemming from a disease state or from medications. Deficiencies of such nutrients as

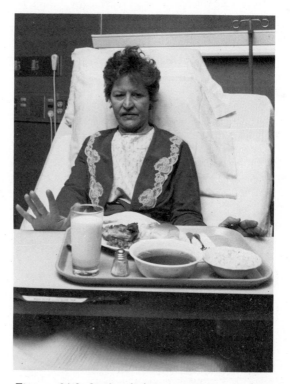

Figure 24-6. Lack of desire to eat may have many causes; the nurse's first task is to determine why a client does not want to eat.

niacin, vitamin A, and zinc have been reported to cause taste deficiencies (Carson and Gormican, 1977). Reductions in taste sensitivity are also widely known during the treatment of cancer.

Nausea that interferes with the ingestion of food may be the result of gastrointestinal disorders, impaired cardiac circulation, infection, or a side effect of certain drugs. A sensation of intra-abdominal pressure or "bloating" resulting from decreased peristalisis in the gastrointestinal tract or following surgery can also decrease the desire to eat.

A psychological dissatisfaction with food selection due to lack of variety or foods not appropriate or familiar to the client's cultural background may also lead to a temporary lack of desire to ingest food in the hospital environment. When the problems of nausea, intra-abdominal pressure, or impaired taste are present in addition to a general dissatisfaction with food selection, the combined effect presents a real challenge that calls for the combined ingenuity and efforts of the nurse and the dietitian. The psychological state of depression in any client often leads to a decreased desire for food. In the young, depression may lead to anorexia nervosa; and in the elderly, to gradual starvation.

Client Objectives

To be able to:

1. Ingest food in the quantity and variety necessary to meet his nutritional requirements.
2. Modify his intake to meet his nutritional requirements.

Dietary Interventions

Clients with cancer, because they experience most, if not all, of the problems with the ingestion of food, provide a good example for nutritional management. Clients who have cancer often experience anorexia, changes in taste perception, and a decreased level of physical energy. The treatment of cancer by radiation therapy, chemotherapy, or surgery produces side effects that directly interfere with the ingestion of food. Radiation therapy generally produces alterations in taste, nausea, vomiting, and diarrhea. Chemotherapy may also produce anorexia, nausea, and vomiting as well as inflammation of the oral cavity (stomatitis) and esophagus (esophagitis). Surgical treatment may result in radical surgery of the head and neck, partial or total removal of the stomach, or partial removal of the intestines. Some resulting problems may be inability to ingest food orally or malabsorption of the nutrients. Inability to ingest food is the next main topic in this chapter; malabsorption is discussed in Chapter 25. Planning must be focused on helping the client understand the probable causes of decreased desire for food and helping him plan foods that will have a stimulating effect on his appetite.

First the nurse may discuss with the client what the client perceives to be causing the decreased desire to ingest food. Has the client been experiencing any physical symptoms that seem to interfere with the ingestion of food? If so, which of these symptoms seem to be most troublesome? The nurse may then explain the physiological causes of some of the symptoms the client is experiencing.

The nurse or dietitian may investigate the client's eating habits by means of a dietary history, which will reveal the general quantity of food consumed, the frequency of eating, and the client's food preferences. Questions may be asked about favorite foods before and after the diagnosis of cancer, if there have been any differences in the amounts of food eaten, and if there any foods the client has a particular aversion to.

The diet used in the nutritional management of cancer is a nutritionally balanced diet based on the normal diet. The diet is modified according to the specific nutritional needs of the client. Maintenance of optimum nutritional status of the client with cancer will improve the response to therapy, reduce the toxicity experienced from therapy, and contribute to the client's well-being (Theologides, 1976). If a nutritionally balanced diet is consumed, it will help the client achieve or maintain ideal weight and prevent or correct any nutritional deficiencies. In this way the symptom of cancer *cachexia* can be avoided. *Cachexia* is a syndrome characterized by anorexia, early satiety, increased BMR, abnormalities in the metabolism of the energy nutrients, and fluid and electrolyte imbalances. This condition is manifested by increased energy expenditure, loss of muscle mass and subcutaneous fat, anemia, and marked physical weakness (Theologides, 1976). The diet may be modified in consistency (liquid to soft), Calories, or individual foods. For some clients a bland or low-residue diet may be ordered. These diets provide foods that are bland in flavor and nonirritating to gastrointestinal mucosa; they are discussed specifically in Chapter 25. The diet for nutritional management of cancer is adequate in Calories and all nutrients and is well tolerated.

Anorexia is often an early manifestation of cancer. The loss of appetite combined with the increased energy requirements caused by growth of the tumor lead to loss of body weight. This weight loss usually worries the client, which may further depress the appetite. The confirmed diagnosis of cancer may lead to depression and more worry, which serve to further depress the appetite and lead to even greater weight loss. The major objective of dietary management of cancer is to maintain the client's nutritional status. A secondary objective is to provide measures to control the undesirable symptoms that interfere with the ingestion of food and to stimulate the appetite.

One of the first steps in cancer intervention is to assure the client that his symptoms and feelings are characteristic of other cancer clients but at the same time to assure him that the nursing and dietary staffs view him as unique and are willing to work closely with him to provide acceptable foods for nutritional support. The client is probably concerned about the altered tastes of foods. He may suffer from decreased taste sensitivity (hypogeusesthesia) or a perverted sense of taste (dysgeusia). Clients with decreased taste sensitivity may describe their food as tasteless. Clients with alterations in taste may have an increased recognition of sweetness, saltiness, or bitterness; they may have a decreased recognition or tolerance for bitterness. They may report that food tastes rancid or spoiled or that a certain taste was predominant such as sourness, saltiness, bitterness, or a metallic taste (Rose, 1978). The client may also report an aversion to eating meat, fish, poultry, eggs, fried foods, and any form of tomatoes. The client needs to be reassured that these disturbances in taste are normal and that a nutritionally balanced diet can be planned omitting the unpalatable items.

Next the client needs to understand the benefits of consuming a nutritionally balanced diet. The nurse should explain that a nutritionally balanced diet will help the client better tolerate the demands imposed by the disease. The effectiveness of the therapy may be enhanced, and the symptoms experienced from the therapy will be less severe. A nutritionally balanced diet will also help improve the general quality of life for the client.

The nurse and the dietitian should both work closely with the client to devise a diet that is not only nutritionally balanced but acceptable. The diet plan should be based as much as possible on the client's food preferences. A nutritionally balanced diet is of no benefit if it is unacceptable to the client and remains on his tray. The goal is to provide foods that will stimulate the client's appetite. The time spent by the nurse and the dietitian working with the client to plan an acceptable diet is well worth the effort. The client should be encouraged to select his own food from the selective menu most hospitals use. For some clients it may be helpful if the selection of

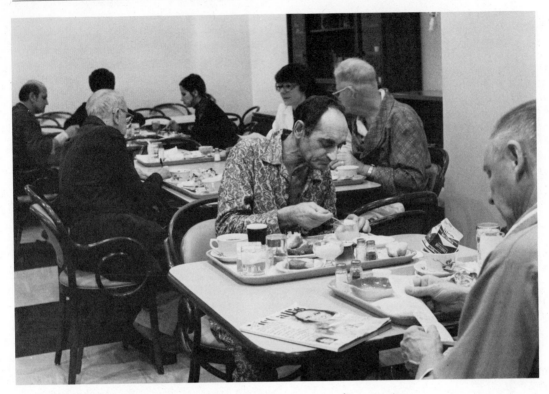

Figure 24-7. Eating with other clients may help to improve the appetite.

food can be made as close to mealtime as possible instead of the day before. The client should be encouraged to select between-meal supplements from a nourishment cart or to eat in the patient dining room if possible (Fig. 24-7). Some clients may need the guidance of the nurse or dietitian to select snacks of nutritional value.

If some of the annoying symptoms associated with cancer can be controlled and minimized, the result will be an increased appetite and an enhanced nutritional status. The decreased appetite and altered taste perception provide a direct interference with the ingestion of food. Although many protein foods, especially cooked meat, fish, or poultry, are not acceptable to most clients with cancer, cold meat salads, cheese, or deviled

eggs may be quite acceptable. Additional protein may be accepted in ice cream, milk shakes, puddings, or custards. If the client is not on a sodium-restricted diet, cured meats such as bacon, corned beef, ham, or luncheon meats might be more acceptable. The client should be encouraged to experiment with seasonings such as spices and herbs, lemon juice, and even extra salt and sugar if no additional dietary restrictions prohibit their use. Appetite may be stimulated by light exercise or a short walk before mealtime. For some clients a small glass of wine or beer about one hour before the meal might serve to stimulate the appetite. Providing small, frequent meals throughout the day is a good way to increase the quantity of food consumed. For many clients with cancer, anorexia seems to increase throughout the day. If the appetite is good in the morning, a hearty, nourishing breakfast should be served that provides at least one-third of the daily protein and Calorie requirements.

Early satiety may result from a feeling of fullness shortly after beginning to eat a meal. This sensation may also be accompanied by nausea, and vomiting may result. The nurse can make several suggestions to the client to reduce these symptoms. The ingestion of small quantities of carbohydrate-containing foods is sometimes helpful. The goal is to reduce the length of time that food remains in the stomach. Because the presence of fats decreases gastric emptying time, fatty and fried foods should be avoided. The volume of food in the stomach can be reduced by not consuming beverages during mealtime, drinking them instead one hour before or after the meal. Nausea may be relieved by eating dry toast or crackers. Cold carbonated beverages may also help to relieve nausea. The client should be instructed to eat slowly and chew the food thoroughly. Resting or lying down after the meal may also help. If the smell of food cooking is nauseating to the client, he should try to stay out of the kitchen as much as possible when food is being prepared. For the client with cancer who must do his own food preparation, simply prepared oven meals or foods cooked in a slow cooker or microwave oven greatly minimize the amount of time spent in the kitchen.

Another symptom experienced by clients being treated by radiation therapy or chemotherapy is a dry or sore mouth or throat. The mouth is dry because of a decreased ability to salivate and swallow as a side effect of radiation therapy. A side effect of chemotherapy is inflammation of the oral cavity. The client who has a dry mouth needs to be encouraged to consume very moist foods. It may be necessary to provide the client with a liquid diet for a few days. The regular hospital liquid diet is often nutritionally inadequate, and it should not be used for more than a few days. If

longer use of liquids is indicated, a nutritionally complete liquid supplement can be included several times daily along with the regular full liquid diet to provide a nutritionally balanced liquid diet. Clients with an inflammation of the oral cavity may experience discomfort consuming citrus fruit juices and tomatoes because of the high acid content of these foods. Cold foods such as ice cream, Popsicles, sherbet, and chilled soft fruits may have a soothing effect on the mouth. For clients who have difficulty swallowing, soft, moist foods and liquids should be provided. The use of liberal amounts of butter or margarine on solid foods may make swallowing easier. Swallowing may also be assisted by using a straw and tilting the head backward.

Diarrhea and gastrointestinal cramping is another symptom associated with cancer and its treatment. The likelihood of diarrhea can be reduced by drinking fluids before or after the meal but not with it and by eating small amounts of food at a meal. The client should be encouraged to refrain from any foods that cause him abdominal discomfort, for instance, carbonated beverages, beer, beans, cabbage, or highly spiced foods. It may be necessary for the client to reduce the fiber content of the diet by decreasing his intake of raw fruits and vegetables, and whole grain breads and cereals. Although constipation is not a frequent problem in the client with cancer, it may be a side effect of chemotherapy. In this case the dietary advice given to the client is to increase the fiber content of the diet by using fresh fruits and vegetables and whole grain breads and cereals and by drinking plenty of liquids including prune juice. A light exercise program or a regular schedule of walking should also help to relieve constipation.

INABILITY TO INGEST FOOD AND FLUIDS

1. Inability to feed self
2. Inadequate fluid intake

3. Fatigue upon eating

4. Difficulty feeding (in infants)

5. Diminished sucking ability (in infants)

6. Dependence on tube feeding management

7. Hiccough

8. Vomiting

9. Hyperemesis

10. Dependence on hyperalimentation management

You Can Lead a Horse to Water But You Can't Make Him Drink is a familiar saying among the farmers of middle America. The futility of providing an adequate diet to an unresponsive client is reflected in the statement. The nurse's efforts that go into planning a diet are futile if the client will not or cannot ingest the food. Inability to ingest food arises from a variety of alterations. Helping a client cope with alterations that prohibit ingestion is a major nursing challenge on which a client's life may depend.

The inability to ingest nutrients may arise from physiological, psychological, or mechanical alterations in the client. The nursing strategies used with each alteration are similar, so only characteristic nursing diagnoses need be discussed. Each client's uniqueness must be considered when planning nursing care. Nursing strategies may be adapted to meet the specific needs of the individual client.

The major assessment parameter leading to a nursing diagnosis centering on the inability to ingest food and fluids is an observation of a client's deteriorating nutritional status when assistance with ingestion is absent. Of course most clients have sought medical attention before significant nutritional deterioration has occurred. Briefly, assessment data will center on the nurse's observation of client difficulty or on the client's reported difficulty in ingesting food and fluids. Usually the alteration will center on client immobility, paralysis, or unconsciousness. Occasionally ingestion will be prevented because of such overt gastrointes-

tinal disturbances as hyperemesis or hiccough. Obstruction of the oral pharnyx is discussed later in this chapter. Whatever the cause, the nurse must be on the alert for difficulties with ingestion that could decrease or totally prevent nutrient consumption.

Client Objectives

To be able to:

1. Ingest nutrients in sufficient quantity and variety to meet his nutritional requirements, using available personal and community resources.

2. Maintain a nourished state, using available resources.

3. Discuss the importance of nutritional care specific to his alteration.

Dietary Interventions

The planning phase of the nursing process dealing with a client's inability to ingest food and fluids centers on overcoming the alteration interfering with ingestion. Long- and short-term goals are set by the nurse to provide a direction for the overall plan of care. Mutually set goals and specific objectives indicate progress and provide a motivating force for the client. More important, they indicate when the nurse's plan of care is not working and needs revision. The long-term goal when dealing with an inability to ingest food centers on maintaining or regaining adequate nutritional status. It is noteworthy that nursing care may not always be directed at correcting the alteration causing decreased ingestion; often intervention centers instead on helping the client adapt to and cope with the alteration. Short-term goals will probably involve the maintenance of oral intake or parenteral Calories in sufficient quantities to maintain nutritional status. Examples of specific objectives for pertinent nursing diagnoses are given in Table 24-2. Of course, the specific objectives used must be individualized for

TABLE 24-2. Short-term Goals for Nursing Diagnoses Centering on the Inability to Ingest Nutrients

Diagnoses Related to	Objectives: The Client Will
Inability to feed self	1. Participate in meal planning 2. Communicate food preferences to nurse 3. Use assistive devices to eat 4. Eat a balanced diet when fed by nurse or significant other
Fatigue	1. Communicate need for rest to nurse 2. Eat small frequent meals that supply adequate nutrients
Impaired consciousness	1. Tolerate nutrients provided by the nurse via parenteral or enteral routes
Dependence on tube feeding or total parenteral nutrition (TPN)	1. State the purpose of the treatment 2. Tolerate nutrients provided by alternate route 3. Communicate any discomfort present

each client. Special techniques used when dysphagia is present are discussed later in this chapter.

Intervention involves carrying out the plans designed to meet the goals. Interventions discussed here center on feeding techniques that may increase client satisfaction with ingestion of nutrients.

Feeding Techniques

When the diagnosis of impaired ingestion is made and the intervention selected involves feeding the client, the nurse must consider more than simply spooning food into the client's mouth. Eating is something most people take for granted; yet feeding another person is not the simple procedure it might appear to be. The success of feeding is affected by the client's ability to chew and swallow; the environment; the client's appetite, food habits, and preferences; the client's feel-

ings about being dependent; the quality and variety of food; and the nurse's general attitude toward feeding clients.

Advance planning and intervention will often determine the amount of food the client ingests and the feeling of success or failure the client has about the meal. The client should be allowed to rest before and after meals. Physical therapy and other procedures should be scheduled carefully around mealtimes. Hurrying or rushing a meal will decrease the client's appetite and the willingness to participate actively in the meal. The client should be made as comfortable as possible for the meal. Pain medication, dressing changes, and personal hygiene activities should be carried out before meals and at a pace that does not overly fatigue the client. Unpleasant or painful treatments should also be carefully scheduled well between meals. The nurse should offer the bedpan or urinal before the client eats, particularly before breakfast. A distended bladder can inhibit ingestion because of discomfort. The client should have sufficient time to arouse himself before a meal; excessive drowsiness may interfere with chewing and swallowing. The environment should also be comfortable for the client. Ventilation, light, clutter, and cleanliness all affect the client's ability to ingest food. If the client has dentures, they should be cleaned and inserted.

Proper positioning of the client is imperative to assure swallowing and prevent reflux or aspiration. If not contraindicated, the client should be assisted to an erect sitting position. The client's lower back and hips should be snug against the chair back and seat, with the feet flat against the floor and legs bent. If the client is confined to bed, he should be assisted to semi-Fowler's or Fowler's position. If a supine position must be maintained, the client should be assisted to lie on his side with his head turned to the side. Never attempt to feed a client while his neck is extended or while he is lying on his back. Such positions precipitate aspiration even in the most alert clients. Aspiration pneumonia is an unfortunate yet common side effect of improper feeding techniques.

Mealtime is customarily a socialization time for most clients. The meal should be made as special as possible. Attractive and personal touches may be added to the tray. In many health care facilities a common dayroom is available where clients can be fed. A social mealtime can be a highlight in an otherwise uneventful day. If at all possible the nurse should sit down while feeding; mealtime provides an opportunity to relate current events and happenings that will help to orient a confused client. The mealtime should be uninterrupted if at all possible. If necessary, cold food can be quickly rewarmed in microwave ovens available in many health care facilities.

The client should be fed at the rate and with an amount of food compatible with his ability to eat and level of energy. Avoid hurrying the client. Food should be offered in small quantities in the order the client prefers. The client's desire in making food choices should be respected. Any decision made by the client reflects his active participation in health care and thus should be encouraged. Care should be taken not to spill food. The client's clothes should always be protected with a napkin. The client's mouth and chin should be frequently wiped.

Whenever possible, utensils used should be those normally used for the food being served. Feeding the client soup with a spoon is much more pleasing than feeding it with an aseptic syringe or other device. A straw or paper cup may help the client drink liquids. Be careful when helping the client drink hot fluids; they feel much hotter when taken with a straw. The student should try drinking a cup of coffee through a straw to experience what a client feels. The client should be encouraged to feed himself as much as possible. Finger foods such as sandwiches, French fries, fruit slices, and cookies can be handled by the client much easier than utensils.

If the client's significant others are present and wish to participate in his care, feeding provides ample opportunity for them to do so. The family may feed the client, assist the nurse in feeding, or bring special food from home as long as permission has been granted. Such contributions to the client's care provide the family with a feeling of usefulness and participation.

After the meal is finished, the tray should be promptly removed. The nurse should note the amount and type of food eaten. If Calorie counts or intake-output records are kept, the food and liquids remaining on the tray should be measured or weighed. A wet washcloth will refresh the client after a meal. Of course, toothbrushing and oral care should be carried out following a meal. This offers a good opportunity for the nurse to teach oral hygiene.

Clients with the most adequate dietary intake are those who are severely handicapped and have to be fed each mealtime and those who are mentally alert and can ask for what they want. Those with the lowest intakes are the depressed, apathetic, or anorectic clients and those whose food preferences limit what they will eat. Clients in the latter category should be considered at risk. Aggressive nursing interventions should be planned to ensure adequate intake.

Special Equipment

A variety of assistive devices and special equipment can make clients increasingly independent while eating. Plates should be placed on a nonslip surface and rimmed with a metal barrier to prevent food from slipping off the plate. Specially shaped spoons, forks, and knives are available that allow a client to grasp them without difficulty. Closed cups with built-in no-spill straws allow the client with impaired muscle function to bring the cup to their mouth and drink without spilling. Splints can support the wrist, hand, or arm when a specific muscle group is impaired.

The most important aid to self-sufficiency, however, is the patience of the nurse. Time and practice will improve the client's ability to eat. With encouragement and consistent reinforcement from the nurse, a client's goals will be more adequately met.

ORAL DISCOMFORT AND/OR OBSTRUCTION

1. Oral tenderness
2. Oral-cavity bleeding
3. Bleeding gums
4. Sensitive teeth
5. Teething pain
6. Predisposition to tooth decay
7. Toothache
8. Oral discomfort
9. Throat soreness
10. Difficulty chewing
11. Difficulty swallowing

Abnormalities present in the mouth or throat that cause the client difficulty in chewing or swallowing will interfere with the ingestion of food. The nature and severity of the disorder will determine the degree of alteration in eating. The abnormality may involve the tenderness of the mouth from inflammation of the mucosa, presence of sores or ulcerations, or bleeding gums. The tenderness of the oral mucosa may be caused by poorly fitting dentures, or it may be a side effect of certain medications or therapy or a result of surgical intervention. The problem may, however, be with the teeth. The client's teeth may be quite sensitive to hot and cold foods and beverages and thus interfere with the enjoyment of eating. The client may have several teeth that are decayed or missing. Clients with poorly fitting dentures with braces or without teeth or dentures can have difficulty chewing. Inability to chew food may also result from a bro-

ken jaw that is immobilized for several weeks for healing. Some clients have no difficulty chewing their food but experience considerable discomfort swallowing it. The pain or difficulty swallowing may arise from inflammation, blockage, or inadequate secretions in the mouth and esophagus. Clients who experience difficulty chewing or swallowing may prefer smaller quantities of food and a modification in its consistency.

Client Objectives

To be able to:

1. Confirm his increased comfort.
2. Maintain appropriate ingestion patterns.

Dietary Interventions

The objective for planning food for the client who experiences difficulty chewing or swallowing food or beverages is to provide the client with foods that minimize the discomfort. The diet should be modified in consistency and perhaps in size and number of feedings. This kind of diet is called a *mechanical soft* or *dental soft diet*. It is the simplest modification of the regular diet and is designed to provide foods that are more easily chewed or swallowed. Because there are many causes of oral discomfort or obstruction and these vary in degree in each client, the specific modifications of the diet must be discussed by the nurse or dietitian with the client. Some knowledge of the major difficulty the client has with chewing or swallowing is necessary before a meal can be planned.

When a mechanical soft diet is ordered, the nurse should consult with the client about the kinds of foods he can best handle. The mechanical soft diet is intended to be a highly individualized dietary modification that excludes only those foods that give the client difficulty chewing or swallowing. The client should always be consulted when planning a mechanical soft diet to ensure that the consistency of foods provided allows for maximal ease in chewing and swallowing. The nurse should explain to the client the reason for the mechanical soft diet, emphasizing that the only restriction is elimination of foods the client finds difficult to chew or swallow. The goal of the diet is to ensure an optimal intake of food in the form best tolerated by the client.

The consistency of food on a mechanical soft diet may be mostly liquids, chopped or pureed food, regular food with a moist consistency, or any combination of these. For maximum client acceptance the food should be provided in the consistency and state closest to the client's regular food. For example, ground or pureed food should not be used unless the client prefers this form. A dish of ground meat and a pureed vegetable can be so psychologically unappealing that many clients will refuse to eat the food and will have little or no appetite for the other foods on the tray. Even clients who have no teeth or who are unable to wear their dentures during hospitalization can comfortably chew and swallow very soft foods in a more natural form. For example, canned fruits are generally soft and are well accepted. Many cooked vegetables are fairly soft. Tender meats such as baked chicken, turkey, roast beef, ground beef, and casseroles are usually easy to chew. Only those foods a particular client experiences difficulty chewing or swallowing should be eliminated. The mechanical soft diet places no restriction on seasonings or method of food preparation. For some clients the mechanical soft diet may not appear to be noticeably different from the regular hospital diet because it is only necessary to eliminate a few foods.

The nurse may make some specific suggestions to the client about ways to minimize chewing and swallowing difficulties. For example, if the client experiences tenderness of the mouth because of inflammation or ulcerations of the gums, he may need to eliminate such foods as raw fruits and vegetables, fried foods, some spicy foods, foods with nuts and seeds, or acidic foods such as citrus fruits and tomatoes. The nurse may also make specific suggestions about oral hygiene, reminding the client that regular brushing and flossing of the teeth and regular dental checkups are necessary to maintain the condition of the teeth. The nurse may suggest between-meal snacks that are considered to be less cariogenic, that is, contributing to dental caries. Such snacks as fresh fruits and vegetables; cheese; nuts; popcorn; milk; pretzels; and sugar-free drinks, candy, and gum help to prevent dental caries.

Dysphagia can be caused by a number of physiological and psychological alterations. CNS damage from cerebrovascular accident, trauma, or progressive degenerative disease frequently causes impaired swallowing. Other causes include radiation therapy, vocal cord paralysis, muscular atrophy, and surgical removal of the glottis or larynx. The problem is identified either by the client or by a direct observation of the client's inability to swallow. A dangerous complication that may occur is aspiration and subsequent development of pneumonia. Because of this possibility, suction equipment should be immediately available for these clients. Many of these clients are nutritionally maintained by nasogastric intubation, TPN or both (see Chap. 23 for an explanation of the nursing responsibilities associated with such intervention).

In the normal eating process, the tongue does most of the work involved. It moves the food to the rear of the mouth to allow swallowing to occur. The muscles involved must have good tone and control. If any of these mechanisms is absent, the client will have difficulty ingesting food. It is possible to stimulate and establish normal ingestion patterns in these people by stimulating the muscle reflexes that remain intact, thus developing coordination and strength.

If the client has a weakness or paralysis of one side of the body, he should be turned toward the unaffected side while eating. This position will provide better postural support for the head and neck area. If the mouth is also involved, the food should be placed on the strong and intact side. This allows the client to have better control over the food. Increased control will also result if the nurse instructs the client to form a bolus by moving the tongue around inside the mouth. The motion places the food back in the larynx and allows more efficient swallowing. It will also prevent food from collecting in the cheek.

If the client's mouth is not affected, placing foods into alternate sides of the mouth will increase oral sensitivity. Control can be better attained if coarse foods are offered rather than pureed foods. Different foods should be offered separately, with the nurse or client naming each food.

If coughing occurs or if swallowing does not occur, pressing down on the client's head with the palm of the hand will decrease laryngeal tension and facilitate swallowing (Buckley, 1976). Swallowing can also be initiated by pressing the chin downward toward the sternum.

It is important not to offer too much food at one time. The food should be cut or offered in small bite-size amounts. As the ability to swallow increases, the amount of food can be increased. The spoon should be immediately removed after placing food in the client's mouth. The nurse should make the client conscious of any drooling that occurs. Eating in front of a mirror will allow the client to observe the muscle movements he uses when eating.

If the client is unable to voluntarily chew, manipulate the jaw in an upward and downward motion, thus simulating chewing movements. Encourage the client to close his lips once the food is in the mouth. If the client cannot do this, the nurse may manually close the client's lips. When lips are sealed, the swallowing reflex is initiated.

Sucking on a straw is a good way to get liquid as well as to exercise facial muscles. Very cold or very hot liquids are not tolerated well if the client's problem involves muscles. Cold liquids may have a numbing effect on already compromised muscles. If the client cannot use a straw, then liquids may be given from a cup. With the client's head at a 90-degree angle, which makes swallowing easier, the cup should be placed at the corners of the lips and tilted slowly, giving only small amounts at one time. If necessary, a portion of the cup rim may be removed to allow for the client's nose.

If the client has a tracheostomy, positioning the head to prevent aspiration is extremely important. It is very easy to aspirate when the chin is elevated, which occurs when the head is tilted back. The nurse should instruct the client to tilt his head forward (Weber, 1974). In addition to causing aspiration, extension of the neck can cause pain or stretch the membranous wall of the tachea if a tracheostomy tube is in place.

General dietary guidelines for the client with dysphagia are as follows: Milk should be avoided because it causes an increase in thick saliva that is difficult to swallow. Foods that are difficult to swallow include: pulp fruits such as prunes, plums, and strawberries; hamburger patties; onions; thick soups; white bread; custards; puddings; and crackers. As previously mentioned, textured foods stimulate swallowing more than smooth foods. For example, all bread should be toasted; bacon should be crisp; and potatoes should be baked. Bitter or acidic foods such as lemon juice or vinegar dressing should be avoided. Lightly sweetened and seasoned foods are more easily handled. Because of the increased risk of nutritional depletion in such clients, a nutritional assessment should be done weekly. A daily Calorie count will provide an accurate basis for nutritional intervention.

Family, client, and significant others all need to be involved in the feeding process. The family can assist greatly in reinforcing progress and specific physical therapy. The dysphagic client will not learn to swallow overnight. Relearning takes time, patience, creativity, and resourcefulness on the part of the nurse.

ALTERATIONS IN INGESTION THAT HAVE ALREADY OCCURRED

1. Obesity
2. Excessive caffeine intake
3. Food poisoning
4. Excessive vitamin and mineral ingestion
5. Food allergies
6. Excessive intake of alcohol

Alteration in the process of ingestion can occur because of the previous ingestion of an excessive amount of food or nutrient supplements or of foods that cause adverse reactions. Dietary intervention differs depending on the type of previous ingestion. Whereas a low dietary intake of specific nutrients results in specific nutritional deficiency diseases, the ingestion of excess quantities of food or nutritional supplements can also result in adverse body reactions. Adverse reactions, even life-threatening reactions, may occur from the ingestion of an allergenic food or from the ingestion of a food contaminated by microorganisms.

Client Objectives

To be able to:

1. Confirm that an alteration in ingestion has occurred.
2. Seek medical intervention if ingestion is life threatening.
3. Discuss future behavior changes that may prevent future ingestion problems.

Dietary Interventions

The major objective in treating the client suffering from adverse affects of previous ingestion is to determine the source of the discomfort and either to decrease the amount of the offending food or remove it from the client's diet. In most cases a specific modification of the diet is not necessary in the treatment. Even though the overall objective of treatment is quite simple, the methods of intervention are relatively specific to the origins of the problem. Dietary intervention for the problem of obesity was already discussed in Chapter 5.

Excess Caffeine Intake

Caffeine is classified as a stimulant drug; it acts on cardiac muscle, the CNS, and gastric secretions (Stephenson, 1977). Caffeine is contained in coffee, tea, cocoa, chocolate, cola beverages, and a number of drugs. It is difficult to define excessive caffeine intake because individual tolerances vary. Sensitivity to caffeine is greater in noncoffee drinkers. Presented with a 50–200 mg dose, they may experience a feeling of nervousness rather than increased alertness; Stephenson (1977) stated that doses of 200–500 mg may be accompanied by headache, tremors, nervousness, and irritability. Heavy coffee drinkers may not experience any of these symptoms from this same dose. One cup (150 ml) of brewed coffee contains approximately 100–150 mg of caffeine, depending on the amount of coffee used in brewing, the method of brewing, and the length of brewing time. Bunker and McWilliams (1979) found that dripolator coffee contains the highest amount of caffeine per cup. This method is the principle employed by the automatic drip coffee makers currently in widespread use. The longer coffee is perked in a percolator, the higher its caffeine content. Stephenson (1977) stated that instant coffee contains less caffeine (60 mg/150 ml) than brewed coffee (85 mg/150 ml). Tea contains considerably less caffeine per cup than coffee. In fact, a cup of instant coffee, a glass of iced tea, a cup of tea, or a can of carbonated beverage all have similar caffeine contents. (Bunker and McWilliams, 1979).

Greden (1974) has suggested that caffeine intakes in excess of 250 mg/day may be excessive. Bunker and McWilliams (1979) point out that caffeine dose is relative to body size; a child who consumes a can of a carbonated beverage receives a dose equivalent to that of four cups of instant coffee consumed by an adult. The nursing mother should be informed that the caffeine from the beverages she consumes passes into her breast milk and may have a stimulating effect on the infant. Manber (1976) found the symptoms of irritability, restlessness, sleeplessness, and nervousness in children and teenagers who consumed large amounts of cola beverages and chocolates.

The client who experiences such symptoms as nervousness, irritability, tremulousness, muscle twitchings, insomnia, sensory disturbances, rapid breathing, palpitations, flushing, arrhythmias, diuresis, and gastrointestinal disturbances from the ingestion of excess caffeine may be instructed to reduce his daily intake of caffeine or to omit it entirely. The purpose of the intervention may be either to reduce the symptoms or to determine if the symptoms are actually linked to caffeine consumption. The reason for eliminating caffeine from the diet may also be because of its harmful effect on a disease process. For example, Stephenson (1977) reported that even small doses of caffeine can produce palpitation, insomnia, restlessness, anxiety, dizziness, headache, nausea, and vomiting in clients with cardiac disease. Also caffeine, as a gastric stimulant, contributes to the development of an ulcer in the ulcer-prone client. Recently Cohen and Booth (1975) found that even decaffeinated coffee has the effect of stimulating gastric acid secretions.

If the client is instructed only to limit the daily intake of caffeine, the nurse might suggest he consume only one cup of regular coffee each day and the rest as decaffeinated coffee. Another suggestion might be that the client have three or four cups of coffee a day distributed at intervals rather than consumed

consecutively. The most restrictive action, however, is the complete elimination of all caffeine-containing beverages and medications. The client is instructed to use decaffeinated coffee and cola beverages that contain no caffeine.

The client should be informed of the possibility of experiencing caffeine withdrawal symptoms, the most common of which is the slow onset of a headache that may be accompanied by nausea and vomiting. Goldstein and Kaizer (1969) reported not only headache but irritability, nervousness, restlessness, inability to work effectively, and lethargy in a group of housewives undergoing caffeine withdrawal. The nurse should instruct the client about substitutions available. Caffeine-free carbonated beverages may be substituted. Although chocolate and cocoa both contain caffeine, *carob powder* can be substituted in home recipes. Decaffeinated coffee, of course, may be substituted for regular coffee.

Excessive Intake of Alcohol

The relationship between nutrition and the excessive consumption of alcoholic beverages is complex; only the effect of the excessive intake on dietary intake is relevant here. The daily consumption of alcohol by the alcoholic replaces much of the desirable intake of food. In simple terms, drinking replaces eating. According to Shaw and Lieber (1977) alcoholism is one of the major causes of nutritional deficiency diseases in the United States. As the consumption of alcohol increases, the consumption of food usually decreases. It is thought that the Calories contributed by the alcohol act to suppress the appetite. The condition of *gastritis,* an inflammation of the lining of the gastrointestinal tract, and the depressed level of consciousness depress the appetite further. Many alcoholics may quit eating altogether when they are on a drinking binge. At other times they eat only very small quantities of food sporadically.

Effective nutritional therapy for the alcoholic requires complete abstinence from alcohol. Nutritional intervention is aimed at providing a nutritionally balanced diet and correcting the existing nutritional deficiencies. A nutritionally balanced diet planned around the basic four food groups is essential. The apparent nutritional deficiencies of the client must be verified by a thorough nutritional assessment including a dietary history, a clinical examination, and laboratory data. The nutritional deficiencies most commonly found in the alcoholic are those of protein, the water-soluble vitamins, magnesium, potassium, and zinc (Stone, 1978). After determining what nutritional deficiencies exist, the nurse should instruct the client on the benefits of a well-balanced diet. Specific emphasis should be placed on planning the diet around foods containing high concentrations of the nutrients that are low in the alcoholic client. For example, many alcoholics' diets are low in thiamine and they also have reduced blood levels of thiamine. A vitamin supplement containing thiamine or several of the B-complex group may be administered temporarily. Improvement of the client's nutritional status should actually help to improve the client's mental attitude and feeling of well-being and enable him to cope with the rehabilitation process. More details about nutritional therapy for the alcoholic client are included in Chapter 27 because the problems of alcoholism are also manifested in metabolism alterations.

Excess Vitamin and Mineral Ingestion

The client diagnosed as having a vitamin or mineral toxicity may present the nurse with a definite challenge. It is quite unlikely that a dietary excess of a vitamin or mineral will result simply from food consumption. Toxicity could result only if the client were particularly overzealous in consuming large amounts daily of certain food such as liver or carrots. Usually a dietary toxicity results from excessive nutrient supplementation. Table 24-3 describes the toxicity symptoms resulting from excess quantities of vitamins and minerals, the levels generally required to produce toxic symptoms, and the current RDAs for each nutrient.

The nurse must seek to educate the client about the basic facts of nutrition including which nutrients are capable of being stored and which are not. Because of their storage potential, excess consumption of the fat-soluble vitamins is most likely to result in toxicity symptoms. It should be explained that harmful symptoms usually do not develop from the water-soluble vitamins because excess intakes are excreted by the kidneys. The

TABLE 24-3.   Recommended and Excess Daily Ingestion of Selected Vitamins and Minerals

Vitamin or Mineral	RDA for Adults	Human Toxicity Level[b]	Potential Danger or Symptoms[b]
Vitamin A	Infants age 6 mo–1 yr, 2,000 IU (400 RE) Children age 1–10, 2,000–3,300 IU (400–700 RE) Men, 5,000 IU (1,000 RE) Women, 4,000 IU (800 RE)	Infants 6 mo–1 yr, 18,000–60,000 IU Children age 1–5, 80,000–500,000 IU Adults, 200,000–275,000 IU per person	Hypercarotenosis (yellowness of the skin but not of the sclera of the eye). Anorexia, headache, blurred vision, irritability, hair loss, muscle soreness after exercise, drying and flaking of the skin, cracking and bleeding of the lips, reddened gingiva, nosebleeds, bone malformations, loss of hair.

TABLE 24-3. *(Continued)*

Vitamin or Mineral	RDA for Adults	Human Toxicity Level[b]	Potential Danger or Symptoms[b]
Vitamin D	Infants–age 18, 400 IU (10 μg) Adults 19–22, 300 IU (7.5 μg) Adults 23 and older, 200 IU (5 μg)	Infants, 3,000–4,000 IU Infants, 20,000–40,000 IU Adults, 75,000–100,000 IU	Loss of appetite, retarded growth. Loss of appetite, nausea, vomiting, intense thirst, diarrhea, irritability, depression, calcification of major body organs (arteries, heart, lungs, kidneys).
Vitamin K[a]	70–140 μg	Unknown	Excess parenteral vitamin K to infants: hemolytic anemia, hyper-bilirubinemia, brain damage.
Vitamin C	Children, 45 mg Adolescents 50 mg Adults, 60 mg	2–8 gm	Oxalate stone formation, decreased absorption of copper, interference with anticoagulants, increased hemolysis of red blood cells, decreased use of vitamin B_{12}.
Folic acid	400 μg	More than 400 μg	Masked symptoms of pernicious anemia.
Fluoride[a]	1.5–4.0 mg	2–8 mg	Mottling or hypoplasia of the enamel; increased bone density and calcification of ligaments of neck and vertebral column.
Selenium[a]	0.5–2.0 mg	1 mg/kg of food (10 ppm)	Chronic dermatitis, excessive fatigue, dizziness.
Chromium[a]	0.5–2.0 mg	Unknown	Imbalances of other trace elements.
Iron	10–18 mg	Specific level unknown; children more suscepti-ble to excesses	Hemochromatosis, liver damage, death in children; interference with use of copper, zinc, man-ganese, and ascorbic acid in adults.
Copper[a]	2–3	Unknown	Vomiting, Wilson's disease (a hereditary disease in which large amounts of copper accumulate in liver, kidney, brain, and cornea).
Manganese[a]	2.5–5.0	Unknown	Interference with iron absorption, behavioral changes, neurological disability, anemia reduced growth rate.
Zinc	15 mg	Unknown; toxic level depends on intake of copper, iron, and phytic acid	Interference with iron and copper metabolism, vomiting, diarrhea.

[a] "Estimated Safe and Adequate Daily Dietary Intake of Additional Selected Vitamins and Minerals," from Food and Nutrition Board, Nat'l Acad. of Science, Nat'l Research Council, *Recommended Dietary Allowances*, 9th Ed. Washington, D.C., 1980.
[b] From National Nutrition Consortium, Inc., *Vitamin-Mineral Safety, Toxicity, and Misuse*. Report of the Committee on Safety, Toxicity, and Misuse of Vitamins and Trace Minerals. Published by the American Dietetic Association, Chicago, Ill., 1978.

minerals also do not generally pose a problem of excess intake because the level of absorption in the body decreases as the level of dietary and supplementary intake increases. This process of educating the client is not always as easy as it may sound because many of the clients engaging in the practice of nutritional supplementation have their personal ideas about nutrition firmly engrained. These clients often come from a background of food faddism or health food use that may be difficult to penetrate. The nurse must attempt to emphasize that no additional health benefits are obtained by consuming quantities of vitamins and minerals in excess of the RDAs. This practice may be beneficial only when a nutritional deficiency is documented with the data from one or more areas of a complete nutritional assessment or during periods of increased nutritional requirements such as during pregnancy, before and after surgery, or during infections and fever. More specific information about periods of increased nutritional requirements and supplements is included in Chapter 27.

Food Poisoning

Some illnesses are actually caused by the ingestion of food contaminated by microorganisms. The three species most commonly associated with food-related illnesses in the United States are *Salmonella, Staphylococcus,* and *Clostridium.* The information about protection against infection of food with these organisms was presented in Chapter 8. The treatment of a client who has contracted a food-related illness is entirely supportive. Nursing care involves the management of acute diarrhea and vomiting along with the maintenance of fluid and electrolyte balance. Nearly all clients with food-related illnesses recover completely in a few days. Many cases of these diseases are simply dismissed as the flu or "the current bug." In most cases the suspected food is not saved or even available for examination by a public health department. Numerous cases go undiagnosed every year. Food-related illnesses pose the most serious health hazards for the elderly whose health status and resistance may be below average and for the infant or young child who can become violently ill in a short time and rapidly become dehydrated by vomiting and diarrhea.

Nursing intervention after the acute stage of the disease involves discussing with the client the probable cause and ways of avoiding future occurrences. The nurse can discuss with the client food safety and sanitation, emphasizing proper refrigeration and freezing temperatures, proper storage of food, prompt storage of leftovers, and the safe temperature for reheated leftovers (see chapter 8).

Food Allergies

Hypersensitivity to food may be manifested in a number of ways, food allergy being only one. Adverse reactions to food may result from absorption of intact food proteins (*antigens*) that cause the body to produce antibodies, thus setting up an allergic reaction. An allergy is not to a food itself but to one of its components such as a protein or another organic component. Adverse reactions may also occur in response to food additives or minute amounts of drugs (such as penicillin) present in milk. According to Freier (1976) food allergy beginning after the first year of life is probably on the increase because of the presence in foods of additives, preservatives, and flavorings. Other adverse reactions to food include the enzyme deficiency in lactose intolerance and the hypersensitivity to the protein gluten in celiac disease. This discussion pertains primarily to interventions for food allergies, although any condition that necessitates the elimination of a major food such as milk or wheat has application here.

The presence of food allergies is determined through observation and experience in clinical practice. Lists of potentially allergic foods differ slightly among allergists because of individual experience. Some of the commonly agreed on food allergies are milk, eggs, wheat, chocolate, fish (especially shellfish), tomatoes, bananas, oranges, strawberries, and nuts. The manifestations of food allergies vary among people but are always consistent for any one person. Food allergies may be manifested by many symptoms, including eczema, asthma, headache, vomiting, diarrhea, dizziness, and seizures. These symptoms may involve the respiratory, gastrointestinal, integumentary and nervous systems.

There are several methods of diagnosing food allergies. A group of these tests are the skin tests (Krause and Mahan, 1979) in which suspected food antigens are, one at a time, placed on the skin (*patch test*) or scratched into the skin (*scratch test*). Todd and Mackaress (1978) describe food allergy test in which the suspected food antigen is inserted under the tongue (*sublingual test*). The results of these tests, however, are not always consistent or definitive.

The most reliable method for diagnosing food allergies is the use of an *elimination diet.* The concept of the elimination diet was first published by Rowe in 1941. The most recent revision of his diets and recipes was published in 1972. The principle of this dietary regimen is to remove all suspected allergenic foods from the diet to see if the client's symptoms dimish. The foods included initially are those known to be the least allergenic. If the symptoms remit after a specified period (usually 10 days), single foods based on a botanical classification are added. If the symptoms reoccur the allergic response is probably due to the food that was most recently added to the diet. This process is continued until all the known food allergies have been identified. A minimum of three months is usually required for the effective diagnosis of food allergies. Before the client begins such a dietary regimen, the nurse should inform him and his family about the time involved and the commitment required. The diets are useful only if they are faithfully followed. Because of the restrictive nature of the diets, supplementation with vitamins and minerals may be neces-

sary during the testing period. A special nonallergenic vitamin and mineral supplement should be provided.

The client is first placed on a cereal-free elimination diet; but if allergy to fruits is also suspected, the initial diet is a fruit-free and cereal-free diet (Robinson and Lawler, 1977). Fruits and then vegetables are added one at a time every few days. Cereals are added next gradually, first rice, then oats, corn, rye, and finally wheat. Milk, eggs, and wheat are added at the end of the test because these foods are the most common sources of food allergy. If an allergy to one of these three foods was suspected initially a simple elimination diet omitting these three foods could be used to observe whether symptoms decreased.

Once the specific food allergy or allergies are known, client and family should have a conference with the dietitian about foods that must be avoided. The nurse can reinforce the information provided by the dietitian. Emphasis should be placed on reading labels, modifying recipes, and obtaining recipes for allergy diets. The most common allergy diets, the wheat-free, egg-free, and milk-free diets, all necessitate careful reading of food labels. If a client has allergies to wheat, milk, *and* eggs, which is sometimes the case, his difficulties in food selection are compounded.

CHINESE RESTAURANT SYNDROME. One other interesting hypersensitivity to food is the Chinese restaurant syndrome. Stanley (1977) reports that the symptoms occur 15–25 minutes after a hearty meal in a Chinese restaurant. The symptoms are described as a burning sensation at the back of the neck spreading to the forearms and anterior chest. This may be accompanied by profuse sweating and a sensation of tightness on both sides of the head in the region of the temples. The cause is an allergic reaction in susceptible persons to the large quantities of monosodium glutamate (5 gm) used in Oriental style cooking. The average non-susceptible person can tolerate up to 25 gm. with no symptoms. The nurse can make some helpful suggestions to the client who experiences this syndrome. She can reassure the client that these symptoms are not harmful and that they should disappear completely in two to three hours. She can encourage the client to consume only moderate amounts of food in a Chinese restaurant so as to lessen or minimize the symptoms. The nurse should definitely caution the client on a low-sodium diet not to consume Chinese food. Besides the monosodium glutamate used in food preparation the soy sauce in Oriental cooking is high in sodium.

CASE STUDY: A Woman Who Has Several Interferences with Ingestion

Olive G. is a 59-year-old woman admitted two weeks ago for a total laryngectomy for cancer of the oral pharynx. She tolerated surgery well and is currently on her tenth postoperative day.

Olive's vital signs have been stable—blood pressure 110–120/70–80, pulse 82, respirations 16–18. She has a tracheostomy tube in place and is receiving humidified air through a tracheostomy collar. At first she had to be suctioned every hour, but now the secretions have decreased and she needs suctioning only once or twice every eight hours. Olive is learning to suction herself, using clean techniques. She anticipates a permanent tracheostomy tube within the next two days.

Olive has gradually increased her activity level so that she can now walk to the bathroom without assistance.

Olive was fed a meat-based *gavage* at the rate of 200 ml every four hours beginning the third postoperative day. After gastrointestinal motility was confirmed and Olive no longer experienced nausea or vomiting, her intravenous therapy was discontinued and a nasogastric tube was inserted. After a week, Olive's nasogastric tube was discontinued, and she was started on a soft diet. She had some difficulty swallowing and tended to aspirate fluids. After a few days, the physician ordered that the nasogastric tube be reinserted. Olive is at present very anxious because she believes she will never be able to eat as long as "I have this tube in my throat." Olive is being weighed daily. Her admission weight was 110 lb (50 kg), marginally underweight for her 5 ft 5 in (165 cm) frame. Her current weight has decreased to 102 lb (46.3 kg).

Olive is eager to learn esophageal speech. Before her surgery she was very active in volunteer organizations. She worked part time as a secretary in a law firm. She has had one year of college. Her husband, a pharmacist, is very concerned about her health. He has verbalized his concerns to the nurses, stating that he will be glad when his wife learns to speak again.

Current treatment of the client centers on speech therapy, preventing infection in her neck wounds, and providing supplemental liquid nutrition.

In spite of all the body image changes she is experiencing, Olive seems to have a positive outlook. The surgeon has told her that he thinks he "got all the cancer" but would like for her to undergo a course of radiation therapy as soon as her wounds heal. Olive will not be discharged until she is able to maintain her weight through dietary intake.

QUESTIONS

1. Referring to the nursing diagnosis classification, what are the three interferences with ingestion that Olive is experiencing?

2. What are the objectives of the dietary management of Olive's condition?

3. What are some practical suggestions that could be made to Olive about her food intake both in the hospital and at home?

4. Why is psychological support from the health team and Olive's family important to her recovery and nutritional status?

BIBLIOGRAPHY

Amos, H. E., and Drake, J. J. P. Problems posed by food additives. *J. Hum. Nutr.* 30:165, 1978.

Barakat, M. R. Pellagra. In G. H. Beaton and J. M. Bengoa, Eds., *Nutrition in Preventive Medicine.* Monograph Series No. 62. Geneva: World Health Org., 1976.

Bennion, M. *Clinical Nutrition.* 1st. Ed. New York: Harper & Row, Pubs., Inc., 1979.

Buckley, J. E. Feeding the patient with dysphagia. *Nurs. Forum* 15(1):69, 1976.

Bunker, M. L., and McWilliams, M. Caffeine content of common beverages. *J. Am. Diet. Assoc.* 74:28, 1979.

Carson, J. A. S., and Gormican, A. Taste acuity and food attitudes of selected patients with cancer. *J. Am. Diet. Assoc.* 70:361, 1977.

Clements, F. W. Endemic goitre. In G. H. Beaton and J. M. Bengoa, Eds., *Nutrition in Preventive Medicine.* Monograph Series No. 62. Geneva: World Health Org., 1976.

Cohen, S., and Booth, G. H., Jr. Gastric acid secretion and lower-esophageal-sphincter pressure in response to coffee and caffeine. *N. Engl. J. Med.* 293:897, 1975.

Copping, A. M. Planning nutrition education in developing countries. *J. Am. Diet. Assoc.* 53:127, 1968.

DeMaeyer, E. M. Protein—energy malnutrition. In G. H. Beaton and J. M. Bengoa, Eds., *Nutrition in Preventive Medicine.* Monograph Series No. 62. Geneva: World Health Org., 1976.

Dickerson, J. W. T., and Wiryanti, J. Pellagra and mental disturbance. *Proc. Nutr. Soc.* 37:167, 1978.

Eade, O. E., and Wright, R. Dietary hypersensitivity: The gastroenterologist's view. *J. Hum. Nutr.* 30:157, 1976.

Ford, J. A. Asian rickets and osteomalacia. *Nursing Times.* 70:49, 1974.

Freier, S. Pediatric gastrointestinal allergy. *J. Hum. Nutr.* 30:187, 1976.

Glad, B. W., Hodges, R. E., Michas, C. A., Moussavian, S. N., and Righi, S. P. Atrophic beriberi: A complication of jejunoileal bypass surgery for morbid obesity. *Am. J. Med.* 65:69, 1978.

Goldsmith, G. A. Curative nutrition: Vitamins. In H. A. Schneider, C. E. Anderson, and D. B. Coursin, Eds., *Nutritional Support of Medical Practice.* New York: Harper & Row, Pubs., Inc., 1977.

Goldstein, A., and Kaizer, S. Psychotropic effects of caffeine in man: A questionnaire study of coffee drinking and its effects in a group of housewives. *Clin. Pharmacol. Ther.* 10:477, 1969.

Gordon, J. E. Synergism of malnutrition and infectious disease. In G. H. Beaton, and J. M. Bengoa, Eds., *Nutri-*

tion in Preventive Medicine. Monograph Series No. 62. Geneva: World Health Org., 1976.

Greden, J. F. Anxiety or caffeinism: A diagnostic dilemma. *Am. J. Psychiatry* 131:1089, 1974.

Gunn, A. D. G. Food poisoning. *Nursing Times* 72:842, 1976.

Herbert, V. The nutritionally and metabolically destructive "nutritional and metabolic antineoplastic diet" of laetrile proponents. *Am. J. Clin. Nutr.* 32:96, 1979.

Hodges, R. E. Scurvy. In G. H. Beaton and J. M. Bengoa, Eds., *Nutrition in Preventive Medicine.* Monograph Series No. 62. Geneva: World Health Org., 1976.

James, W. P. T. Kwashiorkor and marasmus: Old concepts and new developments. *Proc. Roy. Soc. Med.* 70:611, 1977.

Katsura, E., and Oiso, T. Beriberi. In G. H. Beaton and J. M. Bengoa, Eds., *Nutrition in Preventive Medicine.* Monograph Series No. 62. Geneva: World Health Org., 1976.

Kerr, G. R., Wu Lee, M., El-Lozy, M., McGandy, R., and Stare, F. J. Prevalence of the "Chinese restaurant syndrome." *J. Am. Diet. Assoc.* 75:29, 1979.

Krause, M. V., and Mahan, L. K. *Food, Nutrition, and Diet Therapy.* 6th Ed. Philadelphia: W. B. Saunders Co., 1979.

Kimm, S., and Donoso, G. Control of protein calorie malnutrition. In J. Mayer and J. T. Dwyer, Eds., *Food and Nutrition Policy in a Changing World.* New York: Oxford Univ. Press., 1979.

Manber, M. The medical effects of coffee. *Medical World News,* Jan. 1976.

Mitchell, H. S., Rynbergen, H. J., Anderson, L., and Dibble, M. V. *Nutrition in Health and Disease.* 16th Ed. Philadelphia: J. B. Lippincott Co., 1976.

Nat'l Nutrition Consortium, Inc. *Vitamin-Mineral Safety: Toxicity, and Misuse.* Rep. of the Comm. on Safety, Toxicity, and Misuse of Vitamin and Trace Minerals. Chicago: Am. Dietetic Assoc., 1978.

Newell, F. W. Renewed interest in the ancient scourge, xerophthalmia. *Am. J. OF Ophthalmol.* 86:284, 1978.

Olness, K. The ecology of malnutrition in children. *J. Am. Med. Wom. Assoc.* 32(8):279, 1977.

Oomen, H. A. P. C. Xerophthalmia. In G. H. Beaton and J. M. Bengoa, Eds., *Nutrition in Preventive Medicine.* Monograph Series No. 62. Geneva: World Health Org., 1976.

Overton, M. H., and Lukert, B. P. *Clinical Nutrition: A Physiologic Approach.* Chicago: Year Book Medical Pubs., Inc., 1977.

Paunier, L. Rickets and osteomalacia. In G. H. Beaton and J. M. Bengoa, Eds., *Nutrition in Preventive Medicine.* Monograph Series No. 62. Geneva: World Health Org. 1976.

Pennington, J. *Nutritional Diet Therapy.* Palo Alto, Calif.: Bull Pub. Co., 1978.

Ramalingaswami, V., and Tandon, B. N. Approaches to nutrition rehabilitation and supplementary feeding. In J. Mayer and J. T. Dwyer, Eds., *Food and Nutrition Policy in a Changing World.* New York: Oxford Univ. Press, 1979.

Roberts, A. M. Obesity in malnourished children. *Nursing Times* 74(5):194, 1978.

Robinson, C. H., and Lawler, M. R. *Normal and Therapeutic Nutrition.* 15th Ed. New York: Macmillan, Inc., 1977.

Rose, J. C. Nutritional problems in radiotherapy patients. *Am. J. Nurs.* 78:1194, 1978.

Rowe, A. H. *Elimination Diets and the Patient's Allergies: A Handbook of Allergy.* Philadelphia: Lea & Febiger, 1941.

Rowe, A. H., *Food Allergy.* Springfield, Ill.: Charles C. Thomas, Pub., 1972.

Shaw, S., and Lieber, C. S. Alcoholism. H. A. Schneider, C. E. Anderson, and D. B. Coursin, Eds., *Nutritional Support of Medical Practice.* New York: Harper & Row, Pubs., Inc., 1977.

Sommer, A. Assessment of xerophthalmin and the mass vitamin A: Prophylaxis program in El Salvador (Sept. 1973–Dec. 1974). *Environmental Child Health* 22:135, 1976.

Sotaniemi, K. A. Dry beriberi in a slimmer. *Br. Med. J.* 2(6103):1634, 1977.

Spivak, J. L., and Jackson, D. L. Pellagra: An analysis of 18 patients and a review of the literature. *Johns Hopkins Med. J.* 140:295, 1977.

Stanley, W. A. Sin-Cyb-Syn—The Chinese restaurant syndrome. *J. Kans. Med. Soc.* 78:230, 1977.

Stephenson, P. E. Physiologic and psychotropic effects of caffeine on man. *J. Am. Diet. Assoc.* 71:240, 1977.

Stone, O. J. Alcoholic malnutrition and skin infections. *Nutrition Today* 13(6):6, 1978.

Stratigos, J. D., and Katsambas, A. Pellagra: A still existing disease. *Br. J. Dermatol.* 96:99, 1977.

Theologides, A. Why cancer patients have anorexia. *Geriatrics* 31(6):69, 1976.

Thiele, V. F. *Clinical Nutrition.* St. Louis. The C. V. Mosby Co., 1976.

Todd, S., and Mackaress, R. Allergy to food and chemicals: The scope of the problem. *Nursing Times* 74:438, 1978.

Turner, W. Sick of what you ate. *Nursing Times* 67:1299, 1971.

Warin, R. P. Food factors in urticaria. *J. Hum. Nutr.* 30:179, 1976.

Weber, B. Eating with a tracheostomy. *Am. J. Nurs.* 74:1439, 1974.

Williams, J. I., and Cram, D. M. Diet in the management of hyperkinesis: A review of the tests of Feingold's hypothesis. *Can. Psychiatr. Assoc. J.* 23:241, 1978.

Williams, S. R. *Nutrition and Diet Therapy.* 3rd Ed. St. Louis: The C. V. Mosby Co., 1977.

Winick, M. *Nutrition and Cancer.* New York: John Wiley & Sons, Inc., Pubs., 1977.

Woodruff, C. W. Ascorbic acid—scurvy. *Prog. Food Nutr. Sci.* 1:493, 1975.

CHAPTER 25

Alterations in Digestion and Absorption

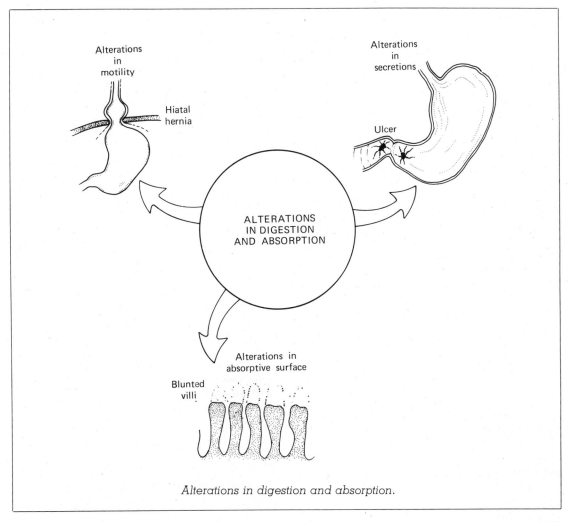

Alterations
in
motility

Hiatal
hernia

Alterations
in
secretions

Ulcer

ALTERATIONS
IN DIGESTION
AND ABSORPTION

Alterations in
absorptive surface

Blunted
villi

Alterations in digestion and absorption.

For most people, eating is a pleasant and satisfying experience. Everyone, however, has at sometime experienced unpleasant symptoms of indigestion after eating certain foods. The symptoms of indigestion associated with the gastrointestinal tract are frequently vague to the nurse who listens to the client describe the symptoms, but to the client experiencing them they are very real. The client will probably describe such symptoms as heartburn, a sensation of bloating, feeling too full, presence of gas, and stomach pain. The client may also state that he "feels sick," is constipated, or has diarrhea. The client may report that some of these symptoms are experienced at the same time each day or after the ingestion of a particular food or beverage. The client's description of the symptoms should give the nurse some clues to the alteration that is occurring in digestion and absorption. Further medical diagnostic tests will need to be used to determine the cause of the symptoms.

Interferences with digestion result from alterations in digestive tract motility or secretions, both necessary for the digestion of food. An abnormality in either secretion or motility affects not only digestion but optimal absorption because the nutrients presented to the small intestine for absorption are not in the prescribed form. Sometimes the defect is in the absorptive surface itself. An inflammatory lesion in the small intestine may lead to increased motility, decreased secretions, and also decreased absorption. An increase in motility causing rapid passage of food through the digestive tract may not allow adequate exposure time to the secretions for adequate digestion. The manifestations of altered digestion and absorption overlap; they can all be discussed in terms of the general symptoms experienced as a result of alterations in motility, secretions, and absorption.

ALTERATIONS IN MOTILITY

1. Biliary colic pain
2. Gastrointestinal spasms

3. Excessive regurgitation
4. Flatulence
5. Indigestion
6. Potential impaired intestinal circulation
7. Pain in esophagus

The movement of food through the digestive tract is *motility*. This movement proceeds at a pace slow enough for adequate digestion and absorption but fast enough to supply nutrients to the body cells. The ingestion of food, however, may result in symptoms of indigestion, or *dyspepsia*. *Indigestion* is an indefinite term used to describe discomfort in the digestive tract. The discomfort may be classified as *organic,* that is, as symptoms of disease within the digestive tract, or as *functional,* that is, resulting from faulty eating habits or dietary indiscretion. The symptoms of indigestion are heartburn (*pyrosis*), regurgitation of gastric acid, a feeling of fullness or bloating after meals (distention), the presence of gas (flatulence), and belching (*eructation*). Alterations in motility in the esophagus or stomach may lead to most of these symptoms. Increased motility of the gastric contents through the small and large intestine results in distention, flatulence, decreased absorption, and diarrhea. This increased motility is often the result of an inflammatory process within the small intestine or colon. Conditions that increase motility of the small intestine primarily affect absorption, so they are discussed later in this chapter. Decreased motility of the lower gastrointestinal (GI) tract results in the opposite problem, constipation. Diarrhea and constipation, being problems of excretion, are discussed in Chapter 28. The symptom of indigestion caused by *gastric reflux* serves as an example here of altered motility of the upper digestive tract.

Role of Food

Foods are often blamed for the symptoms of heartburn, hyperacidity, abdominal fullness, bloating, pain, "gas," rumbling noises in the

GI tract, constipation, and diarrhea. The traditional dietary treatment of gastrointestinal symptoms was based on recommending foods on the basis of certain qualities such as "blandness," high or low residue or fiber, digestibility, gas-forming, or irritant properties. In the early 1960s a committee composed of members from the American Medical Association and the American Dietetic Association was formed to study dietary treatment of GI disease. They found that many of the dietary restrictions for gastrointestinal disorders were based on tradition rather than scientific facts (Weinstein et al., 1961).

Effect of Food on Motility

The diets prescribed for GI disorders are described as bland, low residue, or high or low fiber. *Bland* refers to foods that are soft in texture and nonirritating to the GI mucosa. *Fiber* and *residue* are terms that are sometimes used interchangeably, but they do have different meanings. *Fiber* refers to the skin, seeds, and structural parts of food, including the connective tissue of meat, which are indigestible in humans. Raw fruits and vegetables and whole grain breads and cereals are the principal sources of dietary fiber. *Residue* refers to volume of material present in the colon after digestion. It is composed of undigested fiber, bacterial residues, and sloughed-off mucosa cells. A diet that is high in fiber is also high in residue, but there is one major exception to this rule. Milk is a fiber-free food that leaves a moderate amount of residue in the colon after digestion. This is due to the action of the bacteria in the colon on the milk. Milk fat decreases the motility of the stomach, allowing food to remain there longer (Rynbergen, 1963). Foods with protein and fat leave a moderate amount of residue in the colon. The accumulation of minimal residue in the colon is of primary importance in treating conditions of the lower GI tract. In general, high-fiber foods increase intestinal motility, and low-fiber or low-residue foods decrease motility.

Effect of Food on "Gas" Production

Certain foods have traditionally been associated with the production of gas. Foods labeled as common offenders are baked beans, cabbage, fried foods, onions, and spiced foods (Robinson and Lawler, 1977). Weinstein et al. (1961) reported that the results of human studies of gas production using cabbage revealed no more gas production from cabbage than from other foods. The actual production of human gas is difficult to measure. Also the amount of rectal gas expelled is not necessarily related to the intestinal production of gas (Krause and Mahan, 1979).

The presence of gas may be influenced by the diffusion of nitrogen and oxygen gases from the blood into the intestinal tract. Gas production also results from the presence of nonabsorbable carbohydrates such as *stachyose* and *raffinose*. These indigestible carbohydrates rapidly pass through the small intestine into the colon, where they are used by the bacteria for hydrogen gas production. Levitt (1972) points out that in clients with GI disease an increased proportion of carbohydrate may not be absorbed, providing an increased substrate for increased production of hydrogen by the colonic bacteria. The digestion of fat and protein yields acids that react with bicarbonate in the intestine to produce carbon dioxide, another source of intestinal gas. This could account for gas production in some people after meals high in meat and fat. Production of gas is a highly individual matter; gas production from a certain food may not even consistently occur in the same person.

Client Objectives

To be able to:

1. Exhibit a return to normal motility.
2. Discuss measures that may prevent future problems with motility.
3. Confirm his increased comfort.

Dietary Interventions

Objectives

Altered motility may be the result of faulty dietary habits, stress and nervous tension, or the presence of an organic disease. The symptoms may include general indigestion or diarrhea or constipation. See Table 25-1 for general symptoms that may be clues to kinds of GI disease. There are two major objectives in the dietary treatment of altered motility of the digestive tract. The first is to alleviate the undesirable symptoms. This may be accomplished by establishing good eating habits and eliminating some foods. The second objective is to maintain or restore the client's nutritional status. Because of the symptoms experienced after eating, food intake often declines in clients who suffer from GI disorders. Anxiety about the symptoms and about eating, weight loss, and a gradual decline in nutritional status may occur.

An example of altered motility of the upper digestive tract is the reflux of the gastric contents into the esophagus, causing the symptom of heartburn, or indigestion. Is there a specific GI disease associated with the symptoms, or are the symptoms purely functional with no apparent disease association? Suggestions for the client who experiences indigestion are to get a well-balanced diet and to correct any faulty dietary habits such as large intakes of a single food or beverage or the practice of eating only one large meal each day and snacking the rest of the day. The client should be told about the benefits of three regular meals of approximately equal size eaten at regularly spaced intervals throughout the waking hours. He should be instructed to eat slowly and in a relaxed atmosphere. The nurse should discuss with the client possible ways to reduce emotional tension in his environment and how to find ways to relax throughout the day, especially for a short period after a meal. If the client's indigestion is purely functional and if he makes a conscious effort to follow these suggestions, it is quite likely that the problem will disappear, making a specific dietary modification unnecessary. If the symptoms do not disappear, the nurse may then try to determine specifically which foods seem to cause the client difficulty and instruct him to avoid eating them. A thorough dietary history and interview is quite helpful to the nurse when counseling the client with GI symptoms.

For the client who has gastroesophageal reflux many of the suggestions are the same. Reflux of the gastric contents into the esophagus may lead to an inflammatory process at the lower end of the esophagus. In some cases the lower esophageal sphincter does not close completely between swallows. This allows reflux of the gastric contents back

TABLE 25-1. Dietary History Information That Can Give Clues to Gastrointestinal Disease

Symptom	Possible Disorder
Ingestion of solid food causes distress but liquids do not	
Difficulty in swallowing; food sticks in throat.	Esophageal stricture or tumor.
Epigastric pain when eating.	Esophageal spasm; achalasia.
Pain 2–5 hours after a meal, relieved upon eating.	Gastric ulcer.
Abdominal pain several hours after a fatty meal.	Duodenal ulcer.
Cramps, distention, and flatulence several hours after drinking milk.	Pancreatic or biliary tract disease.
Heartburn after a fatty meal.	Lactose intolerance probably due to lactase deficiency.
	Hiatal hernia; achalasia; esophageal motility problem.

SOURCE: Reprinted with permission from M. V., Krause and L. K. Mahan, *Food, Nutrition, and Diet Therapy*, 6th Ed. Philadelphia: W. B. Saunders Co., 1979.

into the lower part of the esophagus. In the case of *hiatal hernia,* a portion of the stomach protrudes, or herniates, through the diaphragm into the esophagus, also allowing reflux of the gastric contents. Several suggestions can be made that may bring great relief to the client with esophageal reflux. Foods that stimulate the release of the hormone *gastrin* stimulate the lower esophageal sphincter to close between swallows, whereas foods that stimulate the secretion of other hormones such as *cholecystokinin* decrease the pressure so that the lower esophageal sphincter remains open, permitting reflux (Krause and Mahan, 1979). Foods that stimulate gastric secretion should also be restricted to decrease the irritating capacity of the gastric juice. Protein foods stimulate the release of gastrin thus allowing the lower esophageal sphincter to close between swallows. Fatty meals should be avoided because of the stimulation of cholecystokinin. Other substances that decrease the pressure of the lower esophageal sphincter and that should be avoided or restricted are chocolate, coffee, alcohol, peppermint and spearmint oils, and cigarettes (Krause and Mahan, 1979). It is often helpful for the client to avoid large meals and instead eat small amounts at each meal and snacks between meals. Liquids consumed with meals may allow reflux to occur more readily, so the suggestion may be made to consume beverages between meals or to sip small amounts of the beverage. Some clients experience irritation of the esophagus from very hot or very cold beverages, and it may be helpful to avoid these extremes of temperature (Robinson and Lawler, 1977).

The client should be instructed to remain upright after eating; lying down to rest increases the possibility of reflux of the gastric contents. He should also refrain from bending or lifting or excessive exercise right after the meal. Food should also be omitted several hours before bedtime. It may also help for the client to sleep with his head elevated. The client should be encouraged to eat slowly,

chew thoroughly, and eat meals in a relaxed atmosphere at regular times of day. The nurse should emphasize the importance of decreasing daily emotional tension and discourage eating on the run. Chewing gum should be avoided because it leads to swallowed air, which may lead to increased flatulence and discomfort. The overweight client should be encouraged to lose weight because excess abdominal fat is believed to increase reflux and herniation (Robinson and Lawler, 1977).

Fiber-restricted Diet

A fiber-restricted or bland diet may be helpful, at least temporarily, for clients experiencing indigestion or gastric reflux. The bland and fiber-restricted diets are quite similar. The bland diet eliminates foods that are mechanically and chemically irritating. Mechanical stimulation results from foods high in fiber and roughage; chemical stimulation results from foods that cause gastric secretion. The fiber-restricted diet, though designed to restrict foods that are mechanically irritating, often also restricts foods that stimulate gastric secretion and highly spiced foods. The fiber-restricted diet may also be referred to as the low-residue diet, the main difference being that a low-residue diet restricts milk. The general principles of the restricted-fiber diet are:

1. Elimination or restriction of foods high in indigestible carbohydrate (fiber)
2. Inclusion of foods soft in consistency and mild in flavor
3. Elimination of foods thought to cause gastric irritation
4. Exclusion of fried foods

The foods included on a fiber-restricted diet are found in Table 25-2. The client is taught that the fiber content of foods is actually indigestible carbohydrate. Fiber may have an irritating effect on the gastrointestinal mucosa and cause discomfort. A fiber-restricted diet

TABLE 25-2. Restricted-fiber Diet

This diet is modified to provide easily digested foods and to lower the content of indigestible carbohydrate and connective tissue. This modification will be used when a soft diet or a low-residue diet is ordered; additional restrictions can be ordered to suit each patient's preferences and tolerances.

Food Group	Servings per Day	Foods to Include	Foods to Omit
Milk[a]	1 pt or more	Whole milk, skim milk, buttermilk, chocolate milk.	None.
Meat, poultry, fish, cheese	2	Tender lean beef, chicken, lamb, liver, turkey or veal. Crisp bacon and lean pork if tolerated. Cream, cottage, or American cheese.	Highly seasoned meats may cause distress.
Eggs	1	Any style.	None.
Breads and cereals	4 or more	Bread, toast, rolls and crackers made with finely milled whole grain or refined flour.	Breads made with seeds, cracked wheat bread, coarse cereals such as shredded wheat or all-bran.
		Rice, macaroni, spaghetti, noodles.	
		All cooked cereals and refined dry cereals.	Cereals that contain bran, seeds, nuts, or coconut.
Potato	1 or more	White or sweet potatoes, boiled, baked, mashed, creamed, browned, or scalloped.	Potatoes with skins.
Other vegetables	2 or more— at least one green leafy or yellow	Tender cooked vegetables, whole as tolerated.	Raw vegetables, vegetables with tough skins, corn, onion, dried beans, dried peas, and other strong-flavored vegetables not tolerated.
Fruits	2 or more, at least one citrus or tomato	Fruit juice, ripe banana, avocado, citrus fruit sections without membrane, stewed or canned fruit without seeds.	Raw fruit (except banana and avocado), berries.
Fats	3 or more	Butter, margarine, cream, oils, gravy if tolerated.	None.
Soups	As desired	Broth, noodle or rice soup with meat, cream soups.	Soups containing foods not allowed.

TABLE 25-2. *(Continued)*

Food Group	Servings per Day	Foods to Include	Foods to Omit
Beverages	As desired	Tea, coffee, carbonated beverages, fruit beverages.	None.
Desserts	As desired	Cakes, cookies, pudding, custard, ice cream, sherbet, gelatin, cream pie, fruit pie or cobbler made with allowed fruits.	Desserts containing nuts, coconut, or fruits with seeds.
Sweets	As desired	Hard clear candy, gum drops, jelly beans, clear jelly, honey, syrup, plain chocolates.	Candies with nuts, coconut, seeds, skins, jams with seeds or skins.
Seasonings	Moderate amounts as tolerated	All.	None.

SOURCE: Courtesy of Department of Nutrition and Dietetics, Indiana University Medical Center, Indianapolis.
a Milk would be eliminated from the low-residue diet.

should provide more comfort for the client with a motility disorder. Fats, especially fried foods, should be avoided because they may enhance gastric reflux into the esophagus. Highly spiced and strong-flavored foods may need to be restricted because they may lead to GI discomfort. Meats should be prepared by baking, boiling, broiling, roasting, or grilling. The meat selected should be tender or prepared by a long, slow method of cooking until the connective tissue is soft and the meat is tender. The meat may be prepared in the oven in a small amount of liquid in a covered utensil or cooked in an electric slow cooker. Vegetables do not need to be pureed unless the client prefers or this is the only way they can be swallowed. The vegetables should be cooked until tender and then chewed thoroughly by the client. Fruits with tough skins or seeds should be avoided. See Table 25-2 for a list of fruits allowed. Figure 25-1 shows an example of a low-residue menu.

A particular problem of motility that may develop following surgical removal of part or all of the stomach is called the *dumping syndrome*. A series of annoying and unpleasant symptoms become evident about 15 minutes after eating and again after about 2 hours. Fortunately these symptoms do not occur in all clients who have had gastric surgery. For those who do experience these symptoms, there are dietary measures that can reduce or greatly improve tolerance for food.

About 15 minutes after eating, the client has a sensation of fullness in the epigastrium and experiences a cold sweat. These symptoms are experienced because, as a result of the surgery, the remaining portion of the stomach has lost its ability to function as a reservoir. A concentrated mass of food is thus literally dumped in an undigested form into the small intestine, rather than being released in the normal slow, controlled manner as it is ready to leave the stomach. In the body's attempt to dilute this concentrated mixture, water is withdrawn from the intestine. Serotonin, histamine, and *prostaglandins* are released in a response to this hyperosmolar

INDIANA UNIVERSITY HOSPITALS GENERAL MENU	INDIANA UNIVERSITY HOSPITALS GENERAL MENU	INDIANA UNIVERSITY HOSPITALS GENERAL MENU
MORNING	**NOON**	**NIGHT**
FRESHLY SQUEEZED ORANGE JUICE	MINESTRONE SOUP WITH CHEESE PUFF	PINEAPPLE SHERBET PUNCH
	CREAMY CLAM CHOWDER WITH CHEESE PUFF	STRAINED CREAM OF MUSHROOM SOUP
GRAPEFRUIT JUICE	CREAM OF TOMATO SOUP	STRAINED JULIENNE BROTH
	CELERY BROTH	PAN FRIED CATFISH WITH TARTAR SAUCE
HOT ROLLED WHEAT	TUNA AND NOODLE CASSEROLE	BAKED HADDOCK WITH LEMON WEDGE
CORNFLAKES	PORK SAUSAGE PATTY IN GRAVY	ROAST BEEF AU JUS
PUFFED RICE	BEEF (GROUND) IN BROTH	(GROUND) ROAST BEEF AU JUS
		HASHED BROWN POTATOES
SCRAMBLED EGGS	MASHED POTATOES	BUTTERED DICED POTATOES
POACHED EGG	BUTTERED PEAS	
FRIED EGG SUNNY SIDE UP	BUTTERED CABBAGE	BUTTERED ASPARAGUS SPEARS
FRIED EGG OVER LIGHT	BUTTERED BLENDERIZED GREEN PEAS	BUTTERED VEGETABLE MEDLEY
FRIED EGG HARD	FAVORITE RELISHES IN ICE	BUTTERED BLENDERIZED ASPARAGUS
SOFT COOKED EGG IN SHELL	TOSSED GREEN SALAD	CALICO COLESLAW ON LEAF LETTUCE
HARD COOKED EGG IN SHELL	CREAMY SALAD DRESSING	
BROILED BACON STRIP	BRAIDED ROLL WITH MARGARINE	BUTTERCORN ROLL WITH MARGARINE
WARM BEAR CLAW DANISH PASTRY	WHITE BREAD OR TOAST WITH MARGARINE	WHITE BREAD OR TOAST WITH MARGARINE
WHOLE WHEAT TOAST WITH MARGARINE		
WHITE TOAST WITH MARGARINE	WARM APPLE DUMPLING EN SAUCE	CHILLED APRICOT HALVES
WHITE BREAD WITH MARGARINE	PEACH HALVES	CHILLED BLACK BOTTOM PIE
MARGARINE	MARGARINE	MARGARINE
MILK	MILK	MILK
2% MILK	2% MILK	2% MILK
SKIM MILK	SKIM MILK	SKIM MILK
BUTTERMILK	BUTTERMILK	BUTTERMILK
	COTTAGE CHEESE	COTTAGE CHEESE
	CRACKERS	CRACKERS
	CUSTARD	PUDDING
	VANILLA ICE CREAM	VANILLA ICE CREAM
JELLO HOT TEA	JELLO HOT TEA	JELLO HOT TEA
BROTH ICED TEA	ICED TEA	ICED TEA
JELLY LEMON	JELLY LEMON	JELLY LEMON
CREAM FRUIT DRINK	CREAM FRUIT JUICE	CREAM FRUIT JUICE
COFFEE	COFFEE FRUIT DRINK	COFFEE FRUIT DRINK
SANKA	SANKA LEMONADE	SANKA LEMONADE

Figure 25-1. Low-residue diet menu. (Courtesy Indiana University Hospitals)

mixture, and these substances cause the cramping, hypermotility, and diarrhea of this syndrome (Krause and Mahan, 1979).

About two hours later another set of symptoms occurs. The carbohydrate from the concentrated food mass has been rapidly digested and absorbed, leading to a rapid rise in blood glucose level. This glucose load stimulates an overproduction of insulin by the pancreas, causing a rapid fall in blood glucose level below normal. Symptoms of hypoglycemia such as weakness, hunger, nausea, anxiety, perspiration, and shaking occur.

The dietary intervention is aimed at preventing or reducing these symptoms. The diet is high in protein and moderate in fat, with the exclusion of concentrated carbohydrates, especially simple sugars that are rapidly digested. The protein and fat are less rapidly hydrolyzed, and therefore their presence in the diet helps to retard the symptoms. The diet should also be composed of small, frequent feedings or six small meals, and no fluids should be taken with the meals, as they cause the food mass to be dumped into the jejunum even more rapidly. Fluids are allowed between meals. Lying down or resting after a meal may also help reduce the symptoms. The dumping syndrome is more frequently experienced in clients who have had two-thirds or more of the stomach removed. Usually the remaining portion of the stomach will stretch to create a pouch where digestion and preparation for absorption can once again occur.

ALTERATIONS IN SECRETIONS

1. Gastrointestinal-cardiac pain
2. Potential development of stress ulcer
3. Potential gastric distress
4. Heartburn

Hormones, enzymes, and other substances are secreted throughout the digestive tract to assist in the digestion of carbohydrates, proteins, and fats. Any alteration in these secretions will result in alterations in the digestion of the energy nutrients. Secretions are contributed by each major organ along the digestive tract as well as by the accessory organs, the liver, and the pancreas. Alterations in secretions will lead to a disorder in digestion, but the alterations will be manifested as a disorder in absorption. Only those interferences with digestion caused by altered secretions and manifested by gastric pain are discussed. Inadequate secretions from the pancreas and small intestine manifest themselves as altered absorption and are considered under that heading.

Client Objectives

To be able to:

1. Exhibit a return to normal secretory patterns.
2. Discuss behavior changes that may prevent future secretory problems.
3. Confirm his increased comfort.

Dietary Interventions

Bland Diet

Altered secretions may be manifested either in gastric pain or in nutrient malabsorption. The gastric pain may be actual or potential pain from heartburn, a gastric or duodenal ulcer, or gall bladder pain. The dietary objective is to decrease the pain by decreasing the intake of foods that cause the pain. To reduce pain in the region of the gall bladder requires a reduction in the amount of dietary fat because the gall bladder contracts to release bile whenever the hormone cholecystokinin senses the presence of fat in the duodenum. In the case of peptic ulcers the dietary aim is to reduce the secretion of gastric acid, to neutralize the acid that is produced, to protect the lesion from irritation, and to promote healing. The bland diet is the standard diet selected to accomplish these objectives, but there is much debate about its healing effect and what foods should be included. In recent years there has been a gradual shift toward a more liberal approach to bland diet therapy based on recent scientific evidence. In this section the influence of foods on gastric secretions and the effect of foods on the lesion are examined. First, however, it should be helpful to review briefly the principles of the very conservative traditional bland diet.

The foods allowed on a traditional bland diet were believed to be chemically, mechanically, and thermally nonirritating. Hourly feedings of milk or cream were given initially. The diet was gradually advanced through four very restrictive progressive stages as the ulcer healed. This regimen is referred to as the Sippy diet after the doctor who devised it in 1915 (Williams, 1977). Foods believed to be chemically irritating were those, such as coffee, tea, alcohol, citrus juices, fried foods, spices, and flavorings, that stimulated gastric secretion. Mechanically irritating foods were those, such as raw fruits and vegetables and whole grain products, that contained high quantities of indigestible carbohydrate. Gasforming foods were also considered to be mechanically irritating and were excluded from the diet. Very hot or very cold foods or beverages were thought to be thermally irritating and were also excluded. Recent information has revealed that there is little or no scientific basis for the inclusion or exclusion of certain foods on the bland diet. Not all the questions concerning dietary treatment of peptic ulcers have been answered, but enough concrete evidence exists to support the use of a more liberal approach.

One of the major objectives of the bland diet is to reduce gastric secretion. Only a very few foods are actually known to stimulate gastric secretion. Although it was believed for many years that highly spiced foods stimulated gastric secretion and increased pain, in actual experiments it has been shown that very few spices stimulate gastric secretion even when they are applied directly to the mucosa.

A slight reddening of the mucosa was noted with chili powder, cloves, mustard seed, nutmeg, and black pepper (Schneider et al., 1956). A more recent study has shown that garlic, paprika, horseradish, mustard, and a few other spices stimulate gastric secretion only when used alone in fairly large amounts (Demling and Koch, 1974). Known gastric stimulants are caffeine, alcohol, meat extractives, and black pepper. Proteins have an initial buffering effect, which is followed by a stimulation of acid production. Fat tends to inhibit gastric secretion; it is questionable, however, whether the dairy fats generally recommended for use on a bland diet are any more effective in reducing secretion than any other type of fat (Krause and Mahan, 1979).

The next question is whether there are foods that may actually damage a gastrointestinal lesion. The pH of most foods is between 5 and 7. Even highly acidic foods such as orange and grapefruit juice are not as acidic as the gastric secretions. Inclusion of these foods is theoretically irritating only in the case of lesions of the mouth and esophagus. High-fiber foods have been eliminated on the assumption that they cause abrasion and retard healing of ulcers, but there is no evidence that high-fiber foods will irritate a lesion if they are thoroughly masticated (Am. Dietetic Assoc., 1971). The important thing is to reduce the particle size by thorough chewing.

Another consideration is whether any food has the ability to participate in the healing of an ulcer. Milk has been thought to have sufficient buffering capacity actually to help heal ulcers. Milk may raise the pH of the stomach slightly but not to the level of 3.6 needed for actual healing (Odell, 1971). It has been shown that following a bland diet makes no significant difference in the healing of an ulcer (Am. Dietetic Assoc., 1971), but providing foods high in protein, vitamin C, and iron does aid in healing.

The general principles of the current conception of the bland diet are to avoid foods known to stimulate gastric secretion; to include protein foods for a buffering effect; to eat small, frequent meals; to eat in a relaxed atmosphere; and to avoid those foods that cause discomfort. Management of the dietary treatment of a client with a peptic ulcer involves consideration both of the client as an individual and of the activity of the ulcer. The diet should be planned with the client, taking into consideration his particular food tolerances and preferences. Above all, the diet should be realistic for the client to follow. Emphasis should be placed on the foods to be included and not on those to be eliminated.

Intervention should begin with a thorough dietary history of the client. Information should be gathered about the client's normal eating habits and patterns. Questions may be asked about which foods give the client symptoms of digestive discomfort; most clients know which foods these are. These, then, are the first group of foods the client should be told to avoid. Next the nurse should explain to the client which foods are known to stimulate gastric secretion. Because the increased production of acid will continue to irritate and harm the ulcer, thus preventing the healing, these foods must also be omitted, at least temporarily. The nurse may explain that when the healing has progressed the physician may allow the inclusion of moderate amounts of these foods in the diet. The client with an ulcer should never be left with the impression that these foods will have to be omitted permanently. The anxiety produced by this approach may be enough to exacerbate the ulcer and lead to dietary noncompliance and noncooperation. Most hospitals allow the use of decaffeinated coffee despite the fact that studies have demonstrated that it stimulates gastric secretion as much as regular coffee (Cohen and Booth, 1975).

The client should be encouraged to include protein foods for a buffering effect and to eat small, frequent meals. The excess secretion of gastric acid may be explained to the client using the analogy of a dripping faucet. This excess secretion of acid is like a faucet of acid continually dripping in the stomach. Tense situations and worries throughout the day keep the faucet in the "on" position (Taif, 1976). When the stomach is empty, the steady flow of gastric juice continues to erode the gastric lesion and cause pain. Although the ingestion of food stimulates gastric secretion, the presence of food offers some protection to the intestinal wall from the acid. The acid is absorbed and neutralized by the food. Thus the client should be encouraged to eat small amounts of food at regular intervals throughout the day as protection for the intestinal wall. The excess acid will work on the food in the stomach and will not continue to erode the intestinal lining. The client should be encouraged to include a source of protein at each meal or snack for the buffering effect. Some examples of appropriate snacks include milk, toast, custard, cottage cheese, and crackers.

Milk need not be relied on entirely for buffering. Other protein foods such as eggs, cheese, or a small piece of meat may be used for the same effect. The client should be cautioned against the overuse of milk and milk products for two reasons. The first reason is the milk-alkali syndrome that can result from the combination of the high calcium intake from milk with the high levels of alkali from antacids. This combination can produce hypercalcemia, alkalosis, or hyperphosphatemia, which may lead to the development of renal calculi (Bennion, 1979). The excessive consumption of milk and milk products may also lead to an elevation of serum lipids and increase the risk of coronary heart disease.

After the ulcer has healed, the client should be instructed to eat before he gets too hungry. If the client waits too long to eat, the hunger contractions of the stomach will result in a stimulation of gastric secretions. The client should get in the habit of eating a small snack when he knows that a regular meal will be delayed for several hours.

The activity of the client's ulcer is an important consideration in treatment. If the client has suffered hemorrhage from a bleeding ulcer, no food will be allowed until the bleeding has been controlled. The initial feedings may be milk given at two-hour intervals and alternated with foods such as crackers; eggs; custard; toast; simple puddings; or tender, cooked fruits or vegetables (Robinson and Lawler, 1977). Gradual progression in the foods offered may be made as the client's condition improves. A more strict type of bland diet may need to be used during pe-

riods of active ulceration or acute attacks. Some clients also seem to do better medically or psychologically when placed on a fairly restrictive bland diet. The guidelines for the liberal bland diet are shown in Figure 25-2. A sample bland diet menu is shown in Figure 25-3. As stated previously, the menu should be supplemented with between-meal feedings.

In summary, the bland diet should be tailored to the nutritional needs of the individual client. During periods of active ulceration

---

The bland diet is essentially a diet "as tolerated." Each patient's tolerance to food is highly individual. For example, it is improbable that foods high in fiber traumatize the gastrointestinal tract if thoroughly masticated, and therefore they are tolerated by many. So-called strong-flavored or gas-producing foods may be tolerated by some patients when prepared properly. Scientific research has shown that certain foods (underlined below) are harmful and should be avoided by the majority of people with active ulcers or acute gastrointestinal disturbances. The patient should follow this diet plan only in acute phases of disease; thereafter the diet should be advanced to a regular diet "as tolerated" with the guidance of the dietitian.

This is a slight modification of the regular diet in order to:

1. Avoid known stimulants to gastric secretion such as alcohol and strong <u>caffeine-containing beverages</u> (i.e., coffee).
2. Avoid direct mucosal stimulants such as <u>black pepper</u> and <u>chili powder</u>.
3. Emphasize regularity in the meal pattern with unhurried eating habits in order to prepare more properly food for gastric digestion.
4. Provide three or more feedings daily in order to achieve most consistent buffering effects and to minimize gastroduodenal motility.
5. Allow clinical improvement of the patient until the particular illness being treated subsides.

It should be noted that coffee contains the greatest amount of caffeine. Lesser amounts are also found in tea, carbonated beverages, and cocoa. Thus coffee is the only caffeine-containing beverage that is omitted from the regular diet.

Some patients with gastrointestinal disturbances may not be able to tolerate all of the foods allowed on the bland diet. Therefore, the patient's diet will be planned with the guidance of a dietitian. The following food items, as well as others not listed, <u>may</u> cause distress and thus be intolerable to <u>certain</u> people.

MILK—chocolate milk
MEATS, POULTRY, FISH, CHEESE—meat extracts, highly spiced or cured meats (except bacon)
BREADS AND CEREALS—products with coarse bran or seeds
VEGETABLES—raw, onions, those from the cabbage family
FRUITS—raw or those with seeds
SOUPS—meat broths, highly seasoned soups
BEVERAGES—tea, chocolate drinks, carbonated beverages
DESSERTS—pastries, any desserts with dried fruit, seeds, nuts or coconut
SWEETS—jams, preserves, marmalades
SEASONINGS—onion, garlic, cloves, mustard seed

Figure 25-2. Guide for the liberal bland diet. (Courtesy of Department of Nutrition and Dietetics, Indiana University Medical Center, Indianapolis)

INDIANA UNIVERSITY HOSPITALS GENERAL MENU	INDIANA UNIVERSITY HOSPITALS GENERAL MENU	INDIANA UNIVERSITY HOSPITALS GENERAL MENU
MORNING	**NOON**	**NIGHT**
===== FRESHLY SQUEEZED ORANGE JUICE	===== MINESTRONE SOUP WITH CHEESE PUFF	===== PINEAPPLE SHERBET PUNCH
=====	===== CREAMY CLAM CHOWDER WITH CHEESE PUFF	===== STRAINED CREAM OF MUSHROOM SOUP
===== GRAPEFRUIT JUICE	===== CREAM OF TOMATO SOUP	===== STRAINED JULIENNE BROTH
=====	===== CELERY BROTH	===== PAN FRIED CATFISH WITH TARTAR SAUCE
===== HOT ROLLED WHEAT	===== TUNA AND NOODLE CASSEROLE	===== BAKED HADDOCK WITH LEMON WEDGE
===== CORNFLAKES	===== PORK SAUSAGE PATTY IN GRAVY	===== ROAST BEEF AU JUS
===== PUFFED RICE	===== BEEF (GROUND) IN BROTH	===== (GROUND) ROAST BEEF AU JUS
=====	=====	===== HASHED BROWN POTATOES
===== SCRAMBLED EGGS	===== MASHED POTATOES	===== BUTTERED DICED POTATOES
===== POACHED EGG	===== BUTTERED PEAS	=====
===== FRIED EGG SUNNY SIDE UP	===== BUTTERED CABBAGE	===== BUTTERED ASPARAGUS SPEARS
===== FRIED EGG OVER LIGHT	===== BUTTERED BLENDERIZED GREEN PEAS	===== BUTTERED VEGETABLE MEDLEY
===== FRIED EGG HARD	===== FAVORITE RELISHES IN ICE	===== BUTTERED BLENDERIZED ASPARAGUS
===== SOFT COOKED EGG IN SHELL	===== TOSSED GREEN SALAD	===== CALICO COLESLAW ON LEAF LETTUCE
===== HARD COOKED EGG IN SHELL	===== CREAMY SALAD DRESSING	=====
===== BROILED BACON STRIP	===== BRAIDED ROLL WITH MARGARINE	===== BUTTERCORN ROLL WITH MARGARINE
===== WARM BEAR CLAW DANISH PASTRY	===== WHITE BREAD OR TOAST WITH MARGARINE	===== WHITE BREAD OR TOAST WITH MARGARINE
===== WHOLE WHEAT TOAST WITH MARGARINE	=====	=====
===== WHITE TOAST WITH MARGARINE	===== WARM APPLE DUMPLING EN SAUCE	===== CHILLED APRICOT HALVES
===== WHITE BREAD WITH MARGARINE	===== PEACH HALVES	===== CHILLED BLACK BOTTOM PIE
===== MARGARINE	===== MARGARINE	===== MARGARINE
===== MILK	===== MILK	===== MILK
===== 2% MILK	===== 2% MILK	===== 2% MILK
===== SKIM MILK	===== SKIM MILK	===== SKIM MILK
===== BUTTERMILK	===== BUTTERMILK	===== BUTTERMILK
=====	===== COTTAGE CHEESE	===== COTTAGE CHEESE
===== *No Pepper*	===== CRACKERS	===== CRACKERS
=====	===== CUSTARD *No Pepper*	===== PUDDING *No Pepper*
=====	===== VANILLA ICE CREAM	===== VANILLA ICE CREAM
===== JELLO ===== HOT TEA	===== JELLO ===== HOT TEA	===== JELLO ===== HOT TEA
===== BROTH ===== ICED TEA	===== ===== ICED TEA	===== ===== ICED TEA
===== JELLY ===== LEMON	===== JELLY ===== LEMON	===== JELLY ===== LEMON
===== CREAM ===== FRUIT DRINK	===== CREAM ===== FRUIT JUICE	===== CREAM ===== FRUIT JUICE
===== COFFEE =====	===== COFFEE ===== FRUIT DRINK	===== COFFEE ===== FRUIT DRINK
===== SANKA =====	===== SANKA ===== LEMONADE	===== SANKA ===== LEMONADE

Figure 25-3. Bland diet menu. (Courtesy Indiana University Hospitals)

or with a bleeding ulcer, more aggressive therapy should be instituted by using a more restrictive type of bland diet. As the client's condition improves, the foods allowed can be greatly liberalized. When the client is dismissed from the hospital the only restriction of the diet may be to omit those foods that give the client gastric distress and pain. Even though recent scientific information about the effects of food on the gastrointestinal tract has led to liberalization of the bland diet, there are still indications for the use of more conservative therapy during acute attacks. Whether the conservative or liberal bland diet is used, it should not be so restrictive as to be considered "indigestible" by the client.

Low-fat Diet

A low-fat diet is used to ease the pain produced by contraction of the gall bladder when a meal high in fat is ingested. A low-fat diet may contain either 50 gm or 30 gm of fat daily. Fats need to be restricted because they stimulate the secretion of bile by the gall bladder. Contraction of the gall bladder results in pain either because of inflammation or obstruction of the bile ducts. The general principles of the diet are as follows:

1. Elimination of all fried foods and fatty foods
2. Elimination of all sauces and gravies
3. Restricted use of all high-fat meats
4. Elimination of all dairy products containing fat

A sample menu for a low-fat (50 gm) diet is given in Figure 25-4. A low-fat diet may not appear to be too difficult to follow until it is consumed. The first complaint the client usually has is that the food is "dry." The food seems dry because it must be prepared without fat and without any sauces or gravies. Note that the total number of ounces of meat supplied each day is 5 oz. The meat is either baked, boiled, roasted, grilled, or steamed without additional fat. All visible fat has been removed from the meat. This quantity of meat, although quite adequate nutritionally, is considerably less than most clients are use to eating. There are a total of three pats of butter, margarine, or oil allowed during the entire day. One pat of butter or margarine does not stretch very far over all the foods on a tray that could use some. The food on a low-fat diet is dry and unpalatable because it is very restricted in fat. The client who has been on a low-fat diet can greatly appreciate the contribution fat makes to the palatability of a meal. The low-fat diet not only limits the amount of fat but by necessity restricts the quantity of meat because all meat contains some fat. In some cases a 20- or 30-gm fat diet may be ordered. These diets are more restrictive, and often no visible fat (butter or margarine) is provided so that a minimum of 4 oz of meat can be supplied per day.

ALTERATIONS IN ABSORPTIVE SURFACE

1. Inadequate nutrient availability

Any alteration in the absorption process will result in decreased availability of nutrients vital to the body. This alteration in absorption is generally referred to as *malabsorption.* Malabsorption may be described as "starving in the midst of plenty." In other words, malabsorption is an inaccessibility of nutrients, not because of an inadequate intake of food, but because of an alteration in absorption.

Malabsorption is actually a very broad concept that encompasses every aspect of both digestion and absorption. The alterations of secretions and motility are intimately related to altered absorption. Inadequate secretions of digestive enzymes from the stomach, small intestine, or pancreas or an inadequate secretion of bile will result in inadequate digestion of carbohydrate, protein, and fat. Not having been hydrolyzed to the simple forms that can

INDIANA UNIVERSITY HOSPITALS CALORIE CONTROL MENU	INDIANA UNIVERSITY HOSPITALS CALORIE CONTROL MENU	INDIANA UNIVERSITY HOSPITALS CALORIE CONTROL MENU
MORNING	**NOON**	**NIGHT**
FRESHLY SQUEEZED ORANGE JUICE	CELERY BROTH	STRAINED JULIENNE BROTH
GRAPEFRUIT JUICE	D HOMEMADE PORK SAUSAGE PATTY	D BAKED HADDOCK WITH LEMON WEDGE
	CHOPPED SIRLOIN	D ROAST BEEF AU JUS
	SCRAMBLED EGGS	D (GROUND) ROAST BEEF AU JUS
HOT ROLLED WHEAT	D (GROUND) BEEF IN BROTH	
PUFFED RICE	D FLUFFY RICE	D DICED POTATO
CORNFLAKES	D MASHED POTATOES	D WHIPPED POTATOES
	D GREEN PEAS	
SCRAMBLED EGGS	D CHOPPED CABBAGE	D ASPARAGUS SPEARS
POACHED EGG		D VEGETABLE MEDLEY
FRIED EGG SUNNY SIDE UP	D FAVORITE RELISHES IN ICE	
FRIED EGG OVER LIGHT	TOSSED GREEN SALAD	D CALICO COLESLAW ON LEAF LETTUCE
FRIED EGG HARD	ZERO DRESSING	
SOFT COOKED EGG IN SHELL	BRAIDED ROLL	BUTTERCORN ROLL
HARD COOKED EGG IN SHELL	LS BRAIDED ROLL	LS BUTTERCORN ROLL
BROILED BACON STRIP	WHITE TOAST OR BREAD	WHITE TOAST OR BREAD
	LS WHITE TOAST OR BREAD	LS WHITE TOAST OR BREAD
WHOLE WHEAT TOAST		
WHITE TOAST OR BREAD	D PEACH HALVES	D CHILLED APRICOT HALVES
LS WHITE TOAST OR BREAD	D BAKED APPLE WITH CINNAMON	D PEAR HALVES
MARGARINE	MARGARINE	MARGARINE
LS MARGARINE	LS MARGARINE	LS MARGARINE
MILK	MILK	MILK
SKIM MILK	SKIM MILK	SKIM MILK
BUTTERMILK	BUTTERMILK	BUTTERMILK
CREAM	CREAM	CREAM
2% MILK	COTTAGE CHEESE	COTTAGE CHEESE
Jelly	LS COTTAGE CHEESE	LS COTTAGE CHEESE
	2% MILK Jelly	2% MILK Jelly
SALT HOT TEA	SALT HOT TEA	SALT HOT TEA
SALT SUBSTITUTE ICED TEA	SALT SUBSTITUTE ICED TEA	SALT SUBSTITUTE ICED TEA
PEPPER LEMON	PEPPER LEMON	PEPPER LEMON
SUGAR SUBSTITUTE	SUGAR SUBSTITUTE FRUIT JUICE	SUGAR SUBSTITUTE FRUIT JUICE
COFFEE	COFFEE D LEMONADE	COFFEE D LEMONADE
SANKA	SANKA CRACKERS	SANKA CRACKERS

Figure 25-4. Low-fat (50 gm) diet menu. (Courtesy Indiana University Hospitals)

be absorbed, these energy nutrients are excreted through the colon. Increased peristalsis, or motility, results in such a rapid movement of nutrients through the intestinal tract that the exposure time to the intestinal mucosa is not sufficient for optimal absorption to occur. There may also be a defect in the absorptive surface itself, such as an inflammatory condition or a blunting effect on the intestinal villi that greatly decreases the absorptive surface.

The client suffering from some form of malabsorption generally has a poor nutritional status. The client is often severely underweight or has recently lost a large amount of weight. The weight loss is evident because of both inadequate food intake and losses of nutrients through diarrhea. The client experiences anorexia, nausea, intestinal cramping, diarrhea, and sometimes vomiting. Pain is often associated with eating, making the client afraid to eat, which automatically reduces food intake.

Client Objectives

To be able to:

1. Discuss altered intake patterns that provide necessary nutrients for normal growth, development, and maintenance.
2. Ingest a diet that provides necessary nutrients.
3. Maintain adequate nutrition.

Dietary Interventions

The objectives of dietary intervention are to decrease the malabsorption and to improve the client's nutritional status. The general diet for malabsorption disorders is one that is high in Calories, high in protein and carbohydrate, high in vitamins and minerals, but somewhat low in fat content. Specific modifications may also be required in certain disorders. For example, *celiac disease* is a reaction of the intestinal villi to the protein gluten found in several cereal grains, so a specific gluten-restricted diet is used. Dietary treatment of most malabsorption syndromes also uses medium-chain triglycerides (MCT) oil, which is easier for the client to digest and absorb. If the malabsorption is due to a deficiency of a disaccharide digestive enzyme, the diet will simply eliminate those foods that contain the corresponding disaccharide. For example, for clients who have a deficiency of the digestive enzyme lactase, the treatment is to restrict or eliminate milk and milk products.

The general principles of dietary management for alteration in absorption are:

• Calories: higher than normal to compensate for fecal loss.
• Protein: higher than normal to compensate for losses; gluten-free diet used for celiac disease.
• Carbohydrate: generally increased, although starch is poorly tolerated with decreased secretion of pancreatic enzymes; and specific sugars are poorly tolerated with deficiencies of disaccharide enzymes.
• Fat: low to moderate fat to minimize steatorrhea; substitute MCT oil.
• Vitamins and Minerals: large doses to compensate for the losses from malabsorption.
• Feedings: to provide additional Calories and nutrients the number of feedings is increased if the client's appetite is decreased or if the client is underweight.

Malabsorption Related to Increased Motility

Any lesion or inflammatory process in the small intestine will interfere with digestion and also with absorption of the nutrients. An example of this is the condition of regional *enteritis* (*illeitis*). There is abdominal cramping, diarrhea, and steatorrhea. Only one segment of the small intestine may be involved or several segments (Robinson and Lawler, 1977). Because steatorrhea is present, the dietary management of this condition follows the general principles of dietary management for all malabsorption disorders.

The diet should be high in Calories and high in protein (120 gm) to compensate for the losses in the stool. The presence of steatorrhea indicates that fat is poorly tolerated, so the diet is restricted in fat (50 gm). The foods included should be simple, easily digested foods that are low in residue (the principles of the low-residue diet were discussed earlier in this chapter). The client may eat better if the diet is divided into six meals. Encourage the client to eat by emphasizing that the protein in the diet will aid in healing the damaged tissue.

The use of MCT oil may help to improve the absorption of fat and at the same time increase the caloric contect of the diet. This type of fat is digested more readily. These short- and medium-chain fatty acids are water soluble and absorbed directly into the portal circulation. They do not require the presence of pancreatic enzymes or bile, which is important in conditions where these secretions are depressed.

Malabsorption Related to Decreased Secretions
Inadequate digestion and therefore altered absorption may result from decreased pancreatic and intestinal secretions. Decreased pancreatic secretions may be evident in pancreatitis or in cystic fibrosis. In cystic fibrosis there is a decreased secretion of digestive enzymes from the pancreas, resulting in impaired digestion of carbohydrate, protein, and fat. The digestive enzymes produced by the pancreas are trypsin, amylase, and lipase. Fat is the least well tolerated, as evidenced by the large quantities of steatorrhea in the stools. Protein is tolerated quite well, as are simple carbohydrates. Starch should be restricted because of a deficiency of pancreatic amylase. The diet for cystic fibrosis should be high in Calories, high in protein, high in simple sugars, and low-to-moderate in fat. Pancreatic enzyme replacements are given with each meal to aid in the digestion of carbohydrate, protein, and fat. MTC oil is helpful in reducing the fat malabsorption.

A deficiency of one of the disaccharide intestinal enzymes will result in inadequate digestion and absorption of one of the disaccharides—sucrose, maltose, or lactose. One of these enzymes is sucrase isomaltase. A deficiency of sucrase results in an inability to hydrolyze sucrose; deficiency of isomaltase results in a failure to break the branched linkages in the starch molecule (Mitchell et al., 1976). Foods containing sucrose should be severely restricted. A sucrose-free diet is impractical and very difficult because numerous foods besides desserts and table sugar contain sucrose. The student should recall from Chapter 3 that a large number of fruits and vegetables contain sucrose. Even wheat germ and peanuts contain sucrose (Hardinge et al., 1965). Foods containing more than 5% sucrose are usually not well tolerated. The dietitian can supply a list of the foods that should be omitted (Robinson and Lawler, 1977). Glucose-galactase deficiency results in an inability to absorb any carbohydrate that yields glucose or galactose after digestion. This means that only the monosaccharide fructose is tolerated. Fortunately this disorder, found occasionally in infants, is rare. A special infant formula called CHO-free (Syntex Laboratories) is available. By the age of 3 a regular diet is tolerated with the quantities of milk and starch-containing foods restricted. A galactose-free diet may be used. This diet is the same as the lactose-restricted diet with the additional restrictions of beets, peas, and lima beans (Robinson and Lawler, 1977).

The most commonly occurring disaccharide enzyme deficiency, however, is a lactase deficiency resulting in lactose intolerance, sometimes referred to as *milk intolerance*. This condition can be the result of a primary deficiency of the enzyme lactase, or it may occur secondary to inflammatory disease of the small intestine or celiac disease. There are interesting variations in the incidence of lactose intolerance among different racial groups. Welsh (1978) stated that, whereas only 5–15% of white Americans of northern

European extraction have lactose intolerance, 60–95% of adult American blacks, Indians, Mexican-Americans, Jews, and Orientals have lactose intolerance. The exact cause of this decrease or inactivity of lactose is not known.

The digestion of lactose proceeds at a slower rate than the digestion of the other disaccharides. In lactose intolerance the quantity of lactose not digested passes into the colon. The intestinal bacteria continue to act on the unabsorbed lactose, and this produces gas. Some of the symptoms of lactose intolerance are abdominal pain, excessive flatulence, bloating, and diarrhea. These symptoms usually follow the ingestion of milk or milk products. Individual tolerances vary from those clients who must eliminate all milk products and sources of lactose to those who need only restrict their intake of milk as a beverage. Many people who have lactose intolerance are able to tolerate fermented dairy products such as yogurt, cheese, cooked milk, and even chocolate milk.

A lactose tolerance test is used to diagnosis this condition. This test consists of the administration of lactose in the amount that would be present in 1 qt of milk. If the client is lactose intolerant, symptoms will appear, and the blood glucose level will increase less than 25 mg above normal, indicating that the lactose has not been hydrolyzed. Another means of diagnosing this condition is by a breath test for the hydrogen that is produced by the intestinal bacteria acting on the lactose in the colon. Although quite a number of adults seem to have an intolerance for milk, many tolerate it well if the amount consumed at any one time is small, for example ½ to 1 cup per meal.

When working with hospitalized clients, nurses may encounter milk intolerance fairly frequently. It may be following surgery on the GI tract, with patients who have inflammatory diseases of the small intestine, or with clients for whom milk-based tube feedings or nutritional supplements are prescribed. The nurse should be aware that there are commercial liquid feedings and nutritional supplements available that are either low in lactose or lactose free for use with clients who experience intolerance to milk.

Malabsorption Related to Blunted Villi

Another type of malabsorption is caused by a blunting of the intestinal villi. Celiac disease is a genetic disorder that leads to this blunting of the villi and the resulting malabsorption. The number of microvilli on each intestinal villus is greatly reduced, and this reduces both the absorptive and the secretory capacity of the small intestine. The result is inadequate digestion of the energy nutrients and a poor absorption of all nutrients. The most frequent symptom is chronic diarrhea, which is characterized by foamy, bulky, fatty, and foul-smelling stools. This is the steatorrhea found in most cases of malabsorption. There are progressive symptoms of malnutrition and nutrient deficiencies that are secondary to malabsorption. The child with celiac disease resembles the appearance of the child with kwashiorkor with a pot belly and emaciated extremities. The disease usually takes a chronic course with gradual malnutrition. A *celiac crisis* is often precipitated by illness or infection. In adults the disease may be referred to as *nontropical sprue*.

The exact cause of or defect in this disease is still not known. It is known, however, that there is a distinct sensitivity of the client to the *gliadin* portion of the protein gluten, which is found in certain cereal grains. The ingestion of grains containing gluten interferes with normal maturation of the intestinal villi and produces the characteristic flattened appearance. Removal of gluten from the diet results in the return of the intestinal villi to a normal appearance (Krause and Mahan, 1979). Because of this association with gluten, this disease is sometimes referred to as *gluten-induced* or *gluten-sensitive enteropathy*.

The dietary intervention for this disorder is aimed at the removal of most sources of gluten from the diet. This involves the removal of wheat, rye, barley, and oats, because all of these grains contain gluten. The diet is therefore known as the gluten-restricted, or low-gluten, diet. At first this diet may seem to be a simple dietary modification; yet when one considers all the foods and food products that contain wheat flour, implementation becomes much more difficult. Figure 25-5 lists some of the foods that should be eliminated from this diet. The nurse should arrange for the client and his family to consult with the dietitian about implementing this diet. All regular breads and most cereal products including macaroni, noodles, and spaghetti will have to be eliminated. The client must be convinced of the importance of carefully reading ingredients on food labels and avoiding foods containing one of the four grains. The dietitian will be able to supply additional sources of information about the diet and special recipes. The two cereal grains that are allowed are corn and rice. Breads can be prepared using corn or rice flour or other specialty flours such as potato flour, soybean flour, or wheat-starch flour. The diet should also be high in protein and supplemented with vitamins and minerals to cure any nutrient deficiencies and replenish nutrient stores.

General: *Eliminate all foods and food products containing wheat, rye, oats, and barley.*

BREADS and CEREALS
All breads and desserts made from wheat or rye (crackers, cakes, and cookies)
All prepared mixes for muffins, biscuits, waffles, pancakes
Any product containing oatmeal, barley, or buckwheat
Breaded foods and bread crumbs
All wheat and rye cereals (oatmeal, wheat germ, barley and buckwheat)
Macaroni, spaghetti, noodles, dumplings

MEATS
All breaded meats
Cold cuts or processed meat with cereal fillers
Meat loaf prepared with bread crumbs or oatmeal
Croquettes
Bread stuffings

VEGETABLES
Any prepared with cream sauce or breaded

MISCELLANEOUS
Cream sauces with wheat flour
Salad dressings containing flour thickeners
All canned soups except clear broth
All cream soups thickened with wheat flour
Commercial ice cream
Ice cream cones
Puddings thickened with wheat flour
Postum and Ovaltine
Malted milk
Commercial candies containing cereal products
For adults: beer and ale

Figure 25-5. Selected foods to be excluded on a gluten-restricted diet.

CASE STUDY: A Woman with Crohn's Disease

Charlotte is a 46-year-old seamstress who is being treated for Crohn's disease. At 5 ft 6 in (168 cm) she weighs only 89 lb (40.4 kg). She has had two previous surgical operations for the disease, the first, five years ago, the second, two years ago. She has been admitted to the surgical unit of the hospital anticipating another colon resection and perhaps the formation of an ileostomy.

Now on her fourth week of hospitalization, Charlotte is being maintained on a low-residue diet and continuous hyperalimentation and intralipid therapy. She has recently developed a generalized skin rash covering her entire body. The rash is more intense on her arms and legs. The physician, after studying her serum laboratory levels, has concluded that the rash is the result of inadequate zinc levels.

Charlotte is ambulating and able to carry out her activities of daily living. Her husband visits regularly, often accompanied by their 23-year-old daughter.

Charlotte has expressed some impatience over her prolonged hospitalization. She occasionally becomes teary, stating that she hopes that she will not have to undergo another operation. She looks disgustedly at her hyperalimentation bottle, muttering about her forced dependence on it. She understands that she must be "built up" before she can undergo surgery. The current medical orders are:

1. Patient may get out of bed if desired.
2. Low-residue diet.
3. Calorie count, intake, and output.
4. High-Calorie, high-protein diet.
5. Daily weights.
6. Hyperalimentation, 125 cc/hr.
7. Intralipids, 500 cc every Monday, Wednesday, and Friday.
8. Sterile sheets on bed.
9. Nutritional assessment every Monday and Thursday.

QUESTIONS

1. Referring to the nursing diagnosis classification, what alteration in digestion, absorption, or both is Charlotte experiencing?
2. What are the overall objectives of the dietary management of Crohn's disease?
3. What are the general principles of the low-residue diet?
4. What is the rationale for the high-Calorie, high-protein aspect of Charlotte's diet?
5. Why was a Calorie count ordered? What tool could the nurse use to estimate Calories in foods?
6. What practical suggestions should the nurse offer Charlotte about her diet?

BIBLIOGRAPHY

Am. Dietetic Assoc. Position paper on bland diet in the treatment of chronic duodenal ulcer disease. *J. Am. Diet. Assoc.* 59:244, 1971.

Bennion, M. *Clinical Nutrition.* 1st Ed. New York: Harper & Row, Pubs., Inc., 1979.

Carson, H. S., and Roth, H. P. Popular beliefs about the peptic ulcer diet. *J. Am. Diet. Assoc.* 60:306, 1972.

Cohen S., and Booth, G. H., Jr. Gastric acid secretion and lower-esophageal-sphincter pressure in response to coffee and caffeine. *N. Engl. J. Med.* 293:897, 1975.

Demling L., and Koch, H. Condiments. *Acta Hepatogastroenterol.* 21:377, 1974.

Hardinge, M. G., Swarner, J. B., and Crooks, H. Carbohydrates in foods. *J. Am. Diet. Assoc.* 46:197, 1965.

Kramer, P., and Coso, E. K. Is the rationale for gastrointestinal diet therapy sound? *J. Am. Diet. Assoc.* 42:505, 1963.

Krause, M. V., and Mahan, L. K. *Food, Nutrition, and Diet Therapy.* 6th Ed. Philadelphia: W. B. Saunders Co., 1979.

Levitt, M. D. Intestinal gas production. *J. Am. Diet. Assoc.* 60:487, 1972.

Mitchell, H. S., Rynbergen, H. J., Anderson, L., and Dibble, M. V. *Nutrition in Health and Disease.* 16th Ed. Philadelphia: J. B. Lippincott Co., 1976.

Odell, A. C. Ulcer dietotherapy—past and present. *J. Am. Diet. Assoc.* 58:447, 1971.

Overton, M. H., and Lukert, B. P. *Clinical Nutrition: A Physiologic Approach.* Chicago: Year Book Medical Pubs., Inc., 1977.

Pennington, J. *Nurtritional Diet Therapy.* Palo Alto, Calif.: Bull Pub. Co., 1978.

Robinson, C. H., and Lawler, M. R. *Normal and Therapeutic Nutrition.* 15th Ed. New York: Macmillan, Inc., 1977.

Rowe, A. H., and Rowe, A., Jr. *Food Allergy: It's Manifestations and Control and the Elimination Diets.* Springfield, Ill.: Charles C. Thomas, Pub., 1972.

Rynbergen, H. J. In gastrointestinal disease fewer diet restrictions. *Am. J. Nurs.* 63(1):86, 1963.

Schneider, M. A., DeLuca, V., and Gray, S. J. Effect of spice ingestion upon stomach. *Am. J. Gastroenterol.* 26:722, 1956.

Taif, B. Innovations in ulcer therapy. *J. Pract. Nurs.* 26(5):32, 1976.

Thiele, V. F. *Clinical Nutrition.* St. Louis: The C. V. Mosby Co., 1976.

Welsh, J. D. Diet therapy of peptic ulcer disease. *Gastroenterology* 72:740, 1977.

⸺. Diet therapy in adult lactose malabsorption: Present practices. *Am. J. Clin. Nutr.* 31:592, 1978.

Weinstein, L., Olson, R. E., Van Itallie, T. B., Caso, E., Johnson, D., and Ingelfinger, F. J. Diet as related to gastrointestinal function. *J. Am. Med. Assoc.* 176:935, 1961.

Williams, S. R. *Nutrition and Diet Therapy.* 3rd Ed. St. Louis: The C. V. Mosby Co., 1977.

CHAPTER 26

Alterations in Nutrient Transport

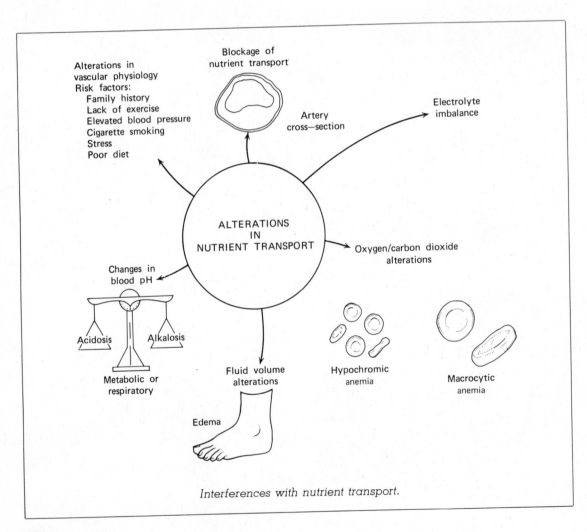

Interferences with nutrient transport.

Nutrients are transported within the body from the absorptive surface of the small intestine to the individual body cells by means of the blood. The heart pumps this nutrient-rich blood through the blood vessels. Any condition that produces an alteration in the flow of nutrients, the quantity of nutrients, or the pumping force of the heart muscle will interfere with the transport of nutrients to the individual cells.

ALTERATIONS IN VASCULAR PHYSIOLOGY

1. Predisposition to cardiovascular disease
2. Lifestyle inappropriate to cardiac disease
3. Predisposition to hypertension
4. Dependence on nursing supervision of controlled hypertension
5. Increased arterial blood pressure
6. Decreased arterial blood pressure

Cardiovascular disease is the leading cause of death in the United States and Canada. The development of alterations in vascular physiology leading to cardiovascular disease is influenced by several risk factors. For this reason cardiovascular disease is often referred to as a *multifactorial disease*. Several of these risk factors can be modified to improve the health of those who have a greater predisposition to the disease. Increased education of the population about the risk factors, increased hypertensive screening, improved antihypertensive therapy, improved emergency medical and cardiac care, and greater interest in physical fitness have all led to the lowering of the incidence of coronary heart disease by 15–20% in the United States from 1975 to 1978 (Mallison, 1978).

The assessment of predisposition to and actual alterations in vascular physiology involves a careful interview and dietary history to determine the risk factors present, laboratory values to determine the levels of cholesterol and lipids in the blood, and a physical examination to detect possible vascular abnormalities.

The risk factors for coronary heart disease may be classified as genetic, medical, and personal. People who have a positive family history of heart disease are much more likely to develop the disease. Age and sex are also considerations. Men over age 35 and women over age 55 have a higher incidence of heart disease. Women seem to be somewhat protected by the regular secretion of female hormones during the childbearing years. This protective advantage is lost, however, with the onset of menopause. The medical conditions that increase the risk of heart disease are obesity, hypertension, diabetes mellitus, and increased levels of serum cholesterol and triglycerides. Other risk factors are a sedentary lifestyle, lack of exercise, stress and tension, cigarette smoking, and a diet high in saturated fat and cholesterol. Of all these risk factors, three stand out as the most significant: hypertension, elevated levels of blood cholesterol, and cigarette smoking. Approximately 80% of the cases of death and disability that result from coronary heart disease occur in people who have one or more of these risk factors present (Vinson, 1975).

Vinson (1975) gives some guidelines for the risks involved when blood pressure, blood cholesterol, and cigarette smoking are at elevated levels. Inasmuch as men have a higher incidence of heart disease than women, the following are increased-risk statistics for men aged 30–62 who participated in the Framingham Massachusetts Heart Study (1949–1971). A man whose systolic blood pressure is over 150 mm Hg ("normal" = 120 mmHg) has more than twice the risk of a heart attack and four times the risk of a stroke than a man whose systolic pressure is under 120 mmHg. The risk of both stroke and heart attack is about three times greater in men whose blood cholesterol levels are 250 mg/100 ml as in men whose cholesterol levels are below 194 mg/100 ml. Smoking more than a pack of cigarettes a day doubles the risk of heart attack and increases the risk of a stroke by five times. The cumulative effect of all three of these factors is shown in Figures 26-1 and 26-2. Fortunately, many of these risk factors can be modified or eliminated from a person's life, including hypertension, cigarette smoking, obesity, sedentary living, and improper diet. A client cannot do anyting to influence his heredity, advancing age, or sex. The client who has a lifestyle inappropriate for his cardiac pathology, along with a family history of heart disease and one or more of the three primary risk factors, should be instructed about the risks involved. The nurse should discuss with the client reasonable ways to modify his habits to reduce the risk. It should be emphasized, however, that making these modifications does not guarantee that heart disease will not develop, but it does reduce the risk significantly.

Client Objectives

To be able to:

1. Discuss altered ingestion patterns that may prevent vascular disease.

2. Plan a diet that provides for adequate nutrition, takes into account alterations necessary for vascular disease, and is satisfying.

3. Consume nutrients that are outlined in such a plan.

Dietary Interventions

Planning the dietary intervention for altered vascular physiology may involve either a pre-

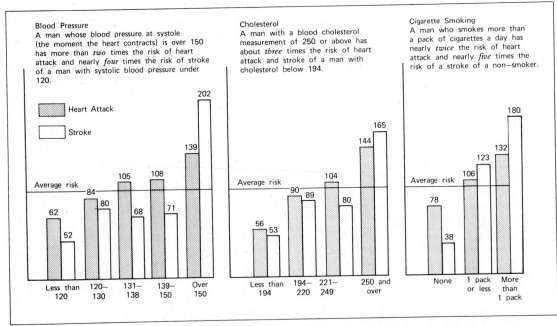

Figure 26-1. Risk factors in heart attack and stroke. These charts show the extent to which particular risk factors increased the risk of heart attack and stroke in the male population, aged 30–62, of Framingham, Mass. For each disease, columns below the black horizontal line indicate lower-than-average risk; columns above the line, higher-than-average risk. (Redrawn with permission from L. J. Vinson, "Modifying the Tide of Coronary Heart Disease." *Nursing Care* 11:12, November 1975.)

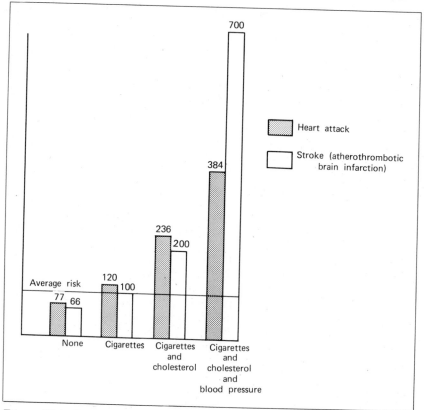

Figure 26-2. This chart shows how a combination of three major risk factors can increase the likelihood of heart attack and stroke. For purposes of illustration, this chart uses an abnormal blood pressure level of 180 systolic, and a cholesterol level of 310 in a 45-year-old man. (Redrawn with permission from L. J. Vinson, "Modifying the Tide of Coronary Heart Disease." *Nursing Care* 11:12, November 1975.)

ventive or therapeutic approach. The general objective is to reduce the risk of death or disability from coronary heart disease. More specifically, the objectives of the diet are to decrease the blood levels of cholesterol and triglycerides, to reduce elevated blood pressure, and to prevent and control edema. There are two major groups of diets that accomplish these objectives. The first is the fat-controlled diet and similar diets for the *hyperlipoproteinemias*. These diets involve a modification in both the total amount and the kind of fat. The emphasis is on avoidance of foods high in cholesterol and saturated fat and the use of low-fat foods that contain a higher proportion of mono- and polyunsaturated fats. The other group of diets is the sodium-restricted diets. There are several levels of sodium restriction ranging from mild to severe restriction.

The American Heart Association believes that sufficient evidence exists to confirm the relationship between dietary saturated fat and cholesterol and the increased incidence of coronary heart disease. Therefore, they recommend that, as a preventive measure, the US population follow a somewhat modified fat-controlled diet to lower serum cholesterol. This belief is also supported by the Task Force on Arteriosclerosis of the National Heart and Lung Institute, the Food and Nutrition Board of the National Research Council, the Council on Food and Nutrition of the American Medical Association, and the Inter-Society Commission on Heart Disease Resources (Vinson, 1975). The American Heart Association recommends that the Calories in the diet be adjusted to attain or maintain ideal body weight. The total fat content of the diet should be decreased, with a reduction in the intake of saturated fat and cholesterol and a substitution of polyunsaturated fat. The intake of simple sugars and salt should also be reduced.

The dietary recommendations of the American Heart Association for use as a preventive measure suggest a restriction of the type and amount of fat as well as the level of sodium intake. In the treatment of coronary heart disease, the fat-controlled diet is often combined with a sodium restriction. As a preventive measure the voluntary limitation of salt intake will not be harmful, for the daily requirement for sodium is quite low. Voluntary restriction of salt intake by adults may even have some benefits such as less fluid retention and decreased dependence on salt. In the therapeutic use of sodium-restricted diets, the level of sodium allowed may vary from 250 mg to 4,000 mg depending on the severity of fluid retention (edema or ascites) or the extent of blood pressure elevation. The fat-controlled and low-sodium diets are used for several interferences with nutrient transport. The rationale and general description of each diet is presented here.

Fat-controlled Diet

The extensive research that has been conducted in heart disease during the past three decades has established a firm relationship between the ingestion of foods high in saturated fat and cholesterol and the incidence of coronary heart disease. The Framingham study determined, among other things, that heart disease is a multifactorial disease and that many variables affect the blood levels of cholesterol (Mallison, 1978). Research has established that there is a definite relationship between the intake of saturated fat and cholesterol and the levels of blood lipids. Populations with high intakes of fat such as the US population were observed to have a higher incidence of coronary heart disease than populations with low intakes of fat such as the Japanese. It was also observed that the populations with low fat intakes had lower serum cholesterol levels than the US population (H. S. Mitchell et al., 1976). The increased intake of polyunsaturated fat has a lowering effect on serum cholesterol; monounsaturated fats do not have an observable effect on blood cholesterol. Yudkin (1972) reported that an increased level of carbohydrate in the diet leads to an increased level of serum triglycerides in some people. This phenomenon seems to be related to the ingestion of simple sugars and possibly fructose. Fructose is a component of sucrose, which is common table sugar.

Although much progress has been made in discovering the relationship of the dietary components to blood lipids and coronary heart disease, many aspects remain unknown. For example, there is no evidence that saturated fat and cholesterol *cause* coronary artery disease. There is no evidence to support the belief that modifying the diet to include less saturated fat and cholesterol and more polyunsaturated fat will prevent or cure coronary heart disease. There is also no evidence at present that the use of a modified-fat diet will lead to a reversal of artherosclerosis (H. S. Mitchell et al., 1976). Although some advise a modified-fat diet beginning in infancy or childhood as a preventive measure, there is no evidence of its beneficial effects.

Also, the long-term effects of a diet high in polyunsaturated fat are not known.

As research has continued, new relationships between dietary substances and heart disease have been unveiled. Some of these substances are dietary fiber, vitamin C, vitamin E, certain trace elements, coffee, and xanthine oxidase. The role of these substances in the cause or prevention of heart disease remains to be determined through additional research.

RATIONALE. The rationale of the fat-controlled diet is that such a diet will lower the blood levels of cholesterol and other lipids and thereby reduce the risk of coronary heart disease. The risk is reduced because there is a decrease in fatty substance being deposited within the arteries. Two other factors besides diet will lower blood lipids. One is weight reduction in those clients who are overweight, and the other is exercise. Weight reduction also helps to reduce strain on the heart. It is well documented today that regular exercise, especially aerobic exercise, improves cardiovascular efficiency and actually strengthens the heart muscle. Therefore, the client who has high blood lipids should be encouraged to lose weight with a low-Calorie diet. The low-Calorie diet is planned quite easily, incorporating the principles of the fat-controlled diet, as this diet is low in fat content. A regular program of exercise provides many benefits for the client with an increased risk of heart disease or one recovering from a heart attack. The physician should recommend an exercise program or the client should seek the physician's approval before beginning a program. Regular exercise improves cardiopulmonary circulation and efficiency, helps reduce levels of blood lipids and decrease blood pressure, and provides many psychological benefits as well. The client's active participation in his own health care is encouraged through both an exercise and a weight reduction program.

A more detailed classification of blood lipids deals with the elevation of the lipoproteins, the transporting form of fat in the blood (discussed in Chap. 11). There are four major kinds of lipoproteins. Lipoproteins are composed of protein, triglycerides, cholesterol, and phospholipids in variable proportions. Abnormalities of the lipoproteins are manifested in elevated levels of the lipoprotein fractions in the blood. These abnormalities are known as the *hyperlipoproteinemias*, of which there were five major types in the original classification by Frederickson (Frederickson et al., 1967). Since then, Type II has been reclassified into Type IIa and Type IIb, for a total of six types (Levy, 1972). The classification is based on the elevation of a specific lipoprotein. Because each of the lipoproteins is composed of a varying proportion of cholesterol and triglycerides as well as protein and phospholipids, the elevated lipoprotein is an elevation in either cholesterol or triglycerides or both. The dietary treatment is aimed specifically at reducing the elevated lipoprotein by modifying Calories, carbohydrate, protein, fat, cholesterol, and alcohol. A summary of the hyperlipoproteinemias and the dietary interventions is found in Table 26-1.

GENERAL PRINCIPLES. The general principles of the fat-controlled diet recommended by the American Heart Association and the diets for the hyperlipoproteinemias recommeded by the National Institutes of Health have many similarities. Both organizations recommend principles of diet planning:

1. Reduce the total proportion of fat in the diet.
2. Decrease the amount of saturated fat.
3. Decrease the cholesterol content of the diet.
4. Increase the intake of polyunsaturated fat.
5. Adjust the Calories to achieve or maintain ideal body weight.

TABLE 26-1. Classification of Hyperlipoproteinemias and Dietary Interventions

Type	Blood Lipid Pattern	Diet
Type I Inability to clear chylomicrons (dietary fat) from the plasma.	Cholesterol, normal or elevated.	Low fat (25–35 gm).
Type IIa Common; excess production or inadequate clearance of β-lipoproteins.	Increased β-lipoproteins (cholesterol elevated).	Modified fat (include high polyunsaturate to saturated fat ratio, very low cholesterol).
Type IIb Excess production or inadequate clearance of β-lipoproteins.	Increased β-lipoproteins (cholesterol elevated).	Adjust Calories to achieve ideal weight; adjust Calories to maintain ideal weight.
Type III Relatively uncommon.	Increased β-lipoproteins (cholesterol elevated); increased triglycerides.	Carbohydrate, 40% of Calories; fat, 40% of Calories; decrease saturated fat; very low cholesterol; increase protein to 18–20%; alcohol may be restricted.
Type IV Associated with diabetes mellitus and premature atherosclerosis; excess production or inadequate clearance of pre-β-lipoproteins.	Incrased pre-β-lipoproteins (increased triglycerides).	Adjust Calories to achieve ideal weight; adjust Calories to maintain ideal weight; carbohydrate, 45% of Calories; concentrated sweets restricted; decrease saturated fat; increase polyunsaturated fat; cholesterol moderately restricted.
Type V Secondary to acute metabolic disorders (pancreatitis, alcoholism, nephrosis); excess of pre-β-lipoproteins and decreased removal of chylomicrons.	Elevated chylomicrons; elevated pre-β-lipoproteins (increased triglycerides).	Adjust Calories to achieve ideal weight; adjust Calories to maintain ideal weight; total fat restricted to 30% of Calories; decrease saturated fat; increase polyunsaturated fat; carbohydrate, 50% of Calories; cholesterol, moderately restricted.

SOURCE: National Heart, Lung, and Blood Institute, *The Dietary Management of Hyperlipoproteinemia: A Handbook for Physicians and Dietitians*, DHEW Publ. No. (NIH) 78-110. Washington, D.C.: Public Health Serv., Nat'l Instit. of Health, 1978.

6. Decrease the intake of simple sugars, and increase the intake of complex carbohydrates.

The recommendations of the fat-controlled diet of the American Heart Association and those for the hyperlipoproteinemias are quite similar, but the diets for the hyperlipo- proteinemias vary slightly depending on the particular lipoprotein that is elevated. The dietary recommendations of the American Heart Association are:

1. Adjust Calories in the diet to achieve and maintain optimal body weight.

2. Reduce the total fat content of the diet to 30–35% of the total Calories, with saturated fat comprising less than 10% of total Calories and polyunsaturated fat comprising up to 10% of total Calories.

3. Restrict dietary cholesterol to approximately 300 mg/day.

4. Decrease intake of simple sugars and increase the intake of fruits, vegetables, and cereals.

5. Avoid excessive use of salt.

Similar recommendations were also made by the Senate Select Committee on Nutrition and Human Needs in the report *Dietary Goals for the United States* (described in Chap. 7). Table 26-2 compares the typical American diet with the recommendations of the American Heart Association and the *U.S. Dietary Goals*. It should be noted that the restrictions in the *U.S. Dietary Goals* are quite similar but even more strict than the recommendations of the American Heart Association.

FOOD RECOMMENDATIONS. When the client with heart disease does not cook for himself, the person responsible for his food prepara-

tion should be present when the dietitian gives the diet instruction or when the nurse discusses the dietary recommendations with the client. Incorporating the principles of the fat-controlled diet into the client's eating habits necessitates translating the principles into actual foods. Even though the client may understand the reasons for the fat-controlled diet and the general principles behind it, he may resist when these principles are translated into foods that are allowed. Simply presenting the client with a list of "allowed" and "not allowed" foods may foster resentment or refusal to modify eating habits.

A better approach may be to explain the food sources of saturated fat, cholesterol, and polyunsaturated fat. On the fat-controlled diet certain foods are recommended for use; some are restricted in use; and some are recommended for avoidance or use in restricted amounts. Some clients may be psychologically able to avoid all foods on the "not allowed list" except for one very favorite food such as sour cream or a favorite variety of cheese made from whole milk. If most of the other provisions of the diet are followed and the client understands why unlimited quantities of the

TABLE 26-2. Comparison of the Typical American Diet, the American Heart Association Recommendations, and the Dietary Goals for the United States

Nutrient	Typical American Diet	American Heart Association Recommendations	US Dietary Goals
Total Calories	Excessive.	Reduce Calories eaten to achieve and maintain ideal body weight.	—
Total fat (percentage of Calories)	40–42%	30–35%	30%
Saturated	15%	10%	10%
Monounsaturated	16–17%	10%	10%
Polyunsaturated	5–6%	10%	10%
Cholesterol	600–700 mg	300 mg	300 mg
Carbohydrate (percentage of Calories)	40–45%	50–55%	58%
Starch	20–25%	Increase.	48%
Simple sugars	15–20%	Decrease.	10%
Protein (percentage of Calories)	12–15%	12–15%	12–15%
Sodium	2,500–6,000 mg	Avoid excessive sodium.	5 gm

favorite food are not allowed, he may be permitted to eat the food in limited quantities occasionally. If the client confides to the nurse a special fondness for such a food, the nurse may want to check with the dietitian about the possibility of allowing the food on a limited basis.

Most foods high in saturated fat and cholesterol are of animal origin. These include foods primarily from the meat and milk groups. A true vegetarian would have very little to be concerned about if placed on a fat-controlled diet. A lactovegetarian would need to restrict the intake of high-fat dairy products, and a lacto-ovo-vegetarian would also need to restrict the number of eggs consumed in a week.

The nurse may begin to explain the fat-controlled diet by naming foods high in saturated fat and cholesterol. All foods of animal origin contain some saturated fat, cholesterol, or both. The objective is not to eliminate all foods of animal origin—because these foods are excellent sources of protein, vitamins, and minerals—but to restrict the intake of those foods of animal origin that are the highest in saturated fat and cholesterol. The amount of meat is also restricted to no more than 6 oz/day—an amount that, though it may seem small to many Americans, more than adequately meets the recommended daily intake from the basic four food groups for all ages. The meats containing the highest amounts of saturated fat and cholesterol are the "red meats"—beef, pork, and lamb. Saturated fat and cholesterol are found in both the visible fat surrounding these meats and the fat (marbling) dispersed throughout. These meats are often restricted to no more than five (3–4 oz) servings a week.

The remainder of the meals in which meat is consumed should consist of the "light meats" such as chicken, turkey, veal, and fish. Egg yolks are quite high in cholesterol, and they are limited to no more than three a week. Egg whites contain no cholesterol, and they may be used as desired. The meats to be se-

verely restricted or completely avoided are duck; goose; glandular and organ meats; and processed meats such as luncheon meats, frankfurters, and bacon. Shellfish are fairly high in cholesterol. Some fat-controlled diets recommend eliminating them, but others permit limited quantities. Peanut butter is neither saturated nor unsaturated. It contains a high proportion of monounsaturated fatty acids, which have no effect on serum cholesterol.

A few important shopping tips should be mentioned concerning the purchase of pork and beef. Some cuts of these meats are higher in saturated fats than others and should be avoided. Pork chops or lean pork loin roasts or ham may be used. Also, fresh or smoked Canadian bacon may be used. The cuts of beef selected should be as lean as possible. Regular hamburger should not be used because it is too high in fat content; hamburger should instead be from the round or chuck portions. The best method is to suggest that the homemaker select a very lean portion of round steak or chuck and have the butcher grind it for hamburger. The steaks allowed should come from the loin or round. These steaks would include round, cube, sirloin, T-bone, porterhouse, and tenderloin. Steaks should be selected with less marbling of the fat than is usually desired. USDA Good beef is preferable to USDA Choice because there is less marbling.

Milk products that are recommended are skimmed and fat free. Low-fat or 2% products may be used by those clients who find skim milk completely intolerable. If this substitution is made, the client should be informed that the low-fat milks do have a higher amount of saturated fat and cholesterol. The client should be advised to use meats that are the lowest in saturated fat and cholesterol to counteract the higher levels supplied by the milk. Low-fat or skim-milk cheeses such as farmer's cheese, mozarella, and sapsago may be used. Cottage cheese and yogurt made from skim or low-fat milk are allowed. All chocolate milk, whole milk, all kinds of cream including sour cream, ice cream, and most cheeses should be avoided or severely restricted.

All fruits and vegetables are allowed with only a few exceptions. Vegetables prepared with a cream sauce or escalloped are to be avoided. Avocados and olives are high in fat content and cholesterol and should be avoided. Potato chips and French-fried potatoes should be avoided because the kind of fat used for frying is generally not known and it is often a saturated fat. Any type of commercial bread is allowed as long as it has not been prepared with extra fat or eggs. Commercial pastries, doughnuts, biscuits, muffins, cornbread, waffles, pancakes, cookies, crackers, cakes, and bakery mixes should all be avoided because the kind of fat is unknown and the proportion of fat in these products is much higher than in regular bread.

The selection of fats, of course, is very important for the client on a fat-controlled diet. As a rule vegetable fats are unsaturated and animal fats are saturated. Some vegetable fats are more desirable because they are more unsaturated. The vegetable fat that is the highest in polyunsaturated fat is safflower oil. It may be purchased in liquid form, but a safflower oil margarine is not yet available. Sunflower and soybean oil are the next highest in polyunsaturated fat, but they are often combined with another more saturated oil or mixed with a hydrogenated oil. The most acceptable margarines now on the market for the fat-controlled diet are manufactured from pure liquid corn oil. This should be the first ingredient listed on the label. The client should be encouraged to use a soft-tub margarine made from liquid safflower or corn oil in preference to a stick margarine because the soft ones have a higher proportion of the preferred oil. The other fats and oils contain varying proportions of polyunsaturated, monounsaturated, and saturated fatty acids. Salad dressings may be selected by reading the label and selecting those made from the allowed oils. A summary of the continuum of food fats is shown in Figure 26-3.

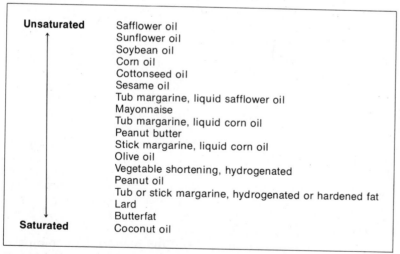

Figure 26-3. Saturation of dietary fats and oils. (Reprinted with permission from M. V. Krause and L. K. Mahan, *Food, Nutrition, and Diet Therapy*, 11th Ed. Philadelphia: W. B. Saunders Co., 1979.)

Most regular desserts should be omitted because a saturated fat has been used in their preparation. Two desserts that *are* allowed on the fat-controlled diet are angel food cake and sherbet. A summary of the fat-controlled diet is presented in Table 26-3. A day's meals following the recommendations of the American Heart Association for the fat-controlled diet are found in Figure 26-4.

PRACTICAL   CONSIDERATIONS.   The   nurse should present a positive approach to the fat-controlled diet by emphasizing the foods that *are* allowed. The client should be instructed concerning what to look for on food labels (Fig. 26-5). Although many commercial foods have been discouraged in the preceding paragraphs, there is a way the client can still have many of these favorite foods in his diet. Most of the baked foods that were restricted because of the kind of fat used may be prepared at home using the allowed fats and oils. The American Heart Association has published an excellent cookbook for the fat-controlled diet (Eshleman and Winston, 1979). It can be used not only by clients on this type of diet but by any person who desires to decrease his intake of saturated fat and cholesterol. It includes recipes for most of the restricted bakery items and breads with allowed-fat substitutions. Also, such foods as potato chips and French-fried potatoes may be prepared at home if they are fried in a polyunsaturated oil. Fried foods and baked products would need to be restricted, however, if the client's diet had a Calorie restriction for weight loss. The cookbook contains many helpful suggestions and substitutions that can be made on a fat-controlled diet.

Fortunately, grocery stores also carry many products that can be substituted for the restricted foods on a fat-controlled diet. There are now several egg substitutes that can be used in place of scrambled eggs or substituted in recipes. There are also some breakfast-meat substitutes made to resemble ham, bacon, and sausage. These substitutes, however, are quite high in sodium content and should not be used by the client who is also on a salt-restricted diet. There are several low-fat cheeses and a specially formulated low-saturated-fat cheese. The client should be cautioned against the use of nondairy creamers because many of them are manufactured from coconut oil. A few nondairy creamers, however, are high in polyunsaturated fat.

The methods of food preparation are important on a fat-controlled diet. The main objective of the diet is to decrease the total amount of fat. This can be accomplished not only by selecting foods lower in fat content but by using food preparation methods that require little or no fat. All the visible fat should be carefully trimmed from the meat before it is cooked. The cooking methods most recommended are roasting, baking, broiling, grilling, and braising (described in Chap. 8). When meat is roasted, it should always be placed on a rack. This allows the fat to drip away from the meat as it cooks. A low roasting temperature (350 F, or 177 C) will help to increase the fat drip-off (Eshleman and Winston, 1979). Broiling and grilling are also good methods of meat preparation because the meat is suspended above the source of heat on a grill or rack.

Braising and stewing are cooking methods that both require the addition of water or other liquid. A larger amount of liquid is usually added during stewing. Long, slow cooking in this moist environment will help to tenderize tough cuts of meat. One slight disadvantage, however, is that the fat from the meat drips directly into the cooking liquid. For this reason it is suggested that the meat be cooked several hours ahead of time or the day before so that the liquid can be refrigerated before it is consumed or used in further steps of food preparation. When the liquid is refrigerated, the fat will solidify on the top so it can be removed quite easily. Skimming the fat while the liquid is still hot is a much less efficient way of removing the fat and is not recommended. Meat drippings may be used

TABLE 26-3. Fat-controlled, Low-cholesterol Diet

Food Groups	Recommended	Avoid or Use Sparingly
Meat, poultry, fish, dried beans, and peas, nuts, eggs	**Chicken, turkey, veal, fish in most of your meat meals for the week.** Shellfish: clams, crab, lobster, oysters, scallops—use a 4-oz serving as a substitute for meat.	Duck, goose. Shrimp is moderately high in cholesterol. Use a 4-oz serving in a meat meal no more than once a week.
	Beef, lamb, pork, ham less frequently. Choose lean ground meat and lean cuts of meat; trim all visible fat before cooking; bake, broil, roast, or stew so that you can discard the fat that cooks out of the meat.	Heavily marbled and fatty meats, spare ribs, mutton, frankfurters, sausages, fatty hamburgers, bacon, luncheon meats. Organ meats: liver, kidney, heart, sweetbreads, are very high in cholesterol. Since liver is very rich in vitamins and iron, it should not be eliminated from the diet completely. Use a 4-oz serving in a meat meal no more than once a week.
	Nuts and dried beans and peas: Kidney beans, lima beans, baked beans, lentils, chick-peas (garbanzos), split peas are high in vegetable protein and may be used in plate of meat occasionally.	
	Egg whites as desired.	Egg yolks: limit to 3 per week including eggs used in cooking. Cakes, batters, sauces, and other foods containing egg yolks.
Vegetables and fruit (fresh, frozen, or canned)	**One serving should be a source of Vitamin C:** Broccoli, cabbage (raw), tomatoes, berries, cantaloupe, grapefruit (or juice), mango, melon, orange (or juice), papaya, strawberries, tangerines.	
	One serving should be a source of Vitamin A—dark green leafy or yellow vegetables, or yellow fruits: Broccoli, carrots, chard, chicory, escarole, greens (beet, collard, dandelion, mustard, turnip), kale, peas, rutabagas, spinach, string beans, sweet potatoes and yams, watercress, winter squash, yellow corn, apricots, cantaloupe, mango, papaya.	
	Other vegetables and fruits are also very nutritious; they should be eaten in salads, main dishes, snacks, and desserts, *in addition* to the recommended daily allowances of high vitamin A and C vegetables and fruits.	If you must limit your Calories use vegetables such as potatoes, corn, or lima beans sparingly. To add variety to your diet, one serving (½ cup of any one of these may be substituted for one serving of bread or cereals.

TABLE 26-3. Fat-controlled, Low-cholesterol Diet (*Continued*)

Food Groups	Recommended	Avoid or Use Sparingly
Bread and Cereals (whole grain, enriched, or restored)	**Breads made with a minimum of saturated fat:** White enriched (including raisin bread), whole wheat, English muffins, French bread, Italian bread, oatmeal bread, pumpernickel, rye bread. Biscuits, muffins, and griddle cakes made at home, using an allowed liquid oil as shortening. Cereal (hot and cold), rice, melba toast, matzo, pretzels. Pasta: macaroni, noodles (except egg noodles), spaghetti.	Butter rolls, commercial biscuits, muffins, donuts, sweet rolls, cakes, crackers, egg bread, cheese bread, commercial mixes containing dried eggs and whole milk.
Milk products	**Milk products that are low in dairy fats:** Fortified skim (nonfat) milk and fortified skim milk powder, low-fat milk. The label on the container should show that the milk is fortified with vitamins A and D. The word *fortified* alone is not enough. Buttermilk made from skim milk, yogurt made from skim milk, canned evaporated skim milk, cocoa made with low-fat milk. Cheeses made from skim or partially skim milk, such as cottage cheese, creamed or un-creamed (uncreamed, perferably); farmer's baker's, or hoop cheese; mozarella and sapsago cheeses. Processed modified-fat cheeses (skim milk and polyunsaturated fat).	**Whole milk and whole milk products:** Chocolate milk; canned whole milk; ice cream; all creams including sour, half and half, whipped; whole milk yogurt. Nondairy cream substitutes (usually contain coconut oil, which is very high in saturated fat). Butter. Cheeses made from cream or whole milk.
Fats and oils (polyunsaturated) An individual allowance should include about 2–4 T daily (depending on how many Calories you can afford) in the form of margarine, salad dressing, and shortening.	**Margarines, liquid oil shortenings, salad dressings and mayonnaise containing any of these polyunsaturated vegetable oils:** Corn oil, cottonseed oil, safflower oil, sesame seed oil, soybean oil, sunflower seed oil. Margarines and other products high in polyunsaturates can usually be identified by their label, which lists a recommended *liquid* vegetable oil as the *first*	**Solid fats and shortenings:** Butter, lard, salt pork fat, meat fat, completely hydrogenated margarines and vegetable shortenings, products containing coconut oil. Peanut oil and olive oil may be used occasionally for flavor, but they are low in polyunsaturates and do not take the place of the recommended oils.

TABLE 26-3. (Continued)

Food Groups	Recommended	Avoid or Use Sparingly
	ingredient, and one or more partially hydrogenated vegetable oils as additional ingredients. Diet margarines are low in Calories because they are low in fat. Therefore it takes twice as much diet margarine to supply the polyunsaturates contained in a recommended margarine.	
Desserts, beverages, snacks, condiments The foods on this list are acceptable because they are low in saturated fat and cholesterol. If you have eaten your daily allowance from the first five lists, however, these foods will be in excess of your nutritional needs, and many of them also may exceed your Calorie limits for maintaining a desirable weight. If you must limit your Calories, limit your portions of the foods on this list as well. Moderation should be observed especially in the use of alcoholic drinks, ice milk, sherbet, sweets, and bottled drinks.	**Low in Calories or no Calories:** Fresh fruit and fruit canned without sugar; tea, coffee (no cream), cocoa powder; water ices; gelatin; fruit whip; puddings made with nonfat milk; low-Calorie drinks; vinegar, mustard, ketchup, herbs, spices. **High in Calories:** Frozen or canned fruit with sugar added; jelly, jam, marmalade, honey; pure sugar candy such as gumdrops, hard candy, mint patties (not chocolate); imitation ice cream made with safflower oil; cakes, pies, cookies, and puddings made with polyunsaturated fat in place of solid shortening; angel food cake; nuts, especially walnuts; peanut butter; bottled drinks; fruit drinks; ice milk; sherbet; wine, beer, whiskey.	Coconut and coconut oil; commercial cakes, pies, cookies, and mixes; frozen cream pies; commercially fried foods such as potato chips and other deep fried snacks; whole milk puddings; chocolate pudding (high in cocoa butter and therefore high in saturated fat); ice cream.

SOURCE: Reprinted with permission, American Heart Association.

if they are refrigerated and the fat is removed. Fat-free gravies may be prepared by using 1 cup of fat-free broth or bouillon and 1 T of cornstarch or flour and shaking in a jar. This thickened broth is now added slowly to the remaining broth that has been heated in a pan. The mixture is stirred until it thickens, and allowed seasonings are added.

Cream sauces may be prepared for vegetables using skim milk and polyunsaturated margarine. Some low-fat cheese may even be added to make a cheese sauce. Whenever frying is necessary the client should be instructed to use the allowed margarine or oil. The nurse will probably want to recommend the *American Heart Association Cookbook* to the client for numerous other helpful suggestions, substitutions, and recipes.

Dining in restaurants may seem to pose difficulties for the client on the fat-controlled diet, but many of these difficulties can be greatly reduced with careful thought and planning. The client should be advised to avoid fried foods, combined foods, and

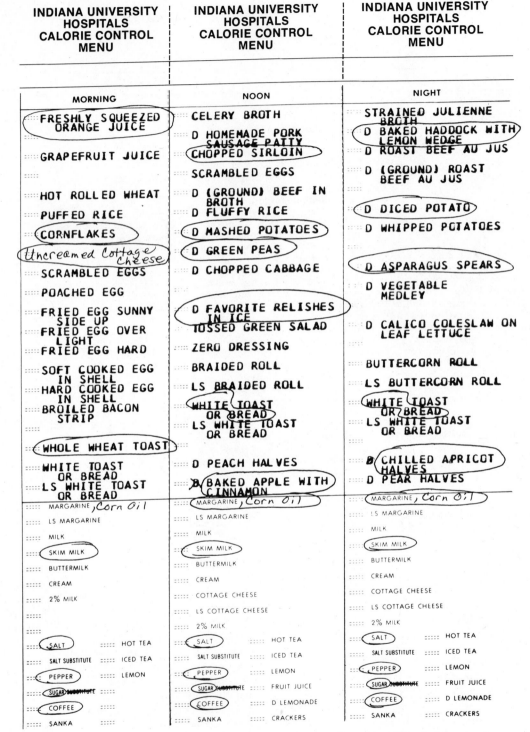

Figure 26-4. Fat-controlled diet menu. (Courtesy Indiana University Hospitals)

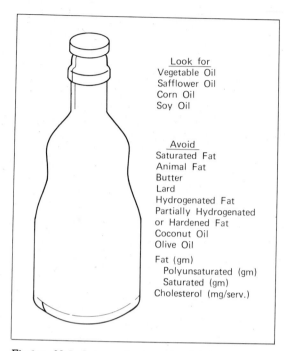

Look for
Vegetable Oil
Safflower Oil
Corn Oil
Soy Oil

Avoid
Saturated Fat
Animal Fat
Butter
Lard
Hydrogenated Fat
Partially Hydrogenated
or Hardened Fat
Coconut Oil
Olive Oil

Fat (gm)
    Polyunsaturated (gm)
    Saturated (gm)
Cholesterol (mg/serv.)

Figure 26-5. Information on food labels helpful for clients on fat-controlled diets.

sauces and gravies in a restaurant. Many restaurants are beginning to offer a more flexible menu that is more suitable for people who are on therapeutic diets. Most restaurants and cafeterias offer both skim milk and margarine. Even if the particular margarine offered is not a corn oil margarine, it is a better choice than butter. It may be better to order food a la carte from the menu. If the client understands the fat-controlled diet, is convinced of its importance, and has a sincere desire to adhere to it, he will be able to select an acceptable menu. Abel and Powell (1971) list the following foods as an example of a satisfactory restaurant meal for someone on a fat-controlled diet:

Clear soup, tomato juice, or fruit cup
Baked or broiled fish, chicken, turkey, or a lean steak (no gravy)

Baked potato or other vegetable without butter
Tossed salad with vinegar and oil dressing
Fruit, sherbet, or gelatin

Sodium-restricted Diets

The low-sodium diet is the most frequently prescribed but the least adhered to of all the therapeutic diets. Physicians may use such vague statements in making verbal recommendations to the client as "cut down on salt"; "don't add any salt at the table"; "avoid very salty foods"; "watch your salt intake"; and "reduce your sodium intake." Nurses may be aware that there are different levels of sodium restrictions and that there is some difference between salt and sodium, but the actual principles of the sodium-restricted diet are so vague to them that they may simply tell the client, "Watch your intake of salt." Dietitians generally have a better knowledge of the sodium-restricted diets, but they may be too dogmatic in their instructions to the client, emphasizing only those foods that must be avoided. Also, eating too much salt or sodium does not generally precipitate severe medical emergencies, but this does not make the benefit of the sodium-restricted diet any less. Medical personnel must be convinced of the benefits of sodium-restricted diets, informed about the general principles and the sodium content of foods, and empathetic to the client's difficulty adjusting to low-sodium foods.

RATIONALE.   The purpose of the low-sodium diet is to decrease the amount of extracellular fluid and sodium. The retention of sodium leads to a retention of fluid in the interstitial spaces. Three signs are related to the retention of sodium and fluid: edema, ascites, and hypertension. Treatment is aimed at reducing the extracellular fluid volume by depleting the body stores of sodium (H. S. Mitchell et al., 1976). The means used to reduce the fluid accumulation is the low-sodium diet, diuretic drugs, or a combination.

GENERAL PRINCIPLES.   Sodium-restricted diets are known by a variety of names: *low salt, salt free, salt poor, mild sodium restriction, moderate sodium restriction, low sodium,* and *no added salt.* Two things are wrong with these vague descriptions of sodium-restricted diets. First, *salt* and *sodium* are not equivalent terms. Second, a level of sodium in milligrams or milliequivalents should be specified for clarity. The terms *salt free* and *sodium free* are complete misnomers because all foods contain some natural salt or sodium with the exception of fruits and some fats and oils. Sodium is an essential nutrient, although the daily requirement is quite low.

Sodium is a component of the compound salt, which is also known as *sodium chloride* (NaCl). The sodium chloride compound is composed of 40% sodium and 60% chloride, so that 1 gm (1,000 mg) of salt contains 400 mg of sodium and 600 mg of chloride. Stated in common household units, 1 t of table salt contains approximately 2,300 mg of sodium (see Fig. 26-6).

The average daily intake of sodium varies greatly depending on the kind and quantity of food consumed and the amount of salt a person adds to the food. South American Indians consume as little as 75 mg of sodium a day; some inhabitants of northern Japan consume in excess of 20 gm a day. By comparison, people in the United States consume between 3 and 6 gm of sodium daily (Robinson and Lawler, 1977). Those, however, who salt their food heavily may be consuming up to 10–12 gm of sodium daily. If these levels were stated in terms of daily "salt intake," the levels would be even higher. For example, a daily intake of 3–6 gm of sodium represents a corresponding intake of 7.5–15 gm of salt. The level of sodium is used more frequently when discussing low-sodium diets because the concern is with the intake of the sodium portion of sodium chloride. There are many other sources of sodium besides salt. The diets should, therefore, be referred to as low-sodium or sodium-restricted diets and never as low-salt or salt-free diets.

The craving for salt is *not* based on the body's need for salt or sodium (Snively et al., 1974). The taste or craving for salt is acquired during the client's lifetime and is controlled by personal food habits, influenced heavily by culture and custom.

The sodium content of foods or diets is specified in either milligrams or grams or milliequivalents. Because many physicians and hospitals use milliequivalents, the nurse should know how to make this conversion readily: 1 mEq of sodium equals 23 mg, which is the gram-atomic weight of sodium. Milligrams are converted to milliequivalents by dividing the number of milligrams of sodium by 23. Milliequivalents are converted to milligrams by multiplying the milliequivalents by 23. The following conversions provide an example:

1000 mg sodium ÷ 23 = 43 mEq sodium
43 mEq sodium × 23 = 989 mg sodium

Because milliequivalents are usually rounded off to the nearest whole number, reconversion to milligrams will yield a few milligrams above or below the original level.

There are four common levels of sodium-restricted diets: *mild sodium restriction* (2500–4000 mg), *moderate sodium restriction* (1000–

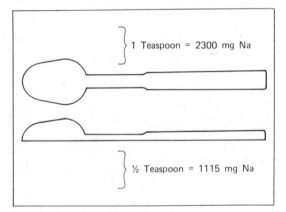

1 Teaspoon = 2300 mg Na

½ Teaspoon = 1115 mg Na

Figure 26-6. Sodium content of 1 t of table salt.

2000 mg), *strict sodium restriction* (500 mg), and *severe sodium restriction* (250 mg). With the increased use and effectiveness of diuretic drugs, the 250 mg sodium diet, which is so very restrictive, is seldom used anymore. If it is ordered, it is used only in severe cases of edema, ascites, or hypertension for a short time during hospitalization. The most common sodium-restricted diet ordered is the 2–3 gm sodium diet. To get a general idea of the foods restricted on each of these diets, it is easiest to begin with the least restrictive diet, the mild sodium restriction (2–3 gm sodium), and proceed to the most restrictive diet (250 mg sodium):

MILD SODIUM RESTRICTION (2500–4500 mg)

- Salt may be used lightly in cooking.
- No salt may be used at the table.
- Only very salty foods are omitted.

MODERATE SODIUM RESTRICTION (1000–2000 mg)

- A total of $\frac{1}{4}$ t/day of salt may be used in cooking or at the table OR regular bread or regular butter or margarine may be substituted for the salt.
- No salty foods are used.

STRICT SODIUM RESTRICTION (500 mg)

- No salt is allowed at the table or in cooking.
- All salty foods are eliminated.
- Only low-sodium breads and cereals are allowed.
- Milk is restricted to 2 cups daily.
- Meat is limited to 5–6 oz daily plus one egg.

SEVERE SODIUM RESTRICTION (250 mg)

- Same as the 500 mg diet above except:
- Meat is limited to 2–4 oz daily.
- Eggs are limited to 3 per week.
- Only low-sodium milk may be used.

FOOD RECOMMENDATIONS. All foods contain some natural sodium, but foods from animal sources contain more sodium than those from plant sources. The cells of meat are surrounded by a physiological saline (salt) solution (H. S. Mitchell et al., 1976). Meat, milk, and eggs that are not processed or prepared with salt still contain significant amounts of sodium. The most significant source of sodium in the diet comes from the salt added during processing and at the table. Plain, unprocessed food does not contain very much sodium. Two cups of milk (240 mg), one egg (25 mg), and 4 oz of meat (100 mg), contribute about 365 mg of sodium. Four servings of regular bread and cereal (480 mg) and three pats of regular margarine (150 mg) add 630 mg of sodium. These basic foods would compose a 1,000 mg sodium diet if low-sodium vegetables were used. The dietitian can make adjustments with the low-sodium diet to allow for client preferences and still maintain the specified level.

A food that is high in sodium content does not necessarily taste "salty." Organ meats are generally higher in sodium content than muscle meats. All shellfish are high in sodium content, but other salt water fish contain about the same amount of sodium as freshwater fish. Cheese, being a concentrated product prepared from milk, is naturally high in sodium. A few vegetables are high in sodium content: artichokes, beet greens, beets, carrots, celery, Swiss chard, dandelion greens, hominy, kale, mustard greens, sauerkraut, spinach, and turnips. These vegetables would need to be eliminated on the 1,000 mg and lower diets. Regular bread contains approximately 120 mg per slice. As most people eat at least two slices per day, regular bread is quite a high source of sodium. By contrast, one slice of homemade white bread prepared without salt contains only 5 mg of sodium. The regular butter or margarine that is spread on bread and added to vegetables is also a significant source of sodium. Each pat or teaspoon of margarine or butter adds 50 mg of sodium to the diet. Perhaps the European custom of eating unsalted margarine or butter is quite advisable.

Sodium compounds are added to foods during processing and in the preparation of food at home. Some of the sodium added during processing is quite obvious in the salt added to crackers and potato chips and the salt used to cure ham. Sodium compounds are added as leavening agents (baking powder and baking soda), as preservatives, and as flavor enhancers. All canned foods with the exception of canned fruit are high in sodium content. A comparison of the sodium content of fresh, canned, and frozen vegetables is found in Table 26-4. A 10-oz can of commercially prepared beef stew may contain as much as 9,000 mg of sodium!

Several of the products used in home food preparation are quite high in sodium and should be avoided. Baking powder and baking soda used in home and commercial baking are high in sodium. Monosodium glutamate is used as a flavor enhancer, and it is a common ingredient in meat tenderizer. Clients on a sodium-restricted diet should be warned against the use of flavor enhancers that contain monosodium glutamates and meat tenderizers. Soy sauce is also quite high in sodium. The client should be advised to read the product labels carefully and to avoid items that list salt, soda, or sodium (chemical symbol is Na) as ingredients.

Sodium content is also high in some water supplies. When the local water supply contains more than 20 mg of sodium per liter, this contribution of sodium to the diet can be significant. The nurse can find out about the sodium content of the water by phoning the state or local department of health (H. S. Mitchell et al., 1976). Water that has been run through a water softener is also higher in sodium content. The softening process involves the exhange of sodium ions for calcium and other ions that contribute to water hardness. It is possible to bypass the cold water faucets and soften only the hot water. The

TABLE 26-4. Effect of Processing on Sodium Content of ½ Cup (100 gm) Portions of Vegetables

Vegetable	Sodium Content (mg)
Asparagus	
Fresh	1
Frozen	1
Regular canned	236
Low-sodium canned	3
Green beans	
Fresh	4
Frozen	1
Regular canned	236
Low-sodium canned	2
Carrots	
Fresh, raw	47
Fresh, cooked	33
Regular canned	236
Low-sodium canned	39
Corn	
Fresh	tr
Frozen	1
Regular canned	236
Low-sodium canned	2
Peas	
Fresh	1
Frozen, with salt	187
Frozen, without salt	115
Regular canned	236
Low-sodium canned	3
Spinach	
Fresh	50
Frozen	49
Regular canned	236
Low-sodium canned	32
Tomatoes	
Fresh	3
Cooked	4
Regular canned	130
Low-sodium canned	3
Tomato juice	
Regular canned	200
Low sodium canned	3

SOURCE: *Composition of Foods: Raw, Processed, and Prepared.* Agricultural Handbook No. 8, USDA, 1963.

nurse should encourage the client to have the sodium content of the household water supply checked. If the client is on a 1,000 mg sodium-restricted diet or less and the sodium content of the home water supply is high, the client should be encouraged to use bottled distilled water for drinking and food preparation.

Other hidden sources of sodium are toothpastes and mouthwashes. The nurse should encourage the client to rinse his mouth thoroughly after using these products. Over-the-counter medications such as aspirin, cough medicines, and laxatives may contain large amounts of sodium. Also, some prescription drugs such as antibiotics, sulfa drugs, and barbiturates may contain sodium. The nurse should caution the client to avoid all medications unless they have been prescribed or advised by a physician. The client should always be instructed to read the labels carefully when purchasing food for the low-sodium diet (see Fig. 26-7).

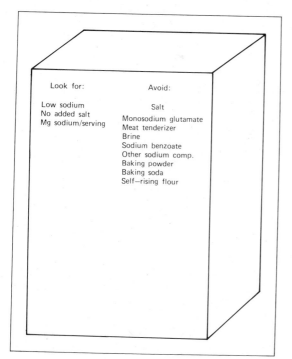

Figure 26-7. Information on food labels helpful for clients on low-sodium diets.

Several types of low-sodium products are available for use by clients on sodium-restricted diets. Low-sodium canned vegetables are available for clients who are on a 1,000 mg of sodium or lower diet. The term *dietetic* on a food label means only that the food has been modified in some way for use on a therapeutic diet. The client must be instructed to read the label further to determine if the product also says "low sodium." Unsalted cottage cheese and Cheddar cheese is also available. Ham cured by a smoking process only may be used. Special low-sodium hams are also available, but these are very expensive. Low-sodium bakery products such as bread, crackers, cakes, and cookies are also available in most stores. The unsalted bread may be kept in the frozen food section because it becomes stale rapidly without salt. Both unsalted butter and margarine are also available. These products, too, are often stored in the freezer. Low-sodium baking powder and baking soda may be purchased and used for preparing baked products at home. Special salt substitutes—potassium, calcium, or ammonium chloride instead of sodium chloride—are available. There are also salt substitutes that are half sodium chloride and half potassium chloride with names like Lo-Salt and Lite-Salt. These products contain only half as much sodium as regular salt. Clients however should be cautioned about the use of these products; they may be allowed in limited quantities on a mildly restrictive diet (2500–4500 mg sodium) but should not be allowed on lower sodium diets.

PRACTICAL CONSIDERATIONS. The two most frequently ordered sodium-restricted diets for home use are the mild (2500–4500 mg) and the moderate (1000–2000 mg) (see Tables 26-5 and 26-6). Within the restrictions of these two diets there is room for flexibility in adjusting the diet to the client's personal food preferences. The nurse who has a good working knowledge of sodium-restricted diets may be able to make simple substitutions for the

TABLE 26-5. Mild Sodium Restriction

Food Groups	Use	Do Not Use
Milk	Regular (whole) milk, evaporated milk, skim milk, buttermilk, reconstituted powdered milk. **If you use skim milk, buttermilk, or powdered milk,** you may add extra fat to your diet to make up for the fat that has been removed from the milk. For each glass, add 2 servings of fat. **Substitutes** for not more than 1 glass of milk a day: 2 oz of meat, poultry, or fish or 6 oz of plain yogurt (¾ of a cup).	**Because of the extra Calories they contain, do not use:** ice cream, sherbet, malted milk, milk shakes, instant cocoa mixes, chocolate milk, condensed milk, all other kinds of milk and fountain drinks.
Meat, poultry, fish	**Fresh, frozen, or canned meat or poultry:** any kind except those listed in the last column. **Fish or shellfish (fresh, frozen, or canned):** any kind except those listed in the last column. **Substitutes** for 1 oz of meat, poultry, or fish: an egg, ¼ cup lightly salted cottage cheese, 1 oz natural American Cheddar or Swiss cheese, 2 T low-sodium dietetic peanut butter.	Salty or smoked meat (bacon, bologna, chipped or corned beef, frankfurters, ham, meats koshered by salting, luncheon meats, salt pork, sausage, smoked tongue). Salty or smoked fish (anchovies, caviar, salted cod, herring, sardines, etc.). Process cheese or cheese spreads unless low-sodium dietetic; cheese such as Roquefort, Camembert, or Gorgonzola; regular peanut butter.
Vegetables	Any fresh, frozen, or canned vegetables or vegetable juices, except those listed in the last column.	Sauerkraut, pickles, or other vegetables prepared in brine or heavily salted.
Fruit	Any kind of fruit or fruit juice—fresh, frozen, canned, or dried—if sugar has not already been added.	**Because of the extra Calories they contain, do not use:** fruits canned or frozen in sugar syrup.
Breads and cereals	Breads, rolls, and lightly salted crackers; lightly salted cooked cereals; dry cereals; matzo; melba toast; macaroni, noodles, spaghetti, rice, barley; lightly salted popcorn; flour. **Substitute** for a serving of bread or cereal: a starchy vegetable.	Breads and rolls with salt topping; regular salted popcorn, potato chips, corn chips, pretzels, etc. **Because of the extra Calories they contain, do not use:** sugar-coated cereals, pastries, cakes, sweet rolls, cookies.
Fat	Butter or margarine, cooking fat or oil, French dressing, mayonnaise, heavy or light cream, unsalted nuts, avocado.	Bacon and bacon fat, salt pork; olives; salted nuts; party spreads and dips and other heavily salted snack foods, such as potato chips and sticks, crackers, etc.
Miscellaneous	**Use as desired:** coffee, tea, coffee substitutes, unsweetened or low-Calorie soft drinks; sugar substitutes; lemons, limes; gelatin; vinegar; cream of tartar; baking powder, baking soda (for baking only); yeast.	Canned soups, stews; any kind of commercial bouillon—cubes, powders, or liquids. **Because of the extra Calories they contain, do not use:** baking chocolate; cocoa and cocoa mixes; fruit-flavored beverage mixes; sugar-sweetened soft drinks, gelatin desserts, custards, and puddings; cornstarch, cornmeal, and tapioca.

SOURCE: Reprinted with permission, American Heart Association.

TABLE 26-6. 1000 mg Sodium-restricted Diet

Food Groups	Use	Do Not Use
Milk	Regular (whole) milk, evaporated milk, skim milk, powdered milk. **If you use skim milk, unsalted buttermilk, or powdered milk,** you may add extra fat to your diet to make up for the fat that has been removed from the milk. For each glass, add 2 servings of fat. **Substitutes** for not more than 1 glass of milk a day: 2 oz of meat, poultry, or fish; or 6 oz of plain yogurt (¾ of a container).	Ice cream, sherbet, malted milk, milk shakes, instant cocoa mixes, chocolate milk, condensed milk, all other kinds of milk and fountain drinks. These foods are high in Calories and the sodium content is unknown.
Meat, poultry, fish	**Fresh, frozen, or dietetic canned meat or poultry:** beef, lamb, pork, veal, fresh tongue, liver, chicken, duck, turkey, rabbit. **Fresh or dietetic canned (not frozen) fish:** any kind except those listed in the last column. **Substitutes** for 1 oz of meat, poultry, or fish: an egg (limit is 1 egg a day), ¼ cup unsalted cottage cheese, 1 oz low-sodium dietetic cheese, 2 T low-sodium dietetic peanut butter.	Brains or kidneys, canned, salted, or smoked meat (bacon, bologna, chipped or corned beef, frankfurters, ham, meats koshered by salting, luncheon meats, salt pork, sausage, smoked tongue). Frozen fish fillets; canned, salted, or smoked fish (anchovies, caviar, salted cod, herring, sardines, etc.); canned tuna or salmon unless low-sodium dietetic; shellfish (clams, crabs, lobsters, oysters, scallops, shrimp, etc.). Cheese which is not dietetic, peanut butter, salted cottage cheese.
Vegetables	Any fresh, frozen, or dietetic canned vegetables or vegetable juices, except those listed in the last column.	Canned vegetables or vegetable juices unless low-sodium dietetic; frozen vegetables if processed with salt; the following vegetables in any form: artichokes, beet greens, beets, carrots, celery, chard, dandelion greens, whole hominy, kale, mustard greens, sauerkraut, spinach, white turnips.
Fruit	Any kind of fruit or fruit juice—fresh, frozen, canned, or dried—if sugar has not already been added. **Substitute** for fruit juice: low-sodium dietetic tomato juice.	Fruits canned or frozen in sugar syrup (because of the extra Calories they contain).
Breads and cereals	Low-sodium breads, rolls, and crackers; unsalted cooked cereals (farina, hominy grits, oatmeal, rolled wheat, wheat meal); dry cereals (puffed rice, puffed wheat, shredded wheat); plain, unsalted matzo; unsalted melba toast; macaroni, noodles, spaghetti, rice, barley; unsalted popcorn; flour. **Substitute** for a serving of bread or cereal: a starchy vegetable.	Regular breads, crackers, etc., commercial mixes, cooked cereals containing a sodium compound (read the label), dry cereals other than those listed or those that have more than 6 mg of sodium in 100 gm of cereal (read the label here too), self-rising cornmeal or self-rising flour, potato chips, pretzels, salted popcorn.

TABLE 26-6. 1000 mg Sodium-restricted Diet (*Continued*)

Food Groups	Use	Do Not Use
Unsalted fat	Unsalted butter or margarine, unsalted cooking fat or oil, unsalted French dressing, unsalted mayonnaise, heavy or light cream, unsalted nuts, avocado.	Regular butter or margarine, commercial salad dressings or mayonnaise unless low-sodium dietetic, bacon and bacon fat, salt pork, olives, salted nuts, party spreads and dips.
Miscellaneous	**Use as desired:** regular and instant coffee, tea, coffee substitutes; lemons, limes; plain unflavored gelatin; vinegar; cream of tartar; potassium bicarbonate; sodium-free baking powder; yeast.	Instant coffee treated with a sodium compound such as sodium hydroxide, instant cocoa mixes, including fruit-flavored powders; fountain beverages, including malted milk; soft drinks, both regular and low Calorie; any kind of commercial bouillon (cubes, powders or liquids); sodium cyclamate and sodium saccharin; commercial candies; commercial gelatin desserts; regular baking powder; baking soda (sodium bicarbonate); rennet tablets; molasses; pudding mixes.

SOURCE: Reprinted with permission, American Heart Association.

client. It is best for the nurse to check with the dietitian concerning substitutions. The dietitian should be willing to make these substitutions if the client's adherence to the diet is improved. Some clients will very willingly use low-sodium bread or margarine if they are allowed to have a food such as cheese that would be eliminated on any sodium-restricted diet.

Hill (1979) suggests that it is more reasonable to allow substitutions if the client understands that upper sodium limits of the diet may not be exceeded. Careful education and explanations about substitutions must be part of the dietary instruction plan and will need to be accomplished with the consultation of the dietitian. It should be pointed out, however, that some clients respond better to a set list of foods that may be consumed, though others respond more positively if specific substitutions are made within the sodium limits of the diet. The nurse is often able to assess the client's level of understanding and willingness to comply with the dietary restrictions. Examples of low-sodium menus are found in Figures 26-8 and 26-9.

For most clients there is a period of adjustment to a reduced amount of salt in the diet. No salt may be used at the table, and little or none may be used in food preparation. Clients who have previously salted their food quite heavily, even before tasting it, will find the new diet extremely severe at first. These clients may describe the food as being tasteless and unappealing; the sense of taste gradually adjusts, however. An encouraging word from the nurse may be all a client will need to persevere through the first difficult weeks. It is also quite important for the client to have a clear understanding of the purpose of the low-sodium diet for his personal medical condition. The student should try to refrain for one day from salting all foods consumed to achieve a better understanding of the sacrifices the client is being asked to make.

The other restricted sources of sodium are foods to which sodium is added during processing and foods with naturally occurring sodium. Extra sodium is added in the form of salt and other sodium compounds during processing. To gain a real appreciation for the foods to be eliminated, the student could omit

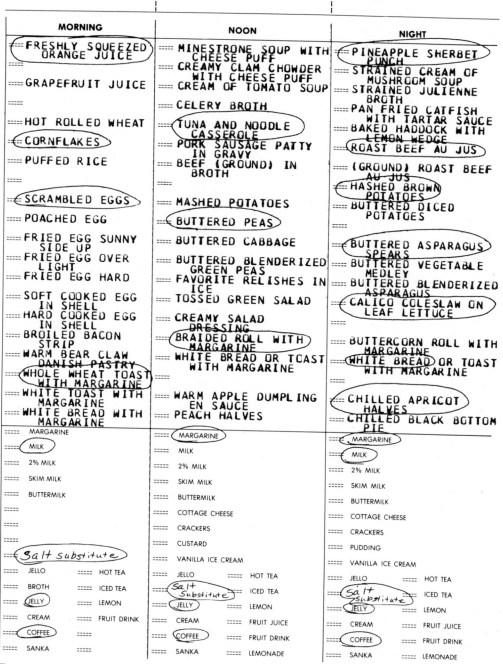

INDIANA UNIVERSITY HOSPITALS GENERAL MENU	INDIANA UNIVERSITY HOSPITALS GENERAL MENU	INDIANA UNIVERSITY HOSPITALS GENERAL MENU
MORNING	**NOON**	**NIGHT**
FRESHLY SQUEEZED ORANGE JUICE	MINESTRONE SOUP WITH CHEESE PUFF	PINEAPPLE SHERBET PUNCH
GRAPEFRUIT JUICE	CREAMY CLAM CHOWDER WITH CHEESE PUFF	STRAINED CREAM OF MUSHROOM SOUP
	CREAM OF TOMATO SOUP	STRAINED JULIENNE BROTH
HOT ROLLED WHEAT	CELERY BROTH	PAN FRIED CATFISH WITH TARTAR SAUCE
CORNFLAKES	TUNA AND NOODLE CASSEROLE	BAKED HADDOCK WITH LEMON WEDGE
PUFFED RICE	PORK SAUSAGE PATTY IN GRAVY	ROAST BEEF AU JUS
	BEEF (GROUND) IN BROTH	(GROUND) ROAST BEEF AU JUS
SCRAMBLED EGGS	MASHED POTATOES	HASHED BROWN POTATOES
POACHED EGG	BUTTERED PEAS	BUTTERED DICED POTATOES
FRIED EGG SUNNY SIDE UP	BUTTERED CABBAGE	BUTTERED ASPARAGUS SPEARS
FRIED EGG OVER LIGHT	BUTTERED BLENDERIZED GREEN PEAS	BUTTERED VEGETABLE MEDLEY
FRIED EGG HARD	FAVORITE RELISHES IN ICE	BUTTERED BLENDERIZED ASPARAGUS
SOFT COOKED EGG IN SHELL	TOSSED GREEN SALAD	CALICO COLESLAW ON LEAF LETTUCE
HARD COOKED EGG IN SHELL	CREAMY SALAD DRESSING	
BROILED BACON STRIP	BRAIDED ROLL WITH MARGARINE	BUTTERCORN ROLL WITH MARGARINE
WARM BEAR CLAW DANISH PASTRY	WHITE BREAD OR TOAST WITH MARGARINE	WHITE BREAD OR TOAST WITH MARGARINE
WHOLE WHEAT TOAST WITH MARGARINE		
WHITE TOAST WITH MARGARINE	WARM APPLE DUMPLING EN SAUCE	CHILLED APRICOT HALVES
WHITE BREAD WITH MARGARINE	PEACH HALVES	CHILLED BLACK BOTTOM PIE
MARGARINE	MARGARINE	MARGARINE
MILK	MILK	MILK
2% MILK	2% MILK	2% MILK
SKIM MILK	SKIM MILK	SKIM MILK
BUTTERMILK	BUTTERMILK	BUTTERMILK
	COTTAGE CHEESE	COTTAGE CHEESE
	CRACKERS	CRACKERS
	CUSTARD	PUDDING
Salt substitute	VANILLA ICE CREAM	VANILLA ICE CREAM
JELLO — HOT TEA	JELLO — HOT TEA	JELLO — HOT TEA
BROTH — ICED TEA	Salt Substitute — ICED TEA	Salt Substitute — ICED TEA
JELLY — LEMON	JELLY — LEMON	JELLY — LEMON
CREAM — FRUIT DRINK	CREAM — FRUIT JUICE	CREAM — FRUIT JUICE
COFFEE —	COFFEE — FRUIT DRINK	COFFEE — FRUIT DRINK
SANKA —	SANKA — LEMONADE	SANKA — LEMONADE

Figure 26-8. Low-sodium diet menu for mild restriction. (Courtesy Indiana University Hospitals)

INDIANA UNIVERSITY HOSPITALS LOW SODIUM MENU	INDIANA UNIVERSITY HOSPITALS LOW SODIUM MENU	INDIANA UNIVERSITY HOSPITALS LOW SODIUM MENU
MORNING	**NOON**	**NIGHT**
FRESHLY SQUEEZED ORANGE JUICE	LS TUNA AND NOODLE CASSEROLE	PINEAPPLE SHERBET PUNCH
GRAPEFRUIT JUICE	LS HOMEMADE PORK SAUSAGE PATTY	LS PAN FRIED CATFISH WITH LEMON WEDGE
	LS SAUSAGE GRAVY	LS BAKED HADDOCK WITH LEMON WEDGE
	LS (GROUND) BEEF IN BROTH	LS ROAST BEEF AU JUS
LS HOT ROLLED WHEAT		LS (GROUND) ROAST BEEF AU JUS
PUFFED RICE	LS MASHED POTATOES	
PUFFED WHEAT	LS GREEN PEAS	LS HASHED BROWN POTATOES
	LS CHOPPED CABBAGE	LS DICED POTATOES
SCRAMBLED EGGS		
POACHED EGG	LS FAVORITE RELISHES IN ICE	LS ASPARAGUS SPEARS
FRIED EGG SUNNY SIDE UP	TOSSED GREEN SALAD	LS VEGETABLE MEDLEY
FRIED EGG OVER LIGHT	LS ZERO DRESSING	
FRIED EGG HARD		LS CALICO COLESLAW ON LEAF LETTUCE
SOFT COOKED EGG IN SHELL	BRAIDED ROLL	
HARD COOKED EGG IN SHELL	LS BRAIDED ROLL	LS BUTTERCORN ROLL
	WHITE TOAST OR BREAD	WHITE TOAST OR BREAD
LS WARM BEAR CLAW DANISH PASTRY	LS WHITE TOAST OR BREAD	LS WHITE TOAST OR BREAD
WHOLE WHEAT TOAST		
WHITE TOAST OR BREAD	LS WARM APPLE DUMPLING EN SAUCE	CHILLED APRICOT HALVES
LS WHITE TOAST OR BREAD	PEACH HALVES	LS CHOCOLATE TART

MARGARINE	MARGARINE	MARGARINE
LS MARGARINE	LS MARGARINE	LS MARGARINE
MILK	MILK	MILK
2% MILK	2% MILK	2% MILK
SKIM MILK	SKIM MILK	SKIM MILK
	LS CRACKERS	LS CRACKERS
	CUSTARD	PUDDING
	VANILLA ICE CREAM	VANILLA ICE CREAM
	COTTAGE CHEESE	COTTAGE CHEESE
SALT SUBSTITUTE HOT TEA	SALT SUBSTITUTE HOT TEA	SALT SUBSTITUTE HOT TEA
ICED TEA	ICED TEA	ICED TEA
JELLY LEMON	JELLY LEMON	JELLY LEMON
CREAM FRUIT DRINK	CREAM FRUIT JUICE	CREAM FRUIT JUICE
COFFEE	COFFEE FRUIT DRINK	COFFEE FRUIT DRINK
SANKA	SANKA LEMONADE	SANKA LEMONADE

Figure 26-9. Low-sodium diet menu for 1,000 mg restriction. (Courtesy Indiana University Hospitals)

for one day all processed foods from the diet. The list in Table 26-6 may be used as a guide. The student should also sample a low-sodium cracker or a slice of low-sodium bread with low-sodium butter or margarine to obtain a clearer perspective on the contribution made by salt to the taste of these simple foods.

Fortunately, however, adjustment to the low-sodium diet is possible, and there are several suggestions that can be made to increase its palatability. The use of spices, herbs, and seasonings is encouraged with the low-sodium diet. Most of these are quite low in sodium content and can be used freely on a sodium-restricted diet. Most physicians will allow the use of one of the salt substitutes as long as there is no evidence of kidney problems. Some clients find a salt substitute quite acceptable and adjust with little or no difficulty to a low-sodium diet. Others complain of a bitter taste or a bitter after taste from the salt substitute; spices and seasonings may be preferable for them as a substitute for salt. Wine, vinegar, or lemon juice may be added to food to enhance the taste.

Following the sodium-restricted diet provides a good opportunity to encourage creativity in cooking through experimentation with herbs and spices. Monosodium glutamate is a flavor enhancer, but it cannot be used because of its high sodium content. All the herbs and spices can be said to be flavor enhancers. After a few weeks of experimentation, the client on the sodium-restricted diet often comments about the subtle flavors of natural foods. The person who prepares the client's meals should try to eat many of the same foods for added encouragement. Many foods have their characteristic flavor because of the presence of one spice or herb. This taste can be captured by increasing the spice or herb and eliminating the salt. The characteristic taste of pizza is oregano; of chili, chili powder; of rye bread, caraway seed. A physician who followed a low-sodium diet after a stroke reported that he and his wife obtained much satisfaction discovering tasty low-sodium foods through the use of seasonings, spices, and herbs; low-sodium baking powder; and salt substitute (Youngstrom, 1971).

Eating out in restaurants does not pose as many difficulties for the client on a mild sodium diet as for one with a moderate or severe restriction. The client with a mild restriction is usually able to select foods from the menu that are similar to those allowed on the diet. Some kind of fruit may be ordered for dessert. It is very difficult for the client with a moderate or severe sodium restriction to select foods from a restaurant menu within the bounds of the diet because so many of the food choices will be of the sodium-containing variety. Broiled meats, the inside slices of a beef roast, or a fruit or vegetable salad may be ordered. Another suggestion is that, if the client expects to be eating a particular meal in a restaurant, he take special care to eat foods very low in sodium at the other two meals. Fortunately, the moderate and severe sodium restrictions are much less common for unhospitalized clients. Most clients are on at least a 2 gm sodium restriction, which allows them safely to enjoy a meal in a restaurant with friends or family.

BLOCKAGE OF NUTRIENT TRANSPORT

1. Impaired lymph circulation
2. Potential airway obstruction
3. Potential peripheral anoxia

The client who has experienced alterations in vascular physiology because of a blockage in nutrient transport due to a disease process requires intensive medical and nursing intervention to support adaptation and survival. Frequently the disease arises from one of three pathophysiological processes: a fatty deposit or calcification along the internal membrane of the vascular wall, a hypertrophy of the muscular portion of the artery, or an obstruction of blood flow by thrombus or embolus. The client's vascular condition is greatly influenced by his metabolic status. It is thought that such conditions as diabetes mellitus, hypothyroidism, hyperuricemia, hyperlipidemia, and obesity contribute to the development of vascular disease (Fabre, 1974).

Client Objectives

To be able to:

1. Discuss alterations in ingestion patterns that may be necessary to prevent further vascular blockage.
2. Consume a diet that will not contribute to further blockage.

Dietary Intervention

A *myocardial infarction* occurs when heart tissue undergoes *necrosis* (death) because of the blockage of an artery that supplies the heart with blood. If a main artery is involved, death may follow immediately. A myocardial infarction is also known as a *coronary*, a *coronary occlusion*, a *coronary thrombosis*, or a *heart attack*. The symptoms include severe chest pain, dyspnea, weakness, and fear of impending death. Cardiac arrhythmias, shock, and cardiac failure may follow. The coronary victim needs immediate emergency assistance and transport by ambulance to a hospital. The American Heart Association is actively involved in training medical personnel and lay people in the principles of CPR as a means of basic cardiac life support. The chances for surviving a heart attack have increased thanks to the use of this technique. Undoubtedly, nursing students will become very familiar with it during their nursing education and professional careers.

On arrival at the hospital, the client is admitted to the coronary care unit, where he can be monitored very closely using specific cardiac monitors and equipment. An intravenous infusion is begun for supportive and replacement therapy of fluid and electrolytes, as needed. Drugs can also be administered through the IV in an emergency. Oral dietary intake during the first few days may be restricted to liquids only or be completely absent, depending on the client's condition. The attending physician will usually write the orders for dietary intake.

Metabolic changes occur during the days following a myocardial infarction. These include the elevation of certain enzymes, which are therefore used to confirm the diagnosis. Other metabolic changes include hyperglycemia and elevated levels of serum free fatty acids and cholesterol. Metabolic acidosis, which is usually present, needs to be carefully monitored and controlled because it can lead to arrhythmais and hypotension, which are life threatening.

Christakis and Winston (1973) have divided nutritional therapy for acute myocardial infarction into three phases: the acute phase, the subacute phase, and the rehabilitative phase. During the acute phase no food may be given by mouth the first 24–48 hours. When feeding is begun, a 500- to 800-Calorie liquid diet is used that contains 1,000–1,500 ml of liquid. A liquid diet is used to prevent gagging on particles of solid food and possible aspiration. Extremes of temperature may be avoided by eliminating very hot and very cold liquids such as coffee, soup, ice cream, and beverages containing ice. Avoidance of these temperature extremes is thought to avert the possible precipitation of arrhythmias by neural mechanisms. Coffee and tea are eliminated because they contain stimulants that may increase the heart rate. A particular effort should be made to help the client avoid liquids such as too much fruit juice or carbonated beverage that may cause abdominal distention. Milk is likely to produce distention in clients who have a known lactose intolerance, and it should be avoided.

After a few days the client may be advanced to a soft diet for the subacute phase. This diet is restricted to 1,000–1,200 Calories to provide enough Calories to meet basal energy requirements but initiate weight loss in the overweight client. It is composed of foods that are easy to digest; that is, they are low in roughage and free from gastric irritants. A bland diet may actually be ordered for use during this phase. Small, frequent feedings may be helpful because the client may have difficulty breathing (dyspnea) or may tire easily during eating. This diet may be low in saturated fat, sodium, and cholesterol. Coffee and tea may be allowed in moderation as long as such symptoms as restlessness and sleeplessness do not occur. A return to regular, solid food may help to reassure the client concerning his recovery.

The rehabilitative phase of the diet contains the type of foods the client will be expected to consume after discharge from the hospital. This diet usually includes a caloric adjustment to provide for weight maintenance or weight loss. A type of fat-controlled diet is usually recommended. It often entails reducing dietary cholesterol to 300 mg/day, decreasing total fat content, especially saturated fat, and substituting polyunsaturated fat. More specific levels of cholesterol and proportions and types of carbohydrates, protein, and fat may be ordered by the physician following the laboratory tests for serum cholesterol, triglyceride, and lipoprotein levels. A fat-controlled diet or a specific dietary prescription for one of the five types of hyperlipoproteinemias may be ordered by the physician. A sodium restriction is often added to this diet order (see Fig. 26-10). The nurse should coordinate with the dietary department to be sure the client is instructed by the dietitian about the diet several days before release from the hospital. The client should understand that following the diet should reduce the chances of a second heart attack. The nurse can reinforce the dietary instruction given by the dietitian by discussing with the client and his family the dietary objectives and practical suggestions for diet implementation (presented earlier in the chapter).

The specific recommendations of Christakis and Winston (1973) are not followed in all coronary care units. Warren et al. (1978) administered a questionnaire to 290 major medical centers concerning the type of diet used for clients during the first 24–72 hours after a myocardial infarction. More than 50% of these institutions observed the following practices in the coronary care unit:

- Served three meals a day to the clients (one-quarter of the clients did receive multiple feedings or snacks).
- Restricted cholesterol or saturated fat.
- Reduced roughage in the diet.
- Prescribed a 2-mg sodium diet.
- Prescribed a bland diet.

From the questionnaire they also found that the institutions were not restricting hot and cold beverages. There did not seem to be any ill effects from this practice. The study revealed that there were wide differences in diet therapy in coronary care units in the United States. The investigators arrived at the following conclusions: caloric intake should be individualized to the client to avoid the extremes of overfeeding or near-starvation diets; the diet should exclude foods likely to cause GI distress; multiple small feedings should be provided; both saturated fat and cholesterol should be restricted; and sodium should be restricted to 2 mg or "no added salt" (3–4 gm of sodium).

Rehabilitation after a myocardial infarction must begin during the initial phase of nursing intervention. Long-term goals should be established early to provide direction for nursing activities. Careful, frequent reinforcement of teaching will provide increasing confidence in both client and family. Of course, as with any illness, the client's level of acceptance of lifestyle changes depends on expectations of his future lifestyle and physical condition, and his acceptance of the illness. At the least, discussion with the client should cover diet, activity level, sexual activity, medications, and resource people available. Many facilities have very well-developed cardiac re-

INDIANA UNIVERSITY HOSPITALS CALORIE CONTROL MENU	INDIANA UNIVERSITY HOSPITALS CALORIE CONTROL MENU	INDIANA UNIVERSITY HOSPITALS CALORIE CONTROL MENU
MORNING	**NOON**	**NIGHT**
(FRESHLY SQUEEZED ORANGE JUICE)	CELERY BROTH	STRAINED JULIENNE BROTH
GRAPEFRUIT JUICE	D HOMEMADE PORK SAUSAGE PATTY	D (BAKED HADDOCK WITH LEMON WEDGE)
	(CHOPPED SIRLOIN)	D ROAST BEEF AU JUS
	SCRAMBLED EGGS	D (GROUND) ROAST BEEF AU JUS
HOT ROLLED WHEAT	D (GROUND) BEEF IN BROTH	
PUFFED RICE	D FLUFFY RICE	(D DICED POTATO)
(CORNFLAKES)	(D MASHED POTATOES)	D WHIPPED POTATOES
	(D GREEN PEAS)	
SCRAMBLED EGGS	D CHOPPED CABBAGE	D ASPARAGUS SPEARS
(POACHED EGG)		(D VEGETABLE MEDLEY)
FRIED EGG SUNNY SIDE UP	(D FAVORITE RELISHES IN ICE)	
FRIED EGG OVER LIGHT	TOSSED GREEN SALAD	(D CALICO COLESLAW ON LEAF LETTUCE)
FRIED EGG HARD	ZERO DRESSING	
SOFT COOKED EGG IN SHELL	(BRAIDED ROLL)	BUTTERCORN ROLL
HARD COOKED EGG IN SHELL	LS BRAIDED ROLL	LS BUTTERCORN ROLL
BROILED BACON STRIP	WHITE TOAST OR BREAD	(WHITE TOAST OR BREAD)
	LS WHITE TOAST OR BREAD	LS WHITE TOAST OR BREAD
(WHOLE WHEAT TOAST)		
WHITE TOAST OR BREAD	(D PEACH HALVES)	(D CHILLED APRICOT HALVES)
LS WHITE TOAST OR BREAD	D BAKED APPLE WITH CINNAMON	D PEAR HALVES
(MARGARINE, Corn Oil)	(MARGARINE, Corn Oil)	(MARGARINE, Corn Oil)
LS MARGARINE	LS MARGARINE	LS MARGARINE
MILK	MILK	MILK
(SKIM MILK)	SKIM MILK	(SKIM MILK)
BUTTERMILK	BUTTERMILK	BUTTERMILK
CREAM	CREAM	CREAM
2% MILK	COTTAGE CHEESE	COTTAGE CHEESE
	LS COTTAGE CHEESE	LS COTTAGE CHEESE
	2% MILK	2% MILK
SALT ::::: HOT TEA	SALT ::::: HOT TEA	SALT ::::: HOT TEA
(SALT SUBSTITUTE) ::::: ICED TEA	(SALT SUBSTITUTE) (ICED TEA)	(SALT SUBSTITUTE) ::::: ICED TEA
PEPPER ::::: LEMON	PEPPER ::::: LEMON	PEPPER ::::: LEMON
(SUGAR SUBSTITUTE)	(SUGAR SUBSTITUTE) ::::: FRUIT JUICE	(SUGAR SUBSTITUTE) ::::: FRUIT JUICE
(COFFEE)	COFFEE ::::: D LEMONADE	(COFFEE) ::::: D LEMONADE
SANKA	SANKA ::::: CRACKERS	SANKA ::::: CRACKERS

Figure 26-10. 1,800-Calorie, Type IV, 2 gm sodium diet menu. (Courtesy Indiana University Hospitals)

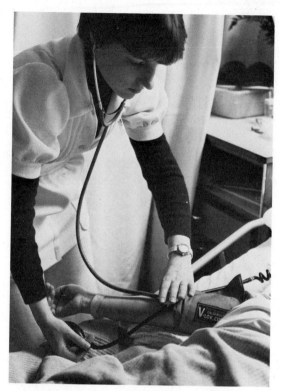

Figure 26-11. Checking the client's blood pressure several times daily is important after a heart attack. (Photo by J. Collins)

habilitation programs that employ a variety of individual and group teaching methods to provide information and counseling to clients and their families.

The client who has been encouraged to alter his diet as part of the treatment for a vascular problem may have many ambivalent feelings. It is normal for the client to grieve over any perceived loss, including loss of a particular lifestyle he may have enjoyed before his heart attack. Often the client feels his life is totally out of his control. While hospitalized he can no longer choose his activity level, leisure activities, hygiene methods, or sleeping times. The desire to regain control may be reflected by an intentional lack of

compliance with the prescribed diet. The client's mental-emotional status should be considered when the nurse is teaching him about any diet. Long-standing food habits are not easily changed. The client's diet should be planned with his participation so it can be adapted to his lifestyle. When existing food habits and eating patterns need to be incorporated into the diet, the dietitian should always be consulted. Of course, the kind of instructions given each client should be individualized to his needs. The client's family and significant others need to be involved from the beginning of counseling. The nurse should encourage the client not only to follow his diet but have his blood pressure checked frequently (Fig. 26-11).

ELECTROLYTE IMBALANCE

1. Potential electrolyte imbalance related to
    a. Potassium infusion
    b. Inadequate fluid intake
    c. Dextrose infusion
    d. T-tube drainage
    e. Colostomy drainage
    f. Adrenal-steroid therapy
    g. Gastric suction
    h. Inadequate sodium intake
    i. Excessive sodium intake
2. Electrolyte imbalance related to
    a. Prolonged emesis and diarrhea
    b. Fistula drainage
    c. Diaphoresis
    d. Diuresis
    e. Malnutrition
    f. Inadequate calcium intake
    g. Excessive calcium intake

A client's fluid and electrolyte balance is threatened by almost every physiological alteration and many medical interventions. Electrolyte disturbances tend to produce very nonspecific symptoms. The nurse is at a distinct advantage in assessing such subtle changes because of constant exposure to the client and his usual behavior patterns. Subtle changes in behavior and psyche may alert the nurse to potential problems that require medical or nursing interventions. Electrolyte disturbances are confirmed with laboratory data. The physiology of fluid and electrolyte homeostasis was discussed in detail in Chapter 11. Here, the topic is dietary interventions used to help regain electrolyte balance.

Clients most at risk for the development of electrolyte imbalance are those who are compromised by such conditions as renal failure, ulcerative colitis, diarrhea, diabetes mellitus, burns, neurological disorders, and hormonal imbalances. Any medical intervention that results in GI fluid loss can precipitate electrolyte imbalance. Examples include nasogastric suction, pumps, drains, fistula repair, colon resection, or ostomies. Clients receiving IV therapy are easily thrown into a fluid or electrolyte imbalance. Older clients and children are particularly susceptible to dehydration.

Client Objectives

To be able to:

1. Follow a diet that provides for adequate nutrient intake and altered electrolyte status.
2. Discuss possible alterations in the diet that may occur with fluctuations in electrolyte status.
3. Plan a diet that meets necessary nutritional alterations and is satisfying.
4. Show a return to normal electrolyte patterns following ingestion of the prescribed diet.

Dietary Interventions

By knowing what type of body fluid is lost, the nurse can anticipate the kind of imbalance most likely to occur. Loss of gastric juices leads to sodium, potassium, magnesium, and chlorine deficits with metabolic alkalemia. Excessive perspiration leads to water and sodium losses. Open wounds lose water, sodium, calcium, and protein; and elevated metabolism, such as occurs during fever, may lead to dehydration and hypernatremia.

Specific data-gathering tools at the nurse's disposal include *accurate* daily weights, intake and output, urine specific gravity, and blood pressure changes. An increased pulse rate may indicate sodium excess or magnesium deficit. A decreased pulse rate occurs with a magnesium excess. A weak, irregular, and rapid pulse may signal a severe potassium deficit. A weak, irregular, slow pulse suggests a severe potassium excess. Tables 26-7 and 26-8 summarize the common signs and symptoms of water and electrolyte imbalance. Table 26-9 describes specific conditions that may lead to a fluid or electrolyte imbalance.

When dealing with clients with potential or actual fluid and electrolyte alterations, the nurse has as a primary objective maintenance of homeostasis. Specific replacement therapy involves medical intervention, but the ability of the client to tolerate and comply with the medical treatment definitely falls within the realm of nursing practice. Specific nursing interventions vary with each electrolyte.

TABLE 26-7. Signs and Symptoms of Water Imbalance

Water Loss	Water Excess
Dizziness	Confusion
Thirst	Nausea
Dry skin and mucous membrane	Muscle cramps
Postural hypotension	Headache
Weight loss	Weight gain
Oliguria	Edema
	Seizures
	Elevated central venous pressure (CVP)
	Bounding pulse
	Hypertension

TABLE 26-8. Signs and Symptoms of Electrolyte Imbalance

Electrolyte	Excess	Deficit
Potassium	Weakness, malaise, nausea, intestinal colic diarrhea, flaccid paralysis, muscle irritability, EKG changes (prolonged P–R interval, wide QRS, S–T depression, tall T wave)	Disturbed muscle function; decreased reflexes; muscle irritability and weakness; speech changes; rapid, weak irregular pulse; paralytic ileus; abdominal distension; EKG changes (S–T segments depression, flattened T wave and U wave
Sodium	Thirst; fever; dry, sticky membranes; flushed skin, oliguria	Weakness, apathy, irritability, decreased skin turgor, tremors, seizures
Calcium	Lethargy, anorexia, nausea, vomiting, constipation, dehydration, cardiac arrhythmias, coma	Tingling around the mouth, twitching, carpopedal spasm, tetany, seizures, cardiac arrhythmias
Magnesium	Flushing; sweating; weak or absent deep tendon reflexes; drowsiness; lethargy; slow, weak pulse; respiratory depression	Insomnia, leg cramps, cardiac arrythmias, muscle weakness, twitching, tetany

Potassium

Hyperkalemia is difficult to correct. Nursing interventions include limiting oral potassium and protein intake, encouraging urinary output, and carrying out medical orders such as administering a *cation exchange resin* or monitoring dialysis. Hypokalemia is treated with potassium supplements. Rapid potassium replacement is ordered by the physician and is usually given intravenously. The nurse must be aware that rapid intravenous infusion of potassium can cause ventricular fibrillation. It

TABLE 26-9. Conditions That May Precipitate Electrolyte Imbalance

Electrolyte	Conditions That Lead to Excesses	Conditions That Lead to Deficits
Potassium	Renal failure, hemmorrhagic shock, Addison's disease, potassium replacement therapy, disorders with cell lysis, burns, crushing injuries, myocardial infarction	Cushing's syndrome, renal disease, congestive heart failure, diuretic therapy, gastric drainage, prolonged vomiting, diarrhea
Sodium	Decreased water intake; therapy with drugs such as diuretics, vasopressin, antihypertensive agents, corticosteroids; diarrhea	Water intoxication, congestive heart failure, renal failure, cirrhosis, burns, diarrhea, vomiting, diuretic therapy
Calcium	Hyperparathyroidism, parathyroid adenoma, multiple myeloma, antacid overuse, Paget's disease, skeletal metastasis of cancer	Parathyroid or thyroid surgery, hemodialysis therapy
Magnesium	Renal failure, excessive use of antacids or cathartics	Malabsorption syndromes, bowel resection, alcoholism, diuretic therapy, prolonged nasogastric suction
Chlorine	Hyperventilation, dehydration, metabolic acidosis	Gastrointestinal suction, congestive heart failure, edema, metabolic alkalosis, renal failure

is wise to monitor the client's EKG continuously for signs of cardiac irritability. Potassium should not be infused faster than 15–20 mEq/liter/hr, nor in greater concentrations than 80 mEq/liter. Peripheral IV therapy is often uncomfortable for the client. Burning at the IV site is common. An icebag at the site may relieve the client's discomfort temporarily.

Oral potassium replacements frequently have a very disagreeable taste and thus are poorly taken by the client, particularly after discharge. Potassium supplements should be given with or after meals with a full glass of water or juice, to minimize GI irritation. If these supplements are in powder or effervescent form, they should be completely dissolved before the client drinks them. Occasionally, potassium supplements can be "hidden" in strong-tasting grape juice. The aftertaste may be decreased by having the juice very cold and by using a straw.

Foods high in potassium may be all that is necessary to replace potassium lost during diuretic therapy. A banana contains 370 mg of potassium/100 mg of banana. Tomatoes, potatoes, avocados, and citrus fruits are also good sources. To increase at-home compliance with the therapy, the nurse needs to explain thoroughly the purposes and effects of potassium therapy both to the client and his significant others.

Sodium

Starvation hyponatremia results from a prolonged decrease in sodium intake in people with impaired ingestion. Hyponatremia in the absence of dehydration or edema occurs in most clients who have lost more than 15% of their body weight. Albumin levels are frequently decreased. Simple sodium replacements will not correct the deficiency. General improved nutrition will correct the problem. If ingestion or absorption is interfered with, as occurs frequently during cancer therapy, hyperalimentation will effectively replace the deficit. True hyponatremia responds to sodium replacement. Careful monitoring for signs of excess during replacement therapy is essential.

Hypernatremia will follow a loss of water or an increase in sodium ingestion. Clients should be taught to read food labels carefully and identify foods with a high sodium content. The general principles of the sodium-restricted diet were discussed earlier in this chapter.

Calcium

Hypocalcemia responds readily to replacement therapy. Parenteral supplements are very irritating to peripheral veins and tissues. Oral supplements are usually given with vitamin D to enhance calcium absorption. Hypercalcemia is treated with rehydration and diuresis. Thiazide diuretics are not used because they inhibit the excretion of calcium. Long-term treatment will usually include corticosteroid therapy. Oral phosphate is added to a low-calcium diet. Phosphate lowers calcium levels by decreasing calcium absorption and promoting deposition of calcium in the bones.

Magnesium

Magnesium is usually ingested in foods such as meats, green vegetables, whole grains, and nuts. Hypomagnesemia is usually treated with injections of magnesium sulfate. If magnesium is being replaced intravenously, the nurse should watch for signs of respiratory depression or heart block. Magnesium intoxication can be reversed by administering calcium gluconate. Teaching the client prudent use of antacids will prevent the onset of hypermagnesemia. Stressing the potential side effects of antacids will alert the client to potential problems with the many over-the-counter preparations available.

OXYGEN/CARBON DIOXIDE ALTERATIONS

1. Oxygen toxicity
2. Oxygen insufficiency
3. Carbon dioxide insufficiency
4. Carbon dioxide toxicity

Shortness of breath is probably one of the most frightening and exhausting experiences people can experience. The feeling of being unable to "get his breath" and fears of suffocation cause the client to focus much of his attention on the problem. When shortness of breath becomes chronic, as in chronic obstructive pulmonary disease, the client's entire lifestyle may be altered. The nutritional implications of such a change in lifestyle follow:

The client with shortness of breath may reveal anxiety, fatigue, restlessness, and irregular or rapid respirations. Chronic shortness of breath is usually secondary to such disease processes as emphysema, myasthenia gravis, and congestive heart failure.

Client Objectives

To be able to:

1. Plan a diet that provides for adequate nutrient intake in the presence of altered oxygen/carbon dioxide status.
2. Consume a diet that meets his nutritional requirements.

Dietary Interventions

The primary purpose of nursing intervention is to provide oxygen to all cells. The nutritional care of the client centers on providing as nutrituous a diet as possible without taking the client's already limited energy reserves. Eating often tends to increase the cleint's shortness of breath. The effort needed to chew and digest food frequently results in such shortness of breath that the client refuses to eat. Loss of weight is common because of the increased metabolic demands resulting from the increased work of breathing. The increased nutritional demands coupled with a decrease in ingestion place the client at risk of malnutrition.

The client may be helped by eating frequent, light meals. Shortening the amount of time it takes to eat will also save energy. Gas-forming foods should be avoided because of the pressure on the diaphragm that results, causing a decreased inspiratory capacity and consequent respiratory distress. Milk and milk products should be avoided because they tend to thicken lung secretions (Malkus, 1976). Fluids such as tea, coffee, bouillon, and water will help to keep secretions thin if taken in quantities greater than 1,500 ml (51 oz)/day.

Nutritional Anemias

Anemia is defined as a reduction in the oxygen-carrying capacity of blood resulting from a decrease in the size or number of red blood cells or the quantity of hemoglobin or both. Some of the symptoms of anemia are directly related to this decreased oxygen-carrying capacity. The anemic client may experience shortness of breath, heart palpitation, physical weakness, and difficulty performing mental work (Pflanzer, 1975). Anemias occur for a number of reasons, and they are associated with many diseases and conditions. Anemias may be caused by impaired or decreased production of blood, increased or excess destruction of blood, or by blood loss.

The nurse will encounter anemias associated with many different diseases. Not all types of anemias are nutritional in their origin, but they all relate to nutrition in a broad sense because the oxygen-carrying capacity of the blood is reduced. Anemais may be classified as either nutritional or nonnutritional. The nutritional anemias are due to a deficiency of any of the nutrients essential for the formation of red blood cells or hemoglobin. The nutrients involved were discussed in Chapter 11; they are protein, iron, vitamin B_{12}, folic acid, vitamin B_6, and vitamin C. The three nutrients of greatest importance in the development of anemias are iron, vitamin B_{12}, and folic acid. Some of the nonnutritional anemias are due to blood loss, excess destruction of red blood cells (hemolytic anemias), congenital defects (sickle cell anemia), inhibition or toxic reactions by drugs, or any diseases that interfere with the production of red blood cells. Only anemias associated with a deficiency of iron, vitamin B_{12}, or folic acid are discussed here.

Anemias may be described and classified by the appearance of the red blood cell, that is, by their size and hemoglobin content. A red blood cell that is smaller than normal is referred to as *microcytic,* whereas one larger than normal is called *macrocytic.* On the basic of hemoglobin content, a red blood cell with an elevated content of hemoglobin is said to be *hyperchromic,* and one with a decreased concentration of hemoglobin is said to be *hypochromic.* Anemias are sometimes referred to using these two sets of descriptive terms. A deficiency of iron produces a microcytic hypochromic anemia commonly known as *iron-deficiency anemia.* This type of anemia is characterized by small, pale red blood cells. A deficiency of folic acid or vitamin B_{12} leads to the development of a macrocytic hyperchromic anemia.

IRON-DEFICIENCY   ANEMIA.   Iron-deficiency anemia viewed from a nutritional perspective has three major causes: blood loss that is acute (hemorrhaging) or chronic (bleeding ulcer or hemorrhoids), a diet deficient in iron, or a diet deficient in total protein content. This association exists between iron and protein because most foods high in protein are also high in iron. This is especially true of meat. Iron-deficiency anemia is one of the nutritional deficiencies that usually accompanies a severe protein deficiency.

Iron-deficiency anemia can be diagnosed by measuring the level of hemoglobin or hematocrit (discussed in Chaps. 11 and 19). The lowering of these blood values may be considered to be a final stage in the development of this anemia. The first stage is the depletion of iron stores. The absorption of iron and the total iron-binding capacity of transferrin both increase in the body's attempt to replenish the iron stores, but to no avail. This second stage is characterized by iron deficiency but without anemia. Continued depletion occurs, and inadequate iron is available for the production of red blood cells. The result is, first, a decreased number of red blood cells being produced, and second the production of an adequate number of small, pale cells (Krause and Mahan, 1979).

The treatment of iron-deficiency anemia involves the use of an iron supplement and an increased dietary intake of iron. The chief treatment is the administration of an iron supplement such as ferrous sulfate, ferrous gluconate, or ferrous fumarate. The most widely used of these is ferrous sulfate. The dose is calculated on the basis of the amount of elemental iron provided. The adult dosage should provide 100–200 mg of elemental iron daily, and children should receive 1.5–2.0 mg/kg of body weight (Krause and Mahan, 1979). The ingestion of an oral iron supplement may lead to gastric irritation. Although iron is better absorbed when the stomach is empty, gastric irritation is increased when the stomach is empty. The side effects can be diminished by having the client take the iron supplement after meals, by gradually increasing his dose during the first few days, and by having him take the iron supplement divided into at least three doses throughout the day. Iron therapy should be continued for about six months, even after hemoglobin levels have returned to normal, to allow for the repletion of the body reserves (Krause and Mahan, 1979).

Iron may be administered by the parenteral route when malabsorption is present, when blood is lost very rapidly, or when the client is unable to tolerate the supplement orally. It is well documented that vitamin C aids in the absorption of iron. The nurse should therefore encourage the client to consume a good source of vitamin C with each dose of the iron supplement. The vitamin C in citrus juices is particularly helpful. If the protein content of the diet has been low, it may be helpful to increase the protein content of the diet to 80–100 gm/day (Robinson and Lawler, 1977). The inclusion of foods high in iron content should also be encouraged. These include meats, especially red meats like beef, liver, dried fruits, dark-green leafy vegetables, and enriched breads and cereals. The student is referred to Chapter 6 and Table 6–8.

PERNICIOUS ANEMIA.   The basic defect in pernicious anemia is inadequate use of vitamin B_{12} owing to a lack of the *intrinsic factor* in the stomach. For vitamin B_{12} to be absorbed, it must first come in contact with the intrinsic factor in the small intestine. In pernicious anemia the intrinsic factor is missing and the concentration of hydrochloric acid in the stomach is low. Although adequate vitamin B_{12} is present from the diet, it is not absorbed. With inadequate vitamin B_{12} available, the maturation of the red blood cell is affected. A reduced number of immature large red blood cells is formed. The symptoms of pernicious anemia often take many years to develop because vitamin B_{12} is stored in fairly large quantities throughout the body. The symptoms often appear in middle and old age. They may also occur after gastric surgery in which the portion of the stomach that produces the intrinsic factor is removed.

General symptoms of pernicious anemia include anorexia, weight loss, weakness, lightheadedness, palpitations, and headache.

More specific symptoms include sore tongue, numbness or tingling in the extremities, poor muscular coordination, poor memory, and hallucinations. In the elderly, unfortunately, these symptoms may be attributed to the aging process, and the person may be hospitalized or even placed in an institution without a diagnosis of the real problem. The client often has pale skin with a yellowish cast, a rapid pulse, incorrdination of the lower extremities, loss of fine finger coordination, and evidence of peripheral nerve degeneration, (Bennion, 1979).

The first treatment of pernicious anemia, demonstrated in 1929, was the consumption of 8 oz of liver daily. Apparently enough vitamin B_{12} was absorbed from this large quantity of liver to alleviate the symptoms. A more practical method of treatment is known today. It consists of injecting therapeutic doses of vitamin B_{12} (30–1,000 μg/day for 1–2 wk) ro replenish body stores. After this initial replacement therapy, monthly injections of 50–1,000 μg must be given for the rest of the client's life (Bennion, 1979). The vitamin replacement for this type of anemia must be given by injection because the vitamin B_{12} from an oral supplement would not be absorbed because of lack of the intrinsic factor. A dietary deficiency of vitamin B_{12} may develop in strict vegetarians because vitamin B_{12} is contained primarily in milk and meat products. In this case the vitamin B_{12} could be taken orally.

FOLIC ACID DEFICIENCY.   Because folic acid and vitamin B_{12} have very similar roles in the formation of red blood cells, a deficiency of folic acid presents an anemia very similar to pernicious anemia. Poor eating habits or inadequate absorption are the most frequent causes of folic-acid deficiency. Treatment involves an oral supplement of 1 mg/day for 2–3 wk to replenish the stores (Krause and Mahan, 1979). The client should be informed about good food sources of this vitamin and the principles of a balanced diet. Long-term replacement therapy is not needed. Foods containing fairly high levels of folate are leafy green vegetables, meat, and whole grain products. Because folate is destroyed by heat, the consumption of fresh, raw fruits and vegetables should be encouraged.

FLUID VOLUME ALTERATIONS

1. Dependence on intravenous infusion management
2. Emergency phase circulatory overload
3. Potential cardiac overload
4. Potential hemorrhage
5. Actual hemorrhage
6. Increased fluid requirements
7. Potential fluid overload

Client Objectives

To be able to:

1. State the purpose of various medical-nursing interventions aimed at reestablishing fluid volume homeostasis.
2. Plan a diet that takes altered fluid requirements into consideration.
3. Use nursing and medical resources to maintain adequate nutrition during emergency phase fluid alterations.

Fluid Restriction

The client may be placed on a fluid restriction when an alteration in fluid balance is present. Usually, a limited fluid intake is necessary for such medical conditions as increased intracranial pressure, cirrhosis, and fluid volume excess that occurs with congestive heart failure or renal shutdown. Discomfort from fluid restriction occurs when the client drinks all the allotted fluid within a short period of time, allowing none for the remainder of the day. The client usually becomes thirsty and may have dry mucous membranes.

Dietary Interventions

A large portion of the discomfort can be prevented by dividing the fluids allowed throughout the day. For example, if the physician has ordered a fluid restriction of 1,200 ml/day, the nurse and the dietitian would divide the fluids based on the client's needs, considering IV therapy, number of medications the client must swallow, type of diet the client is receiving, and client's level of consciousness. One way the total fluid volume may be divided is illustrated in Figure 26-12.

The easiest way to inform the health care team of the fluid restriction is to post a sign above the client's bed. It is necessary to explain to the client and his family the reasons why the fluid restriction has been ordered.

Nursing interventions aimed at dealing with the thirst discomfort include using ice chips instead of water to make up the fluids; frequently brushing the client's teeth and rinsing his mouth; using lemon-glycerin swabs to moisten mucous membranes; giving hard candy to the client to suck on if not contraindicated; and moistening the client's lips with a wet wash cloth.

Increased Fluid Requirements

In the diseased client there are many situations in which large quantities of fluids are lost from the body. This loss greatly increases the client's fluid requirements. Some of the events causing the loss of large volumes of fluid and potential dehydration are diarrhea, vomiting, hemorrhaging, fever, and excess drainage from surgical wounds.

Dietary Interventions

The nurse should constantly be aware of increased fluid needs of the client. Fluids are replaced either orally or through an intravenous infusion or both. If the client is allowed oral intake of fluids, fresh water should be kept by the bedside at all times. The nurse should encourage the client to consume additional fluids and explain why the increased

Nursing Allotment for Fluids:	7 AM to 3 PM	50 cc
	3 PM to 11 PM	50 cc
	11 PM to 7 AM	20 cc
Intravenous Intake (200 cc/hr):		480 cc
Dietary Allotment for Fluids:	Breakfast	200 cc
	Lunch	200 cc
	Dinner	200 cc
TOTAL		1,200 cc

Figure 26-12. Sample fluid restriction.

fluids are necessary and how they will be beneficial. The nurse may inform the dietitian of the client's increased fluid requirements and request that additional fluids be placed on the client's meal tray. This can be easily accomplished by adding soup, gelatin, and a glass of fruit juice to the regular beverages. The student should be reminded that large losses of electrolytes accompany the large fluid losses. Intervention for electrolyte imbalances was discussed earlier in this chapter.

CHANGES IN BLOOD pH

1. Acidosis requiring immediate intervention related to kidney impairment or excessive ingestion of acid
2. Acidosis requiring immediate intervention related to diabetes mellitus
3. Potential acidemia
4. Potential alkalemia
5. Alkalosis requiring immediate intervention

Client Objectives

1. Seek nursing and medical intervention to correct emergency phase serum pH alterations.
2. Discuss preventive measures that may maintain a normal blood pH.

Dietary Interventions

A continual supply of oxygen is necessary for cell survival. Unless oxygen is supplied to and used by the cell, other nutrients cannot be used and metabolism ceases. Supporting the client with an alteration in oxygen levels and its subsequent effect on blood pH is one of the fundamental problems of critical-care nursing. The client's movement into and out of acidemia and alkalemia must be carefully monitored. Medical intervention is directed at maintaining the proper blood pH by correcting the cause of the deficiency. The basic alterations that lead to acid-base imbalance were discussed in Chapter 11.

Nutritional support of clients with altered blood pH is mainly supportive. If the alteration is severe the client will probably be intubated and thus not taking food orally. For those clients who can ingest food, the diet should be palatable and easily digestible. Energy should be conserved for the client's metabolic demands.

CASE STUDY: A Client Who Has Had a Recent myocardial Infarction

Bradford T. is a 52-year-old business executive preparing for discharge from the hospital after a myocardial infarction. Before his heart attack he was a successful businessman with major responsibilities in his corporation. He had mild hypertension (150/90) and hypercholesterolemia (300 mg/100 ml; normal = 220 mg/ml). His serum triglycerides were elevated to 600 mg/100 ml (normal 140 mg/100 ml). On admission, Brad was 5 ft 7 in (170 cm) tall and weighed 190 lb (86.4 kg). He chain smoked while he worked, drank six to eight cups of coffee a day, and got little exercise. He lives with his wife and four children, aged 12, 14, 16, and 18.

He suffered his heart attack while at work, describing the pain as "the worst thing I've ever experienced in my life. I thought my arm was going to fall off." His hospital course was uneventful except for one episode of shortness of breath. Brad's physician has enrolled him in a cardiac rehabilitation course offered through the hospital. He attends classes, eagerly listening to the material being presented by the physician, psychiatrist, nutritionist, and nurse who teach the class.

Discharge orders include a fat-controlled, no-added-salt diet, rest, no smoking, and nitroglycerin for pain. Brad is to return to the rehabilitation class weekly for exercise and group therapy.

QUESTIONS

1. Bradford is experiencing an alteration in which aspect of nutrient transport?

2. What are the major objectives of the diet following a myocardial infarction?

3. What are the general principles of both the fat-controlled and the sodium-restricted diet?

4. What are some common foods to avoid on both the fat-controlled and the sodium-restricted diet?

5. What practical suggestions about food purchasing and preparation should be offered to clients like Brad on a fat-controlled or sodium-restricted diet?

BIBLIOGRAPHY

Abel, E. J., and Powell, R. C. An approach to the dietary management of hyperlipemia. *J. Indiana State Med. Assoc.* 64:827, 1971.

Bennion, M. *Clinical Nutrition.* 1st Ed. New York: Harper & Row, Pubs., Inc., 1979.

Brown, H. B., and Farrand, M. What a dietitian should know about hyperlipidemia. *J. Am. Diet. Assoc.* 63:169, 1973.

Burton, B. J. *Human Nutrition.* 3rd Ed. New York: McGraw-Hill Book Co., 1976.

Christakis, G., and Winston, M. Nutritional therapy in acute myocardial infarction. *J. Am. Diet. Assoc.* 63:233, 1973.

Comm. on Sodium Restricted Diets, Food and Nutrition Board, Nat'l Research Council. *Sodium-Restricted Diets and the Use of Diuretics: Rationale, Complications, and Practical Aspects of Their Use.* Washington, D.C.: Nat'l Acad. of Science, 1979.

Dustan, H. R., Tarazi, R. C., and Bravo, E. L. Diuretic and diet treatment of hypertension. *Arch. Intern. Med.* 133:1007, 1974.

Eshleman, R., and Winston M. *The American Heart Association Cookbook.* 3rd Ed. New York: David McKay Co., Inc., 1979.

Fabre, D., Given, C., Hockenberger, J., and Noland, N. Care of the patients with site actions in adaptation related to transportation of gases and nutrients. Unpublished manuscript, St. Louis University, 1974.

Frederickson, D. S. Dietary management of hyperlipoprotenemia: A handbook for physicians and dietitians. DHEW Publ. No. (NIH) 75-100. Bethesda, Md.: Nat'l Heart and Lung Instit., 1974.

Fredrickson, D. S., Levy, R. I., and Lees, R. S. Fat transport in lipoproteins: An integrated approach to mechanisms and disorders. *N. Engl. J. Med.* 276:34, 1967.

Glueck, C. J., Mattson, F., and Bierman, E. L. Diet and coronary heart disease: Another view. *N. Engl. J. Med.* 298:1471, 1978.

Gordon, E. S. Dietary problems in hypertension. *Geriatrics* 29:139, 1974.

Gotto, A. M. Is atherosclerosis reversible? *J. Am. Diet. Assoc.* 74:551, 1979.

Gotto, A. M., Scott, L., and Manis, E. Prudent eating after 40: Relationship of diet to blood lipids and coronary heart disease. *Geriatrics* 29:109, 1974.

Heap, B. Sodium restricted diets. *Am. J. Nurs.* 60:206, 1960.

Hill, M. Helping the hypertension patient control sodium intake. *Am. J. Nurs.* 79:906, 1979.

Krause, M. V., and Mahan, L. K. *Food, Nutrition, and Diet Therapy.* 6th Ed. Philadelphia: W. B. Saunders Co., 1979.

Kula, J. J. Sodium restricted diets. *Journal of Practical Nursing* 22(11):16, 1972.

Levy, R. I. Dietary and drug treatment of primary hyperlipoprotenemia. *Ann. Int. Med.* 77:267, 1972.

Malkus, B. L. Respiratory care at home. *Am. J. Nurs.* 76:1789, 1976.

Mallison, M. Updating the cholesterol controversy: Verdict—diet does count. *Am. J. Nurs.* 78:1681, 1978.

Mayer, J. Low sodium diets. *Postgrad. Med.* 49:193, 1971.

Mitchell, H. S., Rynbergen, H. J., Anderson, L., and Dibble, M. V. *Nutrition in Health and Disease.* 16th Ed. Philadelphia: J. B. Lippincott, 1976.

Mitchell, S. C. The diet-heart situation. *Postgrad. Med.* 60:197, 1976.

Overton, M. H., and Lukert, B. P. *Clinical Nutrition: A Physiologic Approach.* Chicago: Year Book Medical Pubs. Inc., 1977.

Pennington, J. *Nutritional Diet Therapy.* Palo Alto, Calif.: Bull Pub. Co., 1978.

Pflanzer, R. G. The blood. In E. E. Selkurt, Ed., *Basic Physiology for the Health Sciences.* Boston: Little, Brown and Co., 1975.

Reiser, R. Diet and blood lipids: An overview. *Food and Nutrition News* (Nat'l Livestock and Meat Board, Chicago) 51(2):1–4, 1980.

Robinson, C. H., and Lawler, M. R. *Normal and Therapeutic Nutrition.* 15th Ed. New York: Macmillan, Inc., 1977.

Rosen, E. Nutrition guidelines. *Journal of Practical Nursing* 27:15, 1977.

Snively, W. D., Beshear, D. R., and Roberts, K. T. Sodium restricted diet: Review and current status. *Nurs. Forum* 13:59, 1974.

Strong, J. P., Eggen, D. A., Oalmann, M. C., Richards, M. L., and Tracey, R. E. Pathology and epidemiology of atherosclerosis. *J. Am. Diet. Assoc.* 62:262, 1973.

Thiele, V. F. *Clinical Nutrition.* St. Louis: The C. V. Mosby Co., 1976.

Vinson, L. J. Modifying the American diet to stem the tide of coronary heart disease. *Nursing Care* 8:12, 1975.

Warren, S. E., Alpert, J. S., and Francis, G. S. Diet in the coronary care unit. *Am. Heart J.* 95:130, 1978.

Wiesman, C. K. The art of seasoning low sodium diets. *Nursing Homes* 20:12, 1971.

Williams, S. R. *Nutrition and Diet Therapy.* 3rd Ed. St. Louis: The C. V. Mosby Co., 1977.

Witschi, J. C., Singer, M., Wu Lee, M., and Stare, F. J. Family cooperation and effectiveness in a cholesterol-lowering diet. *J. Am. Diet. Assoc.* 72:384, 1978.

Youngstrom, K. A. Low sodium diet. *J. Kans. Med. Soc.* 72:263, 1971.

Yudkin, J. Sucrose and cardiovascular disease. *Proc. Nutr. Soc.* 31:331, 1972.

CHAPTER 27

Alterations in Metabolism

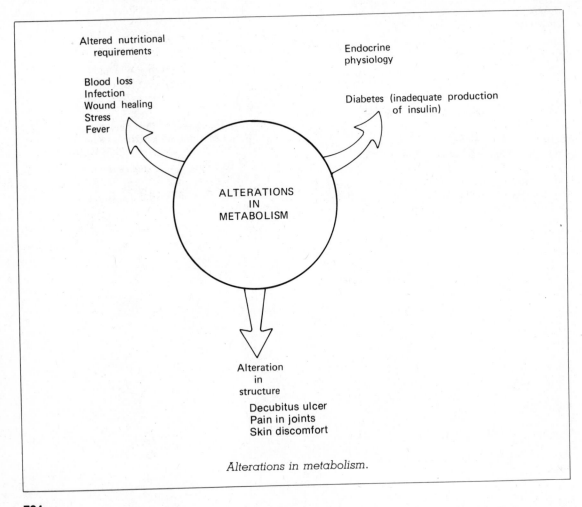

Altered nutritional
requirements

Blood loss
Infection
Wound healing
Stress
Fever

Endocrine
physiology

Diabetes (inadequate production
of insulin)

ALTERATIONS
IN
METABOLISM

Alteration
in
structure

Decubitus ulcer
Pain in joints
Skin discomfort

Alterations in metabolism.

Metabolism is the use of nutrients by the individual body cells for the functions of energy production, repair, and synthesis of necessary compounds. An interference with metabolism may be evidenced by increased nutritional requirements, alterations in the blood pH, or alterations in such body structures as the bones, nerves, or skin. Any alteration in the secretions of the endocrine glands will affect nutrient metabolism. A hereditary deficiency of a specific enzyme will also interfere with specific steps in the metabolism of carbohydrates, proteins, and fats.

ALTERATIONS IN NUTRITIONAL REQUIREMENTS

1. Increased nutritional requirements related to
   a. Blood loss
   b. Increased metabolic rate
   c. Tissue healing
   d. Infection
   e. Fever
2. Decreased protein requirement related to elevated levels of ammonia, blood urea nitrogen, nonprotein nitrogen
3. Alterations in nutritional requirements related to inborn errors of metabolism

Metabolism is a delicate balance between the two processes of anabolism and catabolism. When anabolism exceeds catabolism there is evidence of either physical growth or tissue repair or healing. If a catabolic state predominates there is evidence of inadequate nutritional intake, trauma, or a disease process that has imposed additional metabolic demands on the client.

Chapter 4 explained how body size and composition, age, secretions of the endocrine glands, and health status affect BMR. Basal nutritional requirements are also affected by normal and traumatic stresses. *Stress* may be defined as anything that threatens body homeostasis. Physical growth, pregnancy, and lactation are periods of normal physiological stress. The training of an athlete also imposes some normal physiological stress and increases the BMR. Even severe psychological stress may temporarily increase the BMR. The stress of pregnancy, lactation, and growth were discussed in Unit III. Traumatic stress may be due to immobilization, surgery, fractures, or burns. Clients may suffer one or more of these kinds of trauma. Complications such as fever, infection, hemorrhage, or diarrhea may further increase the nutritional requirements. This section is concerned with the nutritional demands imposed on clients by trauma and its complications.

The metabolic response to stress is catabolism. A summary of the classification of catabolism in different clinical situations is found in Table 27-1. This response is the same following the trauma of surgery, injuries including wounds and bone fractures, infections, and burns. The catabolic response is generally characterized by increased loss of fluid and electrolytes, urinary nitrogen, negative nitrogen balance, and weight loss. The extent of these losses depends on the degree of trauma and the client's previous nutritional status.

There is both an acute phase and an adaptive phase to the catabolic response. In the acute phase there is a release of hormones within the body. Glucagon is released by the pancreas, and glucocorticoid and epinephrine are released by the adrenal glands. The release of these hormones has the effect of decreasing the sensitivity of the tissues to insulin and inhibiting its release (Ryan, 1976), forcing the body to look elsewhere for its supply of glucose. In response, triglycerides are mobilized from the adipose stores to meet the energy demand. Also, protein from the skeletal muscles is mobilized, and large amounts of nitrogen and other minerals appear in the urine (Bennion, 1979). Until recently this catabolism of body protein was thought to have only harmful effects. Now,

TABLE 27-1. Classification of Catabolism

Clinical Situation	Degree of Catabolism	Urea = N (gm/day)	Increase of Resting Metabolic Rate over BMR (%)	Total Caloric Requirement[a] (Calories)
Person in bed	1° (normal)	<5	None	1,800
Uncomplicated surgery	2° (mild)	5–10	0–20	1,800–2,200
Multiple fractures or trauma	3° (moderate)	10–15	20–50	2,200–2,700
Acute major infections or major burns	4° (severe)	>15	50–125	2,700–4,000 or more

SOURCE.   Reprinted with permission from M. V. Krause and L. K. Mahan, *Food, Nutrition, and Diet Therapy*, 6th Ed. Philadelphia: W. B. Saunders Co., 1979; adapted from P. Rutten et al.; "Determination of Optimal Hyperalimentation Infusion Rate." *J. Surg. Res.* 18:477, 1975.
NOTE.   Classification of patients according to the following: (1) obligate nitrogen loss expressed in gm urea-N per 24 hr.; (2) energy expenditure expressed as percentage increase of the resting metabolic expenditure over calculated basal energy expenditure.
   [a] This total caloric resting metabolic requirement includes the amount needed for activity, about 20% since these patients usually are not active, and 10% for specific dynamic action (SDA). This is a rough estimate for a 70-kg man and depends on the patient's size.

however, it is believed that this process supplies the amino acids needed for the internal synthesis of blood proteins to fight infection and replace blood loss, collagen for healing, and necessary enzymes (Krause and Mahan, 1979).

Assessment data include hyperglycemia, increased nitrogen and mineral excretion, loss of appetite, and decreased intestinal motility. This acute catabolic phase usually lasts only a few days and does not have serious consequences for the previously well-nourished client. Administration of glucose intravenously during the acute phase only seems to aggravate the hyperglycemia and does not decrease the protein catabolism (Ryan, 1976). If, however, catabolism is prolonged by a complicated injury, fever, or infection or if the client has been previously weakened by disease or poor nutritional status, prolonged loss of body protein can become a threat to survival. Continued protein catabolism will also result in weakness, reduced immunity, and slower wound healing (Ryan, 1976).

In the adaptive phase levels of hormone return to normal with the exception of gluca-gon. This phase is characterized by a falling level of blood glucose and decreased excretion of urinary nitrogen. Plasma fatty acid levels are still high, and ketones are present in the urine, indicating that large amounts of fat are being used for energy. The adaptive phase is a transition in which nutritional support can be initiated. The client's appetite usually improves during this phase. This transition to a more anabolic state should be promoted by offering food when the blood glucose begins to fall and when GI function returns.

Client Objectives

To be able to:

1. Plan a diet that meets his altered nutritional requirements.
2. Consume a diet that meets his altered nutritional requirements.

Dietary Interventions

Nutritional support is an important part of the medical treatment of trauma and its complications. The general objectives of nutritional therapy are the same for the various kinds of trauma and sepsis. Trauma includes surgery, injuries, fractures, and burns. Fever and infection are complications that often accompany trauma. These processes are catabolic processes that increase the basal nutritional requirements. The overall goal is to provide nutritional support that will change the catabolic process into an anabolic process in which healing of the damaged tissue will begin. The objectives of nutritional therapy to accomplish this goal are to (1) minimize weight loss, (2) reduce the urinary loss of nitrogen, (3) provide adequate Calories and nutrients for healing, and (4) replace those nutrients that have been lost in the catabolic process.

The basic dietary intervention for all these conditions is a high-protein, high-Calorie diet with increased amounts of fluid and additional vitamins and minerals. The specific number of Calories and the amount of protein and other nutrients depends on the severity of the condition, the client's previous nutritional status, and whether two or more of the catabolic processes are present simultaneously. The diet order written in the client's medical chart will usually read "high-protein, high-Calorie diet." The order may also specify high protein between-meal feedings or supplements.

General Principles

Because the RDA's may not be adequate to meet the additional nutritional requirements of a client affected by disease or trauma, a high-protein, high-Calorie diet may be required. This diet is considered by most hospitals to contain 100–125 gm of protein and 2,500–3,000 Calories per day. The usual procedure is to serve the client the regular hospital diet including a dessert, but with the addition of a high-protein, high-Calorie supplement between meals. The protein content of this diet for the adult is based on a range of 0.8–1.5 gm of protein per kilogram of ideal body weight. The RDA for protein for the adult is based on 0.8 gm/kg, so the level of protein is increased by about 50%. This level of protein is usually sufficient for the surgical client or a client with fractures, fever, or infection. Because the level of protein required is only slightly above the RDA, sometimes the physician will not write a specific order for a high-protein, high-Calorie diet. The regular hospital diet contains 90–110 gm of protein daily. Therefore, for the client with uncomplicated minor surgery, simple fractures, or a mild infection or fever, the regular hospital diet is often more than adequate in Calories, protein, and vitamins and minerals. For clients who have had major surgery or who were in poor nutritional status prior to surgery or trauma, a diet high in protein, Calories, and extra vitamins and minerals is highly desirable.

The need for certain vitamins and minerals increases during trauma and infection. Whenever the protein and Calories are increased in the diet, there is a corresponding increase in the requirements for the B-complex vitamins. Because thiamine, riboflavin, and niacin participate directly in the metabolism of carbohydrate, protein, and fat, increased proportions should be provided when the energy nutrients are increased. Increased quantities of the B-complex vitamins will be found in the additional foods supplied to increase Calories and protein, so a separate supplement of these vitamins may not be necessary. Fever increases the requirements for vitamin C and vitamin A. Very little is known about the increased nutritional requirements during stress, but a supplement of these two vitamins is probably desirable with a prolonged fever. There is an increased requirement for vitamin C following surgery or burns to promote new collagen formation for wound healing. Additional vitamin K should be supplied both before and after surgery to assist in normal blood clotting. Vitamin K is usually added to the intravenous solution both before and after surgery. If excessive bleeding or hemorrhage occurs, an iron supplement may be needed.

The burned patient has the highest nutritional requirements of any client. The requirements for protein and Calories are directly proportional to the quantity of body surface area that has been burned. The protein content of the diet for the burned patient is at least two to three times the RDA for protein. The Calorie content of the diet is often from 2,500–5,000 Calories/day. Massive amounts of vitamins are needed in the range of 5 to 10 times the RDA. Doses of vitamin C of 1,000 mg/day are required to aid in collagen formation for wound healing. The nutritional demands imposed on the burned patient often cannot be met by regular food intake, so oral intake must often be supplemented by nasogastric feeding or hyperalimentation in addition to regular intravenous therapy. A summary of the nutritional support of catabolic conditions is found in Table 27-2.

Rationale

The rationale of the high-protein, high-Calorie diet is based on the effect that the nutrients will have on the catabolic processes once the acute phase of trauma has passed. There are three aspects to the rationale. First, surgery, trauma, fever, burns, and infection all increase the BMR. The extra Calories help ensure that the increased energy needs will be met so that excessive weight loss does not occur. Second, a large proportion of the increased Calories are supplied by carbohy-

drate. Most carbohydrates are readily tolerated, and they provide the protein-sparing effect. This means that the carbohydrate will be used first to supply the body's energy needs, thus sparing the dietary protein for its crucial functions of tissue repair and increased synthesis of collagen. Third, the increased protein will be used to repair body tissues and minimize the body's breakdown of its own muscle tissue, thus decreasing the urinary excretion of nitrogen.

Practical Considerations

The foods offered should provide the maximum amount of protein and Calories with the least amount of bulk. They should be soft and easy to digest. Clients with any one of the catabolic conditions often have a decreased appetite. The nurse and dietitian should find out the client's favorite foods and make every effort to include at least some of them. The nurse should clearly explain the rationale for optimal nutritional intake of foods high in Calories and protein as it relates to the client's medical condition. The dietitian or nurse should also encourage the client to consume a nutritional supplement or high-protein snack between meals. This might be a specially prepared eggnog, a milk shake, or a commercial liquid supplement. The client should be encouraged to try different flavors or types of supplements to avoid taste fatigue. An example of a high-Calorie high-protein diet is found in Figure 27-1.

When feeding is begun, the quantity of food offered should be increased gradually

TABLE 27-2. Nutritional Support of Catabolic Conditions

	Calories	Protein
Fever	High-Calorie (40–45 Calories/kg)	High-protein (100–120 gm)
Uncomplicated elective surgery or multiple fractures	1,800–2,700 (40–45 Calories/kg)	100–200 gm (1.0–2.0 gm/kg)
Infection and moderate-to-severe burns	2800–6300 (40–90 Calories/kg)	150–200 gm (2–3 gm/kg)

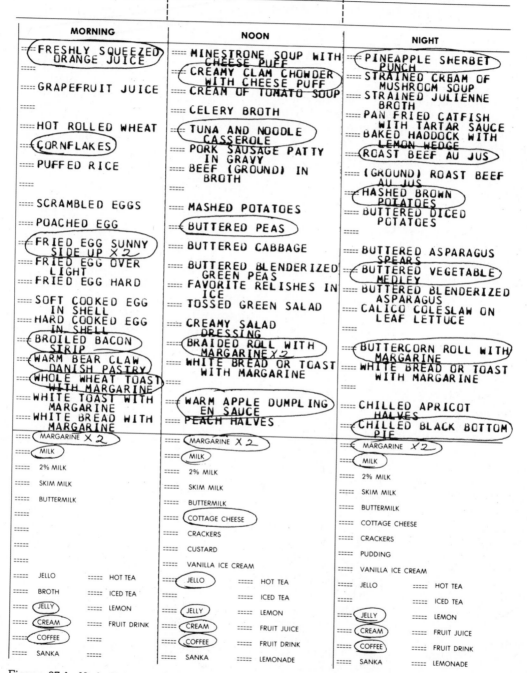

Figure 27-1. High-Calorie high-protein diet. (Courtesy Indiana University Hospitals)

but steadily as tolerated by the client. General appetite usually returns slowly after surgery or other trauma. Some clients may prefer to have their food divided into six smaller meals instead of three meals plus snacks.

The postoperative client usually responds well to a diet as tolerated. The presence of audible bowel sounds indicates the return of intestinal motility and signals that eating may be resumed. The traditional clear, full-liquid, and soft diets may not need to be followed in their strict form. If the physician writes the order "clear liquid, advance to regular as tolerated" or "diet as tolerated," the client is free to select meals in consultation with the nurse or dietitian.

Because of the high nutritional demands imposed on the burned client, several points need to be made about the evaluation of the nutritional support. The client should be weighed daily, if possible. A loss of weight is an indication that caloric intake is not adequate and that body catabolism is excessive. Burned clients should always be on Calorie counts to estimate the quantities of carbohydrate, protein, and fat as well as total Calories that are consumed in a 24-hour period. The correlation between body weight and caloric intake may be assessed. Calorie counts are often done by a member of the dietary staff, but in some hospitals this responsibility may be left to the nursing staff. The nurse assigned to care for burned clients should always check to see who is responsible for this important task. A Calorie count can be accomplished fairly easily using the exchange system (see Chap. 3) to estimate the grams of carbohydrate, protein, and fat in the foods eaten by the client at each meal and between meals. The total grams of carbohydrate, protein, and fat as well as Calories are recorded in the client's chart daily. The high-Calorie foods not listed in the exchange lists can be found in nutritional tables of food composition such as Appendix A of this book. The nurse is often a logical choice to do Calorie counts because she is with the client more

than the dietitian. The nurse must be certain to observe the client's food tray after he has finished eating and before it has been removed by the dietary staff.

The client with fractures has an increased requirement for calcium to replenish the broken bone; but calcium in the diet should not be increased until after mobilization of the client has been resumed, lest it lead to formation of kidney stones. The greatest need of the client with fractures is for increased protein, which helps form the collagen matrix in which the calcium will eventually be deposited.

Liver Disease

Liver disease provides a good example for the incorporation of several dietary modifications in therapy. The dietary modifications are directly related to the physiological state of the client. There are three pathophysiological processes that may occur in the various types of liver disease for which one or more dietary modifications is helpful. The first of these is the inflammation of the liver found in hepatitis. This inflammatory process increases the nutritional requirements. Most of the dietary principles just reviewed also apply to the dietary management of hepatitis. The diet should be a well-balanced one high in Calories and carbohydrate, high in protein, and moderate in fat content. A specific high-protein, high-Calorie diet may not be specified by the physician because the regular hospital menu can be quite high in Calories and protein. Whenever a client's diagnosis is hepatitis, the nurse should recall that a high-Calorie, high-protein diet will help to repair the damaged liver tissue and overcome the negative nitrogen balance. The client's energy needs may be elevated because of the infection and fever present. The high-Calorie, high carbohydrate part of the diet will help meet these increased needs, spare the protein for repair of the liver tissue, and prevent weight loss. The appetite of the client with hepatitis is often greatly reduced, so he will usually need help selecting a menu that provides a high concentration of essential nutrients. The nurse should constantly encourage the client to eat and explain why this type of diet will aid his recovery.

A second pathophysiological condition of liver disease is the gradual loss of functioning liver tissue that occurs in cirrhosis. Cirrhosis may be either acute or chronic. It may result from very severe hepatitis or chronic alcoholism. Some of the liver cells actually die. The third pathophysiological condition is related to the cirrhosis. It is a complication of liver disease called *hepatic coma*. This complication may occur because the damaged liver cells can no longer detoxify the ammonia from protein metabolism into urea. The portal circulation is impaired; the ammonia thus gains entrance into the general circulation and leads to toxification of the CNS. If the symptoms of ascites and hypertension are present in cirrhosis and hepatic coma, the diet must be restricted in sodium.

The dietary intervention for cirrhosis is basically the same as that for hepatitis except that the protein content is not quite as high. The protein content is generally set high enough to regenerate all possible liver tissue but low enough to avoid the complication of hepatic coma. The protein content of the diet for cirrhosis is often between 65 and 85 gm daily. Intakes greater than this may precipitate hepatic coma. This complication may occur when the diseased liver cannot adequately detoxify the ammonia to urea. The client experiencing this complication usually is not in a comatose state; the state could instead be described as one of confusion, disorientation, or stupor. Some of the other symptoms associated with ammonia intoxification are restlessness, irritability, delirium, and drowsiness. The laboratory test indicating impending hepatic coma is for elevated blood levels of ammonia. The dietary management during hepatic coma is the reduction of the dietary protein. The diet should be high in Calories and carbohydrate to prevent the breakdown

of tissue proteins for energy. Catabolism of body tissue would serve only to complicate the problem further because extra ammonia from additional amino acids would be delivered to the liver for conversion to urea. In this way, catabolism of body tissue serves only to aggravate hepatic coma. Another way hepatic coma can be aggravated is by the rupturing of the varicose veins in the esophagus (*esophageal varices*). These varicose veins develop as a complication of portal hypertension. Their rupture can precipitate hepatic coma or even result in death. A bland or low-residue diet is sometimes used to avoid irritation of these veins.

In all instances of liver disease a high-Calorie, high carbohydrate diet is required. The protein level is adjusted according to the client's individual tolerance. If adequate Calories are not consumed at the three meals, appropriate snacks should be encouraged between meals.

Inborn Errors of Metabolism

Another group of physiological disorders is caused by specific defects in the metabolism of nutrients. Considering the intricacies of cellular metabolism and the complexities of protein synthesis and the genetic transfer of information in the formation of a new life at conception, it should not be surprising that the possibilities for inherited metabolic errors are endless. An example of an inborn error of metabolism that is found in all humans and several other species is a deficiency of the enzyme needed to convert L-gulonolactone to ascorbic acid (Thiele, 1976), thus making vitamin C an essential nutrient in the human diet. An inborn error of metabolism is the result of an enzyme deficiency. There are over 600 enzymes that control metabolic reactions, a deficiency in any one of which could cause an inborn error. At present over 300 of these metabolic defects are known. Two-thirds of these represent defects that may occur in the synthesis of hemoglobin, which contains 574 amino acids in its structure (Thiele, 1976).

The remaining 100 are enzyme defects that affect the metabolism primarily of carbohydrate, protein, and lipids, but also of vitamins and minerals.

It is possible to provide here only a brief introduction to managing inborn errors of metabolism by diet therapy. The most common type of metabolic error involves an enzyme deficiency that prevents substrate A from being converted to substrate B; instead there is an accumulation of intermediate products. An example is the metabolic error phenylketonuria. In a few cases the product that cannot be formed is essential, and therapy consists of supplying this missing metabolite. Also in a few cases the action of the enzyme can be enhanced by administering pharmacological doses of specific vitamins (Snyderman, 1975). The effect of the metabolic error on the client varies a great deal. Some inborn errors are incompatible with life. Some result in severe mental retardation and growth retardation if not treated promptly. Some do not produce any serious limitations. Some become evident shortly after birth; others may not become evident until adulthood. Diabetes mellitus and gout may be classified as inborn errors of carbohydrate metabolism, as may the familial hyperlipoproteinemias. Table 27-3 provides a list of inborn errors that respond to dietary management.

The inborn errors of metabolism are all rare disorders, and some are very rare. Specialists working in this field may see only a few cases of any one disorder during a whole career. Two of these disorders that the student may be exposed to are phenylketonuria (PKU) and galactosemia. The incidence of PKU is one in every 10,000 births (Robinson and Lawler, 1977). Galactosemia occurs only about once in every 25,000–50,000 births (Williams, 1977). Most of the other inborn errors of metabolism occur with even less frequency, and the student is referred to other texts such as Krause and Mahan (1979), Robinson and Lawler (1977), and Thiele (1976) for a more complete discussion of these conditions.

The treatment of these metabolic disorders usually occurs in major medical centers with teams of specialists who coordinate their efforts to diagnose and treat the client and educate the family about the disease. The physician and biochemist work together to identify the specific metabolic defect. The nurse and dietitian are concerned with the practical aspects of the client's care. The dietitian is responsible for planning and implementing the specific aspects of the diet to meet the client's nutritional needs. The nurse is involved with the nursing care and participates in the implementation of the dietary management, including discussing the rationale for the diet with the family and offering practical suggestions for its implementation.

The major goal of therapy for inborn errors of metabolism is the prevention of mental retardation and growth failure. Early detection of the disorder and immediate implementation of therapy are the best safeguards. Most states require hospitals to perform a routine screening of all newborns for PKU. This is done shortly after birth by means of the *diaper test,* whereby a drop of ferric chloride is dropped on the diaper to detect the presence of phenylpyruvic acid, an abnormal metabolite found in the urine of clients with PKU (Robinson and Lawler, 1977). Routine screening for galactosemia is not done, for the condition becomes evident within the first few days from such symptoms as anorexia, vomiting, drowsiness, puffiness of the face, edema of the lower extremities, and weight loss.

PHENYLKETONURIA. The main requirement of the diet is the restriction of foods that contain the substances that are cause the metabolic block. In PKU the metabolic defect is the absence of the enzyme phenylalanine hydroxylase, which normally catalyzes the

TABLE 27-3. Dietary Management of Inborn Errors of Metabolism

Error	Treatment
Amino Acid Metabolism Disorders	
Phenylketonuria	Low phenylalanine
Tyrosinemia	Vitamin C, vitamin B_6
Disorders of tryptophan metabolism	Nicotinic acid therapy
1. Hydroxykynureninuria	Nicotinic acid therapy
2. Tryptophanuria	Nicotonic acid therapy
3. Hartnup's disease	Liberal protein with niacin and pyridoxine supplementation.
Maple syrup urine disease	Diet limited in branched-chain amino acids
Isovaleric acidemia	Low-protein diet or restriction of leucine
Glycinemia	Synthetic diet free of both glycine and serine
	High methionine diet
Histidinemia	Restriction of histidine intake
Homocystinuria	Large doses of pyridoxine (B_6)
	Cystine supplement
	Folic acid
Cystinosis	Diets low in methionine and cystine
Lysinemia	Restriction of protein intake
Urea-cycle disorders	Protein-restricted diet
Carbohydrate Metabolism Disorders	
Galactosemia	Elimination of lactose
Fructosemia	Elimination of sucrose and fructose
Disaccharide intolerance	Elimination of the dissaccharides
Glucose-galactose malabsorption	Elimination of glucose and galactose
	Substitution of fructose
Glycogen-storage disease	Small carbohydrate feedings every three hours around the clock
	Decreased fat and substitution of MCT
	Small protein feedings
Vitamin-dependent Disorders	
Resistant rickets	Extremely large doses of 150,000–250,000 IU daily
	Constant monitoring to avoid toxicity
Vitamin B_6 dependency	Large doses of pyridoxine (Vitamin B_6)

conversion of the essential amino acid phenylalanine to tyrosine. When this enzyme is missing, levels of phenylalanine and other metabolites accumulate in the blood. These metabolites are toxic to the brain and prevent normal development of the brain and CNS (Krause and Mahan, 1979). Tyrosine is normally involved with the production of pigments, but because its metabolism is impaired the infant with phenylketonuria often has blond hair, blue eyes, fair skin, and eczema.

The presence of an abnormal metabolite in the urine and on the skin accounts for the characteristic "mousy" or "gamey" odor of these clients.

The dietary management of phenylketonuria involves the restriction of the dietary intake of the amino acid phenylalanine; but because phenylalanine is an essential amino acid it must not be eliminated completely. Nor would it be possible to eliminate it completely, since all animal foods contain all the essential amino acids. The principle of the diet is to limit the intake of phenylalanine to prevent high accumulations but, at the same time, to provide the minimal amount required for normal growth. A special low-phenylalanine formula has been available since the early 1950s that helps in carrying out this principle.

The calculation of the infant or young child's diet is accomplished in a stepwise manner. First, the child's daily Calorie, protein, and phenylalanine requirements are calculated based on the child's age and weight. Next the amount of low-phenylalanine formula to meet the protein and Calorie requirements is calculated. Finally, amounts of other foods are determined to meet the phenylalanine allowance. These three steps determine the foods allowed on the diet. For the very young infant receiving only formula, the low-phenylalanine formula is the basis of the diet, but measured quantities of regular milk or formula must be added to meet the infant's minimum requirement for phenylalanine. The levels of phenylalanine in the diet are continually adjusted according to the laboratory values. The goal is to liberalize the diet as much as possible but to maintain the blood levels of phenylalanine and other metabolites within a safe range. The optimal age for discontinuing the diet is still being debated; dietary treatment of PKU has been in effect for only about 25 years (Justice and Smith, 1975). Most physicians are cautious about discontinuing the diet, but there is general agreement that the diet can be greatly liberalized and in many cases discontinued as the child approaches adolescence.

Many cases of children with PKU who have been successfully treated with a low-phenylalanine diet have been documented. Infants who were diagnosed at birth to have PKU and who have followed a controlled diet during the early childhood years have avoided mental retardation, and they display normal growth and development. Early detection and dietary treatment of PKU has

greatly improved the prognosis for those with this disease. Before the 1950s people with PKU were admitted to institutions and suffered severe mental retardation.

GALACTOSEMIA. The metabolic defect in galactosemia is the absence of the liver enzyme *galactose-1-phosphate uridyl transferase,* which aids in the conversion of galactose to glucose. Galactose-1-phosphate is toxic, and it accumulates in the blood and tissues. The dietary treatment for galactosemia involves a diet restricted in both lactose and galactose. A special galactose-free formula is available for use. Milk and milk products are the foods that are eliminated from the diet. This diet is similar to the one used for lactose intolerance, but it should be more strictly followed because failure to do so will result in mental retardation or possibly even death for the client with galactosemia. A few other foods yield galactose and may be restricted: peas, beets, lima beans, liver, cocoa, and chocolate (Burton, 1976).

ALTERATIONS IN ENDOCRINE PHYSIOLOGY

1. Impending thyroid crisis
2. Potential goiter
3. Predisposition to diabetes
4. Insulin shock
5. Lack of information about diabetes management

The hormones of the endocrine system are important in the regulation of carbohydrates, protein, fat, minerals, and electrolyte metabolism (see Chap. 12). Not only do the secretions of the endocrine glands affect nutrient metabolism, but the nutritional status of the client affects the functioning of the endocrine glands. This section deals with disorders manifested by alterations in endocrine secretions. Alterations in secretions of the endocrine glands may alter metabolism and lead to nutritional imbalances, changes in body weight, and general discomfort for the client. The use of hormone therapy in endocrine disorders is very effective. Nutritional support is necessary only to maintain metabolic balance during the acute phase or to rehabilitate the client after hormonal therapy has begun. Table 27-4 describes the general nutritional therapy used along with hormone therapy for each of the major disorders of the endocrine glands. Disorders of the endocrine function of the pancreas provide a good example of nutritional therapy for an alteration in endocrine function. The two conditions discussed are diabetes mellitus and *functional hyperinsulinism*.

Client Objectives

To be able to:

1. Plan a diet that meets his altered nutritional requirements.
2. Discuss a diet that may prevent endocrine imbalances.

Diabetes Mellitus

The endocrine function of the pancreas involves the secretion of two hormones, insulin and glucagon, which are important in controlling blood glucose. Insulin lowers blood glucose, thus favoring glycogen formation. Glucagon increases blood glucose by favoring the conversion of glycogen to glucose. Any disorder in the amount of insulin released by the pancreas or in the timing of the insulin released will result in abnormalities in carbohydrate metabolism. The body tissues (muscle, liver, and adipose tissue) may also have a resistance to the action of insulin, thus decreasing its effectiveness. The two most common disorders of carbohydrate metabolism are diabetes mellitus and functional hyperinsulinism (hypoglycemia). Uncontrolled diabetes mellitus is characterized by elevated levels of blood glucose both after

fasting and after a meal. In contrast, functional hyperinsulinism is manifested by abnormally low fasting levels of blood, a rise right after a meal, but then a rapid drop in blood sugar below fasting levels two to three hours after a meal.

Diagnosis of abnormal carbohydrate metabolism can be accomplished by the use of an oral glucose tolerance test. The fasting level of blood glucose is measured. The client is then asked to drink a beverage that contains 100 gm of carbohydrate (Glucola). The nurse should caution the client to sip this beverage slowly because it is very concentrated and is quite likely to induce nausea. Blood and urine samples are drawn at regular intervals, usually every hour, and the results are plotted on a graph. Other methods of determining glucose tolerance are the 2-hr postprandial blood sugar and a daily intake of 300 gm of carbohydrate for 3 days before the test.

An abnormal glucose tolerance produces symptoms that are related to the abnormal carbohydrate metabolism. The initial complaints of the client with diabetes mellitus may be increased thirst (*polydipsia*), increased urination (polyuria), increased hunger (*polyphagia*), and weight loss. The laboratory data will reveal an elevation in blood glucose (hyperglycemia) and maybe glucose in the urine (glycosuria). All these symptoms are related to the abnormal metabolism of glucose. The ravenous hunger exists because, although adequate glucose is available, it cannot gain access into the cells because of insufficient insulin. The increased thirst is the body's attempt to dilute the large quantity of glucose in the blood, and it is also a safeguard against the dehydration that will eventually occur. The increased urination is the body's attempt to dilute the large amounts of glucose that must be excreted.

Diabetes is not just an abnormality of carbohydrate metabolism; it is an alteration in carbohydrate, protein, fat, fluid, and electrolyte metabolism. The following description of the metabolism in diabetes mellitus uses many

TABLE 27-4. Nutritional Treatment of Endocrine Disorders

Disorder	General Characteristics	Therapy
Adrenal Gland		
Addison's disease	Decreased hormones of the adrenal cortex; decreased aldosterone causing decreased sodium ion reabsorption and excretion of sodium and chloride ions and water; decreased extracellular fluid; acidosis; increased potassium ion level; decreased glucocorticoid hormones leading to gluconeogenesis leading to hypoglycemia	Replacement hormones or 4–6 gm additional salt daily; high-protein, moderate-carbohydrate diet; frequent feedings; generous fluids; increased vitamin C and B complex
Cushing's syndrome or ACTH therapy	Protein depletion; decreased glucose tolerance; increased hydrochloric acid secretion; depletion of vitamin C from the adrenals	High-protein, moderate-carbohydrate (200–300 gm) diet without concentrated sweets; moderate sodium restriction (2–3 gm); vitamin C supplement
Thyroid Gland		
Hypothyroidism (myxedema in adults, cretinism in children)	Decreased activity of thyroxine or T₃ or both; lowered BMR; rapid rise in weight; increased blood cholesterol level; cold intolerance; lethargy; dry skin; decreased peristalsis	Low-Calorie, high-fiber diet
Hyperthyroidism (exophthalmic goiter or Graves's disease)	Increased BMR; increased carbohydrate and protein metabolism; calcium imbalance; negative nitrogen balance; irritability; hyperexcitability	High-Calorie (4,500–5,000 Calorie), high-protein (100 gm), high-carbohydrate diet; increased vitamins and minerals; administered iodine; decreased stimulants
Endemic goiter	Deficiency of iodine	Administration of 100 μg of iodine daily to adults
Parathyroid Glands		
Tetany Hypocalcemia Alkalosis	Convulsions; cramps; muscle twitchings	High-calcium (1,800–2,400 mg) diet; vitamin D supplement; sometimes magnesium supplement
Pituitary Gland		
Acromegaly	Increased GH	Complicated by diabetes
Pituitary dwarfism	Decreased pituitary hormones; decreased thyroid and adrenal function	None
Diabetes insipidus	ADH	None
Precocious puberty	Abnormally early release of gonadotropic hormones by pituitary	None
Pancreas		
Functional hyperinsulinism (hypoglycemia)	Delayed or excessive release of insulin	Low-carbohydrate (100 gm), high-protein diet; six small meals a day; high-protein snacks; no stimulants
Diabetes mellitus	Elevated blood glucose level; glucose in urine; increased appetite, thirst, and urination	Elimination of concentrated sweets; Calories controlled to maintain or attain ideal weight; specific levels of carbohydrate, protein, and fat

of the principles of intermediary metabolism from Chapter 12. Insulin deficiency leading to hyperglycemia stimulates the secretion of other hormones that stimulate either glycogenolysis or gluconeogenesis, thus enhancing the hyperglycemia even more. Be-

cause the glucose cannot gain entrance into the cells owing to the decreased availability of insulin, the glucose accumulates in the blood (see Fig. 27-2). The body then turns to protein and fat for a source of glucose. Gluconeogenesis is increased, and about 58%

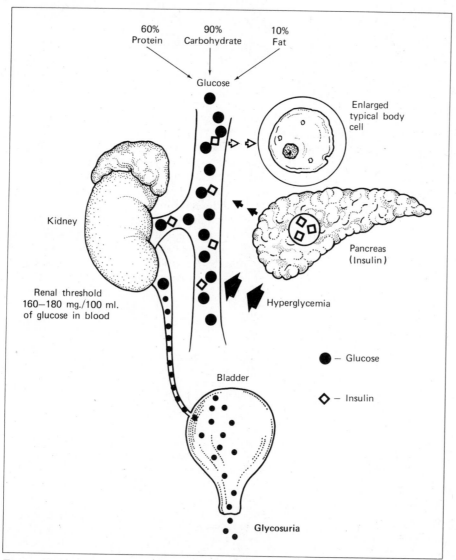

Figure 27-2. Abnormal carbohydrate metabolism from alteration in insulin.

of the protein and 10% of the fat may be converted to glucose. There is, therefore, increased catabolism of protein and fat. There is also an increased release of free fatty acids from the adipose tissue.

There are two basic defects in diabetes that can be used to classify the disease into two types. One defect is in the production of insulin by the *beta cells* of the pancreas, and the other is a resistance of the body tissues to the action of insulin (Arky, 1978). Clients with the first defect require administration of insulin. This type is commonly referred to as *juvenile diabetes*. The second defect, in which there is a tissue resistance to insulin, is called *adult diabetes*. Clients in this group can usually be managed by diet therapy only or with the help of an oral hypoglycemic agent. They do not usually require insulin. The designations of *juvenile* or *adult* diabetes are sometimes misleading because (1) some adult diabetics do require insulin and (2) in some people the symptoms of diabetes may appear in adolescence although their diabetes is of the "adult" type. The terms *ketosis-prone* or *insulin-dependent*, should be used for juvenile diabetes regardless of the age at which it occurs,

and *ketosis-resistant* or *noninsulin-dependent* for adult diabetes regardless of age (Arky, 1978). The terms *growth-onset* and *maturity-onset diabetes* may also be used. There are several differences between the two types in the characteristics of the disease and the medical and dietary treatment. Table 27-5 gives a comparison of these two types of diabetes.

Dietary Intervention

Three methods of treatment are commonly used for diabetes mellitus: diet, exercise, and insulin or oral hypoglycemic agents. Some maturity-onset diabetics may be able to control their diabetes with diet and exercise only. The treatment and education of the client with diabetes requires the knowledge, involvement, and cooperation of every member of the health team. The physician is responsible for the assessment of the client's diabetes and for determining the preferred medical treatment. The physician is usually responsible for ordering a specific diet, but the nurse or dietitian may also be involved. The nurse has the responsibility for teaching the client about the administration of insulin or oral

TABLE 27-5. Comparison of Types of Diabetes

	Juvenile-onset	Mature-onset
Onset	Abrupt	Usually gradual
Weight	Normal or underweight	70% overweight
Stability	Diabetes labile	Diabetes usually relatively stable
Insulin	Necessary for all	$\frac{1}{3}$ must take insulin or use oral agents
Ketoacidosis	Relatively frequent	Infrequent
Insulin sensitivity	Marked	Relatively insensitive
Family history	Very common	Common
Degenerative changes at time of onset	Infrequent	Common
Control of diabetes	Difficult	Easy
Endogenous insulin	None	Present but frequently release in response to glucose is sluggish
Potential response to diet alone	Unsatisfactory	Frequently dramatic
Response to oral agents	None	Good to excellent if diet is followed
Mean age of onset	Under 35	Over 35

medication, encouraging sound general health habits, urging dietary compliance, and answering basic questions related to diet. The dietitian has the major responsibility for planning the diabetic diet with the client; instructing him in the general principles of the diet; and offering practical suggestions for menu planning, food preparation, and eating in restaurants. All members of the health team should encourage the client to adhere to the diabetic diet. One suggestion is that the diabetic diet not be referred to as a "diet" but spoken of as a *meal plan* or *eating plan,* terms that may have a more positive connotation for the client (Flood, 1979). Every attempt should be made to make the diabetic diet seem as close to a regular diet as possible.

GENERAL PRINCIPLES. The general principles of the diabetic diet are those of sound nutrition. The diabetic diet is the most healthful diet to eat; everyone would benefit by adapting its principles to his own eating habits. This positive point should be stressed to the new diabetic client, who may think of this diet as only a list of restrictions.

There are two major objectives in the dietary treatment of diabetes: to achieve or maintain ideal body weight and to achieve a normal level of blood glucose. If these two objectives are achieved over a period of time, the symptoms of diabetes will be minimized, and such long-term degenerative changes as atherosclerosis, retinopathy, and renal problems will be reduced.

It has recently been realized that the most important component of the dietary treatment of diabetes is control of total caloric intake (Arky, 1978); 90% of diabetics are above their ideal weight at the time of diagnosis (C. S. Davidson, 1976). There is a general reduction in glucose tolerance and an increase in blood glucose with obesity. A moderate weight loss of 10 to 15 lb (4.5–6.8 kg) is frequently accompanied by an improvement in glucose tolerance and a decrease in blood glucose levels

(Arky, 1978). In maturity-onset diabetics who have attained their ideal body weight, levels of blood glucose may have returned to normal levels. As long as ideal weight is maintained, their diabetes can be said to be under control.

The second important component of the diabetic diet is the ingestion of carbohydrate. Simple sugars are more rapidly absorbed than starches. More insulin is required in the insulin-dependent diabetic after a high-carbohydrate menu, especially one high in simple sugars (Hamburger et al., 1979). Most diabetes physicians therefore recommend the elimination of simple sugars and concentrated sweets. For the maturity-onset diabetic the nurse might place emphasis on the elimination of concentrated sweets as a means of losing and maintaining weight loss rather than stating that concentrated sweets must be eliminated because the client is a diabetic. Many diabetics resent the elimination of sweets from their diet, but they may respond more positively if weight loss and maintenance of ideal weight are the focus.

The diabetic diet specifies a caloric level based on the client's age, sex, activity level, and present body weight. The main objective of diet therapy is either the attainment or maintenance of ideal body weight. In fact, some physicians believe that diabetic control is better if the client is about 10% under his ideal body weight. The daily allotment of Calories is divided among the energy nutrients of carbohydrate, protein, and fat. A certain percentage of the Calories are contributed by each of these energy nutrients.

The calculation of the diabetic diet is based on the client's personal nutritional needs. The first step is to estimate ideal body weight using the formula based on height and frame size presented in Chapter 4. The next step is to estimate the basal caloric requirement. This can be easily done by multiplying the ideal body weight by 10. A factor for activity may be added according to the following guidelines:

Sedentary caloric requirement
  = Ideal body weight (pounds) × 3
Moderate caloric requirement
  = Ideal body weight (pounds) × 5
Strenuous caloric requirement
  = Ideal body weight (pounds) × 10

The RDA may be used as a guideline for the caloric requirement of children. The protein requirement for an adult is 0.8–1 gm/kg of ideal body weight. The slightly increased amount of protein adds satiety and acceptability to the diet. Other dietary modifications may need to be considered such as raising or lowering the protein or decreasing the sodium content. Because of other complications that may accompany diabetes, the client's diet may need to be restricted in sodium and saturated fat. Some of the particular problems encountered by a client on this combination of diets are discussed later.

The diet prescription or diet order is the way the diabetic diet is written by the physician in the client's chart for communication with the nursing and dietary staffs. The diabetic diet order for a 1,200-Calorie diet may be written any one of the following ways:

• 1,200-Calorie diabetic diet
• 1,200-Calorie diet (120-60-50)
• 1,200-Calorie diabetic diet (120 gm of carbohydrate, 60 gm of protein, 50 gm of fat)
• Diabetic diet 120-60-50

There may also be a remark with the diet order regarding snacks or the desired distribution of carbohydrate in meals. First of all, the amounts specified in the diet prescription are the Calories or grams of carbohydrate, protein, or fat for the entire day, *not* for one meal only. If no snacks nor particular distribution of food throughout the day are mentioned, the amounts may be divided into three equally spaced meals. If three numbers are written together such as 120-60-50, this means that the diet is to contain 120 gm of carbohydrate, 60 gm of protein, and 50 gm of fat. Numbers written this way always refer to the level of carbohydrate, protein, and fat in that order. If no number of grams is specified, but only the level of Calories, it may be assumed that a standard breakdown for the diabetic diet may be used. Table 27-6 gives examples of the calculation of grams of carbohydrate, protein, and fat using two standard breakdowns and 1,200 Calories.

The old standard breakdown for a diabetic diet was 40% of the Calories from carbohydrate and fat and 20% of the Calories from protein. The most recent recommendation is to increase the proportion of carbohydrate from 40% to 50% and to decrease the proportion of fat from 40% to 30%. This change was in response to the increased incidence of atherosclerosis in the diabetic. The revised exchange lists published by the American Diabetes Association and the American Dietetic Association in 1976 reflect this suggested decrease in total fat content as well as restriction or limitation of foods high in saturated fat and cholesterol. Incorporation of the principles of the fat-controlled diet along with those of the diabetic diet is a preventive measure

TABLE 27-6. Sample Calculations of Diabetic Diet

	Old	New
Carbohydrate	40% of Calories: 1,200 × 0.40 = 480 ÷ 4 = 120 gm	50% of Calories 1200 × 0.50 = 600 ÷ 4 = 150 gm
Protein	20% of Calories 1,200 × 0.20 = 240 ÷ 4 = 60 gm	20% of Calories 1200 × 0.20 = 240 ÷ 4 = 60 gm
Fat	40% of Calories: 1,200 × 0.40 = 480 ÷ 9 = 53 gm (50 gm)	30% of Calories 1200 × 0.30 = 360 ÷ 9 = 40 gm

against the premature development of atherosclerosis. This may be particularly important for the growth-onset diabetic client who will be on insulin for the rest of his lifetime. Long-term studies on the effectiveness of this restriction in preventing atherosclerosis in diabetics have not been conducted, but the increased incidence of atherosclerosis in diabetics seems to be enough justification for the incorporation of these principles into the diabetic diet.

The client must learn to understand and follow his meal plan. He should know that his Calorie restriction naturally restricts the amounts of carbohydrate, protein, and fat inasmuch as all three of these nutrients contribute Calories to the diet and that all three of these energy nutrients are also potential sources of glucose. The fact that no additional fat may be added to the diet beyond the amounts specified in the meal plan may limit the methods of food preparation to those that do not use fat. All regular sugar and all sources of concentrated sweets must be eliminated. It should also be stressed to the client that the amount of protein in the diet is also limited. In other words, the client must eat only the amount of meat allowed in the meal plan. The consumption of additional meat will cause the Calorie limits of the diet to be exceeded, and the additional protein is a source of additional glucose. The client is instructed either to measure or to weigh his food. Some of the common aids to measuring are shown in Figure 27-3.

For the convenience of the client the amounts of carbohydrate, protein, and fat in his meal plan are divided into a total number of food exchanges, or portions, that are then distributed among the three meals and sometimes snacks. Dividing the daily allotment of food into exchanges or portions for each meal helps the client understand exactly the amount of food allowed at a meal. This helps in meal planning, shopping, and preparing the food.

The client is encouraged to eat regular meals that are evenly spaced. There should be about four to five hours between meals. No food should be eaten between meals unless a specific snack has been ordered by the physician. The client should be encouraged not to skip any meals or to allow an unnecessary delay in eating. Control of the client's diabetes is based on the regularity of eating. This is especially important for the client who is receiving insulin. The dose of insulin taken must be directly proportional to the amount of food eaten, especially the carbohydrate content. If a meal is skipped or if there is a long delay in eating, the client's blood glucose level may become quite low, and a hypoglycemic reaction (discussed in a more detail later in this chapter) may occur. All the food allowed at a meal should be eaten. Again, this is especially important for the client on insulin. If some food is not eaten, there is also danger of a hypoglycemic reaction before the next meal, because the insulin dosage will have been calculated on the basis of a certain quantity of food being eaten. If inadequate food is eaten, the insulin continues to act to lower blood glucose, but with inadequate glucose available the level of blood glucose is reduced to a level below normal.

The client should be told that it is not permissible to substitute food from one exchange list for food from another exchange list because each exchange list contains a different proportion of carbohydrate, protein, and fat. Substituting exchanges in a meal disrupts the intended balance of carbohydrate, protein, and fat. It should be emphasize, however, that the client may substitute any food within an exchange list for any other food in that same list as long as the total number of exchanges allowed for that meal is not exceeded. Most diabetic diets allow more than one exchange per meal for meat and bread. If the client for example is allowed three meat exchanges for a meal, 3 oz of roast beef may be eaten or the three exchanges may be used for different foods. For example, three meat exchanges might include one hot dog, one slice of

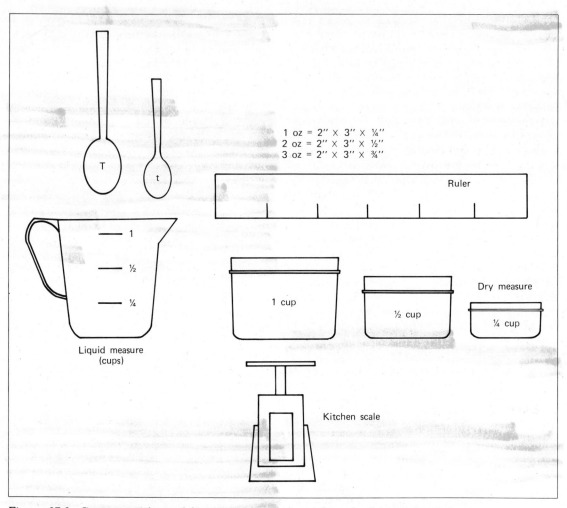

1 oz = 2" × 3" × ¼"
2 oz = 2" × 3" × ½"
3 oz = 2" × 3" × ¾"

Ruler

1

½

¼

Liquid measure
(cups)

1 cup

½ cup

Dry measure

¼ cup

Kitchen scale

Figure 27-3. Common tools used for measuring and weighing food for diabetic diets.

cheese, and ¼ cup of cottage cheese. The client should be instructed not to save food or exchanges from one meal to be eaten at the next meal. This practice also upsets the delicate balance in the control of diabetes with not enough food being consumed at one meal and too much at another.

The control of diabetes involves a balance between diet, exercise, and insulin or oral hypoglycemic agents. The diet is determined for the client, and then dosage of the insulin is determined. With some types of insulin, a variation in the meal distribution is required. It is not the purpose of this text to discuss the different types of insulin, but two basic principles affect the meal distribution. The peak action and the duration of action of the insulin affect the distribution of food. First, carbohydrate from food must be available whenever the insulin has its peak action. Second, enough carbohydrate must be available within the body to last for the duration of the insulin's effect. If inadequate carbohydrate is available at any one of these times, there is an increased likelihood of the client experiencing a low blood glucose level, that is, a hypoglycemic reaction. For example, if the peak action of a type of insulin occurs at 4 PM, a snack should be provided at that time.

Regular exercise has the effect of lowering the requirement for insulin. It is thought that the exercise facilitates the transport of glucose into the cell without the aid of insulin. Therefore most physicians suggest some type of regular exercise program for the diabetic. Any kind of additional exercise that a client engages in, however, requires that a snack be eaten immediately before the activity to guard against a hypoglycemic reaction during the additional exercise.

Sometimes adjustments in food or insulin may need to be made because of different levels of activity on the weekends. The nurse should encourage the client to consult with the physician about adjustments.

DIETARY COUNSELING. One of the best ways to initiate discussion about the diabetic diet is to begin by taking a diet history. This gives the nurse an understanding of the client's regular eating habits and a good idea about the extent of modification that will be needed. It will also provide a basis for initiating diet counseling. It can be very embarrassing for the nurse or dietitian to begin a discussion about the diabetic diet only to be informed by the client that the physician had not told him he was a diabetic. Guideline number one should be to check with the client's physician or the chart to be sure the client has been informed of the diagnosis. Many clients have fears and anxieties about being diabetic, and they may need a period of time to adjust to this diagnosis.

There is a lot for the client to learn about the diabetic diet, and he should not be expected to learn it all in one session. The nurse may prepare the client for the dietitian's initial dietary instruction by explaining diabetes and the general treatment, including diet as an important part. The dietitian should give the client an overview of the principles of the diabetic diet but not expect him to learn too much at that first session. The dietitian may make out some menus for the client to serve as examples. The menus should be based as much as possible on the client's own eating habits. Several sessions on diet should be planned during the client's stay in the hospital. After several sessions the dietitian or nurse may ask the client to write some menus to check his understanding of the exchange system. Many large hospitals now conduct a series of classes for diabetics, including classes taught by a nurse on insulin and general health practices. Classes taught in this manner offer such benefits as clients learning from each other and more time to present the information in a quiet, relaxed atmosphere. A member of the client's family should be present for most if not all of the instructions about the diabetic diet. This is especially important when the client is not the family member in charge of cooking. In the case of a male client, his wife, sister, or mother should be present to hear the instruction.

The first topic that should be discussed with the client is the elimination of all regular sugar and concentrated sweets. Although it may seem a negative way to begin, the exclusion of this source of carbohydrate is the most important aspect of the diabetic diet. The reason for the elimination of foods containing sugar should be outlined simply and clearly to the client. Explain that all sugars contain glucose, which the client's body is unable to use. The glucose therefore accumulates in the blood and causes undesirable symptoms. Bread, milk, fruits, and vegetables also have natural sugars that contain glucose, but they are not present in a concentrated form like in sugar. Elimination of regular table or granulated sugar also means the elimination of all forms of sugar. Cane and beet sugar both

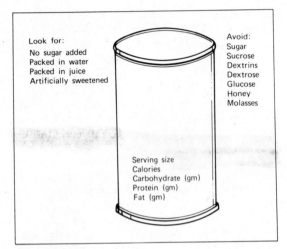

Look for:
No sugar added
Packed in water
Packed in juice
Artificially sweetened

Avoid:
Sugar
Sucrose
Dextrins
Dextrose
Glucose
Honey
Molasses

Serving size
Calories
Carbohydrate (gm)
Protein (gm)
Fat (gm)

Figure 27-4. Information on food labels helpful to clients on diabetic diets.

have the same composition, and both must be eliminated. Other sugars that must be eliminated are brown sugar, powdered sugar, honey, molasses, pancake syrups, jams, jellies, and preserves. Also, all foods prepared with sugar are to be omitted. This, of course, includes cakes, pies, cookies, candies, and other sweet desserts, and many prepared foods made with sugar that come from the store. The client should be taught what to look for on the label, that is, any word on the label that ends in the suffix -ose is quite likely to be a sugar. The client should read the label before purchasing any food item. Figure 27-4 shows some of the terms to look for and avoid when shopping for food to use on the diabetic diet.

The next topic to discuss should be the exchange system of classifying foods into lists that have similar contents of carbohydrate, protein, fat, and Calories (Appendix I). These are the same exchange lists described in Chapter 3. They were developed by a joint commission of the American Diabetes Association and the American Dietetic Association in 1950 for use with diabetics and revised by the same two organizations in 1976. A colorful attractive booklet is available for instruct-

ing clients about the diabetic diet (Fig. 27-5). Since its development the exchange system has found other uses such as in weight-reducing diets.

The concept of an "exchange" should be explained clearly to the client; first of all, that an *exchange* is a portion of food from one of the food lists, of which there are six (milk, vegetables, fruit, bread, meat, and fat) and that one exchange portion is the amount listed beside the food in the list. The diabetic meal plan will allow for a certain number of exchanges from each list at each meal. If two exchanges are allowed at one meal, the client may select two separate foods from that exchange list or twice the amount of a single food. Second, besides reference to the amount of food, the term *exchange* refers to the ability to substitute or trade foods within the same list. Foods from one list may not be substituted for foods on another list because each list has a different content of carbohydrate, protein, fat, and Calories. Substituting in this manner would imbalance the content of the energy nutrients and the Calories in the diet. The ideal situation is for the dietitian to construct an individualized meal plan for the client based on a thorough diet history, the client's personal eating habits, and economic and cultural considerations. A diabetic diet constructed in this manner should lead to better adherence. As previously emphasized, it is a very poor practice simply to hand a client a diet of preprinted exchanges per meal.

The revised exchange lists incorporate the recommendations of the American Heart Association by emphasizing the use of low-fat milk, lean meat, and polyunsaturated fats. They also contain only one vegetable list instead of two. The third major difference is in the meat exchanges. The revised list of meat exchanges is divided into three groups based on fat content: lean meat, medium-fat meat, and high-fat meat. The client is encouraged to select most meats from the lean group. If meats are selected from the medium- or high-fat groups, the client is instructed to

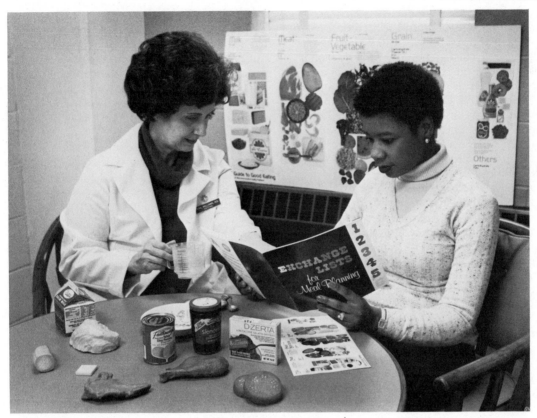

Figure 27-5. The dietitian uses a variety of teaching aids when instructing the client in measuring foods for the diabetic diet. (Photo by J. Collins)

omit one-half a fat exchange or one fat exchange, respectively, for *each* meat exchange allowed. As an example, suppose the client chose to eat a pork tenderloin steak, which is a medium-fat meat. If the client's meal pattern allowed for two meat exchanges at that meal, the client should omit one-half a fat exchange for each meat exchange; that is, the client should omit a total of one fat exchange from the number of fat exchanges allowed in the meal pattern. If the original number of fat exchanges allowed was two, then this number would be reduced to one exchange because of the selection of a medium-fat meat. The purpose of this manipulation of fat is to control

the total amount of fat in the diabetic diet and to encourage the selection of lean meats. This manipulation of fat is often difficult for clients to understand. A similar effect can be obtained by encouraging the client to select meats from either of the first two groups and to restrict his intake of high-fat meats to only a few servings a week. In actual practice, dietitians are treating the meat list as one list with the values of 7 gm of protein and 5 gm of fat for each meat exchange.

Many diabetic clients have, of course, been previously instructed in use of the original exchange lists. Instructing these clients in the use of the revised exchange lists only creates confusion. These clients are accustomed to one meat list and a division of the vegetable list into Group A and Group B vegetables. Such clients should probably not be reinstructed on using the new exchange lists to prevent confusion and anxiety about the diet. Inasmuch as the nurse will come in contact with both versions of the exchange lists in client teaching, she should be familiar with the major differences between the two lists.

The milk exchanges contain all types of fluid milk and plain, unflavored yogurt. It is recommended that the milk consumed be skim or low fat. Consumption of low-fat or skim milk not only reduces the amount of saturated fat in the diet but allows for the inclusion of additional fat exchanges, thereby increasing the palatability of the diet and adding to the flexibility.

The vegetable exchanges offer inclusion of all fresh vegetables and virtually all frozen and canned ones. One vegetable exchange is usually allowed at lunch and dinner. The revised exchange list groups most vegetables into one group of which ½ cup is one exchange. A few raw vegetables may be eaten as desired because their carbohydrate content is quite low. These vegetables are varieties of salad greens and radishes. In the original separated vegetable exchange list, Group A vegetables are low-carbohydrate vegetables that are allowed in quantities of 1 cup cooked or as desired if raw. Group A contains most of the green, leafy and salad vegetables. Group B contains the moderate-carbohydrate vegetables such as beets, carrots, peas, onions, pumpkin, rutabaga, winter squash, and turnips. One serving of a B vegetable is ½ cup.

In addition to the vegetables in this list, several starchy, high-carbohydrate vegetables are found in the bread list, for example, dried beans, corn, lima beans, white potatoes, and sweet potatoes. Also, in the revised exchange list, green peas, pumpkin, and winter squash are in the bread list and not in the vegetable list.

Any type of fresh vegetable may be used on the diabetic diet. All plain frozen vegetables may be used except for those packaged in sauces or butter. Most regular canned vegetables can also be used. It is not necessary to use the special cans of dietetic vegetables. These vegetables are only lower in sodium content and need be used only by clients who are restricted to 1,000 mg of sodium or less each day. Some canned vegetables such as peas, corn, beets, and tomatoes contain added sugar and should be avoided in favor of the fresh or frozen variety. Also, canned sweet potatoes packed in a sugar syrup should be avoided, whereas those that are vacuum packed may be used. The client should be encouraged to get the habit of reading the list of ingredients on the label before purchasing canned or frozen vegetables.

The next list is the fruit exchanges. Any type of fresh fruit may be used on the diabetic diet provided the portion eaten is the same as the amount listed as a fruit exchange. The client should be encouraged to eat fresh fruit in season and to preserve seasonal fruits by home canning or freezing. He must be reminded, however, that sugar may not be added during the processing. The labels of commercially canned or frozen fruit should be read very carefully for sugar content. Most canned fruits are packed in a light or heavy syrup and therefore should not be used. Many frozen fruits are also frozen with sugar and should also be avoided, but some frozen fruits have no sugar added. These unsugared fruits are often found in 1 lb bags. Some fruits frozen in this manner are cherries, strawberries, other berries, and peach slices. Some canned fruits can also be used on a diabetic diet. The label of a canned fruit must state that the fruit is unsweetened, has no sugar added, or is packed in water or natural fruit juice. Red, sour, pitted cherries may be packed in water, pineapple is frequently packed in its own natural juice. Sometime the client must select fruits from the special dietetic canned fruit. Even though the word *dietetic* is on the label, it should not be assumed that all foods labeled dietetic are necessarily suitable for diabetics. The term *dietetic* simply means that a modification has been made in that food. The dietetic food may be modified in Calories, carbohydrate, fat, cholesterol, or sodium. The only way to know for certain what nutrient has been modified is to read the label. Before dietetic canned fruit is purchased, the label should be carefully examined. If the label states that the fruit is unsweetened, has no sugar added, is artificially sweetened, or is packed in water or natural fruit juices, the fruit is acceptable for use on a diabetic diet. Because dietetic fruit is quite expensive, the nurse should encourage the client to use fresh or unsweetened canned or frozen fruit whenever possible. Powdered juice mixes or fruit drinks should not be used because they contain a large amount of sugar.

The bread list contains a variety of bread and cereal products that may be used on the diabetic diet. Most types of breads may be used, but not those that contain a higher-than-usual proportion of sugar such as quick breads or breads with a glaze or icing like cinnamon rolls. Doughnuts, sweet rolls, coffee cakes, and most cakes and cookies are also eliminated because of the high content of sugar and the excess Calories. Most kinds of dry and cooked cereals are allowed with the exception of presweetened cereals and cereals containing dried fruit. Other cereal products such as rice, macaroni, spaghetti, and noodles are allowed, although the amounts permitted are less than the quantities generally consumed by most people. Several varieties of crackers are listed, which may be used as a substitute for bread. In addition to all these foods, portion sizes are given for a few prepared foods such as a biscuit, cornbread, round crackers, a plain muffin, French fries, potato chips, a pancake, or a waffle. Because these foods are higher in fat content than the other foods on the bread list,

a fat exchange should be omitted from the meal at which these foods are consumed. On some exchange lists, equivalent portions are also available for angel food cake, sherbet, ice cream, and vanilla wafers.

The meat list offers a wide range of meats for selection. The restriction pertains to the amount of meat allowed at each meal, the method of preparation, and the type of meat selected. Meat is restricted on the diabetic diet because the protein contained in the meat has the potential of becoming glucose. Large quantities of meat would also add excessive Calories to the diet. The amount of meat allowed is usually two to four meat exchanges at each meal. This represents between 2 and 4 oz of meat, an amount that is more than adequate when compared with the basic four but generally lower than consumed by most people in the United States. The meat must be prepared by some method that does not use fat or add Calories: baking, boiling, broiling, roasting, or grilling. No breading should be used. There are, however, special recipe books that use sauces in the preparation. The carbohydrate, protein, fat, and Calorie content of these sauces has been taken into consideration. The recipe tells how the prepared meat may be substituted into the diet. The diabetic client should be encouraged to select meat either from the low-fat or the medium-fat lists. The overweight diabetic client cannot afford the extra Calories in the high-fat meats. The juvenile-onset diabetic should generally avoid the high-fat meats because of the relationship between the intake of foods high in saturated fat and cholesterol and the increased incidence of atherosclerosis in diabetics.

The final exchange list is the fat list. Fats of both animal and vegetable origin are allowed in the amounts specified in the list. Fats are restricted on the diabetic diet because 10% of the fat has the potential of being converted to glucose but also because each fat exchange adds extra Calories to the diet. Polyunsaturated fat is preferable to saturated fat, and this should be emphasized to the client. Foods may be fried occasionally if the amount of fat used is omitted from the fat exchanges allowed for that meal. A sample of a diabetic menu is found in Figure 27-6. The number of exchanges is provided at the bottom of the figure. Certain foods may be used in unlimited amounts on the diabetic diet because of negligible carbohydrate and Calorie content. These foods are artificially sweetened beverages, coffee, tea, fat-free bouillon, unsweetened unflavored gelatin, unsweetened dill pickles, and cranberries without sugar. All spices and herbs may be used as flavorings as well as lemon juice, lime juice, and vinegar. The use of these foods and flavoring can add to the variety and general acceptability of the diet.

Since the development of the exchange lists, commercial food companies and hospital dietary departments have published additional food lists showing how many prepared foods can be incorporated into the diabetic diet. Commercial food companies have lists available for combination entrees such as beef stew, spaghetti, and canned soups. There are also lists available for using pizzas and frozen prepared dinners. Several of the fast-food restaurants have also converted their products so they can be substituted into the diabetic meal plan.

Several good diabetic cookbooks are available. Once the client has mastered the exchange system, the nurse should encourage him to use the suggestions and recipes in these cookbooks to increase the variety and general acceptability of his diet. The recipes in a good diabetic cookbook should specify the total number of servings in the entire recipe and the amount or proportion that is considered one serving. The recipes should also specify the exchange equivalents of one serving. For example, a recipe for Italian spaghetti might yield four 1-cup servings, each of which is equal to one bread exchange, two meat exchanges, and two fat exchanges.

If spaghetti is included in a meal prepared from a specific recipe, the portion of spaghetti replaces part of the exchanges allowed for that meal. The other foods in the menu are planned according to the number of exchanges remaining.

The diabetic client will need an artificial sweetener of some type as a substitute for regular table sugar. The question which artificial sweetener is best remains unanswered. *Cyclamates,* one of the most acceptable artificial sweeteners, were banned in 1971 from use in the United States. Cyclamates are, however, still available in Canada. An attempt to ban *saccharin* came during 1977 as the result of some studies that reported the development of bladder tumors in rats who were fed large doses of it; instead, the product began to carry a warning on the label concerning the safety of the sweetener. *Sorbitol* and *mannitol* are carbohydrate derivatives that have been used in "dietetic foods." These derivatives are naturally more sweet, so less of them is required. These products are actually carbohydrates, and they do contribute to the carbohydrate and caloric content of the food. Controversy exists about allowing food containing sorbitol and mannitol on the diabetic diet. Questions remain as to the amount absorbed, the effect on blood levels of glucose, and the caloric contribution to the diet.

Some physicians and dietitians are recommending the incorporation of foods with natural sweetness, such as fruits, into the diet. The consumption of fruits, however, would be limited to a specified amount per day. Probably the best advice to give the diabetic client who is concerned about artificial sweeteners is to suggest that he use them only in moderation because overconsumption could cause diarrhea. The search for a safe and pleasant-tasting artificial sweetener continues.

PRACTICAL CONSIDERATIONS. The diabetic diet must become so integrated into the client's eating habits and daily routine that

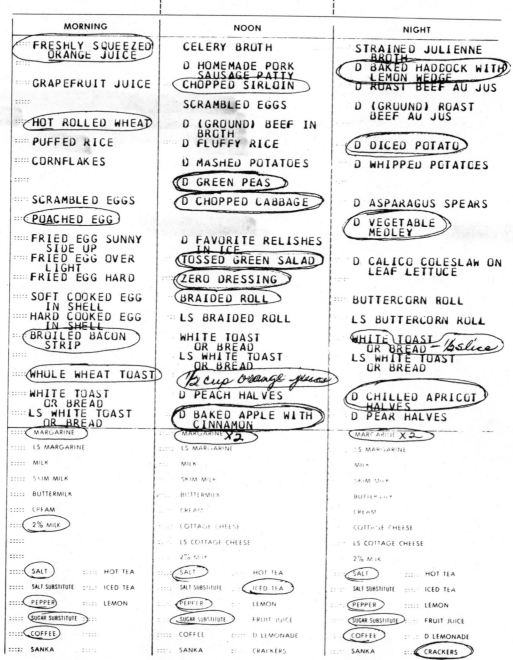

INDIANA UNIVERSITY HOSPITALS CALORIE CONTROL MENU	INDIANA UNIVERSITY HOSPITALS CALORIE CONTROL MENU	INDIANA UNIVERSITY HOSPITALS CALORIE CONTROL MENU
MORNING	**NOON**	**NIGHT**
FRESHLY SQUEEZED ORANGE JUICE	CELERY BROTH	STRAINED JULIENNE BROTH
GRAPEFRUIT JUICE	D HOMEMADE PORK SAUSAGE PATTY	D BAKED HADDOCK WITH LEMON WEDGE
	CHOPPED SIRLOIN	D ROAST BEEF AU JUS
	SCRAMBLED EGGS	D (GROUND) ROAST BEEF AU JUS
HOT ROLLED WHEAT	D (GROUND) BEEF IN BROTH	
PUFFED RICE	D FLUFFY RICE	D DICED POTATO
CORNFLAKES	D MASHED POTATOES	D WHIPPED POTATOES
	D GREEN PEAS	
SCRAMBLED EGGS	D CHOPPED CABBAGE	D ASPARAGUS SPEARS
POACHED EGG		D VEGETABLE MEDLEY
FRIED EGG SUNNY SIDE UP	D FAVORITE RELISHES IN ICE	
FRIED EGG OVER LIGHT	TOSSED GREEN SALAD	D CALICO COLESLAW ON LEAF LETTUCE
FRIED EGG HARD	ZERO DRESSING	
SOFT COOKED EGG IN SHELL	BRAIDED ROLL	BUTTERCORN ROLL
HARD COOKED EGG IN SHELL	LS BRAIDED ROLL	LS BUTTERCORN ROLL
BROILED BACON STRIP	WHITE TOAST OR BREAD	WHITE TOAST OR BREAD — *3 slice*
	LS WHITE TOAST OR BREAD	LS WHITE TOAST OR BREAD
WHOLE WHEAT TOAST	*½ cup orange juice*	
WHITE TOAST OR BREAD	D PEACH HALVES	D CHILLED APRICOT HALVES
LS WHITE TOAST OR BREAD	D BAKED APPLE WITH CINNAMON	D PEAR HALVES
MARGARINE	MARGARINE *X2*	MARGARINE *X2*
LS MARGARINE	LS MARGARINE	LS MARGARINE
MILK	MILK	MILK
SKIM MILK	SKIM MILK	SKIM MILK
BUTTERMILK	BUTTERMILK	BUTTERMILK
CREAM	CREAM	CREAM
2% MILK	COTTAGE CHEESE	COTTAGE CHEESE
	LS COTTAGE CHEESE	LS COTTAGE CHEESE
	2% MILK	2% MILK
SALT HOT TEA	SALT HOT TEA	SALT HOT TEA
SALT SUBSTITUTE ICED TEA	SALT SUBSTITUTE ICED TEA	SALT SUBSTITUTE ICED TEA
PEPPER LEMON	PEPPER LEMON	PEPPER LEMON
SUGAR SUBSTITUTE	SUGAR SUBSTITUTE FRUIT JUICE	SUGAR SUBSTITUTE FRUIT JUICE
COFFEE	COFFEE D LEMONADE	COFFEE D LEMONADE
SANKA	SANKA CRACKERS	SANKA CRACKERS

Figure 27-6. Diabetic 1,800-Calorie diet menu and exchanges. (Courtesy Indiana University Hospitals)

appropriate dietary modifications can be made to allow for changes in levels of exercise or health status with very little or no significant alteration in blood glucose. Whenever the delicate balance among diet, exercise, and insulin or oral medication is upset by an alteration in any one of these factors, the client is likely to experience either an abnormally low blood glucose level (hypoglycemia) or a return to a high blood glucose level (hyperglycemia). An imbalance in the control of diabetes mellitus resulting in either hypo-

glycemia or hyperglycemia if left untreated is a life-threatening condition. Fortunately, both conditions respond to treatment, and the symptoms are easily recognized by the diabetic client, a close friend or family member, or a physician or nurse. A summary of the causes and treatment of both hypoglycemia and hyperglycemia is found in Table 27-7.

Hypoglycemia occurs more frequently. The onset is rapid. It may result from inadequate food, too much insulin, or too much exercise. The result is a rapid drop in the

TABLE 27-7. Warning Signs for Diabetic Reactions

Hypoglycemic Reaction (Insulin Reaction)	Warning Signs	Hyperglycemic Reaction (Diabetic Coma)
Sudden	ONSET	Gradual
Pale, moist, perspiring	SKIN	Flushed, hot, dry
Excited, nervous, trembling, weak, irritable, confused faint, blurred vision	BEHAVIOR	Drowsy, weak
Normal	BREATH	Fruity odor (acetone)
Normal to rapid shallow	BREATHING	Deep, labored
Absent	VOMITING	Present with nausea
Moist, numb, tingling	TONGUE	Dry
Present	HUNGER	Absent
Absent	THIRST	Present (dehydration)
Headache	PAIN	Abdominal
Normal, slight sugar	URINE	Frequent with large amounts of sugar; ketones present
Unconsciousness	CONSCIOUSNESS	Unconsciousness leading to coma
Too much insulin Undereating Vomiting or diarrhea Delayed meal Excessive exercise	CAUSE	Not enough insulin Overeating Infection Illness Surgery Stress Nausea or vomiting
Orange juice (100 ml) Coke Hard candy (Lifesavers, 4–5) Glucagon if unconscious	TREATMENT	Check urine Go to bed Keep warm Force fluids Take usual or increased dose of insulin Call doctor

level of blood glucose to below the normal range. A delay in eating, skipping a meal, or not eating all the food allowed at a meal may lower the level of blood glucose. The client may have any combination of the symptoms of sweating, nervousness, double vision, hunger, trembling, palpitation, or headache. The oral administration of a small amount of easily absorbed carbohydrate will usually bring dramatic results in two to three minutes. This carbohydrate may be in several common forms. A small glass of orange juice with or without some sugar added is the treatment most commonly used in the hospital. This may be administered either by the nursing or the dietary staff, but a note should be made of the amount and the time in the client's chart. Some physicians recommend that their diabetic clients carry Life Saver candies or mints in their pocket or purse specifically for these times. A special product called Instant Glucose is also available. It comes in a tube, and a small amount may be squeezed into the cheek of the diabetic who is semiconscious from a hypoglycemic reaction. Because this substance is absorbed so rapidly, the client will become alert enough so that additional carbohydrate can be administered orally. Instant Glucose has replaced the need to carry glucagon, which was carried by the diabetic for emergencies. A few milligrams of glucagon injected subcutaneously initiates the release of glucose by stimulating glycogenolysis in the liver.

Hyperglycemia involves the elevation of the blood glucose level. This imbalance is a return to the uncontrolled state of diabetes. It may be the result of an inadequate amount of insulin, the increased requirement for insulin imposed by severe illness or stress, or nonadherence to the diabetic diet. Intervention with hyperglycemia or acidosis involves the administration of large doses of insulin to bring the high levels of blood glucose down to a more normal range. The medical intervention with hyperglycemia also involves the administration of fluids and electrolytes to replace the

fluids and to correct the acidosis. The principles of this therapy were discussed in Chapter 23.

To prevent imbalance the nurse should instruct the diabetic client to eat an appropriate snack before participating in unexpected or unusual exercise. The diabetic meal pattern is based on the usual level of physical activity for a specific person. Whenever this normal level of physical activity is exceeded, the client should be encouraged to consume a snack before the unusual physical exercise to provide the additional glucose required for the performance of the activity. If no snack is consumed, the increased level of activity will lower the blood glucose and perhaps precipitate a hypoglycemic reaction. Two examples may make the idea of unusual exercise clearer. A diabetic student decides to participate in a 2-mile bicycle race on Saturday, and a diabetic business executive decides to paint his house on Saturday. Both of these persons will be participating in a level of physical activity in excess of their normal level of energy expenditure. Additional Calories and carbohydrate will be needed to perform these tasks. If a snack or additional food is not consumed prior to the increased exercise, it is quite possible these clients may experience a rapid lowering of blood glucose during the exercise.

The snack should contain sufficient carbohydrate to keep the blood glucose level within the normal range during the exercise and until the next regular meal can be consumed. It should not contain only simple sugars from fruit because this form of carbohydrate is readily used and quickly depleted. The snack should consist of some complex carbohydrate and some protein. Two examples of appropriate snacks are a small sandwich (with one slice of bread) and a small apple. Another example might be ½ cup of milk and a few crackers. The size of the snack should be in proportion to the level of exercise that will occur.

Dining out in restaurants does not pose as

many problems for the client on the diabetic diet as it does for those trying to adhere to other types of diets. The primary prerequisite for eating out is that the diabetic client be very familiar with his diet pattern. The client should be thoroughly acquainted with the types of foods allowed and with portion sizes. For the newly diagnosed diabetic this period of adjustment may take from two weeks to a month, during which time he should be instructed to consume most of his meals at home. If, however, the client's lifestyle or occupation necessitates eating away from home, the nurse or dietitian should help the client plan several "typical" meals he can order using the type of foods usually served in the places where he usually eats.

When eating in a restaurant the client should carefully study the entire menu before making a selection. It is preferable to order meats that have been baked, boiled, roasted, or grilled and to refrain from ordering combination foods such as lasagna and spaghetti. A common problem for the diabetic eating in a restaurant is that the portion size of the meat is too large. Most restaurants provide at least 4 oz and even 6–8 oz in one serving of meat. Many adult diabetics are allowed only 2–4 meat exchanges per meal (2–4 oz). The diabetic should be encouraged to order a small hamburger or a small steak. If another type of meat is desired, the client could share the portion with a friend or eat only the approximate portion specified in his meal pattern and take the rest home for use at another meal.

A baked potato should be ordered whenever possible in place of French fries or home-fried potatoes. Most restaurants serve only a lettuce salad for a vegetable. A mixture of vinegar and oil or a similar type of dressing may be used. The client should ask the waitress to put only a limited quantity of dressing on the salad. Some clients may prefer to bring their own salad dressing in a small container. Some restaurants may even have a low-Calorie dressing available. Fresh fruit or un-

sweetened canned fruit may be ordered for dessert. If fresh fruit is not available the client should ask if unsweetened fruit is available. A small glass of fruit juice if it is unsweetened could also be substituted for the fruit exchange.

Most diabetic clients are limited in the number of bread exchanges per meal, so a decision must be made whether to eat the potato or the bread in a restaurant meal. The number of bread exchanges eaten should conform as closely as possible to the number of bread exchanges allowed per meal. A word of caution is needed here. The diabetic should be told that he should not "save" bread exchanges from one meal for use at the next. Clients on weight-reducing diets can do this because their only concern is the total number of Calories consumed in 24 hours. For the diabetic client the concern is not only with the total number of Calories but, more importantly, with the quantities of carbohydrate, protein, and fat at *each* meal.

For a beverage with his meal, the diabetic may select iced tea, coffee, a sugar-free drink, or milk if it is specified on his meal plan. The only type of milk that may be available, however, is whole milk. The client should always ask what types of milk are available. Low-fat plain yogurt may be available and could be substituted for milk. If only whole milk is available the client should omit one or two fat exchanges from the meal pattern to accommodate the additional fat in the whole milk. As more clients on diabetic, fat-controlled, and weight-reducing diets request low-fat or skim milk in restaurants, more of these establishments will add these to their selection to accommodate these patrons.

A cafeteria is the best choice for the diabetic who is eating away from home. There is usually a wide assortment of fresh fruit and vegetable salads as well as several choices of meats and cooked vegetables, breads, and beverages. Many cafeterias offer a few kinds of unsweetened fruit as well as fresh fruit. Selection of the meat or entree is often the most difficult because many of the items are either fried, breaded, or prepared with a sauce or gravy. Many cafeterias, however, do have a regular feature of roast beef carved on the line, which is an excellent selection for a diabetic.

DIET DURING ILLNESS. The nurse should be sure to instruct the client in what to do when illness occurs. A mild illness such as diarrhea or gastrointestinal upset may present a crisis to the diabetic because of the interference with the balance between diet and insulin. This is especially the case for the insulin-dependent diabetic. These illnesses increase the need for insulin, and they usually interfere with the ingestion of food. Most clients think that if they are consuming little or no food they should not take their regular dose of insulin. Although this belief is quite common, it is erroneous. The body still needs the insulin whether or not the regular amount of food is consumed.

Petrokas (1977) gives some commonsense guidelines for control of diabetes during illness. The nurse should first caution the client not to omit the dose of insulin. The client should be instructed to call the physician at once if vomiting or diarrhea occurs because of the rapid loss of fluid and electrolytes. The client should be told to go to bed and keep warm. A friend or relative should stay with the client if at all possible. The client should be instructed to test his urine more frequently during the day for the presence of sugar and acetone. The physician will want to know this information when he is consulted. Encourage the client to consume liquids every hour to help replace losses from vomiting and diarrhea. If the client is unable to ingest the regular foods on the diabetic diet, he should be encouraged to replace the foods with semiliquid forms of the food or at least to replace the carbohydrate from each meal. If the client is still unable to eat the prescribed diet after four or five modified meals, the physician should be notified.

When diabetics who are receiving insulin do not eat all of the food at a meal, at least the carbohydrate content of the uneaten food should be replaced. If the carbohydrate is not replaced the client may experience a hypoglycemic reaction before the next meal. This practice is referred to as a diabetic replacement. Usually only the carbohydrate portions of food from the bread, milk, fruit, and vegetable lists are replaced. This is most frequently done by using orange juice. The carbohydrate content of the uneaten food is calculated using the exchange system. Since orange juice is a 10% fruit (that is, it contains 10 gm of carbohydrate per 100 ml), the grams of carbohydrate in the uneaten food is multiplied by 10. Thus, for a vegetable containing 5 gm of carbohydrate, 50 ml of orange juice is given. Similarly for a fruit exchange (10 gm) 100 ml; for a milk exchange (12 gm) 120 ml, and for a bread exchange (15 gm) 150 ml of orange juice is given. If the client is nauseated, ginger ale may be substituted. When large quantities of carbohydrate must be replaced, grape juice may be used since it is twice as concentrated as orange juice and only half the quantity is required. The replacement should be offered to the client immediately after the meal. The responsibility for diabetic replacements may be with either the nursing or dietary staff in a hospital. A few hospitals still replace the protein and fat components of the food by considering that 58% of the protein and 10% of the fat can be converted to glucose.

Hypoglycemia (Functional Hyperinsulinism)

Hypoglycemia is not a disease but a symptom of an alteration of carbohydrate metabolism. It is defined as a low level of blood glucose from which the client experiences symptoms. Hypoglycemia can result from an impaired secretion of insulin or excess removal of glucose from the blood or both (Wolfe and

Powers, 1973). It may be the result of an endocrine tumor, severe liver disease, hormonal imbalances, gastric surgery, and the dumping syndrome.

Hypoglycemia can be present in either the fasting state or the fed state. The first type is called *organic hypoglycemia* and is often the result of a hypersecretion of insulin from a tumor of the beta cells, which produce insulin. It may also be the result of other endocrine tumors, liver damage, or starvation. In this type the symptoms of hypoglycemia develop eight or more hours after a meal. The second type is called *reactive hypoglycemia*. No organic lesion is present, but the client experiences hypoglycemic symptoms two to four hours after a meal.

The subject of hypoglycemia has received much attention in the press in recent years. Because the symptoms are nonspecific the condition and its symptoms have been popularized to the point where large numbers of people believe they have this disorder. Some of the symptoms are the same as those of an anxiety reaction, but it is much easier for people to accept the idea that they have "low blood sugar" than to admit the possibility of a psychological or emotional problem.

Dietary Interventions

The nurse should understand the basic physiological mechanisms in reactive hypoglycemia, how the symptoms are related, and the basis of the dietary intervention. In reactive hypoglycemia the blood glucose level falls rapidly two to four hours after eating. The client experiences such symptoms as weakness, hunger, nervousness, trembling, sweating, and sometimes an increased heart rate. In true reactive hypoglycemia the onset of these symptoms corresponds to the rapid drop in blood glucose (below 50 mg/100 ml). Following a meal there is a rapid absorption of carbohydrate into the blood. When the blood glucose level rises, the pancreas overreacts and releases an excessive amount of insulin into the blood. This in turn causes the blood glucose level to fall rapidly below normal. The test for diagnosing this reactive type of hypoglycemia is a five- or six-hour glucose tolerance test so that the blood levels can be plotted on a graph and observed to see if the characteristic drop occurs (Krause and Mahan, 1979).

The dietary intervention is aimed at decreasing the exaggerated reaction of the client to the ingestion of carbohydrate. This is accomplished by decreasing the carbohydrate content of the diet and increasing the protein and fat content. All forms of sugar and concentrated sweets are avoided, so in this respect the diet is like the diabetic diet. The carbohydrate content of the diet is generally 100 gm/day or lower. This is a high enough level to prevent ketosis but not high enough to overstimulate the pancreas. The carbohydrate is supplied by limited amounts of milk, fruits, vegetables, breads, and cereals. The exchange lists are usually used to explain the amounts allowed. The protein content of the diet is increased to 100–150 gm/day, and the remainder of the Calories are supplied by fat. Some of the protein supplied will be used for energy, but the slower rate of absorption will not stimulate the pancreas to produce insulin. The translation of these allowances into foods allowed throughout the day is another important principle of the diet.

The food is distributed so that the client receives three small meals with three high-protein snacks between the meals. The snacks are mainly protein, and very little carbohydrate is allowed. Creativity and imagination are necessary to plan three high-protein snacks daily. Examples might be a boiled egg, cheese, cottage cheese, meat, ham, or nuts. If the client is particularly fond of one of these food items, it is quite permissible to include the same protein food for each snack. A small amount of carbohydrate, such as tomato juice, a few crackers, a small amount of fruit, or a small glass of milk, may also be allowed with the protein snack. Alcohol is usually omitted or restricted because it blocks gluconeogenesis (Krause and Mahan, 1979).

Adherence to this dietary regimen will usually reduce the symptoms of this condition. It should be mentioned that the consumption of fruit juice or the eating of a concentrated sweet will alleviate the symptoms by raising the level of blood glucose. This remedy, however, is only temporary, and the effects may last only a few minutes. The purpose of the low-carbohydrate, high-protein diet with three high-protein snacks is to provide a more even release of glucose into the blood and to the cells for use.

ALTERATIONS IN STRUCTURE

1. Decubitus ulcer
2. Skin discomfort
3. Potential bone demineralization
4. Pain in joints
5. Muscular atrophy
6. Neuromusclar incoordination

The structural body systems are those that provide support and protection to the body. Those structures primarily affected by nutritional disturbances are the bones and skin. Loss of weight decreases the amount of subcutaneous tissue and thus reduces the mechanical padding between the skin and underlying bone, heightening the susceptibility to pressure effects. The loss of padding is coupled with decreased ability to repair tissue during reduced nutritional status. Bone demineralization may be a result of prolonged immobility or altered nutritional intake. Joint pain may result from alterations in uric acid metabolism or joint metabolism.

Client Objectives

To be able to:

1. Maintain (or regain) an intact integumentary system.
2. Ingest nutrients in a quantity and variety that will assist in maintaining skin and bone integrity.

3. Confirm his increased comfort.
4. Follow a diet that is consistent with structural alterations.

Dietary Interventions

Decubitus Ulcers
The aim of nursing care is to prevent *decubitus ulcers* from forming and to reduce the size and promote the healing of those ulcers that are present. Decubitus ulcers form in three predictable stages. The first stage involves a transient circulatory disturbance. Pressure has been sufficient to cause skin redness, which disappears after the pressure is relieved. Cell injury has already begun if redness occurs. Stage two of ulcer formation involves definite superficial circulatory and tissue damage. Redness and induration of tissue occur. Superficial layers of the skin are usually excoriated or blistered. Actual skin breakdown may occur at this stage. Stage three involves necrosis and deep skin breakdown. Subcutaneous tissues, muscles, and bone may be involved in the breakdown. Ulcer formation occurs at all levels of the skin simultaneously. The actual breakdown occurs rather late in the development of the ulcer.

The easiest, most effective, and most economical way to treat decubitus ulcers is to prevent them. The environment can be manipulated by the nurse to prevent skin breakdown before it occurs. Factors that contribute to ulcer formation include heat, moisture, friction injury, poor hygiene, presence of infection, immobility, and general undernutrition. A combination of these factors occurs during the normal aging process and during such conditions as loss of bowel and bladder control, spinal cord or CNS injury, and alterations in nutrient ingestion.

Poor general nutrition will hasten the development of ulcers and slow down their healing. Weight loss and muscle atrophy reduce the effectiveness of subcutaneous tissue as a mechanical pad between the bones and skin. Hypoproteinemia and ascorbic acid deficiency interfere with normal tissue integrity

(Berecek, 1975b). Negative nitrogen balance associated with malnutrition leads to edema and potential decubitus ulcer formation. Tissue repair and healing will not occur during a negative nitrogen balance. Diet therapy centers on a high-Calorie, high-protein diet. Nutritional supplements and Calorie-rich foods will aid in promoting positive nitrogen balances and tissue repair.

Potential Bone Demineralization

Loss of calcium from the bone is related to several clinical conditions: immobility, malnutrition, bone fractures, and osteoporosis. Nutritional principles are involved with each of these conditions, but a specific diet is usually not ordered.

One of the hazards of immobility is mobilization of calcium from the bones. The calcium level becomes elevated in the blood. Diets low in calcium do not seem to reduce the hypercalcemia (Krause and Mahan, 1979), so the dietary intake of calcium should be adequate but not excessive. A return to mobilization or the institution of physical therapy will help to reduce the levels of calcium in the blood.

Calcium is also lost from the bones during fractures. Calcium loss is accompanied by losses of nitrogen, phosphorus, potassium, and sulfur. The diet should be high in protein to restore the protein matrix within the bone. The Calories should be high enough to ensure that the dietary protein will be used for protein synthesis. The calcium content of the diet should be adequate. An excess amount of calcium in the diet could lead to the formation of renal calculi, especially when the client is immobilized. Calcium therapy, if used, should be begun only after the cast has been removed and mobilization has begun (Robinson and Lawler, 1977).

A deficiency of either calcium or vitamin D can lead to bone demineralization or inadequate bone growth. Nutrient deficiencies affecting the bones were discussed in Chapter 13. The dietary intervention is to increase the calcium and vitamin D in the client's diet.

Another condition leading to increased bone demineralization is *osteoporosis*. This word literally means "porous bones," and it usually occurs in the elderly. The exact causes of this disorder are not known, but it may be associated with low dietary intakes of calcium for several decades. The disease seems to be less common in people who have maintained adequate intakes of milk throughout life. A diet that is high in calcium—providing at least 1 qt of milk per day—may help to prevent further bone loss. Vitamin D supplements may help in some cases by increasing the absorption of calcium. In areas where the water supply is fluoridated, the incidence of osteoporosis seems to be less (Robinson and Lawler, 1977), but the exact relation of fluoride to osteoporosis is unknown.

Bone and Joint Pain

Another abnormality of the skeletal system is the bone and joint pain that may result from such conditions as gout or arthritis. Gout results from an accumulation of uric acid in the blood. It is characterized by inflammation, swelling, and pain of the joints. One of the dietary recommendations is to avoid foods that are high in purine content. All types of meat are high in purine because of their protein content. The total protein content of the diet should be reduced by consuming only small servings of meat, poultry, and fish. Other foods that are high in purine content are anchovies, asparagus, organ meats, mushrooms, sardines, dried beans and peas, oatmeal, seafood, and spinach (Robinson and Lawler, 1977). A special diet may not be ordered by the physician, but the client may simply be instructed to lose weight and eat smaller portions of meat. Milk, cheese, and eggs are foods that are high in protein content but low in purines. Another recommendation is to lower the fat content of the diet because fat interferes with the normal excretion of uric acid (Bennion, 1979). Alcohol should be omitted because its consumption is associated with gouty attacks.

There is no specific dietary intervention for arthritis other than a well-balanced diet. Attempts have been made throughout the years to find a diet that would help relieve the painful types of arthritis and rheumatism experienced by so many people. The vitamin supplements and miracle cures offered by food faddists will only be an added expense and disappointment to the client with arthritis. Dietary modifications are aimed at improving the nutritional status of the client. If the client is overweight, weight reduction is recommended. If the client's nutritional status is poor and he is underweight, a high-Calorie, high-protein diet should be selected. The medications used in the treatment of arthritis may necessitate a dietary modification. For example, if steroid therapy is used, a reduction in salt intake may be needed. If gastric irritation is experienced from the ingestion of large amounts of pain medication, a bland diet with protein snacks for buffering might be used.

Neuromuscular Incoordination

Certain diseases not related to nutrition lead to neuromuscular incoordination. These are multiple sclerosis, muscular dystrophy, Parkinson's disease, and epilepsy. Dietary adjustments and nutrient supplements have been tried in these conditions, but no real benefits have been reported. These conditions may interfere with the client's ability to ingest food. The interventions for clients with an inability to ingest food were discussed in Chapter 24. Instruction concerning a well-balanced diet is the only dietary intervention needed.

In the case of Parkinson's disease there is one dietary modification that may be helpful. Most clients with this disease are treated with the amino acid derivative *levodopa*. Vitamin B$_6$ (pyridoxine) interferes with this therapy. The recommendation is that vitamin preparations

containing vitamin B$_6$ be avoided. Also, foods that are high in vitamin B$_6$ should be avoided or restricted. A similar effect could be obtained by reducing the total protein content of the diet (dreyfus, 1977).

One special diet that is sometimes used in the treatment of children with epilepsy is the *ketogenic diet*. It is used for that small group of epileptic children who do not tolerate their medication well or who do not respond to anticonvulsants. The purpose of the diet is to produce ketosis. Ketosis seems to help prevent seizures. The diet is very low in carbohydrate and very high in fat. It is generally unpalatable. Medium-chain triglycerides are used because they are generally more ketogenic (Robinson and Lawler, 1977). The child is hospitalized when the diet is first begun in order to establish the ketosis. This may be accomplished more rapidly by using a period of two to three days of fasting (Krause and Mahan, 1979). It is used only when medication is not effective for one to three years and only with children, especially very young ones with uncontrollable seizures.

CASE STUDY: A Client with a Metabolic Alteration

Billy S. is a 10-year-old boy admitted to the pediatric unit for evaluation of possible diabetes mellitus. Billy's admission weight is 75 lb (34 kg), and his height is 4 ft 7 in (140 cm). Two weeks before this admission Billy had a tonsillectomy and adenoidectomy. After his discharge from the hospital his mother noted that he was eating especially large quantities of food, drinking large amounts of fluids, and getting up several times during the night to void. In spite of his large intake, Billy has lost 6 lb (2.7 kg) in the past two weeks. Billy's admitting blood glucose level was 460. The physician has placed Billy on a sliding-scale insulin coverage as follows:

4+ glucose level in urine—6 units of regular insulin

3+ glucose level in urine—4 units of regular insulin

2+ glucose level in urine—3 units of regular insulin

Billy is to be on a 3,000-Calorie diabetic diet. Billy's mother feels she may have "brought on" the diabetes by giving him colas and sugar-laden drinks after his tonsillectomy. She is rather anxious to learn how to monitor her son's insulin and how to detect its side effects. She does believe that his diet and insulin will be something "to work into our normal routine." Further, she states that Billy should be treated just like any other child; she hopes that her husband and parents do not treat Billy like an invalid.

Billy has told the nutritionist that his favorite foods include peanut butter, tomatoes, chicken, pizza, strawberries, ice cream, and soda pop. He states that he hates spinach, green beans, tunafish, and rye bread.

QUESTIONS

1. What is the specific disorder of endocrine metabolism as described in the nursing diagnosis?

2. What is the primary objective of the dietary intervention for diabetes mellitus?

3. What is the rationale for the use of Billy's diabetic diet?

4. What are the general principles of Billy's 3,000-Calorie diabetic diet?

5. What is the relationship between Billy's daily dose of insulin and his diet?

6. What advice should Billy and his mother be given about including each of his favorite foods in his diabetic diet?

BIBLIOGRAPHY

Arky, R. A. Diet and diabetes mellitus: Concepts and objectives. *Postgrad. Med.* 63:72, 1978.

Balsley, M., Brink, M. F., and Speckman, E. W. Nutrition in disease and stress. *Nursing Digest* 3(2):27, 1975.

Bennion, M. *Clinical Nutrition.* 1st Ed. New York: Harper & Row, Pubs., Inc., 1979.

Berecek, K. Etiology of decubitus ulcers. *Nurs. Clin. North Am.* 10(1):157, 1975a.

———. Treatment of decutitus ulcers. *Nurs. Clin. North Am.* 10(1):171, 1975b.

Boykin, L. Keeping the diabetic on a diet. *Nursing Care* 8:22, 1975.

Burton, B. T. *Human Nutrition.* 3rd Ed. New York: McGraw-Hill Book Co., 1976.

Clowes, G. H. A., O'Donnel, T. F., Blackburn, G. L., and Maki, T. N. Energy metabolism and proteolysis in traumatized and septic man. *Surg. Clin. North Am.* 56:1169, 1976.

Davidson, C. S. Dietary treatment of hepatic diseases. *J. Am. Diet. Assoc.* 62:515, 1973.

Davidson, J. K. Controlling diabetes mellitus with diet therapy. *Postgrad. Med.* 59:114, 1976.

Dreyfus, P. M. Neurologic disease. In H. A. Schneider, C. E. Anderson, and D. B. Coursin, Eds., *Nutritional Support of Medical Practice.* New York: Harper & Row, Pubs., Inc., 1977.

Eisenstein, A. B., Singh, S. P., and Thakor, P. Nutrition and the endocrine glands. *Prog. Food Nutr. Sci.* 1:531, 1975.

Flood, T. M. Diet and diabetes mellitus. *Hosp. Pract.* 14(2):61, 1979.

Fortier, R. R. Nutrition and the burn patient. *Canadian Nurse* 73(8):30, 1977.

Gazzaniga, A. B., Day, A. T., Bartlett, R. H., and Wilson, A. F. Endogenous caloric sources and nitrogen balance. *Arch. Surg.* 111:1357, 1976.

Hamburger, S. C., Covinsky, J. O., and Kelley, K. Diet therapy of diabetes mellitus. *J. Am. Med. Wom. Assoc.* 34:79, 1979.

Justice, P., and Smith, G. F. Phenylketonuria. *Am. J. Nurs.* 75:1303, 1975.

Kaufmann, S. J. In diabetic diets, realism gets results. *Nursing 76* 76(11):751, 1976.

Kavchak-Keyes, M. Treating decubitus ulcers using four proven steps. *Nursing 77* 77(10):44, 1977.

Kenney, J. M. Energy requirements in injury and sepsis. *Acta Anaesthesiol. Scand.* 55(Suppl.):15, 1974.

Krause, M. V., and Mahan, L. K. *Food, Nutrition, and Diet Therapy.* 6th Ed. Philadelphia: W. B. Saunders Co., 1979.

Ladodo, K. S. Peculiarities of dietetic therapy in infants' hereditary disease. *Nutr. Metab.* 21(Suppl. 1):79, 1977.

Lavine, R. L. How to recognize and what to do about hypoglycemia. *Nursing 79* 79(4):52, 1979.

Lenner, R. A. The importance of motivation in the adherence to dietary advice. *Nutr. Metab.* 20:243, 1976.

Luke, B. Your role in dietary therapy of cirrhosis. *RN* 40(10):49, 1977.

Mitchell, H. S., Rynbergen, H. J., Anderson, L. and Dibble, M. V. *Nutrition in Health and Disease.* 16th Ed. Philadelphia: J. B. Lippincott, 1976.

Overton, M. H., and Lukert, B. P. *Clinical Nutrition: A Physiologic Approach.* Chicago: Year Book Medical Pubs., Inc., 1977.

Pennington, J. *Nutritional Diet Therapy.* Palo Alto, Calif.: Bull Pub. Co., 1978.

Petrokas, J. C. Commonsense guidelines for controlling diabetes during illness. *Nursing 77* 77(10):36, 1977.

Robinson, C. H., and Lawler, M. R. *Normal and Therapeutic Nutrition.* 15th Ed. New York: Macmillan, Inc., 1977.

Ryan, N. T. Metabolic adaptations for energy production during trauma and sepsis. *Surg. Clin. North Am.* 56:1073, 1976.

Scrimshaw, N. S. Effect of infection on nutrient requirements. *Am. J. Clin. Nutr.* 30:1536, 1977.

Snyderman, S. E. The dietary therapy of inherited metabolic disease. *Prog. Food Nutr. Sci.* 1:507, 1975.

Soika, C. V. Combatting osteoporosis. *Am. J. Nurs.* 73:1193, 1973.

Stern, J. Inborn errors. *Nutrition* 28:163, 1974.

Taif, B. New concepts in dietary management of diabetes. *Journal of Practical Nursing* 35:16, 1975.

Thiele, V. F. *Clinical Nutrition.* St. Louis: The C. V. Mosby Co., 1976.

West, K. M. Diet therapy of diabetes: An analysis of failure. *Ann. Int. Med.* 79:425, 1973.

Williams, S. R. *Nutrition and Diet Therapy.* 3rd Ed. St. Louis: The C. V. Mosby Co., 1977.

Wolfe, B. M., and Powers, R. Hypoglycemia. *Canadian Nurse* 69:38, 1973.

Woolf, L. I. The dietary treatment of inborn errors of metabolism. *Proc. Nutr. Soc.* 35:31, 1976.

CHAPTER 28

Alterations in Excretion

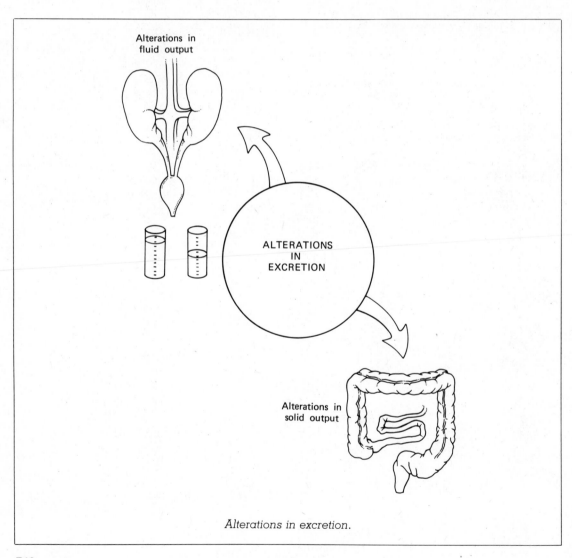

Alterations in fluid output

ALTERATIONS IN EXCRETION

Alterations in solid output

Alterations in excretion.

The final step in the nutritive process is the periodic elimination of nutrient waste. Fluid waste products that have been filtered through the kidneys accumulate in the bladder and are expelled through the urethra. The fluid wastes are composed of water-soluble vitamins, electrolytes, end products of protein metabolism, and water which are in excess or which are by-products of cellular metabolism. Solid waste is composed of undigested and unabsorbed nutrients and fiber as well as intestinal bacteria and their residues. Solid waste accumulates in the colon, where there is final reabsorption of water and sodium. The solid waste accumulates in the rectum and through normal peristaltic movements passes out of the body through the anus. Alterations in excretion may be manifested by altered composition of the urine or feces, altered amounts excreted, or painful or difficult excretion. The overall goal of the therapy is to restore the altered excretion to an amount and composition within a normal range and to eliminate any pain that may be associated with excretion.

ALTERATIONS IN FLUID OUTPUT

1. Dependence on indwelling urinary catheter management
2. Predisposition to development of renal calculi
3. Inadequate urinary output related to urine retention
4. Inadequate urinary output related to inadequate fluid intake
5. Diuresis
6. Painful urination

Client Objectives

To be able to:

1. Maintain an adequate urinary output.
2. Discuss the purpose of selected medical-nursing interventions.

Urinary Catheters

An indwelling urinary catheter is used when a client has difficulty voiding or when an exact measurement of urine output is needed. The most common type is the Foley catheter. The tube is held in place by a saline-filled balloon that is inflated after the catheter tip is passed into the bladder. An indwelling catheter is a focal site for the development of urinary tract infections, for two reasons. The first is that the catheter is a foreign object inside the body. Thus, bacteria and other residue tend to accumulate around the tip. The catheter serves as a means of bacteria getting inside the bladder from the outside of the body. The other reason chronic catheterization may precipitate infection is that the bladder remains empty. Normally, when a bladder is filled and periodically emptied, a "flushing" occurs that washes away the impurities that have managed to collect in the bladder. This flushing mechanism does not occur when a catheter is in place. Because of the potential for infection, a major goal of nursing care is the prevention of infection. Strict adherence to aseptic technique and the maintenance of a closed system will aid in achieving this goal (Wolffe et al., 1979).

Dietary Intervention
Diet therapy is also directed toward the prevention of infection. A large fluid intake (3–4 liters/day, or 102–136 oz—10–13 glasses—per day) is encouraged to assist in flushing bacteria from the bladder. A diet that will help maintain a low urine pH will also inhibit infection because bacteria grow best in an alkaline environment. One food that will help acidify the urine is cranberry juice.

Painful Urination

Clients with a urinary tract infection or renal stones experience painful and difficult urination. Urinary tract infections are much more common in women than in men because of their shorter urethra and its proximity to the anus. Urinary infections may be the result of obstruction within the urinary tract, injury, a chronic inflammation from bacteria, or the presence of kidney stones. On the other hand, the formation of kidney stones may be influenced by urinary tract infections, obstruction, dehydration, or prolonged immobilization. Most renal stones contain calcium and may be precipitated by any condition that increases the excretion of urinary calcium, such as excessive intake of calcium or vitamin D, milk-alkali syndrome, hyperparathyroidism, and prolonged immobilization. Renal stones are also more prevalent in sedentary people than in those who are physically active (Robinson and Lawler, 1977). Both urinary tract infections and renal stones have the potential to cause permanent damage to the kidneys and, eventually, renal failure.

The urine is normally slightly acidic. Acidic urine tends to inhibit bacteria growth; therefore, in urinary tract infections the urine is usually slightly alkaline. Certain types of renal stones are found in either an acidic or an alkaline urine. The reoccurrence of infection or renal stones may be prevented by altering the level of urinary acidity or alkalinity. If the composition of the renal stone can be determined, the dietary and medical treatment can be planned more effectively.

Dietary Interventions

GENERAL PRINCIPLES.   The general objective of treatment is to eliminate the infection, to allow for the passage or removal of the stone, and to prevent reoccurrence of stone formation or infections. The objective of preventive therapy in clients who have a predisposition to renal stones or infections is to decrease the concentration of the urine and to modify its pH. One of the most important aspects of treatment is to encourage the ingestion of large quantities of fluid daily (3,000 ml) to help in flushing the bladder of impurities. The modification of the urinary pH is accomplished primarily by drug therapy; although diet does have an effect on the acidity or alkalinity of the urine, dietary modification alone will not dissolve renal stones. Diet therapy, if used, supports drug therapy by helping to prevent the reoccurrence of the stones or infection (Bennion, 1979). Some foods yield primarily acidic end products; and some, alkaline end products. These end products are due to the mineral components of foods as the minerals are not oxidized during metabolism. They form either an acid or alkaline residue that is excreted in the urine.

The dietary treatment of renal stones or urinary tract infections always involves encouraging the client to consume large quantities of fluid. The acidity or alkalinity of the urine and the composition of the stone determine the diet and medication that will be prescribed (Krause and Mahan, 1979). Stones composed of carbonates, phosphates, and oxalates are most frequently found in an alkaline urine. Uric acid and cystine stones are usually found in acidic urine. The pH of the urine may be altered by the composition of the diet and the type of medication. Controversy exists, however, over the effectiveness and practicality of dietary treatment for renal stones. Because medication is much more effective in altering urinary pH, is it necessary to restrict dietary intake? Some physicians prescribe only drug therapy for the treatment of renal stones; others prescribe a specific diet as supportive therapy. The nurse should be familiar with the general principles of diet therapy whether or not a specific diet is ordered for the treatment of renal stones.

The diet used in the treatment of renal stones is either an acid-ash or alkaline-ash diet. The purpose of these diets is to increase the acidity or alkalinity of the urine. These diets are based on the reaction that ingested food has within the body after it has been metabolized, which is based on the acidity or alkalinity of the ash residue of the food. The alkali-forming elements of the ash are sodium, potassium, calcium, and magnesium;

the acid-forming end products are phosphates and sulfates (Bennion, 1979). Foods that form an alkaline ash are primarily fruits and vegetables; those that form an acid ash are mainly breads, cereals, and meats. The diet may also be increased or decreased in specific constituents based on the composition of the renal stone.

The consumption of a large amount of fluid is always encouraged in the treatment of urinary infections and renal stones, whether or not a specific diet is ordered. Also, for urinary infections, many physicians encourage the consumption of cranberry juice, which helps to acidify the urine. Large doses of vitamin C are usually given as a prophylactic measure in clients prone to urinary tract infection. The ascorbic acid is excreted via the kidneys, causing the urine pH to decrease. This therapy tends to cause GI upset; therefore the medication should be taken with food.

RATIONALE. The major dietary intervention in the treatment of renal stones or urinary infections is for the nurse to encourage the client to drink large quantities of fluid. The total amount of fluid consumed should be at least 3,000–4,000 ml per day. The client should be instructed to drink water after every urination (Fig. 28-1). In the evening the client should drink fluids before going to bed and also in the middle of the night after urinating unless the client has difficulty with *nocturia*. The purpose of this regimen is to maintain diluted urine, thereby avoiding the excretion of a concentrated urine out of which salts may be precipitated (Ing and Kark, 1977).

Cranberry juice has become important in the treatment and prevention of urinary infections and with certain types of calcium stones. It helps to create an acidic urine (Kahn et al., 1967). In addition, an acid-ash diet may be used to create an environment that does not favor the precipitation of mineral elements onto the stone. An acid-ash diet emphasizes the inclusion of foods that leave

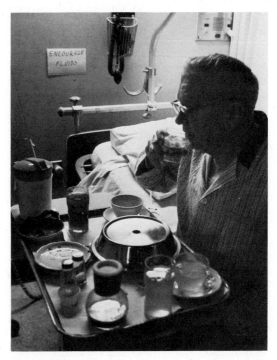

Figure 28-1. Forcing fluids is an important part of the therapy for urinary infections and renal calculi. (Photo by J. Collins)

an acid residue after metabolism. Most fruits and vegetables are restricted because they have an alkaline reaction within the body and leave an alkaline ash. A few foods, however, contain a large quantity of organic acids that are unchanged and leave an acid residue in the urine. These include cranberries, prunes, corn, and plums. Other foods that produce acid within the body are breads, cereals, and meats. A summary of acid-producing, alkali-producing, and neutral foods is found in Table 28-1.

The alkaline-ash diet is used, but less commonly, in the treatment of uric acid and cystine stones. These stones are more common in a highly acidic urine, so the objective is to reduce the acidity of the urine by including foods that leave an alkaline ash. On this diet

TABLE 28-1. Effects of Foods on Urinary Acidity, Alkalinity, or Neutrality

Reaction	Foods
Alkali-producing (due to sodium, potassium, calcium, and magnesium)	Milk, vegetables, most fruits
Neutral	Sugars, fats, beverages
Acid-producing (due to chlorine, sulfate, and phosphate)	Meats, fish, poultry, eggs, cereals, cheese, cranberries, plums, prunes, corn

the intake of milk, fruits, and vegetables is emphasized. In the dietary treatment of specific renal calculi other dietary constituents may be modified. A summary of the dietary modifications for the different types of renal calculi is found in Table 28-2.

Inadequate Urinary Output

Each minute, 1,200 ml of blood is delivered to the kidneys. From this amount about 120 ml of glomerular filtrate is formed. This filtrate is then sent through a series of tubules. Finally, about 1–2 ml of urine is formed, which accumulates in the bladder. The kidneys are involved in filtering the blood, reabsorbing nutrients, and finally excreting waste products from the body. Burton (1977) describes the functions of the kidneys as regulatory, excretory, and endocrine. The kidneys help regulate fluid and electrolyte balance and acid-base balance by filtration through the nephron and by reabsorption of water, electrolytes, and other nutrients. The kidneys are the main organs for the excretion of the end products of protein metabolism. They also perform some endocrine functions. They produce a substance called *renin,* which interacts with angiotensin in the blood to have an effect on blood pressure. The kidneys also secrete the hormone *erythropoietin,* which regulates the production of red blood cells by the bone marrow. In addition, the kidneys are in-

volved in the conversion of vitamin D into an active form.

Fortunately, the kidneys are able to maintain the body's internal equilibrium even when affected by certain diseases and conditions that interfere with their functioning. The kidneys are able to maintain normal functioning even when 60% percent of their functioning units, the nephrons, have been destroyed. When only 10% of the nephrons remain, the excretory and regulatory functions are considerably decreased, and the kidneys are no longer able to excrete a normal quantity of urine or end products of protein metabolism. There is a diminished output of urine (oliguria) or a complete suppression of urine (anuria). Besides an inadequate output of urine, there is also an accumulation in the blood of the end products of protein metabolism, primarily urea and creatinine.

Clues to assessment of renal failure or inadequate urinary output may include diminished urinary output by the client and mental confusion or disorientation. Laboratory data that is helpful to confirm this diagnosis is the levels of blood urea nitrogen (BUN) and serum creatinine and the glomerular filtration rate. The BUN and creatinine levels will be elevated above normal and the glomerular filtration rate will be reduced significantly.

Several types of kidney disorders can lead to permanent damage to the kidneys, loss of functioning tissue, and resulting renal failure. Recurrent or continuous infections such as *pyelonephritis* or *glomerulonephritis* can eventually lead to a loss of functioning tissue. Any obstruction of the flow of blood supplying the kidneys or of the flow of urine can lead to renal failure. Vascular diseases such as hypertension or atherosclerosis may lead to a restricted blood flow to the kidneys and eventual renal failure. Also, the stress of burns, injuries, shock from injury, or surgery may lead to renal failure (Thiele, 1976). In renal failure the kidneys literally shut down and lose their excretory capacity. This shutdown

TABLE 28-2. Possible Dietary Interventions for Prevention and Treating Reoccurrence of Renal Calculi

Type of Calculi	Dietary Intervention
Calcium oxalate stones	Prohibit foods high in calcium and oxalates.[a] Force fluids. Administer vitamin B_6 (pyridoxine). Administer magnesium.
Calcium phosphate stones	Restrict foods high in calcium and phosphorus[b] (a low-phosphorus diet may precipitate formation of citrate stones).
Uric acid stones	Establish a high-alkaline-ash diet (a low-purine diet may also be used or a protein restriction).

[a] Foods high in oxalate are asparagus, spinach, dandelion and beet greens, cranberries, figs, gooseberries, plums, rhubarb, raspberries, black tea, chocolate, cocoa, coffee, gelatin, and pepper. Those moderately high in oxalate and that should be limited to one serving daily are oranges, pineapple, strawberries, beans, Brussel sprouts, potatoes, tomatoes, and beets.
[b] Foods high in phosphorus are milk and milk products, eggs, organ meats, whole grain breads and cereals, nuts, soybeans, meat, and brown and wild rice.

may be the result of acute distress or a chronic condition. The renal failure may be either temporary or permanent. Renal failure associated with acute conditions is often temporary, and regeneration of the nephrons and restoration of function to near normal may be possible. Chronic kidney disorders leading to renal failure have usually caused permanent damage to the nephrons.

A group of related symptoms called the *uremic syndrome* develops as renal function declines. These symptoms are directly related to the retention of the end products of protein metabolism and the fluid and electrolyte imbalances that occur as renal function deteriorates. As the level of kidney function declines, the glomerular filtration rate decreases, the clearance of creatinine and urea decrease, and these protein end products become elevated in the blood. The diluting and concentrating ability of the kidneys is lost, and the metabolism of sodium, potassium, phosphate, and calcium is altered. Sodium is either retained or excreted in excess by the body. There may be protein, pus, and casts in the urine, and the specific gravity is low (Thiele, 1976). Other symptoms that may be present are hypertension and anemia. Clinical symptoms experienced by the client as a result of these imbalances involve primarily the GI system, the skin, and the nervous system. GI symptoms are severe and include anorexia, nausea, vomiting, and diarrhea. Common nervous system symptoms include general weakness, muscle twitchings, disorientation, and convulsions. Intense itching (pruritis) is common, and so is a symptom of "burning feet."

Dietary Interventions

The overall objective in the treatment of renal failure is to maintain renal function at the highest level possible, thus preventing further deterioration of function and improving function if possible. The general objectives of the dietary management are (1) to minimize the work of the diseased kidneys by reducing the end products of protein metabolism and the electrolytes that the kidneys must excrete and (2) to replace those nutrients that are lost from the body in abnormal amounts (Burton, 1974). The diet should have the benefits of correcting fluid and electrolyte and acid-base imbalances, minimizing protein catabolism, and controlling hypertension. Other benefits of the diet should be the elimination of most of the uremic symptoms and an improvement in appetite.

A diet designed to carry out these objectives will be complex. There is no specific diet for renal failure because there are no specific levels of nutrients that are prescribed for all clients. The dietary management of clients with renal disease is based on each client's own laboratory values and symptoms. The diet for renal failure involves the modification of Calories and most of the nutrients. The major dietary components that must be restricted are protein, sodium, potassium, and fluid. The caloric level of the diet must be high enough to prevent any weight loss. Because clients with renal failure have elevated levels of phosphate and low levels of calcium in the blood, the diet may be restricted in phosphorus, or specific phosphate binders may be prescribed. Because the diet is very restrictive it is quite nutritionally inadequate; therefore a multivitamin supplement is usually used.

GENERAL PRINCIPLES AND RATIONALE.   Burton (1977) describes six general principles of the dietary treatment of chronic renal failure along with the rationale for each. Each of the six principles involves the modification of a nutrient or nutrients based on the control of the symptoms associated with renal failure. The most important principle of dietary modification for renal failure is restriction of dietary protein. The basis for this restriction originally came from the research of two Italian doctors working separately on the use of low-protein diets containing the essential amino acids (Giordano, 1963; Giovannetti and Maggiore, 1964). This classic diet has become known as the *Giordano-Giovannetti diet*, the G-G diet, or more commonly, the 20-gm essential amino acid diet. Bailey and Sullivan (1968) modified this diet for food use in the United States. Burton (1974) reported on the principles of this diet. It contains a minimum

amount of protein, which primarily provides the essential amino acids; only minimum quantities of the nonessential amino acids are provided. The assumption is that these nonessential amino acids can be synthesized in the body using the excess endogenous urea in the blood and tissues. The minimum quantities of the essential amino acids are provided by one egg and $\frac{3}{4}$ cup of milk. No meat is allowed on this diet. The proteins from milk and egg were selected because these proteins are of high biological value and contain the highest proportions of essential amino acids. Protein from vegetables, breads, and cereals is kept to a minimum because these foods contain primarily nonessential amino acids.

Clinical experience showed that clients on a 40-gm protein diet progressed just as well as those on a 20-gm protein diet. Their BUN levels were not any higher on the 40-gm protein diet, and psychologically they felt better because the diet contained a small quantity of meat daily along with the milk and egg. In recent years most hospitals have been using a 30- or 40-gm protein diet for clients with renal failure. The 20-gm protein diet is used only for clients who have greatly elevated BUNs or for a short time for those awaiting dialysis. The principles of the 40- or 60-gm protein diet for renal failure are the same as those for the 20-gm diet except that additional amounts of breads, cereals, vegetables, or meat are allowed on the higher protein diets. An example of a 40-gm protein diet with both a potassium and a sodium restriction is shown in Figure 28-2.

The second principle is the regulation of sodium and potassium. The sodium content of the diet is usually restricted in renal failure to avoid sodium retention and edema and to help control hypertension or hyperkalemia. Potassium is often elevated in the blood because of the inability of the kidneys to excrete it. Hyperkalemia increases the risk of cardiac arrhythmias and cardiac arrest. The general guideline for specifying the dietary level of sodium and potassium is determined from

INDIANA UNIVERSITY HOSPITALS LOW PROTEIN MENU	INDIANA UNIVERSITY HOSPITALS LOW PROTEIN MENU	INDIANA UNIVERSITY HOSPITALS LOW PROTEIN MENU
MORNING	**NOON**	**NIGHT**
FRESHLY SQUEEZED ORANGE JUICE	LS HOMEMADE PORK SAUSAGE PATTY CHOPPED SIRLOIN	D BAKED HADDOCK WITH LEMON WEDGE
GRAPEFRUIT JUICE	LS (GROUND) BEEF IN BROTH	*(LS ROAST BEEF AU JUS — 1 oz.)*
Grape Juice (circled)	SCRAMBLED EGGS	LS (GROUND) ROAST BEEF AU JUS
HOT ROLLED WHEAT	LS MASHED POTATOES	LS WHIPPED POTATOES
LS HOT ROLLED WHEAT	*(LS FLUFFY RICE)* (circled)	LS HASHED BROWN POTATOES
CORNFLAKES	LS CHOPPED CABBAGE	LS BUTTERED MACARONI IN LS TOMATO SAUCE
PUFFED RICE	*(LS CANNED BEETS)* (circled)	
	(LS FAVORITE RELISHES IN ICE) (circled)	*(LS ASPARAGUS SPEARS)* (circled)
	TOSSED GREEN SALAD	LS VEGETABLE MEDLEY
(SCRAMBLED EGGS) (circled)	MAYONNAISE	LS CALICO COLESLAW ON LEAF LETTUCE
POACHED EGG		
FRIED EGG SUNNY SIDE UP		LS BUTTERCORN ROLL
FRIED EGG OVER LIGHT	*(BRAIDED ROLL)* (circled)	*(WHITE TOAST)* (circled) OR BREAD
FRIED EGG HARD	LS BRAIDED ROLL	LS WHITE TOAST OR BREAD
SOFT COOKED EGG IN SHELL	WHITE TOAST OR BREAD	LS LP WHEAT STARCH TOAST
HARD COOKED EGG IN SHELL	LS LP WHEAT STARCH TOAST	*Applesauce* (circled)
	LS WARM APPLE DUMPLING EN SAUCE	FRUIT SHERBET
(WHITE TOAST) (circled) OR BREAD	*(PEACH HALVES)* (circled)	CHILLED APRICOT HALVES
LS WHITE TOAST OR BREAD	WARM BAKED APPLE WITH CINNAMON	CHILLED PEAR HALVES
LS LP WHEAT STARCH TOAST	*(LP LEMON CRINKLE COOKIES)* (circled)	LP LEMON CRINKLE COOKIES
MARGARINE *X 3*	*(MARGARINE X 3)* (circled)	*(MARGARINE X 3)* (circled)
LS MARGARINE	LS MARGARINE	LS MARGARINE
(MILK — ½ cup) (circled)	MILK	*(MILK — ½ cup)* (circled)
SKIM MILK	CORNSTARCH COOKIES	*(CORNSTARCH COOKIES)* (circled)
	(CANDY) (circled)	*(CANDY)* (circled)
	SHERBET *½ cup Ice Cream* (circled)	SHERBET
	SKIM MILK	SKIM MILK
	COTTAGE CHEESE	COTTAGE CHEESE
(Salt ¼ tsp.) (circled)	LS COTTAGE CHEESE	LS COTTAGE CHEESE
HOT TEA	HOT TEA	HOT TEA
(PEPPER) ICED TEA	*(PEPPER)* ICED TEA	*(PEPPER)* ICED TEA
(SUGAR) LEMON	*(SUGAR)* LEMON	*(SUGAR)* LEMON
(JELLY) FRUIT DRINK	*(JELLY)* FRUIT JUICE	*(JELLY)* FRUIT JUICE
COFFEE	COFFEE *(FRUIT DRINK)* (circled)	COFFEE FRUIT DRINK
SANKA	SANKA LEMONADE	SANKA *(LEMONADE)* (circled)

Figure 28-2. Sample menu for a 40-gm protein, restricted 2-gm potassium and 2-gm sodium diet for renal disease. (Courtesy Indiana University Hospitals)

continual monitoring of serum and urinary levels of these electrolytes. There is a brief stage in renal failure when the sodium may not need to be restricted. This stage is called the *salt-wasting syndrome*. During this stage the kidneys are unable to conserve sodium, and large amounts are excreted in the urine. If sodium is restricted during this stage, the client could readily become dehydrated, which would enhance the acidosis and uremia and lead to further deterioration of kidney function. This stage lasts only a few days; at the end of it the client once again retains sodium and requires a sodium restriction.

The third principle is that the intake of fluid should be regulated to balance urinary and insensible water loss. The daily ingestion of fluid must be planned according to the kidneys' ability to eliminate fluid. The daily fluid restriction is based on the client's urinary output of the previous 24 hours plus 500–600 ml to allow for fluid loss from the lungs, skin, and feces. For every renal client an accurate daily record of intake and output (I and O) of fluids should be kept.

The fourth principle is regulation of phosphate. Clients with renal failure usually have a high level of serum phosphate. This further aggravates the low level of serum calcium (hypocalcemia). A dietary restriction of phosphate is not usually ordered because dietary phosphate levels are naturally low in restricted protein diets. Instead, aluminum hydroxide preparations are given that bind the phosphate so that it is not absorbed and it will be excreted in the feces.

The fifth principle, and a very important one, is adequate caloric intake. The caloric content of the low-protein diet should be high enough so that the client is able to maintain his ideal body weight. Although this sounds like a simple principle to put into practice, it is surprisingly difficult with the uremic client. Chronic uremia is characterized by a general wasting syndrome similar to the cachexia of the client with high blood levels of ammonia in cirrhosis. The uremic toxins in the blood depress the appetite, and the catabolic state of the illness further increase the caloric demands. The caloric level of the diet should be 35–45 Calories/kg of body weight, or 3,000–4,000 total Calories/day. Because the protein content of the diet is severely restricted, the majority of the Calories must be supplied by carbohydrate and fat. It is very difficult to supply foods high in carbohydrate and fat in a palatable form to a client who has a depressed appetite and may also be nauseated. Adequate caloric intake is essential, however, because if inadequate Calories are consumed the body will break down its own body tissue to meet the energy demands. When body tissues are catabolized the blood urea and potassium levels become elevated beyond the ability of the kidneys to excrete them. If necessary, a client may be maintained on a "no-protein" diet for a short period of time to reduce the uremic symptoms. Figure 28-3 shows the foods allowed on this type of diet.

The sixth principle is vitamin supplementation. Because of the restrictive nature of the low-protein diets, a vitamin supplement should be prescribed for every client on a renal diet. Kopple (1978) suggests the administration of supplements of folic acid, pyridoxine, ascorbic acid, and the water-soluble vitamins. In addition to a vitamin supplement a calcium supplement may be prescribed to counteract the hypocalcemia (Thiele, 1976). Administration of the active form of vitamin D may also help to enhance calcium absorption.

PRACTICAL CONSIDERATIONS. The dietary management of renal disease is an important means of life support. Careful adherence to the diet can reduce the distressing symptoms of uremia, prolong life, and improve its quality. For the client on chronic dialysis, dietary compliance can reduce the frequency with which dialysis is required. The diet, however, is very complex because the combination of nutrients is restricted and very limited in food

A diet supplying no protein may be of value during periods of ammonia toxicity or renal failure. The diet is inadequate in all nutrients and should be used for as brief a period as possible. Sufficient Calories should be supplied to prevent the breakdown and metabolism of the client's protein stores.

NO-PROTEIN DIET

Fruit juice
Synthetic juice
Butter balls with powdered sugar
Borst pudding
Hard candy
Carbonated beverages
Sugar
Coffee and tea

NO-PROTEIN, NO-SODIUM, NO-POTASSIUM DIET

Synthetic juice
Borst pudding
Salt-free butter balls with powdered sugar
Hardy candy
Sugar (no brown sugar)

Recipe for Borst Pudding

Cornstarch, 90 gm
Dextrose, 180 gm
Unsalted butter, 150 gm
Water, 1 qt

Cook mixture until clear.
100 gm of borst pudding provides:
18.6 gm of carbohydrate
9.5 gm of fat
159.5 Calories

Figure 28-3. No-protein diet. (Courtesy of Department of Nutrition and Dietetics, Indiana University Medical Center, Indianapolis)

choice. Biller (1977) stated that food is an obsession for people who suffer from renal disease. The restrictive nature of the diet only adds to the considerable psychological strain on the client created by the diagnosis of renal failure. Initial refusal to follow the diet may be the client's attempt to deny the severity of the illness. Most clients can be motivated to follow the diet when they are told that adherence to it will help to relieve the distressing symptoms of edema, anorexia, nausea, and vomiting. The client's psychological state and attitude are important in both the medical and dietary treatment of renal disease. Severe dietary restrictions coupled with hospitalization, the general stress of the illness, and the anxiety about renal transplant or chronic dialysis all impose severe psychological stress. Biller (1977) notes that the suicide rate in dialysis clients is 400 times greater than in the general population.

Although the restriction in protein, sodium, and potassium content of the diet may at first seem benign, it makes most of the foods a normal person enjoys taboo for the client with renal disease. The restrictions in protein, sodium, and potassium greatly limit the total quantity of food allowed, causing concern about the total number of Calories. There is also concern about imbalances among calcium, phosphorous, iron and about other possible vitamin and mineral deficiencies.

The team approach is very important in the dietary management of the renal client. Physician, dietitian, and nurse all have specific functions associated with the client's diet. Each member of the team should also offer psychological support concerning the diet (Fig. 28-4). The physician prescribes the specific restrictions of the diet based on the client's blood values and level of remaining renal function. He should also explain the role of the diet as an important means of nutritional support. The health team should show some sensitivity about the restrictive nature of the diet but emphasize nonetheless the benefits to be realized, such as decreased symptoms of uremia.

It is the responsibility of the dietitian to carry out the physician's diet order. This is accomplished by translating the diet order into foods allowed at each meal. A group of exchange lists similar to those for diabetic and weight reducing diets has been developed

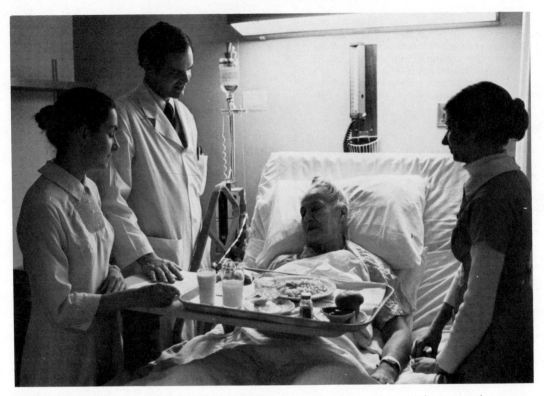

Figure 28-4. The support and encouragement of the medical team (nurse, doctor, and dietitian) is important when counseling the client with renal disease about his diet. (Photo by J. Collins)

for use with renal diets. The difference is that the exchange lists for renal disease were developed by considering the protein, sodium, and potassium content of foods. Some of the lists are divided into two separate lists because foods within the lists may vary in potassium and protein content. Renal exchange lists are found in Table 28-3.

The nurse's role in the dietary management of a client with renal disease is to reinforce the instructions of the physician and the dietitian, to offer practical suggestions about the diet, to observe the client's food consumption and adherence to the diet, and to offer psychological support. The major dietary in-

struction of the client about the diet is the responsibility of the dietitian. It would be helpful if the nurse, who is primarily responsible for the client's care, could attend the diet instruction. The client cannot be expected to learn all there is to know about the diet during one session. The dietitian should plan for several instructional periods, if possible. The nurse can reinforce the teaching of the dietitian between instructional sessions. The nurse may observe the client's eating habits and mealtimes and report to the dietitian any foods that are not consistently eaten. Mealtime may also be used by the nurse to explain dietary restrictions further by using the food

TABLE 28-3. Food Exchange Lists for Renal Diets

MILK EXCHANGES

	Amount	Protein (gms)	Na (mg)	K (mg)	P (mg)	Calories
Milk, whole	½ cup	4	64	172	117	84
Milk, skim	½ cup	4	64	179	117	45
Milk, evaporated	¼ cup	4	75	191	119	87
Half and half	1 oz	—	14	38	25	40
Sour cream	1 oz	—	12	17	23	57
Ice Cream, Vanilla, 12% butterfat	4 oz	5	48	134	118	248

Avoid milk shakes, malted milk, and buttermilk (too high in sodium).

VEGETABLE EXCHANGES

All vegetables contain potassium but some have more than others. The vegetables allowed on the diet are those which are low in protein and relatively low in potassium. The vegetables have been divided into two groups according to potassium content. You are allowed four servings of vegetables from group I daily. For instance, 1 oz of lettuce and 1 oz of tomatoes for lunch and 4 oz of low-sodium canned green beans and 1 oz of cucumbers for supper. The items in group II may be eaten only twice a week. For instance, 4 oz of fresh asparagus spears on Monday and one medium ear of corn on Friday.

All food should be fresh, dietetic canned, or frozen without salt or sodium compounds. Some vegetables have been eliminated entirely because of high potassium and sodium content.

Eat only the vegetables listed.

Group I	Amount	Protein (gms)	Na (mg)	K (mg)
Asparagus, low-sodium canned	½ cup	4	4	168
Beans, green				
Fresh or frozen	½ cup	—	4	172
Low-sodium canned	½ cup	—	4	108
Cabbage				
Cooked	½ cup	—	16	168
Fresh	¼ cup	—	10	140
Carrots				
Raw	¼ cup	—	18	124
Raw	1 oz	—	14	102
Corn, low-sodium canned	½ cup	4	4	108
Cucumber	2 oz	—	4	90
Eggplant	½ cup	—	—	168
Mustard greens	½ cup	4	12	176
Okra	½ cup	4	4	184
Onions, cooked	½ cup	—	8	124
Peas				
Fresh	½ cup	4	1	152
Low-sodium canned	½ cup	4	4	108
Radishes, raw	2 small	—	4	64
Rutabagas	½ cup	—	4	188
Squash, summer	½ cup	—	—	156

TABLE 28-3. Food Exchange Lists for Renal Diets (Continued)

| | Group I | Protein | Na | K |
	Amount	(gms)	(mg)	(mg)

For salads; use these vegetables that are relatively low in potassium.

		Protein (gms)	Na (mg)	K (mg)
Lettuce	1 oz	—	3	49
Romaine	1 oz	—	2	48
Onions				
Young green	2	—	1	39
Raw	½ oz	—	1	24
Radishes, raw	2 small	—	4	64
Tomatoes, raw	1 oz·	—	1	36
Pepper, green	¼ oz	—	1	15

| | Group II | Protein | Na | K |
	Amount	(gms)	(mg)	(mg)
Asparagus, fresh or frozen spears	½ cup	4	—	244
Beans, lima, low-sodium canned	½ cup	4	4	248
Broccoli spears	½ cup	4	12	248
Cauliflower	½ cup	4	8	232
Collards	½ cup	4	16	264
Corn, medium ear	1 Ear	4	—	240
Tomatoes, low-sodium canned	½ cup	1	4	260

FRUIT EXCHANGES

All fruits and juices contain potassium but some have more than others. Use only the foods listed below. Those containing highest potassium values, such as grapefruit, raw figs, grape juice, and frozen strawberries, should be used less frequently or in small amounts. The following fruits should be avoided entirely: apricots, avocados, bananas, cantaloupe, dates, honeydew melon, oranges, fresh plums, and rhubarb.

	Amount	Protein (gms)	Na (mg)	K (mg)
Apple	1 small	—	1	110
Apple juice	½ cup	—	1	126
Applesauce	½ cup	—	3	83
Blackberries	½ cup	—	1	123
Blueberries	½ cup	—	—	56
Cherries				
Raw sweet	½ cup	—	1	109
Canned sweet	¼ cup	1	1	101
Cranberries, raw	1 cup	—	2	82

The next two items are low in potassium and you can use larger quantities within the limits of your fluid allowance:

		Protein (gms)	Na (mg)	K (mg)
Cranberry sauce	2 T	—	—	12
Cranberry juice cocktail	½ cup	—	1	13
Figs				
Raw	2 medium	1	2	147
Canned	2 medium	—	2	104
Fruit cocktail	¼ cup	—	3	94
Grapefruit				
Raw	¼	—	1	97
Canned	½ cup	—	1	151

TABLE 28-3. *(Continued)*

	Amount	Protein (gms)	Na (mg)	K (mg)
Grapefruit-pineapple juice	½ cup	—	1	112
Grapes	22 grapes	1	3	100
Grape juice	½ cup	1	3	147
Lemonade, sweetened	½ cup	—	—	20
Lemon juice, fresh	1 T	—	—	21
Peaches, canned	2 halves	—	4	154
Pears, canned	2 halves	—	2	100
Pear nectar	½ cup	1	1	49
Pineapple				
Canned crushed	¼ cup	—	1	96
Canned sliced	1 slice	—	1	117
Pineapple juice	⅓ cup	—	1	124
Plums, canned	2 medium	—	1	115
Prunes, dried, cooked	2 prunes	—	2	104
Raspberries				
Red, frozen	½ cup	1	1	128
Red, raw	¼ cup	1	1	100
Red, canned	½ cup	1	1	103
Strawberries				
Raw	10 large	—	—	124
Frozen	½ cup	—	2	125
Tangerine	1	1	2	126
Watermelon cubes	½ cup	1	—	110

BREAD EXCHANGES

Foods in this list may make significant contributions to the protein content of the diet and should be used only in the amount allowed in your meal plan.

	Amount	Protein (gms)	Na (mg)	K (mg)	Calories
Bread	1 slice				
French or Vienna		1	75	12	37
Raisin		2	84	54	60
Rye		2	128	33	55
Unsalted		2	6	27	63
White		2	117	24	60
Whole wheat		2	117	24	55
Cake, Angel Food	1-oz slice	3	113	35	110
Cereals					
Unsalted, cooked	½ cup				
Farina		2	—	11	53
Grits		2	—	13	60
Oatmeal		3	2	72	75
Whole wheat		2	2	57	54
Unsalted, dry	1 oz				
Corn flakes		2	1	24	77
Puffed rice		2	2	28	113
Rice flakes		2	2	28	113
Crackers, salt-free	2	1	—	8	32
Potatoes and substitutes					
Macaroni	½ cup	3	1	43	78
Noodles	½ cup	4	2	35	100
Rice	½ cup	2	1	24	100
*Potatoes	½ cup	2	2	140	70

TABLE 28-3. Food Exchange Lists for Renal Diets (Continued)

	Amount	Protein (gms)	Na (mg)	K (mg)	Calories
Spaghetti	½ cup	3	1	43	78
Sweet potato, candied	½ cup	4	12	212	188
Rolls					
Hamburger	1	3	255	53	117
Plain	1	3	192	36	115
Sweet	1	4	167	53	135
Hard Roll	1	5	325	50	160

* See directions for preparing potatoes after "Fat Exchanges."

Avoid

Quick-cooking or instant cereals, and dry cereals other than those listed, salted crackers, pretzels, popcorn, self-rising cornmeal and flour, commercial mixes (biscuits, muffins, pancakes, cookies, cakes, etc.). Do not use baked potatoes, instant or canned white and sweet potatoes, instant or quick-cooking rice, potato chips, corn chips, and bread made with salt, soda, or baking powder unless specified in your meal plan.

MEAT EXCHANGES

The major source of protein in the diet should come from this group. All of these foods are good sources of the essential amino acids.

Due to their high sodium content, some meats should be avoided and are not listed. These are spiced, smoked, cured, or pickled meat such as luncheon meat, sausage, bacon, ham, dried meat, and sandwich spreads.

Flounder, sole, some shellfish, and halibut should be avoided because of their high potassium content.

Some meats have a higher protein content than others, e.g.:

1 oz Swiss steak	11 gms protein
1 oz turkey	9 gms protein
1 oz pork chops or lamb chops	5 gms protein
1 oz oyster	2 gms protein

When planning your menu for the day, use high-protein meat for lunch and low-protein meat for supper or vice versa in order to balance your daily allowance.

Weigh the cooked meat to determine the correct portion for use.

The meats and meat substitutes listed on the following pages are equal to one meat exchange.

	Amount	Protein (gms)	Na (mg)	K (mg)	Calories
Cheese, low-sodium	1 oz	8	3	120	115
Cottage cheese, low-sodium	¼ cup	7	10	36	43
Egg	1	6	61	65	80
Hamburger	1 oz	7	17	103	82
Roast, rib	1 oz	5	17	103	130
Roast, round	1 oz	8	17	103	73
Steak, sirloin	1 oz	7	17	103	109
Steak, Swiss, low-sodium	1 oz	11	32	103	142
Chicken breast	1 oz	8	15	76	47
Chicken leg	1 oz	6	13	65	43
Chicken livers	1 oz	7	17	42	47
Duck	1 oz	6	22	85	50
Lamb chops	1 oz	5	20	82	83
Lamb, roast	1 oz	7	20	82	78
Liver, beef	1 oz	7	52	106	64

TABLE 28-3. (Continued)

	Amount	Protein (gms)	Na (mg)	K (mg)	Calories
Meat Loaf, low-sodium	1 oz	8	20	107	66
Pork chops	1 oz	5	18	109	75
Pork roast	1 oz	7	18	109	103
Tongue beef	1 oz	6	17	46	68
Turkey	1 oz	9	36	103	54
Veal	1 oz	8	22	140	77
Codfish	1 oz	9	33	122	51
Haddock	1 oz	5	18	91	24
Oysters	1 oz	2	20	34	18
Perch	1 oz	3	19	65	65
Salmon	1 oz	8	32	124	51
Salmon loaf, low-sodium	1 oz	5	13	97	57
Shrimp	1 oz	6	42	66	27
Tuna, low-sodium	1 oz	8	11	79	36

FAT EXCHANGES

These foods contribute to the caloric content of the diet and should be used as much as possible. This will enable you to maintain your normal weight. It is not necessary to measure *unsalted* butter, margarine, oil, salad dressing and Cremora because they contain only small amounts of protein, sodium, and potassium. To get more Calories, try to use butter or margarine on cooked cereals, breads, potatoes, vegetables, etc. Also fried foods of all kinds give you extra Calories.

The following dairy products should be measured:

	Amount	Na (mg)	K (mg)	Calories
Butter, regular (salted)	1 t	49	1	36
Cream, light	2 T	13	37	70
Half and half	2 T	14	39	40
Cream, sour	2 T	12	17	57
Cream, whipping	2 T	10	26	90
Margarine (regular)	1 t	49	1	36

DIRECTIONS FOR PREPARING POTATOES

1. Peel a small potato (approximately 100–120 gm) and dice—or slice into $\frac{1}{4}$ in slices.
2. Put peeled potato into 2 qt of water and soak overnight.
3. The following day, drain all water (this is important because the potassium is now in the water). Add 2 qt of fresh water.
4. Bring to boil and simmer on top of stove in a covered saucepan for 30 minutes. Discard the liquid.
5. These potatoes can then be French fried, cottage fried, mashed, or oven browned.

TABLE 28-3. Food Exchange Lists for Renal Diets (*Continued*)

BEVERAGES

Select all beverages including water according to your fluid allowance. Ice and juices from canned fruits and vegetables are sources of fluid.

	Amount	Na (mg)	K (mg)	Calories
Coffee	6 oz cup	3	66	—
Coffee, decaffeinated, dry	1 T	1	50	—
Tea	6 oz cup	—	45	—
Ginger ale	12 oz can	24	—	120
Beer	12 oz can	12	66	174
Gin, rum, vodka, whiskey (86 Proof)	1 shot or jigger (1½ oz)	1	1	102
Wine, dessert varieties (apple, muscatel, sherries, port, Tokay, aperitifs)	1 3-oz glass	4	67	123
Wine, table varieties (Burgundy, Champagne, claret, Chianti, rosé, sauterne)	1 4-oz glass	6	110	102

CONDIMENTS, FLAVORING, AND MISCELLANEOUS ITEMS ALLOWED

The following suggestions may help to make meals more appealing:

Allspice: meat, soup
Anise: bread
Basil: salad, egg dishes, tomatoes
Bayleaf: meat, fish, soup
Candy—assorted hard candy
Caraway seed: meat, vegetables, cheese, slaw
Chili powder
Chives: salad, soup, fish sauces, egg dishes
Cinnamon: certain desserts
Cloves: meat, fruits, desserts
Cornstarch
Curry (salt free): meat, vegetables
Dill: meat, fish, vegetables, soup
Gum drops
Garlic: meat, salad
Gelatin, dry, plain
Ginger: meat
Honey
Jam, jelly
Mace: meat, sauces, cakes, sweets
Marjoram, sweet: meat, vegetables, salad, fruit
Marshmallows (limit to 10 per day)
Mint: beverages, meat, confections, desserts, garnish
Mustard, dry: meat, fish, salad
Nutmeg: cake, desserts
Onion: meat, salad, vegetables

TABLE 28-3. (*Continued*)

Oregano: meat, tomato sauce, salad greens and dressings
Parsley: salad, soup, meat, vegetables, garnish
Paprika: meat, fish
Pepper, black, white, and red: meat, vegetables, salad, dressings
Poppy seeds: meat, macaroni products
Rosemary: salad, meat, fish
Saffron: meat, fish, rice
Sage
Sugar, granulated and powdered
Syrup
Tapioca, dry
Thyme: stuffing, soup, meat
Vanilla extract
Vinegar, white or cider: salads, vegetables
Yeast, bakers
Lemon extract
Lemon juice

CONDIMENTS, FLAVORINGS, AND MISCELLANEOUS ITEMS TO AVOID

Baking powder
Baking soda
Barbecue sauce
Bouillon in any form
Brown sugar
Catsup
Celery leaves, dried or fresh
Celery seeds
Chili sauce
Chocolate, sweet and bitter
Cocoa
Coconut
Cooking wine
Garlic salt
Horseradish
Meat extracts
Meat sauces
Meat tenderizers
Molasses
Monosodium glutamate
Mustard, prepared
Nuts
Olives
Onion salt
Pickles and pickle relish
Pudding—mixes
Salt or salt substitute
Soy sauce
Steak sauce
Worchestershire sauce
Yeast, brewer's

SOURCE. From W. O. Jones, *Diet Guide for Patients on Chronic Dialysis.* Artificial Kidney–Chronic Uremia Program. Natl Instit. of Arthritis, Metabolism, and Digestive Disease, DHEW Publ. No. (NH) 76-685. Washington, D.C., 1977.

on the client's tray as an example. The client may have specific questions about the diet that the nurse or the dietitian can answer.

The nurse should be familiar with the exchange lists used for the dietary treatment of renal disease (see Table 28-3). These lists will vary among hospitals, but their purpose and use are still the same. The dietitian constructs an exchange type of diet based on the physician's diet order. The daily allowances for protein, sodium, and potassium are apportioned among the three meals. The allotments for each meal are divided into a specific number of exchanges allowed for each meal. The development of the exchange lists for renal disease has made meal planning for the renal diet much simpler for the dietitian and much easier for the client and his family to comprehend.

The nurse should be aware of some of the special products and suggested methods of food preparation. The foods that are the most severely restricted in renal disease are milk and meats because they are high in protein. Both fruits and vegetables are divided into two groups because of the differences in potassium content. Canned fruits and vegetables are often recommended because they are lower in potassium content than fresh or frozen ones. The sodium content of the canned vegetables is often too high to use, so low-sodium canned vegetables must be substituted. Certain foods are generally avoided or severely restricted on a renal diet because of the high potassium content; some of them are oranges, bananas, potatoes, cocoa, and chocolate. Coffee, tea, and cola beverages may also be omitted or severely restricted. A salt substitute is usually not recommended for use by a client with renal disease because of its potassium content. The sodium and potassium content of some common foods is found in Appendix G.

A limited number of breads and cereals are allowed each day. On a diet that allows 20–40 gm of protein, a special kind of bread called *wheat starch bread* may be used. It is prepared from wheat flour that has had the gluten (protein) portion removed, leaving only the starch portion. Bread derives its light texture from its protein component, so wheat starch bread lacks this quality. It is compact and heavy, and many clients find it unpalatable. The acceptability may be improved by toasting. When it is used, it is served at each meal with butter or margarine and jelly. This bread is higher in Calories than regular bread and provides a way to incorporate additional Calories in the diet.

The Calories in the diet can be increased by adding servings of pure fats and carbohydrates. Unsalted butter or margarine and cooking oil can be used as desired. At least 3 t of fats are included on the tray at each meal to add Calories. The ingestion of pure carbohydrates should be encouraged with meals and between meals for additional Calories. The nurse should encourage the client to eat candies made from pure carbohydrates between meals. These candies may be hard sugar candy, gum drops, marshmallows, or jelly beans. This is one of the few times when a nurse encourages a client to eat candy. Desserts may be specially prepared using the wheat starch flour or special carbohydrate supplements.

During the period of the salt-wasting syndrome, additional sodium is added to the diet. Specific foods such as regular butter or margarine, a salt packet, a bouillon cube, olives, or dill pickles may be added. Specific amounts of one or more of these foods are added to the client's meal tray. The client or the nurse may think the dietitian has made a mistake; but if the nurse checks the client's chart, she will probably find that the physician has increased the level of sodium in the diet order. This sudden addition of salt or salty foods is often difficult for the client to understand. The nurse should explain the physiological reason, why it is important for the client to consume this extra salt, and that it is quite likely that the sodium will be restricted again in a few days.

Diet during Dialysis

The only method of treating renal failure discussed thus far has been diet. The two other general methods of treatment are *renal dialysis* and *transplantation*. If dialysis is used, the process will need to be repeated several times weekly for the rest of the client's life. If a successful transplant is performed, the client will be able to live a normal life with no further dietary restrictions.

When the glomerular filtration rate is reduced to 1.5 ml/min (Overton and Lukert, 1977), the clients kidneys are no longer able to excrete urine or filter protein end products, sodium, or potassium; so these substances accumulate in the blood. If they are not removed by dialysis, renal function will continue to deteriorate and death will follow. Bennion (1979) defines *dialysis* as "the diffusion of dissolved particles across a semipermeable membrane from one fluid compartment to another". Two basic types of dialysis have been used for clients with renal disease. One of these is *peritoneal dialysis*, which uses the peritoneum as the semipermeable membrane. A dialyzing solution is introduced into the peritoneal cavity through a small catheter placed in the abdominal wall. An exchange of solutes and fluid occurs and the *dialysate* is removed after a specified period of time. This process is continued until blood values are reduced to near-normal levels. The second method of dialysis is called *hemodialysis*. The basic principle of hemodialysis is depicted in Figure 28-5. This method employs the use of the artificial kidney machine (Fig. 28-6). The client's blood is pumped outside the body through a semipermeable membrane in the machine, which has a dialysate solution surrounding it (Bennion, 1979). The client's blood is cleansed of the excess protein metabolites, sodium, and potassium through the simple principle of diffusion. The dialysate solution contains a concentration of solutes similar to that of the extracellular fluid. Because the concentration of solutes in the client's blood is higher than the concentration in the dialysate solution, the excess solutes will diffuse from this area of high concentration into the lower concentration of the dialysate. Excess fluid is also pulled from the client's blood by *ultrafiltration* (a negative pressure) (Bennion, 1979).

The aim of dietary management during dialysis is to supply the amount of protein, sodium, and potassium that can be held in equilibrium by the process of dialysis. During dialysis the blood levels of amino acids and albumin are reduced, as are the toxic levels of the blood urea nitrogen. The blood levels of the water-soluble amino acids as well as the excess levels of sodium and potassium are removed. The diet must replace all the substances lost during dialysis. In comparison with the strict diet used in chronic renal failure, the diet used in dialysis is more liberal. The allowed levels of protein, sodium, and potassium are higher, and thus the diet is more palatable. Burton (1974) suggests that the protein content of the diet during hemodialysis be 1 gm per kilogram of ideal body weight with at least 75% of this amount being supplied by proteins of high biological value. He further suggests that the diet be restricted to about 1,500–2,000 mg of sodium and about 2,000 mg of potassium. Fluid content of the diet also needs to be restricted to the 24-hour urinary output plus 300–500 ml. If a client says he is thirsty, he is probably ingesting too much sodium. In anuric clients, dietary compliance can be assessed by recording the weight gain between dialysis. An example of a diet used during dialysis is found in Figure 28-7.

Hemodialysis has been used primarily for long-term dialysis despite the high costs. Peritoneal dialysis was associated with frequent infections and progressive wasting and malnutrition when it was used for long-term dialysis. Blumenkrantz et al. (1978) reports that an improved method of peritoneal dialysis has been tested that uses an implantable catheter with an inexpensive method of peritoneal dialysis. There is less evidence of

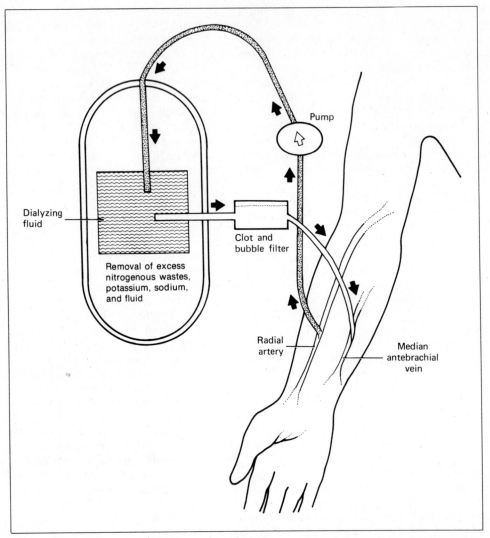

Figure 28-5. Hemodialysis, the purpose of which is to allow the client's blood to circulate outside the body through a filter in the dialysis machine. The filter removes the toxic end products of protein metabolism and also the excessive levels of sodium and potassium.

infection and a greatly reduced loss of valuable body protein during this process. The suggested levels of protein, sodium, and potassium allowed with this new type of peritoneal dialysis are even more liberal than the levels allowed with hemodialysis.

Blumenkrantz, et al. (1978) recommend a protein intake of 1.0–1.5 gm per kilogram of ideal body weight, to consist primarily of high-biological-value protein; 2,000–3,000 mg of sodium, and 3,000–3,500 mg of potassium. If this new method continues to prove

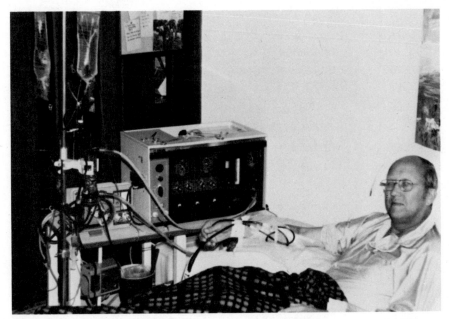

Figure 28-6. This client is performing self-dialysis at home by means of a kidney machine.

effective, it will provide a diet even closer to a regular diet as well as a method of long-term dialysis that is much less expensive and that can be conducted overnight.

ALTERATIONS IN SOLID WASTE EXCRETION

1. Painful defecation
2. Fecal impaction
3. Constipation
4. Diarrhea
5. Dependence on nursing intervention for ostomy care

An alteration in solid waste excretion may be manifested either by constipation or in diarrhea. These alterations may be the result of faulty dietary or health habits, the stress imposed by illness or disease, or drug therapy or other medical treatment. Because constipa-tion and diarrhea are both alterations from normal excretion, they can impose both psy-chological and physiological stress on the client. The nurse has a major responsibility to assist the client to maintain or regain normal excretion of solid waste during hospitalization as well as to offer suggestions for the mainte-nance of a good nutritional and eliminational status after discharge.

Client Objectives

To be able to:

1. Maintain an adequate solid waste output.
2. Plan a diet that may help correct his altera-tions in solid waste excretion.

Constipation

Constipation is a frequent chronic complaint of many clients in the hospital. It may be re-lated to such factors as decreased physical ac-

INDIANA UNIVERSITY HOSPITALS LOW PROTEIN MENU	INDIANA UNIVERSITY HOSPITALS LOW PROTEIN MENU	INDIANA UNIVERSITY HOSPITALS LOW PROTEIN MENU
MORNING	**NOON**	**NIGHT**
FRESHLY SQUEEZED ORANGE JUICE	LS HOMEMADE PORK SAUSAGE PATTY	D BAKED HADDOCK WITH LEMON WEDGE
	~~CHOPPED SIRLOIN -3oz.~~	~~LS ROAST BEEF -3oz~~ AU JUS
GRAPEFRUIT JUICE	LS (GROUND) BEEF IN BROTH	LS (GROUND) ROAST BEEF AU JUS
~~Grape Juice~~	~~SCRAMBLED EGGS~~	LS WHIPPED POTATOES
~~HOT ROLLED WHEAT~~	~~LS Peas~~	
LS HOT ROLLED WHEAT	LS MASHED POTATOES	LS HASHED BROWN POTATOES
CORNFLAKES	~~LS FLUFFY RICE~~	~~LS BUTTERED MACARONI IN LS TOMATO SAUCE~~
PUFFED RICE	LS CHOPPED CABBAGE	
	LS CANNED BEETS	~~LS ASPARAGUS SPEARS~~
	LS FAVORITE RELISHES IN ICE	LS VEGETABLE MEDLEY
SCRAMBLED EGGS	~~TOSSED GREEN SALAD~~	LS CALICO COLESLAW ON LEAF LETTUCE
POACHED EGG	MAYONNAISE	
~~FRIED EGG SUNNY SIDE UP~~		LS BUTTERCORN ROLL
FRIED EGG OVER LIGHT	~~BRAIDED ROLL~~	~~WHITE TOAST~~ OR BREAD
FRIED EGG HARD	LS BRAIDED ROLL	LS WHITE TOAST OR BREAD
SOFT COOKED EGG IN SHELL	WHITE TOAST OR BREAD	LS LP WHEAT STARCH TOAST
HARD COOKED EGG IN SHELL	LS LP WHEAT STARCH TOAST	
	LS WARM APPLE DUMPLING EN SAUCE	FRUIT SHERBET
~~WHITE TOAST~~ OR BREAD	~~PEACH HALVES~~	CHILLED APRICOT HALVES
LS WHITE TOAST OR BREAD	WARM BAKED APPLE WITH CINNAMON	~~CHILLED PEAR HALVES~~
LS LP WHEAT STARCH TOAST	LP LEMON CRINKLE COOKIES	LP LEMON CRINKLE COOKIES
~~MARGARINE X 3~~	~~MARGARINE X 3~~	~~MARGARINE X 3~~
LS MARGARINE	LS MARGARINE	LS MARGARINE
~~MILK - ½ cup~~	~~MILK - ½ cup~~	~~MILK - ½ cup~~
SKIM MILK	CORNSTARCH COOKIES	CORNSTARCH COOKIES
	CANDY	CANDY
	~~SHERBET - ½ cup~~	SHERBET
	SKIM MILK	SKIM MILK
	COTTAGE CHEESE	COTTAGE CHEESE
	LS COTTAGE CHEESE	LS COTTAGE CHEESE

		HOT TEA			HOT TEA		HOT TEA
PEPPER		ICED TEA	PEPPER		ICED TEA	PEPPER	ICED TEA
SUGAR		LEMON	SUGAR		LEMON	SUGAR	LEMON
~~JELLY~~		FRUIT DRINK	~~JELLY~~		FRUIT JUICE	~~JELLY~~	FRUIT JUICE
COFFEE			COFFEE		~~FRUIT DRINK~~	COFFEE	FRUIT DRINK
SANKA			SANKA		LEMONADE	SANKA	~~LEMONADE~~

Figure 28-7. Sample menu for an 80-gm protein, restricted to 2-gm sodium and 2.5-gm potassium diet for the client receiving dialysis. (Courtesy Indiana University Hospitals)

tivity, inadequate fluid and fiber intake, stress from disease, suppression of the urge to defecate, or drug therapy. The client may complain of a decreased frequency of bowel movements, the difficult passage of a small and hard stool, or the sensation of incomplete fecal elimination. Inactivity and stress are so often manifested in the hospitalized client by the complaint of constipation that nurses may consider the use of laxatives, enemas, and stool softeners routine practice. Nurses often do not consider using instead the practice of increasing fluids and dietary fiber, which is a natural way to eliminate constipation. Even though they know that a daily bowel movement is not necessary for all adults, they may condone the use of laxatives when clients are concerned about their personal bowel habits. Assessment data should be gathered concerning the client's normal bowel habits before hospitalization and what, if any, aids were used.

Dietary Interventions

The first step in planning the treatment for constipation is to determine the factors contributing to the development of this state. Temporary or long-term constipation may be due to poor health habits associated with eating, rest, and elimination; inadequate fluid or fiber intake; interference with the urge to defecate; change in the activities of daily living; overuse of laxatives; decreased intestinal muscle tone; painful elimination because of hemorrhoids; intestinal spasms or other organic disorders of the colon; or the ingestion of drugs that produce constipation as a side effect. With this knowledge the nurse has a better understanding of the problem and whether it is of a temporary or chronic nature.

The objective of the dietary management of constipation is to provide foods with an increased fiber content that will stimulate the peristalsis and motility of the colon, thus allowing for the passage of feces with no straining or discomfort. The diet used in the treatment of constipation is the high-fiber diet with increased fluids. An increase in the client's exercise or physical activity level should also be encouraged when possible.

GENERAL PRINCIPLES AND RATIONALE. Although there is much controversy surrounding the use of the high-fiber diet, it has been recognized for many years to be effective in relieving constipation. The two basic characteristics of the high-fiber diet are that it specifies (1) the inclusion of foods that are high in fiber content and (2) reduced consumption of refined foods. An aid to eliminating constipation is to encourage the client to consume at least 8–10 glasses (2,500–3,000 ml) of water a day. Another aid to elimination for some clients is the consumption of prunes or prune juice. Prune juice is not particularly high in fiber, but it stimulates intestinal motility by a pharmacological means. Prunes contain a laxative substance called *dihydroxyphenyl isatin* (Krause and Mahan, 1979).

The general principle of the high-fiber diet is to increase the fiber content. The studies by Burkitt (1973, 1979) comparing the high-fiber dietary intake of Africans and their almost nonexistent incidence of colon cancer and other colon diseases with the much lower fiber diet of the US population and their higher incidence of colon disease still leave many questions unanswered. The publicity about fiber has led, however, to a renewed interest in this aspect of nutrition. Consuming a diet higher in fiber will do no harm, and it may have beneficial effects, especially for people suffering from constipation.

Dietary fiber refers to all undigestible carbohydrates and lignin that come from the cell walls of plants (Pollman et al., 1978). Crude fiber, however, is only cellulose and lignin. At present, the majority of dietary tables list crude fiber. The values for crude fiber, however, generally underestimate the quantity of fiber present in foods of plant origin. Figures for dietary fiber are becoming more available, but the student should remember that many figures for the fiber content of food are still listed as crude fiber. Table 28-4 lists the crude-fiber content of some common foods.

TABLE 28-4. Fiber Content of Selected Foods

Food	Crude Fiber (gm/100 gm)
Wheat bran	9.1
Wheat germ	2.5
Nuts	
Almonds	2.6
Peanuts	2.4
Pecans	2.3
Breads and cereals	
Whole wheat bread	1.6
White bread	0.2
Cornmeal, whole	1.6
Cornmeal, degermed	0.6
Brown rice	0.3
White rice	0.1
Whole grain wheat flour	2.3
White wheat flour	0.3
Vegetables	
Lima beans	1.8
Green beans	1.0
Beets	0.8
Cabbage	0.8
Carrots	0.6
Celery	0.6
Collards	1.0
Lettuce	0.7
Peas	2.0
Baked potatoes	0.6
Mashed potatoes	0.4
Spinach	0.6
Tomatoes	0.5
Fruits	
Apples, raw	1.0
Apples, dried	3.1
Applesauce	0.6
Apricots, raw	0.6
Apricots, dried	3.0
Grapefruit	0.2
Grapes	0.6
Orange	0.5
Pears, fresh	1.4
Prunes, cooked	0.8
Raisins	0.9
Strawberries	1.3

SOURCE: From *Composition of Foods; Raw, Processed, Prepared.* Agricultural Handbook No. 8. USDA, 1963.

The chief function of fiber is to increase the bulk of the diet. Fiber performs as a bulk agent because it has the ability to absorb water. This property allows the stools to be softer and bulkier, which in turn allows them to be evacuated with less effort (Pollman et al., 1978).

Opinions vary about the significance of decreased intestinal transit times with the ingestion of a high-fiber diet. *Intestinal transit time* is the length of time from the ingestion of a meal to its evacuation from the rectum. Generally, it is expected that increased quantities of dietary fiber will lead to a decreased intestinal transit time. This has been observed by Burkitt (1972). From a review of the literature Pollman et al. (1978) state that there is general disagreement about the effect of increased dietary fiber and transit time.

Another theory of the cause of colon disease is that it may be due to abnormally high pressures within the colon. These pressures are higher in clients who are predisposed to *diverticulosis*, which is an outpouching of the mucosa of the colon wall, often because of a weakness in the wall. If this pouch becomes inflamed, the condition is known as *diverticulitis* (see Fig. 28-8). This abnormally high pressure may be increased even further by a diet low in fiber and by straining. Burkitt (1972; 1973) has suggested that the increased pressures that are aggravated by straining may be causative factors in the development of hiatal hernias, varicose veins, deep vein thrombosis, and hemorrhoids. A high-fiber diet leads to the formation of a larger, bulkier stool that distends the colon and decreases the pressure (Goldstein, 1972). Also, the bacteria in the colon attack the dietary fiber, forming volatile fatty acids that stimulate evacuation.

PRACTICAL CONSIDERATIONS. The high-fiber diet is similar to the regular diet except that it contains additional fiber. A high-fiber menu is found in Figure 28-9. There is no set dietary requirement for fiber. The average US diet

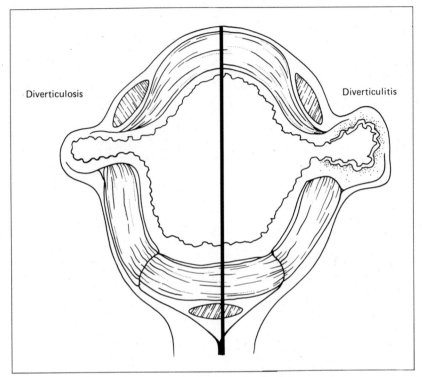

Figure 28-8. *Diverticula* are outpouchings of the mucosal wall of the colon; the presence of the pouches is known as *diverticulosis*. A high-fiber diet is often used to prevent the occurrence of additional pouches. If these pouches become inflamed, the condition is known as *diverticulitis*. A low-residue diet should be used to prevent irritation during this inflammation.

contains about 2–4 gm of fiber daily (Guthrie, 1979). The fiber content of the diet can be modified a small or a moderate amount depending on the amount and type of fiber added. Connell (1976) states that the addition of 2 gm of fiber per day is required to effect a significant change in fecal volume. Burkitt and Meisner (1979) recommend a daily intake of 6–10 gm of dietary fiber. These recommendations represent only minor changes in the diet. For example, an additional 2 gm of fiber daily can be obtained by eating 1 cup of a bran cereal or two to three raw carrots. Krause and Mahan (1979) state that about 800 gm of fruits and vegetables are needed to produce a daily bowel movement. This is equivalent to about four pieces of fresh fruit and a large salad. The amount of residue needed to relieve constipation is an individual matter. Bennion (1979) suggests that five to six servings of fruits and vegetables and four to six servings of whole grain breads and cereals daily should be sufficient.

Adequate fiber can be obtained by the addition of regular foods high in fiber or the addition of a small amount of bran. Painter (1975) recommended the addition of 12–14 gm of bran (2.5 gm of fiber) to help relieve the symptoms of constipation. He advocates the use of 1 heaping t of bran before each meal.

MORNING	NOON	NIGHT
(FRESHLY SQUEEZED ORANGE JUICE)	(MINESTRONE SOUP WITH CHEESE PUFF)	(PINEAPPLE SHERBET PUNCH)
	CREAMY CLAM CHOWDER WITH CHEESE PUFF	STRAINED CREAM OF MUSHROOM SOUP
GRAPEFRUIT JUICE	CREAM OF TOMATO SOUP	STRAINED JULIENNE BROTH
	CELERY BROTH	PAN FRIED CATFISH WITH TARTAR SAUCE
(HOT ROLLED WHEAT)	(TUNA AND NOODLE CASSEROLE)	BAKED HADDOCK WITH LEMON WEDGE
CORNFLAKES	PORK SAUSAGE PATTY IN GRAVY	(ROAST BEEF AU JUS)
PUFFED RICE	BEEF (GROUND) IN BROTH	(GROUND) ROAST BEEF AU JUS
		HASHED BROWN POTATOES
(SCRAMBLED EGGS)	MASHED POTATOES	BUTTERED DICED POTATOES
POACHED EGG	(BUTTERED PEAS)	
FRIED EGG SUNNY SIDE UP	BUTTERED CABBAGE	BUTTERED ASPARAGUS SPEARS
FRIED EGG OVER LIGHT	BUTTERED BLENDERIZED GREEN PEAS	(BUTTERED VEGETABLE MEDLEY)
FRIED EGG HARD	FAVORITE RELISHES IN ICE	BUTTERED BLENDERIZED ASPARAGUS
SOFT COOKED EGG IN SHELL	(TOSSED GREEN SALAD)	(CALICO COLESLAW ON LEAF LETTUCE)
HARD COOKED EGG IN SHELL	(CREAMY SALAD DRESSING)	
BROILED BACON STRIP	BRAIDED ROLL WITH MARGARINE	BUTTERCORN ROLL WITH MARGARINE
WARM BEAR CLAW DANISH PASTRY	WHITE BREAD OR TOAST WITH MARGARINE	WHITE BREAD OR TOAST WITH MARGARINE
(WHOLE WHEAT TOAST WITH MARGARINE)	(Whole Wheat Bread)	(Whole Wheat Bread)
WHITE TOAST WITH MARGARINE	WARM APPLE DUMPLING EN SAUCE	CHILLED APRICOT HALVES
WHITE BREAD WITH MARGARINE	PEACH HALVES (Fresh Apple)	CHILLED BLACK BOTTOM PIE (Fresh Pear)
MARGARINE	(MARGARINE)	(MARGARINE)
(MILK)	(MILK)	(MILK)
2% MILK	2% MILK	2% MILK
SKIM MILK	SKIM MILK	SKIM MILK
BUTTERMILK	BUTTERMILK	BUTTERMILK
	COTTAGE CHEESE	COTTAGE CHEESE
	(CRACKERS)	CRACKERS
	CUSTARD	PUDDING
	VANILLA ICE CREAM	VANILLA ICE CREAM
JELLO — HOT TEA	JELLO — HOT TEA	JELLO — HOT TEA
BROTH — ICED TEA	— (ICED TEA)	— ICED TEA
(JELLY) — LEMON	JELLY — LEMON	JELLY — LEMON
CREAM — FRUIT DRINK	CREAM — FRUIT JUICE	CREAM — FRUIT JUICE
(COFFEE) —	COFFEE — FRUIT DRINK	(COFFEE) — FRUIT DRINK
SANKA —	SANKA — LEMONADE	SANKA — LEMONADE

Figure 28-9. A sample high-fiber diet. (Courtesy Indiana University Hospitals)

This dose is increased by 1 t before each meal after two weeks if the symptoms of constipation persist. The bran may be further increased by 1 t per meal per week if necessary until a soft stool is passed, without straining, at least once a day. Many authorities disagree about the necessity of passing a daily stool. Until more conclusive evidence is available, many physicians and dietitians recommend a simple increase in daily dietary fiber through the inclusion of more fresh fruits and vegetables and more whole grain breads and cereals. Clients who are instructed to ingest bran should be warned that bran may produce a feeling of discomfort owing to flatulence (Painter, 1975).

Some interesting studies have been conducted using the high-fiber diet on elderly clients. Zimring (1978) reported a study conducted on clients in an extended care facility. Before the study, 15 clients received laxatives, suppositories, stool softeners, or enemas. All these constipation aids were discontinued during the study unless they were required. The clients received bran each morning for two months. During the study, only 6 of the 15 required any aid for constipation (other than the diet), and these 6 required aid only once during the two-month study.

Another study was conducted by a nurse in a hospital geriatric unit (Bass, 1977). In this 10-week study, 17 clients who frequently required the use of a laxative, stool softener, or enema were given diets that were higher in fiber. Each week a different high-fiber dietary modification was used. The dietary changes were minimal. The first week rye or whole wheat bread was substituted for white bread at two meals. The second week whole grain cereals were included at breakfast on three days. During the third week one serving of a raw fruit or raw vegetable was included; and during the fourth week whole grain cereals were used daily. At bedtime 4 oz of prune juice was given because many of the clients were accustomed to this practice. There was a 27% decrease in the number of laxatives given to these clients even with the modest dietary changes.

Dependence on Ostomy Care

A client who has had surgery involving the formation of an ostomy is challenged with a large number of changes that may significantly alter his lifestyle. The health care team can greatly aid the client and his family in facing these adaptations. The postsurgical assessment of the client with an ostomy involves the person as a whole. Specific areas to be assessed include the client's psychosocial adaptation and acceptance of the ostomy; the specific type of ostomy present; the type, amount, and frequency of drainage; the condition of the skin around the stoma; and any situations the client perceives as problems.

Dietary Interventions

Planning the nursing care of the client with an ostomy centers on three major areas: specific diet therapy, care of the skin, and lifestyle changes that may occur. The student may refer to a medical-surgical textbook for techniques of skin care for ostomy cases. Lewis (1977) describes four major areas to consider when teaching the client about diet: the client's nutritional requirements, the type of ostomy and its relationship to nutrient use, the effect of specific foods on establishing and maintaining bowel control, and the presence of concurrent disease or alterations.

The healthy client with an ostomy has the same general nutritional needs as other people of the same age and sex. The client should be encouraged to return to a nutritionally adequate diet with his own preferences as soon as possible. The return to this "normalcy" will aid the ostomate both physically and psychologically. Immediately following surgery the client's nitrogen balance may be negative, and he may need a nutritional supplement.

The client who has an ileostomy has had a large portion of the small intestine resected.

As discussed in Unit II, most absorption takes place in the jejunum; therefore an ileostomy does not necessarily predispose the client to malnutrition or malabsorption. The two nutrients specifically absorbed in the ileum are vitamin B_{12} and bile salts. Vitamin B_{12} can be replaced by the physician through regular intramuscular administration. A bile salt deficiency will cause the client to have difficulty digesting and absorbing fats. Steatorrhea and a watery fecal discharge indicate that a bile salt deficiency may be present. The problem may be corrected by limiting fat intake, but when this is done the hazard of malabsorption of the fat soluble vitamins (A, D, E, and K) is present. Corn on the cob may cause a blockage or dysfunction in the ostomy because of decreased digestion of cellulose. In addition, ileostomates usually do not tolerate large amounts of foods containing cellulose, such as bamboo shoots or peanuts. Because the colon has been removed, the bacteria that digest cellulose are no longer present.

When weight loss is a major problem with the iliostomate, the dietitian may supplement the client's diet with MCT that can be digested and absorbed without bile. Low-residue supplements containing sugars, amino acids, essential fatty acids, vitamins, and minerals are easily digested and absorbed. The dietitian will be able to supply the nurse and the client with information concerning commercially available supplements that will meet the individual needs of the client.

The nurse should be aware that, when a client intially loses large amounts of fluid through the ostomy, he is also losing large amounts of electrolytes. Usually the client's bowel will gradually adapt and increase its absorptive capacity. The region where the ostomy is performed will affect the consistency of the discharge (see Fig. 28-10). During the adjustment phase it may help to control excess fluid and electrolyte loss through a decrease in the intake of foods high in fiber and sugar. The nurse should reassure the client

that these foods can gradually be reintroduced into the diet after his bowel begins to adapt. In addition, she should caution the client to avoid salt tablets, for these may act as a cathartic and prolong or worsen diarrhea. Beverages containing both fluids and electrolytes may be used to supplement the client's intake during the adjustment phase.

After the adjustment phase, the client may be encouraged to follow such dietary habits as eating at regular times, chewing food thoroughly, chewing with the mouth closed to avoid excessive air swallowing, eating in moderate amounts, and drinking six to eight glasses of water a day. The nurse should reinforce the fact that restricting fluids will not decrease the fluidity of the discharge. Furthermore, diarrhea may be helped by eating strained bananas or applesauce.

A client's bowel patterns are not changed through surgery; therefore, a tolerance or intolerance to specific foods will not vary significantly after surgery. If a food did not cause gas, constipation, or diarrhea before surgery, it will most likely be well tolerated after surgery. Adding new foods to the diet one at a time will help determine which ones may be troublesome. Milk intolerance may be a particular problem to the ostomate. Fermented forms of milk such as buttermilk, yogurt, or cheese may be more easily tolerated by the ostomate with a lactose intolerance. Foods that have been reported to cause excessive watery discharge include raw fruits, highly spiced foods, fried foods, corn, and prune juice (Lewis, 1977). Hard stools may be the result of low fiber intake or a side effect of such medications as calcium antacids.

Gas and odor problems frequently worry the ostomate. Gas may be caused by swallowing air, eating too rapidly, or having irregular eating habits. Peas, beans, cabbage, fish, onions, radishes, and cucumbers are believed to cause gas. (Gill et al., 1972). Odor problems may be a result of the client's punching holes in the top of the appliance for gas release. Continuous odor release can be controlled by

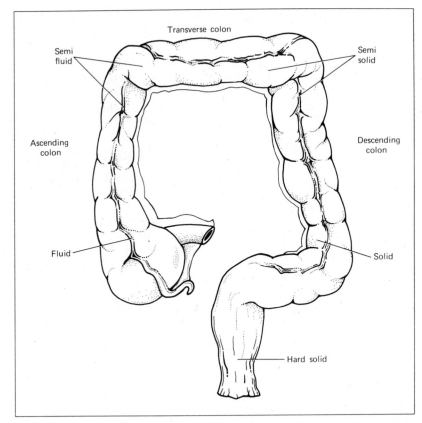

Figure 28-10. Water reabsorption occurs mainly in the terminal portion of the colon. Excessive motility in the colon results in diarrhea in which there is an inadequate reabsorption of water. If surgery is required on the colon to establish an ostomy, the region where the ostomy is established will influence the consistency of the solid waste.

punching a small hole in the top of the pouch and covering it with tape. The client can remove the tape in the privacy of the bathroom to allow gas to escape (Yahle, 1975). There are many deodorants on the market manufactured specifically for ostomates. Placing an aspirin in the bag should never be done to control odor. If the aspirin should come into contact with the stomach, tissue sloughing or bleeding may occur. The doctor may order bismuth subgallate to be taken three times a day to aid in odor control.

In conclusion, the client's diet will be best determined by his individual tolerances and habits. The members of the health care team need to match the client's nutritional needs to his food preferences.

The client with an ostomy may need to be reassured that his lifestyle will not necessarily be altered by the ostomy. Physical activity is generally not limited except for lifting heavy objects. Once a schedule has been established, the care of the ostomy need not interfere with the day's schedule. Personal habits such as bathing, swimming, clothing, travel, social life, or sexual patterns usually will not be significantly altered.

Frequently the degree of client acceptance and adaptation to the ostomy will influence his success in ostomy management. The possibility of cancer or disfigurement and the degree of loss perceived by the client need to be carefully assessed by the nurse and dietitian before learning can occur.

Diarrhea

Diarrhea is one of the most common alterations in elimination. It may be defined as increased frequency (more than three bowel movements per day), increased fluidity, or increased total weight of stools (greater than 200 gm/day in people on a regular Western diet). Diarrhea usually occurs when the gut is in a state of hypermotility. If the process continues over time, the total absorptive time is decreased, resulting in the loss of fluid and electrolytes. Factors leading to diarrhea include various diseases such as ulcerative colitis, Crohn's disease, malabsorption, or an infectious process. In addition, diarrhea may be secondary to the overuse of laxatives or enemas; prolonged stress; antibiotic therapy; or surgical intervention.

Assessment of the client with diarrhea will center on the subjective and objective symptoms he is experiencing. The symptoms may include cramping; frequent watery, loose stools; weakness and nausea; hyperactive gurgling bowel sounds; and loss of appetite. Signs of dehydration such as diminished skin turgor may also appear. The client should be questioned about his normal bowel patterns and recent dietary intake.

Dietary Interventions

Nursing care of the client with diarrhea is primarily supportive. The goals of treatment may include the reduction of the number of stools, the maintenance of fluid and electrolyte balance, and the provision for rest and comfort. Skin breakdown is a frequent com-

plication of diarrhea; therefore nursing actions should also be directed at maintaining skin integrity.

Diet therapy consists primarily of decreasing the stimulus to the gut. In severe cases the client is given no food by mouth and maintained on IV therapy. In milder forms, the client is placed on a clear or full-liquid diet. A decrease in the total residue taken in by the client will tend to decrease motility. Hot or cold liquids also tend to increase GI motility and thus should be avoided. Bland fluids may be tolerated and at the same time supply nutrients as well as fluid.

Nursing interventions focus on reducing stress in the environment, decreasing the general activity level of the client, and making the appropriate dietary modification. Providing a bedside commode may help the client feel more secure if he is having frequent diarrhea. Frequent reassessment is necessary to monitor fluid and electrolyte balance.

Chronic diarrhea can lead to weight loss and malnutrition. Malabsorption may cause a caloric deficit and specific deficiencies in vitamins and minerals. Clients who excrete more than 7 gm of fat in 24 hours while on a daily diet that provides 70–80 gm of fat are considered to have malabsorption. Frequent small feedings will sometimes provide a greater caloric intake than the traditional three-meal-a-day diet. Vitamin, Calorie, and protein supplements may be necessary if continued weight loss occurs. For the hospitalized client, nutritional needs can be met by total parenteral nutrition (see Chap. 23).

CASE STUDY: A Patient with Chronic Renal Failure

Sara B. is a 42-year-old secretary in chronic renal failure. She has been transferred to a university medical center for hemodialysis three times a week. Sara's history reveals an almost lifelong battle with hypertension. She had no renal symptoms until three months ago when, following an attack of influenza, she suddenly developed generalized edema. A medical diagnosis of chronic renal failure was made after a work-up involving a cystoscopy, an intravenous urogram, and various renal function tests. She is being treated with a high-carbohydrate, low-protein (60 gm), low-sodium (1 gm), potassium-restricted (1500 mg) diet; a 1,000 ml fluid restriction; methyldopa (Aldomet); furosemide (Lasix); and aluminum hydroxide gel (Amphogel).

The admitting nursing assessment notes erosions of Sara's mucosa, generalized bruising, and an ammonia odor on her breath. Sara states she is having headaches, dizzy spells, and poor appetite. Vital signs are: pulse, 102; respirations, 28; blood pressure, 210/110; and oral temperature, 37.2 C (99 F). She is 5 ft 4 in (163 cm) tall and weighs 212 lb (96.4 kg), and has experienced a weight gain of 10 lb (4.54 kg) in the last week. On admission her laboratory values for creatinine, potassium, and blood urea nitrogen were elevated.

QUESTIONS

1. What is the specific nursing diagnosis for Sara evidenced by an alteration in fluid output?

2. What are the specific objectives of the diet prescribed for Sara?

3. What are the general principles of the different nutritional components of Sara's diet?

4. Why is psychological support from the health team and the client's family important to Sara's adherence to the diet?

5. Why is the physician or nurse so concerned about rapid weight gain by Sara or any client with chronic renal failure?

6. How are the blood levels of sodium, potassium, and blood urea nitrogen related to the dietary modifications of sodium, potassium, protein, and Calories?

BIBLIOGRAPHY

Bailey, G. L., and Sullivan, N. R. Selected protein diet in terminal uremia. *J. Am. Diet. Assoc.* 52:125, 1968.

Bass, L. More fiber—less constipation. *Am. J. Nurs.* 77:254, 1977.

Beckett, J., and Shealey, F. Role of the nurse in managing the patient's diet. *Nursing Mirror* 139(11):69, 1974.

Bennion, M. *Clinical Nutrition.* 1st Ed. New York: Harper & Row, Pubs., Inc., 1979.

Biller, D. C. Patient's point of view: Diet in chronic renal failure. *J. Am. Diet. Assoc.* 71:633, 1977.

Blackburn, S. L. Dietary compliance of chronic hemodialysis patients. *J. Am. Diet. Assoc.* 70:31, 1977.

Blumenkrantz, M. J., Roberts, C. E., Card, B., Colburn, J. W., and Kopple, J. D. Nutrition management of the adult patient undergoing peritoneal dialysis. *J. Am. Diet. Assoc.* 73:251, 1978.

Burkitt, D. P. Effect of dietary fiber on stools and transit times and its roles in the causation of disease. *Lancet* 2:1408, 1972.

_____. Epidemiology of large bowel disease. The role of fiber. *Proc. Nutr. Soc.* 33:145, 1973.

Burkitt, D. P., and Meisner, P. How to manage constipation with high fiber diet. *Geriatrics* 34:33, 1979.

Burton, B. T. Current concepts of nutrition and diet in disease of the kidney. *J. Am. Diet. Assoc.* 65:623, 1974.

_____. Nutritional implications of renal disease: I. Current overview and general principles. *J. Am. Diet. Assoc.* 70:479, 1977.

Chermoff, R., and Dean, J. A. Medical and nutritional aspects of intractable diarrhea. *J. Am. Diet. Assoc.* 76:161, 1980.

Connell, A. M. Dietary fiber and diverticular disease. *Hosp. Pract.* 11(3):119, 1976.

Corea, A. L. Current trends in diet and drug therapy for the dialysis patient. *Nurs. Clin. North Am.* 10:469, 1975.

Danovitch, G. M. Bourgoignie, J., and Bricker, N. S. Reversibility of the "salt-losing" tendency of chronic renal failure. *N. Engl. J. Med.* 296:14, 1977.

Dericks, V., and Donovan, C. The ostomy patient really needs you. *Nursing 76* 76(9):30, 1976.

Frowell, H. C. Dietary fiber and diseases of the large bowel. *Practitioner* 219:350, 1977.

_____. The development of the concept of dietary fiber in human nutrition. *Am. J. Clin. Nutr.* 3(Suppl.):3, 1978.

Gill, N., Hogern, W., Rowbotham, J., and Schuster, M. Helping your ostomate patient cope. *Patient Care* 6(4):46, 1972.

Giordano, C. Use of exogenous and endogenous urea for protein synthesis in normal and uremic subjects. *J. Lab. Clin. Med.* 62:231, 1963.

_____. The role of diet in renal disease. *Hosp. Pract.* 12:113, 1977.

Giovannetti, S., and Maggiore, Q. A low nitrogen diet with proteins of high biological value for severe chronic uremia. *Lancet* 1:1000, 1964.

Goldstein, F. Diet and colonic disease. *J. Am. Diet. Assoc.* 60:499, 1972.

Guthrie, H. A. *Introductory Nutrition.* 4th Ed. St. Louis: The C. V. Mosby Co., 1979.

Habeeb, M. C., and Kallstrom, M. D. Bowel program for institutionalized adults. *Am. J. Nurs.* 76:606, 1976.

Ing, J. S., and Kark, R. M. Renal disease. In H. A. Schneider, C. E, Anderson, and D. B. Coursin, Eds., *Nutritional Support of Medical Practice.* New York: Harper & Row Pubs., Inc., 1977.

Joseph, M. Dietary needs of patients with renal failure. *Nursing Journal of India* 64:15, 1973.

Kahn, H. D., Panariello, V. A., Saeli, J., Sampson, J. R., and Schwartz, E. T. Effect of cranberry juice on urine. *J. Am. Diet. Assoc.* 51:251, 1967.

Kopple, J. D. Nutritional management of chronic renal failure. *Postgrad. Med.* 64:135, 1978.

Krause, M. V., and Mahan, L. K. *Food, Nutrition, and Diet Therapy.* 6th Ed. Philadelphia: W. B. Saunders Co., 1979.

Lenneberg, E., and Mendelssohn, A. *Colostomies: A Guide.* Los Angeles: United Ostomy Assoc., 1971.

Lewis, C. Diet planning for ostomates. *Patient Care* 11(13):152, 1977.

Mitchell, H. S., Rynbergen, H. J., Anderson, L., and Dibble, M. V. *Nutrition in Health and Disease.* 16th Ed. Philadelphia: J. B. Lippincott Co., 1976.

Overton, M. H., and Lukert, B. P. *Clinical Nutrition: A Physiologic Approach.* Chicago: Year Book Medical Pubs., Inc., 1977.

Painter, N. S. Trouble down below: Diverticular disease. *Emergency Medicine* 7:111, 1975.

Pennington, J. *Nutritional Diet Therapy.* Palo Alto, Calif.: Bull Pub. Co., 1978.

Plumley, P. F., and Francis, B. Dietary management of diverticular disease. *J. Am. Diet. Assoc.* 63:527, 1973.

Pollman, J. W., Morris, J. J., and Rose, P. N. Is fiber the answer to constipation problems in the elderly: A review of literature. *Int. J. Nurs. Stud.* 15:107, 1978.

Robinson, C. H., and Lawler, M. R. *Normal and Therapeutic Nutrition.* 15th Ed. New York: Macmillan, Inc., 1977.

Sargent, J. A., and Gotch, F. A. The predialysis patient with renal disease. *J. Am. Diet. Assoc.* 75:547, 1979.

Sargent, J. A., Gotch, F. A., Henry, R. R., and Bennett, K. The dialyzed patient. *J. Am. Diet. Assoc.* 75:551, 1979.

Smith, L. H., Van Den Berg, C. J., and Wilson, D. M. Nutrition and urolitheasis. *N. Engl. J. Med.* 298:87, 1978.

Swendseid, M. E. Nutritional needs of patients with renal disease. *J. Am. Diet. Assoc.* 70:488, 1977.

Thiele, V. F. *Clinical Nutrition.* St. Louis: The C. V. Mosby Co., 1976.

Wentworth, A., and Cox B. Nursing the patient with a continent ileostomy. *Am. J. Nurs.* 76(9):1424, 1976.

Williams, S. R. *Nutritional and Diet Therapy.* 3rd Ed. St. Louis: The C. V. Mosby Co., 1977.

Wolffe, L. V., Weitzel, M. H., and Fuerst, E. V. *Fundamentals of Nursing.* 6th Ed. Philadelphia: J. B. Lippincott Co., 1979.

Yahle, M. E. An ostomy information clinic. *Nurs. Clin. North Am.* 11(3):457, 1975.

Zimring, J. G. High fiber diet versus laxatives in geriatric patients. *N.Y. State J. of Med.* 78:2223, 1978.

APPENDICES

GLOSSARY

INDEX

APPENDIX A

Nutritive Values of the Edible Parts of Foods

Food, approximate measure, and weight (in grams)			Food energy	Pro-tein	Fat (total lipid)	Satu-rated (total)	Unsaturated		Carbo-hydrate	Cal-cium	Iron	Vita-min A value	Thia-mine	Ribo-flavin	Niacin	Ascor-bic acid
							Oleic	Linoleic								
		gm.	(Calo-ries)	(gm.)	(gm.)	(gm.)	(gm.)	(gm.)	(gm.)	(mg.)	(mg.)	(I.U.)	(mg.)	(mg.)	(mg.)	(mg.)
Milk, cream, cheese (related products)																
Milk, cow's																
Fluid, whole (3.5% fat)	1 cup	244	160	9	9	5	3	Trace	12	288	0.1	350	0.08	0.42	0.1	2
Fluid, nonfat (skim)	1 cup	246	90	9	Trace	—	—	—	13	298	.1	10	.10	.44	.2	2
Buttermilk, cultured, from skim milk	1 cup	246	90	9	Trace	—	—	—	13	298	.1	10	.09	.44	.2	2
Evaporated, unsweet-ened, undiluted	1 cup	252	345	18	20	11	7	1	24	635	.3	820	.10	.84	.5	3
Condensed, sweetened, undiluted	1 cup	306	980	25	27	15	9	1	166	802	.3	1,090	.23	1.17	.5	3
Dry, whole	1 cup	103	515	27	28	16	9	1	39	936	.5	1,160	.30	1.50	.7	6
Dry, nonfat, instant	1 cup	70	250	25	Trace	—	—	—	36	905	.4	20	.24	1.25	.6	5
Milk, goat's																
Fluid, whole	1 cup	244	165	8	10	6	2	Trace	11	315	.2	390	.10	.27	.7	2
Cream																
Half-and-half (cream and milk)	1 cup	242	325	8	28	16	9	1	11	261	.1	1,160	.08	.38	.1	2
	1 tbsp.	15	20	Trace	2	1	1	Trace	1	16	Trace	70	Trace	.02	Trace	Trace
Light, coffee or table	1 cup	240	505	7	49	27	16	1	10	245	.1	2,030	.07	.36	.1	2
	1 tbsp.	15	30	Trace	3	2	1	Trace	1	15	Trace	130	Trace	.02	Trace	Trace
Whipping, unwhipped (volume about double when whipped)																
Light	1 cup	239	715	6	75	41	25	2	9	203	.1	3,070	.06	.30	.1	2
	1 tbsp.	15	45	Trace	5	3	2	Trace	1	13	Trace	190	Trace	.02	Trace	Trace
Heavy	1 cup	238	840	5	89	49	29	3	7	178	.1	3,670	.05	.26	.1	2
	1 tbsp.	15	55	Trace	6	3	2	Trace	Trace	11	Trace	230	Trace	.02	Trace	Trace

Continued.

Food	Measure	Grams	Food energy (cal.)	Protein (g)	Fat (g)	Saturated (g)	Oleic (g)	Linoleic (g)	Carbohydrate (g)	Calcium (mg)	Iron (mg)	Vitamin A (I.U.)	Thiamine (mg)	Riboflavin (mg)	Niacin (mg)	Ascorbic acid (mg)
Cheese																
Blue or Roquefort type	1 oz.	28	105	6	9	5	3	Trace	1	89	.1	350	.01	.17	.1	0
Cheddar or American																
Ungrated	1 inch cube	17	70	4	5	3	2	Trace	Trace	128	.2	220	Trace	.08	Trace	0
Grated	1 cup	112	445	28	36	20	12	1	2	840	1.1	1,470	.03	.51	.1	0
	1 tbsp.	7	30	2	2	1	1	Trace	Trace	52	.1	90	Trace	.03	Trace	0
Cheddar, process	1 oz.	28	105	7	9	5	3	Trace	1	219	.3	350	Trace	.12	Trace	0
Cheese foods, Cheddar	1 oz.	28	90	6	7	4	2	Trace	2	162	.2	280	.01	.16	Trace	0
Cottage cheese, from skim milk																
Creamed	1 cup	225	240	31	9	5	3	Trace	7	212	0.7	380	0.07	0.56	0.2	0
	1 oz.	28	30	4	1	1	Trace	Trace	1	27	.1	50	.01	.07	Trace	0
Uncreamed	1 cup	225	195	38	1	Trace	Trace	—	6	202	.9	20	.07	.63	.2	0
	1 oz.	28	25	5	Trace	—	—	Trace	1	26	.1	Trace	.01	.08	Trace	0
Cream cheese	1 oz.	28	105	2	11	6	4	Trace	1	18	.1	440	Trace	.07	Trace	0
	1 tbsp.	15	55	1	6	3	2	Trace	Trace	9	Trace	230	Trace	.04	Trace	0
Swiss (domestic)	1 oz.	28	105	8	8	4	3	Trace	1	262	.3	320	Trace	.11	Trace	0
Milk beverages																
Cocoa	1 cup	242	235	9	11	6	4	Trace	26	286	.9	390	.09	.45	.4	2
Chocolate-flavored milk drink (made with skim milk)	1 cup	250	190	8	6	3	2	Trace	27	270	.4	210	.09	.41	.2	2
Malted milk	1 cup	270	280	13	12	—	—	—	32	364	.8	670	.17	.56	.2	2
Milk desserts																
Cornstarch pudding, plain (blanc mange)	1 cup	248	275	9	10	5	3	Trace	39	290	.1	390	.07	.40	.1	2
Custard, baked	1 cup	248	285	13	14	6	5	1	28	278	1.0	870	.10	.47	.2	1
Ice cream, plain, factory packed																
Slice or cut brick, ⅛ of quart brick	1 slice or cut brick	71	145	3	9	5	3	Trace	15	87	.1	370	.03	.13	.1	1
Container	3½ fld. oz.	62	130	2	8	4	3	Trace	13	76	.1	320	.03	.12	.1	1
Container	8 fld. ozs.	142	295	6	18	10	6	1	29	175	.1	740	.06	.27	.1	1
Ice milk	1 cup	187	285	9	10	6	3	Trace	42	292	.2	390	.09	.41	.2	2
Yogurt, from partially skimmed milk	1 cup	246	120	8	4	2	1	Trace	13	295	.1	170	.09	.43	.2	2

¹Reprinted from Nutritive value of foods, U.S. Department of Agriculture, Home and Garden Bulletin No. 72.
Dashes show that no basis could be found for imputing a value although there was some reason to believe that a measurable amount of the constituent might be present.

Food, approximate measure, and weight (in grams)		weight (gm.)	Food energy (Calories)	Protein (gm.)	Fat (total lipid) (gm.)	Fatty acids Saturated (total) (gm.)	Fatty acids Unsaturated Oleic (gm.)	Fatty acids Unsaturated Linoleic (gm.)	Carbohydrate (gm.)	Calcium (mg.)	Iron (mg.)	Vitamin A value (I.U.)	Thiamine (mg.)	Riboflavin (mg.)	Niacin (mg.)	Ascorbic acid (mg.)
Eggs																
Eggs, large, 24 ounces per dozen																
Raw																
Whole, without shell	1 egg	50	80	6	6	2	3	Trace	Trace	27	1.1	590	.05	.15	Trace	0
White of egg	1 white	33	15	4	Trace	—	—	—	Trace	3	Trace	0	Trace	.09	Trace	0
Yolk of egg	1 yolk	17	60	3	5	2	2	Trace	Trace	24	.9	580	.04	.07	Trace	0
Cooked																
Boiled, shell removed	2 eggs	100	160	13	12	4	5	1	1	54	2.3	1,180	.09	.28	.1	0
Scrambled, with milk and fat	1 egg	64	110	7	8	3	3	Trace	1	51	1.1	690	.05	.18	Trace	0
Meat, poultry, fish, shellfish (related products)																
Bacon, broiled or fried, crisp	2 slices	16	100	5	8	3	4	1	1	2	.5	0	.08	.05	.8	—
Beef, trimmed to retail basis², cooked																
Cuts braised, simmered, or pot-roasted																
Lean and fat	3 oz.	85	245	23	16	8	7	Trace	0	10	2.9	30	.04	.18	3.5	—
Lean only	2.5 oz.	72	140	22	5	2	2	Trace	0	10	2.7	10	.04	.16	3.3	—
Hamburger (ground beef), broiled																
Lean	3 oz.	85	185	23	10	5	4	Trace	0	10	3.0	20	.08	.20	5.1	—
Regular	3 oz.	85	245	21	17	8	8	Trace	0	9	2.7	30	.07	.18	4.6	—
Roast, oven-cooked, no liquid added																
Relatively fat, such as rib																
Lean and fat	3 oz.	85	375	17	34	16	15	1	0	8	2.2	70	.05	.13	3.1	—
Lean only	1.8 oz.	51	125	14	7	3	3	Trace	0	6	1.8	10	.04	.11	2.6	—
Relatively lean, such as heel of round																
Lean and fat	3 oz.	85	165	25	7	3	3	Trace	0	11	3.2	10	.06	.19	4.5	—
Lean only	2.7 oz.	78	125	24	3	1	1	Trace	0	10	3.0	Trace	.06	.18	4.3	—
Steak, broiled																
Relatively fat, such as sirloin																
Lean and fat	3 oz.	85	330	20	27	13	12	1	0	9	2.5	50	.05	.16	4.0	—
Lean only	2.0 oz.	56	115	18	4	2	2	Trace	0	7	2.2	10	.05	.14	3.6	—
Relatively lean, such as round																
Lean and fat	3 oz.	85	220	24	13	6	6	Trace	0	10	3.0	20	.07	.19	4.8	—
Lean only	2.4 oz.	68	130	21	4	2	2	Trace	0	9	2.5	10	.06	.16	4.1	—

Food	Measure	Weight (g)	Food energy	Protein (g)	Fat (g)	Saturated	Oleic	Linoleic	Carbohydrate (g)	Calcium (mg)	Iron (mg)	Vitamin A (I.U.)	Thiamine (mg)	Riboflavin (mg)	Niacin (mg)	Ascorbic acid (mg)
Beef, canned																
Corned beef	3 oz.	85	185	22	10	5	4	Trace	0	17	3.7	20	.01	.20	2.9	—
Corned beef hash	3 oz.	85	155	7	10	5	4	Trace	9	11	1.7	—	.01	.08	1.8	—
Beef, dried or chipped	2 oz.	57	115	19	4	2	2	Trace	0	11	2.9	—	.04	.18	2.2	—
Beef and vegetable stew	1 cup	235	210	15	10	5	4	Trace	15	28	2.8	2,310	.13	.17	4.4	15
Beef potpie, baked: individual pie, 4¼-inch diameter, weight before baking about 8 oz.	1 pie	227	560	23	33	9	20	2	43	32	4.1	1,860	.25	.27	4.5	7
Chicken, cooked																
Flesh only, broiled	3 oz.	85	115	20	3	1	1	1	0	8	1.4	80	0.05	0.16	7.4	—
Breast, fried, ½ breast																
With bone	3.3 oz.	94	155	25	5	1	2	1	1	9	1.3	70	.04	.17	11.2	—
Flesh and skin only	2.7 oz.	76	155	25	5	1	2	1	1	9	1.3	70	.04	.17	11.2	—
Drumstick, fried																
With bone	2.1 oz.	59	90	12	4	1	2	1	Trace	6	.9	50	.03	.15	2.7	—
Flesh and skin only	1.3 oz.	38	90	12	4	1	2	1	Trace	6	.9	50	.03	.15	2.7	—
Chicken, canned, boneless	3 oz.	85	170	18	10	3	4	2	0	18	1.3	200	.03	.11	3.7	3
Chicken potpie—See Poultry potpie																
Chile con carne, canned																
With beans	1 cup	250	335	19	15	7	7	Trace	30	80	4.2	150	.08	.18	3.2	—
Without beans	1 cup	255	510	26	38	18	17	1	15	97	3.6	380	.05	.31	5.6	—
Heart, beef, lean, braised	3 oz.	85	160	27	5	—	—	—	1	5	5.0	20	.21	1.04	6.5	1
Lamb, trimmed to retail basis,[2] cooked																
Chop, thick, with bone, broiled	1 chop, 4.8 oz.	137	400	25	33	18	12	1	0	10	1.5	—	.14	.25	5.6	—
Lean and fat	4.0 oz.	112	400	25	33	18	12	1	0	10	1.5	—	.14	.25	5.6	—
Lean only	2.6 oz.	74	140	21	6	3	2	Trace	0	9	1.5	—	.11	.20	4.5	—
Leg, roasted																
Lean and fat	3 oz.	85	235	22	16	9	6	Trace	0	9	1.4	—	.13	.23	4.7	—
Lean only	2.5 oz.	71	130	20	5	3	2	Trace	0	9	1.4	—	.12	.21	4.4	—
Shoulder, roasted																
Lean and fat	3 oz.	85	285	18	23	13	8	1	0	9	1.0	—	.11	.20	4.0	—
Lean only	2.3 oz.	64	130	17	6	3	2	Trace	0	8	1.0	—	.10	.18	3.7	—
Liver, beef, fried	2 oz.	57	130	15	6	—	—	—	3	6	5.0	30,280	.15	2.37	9.4	15

[2]Outer layer of fat on the cut was removed to within approximately ½ inch of the lean. Deposits of fat within the cut were not removed.

Continued.

Food, approximate measure, and weight (in grams)			Food energy	Protein	Fat (total lipid)	Fatty acids			Carbohydrate	Calcium	Iron	Vitamin A value	Thiamine	Riboflavin	Niacin	Ascorbic acid
						Saturated (total)	Unsaturated Oleic	Unsaturated Linoleic								
		gm.	(Calories)	(gm.)	(gm.)	(gm.)	(gm.)	(gm.)	(gm.)	(mg.)	(mg.)	(I.U.)	(mg.)	(mg.)	(mg.)	(mg.)
Pork, cured, cooked																
Ham, light cure, lean and fat, roasted	3 oz.	85	245	18	19	7	8	2	0	8	2.2	0	.40	.16	3.1	—
Luncheon meat																
Boiled ham, sliced	2 oz.	57	135	11	10	4	4	1	0	6	1.6	0	.25	.09	1.5	—
Canned, spiced or unspiced	2 oz.	57	165	8	14	5	6	1	1	5	1.2	0	.18	.12	1.6	—
Pork, fresh, trimmed to retail basis,[2] cooked																
Chop, thick, with bone	1 chop, 3.5 oz.	98	260	16	21	8	9	2	0	8	2.2	0	.63	.18	3.8	—
Lean and fat	2.3 oz.	66	260	16	21	8	9	2	0	8	2.2	0	.63	.18	3.8	—
Lean only	1.7 oz.	48	130	15	7	2	3	1	0	7	1.9	0	.54	.16	3.3	—
Roast, oven-cooked, no liquid added																
Lean and fat	3 oz.	85	310	21	24	9	10	2	0	9	2.7	0	.78	.22	4.7	—
Lean only	2.4 oz.	68	175	20	10	3	4	1	0	9	2.6	0	.73	.21	4.4	—
Cuts, simmered																
Lean and fat	3 oz.	85	320	20	26	9	11	2	0	8	2.5	0	.46	.21	4.1	—
Lean only	2.2 oz.	63	135	18	6	2	3	1	0	8	2.3	0	.42	.19	3.7	—
Poultry potpie (based on chicken potpie). Individual pie, 4¼-inch diameter, weigh before baking	1 pie	227	535	23	31	10	15	3	42	68	3.0	3,020	.25	.26	4.1	5
Sausage																
Bologna, slice, 4.1 by 0.1 inch	8 slices	227	690	27	62	—	—	—	2	16	4.1	—	.36	.49	6.0	—
Frankfurter, cooked	1	51	155	6	14	—	—	—	1	3	.8	—	.08	.10	1.3	—
Pork, links or patty, cooked	4 oz.	113	540	21	50	18	21	5	Trace	8	2.7	0	.89	.39	4.2	—
Tongue, beef, braised	3 oz.	85	210	18	14	—	—	—	Trace	6	1.9	—	.04	.25	3.0	—
Turkey potpie. See Poultry potpie																
Veal, cooked																
Cutlet, without bone, broiled	3 oz.	85	185	23	9	5	4	Trace	—	9	2.7	—	.06	.21	4.6	—
Roast, medium fat, medium done; lean and fat	3 oz.	85	230	23	14	7	6	Trace	0	10	2.9	—	.11	.26	6.6	—

Fish and shellfish

Food	Measure	Grams	Calories	Protein	Fat	Saturated	Oleic	Linoleic	Carbohydrate	Calcium	Iron	Vitamin A	Thiamine	Riboflavin	Niacin	Ascorbic acid
Bluefish, baked or broiled	3 oz.	85	135	22	4	—	—	—	0	25	.6	40	.09	.08	1.6	—
Clams																
Raw, meat only	3 oz.	85	65	11	1	—	—	—	2	59	5.2	90	.08	.15	1.1	8
Canned, solids and liquid	3 oz.	85	45	7	1	—	—	—	2	47	3.5	—	.01	.09	.9	—
Crabmeat, canned	3 oz.	85	85	15	2	—	—	1	1	38	.7	—	.07	.07	1.6	—
Fish sticks, breaded, cooked, frozen; stick 3.8 by 1.0 by 0.5 inch	10 sticks or 8 oz. package	227	400	38	20	5	4	10	15	25	.9	—	.09	.16	3.6	—
Haddock, fried	3 oz.	85	140	17	5	1	3	—	5	34	1.0	—	0.03	0.06	2.7	2
Mackerel																
Broiled, Atlantic	3 oz.	85	200	19	13	—	—	—	0	5	1.0	450	.13	.23	6.5	—
Canned, Pacific, solids and liquid[3]	3 oz.	85	155	18	9	—	—	—	0	221	1.9	20	.02	.28	7.4	—
Ocean perch, breaded (egg and bread-crumbs), fried	3 oz.	85	195	16	11	—	—	—	6	28	1.1	—	.08	.09	1.5	—
Oysters, meat only. Raw, 13-19 medium selects	1 cup	240	160	20	4	—	—	—	8	226	13.2	740	.33	.43	6.0	—
Oyster stew, 1 part oysters to 3 parts milk by volume, 3-4 oysters	1 cup	230	200	11	12	—	—	—	11	269	3.3	640	.13	.41	1.6	—
Salmon, pink, canned	3 oz.	85	120	17	5	1	1	Trace	0	[4]167	.7	60	.03	.16	6.8	—
Sardines, Atlantic, canned in oil, drained solids	3 oz.	85	175	20	9	—	—	—	0	372	2.5	190	.02	.17	4.6	—
Shad, baked	3 oz.	85	170	20	10	—	—	—	0	20	.5	20	.11	.22	7.3	—
Shrimp, canned, meat only	3 oz.	85	100	21	1	—	—	—	1	98	2.6	50	.01	.03	1.5	—
Swordfish, broiled with butter or margarine	3 oz.	85	150	24	5	—	—	—	0	23	1.1	1,780	.03	.04	9.3	—
Tuna, canned in oil, drained solids	3 oz.	85	170	24	7	—	—	—	0	7	1.6	70	.04	.10	10.1	—

Mature dry beans and peas, nuts, peanuts (related products)

Food	Measure	Grams	Calories	Protein	Fat	Saturated	Oleic	Linoleic	Carbohydrate	Calcium	Iron	Vitamin A	Thiamine	Riboflavin	Niacin	Ascorbic acid
Almonds, shelled	1 cup	142	850	26	77	6	52	15	28	332	6.7	0	.34	1.31	5.0	Trace

[2] Outer layer of fat on the cut was removed to within approximately ½ inch of the lean. Deposits of fat within the cut were not removed.
[3] Vitamin values based on drained solids.
[4] Based on total contents of can. If bones are discarded, value will be greatly reduced.

Continued.

Food, approximate measure, and weight (in grams)			Food energy	Protein	Fat (total lipid)	Fatty acids: Saturated (total)	Fatty acids: Unsaturated: Oleic	Fatty acids: Unsaturated: Linoleic	Carbohydrate	Calcium	Iron	Vitamin A value	Thiamine	Riboflavin	Niacin	Ascorbic acid
		gm.	(Calories)	(gm.)	(gm.)	(gm.)	(gm.)	(gm.)	(gm.)	(mg.)	(mg.)	(I.U.)	(mg.)	(mg.)	(mg.)	(mg.)
Beans, dry																
Common varieties, such as Great Northern, navy, and others, canned:																
Red	1 cup	256	230	15	1	—	—	—	42	74	4.6	Trace	.13	.10	1.5	—
White, with tomato sauce																
With pork	1 cup	261	320	16	7	3	3	1	50	141	4.7	340	.20	.08	1.5	5
Without pork	1 cup	261	310	16	1	—	—	—	60	177	5.2	160	.18	.09	1.5	5
Lima, cooked	1 cup	192	260	16	1	—	—	—	48	56	5.6	Trace	.26	.12	1.3	Trace
Brazil nuts	1 cup	140	915	20	94	19	45	24	15	-260	4.8	Trace	1.34	.17	2.2	—
Cashew nuts, roasted	1 cup	135	760	23	62	10	43	4	40	51	5.1	140	.58	.33	2.4	—
Coconut																
Fresh, shredded	1 cup	97	335	3	34	29	2	Trace	9	13	1.6	0	.05	.02	.5	3
Dried, shredded, sweetened	1 cup	62	340	2	24	21	2	Trace	33	10	1.2	0	.02	.02	.2	0
Cowpeas or blackeye peas, dry, cooked	1 cup	248	190	13	1	—	—	—	34	42	3.2	20	.41	.11	1.1	Trace
Peanuts, roasted, salted																
Halves	1 cup	144	840	37	72	16	31	21	27	107	3.0	—	.46	.19	24.7	0
Chopped	1 tbsp.	9	55	2	4	1	2	1	2	7	.2	—	.03	.01	1.5	0
Peanut butter	1 tbsp.	16	95	4	8	2	4	2	3	9	.3	—	.02	.02	2.4	0
Peas, split, dry, cooked	1 cup	250	290	20	1	—	—	—	52	28	4.2	100	.37	.22	2.2	—
Pecans																
Halves	1 cup	108	740	10	77	5	48	15	16	79	2.6	140	.93	.14	1.0	2
Chopped	1 tbsp.	7.5	50	1	5	Trace	3	1	1	5	.2	10	.06	.01	.1	Trace
Walnuts, shelled																
Black or native, chopped	1 cup	126	790	26	75	4	26	36	19	Trace	7.6	380	.28	.14	.9	—
English or Persian																
Halves	1 cup	100	650	15	64	4	10	40	16	99	3.1	30	.33	.13	.9	3
Chopped	1 tbsp.	8	50	1	5	Trace	1	3	1	8	.2	Trace	.03	.01	.1	Trace
Vegetables and vegetable products																
Asparagus																
Cooked, cut spears	1 cup	175	35	4	Trace	—	—	—	6	37	1.0	1,580	.27	.32	2.4	46
Canned spears, medium																
Green	6 spears	96	20	2	Trace	—	—	—	3	18	1.8	770	.06	.10	.8	14
Bleached	6 spears	96	20	2	Trace	—	—	—	4	15	1.0	80	.05	.06	.7	14

Beans																
Lima, immature, cooked	1 cup	160	180	12	1	—	—	—	32	75	4.0	450	.29	.16	2.0	28
Snap, green																
Cooked																
In small amount of water, short time	1 cup	125	30	2	Trace	—	—	—	7	62	.8	680	.08	.11	.6	16
In large amount of water, long time	1 cup	125	30	2	Trace	—	—	—	7	62	0.8	680	0.07	0.10	0.4	13
Canned																
Solids and liquid	1 cup	239	45	2	Trace	—	—	—	10	81	2.9	690	.08	.10	.7	9
Strained or chopped (baby food)	1 oz.	28	5	Trace	Trace	—	—	—	1	9	.3	110	.01	.02	.1	Trace
Bean sprouts. See Sprouts																
Beets, cooked, diced	1 cup	165	50	2	Trace	—	—	—	12	23	.8	40	.04	.07	.5	11
Broccoli spears, cooked	1 cup	150	40	5	Trace	—	—	—	7	132	1.2	3,750	.14	.29	1.2	135
Brussels sprouts, cooked	1 cup	130	45	5	1	—	—	—	8	42	1.4	680	.10	.18	1.1	113
Cabbage																
Raw																
Finely shredded	1 cup	100	25	1	Trace	—	—	—	5	49	.4	130	.05	.05	.3	47
Coleslaw	1 cup	120	120	1	9	5	2	2	9	52	.5	180	.06	.06	.3	35
Cooked																
In small amount of water, short time	1 cup	170	35	2	Trace	—	—	—	7	75	.5	220	.07	.07	.5	56
In large amount of water, long time	1 cup	170	30	2	Trace	—	—	—	7	71	.5	200	.04	.04	.2	40
Cabbage, celery or Chinese																
Raw, leaves and stalk, 1-inch pieces	1 cup	100	15	1	Trace	—	—	—	3	43	.6	150	.05	.04	.6	25
Cabbage, spoon (or pakchoy), cooked	1 cup	150	20	2	Trace	—	—	—	4	222	.9	4,650	.07	.12	1.1	23
Carrots																
Raw																
Whole, 5½ by 1 inch, (25 thin strips)	1	50	20	1	Trace	—	—	—	5	18	.4	5,500	.03	.03	.3	4
Grated	1 cup	110	45	1	Trace	—	—	—	11	41	.8	12,100	.06	.06	.7	9
Cooked, diced	1 cup	145	45	1	Trace	—	—	—	10	48	.9	15,220	.08	.07	.7	9
Canned, strained or chopped (baby food)	1 oz.	28	10	Trace	Trace	—	—	—	2	7	.1	3,690	.01	.01	.7	1
Cauliflower, cooked, flowerbuds	1 cup	120	25	3	Trace	—	—	—	5	25	.8	70	.11	.10	.7	66

Food, approximate measure, and weight (in grams)		gm.	Food energy	Pro-tein	Fat (total lipid)	Fatty acids Satu-rated (total)	Unsaturated Oleic	Linoleic	Carbo-hydrate	Cal-cium	Iron	Vita-min A value	Thia-mine	Ribo-flavin	Niacin	Ascor-bic acid
		gm.	(Calo-ries)	(gm.)	(gm.)	(gm.)	(gm.)	(gm.)	(gm.)	(mg.)	(mg.)	(I.U.)	(mg.)	(mg.)	(mg.)	(mg.)
Celery, raw																
Stalk, large outer, 8 by about 1½ inches, at root end	1 stalk	40	5	Trace	Trace	—	—	—	2	16	.1	100	.01	.01	.1	4
Pieces, diced	1 cup	100	15	1	Trace	—	—	—	4	39	.3	240	.03	.03	.3	9
Collards, cooked	1 cup	190	55	5	1	—	—	—	9	289	1.1	10,260	.27	.37	2.4	87
Corn, sweet																
Cooked, ear 5 by 1¾ inches[5]	1 ear	140	70	3	1	—	—	—	16	2	.5	[6]310	.09	.08	1.0	7
Canned, solids and liquid	1 cup	256	170	5	2	—	—	—	40	10	1.0	[6]690	.07	.12	2.3	13
Cowpeas, cooked, imma-ture seeds	1 cup	160	175	13	1	—	—	—	29	38	3.4	560	.49	.18	2.3	28
Cucumbers, 10 oz., 7½ by about 2 inches																
Raw, pared	1	207	30	1	Trace	—	—	—	7	35	.6	Trace	.07	.09	.4	23
Raw, pared, center slice ⅛-inch thick	6 slices	50	5	Trace	Trace	—	—	—	2	8	.2	Trace	.02	.02	.1	6
Dandelion greens, cooked	1 cup	180	60	4	1	—	—	—	12	252	3.2	21,060	.24	.29	—	32
Endive, curly (including escarole)	2 oz.	57	10	1	Trace	—	—	—	2	46	1.0	1,870	.04	.08	.3	6
Kale, leaves including stems, cooked	1 cup	110	30	4	1	—	—	—	4	147	1.3	8,140	—	—	—	68
Lettuce, raw																
Butterhead, as Boston types; head, 4-inch diameter	1 head	220	30	3	Trace	—	—	—	6	77	4.4	2,130	.14	.13	.6	18
Crisphead, as Iceberg; head, 4¾-inch diameter	1 head	454	60	4	Trace	—	—	—	13	91	2.3	1,500	.29	.27	1.3	29
Looseleaf, or bunching varieties, leaves	2 large	50	10	1	Trace	—	—	—	2	34	.7	950	.03	.04	.2	9
Mushrooms, canned, solids and liquid	1 cup	244	40	5	Trace	—	—	—	6	15	1.2	Trace	.04	.60	4.8	4
Mustard greens, cooked	1 cup	140	35	3	1	—	—	—	6	193	2.5	8,120	.11	.19	.9	68
Okra, cooked, pod 3 by ⅝ inch	8 pods	85	25	3	Trace	—	—	—	5	78	.4	420	.11	.15	.8	17

Food	Measure	Grams	Food energy	Protein	Fat	Saturated	Oleic	Linoleic	Carbohydrate	Calcium	Iron	Vit. A	Thiamine	Riboflavin	Niacin	Ascorbic acid
Onions																
Mature																
Raw, onion 2½-inch diameter	1	110	40	2	Trace	—	—	—	10	30	0.6	40	0.04	0.04	0.2	11
Cooked	1 cup	210	60	3	Trace	—	—	—	14	50	.8	80	.06	.06	.4	14
Young green, small, without tops	6	50	20	1	Trace	—	—	—	5	20	.3	Trace	.02	.02	.2	12
Parsley, raw, chopped	1 tbsp.	3.5	1	Trace	Trace	—	—	—	Trace	7	.2	300	Trace	.01	Trace	6
Parsnips, cooked	1 cup	155	100	2	1	—	—	—	23	70	.9	50	.11	.13	.2	16
Peas, green																
Cooked	1 cup	160	115	9	1	—	—	—	19	37	2.9	860	.44	.17	3.7	33
Canned, solids and liquid	1 cup	249	165	9	1	—	—	—	31	50	4.2	1,120	.23	.13	2.2	22
Canned, strained (baby food)	1 oz.	28	15	1	Trace	—	—	—	3	3	.4	140	.02	.02	.4	3
Peppers, hot, red, without seeds, dried (ground chili powder, added seasonings)	1 tbsp.	15	50	2	2	—	—	—	8	40	2.3	9,750	.03	.17	1.3	2
Peppers, sweet																
Raw, medium, about 6 per pound																
Green pod without stem and seeds	1 pod	62	15	1	Trace	—	—	—	3	6	.4	260	.05	.05	.3	79
Red pod without stem and seeds	1 pod	60	20	1	Trace	—	—	—	4	8	.4	2,670	.05	.05	.3	122
Canned, pimentos, medium	1 pod	38	10	Trace	Trace	—	—	—	2	3	.6	870	.01	.02	.1	36
Potatoes, medium (about 3 per pound raw)																
Baked, peeled after baking	1	99	90	3	Trace	—	—	—	21	9	.7	Trace	.10	.04	1.7	20
Boiled																
Peeled after boiling	1	136	105	3	Trace	—	—	—	23	10	.8	Trace	.13	.05	2.0	22
Peeled before boiling	1	122	80	2	Trace	—	—	—	18	7	.6	Trace	.11	.04	1.4	20
French-fried, piece 2 by ½ by ½ inch																
Cooked in deep fat	10 pieces	57	155	2	7	2	2	4	20	9	.7	Trace	.07	.04	1.8	12
Frozen, heated	10 pieces	57	125	2	5	1	1	2	19	5	1.0	Trace	.08	.01	1.5	12
Mashed																
Milk added	1 cup	195	125	4	1	—	—	—	25	47	.8	50	.16	.10	2.0	19
Milk and butter added	1 cup	195	185	4	8	4	3	Trace	24	47	.8	330	.16	.10	1.9	18

[5] Measure and weight apply to entire vegetable or fruit including parts not usually eaten.
[6] Based on yellow varieties; white varieties contain only a trace of cryptoxanthin and carotenes, the pigments in corn that have biological activity.

Continued.

783

Food, approximate measure, and weight (in grams)		gm.	Food energy (Calories)	Protein (gm.)	Fat (total lipid) (gm.)	Fatty acids Saturated (total) (gm.)	Fatty acids Unsaturated Oleic (gm.)	Fatty acids Unsaturated Linoleic (gm.)	Carbohydrate (gm.)	Calcium (mg.)	Iron (mg.)	Vitamin A value (I.U.)	Thiamine (mg.)	Riboflavin (mg.)	Niacin (mg.)	Ascorbic acid (mg.)
Potato chips, medium, 2-inch diameter	10 chips	20	115	1	8	3	2	4	10	8	.4	Trace	.04	.01	1.0	3
Pumpkin, canned	1 cup	228	75	2	1	—	—	—	18	57	.9	14,590	.07	.12	1.3	12
Radishes, raw, small, without tops	4	40	5	Trace	Trace	—	—	—	1	12	.4	Trace	.01	.01	.1	10
Sauerkraut, canned, solids and liquid	1 cup	235	45	2	Trace	—	—	—	9	85	1.2	120	.07	.09	.4	33
Spinach																
Cooked	1 cup	180	40	5	1	—	—	—	6	167	4.0	14,580	.13	.25	1.0	50
Canned, drained solids	1 cup	180	45	5	1	—	—	—	6	212	4.7	14,400	.03	.21	.6	24
Canned, strained or chopped (baby food)	1 oz.	28	10	1	Trace	—	—	—	2	18	.2	1,420	.01	.04	.1	2
Sprouts, raw																
Mung bean	1 cup	90	30	3	Trace	—	—	—	6	17	1.2	20	.12	.12	.7	17
Soybean	1 cup	107	40	6	2	—	—	—	4	46	.7	90	.17	.16	.8	4
Squash																
Cooked																
Summer, diced	1 cup	210	30	2	Trace	—	—	—	7	52	.8	820	.10	.16	1.6	21
Winter, baked, mashed	1 cup	205	130	4	1	—	—	—	32	57	1.6	8,610	.10	.27	1.4	27
Canned, winter, strained and chopped (baby food)	1 oz.	28	10	Trace	Trace	—	—	—	2	7	.1	510	.01	.01	.1	1
Sweetpotatoes																
Cooked, medium, 5 by 2 inches, weight raw about 6 oz.																
Baked, peeled after baking	1	110	155	2	1	—	—	—	36	44	1.0	8,910	.10	.07	.7	24
Boiled, peeled after boiling	1	147	170	2	1	—	—	—	39	47	1.0	11,610	.13	.09	.9	25
Candied, 3½ by 2¼ inches	1	175	295	2	6	2	3	1	60	65	1.6	11,030	.10	.08	.8	17
Canned, vacuum or solid pack	1 cup	218	235	4	Trace	—	—	—	54	54	1.7	17,000	.10	.10	1.4	30

Food	Measure	Grams	Calories	Protein	Fat	Saturated	Oleic	Linoleic	Carbohydrate	Calcium	Iron	Vitamin A	Thiamine	Riboflavin	Niacin	Ascorbic acid
Tomatoes																
Raw, medium, 2 by 2½ inches, about 3 per pound	1	150	35	2	Trace	—	—	—	7	20	.8	1,350	.10	.06	1.0	⁷34
Canned	1 cup	242	50	2	Trace	—	—	—	10	15	1.2	2,180	.13	.07	1.7	40
Tomato juice, canned	1 cup	242	45	2	Trace	—	—	—	10	17	2.2	1,940	.13	.07	1.8	39
Tomato catsup	1 tbsp.	17	15	Trace	Trace	—	—	—	4	4	.1	240	.02	.01	.3	3
Turnips, cooked, diced	1 cup	155	35	1	Trace	—	—	—	8	54	.6	Trace	.06	.08	.5	33
Turnip greens																
Cooked																
In small amount of water, short time	1 cup	145	30	3	Trace	—	—	—	5	267	1.6	9,140	.21	.36	.8	100
In large amount of water, long time	1 cup	145	25	3	Trace	—	—	—	5	252	1.4	8,260	.14	.33	.8	68
Canned, solids and liquid	1 cup	232	40	3	1	—	—	—	7	232	3.7	10,900	.04	.21	1.4	44
Fruits and fruit products																
Apples, raw, medium, 2½-inch diameter, about 3 per pound⁵	1	150	70	Trace	Trace	—	—	—	18	8	.4	50	.04	.02	.1	3
Apple brown betty	1 cup	230	345	4	8	4	3	Trace	68	41	1.4	230	.13	.10	.9	3
Apple juice, bottled or canned	1 cup	249	120	Trace	Trace	—	—	—	30	15	1.5	—	.01	.04	.2	2
Applesauce, canned																
Sweetened	1 cup	254	230	1	Trace	—	—	—	60	10	1.3	100	.05	.03	.1	3
Unsweetened or artificially sweetened	1 cup	239	100	Trace	Trace	—	—	—	26	10	1.2	100	.04	.02	.1	2
Applesauce and apricots, canned, strained or junior (baby food)	1 oz.	28	25	Trace	Trace	—	—	—	6	1	.1	170	Trace	Trace	Trace	1
Apricots																
Raw, about 12 per pound⁵	3 apricots	114	55	1	Trace	—	—	—	14	18	.5	2,890	.03	.04	.7	10
Canned in heavy syrup																
Halves and syrup	1 cup	259	220	2	Trace	—	—	—	57	28	.8	4,510	.05	.06	.9	10
Halves (medium) and syrup	4 halves; 2 tbsp. syrup	122	105	1	Trace	—	—	—	27	13	.4	2,120	.02	.03	.4	5

⁵Measure and weight apply to entire vegetable or fruit including parts not usually eaten.

⁷Year-round average. Samples marketed from November through May average around 15 milligrams per 150-gram tomato; from June through October, around 39 milligrams.

Food, approximate measure, and weight (in grams)	gm.	Food energy	Pro-tein	Fat (total lipid)	Fatty acids Satu-rated (total)	Unsaturated Oleic	Linoleic	Carbo-hydrate	Cal-cium	Iron	Vita-min A value	Thia-mine	Ribo-flavin	Niacin	Ascor-bic acid
	gm.	(Calo-ries)	(gm.)	(gm.)	(gm.)	(gm.)	(gm.)	(gm.)	(mg.)	(mg.)	(I.U.)	(mg.)	(mg.)	(mg.)	(mg.)
Apricots—cont'd															
Dried															
Uncooked, 40 halves, small, 1 cup	150	390	8	1	—	—	—	100	100	8.2	16,350	.02	.23	4.9	19
Cooked, unsweetened, fruit and liquid, 1 cup	285	240	5	1	—	—	—	62	63	5.1	8,550	.01	.13	2.8	8
Apricot nectar, canned, 1 cup	250	140	1	Trace	—	—	—	36	22	.5	2,380	.02	.02	.5	7
Avocados, raw															
California varieties, mainly Fuerte															
10-ounce avocado, about 3½ by 4¼ inches, peeled, pitted, ½	108	185	2	18	4	8	2	6	11	.6	310	.12	.21	1.7	15
½-inch cubes, 1 cup	152	260	3	26	5	12	3	9	15	.9	440	.16	.30	2.4	21
Florida varieties															
13 oz. avocado, about 4 by 3 inches, peeled, pitted, ½	123	160	2	14	3	6	2	11	12	.7	360	.13	.24	2.0	17
½-inch cubes, 1 cup	152	195	2	17	3	8	2	13	15	.9	440	.16	.30	2.4	21
Bananas, raw, 6 by 1½ inches, about 3 per pound[5], 1	150	85	1	Trace	—	—	—	23	8	.7	190	.05	.06	.7	10
Blackberries, raw, 1 cup	144	85	2	1	—	—	—	19	46	1.3	290	.05	.06	.5	30
Blueberries, raw, 1 cup	140	85	1	1	—	—	—	21	21	1.4	140	.04	.08	.6	20
Cantaloups, raw; medium, 5-inch diameter, about 1⅔ pounds[5], ½	385	60	1	Trace	—	—	—	14	27	.8	[8] 6,540	.08	.06	1.2	63
Cherries															
Raw, sweet, with stems[5], 1 cup	130	80	2	Trace	—	—	—	20	26	.5	130	.06	.07	.5	12
Canned, red, sour, pitted, heavy syrup, 1 cup	260	230	2	1	—	—	—	59	36	.8	1,680	.07	.06	.4	13
Cranberry juice cocktail, canned, 1 cup	250	160	Trace	Trace	—	—	—	41	12	.8	Trace	.02	.02	.1	(9)

Food	Measure	Weight (g)	Food energy (cal.)	Protein (g)	Fat (g)				Carbohydrate (g)	Calcium (mg)	Iron (mg)	Vitamin A (I.U.)	Thiamine (mg)	Riboflavin (mg)	Niacin (mg)	Ascorbic acid (mg)
Cranberry sauce, sweetened, canned, strained	1 cup	277	405	Trace	1	—	—	—	104	17	.6	40	.03	0.3	.1	5
Dates, domestic, natural and dry, pitted, cut	1 cup	178	490	4	1	—	—	—	130	105	5.3	90	.16	.17	3.9	0
Figs																
Raw, small, 1½-inch diameter, about 12 per pound	3 figs	114	90	1	Trace	—	—	—	23	40	.7	90	.07	.06	.5	2
Dried, large, 2 by 1 inch[5]	1 fig	21	60	1	Trace	—	—	—	15	26	.6	20	.02	.02	.1	0
Fruit cocktail, canned in heavy syrup, solids and liquid	1 cup	256	195	1	1	—	—	—	50	23	1.0	360	.04	.03	1.1	5
Grapefruit																
Raw, medium, 4¼-inch diameter, size 64																
White[5]	½	285	55	1	Trace	—	—	—	14	22	.6	10	.05	.02	.2	52
Pink or red[5]	½	285	60	1	Trace	—	—	—	15	23	.6	640	.05	.02	.3	52
Raw sections, white	1 cup	194	75	1	Trace	—	—	—	20	31	.8	20	.07	.03	.3	72
Canned, white																
Syrup pack, solids and liquid	1 cup	249	175	1	Trace	—	—	—	44	32	.7	20	.07	.04	.5	75
Water pack, solids and liquid	1 cup	240	70	1	Trace	—	—	—	18	31	.7	20	.07	.04	.5	72
Grapefruit juice																
Fresh	1 cup	246	95	1	Trace	—	—	—	23	22	.5	([10])	.09	.04	.4	92
Canned, white																
Unsweetened	1 cup	247	100	1	Trace	—	—	—	24	20	1.0	20	.07	.04	.4	84
Sweetened	1 cup	250	130	1	Trace	—	—	—	32	20	1.0	20	.07	.04	.4	78
Frozen, concentrate, unsweetened																
Undiluted, can, 6 fluid oz.	1 can	207	300	4	1	—	—	—	72	70	.8	60	.29	.12	1.4	286
Diluted with 3 parts water, by volume	1 cup	247	100	1	Trace	—	—	—	24	25	.2	20	.10	.04	.5	96
Frozen, concentrate, sweetened																
Undiluted, can, 6 fluid oz.	1 can	211	350	3	1	—	—	—	85	59	.6	50	.24	.11	1.2	245
Diluted with 3 parts water, by volume	1 cup	249	115	1	Trace	—	—	—	28	20	.2	20	.08	.03	.4	82

Continued.

[5] Measure and weight apply to entire vegetable or fruit including parts not usually eaten.
[8] Value based on varieties with orange-colored flesh; for green-fleshed varieties value is about 540 I.U. per ½ melon.
[9] About 5 milligrams per 8 fluid ounces is from cranberries. Ascorbic acid is usually added to approximately 100 milligrams per 8 fluid ounces.
[10] For white-fleshed varieties value is about 20 I.U. per cup; for red-fleshed varieties, 1,080 I.U. per cup.

Food, approximate measure, and weight (in grams)		gm.	Food energy	Protein	Fat (total lipid)	Fatty acids			Carbohydrate	Calcium	Iron	Vitamin A value	Thiamine	Riboflavin	Niacin	Ascorbic acid
						Saturated (total)	Unsaturated Oleic	Unsaturated Linoleic								
			(Calories)	(gm.)	(gm.)	(gm.)	(gm.)	(gm.)	(gm.)	(mg.)	(mg.)	(I.U.)	(mg.)	(mg.)	(mg.)	(mg.)
Grapefruit juice—cont'd																
Dehydrated																
Crystals, can, net weight 4 oz.	1 can	114	430	5	1	—	—	—	103	99	1.1	90	.41	.18	2.0	399
Prepared with water (1 pound yields about 1 gal.)	1 cup	247	100	1	Trace	—	—	—	24	22	.2	20	.10	.05	.5	92
Grapes, raw																
American type (slip skin), such as Concord, Delaware, Niagara, Catawba, and Scuppernong[5]	1 cup	153	65	1	1	—	—	—	15	15	.4	100	.05	.03	.2	3
European type (adherent skin), such as Malaga, Muscat, Thompson Seedless, Emperor, and Flame Tokay[5]	1 cup	160	95	1	Trace	—	—	—	25	17	.6	140	.07	.04	.4	6
Grape juice, bottled or canned	1 cup	254	165	1	Trace	—	—	—	42	28	.8	—	.10	.05	.6	Trace
Lemons, raw, medium, 2½-inch diameter, size 150[5]	1 lemon	106	20	1	Trace	—	—	—	6	18	.4	10	.03	.01	.1	38
Lemon juice																
Fresh	1 cup	246	60	1	Trace	—	—	—	20	17	.5	40	.08	.03	.2	113
	1 tbsp.	15	5	Trace	Trace	—	—	—	1	1	Trace	Trace	Trace	Trace	Trace	7
Canned, unsweetened	1 cup	245	55	1	Trace	—	—	—	19	17	.5	40	.07	.03	.2	102
Lemonade concentrate, frozen, sweetened																
Undiluted, can, 6 fluid oz.	1 can	220	430	Trace	Trace	—	—	—	112	9	.4	40	.05	.06	.7	66
Diluted with 4½ parts water, by volume	1 cup	248	110	Trace	Trace	—	—	—	28	2	.1	10	.01	.01	.2	17
Lime juice																
Fresh	1 cup	246	65	1	Trace	—	—	—	22	22	.5	30	.05	.03	.03	80
Canned	1 cup	246	65	1	Trace	—	—	—	22	22	.5	30	.05	.03	.3	52

Food	Measure															
Limeade concentrate, frozen, sweetened																
Undiluted, can, 6 fluid oz.	1 can	218	410	Trace	Trace	—	—	—	108	11	.2	Trace	.02	.02	.3	26
Diluted with 4⅓ parts water, by volume	1 cup	248	105	Trace	Trace	—	—	—	27	2	Trace	Trace	Trace	Trace	Trace	6
Oranges, raw																
California, Navel (winter), 2⅘-inch diameter, size 88[5]	1 orange	180	60	2	Trace	—	—	—	16	49	.5	240	.12	.05	.5	75
Florida, all varieties, 3-inch diameter[5]	1	210	75	1	Trace	—	—	—	19	67	.3	310	.16	.06	.6	70
Orange juice																
Fresh																
California, Valencia (summer)	1 cup	249	115	2	1	—	—	—	26	27	.7	500	.22	.06	.9	122
Florida varieties																
Early and mid-season	1 cup	247	100	1	Trace	—	—	—	23	25	.5	490	.22	.06	.9	127
Late season, Valencia	1 cup	248	110	1	Trace	—	—	—	26	25	.5	500	.22	.06	.9	92
Canned, unsweetened	1 cup	249	120	2	Trace	—	—	—	28	25	1.0	500	.17	.05	.6	100
Frozen concentrate																
Undiluted, can, 6 fluid oz.	1 can	210	330	5	Trace	—	—	—	80	69	.8	1,490	.63	.10	2.4	332
Diluted with 3 parts water, by volume	1 cup	248	110	2	Trace	—	—	—	27	22	.2	500	.21	.03	.8	112
Dehydrated																
Crystals, can, net weight 4 oz.	1 can	113	430	6	2	—	—	—	100	95	1.9	1,900	.76	.24	3.3	406
Prepared with water, 1 lb. yields about 1 gal.	1 cup	248	115	1	Trace	—	—	—	27	25	.5	500	.20	.06	.9	108
Orange and grapefruit juice																
Frozen concentrate																
Undiluted, can, 6 fluid oz.	1 can	209	325	4	1	—	—	—	78	61	.8	790	.47	.06	2.3	301
Diluted with 3 parts water, by volume	1 cup	248	110	1	Trace	—	—	—	26	20	.3	270	.16	.02	.8	102
Papayas, raw, ½-inch cubes	1 cup	182	70	1	Trace	—	—	—	18	36	.5	3,190	.07	.08	.5	102

[5]Measure and weight apply to entire vegetable or fruit including parts not usually eaten.

Continued.

789

Food, approximate measure, and weight (in grams)	gm.	Food energy (Calories)	Protein (gm.)	Fat (total lipid) (gm.)	Fatty acids Saturated (total) (gm.)	Fatty acids Unsaturated Oleic (gm.)	Fatty acids Unsaturated Linoleic (gm.)	Carbohydrate (gm.)	Calcium (mg.)	Iron (mg.)	Vitamin A value (I.U.)	Thiamine (mg.)	Riboflavin (mg.)	Niacin (mg.)	Ascorbic acid (mg.)
Peaches															
Raw															
Whole, medium, 2-inch diameter, about 4 per pound[5]	114	35	1	Trace	—	—	—	10	9	.5	[11]1,320	.02	.05	1.0	7
Sliced	1 cup 168	65	1	Trace	—	—	—	16	15	.8	[11]2,230	.03	.08	1.6	12
Canned, yellow-fleshed, solids and liquid															
Syrup pack, heavy															
Halves or slices	1 cup 257	200	1	Trace	—	—	—	52	10	.8	1,100	.02	.06	1.4	7
Halves (medium) and syrup	2 halves and 2 tbsp. syrup 117	90	Trace	Trace	—	—	—	24	5	.4	500	.01	.03	.7	3
Water pack	1 cup 245	75	1	Trace	—	—	—	20	10	.7	1,100	.02	.06	1.4	7
Strained or chopped (baby food)	1 oz. 28	25	Trace	Trace	—	—	—	6	2	.1	140	Trace	.01	.2	1
Dried															
Uncooked	1 cup 160	420	5	1	—	—	—	109	77	9.6	6,240	.02	.31	8.5	28
Cooked, unsweetened, 10-12 halves and 6 tbsp. liquid	1 cup 270	220	3	1	—	—	—	58	41	5.1	3,290	.01	.15	4.2	6
Frozen															
Carton, 12 oz., not thawed	1 carton 340	300	1	Trace	—	—	—	77	14	1.7	2,210	.03	.14	2.4	[12]135
Can, 16 oz., not thawed	1 can 454	400	2	Trace	—	—	—	103	18	2.3	2,950	.05	.18	3.2	[12]181
Peach nectar, canned	1 cup 250	120	Trace	Trace	—	—	—	31	10	.5	1,080	.02	.05	1.0	1
Pears															
Raw, 3 by 2½-inch diameter[5]	182	100	1	1	—	—	—	25	13	.5	30	.04	.07	.2	7
Canned, solids and liquid															
Syrup pack, heavy															
Halves or slices	1 cup 255	195	1	Trace	—	—	—	50	13	.5	Trace	.03	.05	.3	4
Halves (medium) and syrup	2 halves and 2 tbsp. syrup 117	90	Trace	Trace	—	—	—	23	6	.2	Trace	.01	.02	.2	2

Food	Measure	Weight (g)	Food energy	Protein	Fat			Carbohydrate	Calcium	Iron	Vitamin A	Thiamine	Riboflavin	Niacin	Ascorbic acid
Water pack	1 cup	243	80	Trace	Trace	—	—	20	12	.5	Trace	.02	.05	.3	4
Strained or chopped (baby food)	1 oz.	28	20	Trace	Trace	—	—	5	2	.1	10	Trace	.01	.1	1
Pear nectar, canned	1 cup	250	130	1	Trace	—	—	33	8	.2	Trace	.01	.05	Trace	1
Persimmons, Japanese or kaki, raw, seedless, 2½-inch diameter[5]	1	125	75	1	Trace	—	—	20	6	.4	2,740	.01	.02	.1	11
Pineapple															
Raw, diced	1 cup	140	75	1	Trace	—	—	19	24	.7	100	.12	.04	.3	24
Canned, heavy syrup pack, solids and liquid															
Crushed	1 cup	260	195	1	Trace	—	—	50	29	.8	120	.20	.06	.5	17
Sliced, slices and juice	2 small or 1 large and 2 tbsp. juice	122	90	Trace	Trace	—	—	24	13	.4	50	.09	.03	.2	8
Pineapple juice, canned	1 cup	249	135	1	Trace	—	—	34	37	.7	120	.12	.04	.5	22
Plums, all except prunes															
Raw, 2-inch diameter, about 2 ounces[5]	1	60	25	Trace	Trace	—	—	7	7	.3	140	.02	.02	.3	3
Canned, syrup pack (Italian prunes)															
Plums (with pits) and juice[5]	1 cup	256	205	1	Trace	—	—	53	22	2.2	2,970	.05	.05	.9	4
Plums (without pits) and juice	3 plums and 2 tbsp. juice	122	100	Trace	Trace	—	—	26	11	1.1	1,470	.03	.02	.5	2
Prunes, dried, "softenized," medium															
Uncooked[5]	4	32	70	1	Trace	—	—	18	14	1.1	440	.02	.04	.4	1
Cooked, unsweetened, 17-18 prunes and ⅓ cup liquid[5]	1 cup	270	295	2	1	—	—	78	60	4.5	1,860	.08	.18	1.7	2
Prunes with tapioca, canned, strained or junior (baby food)	1 oz.	28	25	Trace	Trace	—	—	6	2	.3	110	.01	.02	.1	1
Prune juice, canned	1 cup	256	200	1	Trace	—	—	49	36	10.5	—	.02	.03	1.1	4
Raisin, dried	1 cup	160	460	4	Trace	—	—	124	99	5.6	30	.18	.13	.9	2

[5]Measure and weight apply to entire vegetable or fruit including parts not usually eaten.

[11]Based on yellow-fleshed varieties; for white-fleshed varieties value is about 50 I.U. per 114-gram peach and 80 I.U. per cup of sliced peaches.

[12]Average weighted in accordance with commercial freezing practices. For products without added ascorbic acid, value is about 37 milligrams per 12-ounce carton and 50 milligrams per 16-ounce can; for those with added ascorbic acid, value is about 139 milligrams per 12 ounces and 186 milligrams per 16 ounces.

Continued.

Food, approximate measure, and weight (in grams)		weight (gm.)	Food energy (Calories)	Protein (gm.)	Fat (total lipid) (gm.)	Fatty acids Saturated (total) (gm.)	Unsaturated Oleic (gm.)	Unsaturated Linoleic (gm.)	Carbohydrate (gm.)	Calcium (mg.)	Iron (mg.)	Vitamin A value (I.U.)	Thiamine (mg.)	Riboflavin (mg.)	Niacin (mg.)	Ascorbic acid (mg.)
Raspberries, red																
Raw	1 cup	123	70	1	1	—	—	—	17	27	1.1	160	.04	.11	1.1	31
Frozen, 10 oz. carton, not thawed	1 carton	284	275	2	1	—	—	—	70	37	1.7	200	.06	.17	1.7	59
Rhubarb, cooked, sugar added	1 cup	272	385	1	Trace	—	—	—	98	212	1.6	220	.06	.15	.7	17
Strawberries																
Raw, capped	1 cup	149	55	1	1	—	—	—	13	31	1.5	90	.04	.10	1.0	88
Frozen, 10-oz. carton, not thawed	1 carton	284	310	1	1	—	—	—	79	40	2.0	90	.06	.17	1.5	150
Frozen, 16-ounce can, not thawed	1 can	454	495	2	1	—	—	—	126	64	3.2	150	.09	.27	2.4	240
Tangerines, raw, medium, 2½-inch diameter, about 4 per pound[5]	1	114	40	1	Trace	—	—	—	10	34	.3	350	.05	.02	.1	26
Tangerine juice																
Canned, unsweetened	1 cup	248	105	1	Trace	—	—	—	25	45	.5	1,040	.14	.04	.3	56
Frozen concentrate Undiluted, can, 6 fluid oz.	1 can	210	340	4	1	—	—	—	80	130	1.5	3,070	.43	.12	.9	202
Diluted with 3 parts water, by volume	1 cup	248	115	1	Trace	—	—	—	27	45	.5	1,020	.14	.04	.3	67
Watermelon, raw, wedge, 4 by 8 inches (1/16 of 10 by 16-inch melon, about 2 pounds with rind)[5]	1 wedge	925	115	2	1	—	—	—	27	30	2.1	2,510	.13	.13	.7	30
Barley, pearled, light, uncooked	1 cup	203	710	17	2	Trace	1	1	160	32	4.1	0	.25	.17	6.3	0
Biscuits, baking powder with enriched flour, 2½-inch diameter	1	38	140	3	6	2	3	1	17	46	.6	Trace	.08	.08	.7	Trace
Bran flakes (40 percent bran) added thiamine	1 oz.	28	85	3	1	—	—	—	23	20	1.2	0	.11	.05	1.7	0

Food	Measure															
Bread																
Boston brown bread, slice, 3 by ¾ inch	1 slice	48	100	3	1	—	—	—	22	43	.9	0	.05	.03	.6	0
Cracked-wheat bread																
Loaf, 1-pound, 20 slices	1 loaf	454	1,190	39	10	2	5	2	236	399	5.0	Trace	.53	.42	5.8	Trace
Slice	1	23	60	2	1	—	—	—	12	20	.3	Trace	.03	.02	.3	Trace
French or Vienna bread																
Enriched, 1-pound loaf	1 loaf	454	1,315	41	14	3	8	2	251	195	10.0	Trace	1.26	.98	11.3	Trace
Unenriched, 1-pound loaf	1 loaf	454	1,315	41	14	3	8	2	251	195	3.2	Trace	.39	.39	3.6	Trace
Italian bread																
Enriched, 1-pound loaf	1 loaf	454	1,250	41	4	Trace	1	2	256	77	10.0	0	1.31	.93	11.7	0
Unenriched, 1-pound loaf	1 loaf	454	1,250	41	4	Trace	1	2	256	77	3.2	0	.39	.27	3.6	0
Raisin bread																
Loaf, 1-pound, 20 slices	1 loaf	454	1,190	30	13	3	8	2	243	322	5.9	Trace	.24	.42	3.0	Trace
Slice	1	23	60	2	1	—	—	—	12	16	.3	Trace	.01	.02	.2	Trace
Rye bread																
American, light (⅓ rye, ⅔ wheat)																
Loaf, 1-pound, 20 slices	1 loaf	454	1,100	41	5	—	—	—	236	340	7.3	0	.81	.33	6.4	0
Slice	1	23	55	2	Trace	—	—	—	12	17	.4	0	.04	.02	.3	0
Pumpernickel, loaf, 1 pound	1 loaf	454	1,115	41	5	—	—	—	241	381	10.9	0	1.05	.63	5.4	0
White bread, enriched																
1 to 2 percent nonfat dry milk																
Loaf, 1-pound, 20 slices	1 loaf	454	1,225	39	15	3	8	2	229	318	10.9	Trace	1.13	.77	10.4	Trace
Slice	1 slice	23	60	2	1	Trace	Trace	Trace	12	16	.6	Trace	.06	.04	.5	Trace
3 to 4 percent nonfat dry milk[13]																
Loaf, 1-pound	1	454	1,225	39	15	3	8	2	229	381	11.3	Trace	1.13	.95	10.8	Trace
Slice, 20 per loaf	1	23	60	2	1	Trace	Trace	Trace	12	19	.6	Trace	.06	.05	.6	Trace
Slice, toasted	1	20	60	2	1	Trace	Trace	Trace	12	19	.6	Trace	.05	.05	.6	Trace
Slice, 26 per loaf	1	17	45	1	1	Trace	Trace	Trace	9	14	.4	Trace	.04	.04	.4	Trace

[5]Measure and weight apply to entire vegetable or fruit including parts not usually eaten.
[13]When the amount of nonfat dry milk in commercial white bread is unknown, values for bread with 3 to 4% nonfat dry milk are suggested.

Food, approximate measure, and weight (in grams)		gm.	Food energy	Pro-tein	Fat (total lipid)	Fatty acids			Carbo-hydrate	Cal-cium	Iron	Vita-min A value	Thia-mine	Ribo-flavin	Niacin	Ascor-bic acid
						Satu-rated (total)	Unsaturated Oleic	Unsaturated Linoleic								
		(gm.)	(Calo-ries)	(gm.)	(gm.)	(gm.)	(gm.)	(gm.)	(gm.)	(mg.)	(mg.)	(I.U.)	(mg.)	(mg.)	(mg.)	(mg.)
Bread—cont'd																
White bread, enriched—cont'd																
5 to 6 percent nonfat dry milk																
Loaf, 1-pound, 20 slices	1 loaf	454	1,245	41	17	4	10	2	228	435	11.3	Trace	1.22	.91	11.0	Trace
Slice	1	23	65	2	1	Trace	Trace	Trace	12	22	.6	Trace	.06	.05	.6	Trace
White bread, unenriched																
1 to 2 percent nonfat dry milk																
Loaf, 1-pound, 20 slices	1 loaf	454	1,225	39	15	3	8	2	229	318	3.2	Trace	.40	.36	5.6	Trace
Slice	1	23	60	2	1	Trace	Trace	Trace	12	16	.2	Trace	.02	.02	.3	Trace
3 to 4 percent nonfat dry milk[13]																
Loaf, 1-pound	1 loaf	454	1,225	39	15	3	8	—	229	381	3.2	Trace	.31	.39	5.0	Trace
Slice, 20 per loaf	1 slice	23	60	2	1	Trace	Trace	Trace	12	19	.2	Trace	.02	.02	.3	Trace
Slice, toasted	1 slice	20	60	2	1	Trace	Trace	Trace	12	19	.2	Trace	.01	.02	.3	Trace
Slice, 26 per loaf	1 slice	17	45	1	1	Trace	Trace	Trace	9	14	.1	Trace	.01	.01	.2	Trace
5 to 6 percent nonfat dry milk																
Loaf, 1-pound, 20 slices	1 loaf	454	1,245	41	17	4	10	2	228	435	3.2	Trace	.32	.39	4.1	Trace
Slice	1	23	65	2	1	Trace	Trace	Trace	12	22	.2	Trace	.02	.03	.2	Trace
Whole-wheat bread, made with 2 percent nonfat dry milk																
Loaf, 1-pound, 20 slices	1 loaf	454	1,105	48	14	3	6	3	216	449	10.4	Trace	1.17	.56	12.9	Trace
Slice	1	23	55	2	1	Trace	Trace	Trace	11	23	.5	Trace	.06	.03	.7	Trace
Slice, toasted	1	19	55	2	1	Trace	Trace	Trace	11	22	.5	Trace	.05	.03	.6	Trace
Breadcrumbs, dry, grated	1 cup	88	345	11	4	1	2	1	65	107	3.2	Trace	.19	.26	3.1	Trace
Cakes[14]																
Angelfood cake; sector, 2-inch (1/12 of 8-inch-diameter cake)	1 sector	40	110	3	Trace	—	—	—	24	4	.1	0	Trace	.06	.1	0
Chocolate cake, choco-late icing; sector, 2-inch (1/16 of 10-inch-diameter layer cake)	1 sector	120	445	5	20	8	10	1	67	84	1.2	190[15]	.03	.12	.3	Trace

Food	Measure															
Fruitcake, dark (made with enriched flour); piece, 2 by 2 by 1/2 inch	1 piece	30	115	1	5	1	3	1	18	22	.8	[15]40	.04	.04	.2	Trace
Gingerbread (made with enriched flour); piece, 2 by 2 by 2 inches	1 piece	55	175	2	6	1	4	Trace	29	37	1.3	50	.06	.06	.5	0
Plain cake and cupcakes, without icing Piece, 3 by 2 by 1½ inches	1	55	200	2	8	2	5	1	31	35	.2	[15]90	.01	.05	.1	Trace
Cupcake, 2¾-inch diameter		40	145	2	6	1	3	Trace	22	26	.2	[15]70	.01	.03	.1	Trace
Plain cake and cupcakes, with chocolate icing Sector, 2-inch (1/16 of 10-inch-layer cake)	1	100	370	4	14	5	7	1	59	63	.6	[15]180	.02	.09	.2	Trace
Cupcake, 2¾-inch diameter	1	50	185	2	7	2	4	Trace	30	32	.3	[15]90	.01	.04	.1	Trace
Poundcake, old-fashioned (equal weights flour, sugar, fat, eggs); slice, 2¾ by 3 by 5/8 inch	1 slice	30	140	2	9	2	5	1	14	6	.2	[15]80	.01	.03	.1	0
Sponge cake; sector, 2-inch (1/12 of 8-inch-diameter cake)	1	40	120	3	2	1	1	Trace	22	12	.5	180	.02	.06	.1	Trace
Cookies Plain and assorted, 3-inch diameter	1 cooky	25	120	1	5	—	—	—	18	9	.2	20	.01	.01	.1	Trace
Fig bars, small	1	16	55	1	1	—	—	—	12	12	.2	20	.01	.01	.1	Trace
Corn, rice and wheat flakes, mixed, added nutrients	1 oz.	28	110	2	Trace	—	—	—	24	11	.5	0	.11	—	.9	0
Corn flakes, added nutrients Plain	1 oz.	28	110	2	Trace	—	—	—	24	5	.4	0	.12	.02	.6	0
Sugar-covered	1 oz.	28	110	1	Trace	—	—	—	26	3	.3	0	.12	.01	.5	0

Continued.

[12]When the amount of nonfat dry milk in commercial white bread is unknown, values for bread with 3 to 4% nonfat dry milk are suggested.

[14]Unenriched cake flour and vegetable cooking fat used unless otherwise specified.

[15]If the fat used in the recipe is butter or fortified margarine, the vitamin A value for chocolate cake with chocolate icing will be 490 I.U. per 2-inch sector; 100 I.U. for fruitcake; for plain cake without icing, 300 I.U. per piece; 220 I.U. per cupcake; for plain cake with icing, 440 I.U. per 2-inch sector; 220 I.U. per cupcake; and 300 I.U. for poundcake.

Food, approximate measure, and weight (in grams)		Food energy	Protein	Fat (total lipid)	Fatty acids Saturated (total)	Unsaturated Oleic	Linoleic	Carbohydrate	Calcium	Iron	Vitamin A value	Thiamine	Riboflavin	Niacin	Ascorbic acid
	gm.	(Calories)	(gm.)	(gm.)	(gm.)	(gm.)	(gm.)	(gm.)	(mg.)	(mg.)	(I.U.)	(mg.)	(mg.)	(mg.)	(mg.)
Corn grits, degermed, cooked															
Enriched 1 cup	242	120	3	Trace	—	—	—	27	2	[16].7	[17]150	[16].10	[16].07	[16]1.0	0
Unenriched 1 cup	242	120	3	Trace	—	—	—	27	2	.2	[17]150	.05	.02	.5	0
Cornmeal, white or yellow, dry															
Whole ground, unbolted 1 cup	118	420	11	5	1	2	2	87	24	2.8	[17]600	.45	.13	2.4	0
Degermed, enriched 1 cup	145	525	11	2	Trace	2	1	114	9	[16]4.2	[17]640	[16].64	[16].38	[16]5.1	0
Corn muffins, made with enriched degermed cornmeal and enriched flour; muffin, 2¾-inch diameter 1 muffin	48	150	3	5	2	2	Trace	23	50	.8	[18]80	.09	.11	.8	Trace
Corn, puffed, pre-sweetened, added nutrients 1 oz.	28	110	1	Trace	—	—	—	26	3	.5	0	.12	.05	.6	0
Corn, shredded, added nutrients 1 oz.	28	110	2	Trace	—	—	—	25	1	.7	0	.12	.05	.6	0
Crackers															
Graham, plain 4 small or 2 medium	14	55	1	1	—	—	—	10	6	.2	0	.01	.03	.2	0
Saltines, 2 inches squares 2 crackers	8	35	1	1	—	—	—	6	2	.1	0	Trace	Trace	.1	0
Soda, Cracker, 2½ inches square 2 crackers	11	50	1	1	Trace	1	Trace	8	2	.2	0	Trace	Trace	.1	0
Oyster crackers 10 crackers	10	45	1	1	Trace	1	Trace	7	2	.2	0	Trace	Trace	.1	0
Cracker meal 1 tbsp.	10	45	1	1	Trace	1	Trace	7	2	.1	0	.01	Trace	.1	0
Doughnuts, cake type 1 doughnut	32	125	1	6	1	4	Trace	16	13	[19].4	30	[19].05	[19].05	[19].4	Trace
Farina, regular, enriched, cooked 1 cup	238	100	3	Trace	—	—	—	21	10	[16].7	0	[16].11	[16].07	[16]1.0	0
Macaroni, cooked															
Enriched, Cooked, firm stage (8 to 10 minutes; undergoes additional cooking in a food mixture) 1 cup	130	190	6	1	—	—	—	39	14	[16]1.4	0	[16].23	[16].14	[16]1.9	0

Cooked until tender	1 cup	140	155	5	1	—	—	—	32	11	[16]1.3	0	[16].19	[16].11	[16]1.5	0
Unenriched																
Cooked, firm stage (8 to 10 minutes; undergoes additional cooking in a food mixture)	1 cup	130	190	6	1	—	—	—	39	14	.6	0	.02	.02	.5	0
Cooked until tender	1 cup	140	155	5	1	—	—	—	32	11	.6	0	.02	.02	.4	0
Macaroni (enriched) and cheese, baked	1 cup	220	470	18	24	11	10	1	44	398	2.0	950	.22	.44	2.0	Trace
Muffins, with enriched white flour; muffin, 2¾-inch diameter	1	48	140	4	5	1	3	Trace	20	50	.8	50	.08	.11	.7	Trace
Noodles (egg noodles), cooked																
Enriched	1 cup	160	200	7	2	1	1	Trace	37	16	[16]1.4	110	[16].23	[16].14	[16]1.8	0
Unenriched	1 cup	160	200	7	2	1	1	Trace	37	16	1.0	110	.04	.03	.7	0
Oats (with or without corn) puffed, added nutrients	1 oz.	28	115	3	2	Trace	1	1	21	50	1.3	0	.28	.05	.5	0
Oatmeal or rolled oats, regular or quick-cooking, cooked	1 cup	236	130	5	2	Trace	1	1	23	21	1.4	0	.19	.05	.3	0
Pancakes (griddlecakes), 4-inch diameter																
Wheat, enriched flour (home recipe)	1 cake	27	60	2	2	Trace	1	Trace	9	27	.4	30	.05	.06	.3	Trace
Buckwheat (buckwheat pancake mix, made with egg and milk)	1 cake	27	55	2	2	Trace	1	1	6	59	.4	60	.03	.04	.2	Trace
Piecrust, plain, baked																
Enriched flour																
Lower crust, 9-inch shell	1	135	675	8	45	10	29	3	59	19	2.3	0	.27	.19	2.4	0
Double crust, 9-inch pie	1	270	1,350	16	90	21	58	7	118	38	4.6	0	.55	.39	4.9	0

[16]Iron, thiamine, riboflavin, and niacin are based on the minimum levels of enrichment specified in standards of identity promulgated under the Federal Food, Drug, and Cosmetic Act.

[17]Vitamin A value based on yellow product. White product contains only a trace.

[18]Based on recipe using white cornmeal; if yellow cornmeal is used, the vitamin A value is 140 I.U. per muffin.

[19]Based on product made with enriched flour. With unenriched flour, approximate values per doughnut are: Iron, 0.2 milligram; thiamine, 0.01 milligram; riboflavin, 0.03 milligram; niacin, 0.2 milligram.

Continued.

Food, approximate measure, and weight (in grams)		gm.	Food energy	Protein	Fat (total lipid)	Fatty acids			Carbohydrate	Calcium	Iron	Vitamin A value	Thiamine	Riboflavin	Niacin	Ascorbic acid
						Saturated (total)	Unsaturated Oleic	Unsaturated Linoleic								
		gm.	(Calories)	(gm.)	(gm.)	(gm.)	(gm.)	(gm.)	(gm.)	(mg.)	(mg.)	(I.U.)	(mg.)	(mg.)	(mg.)	(mg.)
Piecrust, plain, baked—cont'd																
Unenriched flour																
Lower crust, 9-inch shell	1	135	675	8	45	10	29	3	59	19	.7	0	.04	.04	.6	0
Double crust, 9-inch pie	1	270	1,350	16	90	21	58	7	118	38	1.4	0	.08	.07	1.3	0
Pies (piecrust made with unenriched flour); sector, 4-inch, 1/7 of 9-inch-diameter pie																
Apple	1 sector	135	345	3	15	4	9	1	51	11	.4	40	.03	.02	.5	1
Cherry	1 sector	135	355	4	15	4	10	1	52	19	.4	590	.03	.03	.6	1
Custard	1 sector	130	280	8	14	5	8	1	30	125	.8	300	.07	.21	.4	0
Lemon meringue	1 sector	120	305	4	12	4	7	1	45	17	.6	200	.04	.10	.2	4
Mince	1 sector	135	365	3	16	4	10	1	56	38	1.4	Trace	.09	.05	.5	1
Pumpkin	1 sector	130	275	5	15	5	7	1	32	66	.6	3,210	.04	.13	.6	Trace
Pizza (cheese); 5½-inch sector; ⅛ of 14-inch-diameter pie	1 sector	75	185	7	6	2	3	Trace	27	107	.7	290	.04	.12	.7	4
Popcorn, popped, with added oil and salt	1 cup	14	65	1	3	2	Trace	Trace	8	1	.3	—	.01		.2	0
Pretzels, small stick	5 sticks	5	20	Trace	Trace	—	—	—	4	1	0	0	Trace	Trace	Trace	0
Rice, white (fully milled or polished), enriched, cooked																
Common commercial varieties, all types	1 cup	168	185	3	Trace	—	—	—	41	17	[20]1.5	0	[20].19	[20].01	[20]1.6	0
Long grain, parboiled	1 cup	176	185	4	Trace	—	—	—	41	33	[20]1.4	0	[20].19	[20].02	[20]2.0	0
Rice, puffed, added nutrients (without salt)	1 cup	14	55	1	Trace	—	—	—	13	3	.3	0	.06	.01	.6	0
Rice flakes, added nutrients	1 cup	30	115	2	Trace	—	—	—	26	9	.5	0	.10	.02	1.6	0
Rolls																
Plain, pan; 12 per 16 ounces																
Enriched	1 roll	38	115	3	2	Trace	1	Trace	20	28	.7	Trace	.11	.07	.8	Trace
Unenriched	1 roll	38	115	3	2	Trace	1	Trace	20	28	.3	Trace	.02	.03	.3	Trace
Hard, round; 12 per 22 oz.	1 roll	52	160	5	2	Trace	1	Trace	31	24	.4	Trace	.03	.05	.4	Trace
Sweet, pan; 12 per 18 oz.	1 roll	43	135	4	4	1	2	Trace	21	37	.3	30	.03	.06	.4	Trace

Food	Measure	Weight (g)	Food energy (cal)	Protein (g)	Fat (g)	Saturated fatty acids (g)	Oleic (g)	Linoleic (g)	Carbohydrate (g)	Calcium (mg)	Iron (mg)	Vitamin A (IU)	Thiamine (mg)	Riboflavin (mg)	Niacin (mg)	Ascorbic acid (mg)
Rye wafers, whole-grain, 1⅞ by 3½ inches	2 wafers	13	45	2	Trace	—	—	—	10	7	.5	0	.04	.03	.2	0
Spaghetti																
Cooked, tender stage (14 to 20 minutes)																
Enriched	1 cup	140	155	5	1	—	—	—	32	11	[16]1.3	0	[16].19	[16].11	[16]1.5	0
Unenriched	1 cup	140	155	5	1	—	—	—	32	11	.6	0	.02	.02	.4	0
Spaghetti with meat balls in tomato sauce (home recipe)	1 cup	250	335	19	12	4	6	1	39	125	3.8	1,600	.26	.30	4.0	22
Spaghetti in tomato sauce with cheese (home recipe)	1 cup	250	260	9	9	2	5	1	37	80	2.2	1,080	.24	.18	2.4	14
Waffles, with enriched flour, ½ by 4½ by 5½ inches	1	75	210	7	7	2	4	1	28	85	1.3	250	.13	.19	1.0	Trace
Wheat, puffed																
With added nutrients (without salt)	1 oz.	28	105	4	Trace	—	—	—	22	8	1.2	0	.15	.07	2.2	0
With added nutrients, with sugar and honey	1 oz.	28	105	2	1	—	—	—	25	7	.9	0	.14	.05	1.8	0
Wheat, rolled; cooked	1 cup	236	175	5	1	—	—	—	40	19	1.7	0	.17	.06	2.1	0
Wheat, shredded, plain (long, round, or bite-size)	1 oz.	28	100	3	1	—	—	—	23	12	1.0	0	.06	.03	1.2	0
Wheat and malted barley flakes, with added nutrients	1 oz.	28	110	2	Trace	—	—	—	24	14	.7	0	.13	.03	1.1	0
Wheat flakes, with added nutrients	1 oz.	28	100	3	Trace	—	—	—	23	12	1.2	0	.18	.04	1.4	0
Wheat flours																
Whole-wheat, from hard wheats, stirred	1 cup	120	400	16	2	Trace	1	1	85	49	4.0	0	.66	.14	5.2	0
All-purpose or family flour																
Enriched, sifted	1 cup	110	400	12	1	Trace	Trace	Trace	84	18	[16]3.2	0	[16].48	[16].29	[16]3.8	0
Unenriched, sifted	1 cup	110	400	12	1	Trace	Trace	Trace	84	18	.9	0	.07	.05	1.0	0
Self-rising, enriched	1 cup	110	385	10	1	Trace	Trace	Trace	82	292	[16]3.2	0	[16].49	[16].29	[16]3.9	0
Cake or pastry flour, sifted	1 cup	100	365	8	1	Trace	Trace	Trace	79	17	.5	0	.03	.03	.7	0
Wheat germ, crude, commercially milled	1 cup	68	245	18	7	1	2	4	32	49	6.4	0	1.36	.46	2.9	0

[16] Iron, thiamine, riboflavin, and niacin are based on the minimum levels of enrichment specified in standards of identity promulgated under the Federal Food, Drug, and Cosmetic Act. *Continued.*

[20] Iron, thiamine, and niacin are based on the minimum levels of enrichment specified in standards of identity promulgated under the Federal Food, Drug, and Cosmetic Act. Riboflavin is based on unenriched rice. When the minimum level of enrichment for riboflavin specified in the standards of identity becomes effective the value will be 0.12 milligram per cup of parboiled rice and of white rice.

Food, approximate measure, and weight (in grams)			Food energy	Protein	Fat (total lipid)	Fatty acids			Carbohydrate	Calcium	Iron	Vitamin A value	Thiamine	Riboflavin	Niacin	Ascorbic acid
						Saturated (total)	Unsaturated Oleic	Unsaturated Linoleic								
		gm.	(Calories)	(gm.)	(gm.)	(gm.)	(gm.)	(gm.)	(gm.)	(mg.)	(mg.)	(I.U.)	(mg.)	(mg.)	(mg.)	(mg.)
Fats, oils																
Butter, 4 sticks per pound																
Sticks, 2	1 cup	227	1,625	1	184	101	61	6	1	45	0	[21] 7,500	—	—	—	0
Stick, ⅛	1 tbsp.	14	100	Trace	11	6	4	Trace	Trace	3	0	[21] 460	—	—	—	0
Pat or square (64 per pound)	1	7	50	Trace	6	3	2	Trace	Trace	1	0	[21] 230	—	—	—	0
Fats, cooking																
Lard	1 cup	220	1,985	0	220	84	101	22	0	0	0	0	0	0	0	0
Lard	1 tbsp.	14	125	0	14	5	6	1	0	0	0	0	0	0	0	0
Vegetable fats	1 cup	200	1,770	0	200	46	130	14	0	0	0	—	0	0	0	0
Vegetable fats	1 tbsp.	12.5	110	0	12	3	8	1	0	0	0	—	0	0	0	0
Margarine, 4 sticks per pound																
Sticks, 2	1 cup	227	1,635	1	184	37	105	33	1	45	0	[22] 7,500	—	—	—	0
Stick, ⅛	1 tbsp.	14	100	Trace	11	2	6	2	Trace	3	0	[22] 460	—	—	—	0
Pat or square (64 per pound)	1 pat	7	50	Trace	6	1	3	1	Trace	1	0	[22] 230	—	—	—	0
Oils, salad or cooking																
Corn	1 tbsp.	14	125	0	14	1	4	7	0	0	0	—	0	0	0	0
Cottonseed	1 tbsp.	14	125	0	14	4	3	7	0	0	0	—	0	0	0	0
Olive	1 tbsp.	14	125	0	14	2	11	1	0	0	0	—	0	0	0	0
Soybean	1 tbsp.	14	125	0	14	2	3	7	0	0	0	—	0	0	0	0
Salad dressings																
Blue cheese	1 tbsp.	16	80	1	8	2	2	4	1	13	Trace	30	Trace	.02	Trace	Trace
Commercial, mayonnaise type	1 tbsp.	15	65	Trace	6	1	1	3	2	2	Trace	30	Trace	Trace	Trace	—
French	1 tbsp.	15	60	Trace	6	1	1	3	3	2	.1	—	—	—	—	—
Home cooked, boiled	1 tbsp.	17	30	1	2	1	1	Trace	3	15	.1	80	.01	.03	Trace	Trace
Mayonnaise	1 tbsp.	15	110	Trace	12	2	3	6	Trace	3	.1	40	Trace	.01	Trace	Trace
Thousand island	1 tbsp.	15	75	Trace	8	1	2	4	2	2	.1	50	Trace	Trace	Trace	Trace
Sugars, sweets																
Candy																
Caramels	1 oz.	28	115	1	3	2	1	Trace	22	42	.4	Trace	.01	.05	Trace	Trace
Chocolate, milk, plain	1 oz.	28	150	2	9	5	3	Trace	16	65	.3	80	.02	.09	.1	Trace
Fudge, plain	1 oz.	28	115	1	3	2	1	Trace	21	22	.3	Trace	.01	.03	.1	Trace

Food	Measure	Weight (g)	Food energy (Cal.)	Protein (g)	Fat (g)	Saturated fatty acids (g)	Unsaturated fatty acids (g)	Carbohydrate (g)	Calcium (mg)	Iron (mg)	Vitamin A (I.U.)	Thiamine (mg)	Riboflavin (mg)	Niacin (mg)	Ascorbic acid (mg)
Hard candy	1 oz.	28	110	0	Trace	—	—	28	6	.5	0	0	0	0	0
Marshmallows	1 oz.	28	90	1	Trace	—	—	23	5	.5	0	0	Trace	Trace	0
Chocolate sirup, thin type	1 tbsp.	20	50	Trace	Trace	—	Trace	13	3	.3	—	Trace	.01	.1	Trace
Honey, strained or extracted	1 tbsp.	21	65	Trace	0	—	—	17	1	.1	0	Trace	.01	.1	Trace
Jams and preserves	1 tbsp.	20	55	Trace	Trace	—	—	14	4	.2	Trace	Trace	.01	Trace	Trace
Jellies	1 tbsp.	20	55	Trace	Trace	—	—	14	4	.3	Trace	Trace	.01	Trace	1
Molasses, cane															
Light (first extraction)	1 tbsp.	20	50	—	—	—	—	13	33	.9	—	.01	.01	Trace	—
Blackstrap (third extraction)	1 tbsp.	20	45	—	—	—	—	11	137	3.2	—	.02	.04	.4	—
Sirup, table blends (chiefly corn, light and dark)	1 tbsp.	20	60	0	0	—	—	15	9	.8	0	0	0	0	0
Sugars (cane or beet)															
Granulated	1 cup	200	770	0	0	—	—	199	0	.2	0	0	0	0	0
	1 tbsp.	12	45	0	0	—	—	12	0	Trace	0	0	0	0	0
Lump, 1⅛ by ¾ by ⅜	1 lump	6	25	0	0	—	—	6	0	Trace	0	0	0	0	0
Powdered, stirred before measuring	1 cup	128	495	0	0	—	—	127	0	.1	0	0	0	0	0
	1 tbsp.	8	30	0	0	—	—	8	0	Trace	0	0	0	0	0
Brown, firm-packed	1 cup	220	820	0	0	—	—	212	187	7.5	0	.02	.07	.4	0
	1 tbsp.	14	50	0	0	—	—	13	12	.5	0	Trace	Trace	Trace	0
Miscellaneous items															
Beer (average 3.6 percent alcohol by weight)	1 cup	240	100	1	0	—	—	9	12	Trace	—	.01	.07	1.6	—
Beverages, carbonated															
Cola type	1 cup	240	95	0	0	—	—	24	—	—	0	0	0	0	0
Ginger ale	1 cup	230	70	0	0	—	—	18	—	—	0	0	0	0	0
Bouillon cube, ⅝ inch	1 cube	4	5	1	Trace	—	—	Trace	—	—	—	—	—	—	—
Chili powder. See Vegetables, peppers															
Chili sauce (mainly tomatoes)	1 tbsp.	17	20	Trace	Trace	—	—	4	3	.1	240	.02	.01	.3	3
Chocolate															
Bitter or baking	1 oz.	28	145	3	15	8	6	8	22	1.9	20	.01	.07	.4	0
Sweet	1 oz.	28	150	1	10	6	4	16	27	.4	Trace	.01	.04	.1	Trace
Cider. See Fruits, apple juice															

Continued.

[21] Year-round average.

[22] Based on the average vitamin A content of fortified margarine. Federal specifications for fortified margarine require a minimum of 15,000 I.U. of vitamin A per pound.

Food, approximate measure, and weight (in grams)		gm.	Food energy (Calories)	Protein (gm.)	Fat (total lipid) (gm.)	Fatty acids Saturated (total) (gm.)	Fatty acids Unsaturated Oleic (gm.)	Fatty acids Unsaturated Linoleic (gm.)	Carbohydrate (gm.)	Calcium (mg.)	Iron (mg.)	Vitamin A value (I.U.)	Thiamine (mg.)	Riboflavin (mg.)	Niacin (mg.)	Ascorbic acid (mg.)
Gelatin, dry																
Plain	1 tbsp.	10	35	9	Trace	—	—	—	—	—	—	—	—	—	—	—
Dessert powder, 3-oz. package	½ cup	85	315	8	0	—	—	—	75	—	—	—	—	—	—	—
Gelatin dessert, ready-to-eat																
Plain	1 cup	239	140	4	0	—	—	—	34	—	—	—	—	—	—	—
With fruit	1 cup	241	160	3	Trace	—	—	—	40	—	—	—	—	—	—	—
Olives, pickled																
Green	4 medium or 3 extra large or 2 giant	16	15	Trace	2	Trace	2	Trace	Trace	8	.2	40	—	—	—	—
Ripe: Mission	3 small or 2 large	10	15	Trace	2	Trace	2	Trace	Trace	9	.1	10	Trace	Trace	—	—
Pickles, cucumber																
Dill, large, 4 by 1¾ inches	1	135	15	1	Trace	—	—	—	3	35	1.4	140	Trace	.03	Trace	8
Sweet, 2¾ by ¾ inches	1	20	30	Trace	Trace	—	—	—	7	2	.2	20	Trace	Trace	Trace	1
Popcorn. See Grain products																
Sherbet, orange	1 cup	193	260	2	2	—	—	—	59	31	Trace	110	.02	.06	Trace	4
Soups, canned; ready-to-serve (prepared with equal volume of water)																
Bean with pork	1 cup	250	170	8	6	1	2	2	22	62	2.2	650	.14	.07	1.0	2
Beef noodle	1 cup	250	70	4	3	1	1	1	7	8	1.0	50	.05	.06	1.1	Trace

Beef bouillon, broth, consomme	1 cup	240	30	5	0	0	0	0	3	Trace	.5	Trace	Trace	.02	1.2	—
Chicken noodle	1 cup	250	65	4	2	Trace	1	1	8	10	.5	50	.02	.02	.8	Trace
Clam chowder	1 cup	255	85	2	3	—	—	—	13	36	1.0	920	.03	.03	1.0	—
Cream soup (mushroom)	1 cup	240	135	2	10	1	3	5	10	41	.5	70	.02	.12	.7	Trace
Minestrone	1 cup	245	105	5	3	—	1	—	14	37	1.0	2,350	.07	.05	1.0	—
Pea, green	1 cup	245	130	6	2	1	1	Trace	23	44	1.0	340	.05	.05	1.0	7
Tomato	1 cup	245	90	2	2	Trace	1	1	16	15	.7	1,000	.06	.05	1.1	12
Vegetable with beef broth	1 cup	250	80	3	2	—	—	—	14	20	.8	3,250	.05	.02	1.2	—
Starch (cornstarch)	1 cup	128	465	Trace	Trace	—	—	—	112	0	0	0	0	0	0	0
	1 tbsp.	8	30	Trace	Trace	—	—	—	7	0	0	0	0	0	0	0
Tapioca, quick-cooking granulated, dry, stirred before measuring	1 cup	152	535	1	Trace	—	—	—	131	15	.6	0	0	0	0	0
	1 tbsp.	10	35	Trace	Trace	—	—	—	9	1	Trace	0	0	0	0	0
Vinegar	1 tbsp.	15	2	0	—	—	—	—	1	1	.1	—	—	—	—	—
White sauce, medium	1 cup	265	430	10	33	18	11	1	23	305	.5	1,220	.12	.44	.6	Trace
Yeast																
Baker's																
Compressed	1 oz.	28	25	3	Trace	—	—	—	3	4	1.4	Trace	.20	.47	3.2	Trace
Dry active	1 oz.	28	80	10	Trace	—	—	—	11	12	4.6	Trace	.66	1.53	10.4	Trace
Brewer's, dry, debittered	1 tbsp.	8	25	3	Trace	—	—	—	3	17	1.4	Trace	1.25	.34	3.0	Trace
Yogurt. See Milk, cream, cheese; related products																

SOURCE: *Nutritive Value of Foods.* Home & Garden Bull. No. 72, rev., Table 2, pp. 4–30. USDA, 1977. (Superintendent of Documents, US Govt. Printing Office, Washington, D.C., Stock No. 001-000-03667-0.)

APPENDIX B

Mean Heights and Weights and Recommended Energy Intake

Category	Age (Years)	Weight (kg)	Weight (lb)	Height (cm)	Height (in)	Energy Needs (with Range) (Calories)	(MJ)
Infants	0.0–0.5	6	13	60	24	kg × 115 (95–145)	kg × .48
	0.5–1.0	9	20	71	28	kg × 105 (80–135)	kg × .44
Children	1–3	13	29	90	35	1,300 (900–1,800)	5.5
	4–6	20	44	112	44	1,700 (1,300–2,300)	7.1
	7–10	28	62	132	52	2,400 (1,650–3,300)	10.1
Males	11–14	45	99	157	62	2,700 (2,000–3,700)	11.3
	15–18	66	145	176	69	2,800 (2,100–3,900)	11.8
	19–22	70	154	177	70	2,900 (2,500–3,300)	12.2
	23–50	70	154	178	70	2,700 (2,300–3,100)	11.3
	51–75	70	154	178	70	2,400 (2,000–2,800)	10.1
	76+	70	154	178	70	2,050 (1,650–2,450)	8.6
Females	11–14	46	101	157	62	2,200 (1,500–3,000)	9.2
	15–18	55	120	163	64	2,100 (1,200–3,000)	8.8
	19–22	55	120	163	64	2,100 (1,700–2,500)	8.8
	23–50	55	120	163	64	2,000 (1,600–2,400)	8.4
	51–75	55	120	163	64	1,800 (1,400–2,200)	7.6
	76+	55	120	163	64	1,600 (1,200–2,000)	6.7
Pregnancy						+ 300	
Lactation						+ 500	

SOURCE: *Recommended Dietary Allowances*, 9th Ed., 1979. Food and Nutrition Board, Natl Acad. of Sciences–Natl Research Council, Washington, D.C. Reproduced with the permission of the National Academy of Sciences, Washington, D.C.

NOTE: The data in this table have been assembled from the observed median heights and weights of children, together with desirable weights for adults for the mean heights of men (70 in) and women (64 in) between the ages of 18 and 34 years as surveyed in the US population (HEW/NCHS data).

The energy allowances for the young adults are for men and women doing light work. The allowances for the two older age groups represent mean energy needs over these age spans, allowing for a 2% decrease in basal (resting) metabolic rate per decade and a reduction in activity of 200 Calories/day for men and women between 51 and 75 years, 500 Calories for men over 75 years, and 400 Calories for women over 75. The customary range of daily energy output is shown for adults in parentheses and is based on a variation in energy needs of ±400 Calories at any one age, emphasizing the wide range of energy intakes appropriate for any group of people.

Energy allowances for children through age 18 are based on median energy intakes of children these ages followed in longitudinal growth studies. The values in parentheses are tenth and ninetieth percentiles of energy intake, to indicate the range of energy consumption among children of these ages.

APPENDIX C

Estimated Safe and Adequate Daily Dietary Intakes of Additional Selected Vitamins and Minerals

		Vitamins			Trace Elements[a]						Electrolytes		
	Age (Years)	Vitamin K (µg)	Biotin (µg)	Pantothenic Acid (mg)	Copper (mg)	Manganese (mg)	Fluorine (mg)	Chromium (mg)	Selenium (mg)	Molybdenum (mg)	Sodium (mg)	Potassium (mg)	Chlorine (mg)
Infants	0–0.5	12	35	2	0.5–0.7	0.5–0.7	0.1–0.5	0.01–0.04	0.01–0.04	0.03–0.06	115–350	350–925	275–700
	0.5–1	10–20	50	3	0.7–1.0	0.7–1.0	0.2–1.0	0.02–0.06	0.02–0.06	0.04–0.08	250–750	425–1,275	400–1,200
Children	1–3	15–30	65	3	1.0–1.5	1.0–1.5	0.5–1.5	0.02–0.08	0.02–0.08	0.05–0.1	325–975	550–1,650	500–1,500
and	4–6	20–40	85	3–4	1.5–2.0	1.5–2.0	1.0–2.5	0.03–0.12	0.03–0.12	0.06–0.15	450–1,350	775–2,325	700–2,100
Adolescents	7–10	30–60	120	4–5	2.0–2.5	2.0–3.0	1.5–2.5	0.05–0.2	0.05–0.2	0.1–0.3	600–1,800	1,000–3,000	925–2,775
	11+	50–100	100–200	4–7	2.0–3.0	2.5–5.0	1.5–2.5	0.05–0.2	0.05–0.2	0.15–0.5	900–2,700	1,525–4,575	1,400–4,200
Adults		70–140	100–200	4–7	2.0–3.0	2.5–5.0	1.5–4.0	0.05–0.2	0.05–0.2	0.15–0.5	1,100–3,300	1,875–5,625	1,700–5,100

SOURCE: Recommended Dietary Allowances, 9th Ed. Food and Nutrition Board, Natl Acad. of Sciences—Natl Research Council, Washington, D.C. Reproduced with the permission of the National Academy of Sciences, Washington, D.C.

NOTE: Because there is less information on which to base allowances, these figures are not given in the main table of the RDA and are provided here in the form of ranges of recommended intakes.

[a] Since the toxic levels for many trace elements may be only several times usual intakes, the upper levels for the trace elements given in this table should not be habitually exceeded.

APPENDIX D

Canadian Dietary Standard
Recommended Daily Nutrient Intakes—Revised 1974 Committee for Revision of the
Canadian Dietary Standard, Bureau of Nutritional Sciences, Health and
Welfare Canada

Age (yr)	Sex	Weight (kg)	Height (cm)	Energy[a] (kcal)	Pro-tein (gm)	Water-soluble vitamins Thia-mine (mg)	Nia-cin[e] (mg)	Ribo-flavin (mg)	Vit B_6[f] (mg)	Folate[g] (μg)
0–6 mo	Both	6	—	kg × 117	kg × 2.2 (2.0)[d]	0.3	5	0.4	0.3	40
7–11 mo	Both	9	—	kg × 108	kg × 1.4	0.5	6	0.6	0.4	60
1–3	Both	13	90	1,400	22	0.7	9	0.8	0.8	100
4–6	Both	19	110	1,800	27	0.9	12	1.1	1.3	100
7–9	M	27	129	2,200	33	1.1	14	1.3	1.6	100
	F	27	128	2,000	33	1.0	13	1.2	1.4	100
10–12	M	36	144	2,500	41	1.2	17	1.5	1.8	100
	F	38	145	2,300	40	1.1	15	1.4	1.5	100
13–15	M	51	162	2,800	52	1.4	19	1.7	2.0	200
	F	49	159	2,200	43	1.1	15	1.4	1.5	200
16–18	M	64	172	3,200	54	1.6	21	2.0	2.0	200
	F	54	161	2,100	43	1.1	14	1.3	1.5	200
19–35	M	70	176	3,000	56	1.5	20	1.8	2.0	200
	F	56	161	2,100	41	1.1	14	1.3	1.5	200
36–50	M	70	176	2,700	56	1.4	18	1.7	2.0	200
	F	56	161	1,900	41	1.0	13	1.2	1.5	200
51+	M	70	176	2,300[b]	56	1.4	18	1.7	2.0	200
	F	56	161	1,800[b]	41	1.0	13	1.2	1.5	200
Pregnant				+300[c]	+20	+0.2	+2	+0.3	+0.5	+50
Lactating				+500	+24	+0.4	+7	+0.6	+0.6	+50

SOURCE: Canadian Council on Nutrition, "Dietary Standards for Canada." *Can. Bull. Nutr.* **6**:1, 1964 (suppl. 1974).

[a] Recommendations assume characteristic activity pattern for each age group.

[b] Recommended energy allowance for age 66+ years reduced to 2,000 for men and 1,500 for women.

[c] Increased energy allowance recommended during second and third trimesters. An increase of 100 calories per day is recommended during first trimester.

[d] Recommended protein allowance of 2.2 gm/kg of body weight for infants age 0 to 2 months and 2.0 gm/kg of body weight for those age 3 to 5 months. Protein recommendation for infants, 0 to 11 months, assumes consumption of breast milk or protein of equivalent quality.

[e] Approximately 1 mg of niacin is derived from each 60 mg of dietary tryptophan.

[f] Recommendations are based on the estimated average daily protein intake of Canadians.

[g] Recommendation given in terms of free folate.

Vit B$_{12}$ (μg)	Ascorbic Acid (mg)	Fat-soluble vitamins			Minerals					
		Vit A (μg RE)[i]	Vit D (μg choelcal-ciferol)[j]	Vit E (mg α-to-coph-erol)	Ca (mg)	P (mg)	Mg (mg)	I (μg)	Fe (mg)	Zn (mg)
0.3	20[h]	400	10	3	500[l]	250[l]	50[l]	35[l]	7[l]	4[l]
0.3	20	400	10	3	500	400	50	50	7	5
0.9	20	400	10	4	500	500	75	70	8	5
1.5	20	500	5	5	500	500	100	90	9	6
1.5	30	700	2.5[k]	6	700	700	150	110	10	7
1.5	30	700	2.5[k]	6	700	700	150	100	10	7
3.0	30	800	2.5[k]	7	900	900	175	130	11	8
3.0	30	800	2.5[k]	7	1,000	1,000	200	120	11	9
3.0	30	1,000	2.5[k]	9	1,200	1,200	250	140	13	10
3.0	30	800	2.5[k]	7	800	800	250	110	14	10
3.0	30	1,000	2.5[k]	10	1,000	1,000	300	160	14	12
3.0	30	800	2.5[k]	6	700	700	250	110	14	11
3.0	30	1,000	2.5[k]	9	800	800	300	150	10	10
3.0	30	800	2.5[k]	6	700	700	250	110	14	9
3.0	30	1,000	2.5[k]	8	800	800	300	140	10	10
3.0	30	800	2.5[k]	6	700	700	250	100	14	9
3.0	30	1,000	2.5[k]	8	800	800	300	140	10	10
3.0	30	800	2.5[k]	6	700	700	250	100	9	9
+1.0	+20	+100	+2.5[k]	+1	+500	+500	+25	+15	+1[m]	+3
+0.5	+30	+400	+2.5[k]	+2	+500	+500	+75	+25	+1[m]	+7

[h] Considerably higher levels may be prudent for infants during the first week of life to guard against neonatal tyrosinemia.

[i] One μg Retinol Equivalent (1 μg RE) corresponds to a biological activity in humans equal to 1 μg of retinol (3.33 IU) and 6 μg of β-carotene (10 IU).

[j] One μg cholecalciferol is equivalent to 40 IU vitamin D activity.

[k] Most older children and adults receive enough vitamin D from irradiation but 2.5 μg daily is recommended. This recommended allowance increases to 5.0 μg daily for pregnant and lactating women and for those who are confined indoors or otherwise deprived of sunlight for extended periods.

[l] The intake of breast-fed infants may be less than the recommendation but is considered to be adequate.

[m] A recommended total intake of 15 mg daily during pregnancy and lactation assumes the presence of adequate stores of iron. If stores are suspected of being inadequate, additional iron as a supplement is recommended.

APPENDIX E

Desirable Weights for Women of Age 25 and Over

Height (with Shoes, 2-in Heels)		Weights in Pounds according to Frame (as Ordinarily Dressed)		
Feet	*Inches*	*Small Frame*	*Medium Frame*	*Large Frame*
4	10	92–98	96–107	104–119
4	11	94–101	98–110	106–122
5	0	96–104	101–113	109–125
5	1	99–107	104–116	112–128
5	2	102–110	107–119	115–131
5	3	105–113	110–122	118–134
5	4	108–116	113–126	121–138
5	5	111–119	116–130	125–142
5	6	114–123	120–135	129–146
5	7	118–127	124–139	133–150
5	8	122–131	128–143	137–154
5	9	126–135	132–147	141–158
5	10	130–140	136–151	145–163
5	11	134–144	140–155	149–168
6	0	138–148	144–159	153–173

SOURCE: From the Metropolitan Life Insurance Company. Derived from data of the Body Build and Blood Pressure Study, 1959, Society of Actuaries.

APPENDIX F

Desirable Weights for Men of Age 25 and Over

Height (with Shoes, 1-in Heels)		Weight in Pounds according to Frame (as Ordinarily Dressed)		
Feet	Inches	Small Frame	Medium Frame	Large Frame
5	2	112–120	118–129	126–141
5	3	115–123	121–133	129–144
5	4	118–126	124–136	132–148
5	5	121–129	127–139	135–152
5	6	124–133	130–143	138–156
5	7	128–137	134–147	142–161
5	8	132–141	138–152	147–166
5	9	136–145	142–156	151–170
5	10	140–150	146–160	155–174
5	11	144–154	150–165	159–179
6	0	148–158	154–170	164–184
6	1	152–162	158–175	168–189
6	2	156–167	162–180	173–194
6	3	160–171	167–185	178–199
6	4	164–175	172–190	182–204

SOURCE: From the Metropolitan Life Insurance Company. Derived from data of the Body Build and Blood Pressure Study, 1959, Society of Actuaries.

APPENDIX G

Sodium and Potassium Content of Foods

Food	Approximate Amount	Weight (gm)	Sodium (mEq)	Potassium (mEq)
Meat Group				
Meat (cooked)				
Beef	1 oz	30	0.8	2.8
Ham	1 oz	30	14.3	2.6
Lamb	1 oz	30	0.9	2.2
Pork	1 oz	30	0.9	3.0
Veal	1 oz	30	1.0	3.8
Liver	1 oz	30	2.4	3.2
Sausage, pork	2 links	40	16.5	2.8
Beef, dried	2 slices	20	37.0	1.0
Cold cuts	1 slice	45	25.0	2.7
Frankfurters	1	50	24.0	3.0
Fowl				
Chicken	1 oz	30	1.0	3.0
Goose	1 oz	30	1.6	4.6
Duck	1 oz	30	1.0	2.2
Turkey	1 oz	30	1.2	2.8
Egg	1	50	2.7	1.8
Fish	1 oz	30	1.0	2.5
Salmon				
Fresh	$\frac{1}{4}$ cup	30	0.6	2.3
Canned	$\frac{1}{4}$ cup	30	4.6	2.6
Tuna				
Fresh	$\frac{1}{4}$ cup	30	0.5	2.2
Canned	$\frac{1}{4}$ cup	30	10.4	2.3
Sardines	3 medium	35	12.5	4.5
Shellfish				
Clams	5 small	50	2.6	2.3
Lobster	1 small tail	40	3.7	1.8
Oysters	5 small	70	2.1	1.5
Scallops	1 large	50	5.7	6.0
Shrimp	5 small	30	1.8	1.7
Cheese				
Cheese, American or Cheddar type	1 slice	30	9.1	0.6
Cheese foods	1 slice	30	15.0	0.8
Cheese spreads	2 T	30	15.0	0.8
Cottage cheese	$\frac{1}{4}$ cup	50	5.0	1.1
Peanut butter	2 T	30	7.8	5.0
Peanuts, unsalted	25	25	—	4.5
Fat Group				
Avocado	$\frac{1}{8}$	30	—	4.6
Bacon	1 slice	5	2.2	0.6

Sodium and Potassium Content of Foods (Continued)

Food	Approximate Amount	Weight (gm)	Sodium (mEq)	Potassium (mEq)
Butter or margarine	1 t	5	2.2	—
Cooking fat	1 t	5	—	—
Cream				
Half and half	2 T	30	0.6	1.0
Sour	2 T	30	0.4	—
Whipped	1 T	15	0.3	1.0
Cream cheese	1 T	15	1.7	—
Mayonnaise	1 t	5	1.3	—
Nuts				
Almonds, slivered	5 (2 t)	6	—	0.8
Pecans	4 halves	5	—	0.8
Walnuts	5 halves	10	—	1.0
Oil, salad	1 t	5	—	—
Olives, green	3 medium	30	31.3	0.4
Bread Group				
Bread	1 slice	25	5.5	0.7
Biscuit	1 (2 in diameter)	35	9.6	0.7
Muffin	1 (2 in diameter)	35	7.3	1.2
Cornbread	1 (1½ in cube)	35	11.3	1.7
Roll	1 (2 in diameter)	25	5.5	0.6
Bun	1	30	6.6	0.7
Pancake	1 (4 in diameter)	45	8.8	1.1
Waffle	½ square	35	8.5	1.0
Cereals				
Cooked	⅔ cup	140	8.7	2.0
Dry, flake	⅔ cup	20	8.7	0.6
Dry, puffed	1½ cups	20	—	1.5
Shredded wheat	1 biscuit	20	—	2.2
Crackers				
Graham	3	20	5.8	2.0
Melba toast	4	20	5.5	0.7
Oyster	20	20	9.6	0.6
Ritz	6	20	9.5	0.5
Rye-Krisp	3	30	11.5	3.0
Saltines	6	20	9.6	0.6
Soda	3	20	9.6	0.6
Dessert				
Commercial gelatin	½ cup	100	2.2	—
Ice cream	½ cup	75	2.0	3.0
Sherbet	⅓ cup	50	—	—
Angel food cake	1½ in × 1½ in	25	3.0	0.6
Sponge cake	1½ in × 1½ in	25	1.8	0.6
Vanilla wafers	5	15	1.7	—
Floor products				
Cornstarch	2 T	15	—	—
Macaroni	¼ cup	50	—	0.8
Noodles	¼ cup	50	—	0.6
Rice	¼ cup	50	—	0.9
Spaghetti	¼ cup	50	—	0.8
Tapioca	2 T	15	—	—

Sodium and Potassium Content of Foods (Continued)

Food	Approximate Amount	Weight (gm)	Sodium (mEq)	Potassium (mEq)
*Vegetable Group**				
Artichokes	1 large bud	100	1.3	7.7
Asparagus				
Cooked	½ cup	100	—	4.7
Canned†	½ cup	100	10.0	3.6
Frozen	½ cup	100	—	5.5
Beans, dried (cooked)	½ cup	90	—	10.0
Beans, lima	½ cup	90	—	9.5
Bean sprouts	½ cup	100	—	4.0
Beans, green or wax				
Fresh or frozen	½ cup	100	—	4.0
Canned†	½ cup	100	10.0	2.5
Beet greens	½ cup	100	3.0	8.5
Beets	½ cup	100	1.8	5.0
Broccoli	½ cup	100	—	7.0
Brussels sprouts	⅔ cup	100	—	7.6
Cabbage, cooked	½ cup	100	0.6	4.2
Raw	1 cup	100	0.9	6.0
Carrots, cooked	½ cup	100	1.4	5.7
Raw	1 large	100	2.0	8.8
Cauliflower, cooked	1 cup	100	0.4	5.2
Celery, raw	1 cup	100	5.4	9.0
Chard, Swiss	⅗ cup	100	3.7	8.0
Collards	½ cup	100	0.8	6.0
Corn				
Canned†	⅓ cup	80	8.0	2.0
Fresh	½ ear	100	—	2.0
Frozen	⅓ cup	80	—	3.7
Cress, garden (cooked)	½ cup	100	0.5	7.2
Cucumber	1 medium	100	0.3	4.0
Dandelion greens	½ cup	100	2.0	6.0
Eggplant	½ cup	100	—	3.8
Hominy (dry)	¼ cup	36	4.1	—
Kale, cooked	¾ cup	100	2.0	5.6
Frozen	½ cup	100	1.0	5.0
Kohlrabi	⅔ cup	100	—	6.6
Leeks, raw	3–4	100	—	9.0
Lettuce	Varies	100	0.4	4.5
Mushrooms, raw	4 large	100	0.7	10.6
Mustard greens	½ cup	100	0.8	5.5
Okra	½ cup	100	—	4.4
Onions, cooked	½ cup	100	—	2.8
Parsnips	⅔ cup	100	0.3	9.7
Peas				
Canned†	½ cup	100	10.0	1.2
Dried	½ cup	90	1.5	6.8
Fresh	½ cup	100	—	2.5
Frozen	½ cup	100	2.5	1.7
Pepper, green or red				
Cooked	½ cup	100	—	5.5
Raw	1	100	0.5	4.0
Popcorn	1 cup	15	—	--
Potato				
Potato chips	1 oz	30	13.0	3.7
White, baked	½ cup	100	—	13.0

Sodium and Potassium Content of Foods (*Continued*)

Food	Approximate Amount	Weight (gm)	Sodium (mEq)	Potassium (mEq)
White, boiled	½ cup	100	—	7.3
Sweet, baked	¼ cup	50	0.4	4.0
Pumpkin	½ cup	100	—	6.3
Radishes	10	100	0.8	8.0
Rutabagas	½ cup	100	—	4.4
Sauerkraut	⅔ cup	100	32.0	3.5
Spinach	½ cup	100	2.2	8.5
Squash	½ cup	100	—	3.5
Squash, winter				
Baked	½ cup	100	—	12.0
Boiled	½ cup	100	—	6.5
Tomatoes	½ cup	100	—	6.5
Tomato juice‡	½ cup	100	9.0	5.8
Turnip greens	½ cup	100	0.7	3.8
Turnips	½ cup	100	1.5	4.8
Milk Group				
Whole milk	1 cup	240	5.2	8.8
Evaporated whole milk	½ cup	120	6.0	9.2
Powdered whole milk	¼ cup	30	5.2	10.0
Buttermilk	1 cup	240	13.6	8.5
Skim milk	1 cup	240	5.2	8.8
Powdered skim milk	¼ cup	30	6.9	13.5
Fruit				
Figs				
Canned	½ cup	120	—	4.6
Dried	1 small	15	—	2.5
Fresh	1 large	60	—	3.0
Fruit cocktail	½ cup	120	—	5.0
Grapes				
Canned	⅓ cup	80	—	2.2
Fresh	15	80	—	3.2
Juice				
Bottled	¼ cup	60	—	2.8
Frozen	⅓ cup	80	—	2.4
Grapefruit				
Fresh	½ medium	120	—	3.6
Juice	½ cup	120	—	4.1
Sections	¾ cup	150	—	5.1
Mandarin orange	¾ cup	200	—	6.5
Mango	½ small	70	—	3.4
Melon				
Cantaloupe	½ small	200	—	13.0
Honeydew	¼ medium	200	—	13.0
Watermelon	½ slice	200	—	5.0
Nectarine	1 medium	80	—	6.0
Orange				
Fresh	1 medium	100	—	5.1
Juice	½ cup	120	—	5.7
Sections	½ cup	100	—	5.1
Papaya	½ cup	120	—	7.0
Peach				
Canned	½ cup	120	—	4.0
Dried	2 halves	20	—	5.0

Sodium and Potassium Content of Foods (*Continued*)

Food	Approximate Amount	Weight (gm)	Sodium (mEq)	Potassium (mEq)
Peach (*Continued*)				
Fresh	1 medium	120	—	6.2
Nectar	½ cup	120	—	2.4
Pear				
Canned	½ cup	120	—	2.5
Dried	2 halves	20	—	3.0
Fresh	1 small	80	—	2.6
Nectar	⅓ cup	80	—	0.9
Pineapple				
Canned	½ cup	120	—	3.0
Fresh	½ cup	80	—	3.0
Juice	⅓ cup	80	—	3.0
Plums				
Canned	½ cup	120	—	4.5
Fresh	2 medium	80	—	4.1
Prunes	2 medium	15	—	2.6
Juice	¼ cup	60	—	3.6
Raisins	1 T	15	—	2.9
Rhubarb	½ cup	100	—	6.5
Tangerines				
Fresh	2 small	100	—	3.2
Juice	½ cup	120	—	5.5
Sections	½ cup	100	—	3.2

SOURCE: Reproduced with permission from *Mayo Clinic Diet Manual*, 4th ed. Philadelphia: W. B. Saunders Company, 1971.

* Value for products without added salt.

† Estimated average based on addition of salt, approximately 0.6% of the finished product.

NOTE: To convert mEq. to mg multiply mEq. by 23 (sodium) or 39 (potassium) mEq. × 23 = mg of Sodium mEq. × 39 = mg of Potassium.

APPENDIX H

Fatty Acid and Cholesterol Content of Foods

Food	Approximate Amount	Weight (gm)	Total Fat (gm)	Saturated Fat (gm)	Unsaturated Fatty Acids Oleic (gm)	Linoleic (gm)	Cholesterol (mg)
Meat Group							
Beef	1 oz	30	7.5	3.6	3.3	Trace	27
Veal	1 oz	30	3.6	1.8	1.5	Trace	27
Lamb	1 oz	30	6.3	3.6	2.4	Trace	27
Pork, ham	1 oz	30	7.8	3.0	3.3	Trace	27
Liver	1 oz	30	1.5	0.4	Trace	Trace	75
Beef, dried	2 slices	20	1.2	0.6	0.6	—	18
Pork sausage	2 links	40	17.6	6.4	7.6	1.6	45
Cold cuts	1 slice	45	9.7	2.4	2.7	0.6	30
Frankfurters	1	50	17.4	9.0	8.0	0.4	50
Fowl	1 oz	30	3.6	1.2	1.2	0.6	23
Eggs	1	50	6.0	2.0	2.5	0.5	253
Fish	1 oz	30	2.7	0.5	1.7	0.5	21
Salmon and tuna	¼ cup	30	5.1	1.4	1.5	1.2	—
Shellfish	1 oz	30	1.9	0.6	1.0	0.3	45
Cheese	1 oz	30	9.0	5.1	3.0	—	45
Cottage cheese	¼ cup	50	2.1	1.0	0.5	—	5
Peanut butter	2 T	30	15.0	2.7	7.5	4.2	—
Peanuts	25	25	12.0	2.5	5.0	3.2	—
Fat Group							
Avocado	⅛	30	5.1	0.9	2.4	0.6	—
Bacon	1 strip	5	2.6	0.9	1.0	0.3	5
Butter	1 t	5	4.0	2.3	1.2	—	12
Margarine	1 t	5	4.0	1.1	2.5	0.4	—
Special margarine	1 t	5	4.0	0.6	2.3	1.1	—
Coconut oil	1 t	5	5.0	4.4	0.5	0.1	—
Corn oil	1 t	5	5.0	0.5	1.8	2.7	—
Cottonseed oil	1 t	5	5.0	1.3	1.2	2.5	—
Olive oil	1 t	5	5.0	0.6	4.0	0.4	—
Peanut oil	1 t	5	5.0	0.9	1.6	1.5	—
Safflower oil	1 t	5	5.0	0.4	1.0	3.6	—
Sesame oil	1 t	5	5.0	0.9	1.0	2.1	—
Soybean oil	1 t	5	5.0	0.8	1.6	2.6	—
Vegetable fat	1 t	5	5.0	1.0	2.6	0.4	—
Half and half	2 T	30	3.6	1.8	1.8	—	12
Cream substitute, dried	1 T	2	0.5	0.3	0.2	—	—
Whipping cream	1 T	15	5.6	3.2	2.2	0.2	18
Cream cheese	1 T	15	5.3	3.0	2.2	0.1	18

Food	Approximate Amount	Weight (gm)	Total Fat (gm)	Saturated Fat (gm)	Unsaturated Fatty Acids		Cholesterol (mg)
					Oleic (gm)	Linoleic (gm)	
Mayonnaise	1 t	5	4.0	0.7	1.3	2.0	8
French dressing	1 T	15	5.0	1.1	1.1	3.0	—
Nuts							
Almonds	5	6	3.5	0.3	2.5	0.7	—
Pecans	4	5	3.6	0.3	2.6	0.7	—
Walnuts	5	10	6.5	0.4	2.0	4.0	—
Olives	3	30	4.2	0.6	3.0	0.3	—
Milk Group							
Milk, whole	1 cup	240	8.5	4.9	3.6	—	27
2% milk	1 cup	240	4.9	2.4	2.5	—	15
Skim milk	1 cup	240	—	—	—	—	7
Cocoa (skim milk)	1 cup	240	1.9	0.7	1.2	—	—
Chocolate milk	1 cup	240	8.5	2.5	6.0	—	—
Bread Group							
Bread	1 slice	25	0.8	0.3	0.5	—	—
Biscuit	1	35	6.5	2.3	3.4	0.8	17
Muffin	1	35	3.5	0.7	2.4	0.4	16
Cornbread	1 (1½ in cube)	35	4.0	1.4	2.1	0.4	16
Roll	1	28	1.3	0.3	0.7	0.3	—
Pancake	1 (4 in diam)	45	3.2	0.9	1.9	0.4	38
Waffle	1	35	3.4	1.0	2.1	0.4	28
Sweet roll	1	35	8.2	2.4	5.1	0.7	25
French toast	1 slice	65	8.1	3.9	3.4	0.8	130
Doughnut	1	30	6.0	1.3	4.4	0.3	27
Cereal, cooked	⅔ cup	140	1.4	—	1.4	0.3	—
Crackers (saltines)	6	20	2.4	0.6	1.4	—	—
Popcorn (unbuttered)	1 cup	15	0.7	0.1	0.2	0.4	—
Potatoes							
Potato chips	1-oz bag	30	12.0	3.0	4.0	6.0	—
French fried							
In corn oil	10	50	6.2	0.4	2.3	3.5	—
In hydrogenated fat	10	50	6.2	1.6	4.0	0.6	—
Mashed potato	½ cup	100	4.3	2.0	2.3	—	—
Soup, cream	½ cup	100	4.2	1.0	2.2	1.0	9
Dessert							
Ice milk	½ cup	75	2.5	1.5	—	—	5
Ice cream	½ cup	75	9.0	5.0	3.9	—	43
Sherbet	⅓ cup	50	0.6	0.4	0.2	—	—
Low-fat cookies	5	15	1.8	0.3	—	—	—
Cake	1 piece	50	14.0	2.0	—	0.5	45
Fruit pie	⅙ pie (9 in)	160	15.0	4.0	9.5	1.4	11
Miscellaneous							
Gravy	¼ cup	60	13.8	6.8	6.6	0.4	18
White sauce	¼ cup	60	8.2	4.6	3.6	—	29
Coconut	1 oz	28	10.9	9.5	1.4	—	—
Chocolate sauce	1 oz	30	3.8	2.0	1.8	—	—

SOURCE: Reproduced with permission from *Mayo Clinic Diet Manual*, 4th ed. Philadelphia: W. B. Saunders Co., 1971.

APPENDIX I

Exchange Lists for Meal Planning

LIST 1. Milk Exchanges (Includes **Nonfat**, Low-fat, and Whole Milk)

One exchange of milk contains 12 gm of carbohydrate, 8 gm of protein, and a trace of fat.

This list shows the kinds and amounts of milk or milk products to use for one milk exchange. Those which appear in **bold type** are **nonfat**. Low-fat and whole milk contain saturated fat.

Nonfat fortified milk	
Skim or nonfat milk	1 cup
Powdered (nonfat dry, before adding liquid)	⅓ cup
Canned, evaporated—skim milk	½ cup
Buttermilk made from skim milk	1 cup
Yogurt made from skim milk (plain, unflavored)	1 cup
Lowfat fortified milk	
1% fat fortified milk (omit ½ fat exchange)	1 cup
2% fat-fortified milk (omit 1 fat exchange)	1 cup
Yogurt made from 2% fortified milk (plain, unflavored) (omit 1 fat exchange)	1 cup
Whole milk (omit 2 fat exchanges)	
Whole milk	1 cup
Canned, evaporated whole milk	½ cup
Buttermilk made from whole milk	1 cup
Yogurt made from whole milk (plain, unflavored)	1 cup

LIST 2. Vegetable Exchanges

One exchange of vegetables contains about 5 gm of carbohydrate and 2 gm of protein.

This list shows the kinds of **vegetables** to use for one vegetable exchange. One Exchange is ½ cup.

Asparagus	Greens:
Bean sprouts	Mustard
Beets	Spinach
Broccoli	Turnip
Brussels sprouts	Mushrooms
Cabbage	Okra
Carrots	Onions
Cauliflower	Rhubarb
Celery	Rutabaga
Cucumbers	Sauerkraut
Eggplant	String beans, green or yellow
Green pepper	Summer Squash
Greens:	Tomatoes
Beet	Tomato juice
Chards	Turnips
Collards	Vegetable juice cocktail
Dandelion	Zucchini
Kale	

The following **raw vegetables** may be used as desired:

Chicory	Lettuce
Chinese Cabbage	Parsley
Endive	Radishes
Escarole	Watercress

Starchy Vegetables are found in the bread exchange list.

LIST 3. Fruit Exchanges

One exchange of fruit contains 10 gm of carbohydrate.
This list shows the kinds and amounts of **fruits** to use for one fruit exchange.

Apple	1 small	Mango	$\frac{1}{2}$ small
Apple juice	$\frac{1}{3}$ cup	Melon	
Applesauce (unsweetened)	$\frac{1}{2}$ cup	Cantaloupe	$\frac{1}{4}$ small
Apricots, fresh	2 medium	Honeydew	$\frac{1}{8}$ medium
Apricots, dried	4 halves	Watermelon	1 cup
Banana	$\frac{1}{2}$ small	Nectarine	1 small
Berries		Orange	1 small
Blackberries	$\frac{1}{2}$ cup	Orange juice	$\frac{1}{2}$ cup
Blueberries	$\frac{1}{2}$ cup	Papaya	$\frac{3}{4}$ cup
Raspberries	$\frac{1}{2}$ cup	Peach	1 medium
Strawberries	$\frac{3}{4}$ cup	Pear	1 small
Cherries	10 large	Persimmon, native	1 medium
Cider	$\frac{1}{3}$ cup	Pineapple	$\frac{1}{2}$ cup
Dates	2	Pineapple juice	$\frac{1}{3}$ cup
Figs, fresh	1	Plums	2 medium
Figs, dried	1	Prunes	2 medium
Grapefruit	$\frac{1}{2}$	Prune juice	$\frac{1}{4}$ cup
Grapefruit Juice	$\frac{1}{2}$ cup	Raisins	2 T
Grapes	12	Tangerine	1 medium
Grape Juice	$\frac{1}{4}$ cup		

Cranberries may be used as desired if no sugar is added.

LIST 4. Bread Exchanges (Includes Bread, Cereal, and Starchy Vegetables)

One exchange of bread contains 15 gm of carbohydrate and 2 gm of protein.

This list shows the kinds and amounts of breads, cereals, starchy vegetables, and prepared foods to use for one bread exchange. Those which appear in **bold type** are low-fat.

Cereal

Bran flakes	½ cup
Other ready-to-eat unsweetened cereal	¾ cup
Puffed cereal (unfrosted)	1 cup
Cereal (cooked)	½ cup
Grits (cooked)	½ cup
Rice or barley (cooked)	½ cup
Pasta (cooked),	½ cup
Spaghetti, noodles, macaroni	
Popcorn (popped, no fat added)	3 cup
Cornmeal (dry)	2 T
Flour	2½ T
Wheat germ	¼ cup

Crackers

Arrowroot	3
Graham, 2½ in sq	2
Matzoth, 4 in × 6 in	½
Oyster	20
Pretzels, 3⅛ in long × ⅛ in dia	25
Rye wafers, 2 in × 3½ in	3
Saltines	6
Soda, 2½ in sq	4

Dried beans, peas, and lentils

Beans, Peas, Lentils (dried and cooked)	½ cup
Baked beans, no pork (canned)	¼ cup

Starchy vegetables

Corn	⅓ cup
Corn on cob	1 small
Lima beans	½ cup
Parsnips	⅔ cup
Peas, green (canned or frozen)	½ cup
Potato, white	1 small
Potato (mashed)	½ cup
Pumpkin	¾ cup
Winter squash, Acorn, or butternut	½ cup
Yam or sweet potato	¼ cup

Prepared Foods

Biscuit 2 in dia (omit 1 fat exchange)	1
Corn bread, 2 in × 2 in × 1 in (omit 1 fat exchange)	1
Corn muffin, 2 in dia (omit 1 fat exchange)	1
Crackers, round butter type (omit 1 fat exchange)	5
Muffin, plain small (omit 1 fat exchange)	1
Potatoes, french fried, length 2 in to 3½ in (omit 1 fat exchange)	8
Potato or corn chips (omit 2 fat exchanges)	15
Pancake, 5 in × ½ in (omit 1 fat exchange)	1
Waffle, 5 in × ½ in (omit 1 fat exchange)	1

LIST 5. Meat Exchanges: Lean Meat

One exchange of lean meat (1 oz) contains 7 gm of protein and 3 gm of fat.

This list shows the kinds and amounts of **lean meat** and other protein-rich foods to use for one low-fat meat exchange.

Beef:	Baby beef (very lean), chipped beef, chuck, flank steak, tenderloin, plate ribs, plate skirt steak, round (bottom, top), all cuts rump, sirloin, tripe	1 oz
Lamb:	Leg, rib, sirloin, loin (roast and chops), shank, shoulder	1 oz
Pork:	Leg (whole rump, center shank), ham, smoked (center slices)	1 oz
Veal:	Leg, loin, rib, shank, shoulder, cutlets	1 oz
Poultry:	Meat without skin of chicken, turkey, cornish hen, Guinea hen, pheasant	1 oz
Fish:	Any fresh or frozen	1 oz
	canned salmon, tuna, mackerel, crab and lobster,	¼ cup
	clams, oysters, scallops, shrimp,	5 or 1 oz
	sardines, drained	3
Cheeses containing less than 5% butterfat		1 oz
Cottage cheese, dry and 2% butterfat		¼ cup
Dried beans and peas (omit 1 bread exchange)		½ cup

LIST 5. Meat Exchanges: Medium-fat Meat

For each exchange of medium-fat meat omit ½ fat exchange.

This list shows the kinds and amounts of medium-fat meat and other protein-rich foods to use for one medium-fat meat exchange.

Beef: ground (15% fat), corned beef (canned), rib eye, round (ground commercial)	1 oz
Pork: loin (all cuts tenderloin), shoulder arm (picnic), shoulder blade, Boston butt, Canadian bacon, boiled ham	1 oz
Liver, heart, kidney, and sweetbreads (these are high in cholesterol)	1 oz
Cottage cheese, creamed	¼ cup
Cheese: Mozzarella, ricotta, farmer's cheese, Neufchatel, Parmesan	1 oz
	3 T
Egg (high in cholesterol)	1
Peanut Butter (omit 2 additional fat exchanges)	2 Tbs

LIST 5. Meat Exchanges: High-fat Meat

For each exchange of high-fat meat omit 1 fat exchange.

This list shows the kinds and amounts of high-fat meat and other protein-rich foods to use for one high-fat meat exchange.

Beef:	Brisket, corned beef (brisket), ground beef (more than 20% fat), hamburger (commercial), chuck (ground commercial), roasts (rib), steaks (club and rib)	1 oz
Lamb:	Breast	1 oz
Pork:	Spare ribs, loin (back ribs), pork (ground), country-style ham, deviled ham	1 oz
Veal:	Breast	1 oz
Poultry:	Capon, duck (domestic), goose	1 oz
Cheese:	Cheddar types	1 oz
Cold cuts		4½ in × ⅛ in slice
Frankfurter		1 small

LIST 6. Fat Exchanges

One exchange of fat contains 5 gm of fat.

This list shows the kinds and amounts of fat-containing foods to use for one fat exchange. To plan a diet low in saturated fat select only those exchanges which appear in **bold type.** They are **polyunsaturated.**

Margarine, soft, tub or stick[a]	1 t
Avocado (4 in dia)[b]	⅛
Oil, corn, cottonseed, safflower, soy, sunflower	1 t
Oil, olive[b]	1 t
Oil, peanut[b]	1 t
Olives[b]	5 small
Almonds[b]	10 whole
Pecans[b]	2 large whole
Peanuts[b]	
Spanish	20 whole
Virginia	10 whole
Walnuts	6 small
Nuts, other[b]	6 small
Margarine, regular stick	1 t
Butter	1 t
Bacon fat	1 t
Bacon, crisp	1 strip
Cream, light	2 T
Cream, sour	2 T
Cream, heavy	1 T
Cream cheese	1 T
French dressing[c]	1 T
Italian dressing[c]	1 T
Lard	1 t
Mayonnaise[c]	1 t
Salad dressing, mayonnaise type[c]	2 t
Salt pork	¾-in cube

[a] Made with corn, cottonseed, safflower, soy or sunflower oil only.
[b] Fat content is primarily monounsaturated.
[c] If made with corn, cottonseed, safflower, soy or sunflower oil can be used on fat-modified diet.

SOURCE: The exchange lists are based on material in *Exchange Lists for Meal Planning* prepared by committees of the American Diabetes Association, Inc., and The American Dietetic Association in cooperation with the National Institute of Arthritis, Metabolism, and Digestive Diseases and the National Heart and Lung Institute, National Institutes of Health, US Dept. of Health, Education, and Welfare, 1977.

APPENDIX J

Pathophysiological Conditions and Associated Nutritional Nursing Diagnoses and Dietary Interventions

The index that follows contains symptoms and diseases and also the nutritional nursing diagnoses and dietary interventions which are commonly associated with them. It is intended as a ready reference for the student in applying the nursing process to nutritional care of clients. *The broad nursing diagnoses in this index are intended only as examples for educational purposes; in dealing with actual clients each one's condition must be individually assessed and diagnosed.*

Only frequently encountered *pathophysiological conditions* (symptoms or diseases) have been included in this index. After each definition, one or more of the major nursing diagnoses are given, followed by a dietary intervention, if any. Each nursing diagnosis describes how the associated condition represents an alteration in the nutritive process. The reader is reminded that a specific disease may cause an alteration in more than one step of the nutritive process and that a client may have two or more alterations simultaneously.

In most cases only one of several possible nursing diagnoses is listed. The student is encouraged to develop specific nutritional nursing diagnoses for each client. Examples of more specific nursing diagnoses are found in Chapter 21.

Dietary interventions are given only for conditions that are known to be treatable by diet therapy. Only basic features of therapeutic diets are listed because the physician is responsible for writing specific diet orders and the dietitian for instructing clients about the details of their diets. The reader may refer back to the appropriate chapters in Unit V for a discussion of each dietary intervention. For diseases requiring the same dietary intervention, cross-references have been provided. Note that nursing interventions have not been given for nutritional deficiency diseases (scurvy, pellagra, etc.) because the intervention in each case is simply to add the missing nutrient to the diet.

Achalasia Failure of the smooth muscle of the gastrointestinal tract to relax where one part is connected to the next such as occurs with the lower esophagus. Symptoms include regurgitation, esophageal pain, and dyspepsia.
Nursing diagnosis Alteration in digestion manifested by an alteration in motility.
Dietary intervention See Hiatal hernia.

Acidemia A condition resulting from the accumulation of acid (a lowering of pH) or a decrease in the alkali (base) reserve.

Nursing diagnosis Alteration in nutrient transport manifested by changes in blood pH.

Adrenocortical insufficiency (Addison's disease) A metabolic disorder owing to impaired function of the adrenal cortex. Decreased secretion of aldosterone and cortisol result in rapid weight loss, anorexia, anemia, weakness, emaciation, hypoglycemia, low blood pressure, and electrolyte imbalance.
Nursing diagnosis Alteration in metabolism manifested by an alteration in endocrine physiology; an

alteration in nutrient transport manifested by electrolyte imbalance.

Dietary invervention   High protein, moderate carbohydrate, high sodium, frequent feedings, liberal fluids.

Adrenocorticotropic hormone (ACTH) therapy   The administration of ACTH and steroids of the adrenal cortex for the treatment of numerous diseases including arthritis, allergy, dermatitis, and gastrointestinal diseases.

Nursing diagnosis   Alteration in metabolism manifested by alterations in endocrine physiology.

Dietary intervention   Same as for adrenocortical insufficiency but with a mild (2–3 gm) sodium restriction.

Alkalemia   A condition resulting from the accumulation of base or a loss of acid (a rise in pH).

Nursing diagnosis   Alteration in nutrient transport manifested by changes in blood pH.

Allergy, food   An allergic response to the ingestion of a particular food. Symptoms may appear within a few minutes or after several days and may be mild to quite severe.

Nursing diagnosis   Interference with ingestion manifested by alteration in ingestion that has already occurred.

Dietary intervention   Exclusion of the offending food or foods if known; also the exclusion of foods containing the allergen (such as wheat, milk, or eggs). If allergen is unknown a series of elimination diets may be used to isolate the offending food.

Anemia, folic acid –deficiency   A type of nutritional anemia resulting from a deficiency of folic acid.

Nursing diagnosis   Alteration in nutrient transport manifested by oxygen/carbon dioxide alterations.

Dietary intervention   Diet high in protein and foods high in folic acid and supplemented with folic acid and vitamin C.

Anemia, iron-deficiency   A type of anemia resulting from a deficiency of dietary iron or chronic blood loss, impaired iron absorption, or an increase in blood volume during pregnancy.

Nursing diagnosis   Alteration in nutrient transport manifested by oxygen/carbon dioxide alterations.

Dietary intervention   Diet high in good-quality protein and iron, usually accompanied by iron and vitamin C supplementation.

Anemia, pernicious   A type of nutritional anemia resulting from a dietary deficiency of vitamin B_{12},

lack of the intrinsic factor, or faulty absorption of vitamin B_{12}.

Nursing diagnosis   Alteration in nutrient transport manifested by oxygen/carbon dioxide alterations.

Dietary intervention   Vitamin B_{12} supplementation plus a high-protein diet.

Anorexia   A decreased desire for food.

Nursing diagnosis   Interference with ingestion manifested by a lack of desire to ingest food and fluids.

Anorexia nervosa   A psychological state characterized by extreme weight loss and severe rejection of food.

Nursing diagnosis   Interference with ingestion manifested by a lack of desire to ingest food and fluids.

Dietary intervention   Small quantities of attractive, palatable food; gradual increase in Calories. Tube feeding, intravenous feeding, or hyperalimentation may be necessary to supplement oral intake.

Arteriosclerosis   A thickening and hardening of the inner walls of the arteries resulting in a loss of elasticity.

Nursing diagnosis   Alteration in nutrient transport manifested by alterations in vascular physiology.

Arthritis   An acute or chronic inflammation of a joint.

Nursing diagnosis   Alteration in metabolism manifested by an alteration in structure (pain in joints).

Dietary intervention   No specific diet, only a well-balanced, nutritionally adequate diet; low-Calorie diet if client is overweight; high-Calorie, high-protein diet if client is underweight.

Ascites   An accumulation of fluid in the peritoneal cavity related to portal hypertension, low levels of serum protein, or sodium retention.

Nursing diagnosis   Alteration in nutrient transport manifested by fluid volume alterations.

Dietary intervention   Rigid sodium restriction (250–500 mg/day) and sometimes a fluid restriction. As diuresis occurs the sodium restriction is liberalized.

Atherosclerosis   A thickening of the inner walls of the arteries by the depositing of fatty substances, such as cholesterol, phospholipids, and triglycerides. Other substances such as complex carbohydrates, calcium, and fibrin are also deposited. This accumulation of material, called *plaque,* leads to a narrowing of the opening (lumen) and decreases blood flow.

Nursing diagnosis Alteration in nutrient transport manifested by alterations in vascular physiology.

Dietary intervention Decrease in Calories, decrease in cholesterol to 250–300 mg/day, decrease in saturated fat, and increase in polyunsaturated fat (fat-controlled diet).

Atonic constipation A form of constipation that results because of a lack of tone of the colon. The urge to defecate is lacking, and the feces are large and hard.

Nursing diagnosis Alteration in excretion manifested by an alteration in solid waste output.

Dietary intervention High-fiber diet with liberal fluids (8–10 glasses daily).

Azotemia The retention of urea and other end products of protein metabolism in the blood.

Nursing diagnosis Alteration in metabolism manifested by an alteration in nutritional requirements (decreased protein use).

Dietary intervention See diet for Uremia.

Beriberi A nutritional deficiency disease resulting from deficiency of thiamine.

Nursing diagnosis Interference with ingestion manifested by the inaccessibility of nutrients.

Botulism A severe kind of food poisoning, usually fatal, caused by the toxin of *Clostridium botulinum* found in improperly canned food.

Nursing diagnosis Interference with ingestion manifested by an alteration in ingestion that has already occurred.

Burns Injury to or destruction of body tissue caused by excessive heat, caustics, friction, electricity, or radiation.

Nursing diagnosis Alteration in metabolism manifested by an alteration in nutritional requirements (increased nutritional requirements).

Dietary intervention High-protein, high-Calorie diet with between-meal feedings or supplements. Diet also high in vitamins and minerals, especially vitamin C. Tube feeding may be necessary in addition to regular feeding.

Calculus An abnormal stony mass, usually composed of mineral salts, which is found in the ducts and passages of the body.

Nursing diagnosis Alteration in excretion manifested by an alteration in fluid output.

Dietary intervention See diets for Cholelithiasis and Nephrolithiasis.

Cancer A cellular tumor characterized by uncontrollable growth.

Nursing diagnosis Interference with ingestion manifested by a lack of desire to or an inability to ingest food and fluids or by oral discomfort and/or obstruction.

Dietary intervention Appetizing food according to the client's food preferences; bland or low-residue diet with cancer of the GI tract; small, frequent feedings; mechanical soft diet if there is difficulty swallowing or chewing.

Celiac disease A disease that leads to a blunting of the villi of the small intestine and malabsorption of nutrients; believed to be due to a sensitivity to the gliadin portion of the protein gluten in cereal grains.

Nursing diagnosis Alteration in absorption manifested by an alteration in absorptive surface.

Dietary intervention Gluten-restricted diet, high Calories, high protein, moderate fat; use of MCT oil, supplementary vitamins and minerals.

Chemotherapy The treatment of disease, especially cancer, by chemical agents.

Nursing diagnosis Interference with ingestion manifested by a lack of desire to ingest food or fluids or by oral discomfort.

Dietary intervention Appetizing food according to client's food preferences; small, frequent feedings.

Cholecystectomy Surgical removal of the gall bladder.

Nursing diagnosis Alteration in digestion manifested by an alteration in secretion.

Dietary intervention Low-fat diet for about 1 month; fat content gradually increased as tolerated.

Cholecystitis Inflammation of the gall bladder.

Nursing diagnosis Alteration in digestion manifested by an alteration in motility (biliary colic pain) and secretion.

Dietary intervention All food withheld during an acute attack, then clear liquid for several days, advancing to a very low-fat (20–30 gm/day) diet; in the chronic condition, a low-fat (50 gm) diet; weight reduction if overweight.

Cholelithiasis The presence or formation of gall stones.

Nursing diagnosis Alteration in digestion manifested by an alteration in motility (biliary colic pain) and secretion.

Dietary intervention Low-fat diet (50 gm/day).

Chronic renal failure See Renal failure.

Cirrhosis A progressive disease of the liver in

which there is a loss of functioning liver cells owing to replacement by fibrous connective tissue.
Nursing diagnosis Alteration in metabolism manifested by an alteration in nutritional requirements (decreased protein use).
Dietary intervention High Calories, high protein (100–150 gm/day), high carbohydrate, moderate fat; for advanced cirrhosis, lower protein content (60–80 gm/day) because of impending coma. With ascites, sodium may be reduced to 250–500 mg/day. Vitamin and mineral supplementation.

Cleft palate A condition present at birth in which there is incomplete closure of the mouth. Food may pass from the mouth (oral cavity) into the nasal cavity.
Nursing diagnosis Interference with ingestion manifested by oral discomfort and/or obstruction.
Dietary intervention Newborns fed with medicine dropper or bottle with a large-hole nipple; liquids in small quantities; avoidance of spicy and acid foods that may irritate the mouth; use of pureed food mixed with milk and fed through a bottle; small, frequent feedings.

Colitis An inflammation of the colon or large bowel.
Nursing diagnosis Alteration in excretion manifested by an alteration in solid waste output.
Dietary intervention See diet for Ulcerative colitis.

Colostomy The surgical establishment of an opening from a section of the colon to the outside of the body.
Nursing diagnosis Alteration in excretion manifested by an alteration in solid waste output.
Dietary intervention Clear liquid after surgery, advanced to low-residue diet and then to a regular diet as tolerated.

Congestive heart failure A type of heart failure in which the pumping mechanism of the heart is impaired as a result of muscle damage or fluid overload. The blood backs up into the pulmonary circulation, preventing adequate oxygen and carbon dioxide exchange.
Nursing diagnosis Alteration in nutrient transport manifested by oxygen/carbon dioxide alterations.
Dietary intervention Weight loss if overweight; sodium restriction (500–100 mg); cholesterol may be restricted and polyunsaturated fats and complex carbohydrates encouraged; small frequent feedings; soft, easily digested foods; omission of foods that might cause GI distress. Very hot or iced

beverages and caffeine beverages may be eliminated during an acute attack.

Constipation Difficult or infrequent elimination of feces.
Nursing diagnosis Alteration in excretion manifested by an alteration in solid waste output.
Dietary intervention High-fiber diet with liberal fluids.

Coronary heart disease A condition characterized by decreased coronary circulation owing to a narrowing of the lumen or complete occlusion of the coronary arteries. See Atherosclerosis, Myocardial infarction, and Congestive heart failure.
Nursing diagnosis Alteration in nutrient transport manifested by an alteration in vascular physiology.

Crohn's disease Regional enteritis or ileitis.
Nursing diagnosis Alteration in absorption manifested by an alteration in absorptive surface; alteration in excretion manifested by an alteration in solid waste output.
Dietary intervention See diet for Regional enteritis.

Cystic fibrosis A congenital disorder characterized by a general dysfunction of the exocrine glands resulting in thick mucus secretions and excess levels of sodium and chlorine.
Nursing diagnosis Alteration in digestion manifested by an alteration in secretion.
Dietary intervention High Calories, high protein, low to moderate fat, increased salt intake; use of MCT oil and simple sugars; pancreatic enzyme replacement with meals; vitamin and mineral supplementation.

Decubitus ulcer An area where the skin and/or underlying tissue has been destroyed owing to an insufficient blood supply to the area caused by prolonged pressure; commonly called a *bed sore*.
Nursing diagnosis Alteration in metabolism manifested by an alteration in structure.
Dietary intervention High-Calorie, high-protein diet; between-meal feedings or supplements.

Diabetes mellitus A metabolic disorder characterized by an impairment of the body's ability to use carbohydrate.
Nursing diagnosis Alteration in metabolism manifested by an alteration in endocrine physiology.
Dietary intervention Total caloric intake adjusted to maintain or attain ideal weight; elimination of concentrated carbohydrates; moderate fat intake with possible recommendation to decrease intake of foods high in cholesterol and saturated fat and to

substitute polyunsaturated fat. Levels of carbohydrate, protein, and fat controlled by the number of exchanges allowed per meal.

Diabetic acidosis   A complication of diabetes mellitus characterized by elevated levels of glucose in the blood and urine.

Nursing diagnosis   An alteration in nutrient transport manifested by a change in blood pH.

Dietary intervention   Initial administration of insulin, electrolytes, and fluids to replace fluids and reduce hyperglycemia and glycosuria; IV fluid replacement followed by clear liquids and a return to a diabetic diet.

Diabetic coma   A state of unconsciousness in diabetics precipitated by acidosis.

Nursing diagnosis   An alteration in nutrient transport manifested by a change in blood pH.

Dietary intervention   See diet for Diabetic acidosis.

Diabetic reaction   A complication of diabetes mellitus characterized by a low level of blood glucose (hypoglycemia). It may be precipitated by a delay in eating, the administration of too much insulin, or increased exercise. It is also called *insulin shock* or *insulin reaction*.

Nursing diagnosis   Alteration in metabolism manifested by an alteration in endocrine physiology.

Dietary intervention   Administration of a concentrated carbohydrate such as orange juice, sugar, cola beverage, syrup, or honey.

Dialysis   *See* Hemodialysis.

Diarrhea   The frequent passage of loose, unformed stool.

Nursing diagnosis   Alteration in absorption manifested by an alteration in motility; alteration in excretion manifested by an alteration in solid waste output.

Dietary intervention   Food withheld in severe diarrhea, then clear fluids advanced to a low-residue diet. Liberal intake of fluids and electrolytes, especially sodium and potassium.

Disaccharide intolerance   An inability to absorb a disaccharide owing to a deficiency or lack of the corresponding digestive enzyme (disaccharidase).

Nursing diagnosis   Alteration in digestion and absorption manifested by an alteration in secretion.

Dietary intervention   Exclusion of the offending disaccharide and foods containing it from the diet.

Diverticular disease   Disease relating to the presence of a diverticulum (diverticula, *pl*) in the colon. A *diverticulum* is a pouch formed by herniation of

the mucosal membrane of the colon. *Diverticulosis* refers to the presence of these pouches, and *diverticulitis* refers to the inflammatory condition of these pouches.

Nursing diagnosis   Alteration in excretion manifested by an alteration in solid waste output.

Dietary intervention   For diverticulosis, a high-fiber diet; for diverticulitis, a clear liquid diet during acute attacks, followed by progression to a very low-residue or a low-residue diet.

Dumping syndrome   A complication following a gastrectomy; uncomfortable symptoms such as epigastric pain, nausea, weakness, pallor, sweating, and rapid pulse occur during or shortly after a meal.

Nursing diagnosis   Alteration in digestion and absorption manifested by an alteration in motility.

Dietary intervention   High-protein, low-carbohydrate, moderate-fat diet served in small, frequent meals (4–6) with no fluids allowed during the meal; liquids allowed between meals.

Dysgeusia   An altered sense of taste associated with a decrease in taste acuity.

Nursing diagnosis   Interference with ingestion manifested by a lack of desire to ingest food and fluids.

Dysosmia   An impaired sense of smell.

Nursing diagnosis   Interference with ingestion manifested by a lack of desire to ingest food and fluids.

Dyspepsia   A wide variety of gastric symptoms commonly referred to as *indigestion*.

Nursing diagnosis   Interference with ingestion manifested by an alteration in ingestion that has already occurred.

Dietary intervention   Bland diet.

Dysphagia   Difficulty swallowing.

Nursing diagnosis   An interference with ingestion manifested by oral discomfort and/or obstruction.

Dietary intervention   Mechanical soft diet.

Edema   The accumulation of excess amounts of fluid in the intercellar tissue spaces.

Nursing diagnosis   Alteration in nutrient transport manifested by fluid volume alterations or by blockage of nutrient transport.

Dietary intervention   Sodium-restricted diet, severe (250 mg/day) to mild (200–4,000 mg/day).

Emphysema   The abnormal presence of air or gas in the body tissues. Usually used to refer to pulmonary emphysema, a lung disorder in which

there is a loss of elasticity in the alveoli so that inspired air becomes trapped.
Nursing diagnosis Alteration in nutrient transport manifested by oxygen/carbon dioxide alterations.
Dietary intervention Soft, high-Calorie diet with small, frequent feedings.

Enteritis An inflammation of the intestinal mucosa, especially the small intestine. *See* Ileitis.
Nursing diagnosis Alteration in absorption manifested by alterations in absorptive surface; alteration in excretion manifested by solid waste output.
Dietary intervention *See* diet for Regional enteritis.

Epilepsy A disorder of the nervous system characterized by episodes of motor, sensory, or psychical dysfunction with or without unconsciousness and/or convulsions.
Nursing diagnosis Alteration in metabolism manifested by an alteration in structure.
Dietary intervention Usually a nutritionally balanced diet; in some cases a ketogenic diet with high fat and low carbohydrate.

Esophagitis Inflammation of the esophagus.
Nursing diagnosis Interference with ingestion manifested by oral discomfort and/or obstruction or by the inability to ingest food and fluids.
Dietary intervention Soft or bland diet.

Failure to thrive Failure of infants to grow at a normal rate owing to such factors as high caloric requirements, excessive losses in vomiting and diarrhea, or deprivation of maternal love.
Nursing diagnosis Interference with ingestion manifested by inaccessibility of nutrients or by a lack of desire to ingest food and fluids; alteration in absorption manifested by increased motility; alteration in excretion manifested by an alteration in solid waste output.

Fever An elevation in body temperature above normal.
Nursing diagnosis An alteration in metabolism manifested by an alteration in nutritional requirements (increased nutritional requirements).
Dietary intervention High-Calorie, high-protein diet with between-meal feedings and liberal fluids; increased vitamin A, C, and B complex intake; replacement of sodium and potassium losses.

Flatulence (excessive) Distention of the stomach or intestines with air or gases.
Nursing diagnosis Alteration in digestion manifested by an alteration in motility.

Food allergy A distinct susceptibility to a specific allergen present in a food.
Nursing diagnosis Interference with ingestion manifested by an alteration in ingestion that has already occurred.
Dietary intervention Exclusion of the offending food.

Food-borne illness An illness caused by the ingestion of food contaminated with bacteria, parasites, chemical poisons, or radioactive fallout.
Nursing diagnosis Interference with ingestion manifested by an alteration in ingestion that has already occurred.

Fracture The breaking of a bone.
Nursing diagnosis Alteration in metabolism manifested by an alteration in nutritional requirements (increased nutritional requirements).
Dietary intervention High-Calorie, high-protein diet with supplementation of calcium, phosphorus, and vitamin C.

Functional hyperinsulinism An oversecretion of insulin following the ingestion of carbohydrate, which leads to a lowering of blood glucose and the symptoms of hypoglycemia.
Nursing diagnosis Alteration in metabolism manifested by an alteration in endocrine physiology.
Dietary intervention Low-carbohydrate, high-protein, moderate-fat diet with high-protein snacks between meals; avoidance of concentrated carbohydrates.

Galactosemia An inborn error of metabolism characterized by the presence of galactose in the blood caused by inability to convert galactose to glucose because of an enzyme deficiency.
Nursing diagnosis Alteration in metabolism manifested by an alteration in nutritional requirements related to inborn errors of metabolism.
Dietary intervention A galactose-free diet in which milk and milk products are not allowed.

Gallstones Stones in the gall bladder or biliary ducts. *See* Cholelithiasis.

Gastrectomy Surgical removal of part or all of the stomach.
Nursing diagnosis Alteration in digestion manifested by an alteration in motility and an alteration in secretion.
Dietary intervention *See* diet Dumping syndrome.

Gastritis An inflammation of the lining of the stomach.
Nursing diagnosis Alteration in digestion man-

ifested by an alteration in motility and an alteration in secretion.

Dietary intervention See diet for Peptic ulcer.

Gastroesophageal reflux The regurgitation of a portion of the stomach contents back into the esophagus causing the symptoms of indigestion.

Nursing diagnosis Alteration in digestion manifested by an alteration in motility.

Dietary intervention See diet for Hiatal hernia.

Gastrostomy The surgical establishment of an opening from the stomach to the outside of the body, usually for the purpose of feeding.

Nursing diagnosis Interference with ingestion manifested by the inability to ingest food and fluids or by an alteration in motility.

Dietary intervention Tube feeding administered directly into the stomach through a gastrostomy tube.

Glomerulonephritis Inflammatory disease of the glomeruli portion of the kidneys. Symptoms may include the presence of blood or albumin in the urine, retention of nitrogenous constituents, edema, or hypertension.

Nursing diagnosis Alteration in excretion manifested by an alteration in fluid output.

Dietary intervention High carbohydrate (300–400 gm/day), moderate protein (60–80 gm/day based on 0.9–1.0 gm/kg), moderate fat, 500–1,000 mg sodium; fluid restricted to 500–700 ml per day.

Gluten-induced enteropathy A disease of the proximal part of the small intestine characterized by pathological changes in the intestinal mucosa and the malabsorption of nutrients owing to the ingestion of foods containing gluten. *See* Celiac disease.

Nursing diagnosis Alteration in absorption manifested by an alteration in absorptive surface.

Dietary intervention See diet for Celiac disease.

Goiter An enlargement of the thyroid gland resulting from a deficiency of iodine.

Nursing diagnosis Interference with ingestion manifested by the inaccessibility of nutrients or by oral discomfort and/or obstruction; alteration in metabolism manifested by an alteration in endocrine physiology.

Gout A metabolic disorder characterized by elevated levels of uric acid in the blood and manifested by severe joint pain.

Nursing diagnosis Alteration in metabolism manifested by an alteration in structure.

Dietary intervention Weight reduction for the

obese; avoidance of foods high in purines; exclusion of alcohol. A diet high in carbohydrate and low in fat will aid the excretion of uric acid.

Heartburn (pyrosis) A burning sensation in the epigastric region, often accompanied by the regurgitation of acid and the presence of gas in the stomach.

Nursing diagnosis Alteration in digestion manifested by alterations in motility and secretions; interference with ingestion manifested by a lack of desire to ingest food and fluids.

Dietary intervention Soft or bland diet divided into six small meals.

Hemodialysis The process of removing excess levels of nitrogenous wastes and excess sodium and potassium from the blood of a person with chronic renal failure.

Nursing diagnosis Alteration in excretion manifested by an alteration in fluid output.

Dietary intervention 60–80 gm of protein, 1,500–2,000 mg of potassium, 1,500–2,000 mg of sodium, high carbohydrate, and high Calories; fluid restriction (approx. 300–500 ml plus the amount lost in the urine).

Hemorrhage An excessive loss of blood.

Nursing diagnosis Alteration in metabolism manifested by an alteration in nutritional requirements (increased nutritional requirements); alteration in transport manifested by fluid volume alterations.

Dietary intervention Diet high in protein and iron.

Hemorrhoids The presence of enlarged veins in the lower part of the rectum and around the anus.

Nursing diagnosis Alteration in excretion manifested by alteration in solid waste output.

Dietary intervention Low-fiber diet with a high-fluid intake.

Hepatic coma A complication of liver disease in which ammonia is not detoxified by the liver and gains entrance to the general circulation, causing toxification of the CNS.

Nursing diagnosis Alteration in metabolism manifested by an alteration in nutritional requirements (decreased protein use); alteration in nutrient transport manifested by fluid volume alterations.

Dietary intervention High Calories; high carbohydrate; no protein, adding protein in 10-gm intervals as the condition improves; moderate fat; soft foods to avoid rupture of esophageal varices.

Hepatitis Inflammation of the liver.

Nursing diagnosis Alteration in metabolism man-

ifested by an alteration in nutritional requirements (increased nutritional requirements).
Dietary intervention   High Calories, high protein, high carbohydrate, moderate fat.

Hiatal hernia   The protrusion of the upper part of the stomach through the esophageal hiatus of the diaphragm.
Nursing diagnosis   Alteration in digestion manifested by an alteration in motility; interference with ingestion manifested by a lack of desire to ingest food and fluids.
Dietary intervention   Bland (or low-residue) diet divided into small, frequent feedings.

Hypercalcemia   Excessive levels of calcium in the blood.
Nursing diagnosis   Alteration in nutrient transport manifested by electrolyte imbalance.

Hypercholesterolemia   An elevated level of cholesterol in the blood.
Nursing diagnosis   Alteration in nutrient transport manifested by alteration in vascular physiology or by blockage of transport.
Dietary intervention   Weight reduction; reduced intake of foods high in saturated fat and cholesterol; replacement with polyunsaturated fat.

Hyperinsulinism   The excessive release of insulin.
Nursing diagnosis   Alteration in metabolism manifested by an alteration in endocrine physiology.
Dietary intervention   *See* diet for Functional hyperinsulinism.

Hyperlipoproteinemias   An elevation of one or more of the four lipoproteins in the blood that carry cholesterol or triglycerides.
Nursing diagnosis   Alteration in nutrient transport manifested by an alteration in vascular physiology; alteration in metabolism manifested by an alteration in nutritional requirements related to inborn errors.
Dietary intervention   Diet aimed at reduction of cholesterol and triglyceride levels by restrictions of Calories, dietary fat, cholesterol, carbohydrate, and alcohol. *See* Chapter 26 for specific diets for each of the five types of hyperlipoproteinemias.

Hypertension   High blood pressure.
Nursing diagnosis   Alteration in nutrient transport manifested by an alteration in vascular physiology.
Dietary intervention   Sodium-restricted (2,000–4,000 mg/day) diet.

Hyperthyroidism   An endocrine disorder caused by excessive thyroid gland secretion.

Nursing diagnosis   Alteration in metabolism manifested by an alteration in endocrine physiology.
Dietary intervention   High-Calorie, high-protein diet with supplements of calcium, phosphorus, vitamin D, B-complex vitamins, and vitamins A and C.

Hypertriglyceridemia   An elevation of triglycerides in the blood.
Nursing diagnosis   Alteration in nutrient transport manifested by an alteration in vascular physiology.
Dietary intervention   Reduction in total dietary fat and in the quantity of simple sugars; substitution of complex carbohydrates (starch) for simple sugars.

Hyperuricemia   An elevation of uric acid in the blood.
Nursing diagnosis   Alteration in metabolism manifested by an alteration in structure.
Dietary Intervention   Restriction of foods high in purines.

Hypervitaminosis   A toxicity produced by the excessive ingestion of vitamins.
Nursing diagnosis   Interference with ingestion manifested by an alteration in ingestion that has already occurred.

Hypoalbuminemia   A low level of albumin in the blood.
Nursing diagnosis   Alteration in metabolism manifested by an alteration in nutritional requirements. (decreased protein use).
Dietary intervention   Increased amount of high-quality dietary protein.

Hypochlorhydria   A deficiency of hydrochloric acid in the gastric juice.
Nursing diagnosis   Alteration in digestion manifested by an alteration in secretion.

Hypogeusesthesia   A diminished sense of taste.
Nursing diagnosis   Interference with ingestion manifested by a lack of desire to ingest food and fluids.

Hypoglycemia   A low level of blood glucose.
Nursing diagnosis   Alteration in metabolism manifested by an alteration in endocrine physiology.
Dietary intervention   For fasting hypoglycemia a high carbohydrate intake with between-meals feedings; for stimulative hypoglycemia or functional hyperinsulinism, a restriction of dietary carbohydrate.

Hypokalemia   A low level of potassium in the blood.

Nursing diagnosis Alteration in nutrient transport manifested by electrolyte imbalance.
Dietary intervention Ingestion encouraged of foods high in potassium.

Hyposmia A decreased sense of smell.
Nursing diagnosis Interference with ingestion manifested by a lack of desire to ingest food or fluids.

Hypothyroidism An endocrine disorder resulting from a decrease in activity of the thyroid gland.
Nursing diagnosis Alteration in metabolism manifested by an alteration in endocrine physiology.
Dietary intervention Reduction in caloric intake to control weight.

Ileitis An inflammatory condition of the ileum portion of the small intestine.
Nursing diagnosis Alteration in excretion manifested by an alteration in solid waste output.
Dietary intervention *See* diet for Regional enteritis.

Ileostomy The surgical establishment of an artificial opening from the ileum to the outside of the body.
Nursing diagnosis Alteration in excretion manifested by an alteration in solid waste output.
Dietary intervention High-protein, high-Calorie diet low in fiber, with variety of foods gradually increased as tolerated.

Inborn errors of metabolism A metabolic disorder of a hereditary nature resulting from an enzyme deficiency.
Nursing diagnosis Alteration in metabolism manifested by an alteration in nutritional requirements (inborn errors of metabolism).

Indigestion Faulty or incomplete digestion of food leading to unpleasant symptoms following a meal.
Nursing diagnosis Alteration in digestion manifested by alterations in motility and secretions.
Dietary intervention Slow eating; relaxation before, during, and after meals; avoidance of overeating, especially foods that are difficult to digest.

Infection The invasion of the body by pathogenic microorganisms and the response of the tissues to them. *See also* Sepsis.
Nursing diagnosis Alteration in metabolism manifested by an alteration in nutritional requirements (increased nutritional requirement).
Dietary intervention High-Calorie, high-protein diet with between-meal feedings and vitamin and mineral supplementation.

Insulin shock *See* Diabetic reaction.
Iron-deficiency anemia *See* Anemia, iron-deficiency.
Irritable colon Irregular contractions of the bowel with either excessive motility or loss of rectal sensibility, which can cause either diarrhea or constipation. Also called *spastic colitis* or *spastic colon.*
Nursing diagnosis Alteration in excretion manifested by an alteration in solid waste output.
Dietary intervention Low-residue diet with a high fluid intake.

Jaundice A yellow discoloration of the skin and mucous membranes owing to the accumulation of bile pigments in the blood.
Nursing diagnosis Alteration in metabolism manifested by an alteration in structure (skin).
Dietary intervention High-Calorie, high-protein, low-fat diet.

Kwashiorkor A deficiency disease resulting from an inadequate intake of protein.
Nursing diagnosis Interference with ingestion manifested by inaccessibility of nutrients.

Lactase deficiency A deficiency of the digestive enzyme lactase.
Nursing diagnosis Alteration in digestion manifested by an alteration in secretion.
Dietary intervention A reduction in the ingestion of milk and milk-containing products.

Lactose intolerance Malabsorption of lactose owing to a deficiency of the enzyme lactase.
Nursing diagnosis Alteration in absorption manifested by an alteration in secretion.
Dietary intervention Lactose-free diet.

Liver disease *See* Hepatitis, Cirrhosis, and Hepatic coma.

Malabsorption syndrome A set of symptoms that indicates defective absorption of nutrients.
Nursing diagnosis Alteration in absorption manifested by an alteration in secretion, an alteration in motility, or an alteration in absorptive surface.
Dietary intervention High Calories, high protein, low-to-moderate fat, vitamin and mineral supplementation; a low-residue diet for persistent diarrhea; the use of MCT oil as a source of fat and Calories.

Marasmus Severe undernutrition resulting from a deficiency of both Calories and protein.
Nursing diagnosis Interference with ingestion manifested by the inaccessibility of nutrients.

Multiple sclerosis A disorder of the CNS in which there is degeneration of the myelin sheath of the brain and spinal cord.
Nursing diagnosis Alteration in metabolism manifested by an alteration in structure; interferences with ingestion manifested by the inability to ingest food and fluids.
Dietary intervention Nutritionally balanced, adequate diet.

Muscular dystrophy A disorder of skeletal muscle in which there is progressive atrophy of the muscle.
Nursing diagnosis Alteration in metabolism manifested by an alteration in structure; interferences with ingestion manifested by the inability to ingest food and fluids.
Dietary intervention Nutritionally balanced, adequate diet.

Myocardial infarction An area of necrosis in the heart muscle caused by an interruption of the blood supply; commonly called a *heart attack*.
Nursing diagnosis Alteration in nutrient transport manifested by blockage of nutrient transport.
Dietary intervention For the acute phase; a 500 to 800-Calorie liquid diet with a volume of 1,000–1,500 ml; for the subacute phase; a 1000- to 1,200-Calorie soft or bland diet with cholesterol restricted to 300 mg/day; for the rehabilitative phase; attainment and maintenance of ideal weight and a fat-controlled diet with a sodium restriction.

Nephritis Inflammation of the kidney. *See also* Glomerulonephritis and Pyelonephritis.
Nursing diagnosis Alteration in excretion manifested by an alteration in fluid output.
Dietary intervention Normal protein (0.9–1 gm/kg body weight) unless signs of nitrogen retention (uremia) occur; sodium restriction (1,000–2,000 mg/day); fluid restricted to urinary output plus 500 ml; adequate Calories for protein sparing.

Nephrolithiasis A condition marked by the presence of renal calculi in the kidney or bladder.
Nursing diagnosis Alteration in excretion manifested by an alteration in fluid output.
Dietary intervention Diet aimed at the prevention or reduction of the formation of specific types of stones, e.g., a calcium- and phosphorus-restricted diet, an acid-ash or alkaline-ash diet, an oxalate-restricted diet, or a purine-restricted diet; forced fluids.

Nephrosclerosis A hardening of the renal arteries, usually accompanying renal hypertension.
Nursing diagnosis Alteration in excretion manifested by alteration in fluid output.
Dietary intervention Weight reduction for the obese; a sodium-restricted (250–500 mg) diet; decreased dietary protein intake, should nitrogen retention occur.

Nephrosis A gradual degeneration of the kidney. *See* Nephrotic syndrome.
Nursing diagnosis Alteration in excretion manifested by an alteration in fluid output.

Nephrotic syndrome A set of symptoms characterized by large amounts of proteinuria and massive edema.
Nursing diagnosis Alteration in excretion manifested by an alteration in fluid output.
Dietary intervention High-protein (120–150 gm/day), sodium-restricted (1,000–2,000 mg/day) diet.

Neuropathy Any disorder of the peripheral nerves.
Nursing diagnosis Alteration in metabolism manifested by an alteration in structure.

Nutritional deficiency diseases A disease that results from a deficiency of an essential nutrient, either from a deficient dietary intake or from impaired absorption or use within the body.
Nursing diagnosis Interference with ingestion manifested by the inaccessibility of nutrients or by the inability to ingest food and fluids.

Obesity An accumulation of body fat to about 20% or more above ideal body weight.
Nursing diagnosis Interference with ingestion manifested by an alteration in ingestion that has already occurred.
Dietary intervention Reduction of caloric intake below energy requirement but sufficient to allow for a safe weight loss.

Osteomalacia An inadequate mineral content of the bones resulting from a deficiency of vitamin D, calcium, and/or phosphorus; also called *adult rickets*.
Nursing diagnosis Interference with ingestion manifested by inaccessibility of nutrients.

Overweight The accumulation of body fat to about 10–20% above ideal body weight.
Nursing diagnosis Interference with ingestion manifested by an alteration in ingestion that has already occurred.
Dietary intervention A reduction in caloric intake.

Pancreatic insufficiency   A deficiency of pancreatic secretions.
Nursing diagnosis Alteration in digestion manifested by an alteration in secretions.

Pancreatitis   Inflammation of the pancreas.
Nursing diagnosis Alteration in digestion manifested by an alteration in secretions.
Dietary intervention For acute attacks, no oral feeding; otherwise, a clear liquid diet or an elemental liquid diet; in less severe attacks, easily digested foods that are very low in fat.

Parkinson's disease   A neurological disorder characterized by muscular tremors and rigidity; affects walking, speaking, chewing, and swallowing.
Nursing diagnosis Alteration in metabolism manifested by an alteration in structure.
Dietary intervention Low-protein diet of high-quality protein to enhance the drug therapy.

Pellagra   A nutritional deficiency disease resulting from a lack of niacin.
Nursing diagnosis Interference with ingestion manifested by the inaccessibility of nutrients.

Peptic ulcer   A sore or ulceration of the mouth, esophagus, or duodenum caused by the action of gastric juice.
Nursing diagnosis Alteration in digestion manifested by an alteration in secretions.
Dietary intervention Bland diet with between-meal feedings.

Penicious anemia   *See* Anemia, pernicious.

Pernicious vomiting (hyperemesis)   Excessive vomiting.
Nursing diagnosis Interference with ingestion manifested by a lack of desire to ingest food and fluids and by the inability to ingest food and fluids.
Dietary intervention IV administration of glucose for 1–2 days; after vomiting diminishes, simple carbohydrate foods such as dry toast and crackers as tolerated; fluids between meals and not with meals.

Phenylketonuria   An inherited inborn error of metabolism resulting from the lack of the enzyme phenylalanine hydroxylase, which is required to convert phenylalanine to tyrosine.
Nursing diagnosis Alteration in metabolism manifested by an alteration in nutritional requirements (inborn errors of metabolism).
Dietary intervention Phenylalanine-restricted diet.

Proteinuria   The excretion of protein in the urine.

Nursing diagnosis Alteration in excretion manifested by an alteration in fluid output; alterations in metabolism manifested by decreased protein use.
Dietary intervention Dietary protein increased by the amount lost in the urine.

Pyelonephritis   An inflammation of the kidney and its pelvis caused by the invasion of bacteria from the urinary tract.
Nursing diagnosis Alteration in excretion manifested by an alteration in fluid output.
Dietary intervention Emphasis on the inclusion of foods that leave an acid ash such as cereals, meats, cranberries, and plums; forced fluids.

Radiation therapy   The treatment of cancer by means of x-radiation.
Nursing diagnosis Interference with ingestion manifested by a lack of desire to ingest food and fluids or by oral discomfort.
Dietary intervention Appetizing food according to the client's food preferences; small, frequent feedings.

Regional enteritis (or ileitis)   Crohn's disease; a chronic inflammatory disease process of the intestines, particularly the ileum.
Nursing diagnosis Alteration in excretion manifested by an alteration in solid waste output; alteration in absorption manifested by an alteration in the absorptive surface.
Dietary intervention High Calories, high protein, low residue, with vitamin and mineral supplementation.

Renal calculi   Kidney stones (*See* Calculus).

Renal failure   A loss of functioning nephrons in the kidney to the point where the kidneys are no longer able to filter the blood and maintain the normal composition of constituents in the blood.
Nursing diagnosis Alteration in excretion manifested by an alteration in fluid output.
Dietary intervention Low protein (20–40 gm/day), sodium restriction (500–1,500 mg/day), potassium restriction (1,100–2,000 mg/day), fluid restriction (800–1000 ml/day), high Calories, high carbohydrate, vitamin and mineral supplementation.

Rickets   A nutritional deficiency disease caused by a lack of vitamin D or a disturbance in calcium-phosphorus metabolism.
Nursing diagnosis Interference with ingestion manifested by the inaccessibility of nutrients.

Scurvy A nutritional deficiency disease caused by a lack of vitamin C.
Nursing diagnosis Interference with ingestion manifested by the inaccessibility of nutrients.

Sepsis Infection caused by the products or toxins of pathogenic bacteria.
Nursing diagnosis Alteration in metabolism manifested by alteration in nutritional requirements (increased nutritional requirements)
Dietary intervention High-Calorie, high-protein diet with between-meal feedings or supplements and vitamin and mineral supplementation, particularly vitamins A and C.

Spastic colon *See* Irritable colon.

Sprue A chronic disease characterized by diarrhea, steatorrhea, malabsorption, weight loss, and anemia.
Nursing diagnosis Alteration in absorption manifested by an alteration in the absorptive surface or by an alteration in secretion.
Dietary intervention *See* diet for Celiac disease.

Steatorrhea The presence of fat in the stool.
Nursing diagnosis Alteration in absorption manifested by an alteration in the absorptive surface or by an alteration in secretion.
Dietary intervention *See* diet for Malabsorption syndrome.

Stress Any stimulus that interferes with the homeostasis of an organism. Stress factors may be physiological, pathological, physical, or psychological.
Nursing diagnosis Alteration in metabolism manifested by an alteration in nutritional requirements (increased nutritional requirements).
Dietary intervention High-Calorie, high-protein diet with between-meal feedings or supplements and vitamin and mineral supplementation.

Surgery The treatment of disease by operative procedures.
Nursing diagnosis Alteration in metabolism manifested by an alteration in nutritional requirements (increased nutritional requirements); interferences with ingestion manifested by inability to ingest food and fluids.
Dietary intervention High-Calorie, high-protein diet with between-meal feedings or supplements if needed and supplements of iron, vitamin C, B-complex vitamins, and vitamin K.

Tonsillectomy Surgical removal of a tonsil or tonsils.

Nursing diagnosis Interference with ingestion manifested by inability to ingest food and fluids and by oral discomfort and/or obstruction.
Dietary intervention Cold liquids, fruit juices, and sherbet following surgery progressing to soft foods and gradual resumption of a regular diet as tolerated.

Toxemia of pregnancy A series of pathological conditions that are metabolic disturbances; they include pernicious vomiting; edema, hypertension, albuminuria; finally, convulsions and coma.
Nursing diagnosis Interference with ingestion manifested by lack of desire to ingest food and fluids or by inability to ingest food and fluids; alteration in nutrient transport manifested by electrolyte imbalance and by fluid volume alterations; alteration in metabolism manifested by an alteration in nutritional requirements (decreased protein use).
Dietary intervention Sodium-restricted diet.

Toxicity of vitamins and minerals The ingestion of excess quantities of vitamins and/or minerals, resulting in symptoms of toxicity.
Nursing diagnosis Interference with ingestion manifested by an alteration in ingestion that has already occurred.

Trauma A wound or injury.
Nursing diagnosis Alteration in metabolism manifested by an alteration in nutritional requirements (increased nutritional requirements); interference with ingestion manifested by inability to ingest nutrients; alteration in absorption manifested by an alteration in motility.
Dietary intervention High-Calorie, high-protein, high-carbohydrate diet with between-meal feedings or supplements and vitamin and mineral supplementation.

Ulcerative colitis A chronic inflammation and ulceration in the colon.
Nursing diagnosis Alteration in excretion manifested by an alteration in solid waste output.
Dietary intervention High-Calorie, high-protein, low-residue diet with between-meal feedings and supplements and vitamin and mineral supplementation; during acute attacks, possible use of an elemental or minimal-residue diet.

Undernutrition A state of nutritional status caused by a deficiency in nutrients and/or Calories.
Nursing diagnosis Interference with ingestion manifested by the inaccessibility of nutrients.

Underweight   A decrease in body weight to more than 10% below the ideal weight for a given age, sex, and height.
Nursing diagnosis   Interference with ingestion manifested by the inaccessibility of nutrients, by a lack of desire to ingest food and fluids, by inability to ingest food and fluids, or by oral obstruction and/or discomfort.
Dietary intervention   Calorie increase achieved by gradual increase in the quantity of food and addition of high-Calorie feedings between meals.

Uremia   A toxic condition produced by the retention of urinary constituents in the blood.
Nursing diagnosis   Alteration in metabolism manifested by an alteration in nutritional requirements (decreased protein use); alteration in nutrient transport manifested by electrolyte imbalance.
Dietary intervention   High Calories, high carbohydrate, low protein (20–40 gm/day). Protein must be of high biological quality and include one egg and ¾ cup milk to provide the essential amino acids.

Urinary calculi   A stone in any part of the urinary tract formed by the precipitation of insoluble constituents in the urine.
Nursing diagnosis   Alteration in excretion manifested by an alteration in fluid output.
Dietary intervention   *See* diet for Nephrolithiasis.

Urinary tract infection   An infection within the urinary tract resulting from the presence of pathogenic bacteria.
Nursing diagnosis   Alteration in excretion manifested by an alteration in fluid output.
Dietary intervention   Forced fluids; consumption of foods to acidify the urine such as cranberries and plums.

Xerophthalmia   A serious eye disease thats results from a deficiency of vitamin A.
Nursing diagnosis   Interference with ingestion manifested by the inaccessibility of nutrients.

GLOSSARY

Absorption The step in the nutritive process in which the end products of digestion pass through the walls of the intestinal tract.

Acetoacetic acid An intermediate product of normal fatty acid metabolism. An accumulation of this acid in the blood indicates incomplete fatty acid oxidation.

Acetone An intermediate in fatty acid metabolism formed by the removal of carbon dioxide from acetoacetic acid. It accumulates in the blood and urine when fatty acid degradation is incomplete or excessive.

Acetylcholine An important compound in the body that has many physiological functions, such as the transmission of nerve impulse.

Acetyl-CoA (acetylcoenzyme A) An important compound in the Krebs cycle, formed by a combination of acetic acid and coenzyme A. It is also an important intermediate in fatty acid oxidation and synthesis.

Achlorhydria The absence of hydrochloric acid in the gastric secretions.

Acid Any substance that liberates hydrogen ions when placed in an aqueous solution.

Acid-base balance The equalization of acidic and basic components in the body fluids to levels that are compatible with life.

Acidosis A condition resulting from the accumulation of too many acids or the loss of two much alkali from the body.

Acrolein An irritating liquid that results from the decomposition of glycerin.

Acromegaly A chronic condition resulting from the hypersecretion of growth hormone during adulthood.

Actin One of the two proteins of the muscle fibril. When combined with myosin in actomyosin it is involved with muscular contraction and relaxation.

Active transport An energy requiring mechanism by which substances are transported across cell membranes.

Adenine A purine that is an essential component of the nucleic acids RNA and DNA.

Adenosine diphosphate (ADP) A high energy phosphate compound composed of adenine, ribose, and two molecules of phosphate.

Adenosine monophosphate (AMP) A compound composed of one molecule each of adenine, ribose, and phosphoric acid.

Adenosine triphosphate (ATP) A high-energy compound for the storage and release of energy within the cell, containing an adenine and molecule and three phosphate molecules.

Adipose Fatty tissue that acts as a storage reservoir for excess body fat.

Aerobic Functioning in the presence of oxygen.

Afferent fibers Sensory fibers carrying nerve impulses from the periphery to the central nervous system.

Albumin A protein in body tissues and fluids.

Aldehyde A group of organic compounds containing a carbon-hydrogen-oxygen group.

Aldosterone A hormone secreted by the adrenal cortex. It helps regulate electrolyte balance by causing the reabsorption of sodium and water and the excretion of potassium.

Alkalosis A condition, resulting from the loss of excess acids or the accumulation of too much base, in which the alkalinity of the body increases beyond normal.

Allergen An agent or substance capable of producing an allergic reaction.

Alimentary tract The digestive tract extending from the mouth to the anus.

Alopecia Loss of hair.

Amino acid A chemical compound that contains an amino and a carboxyl (acid) group. Amino acids are the individual components of protein.

Amniotic fluid The fluid surrounding the developing fetus, which serves to protect it.

Amphetamine A drug that is an appetite depressant and a central nervous system stimulant.

Amylase An enzyme that catalyzes the hydrolysis of starch.

Amylopectin Branched glucose chains of the polysaccharide starch.

Amylose Unbranched glucose chains of the polysaccharide starch.

Anabolism The synthesis or manufacture of complex substances from simple substances.

Anaerobic Functioning in the absence of oxygen.

Anaphylaxis A hypersensitivity to a substance or foreign protein; characterized by widespread systemic involvement.

Anastomosis The surgical joining of two internal parts of the body.

Anemia A condition in which there is a reduction of circulating red blood cells or hemoglobin.

Angiotensin A vasoconstrictor substance present in the blood; it stimulates the secretion of aldosterone by the adrenal cortex.

Anion A negatively charged ion.

Anorexia A decreased desire for food.

Antepartum The time before birth.

Anthropometric The type of measurements that deal with the size, weight, and proportions of the human body.

Anthropometry The science concerned with the measurement of the size, weight, and proportions of the human body.

Antibody A substance produced in the body in response to the invasion by a foreign substance called an *antigen*.

Anticoagulant A substance that prevents or inhibits coagulation by interfering with the clotting mechanism.

Antiemetic An agent that prevents or alleviates vomiting.

Antigen A foreign substance that causes the body to produce antibodies.

Antioxidant A substance capable of preventing or retarding oxidation of another substance.

Antivitamin A substance that interferes with the metabolism or synthesis of a vitamin.

Anuria Absence of urinary excretion.

Apathy Lack of interest and emotion.

Appetite A psychological desire for food based on pleasant past experiences with food.

Arachidonic acid An unsaturated fatty acid containing 200 carbons and 4 double bonds. It is synthesized in the body from the essential fatty acid linoleic acid.

Ariboflavinosis A deficiency of riboflavin.

Arrhythmia A variation in the normal rhythm of the heartbeat.

Arteiole A minute artery branch adjacent to a capillary.

Ascorbic acid Another name for vitamin C.

-Ase Suffix used to denote an enzyme.

Asymptomatic Without symptoms.

Ataxia Loss of ability to coordinate muscular movements.

Atrophy Wasting; a general decrease in size of a cell, tissue, organ, or body.

Auscultation A physical assessment techniqe involving listening to body sounds, usually with a stethoscope.

Azotemia The symptoms caused by an elevation of nitrogenous constituents in the blood.

Basal metabolic rate (BMR) The amount of human energy expended per unit of time or per unit of body size when the body is at rest and is in a postabsorptive state (12 hours after the ingestion of food).

Basal metabolism The amount of energy needed to sustain the involuntary activities of the body.

Base A substance that will accept or bind with hydrogen ions in an aqueous solution.

Basic four food groups Four groups of foods and the recommended number of daily servings of each, which serve as a guide to good eating. The four food groups are: milk, meat, fruits and vegetables, and grain.

Benign Not fatal nor endangering to life; the opposite of malignant.

Beriberi A nutritional deficiency disease caused by a deficiency of thiamine.

Beta-hydroxybutyric acid An intermediate compound in the oxidation of fatty acids. It is composed of four carbons.

Bicarbonate ion An acid salt of carbonic acid. The bicarbonate ion is HCO_3^-.

Bile acids Acids formed in the liver and secreted in the bile.

Bio- A prefix meaning *life*.

Biological value The relative nutritional value of a protein based on its content of essential amino acids.

Biopsy The removal and examination of a piece of living tissue for the purpose of diagnosis.

Biotin One of the members of the B-complex group of vitamins.

Bitot's spots Gray or silver triangular spots on the conjunctiva caused by a vitamin A deficiency.

Bolus A mass of food entering the esophagus.

Bone density The amount of mineral composition of the bone.

Bone matrix The protein framework in which the minerals are deposited.

Botulism A severe, sometimes fatal form of poisoning caused by a toxin of *Clostridium botulinum* in improperly canned food.

Brush border The microvilli on the surface of an intestinal epithelial cell, which greatly increases the surface area of the small intestine.

Buffer A chemical that tends to stabilize the pH of a solution despite the addition of acids or bases. Buffers are very important in regulating the acid-base balance of the body.

Cachexia A syndrome in clients with chronic diseases or terminal illnesses; it is characterized by extreme weight loss, weakness, and severe wasting of body tissues.

Caffeine A substance found in coffee, tea, and cola beverages; it acts as a cardiac and renal stimulant.

Calciferol Vitamin D_2 of plant origin formed by irradiation of ergosterol.

Calcification The deposition of calcium salts in the tissues of the body. Calcification of the bones is a normal physiological process, but calcification of such tissues as the arteries, kidneys, and lungs is pathological.

Calcitonin A hornome secreted by the thyroid gland; it inhibits the release of calcium from the bones and into the blood.

Calculus An abnormal stony mass in the body; composed of organic material and mineral salts. It is commonly referred to as a *stone*.

Caliper An instrument used to measure the thickness or diameter of various parts of the body.

Calorie A unit of heat. The small Calorie is the amount of heat required to raise the temperature of 1 gm of water 1 C. The large Calorie (kilocalorie) is the amount of heat required to raise the temperature of 1 kg of water 1 C.

Calorimeter An apparatus used to measure the amount of heat produced by a food or person.

Calorimetry The science of measuring the production of heat.

Capillary A minute blood vessel that connects arterioles to venules.

Carbohydrates Chemical substances composed of carbon, hydrogen, and oxygen; commonly referred to as *starches* and *sugars*.

Carbonic acid The acid that is formed when carbon dioxide is dissolved in water.

Carboxyl group The group found in most organic acids (—COOH).

Carboxylase An enzyme that contains thiamine and catalyzes the removal of the carboxyl group.

Carboxypeptidase An intestinal enzyme that catalyzes the hydrolysis of polypetides.

Carcinoma A malignant tumor; cancer.

Cardiogenic failure Heart failure.

Caries Tooth decay.

Cariogenic Conducive to producing decay.

Carotene The precursor of vitamin A; found in plants.

Cartilage A type of connective tissue in which cells are embedded in a matrix of collagen fibers.

Cathartics An agent that promotes defecation.

Casein The principal protein in milk.

Catabolism The process of breaking down complex substances into simpler ones.

Catalyst A substance that speeds up a chemical reaction without itself undergoing any change.

Catheter A slender tube inserted into the body for the purpose of removing fluid, especially into the bladder through the urethra for the removal of urine.

Cation A postively charged ion.

Cecum The blind pouch located between the ileum and the first part of the colon from which the appendix is suspended.

Cell The basic structural and functional unit of life.

Cellulose An indigestible carbohydrate that composes the structural part of plants.

Cementum The bony tissue covering the root of the tooth.

Cephalic phase The initial phase of digestion in which the thought, sight, or smell of food initiates salivary and gastric secretion.

Cephalin A phospholipid found in brain and nervous tissue.

Cerebrospinal fluid The colorless fluid formed from blood plasma which serves to transport nutrients and waste products and provides a protective cushion for the brain and spinal cord.

Cheilosis Bilateral cracks or fisures at the corners of the mouth resulting from a deficiency of riboflavin.

Chlorophyll The green pigment in plants that, in the presence of light, manufactures carbohydrates from carbon dioxide and water by the process of photosynthesis.

Cholecalciferol A form of vitamin D formed from the irradiation of 7-dehydrocholesterol; vitamin D_3.

Cholecystokinin A hormone produced in the duodenum in response to the presence of fat; it stimulates contraction of the gall bladder and the release of bile.

Cholesterol A fat-related compound found in animal foods and present within human tissues.

Choline A substance necessary for the transport of fat in the body.

Chondroitin sulfate A mucopolysaccharide found in skin and cartilage.

Chylomicron A lipoprotein composed mainly of lipid surrounded by a protein coating.

Chyme The semifluid mass produced by the gastric digestion of food.

Chymotrypsin A digestive enzyme secreted by the pancreas for the hydrolysis of protein.

Citric acid An organic acid that is a key compound in the Krebs cycle.

Citric acid cycle *See* Krebs cycle and Tricarboxylic acid cycle.

Clostridium A genus of anaerobic sporeforming bacteria. Examples of two members are *Clostridium botulinum*, which can cause botulism, and *Clostridium perfringens*, which causes gangrene.

Cobalamin The many forms of vitamin B_{12}, which all contain cobalt.

Cocarboxylase A coenzyme of carboxylase; contains thiamine.

Coenzyme An organic molecule required for the action of an enzyme. Coenzymes are usually organic molecules related to a vitamin, such as thiamine, riboflavin, niacin, pyridoxine, folic acid, and pantothenic acid.

Coenzyme A (CoA) An important coenzyme containing pantothenic acid; helps form active acetate for entrance into the Krebs cycle. It is also involved with fatty acid synthesis and oxidation.

Collagen A protein found in the organic matrix of bone, cartilage, and connective tissue.

Colonic Pertaining to the colon or the part of the large intestine extending from the cecum to the rectum.

Colostomy The establishment of an artificial opening from a region of the colon to the outside of the body.

Colostrum The first milk secreted by the mammary gland a few days after birth of a baby.

Coma An abnormal state of unconsciousness from which a patient cannot be aroused.

Congenital Existing at or before birth.

Conjunctiva The mucous membrane covering the eyeball and lining of the eyelids.

Connective tissue All the tissues that bind together and support the various structures of the body.

Cortex The outer layers of an organ.

Cortisone 1. A hormone secreted by the adrenal cortex; it regulates carbohydrate metabolism. 2. A steroid used in the treatment of arthritis and other disorders.

Costochondral beading Sharp projections formed at the end of the ribs as a result of deficiency of vitamin C.

Craniotabes An abnormal softening of the bones of the skull associated with a reduced mineralization of the skull.

Creatine A constituent of muscle; as creatine phosphate it is essential for muscle contraction.

Creatinine An end product of creatine metabolism in muscle tissue.

Cretinism A disease produced in the offspring from a chronic iodine deficiency in the mother.

Crude fiber   Indigestible plant fiber, primarily cellulose and lignin.

Cyanosis   A bluish discoloration of the skin and mucous membranes.

-Cyte   A suffix meaning *cell*.

Cytochromes   A group of respiratory enzymes concerned with the transfer of electrons for the release of energy.

Cytoplasm   The protoplasm of the cell outside the nucleus.

Deamination   Removal of the amino group from an amino acid.

Debility   Bodily weakness; general loss of strength.

Decarboxylation   Removal of carbon dioxide (carboxyl group) from a molecule by a specific enzyme (decarboxylase).

Defecation   Elimination of solid waste material from the anus.

Dehydrocholesterol, 7-   A derivative of cholesterol in the skin that is converted to vitamin D in the presence of sunlight.

Dehydrogenases   Enzymes that catalyze the transfer of hydrogen from a carrier to an acceptor.

Dementia   A mental disorder characterized by mental deterioration.

Dentin   The main substance of the tooth; it surrounds the pulp and is covered by the enamel and cementum.

Deoxyribonucleic acid (DNA)   A nucleic acid that contains the code for protein synthesis.

Dermatitis   An inflammation of the skin.

Dermatosis   Any disorder of the skin.

Detoxification   The conversion within the body of toxic substances into less toxic forms that can be excreted.

Dextrin   An intermediate product in the hydrolysis of starch.

Dextrose   Another term for glucose.

Dialysis   Removal of substances in solution by selective diffusion through a semipermeable membrane.

Diaphoresis   Profuse perspiration.

Diarrhea   The frequent passage of loose, unformed stool.

Diffusion   The movement of molecules from a region of higher to lower concentration.

Digestion   The breakdown of food mechanically and chemically into simpler units that can be absorbed.

Diglyceride   A fat composed of two fatty acids attached to a glycerol molecule.

Disaccharide   A sugar composed of two monosaccharides.

Distention   A feeling of fullness or bloating after a meal.

Diuresis   An increased excretion of urine.

Diuretic   A substance that promotes the excretion of urine.

Duodenum   The first portion of the small intestine extending from the stomach to the jejunum.

Dys-   A prefix meaning *bad*.

Dyscrasia   A morbid condition, especially one that involves an imbalance of components of the blood or lymph.

Dysgeusia   A perverted sense of taste.

Dysosmia   An impaired sense of smell.

Dyspepsia   Feelings of physical discomfort following the ingestion of food; indigestion.

Dysphagia   Difficulty swallowing.

Dyspnea   Difficult or labored breathing.

Edema   An abnormal accumulation of fluid in the intercellular spaces of the body.

Efferent fibers   Motor fibers carrying impulses from the central nervous system to the muscles.

Elastin   The protein constituent of yellow, elastic fibers in ligaments and blood vessels.

Electrolyte   Any compound that releases charged particles when dissolved in water.

Emaciation   Wasting away of body tissue.

Embryo   The developing human organism from one week after conception until the end of the second month.

Emesis   Vomiting.

-Emia   A suffix referring to a condition of the blood.

Enamel   The hard outer covering of the tooth.

Endemic   Occurring infrequently but constantly in a particular region.

Endocrine gland   Ductless gland that secretes hormones directly into the bloodstream.

Endogenous   Originating within the cells or tissues of the body.

Endoplasmic reticulum   A system of membranes or channels in the cell that provide a method of transportation for substances within the cell.

Energy   Capacity to do work. Energy is derived from the use of foods. The body requires energy for physical activity, maintenance of body temperature, and metabolic reactions.

Energy balance   A balance between energy consumption in foods and energy expenditure so that a person maintains his ideal body weight.

Enrichment   The replacement in bread and cereal products of thiamine, riboflavin, niacin, and iron removed during processing.

Enteric   Pertaining to the intestines.

Enzyme   A protein substance produced by living tissue; it initiates or speeds up metabolic reactions.

Epidemiology   The scientific study of the frequency and distribution of human diseases.

Epidermis   The outer layer of the skin.

Epigastric   Pertaining to the upper and middle part of the abdomen in front of the stomach.

Epinephrine   The hormone secreted by the medulla of the adrenal gland; it increases blood pressure, heart rate, and the level of blood glucose.

Epistaxis   Hemorrhage from the nose; nosebleed.

Epithelial   Tissues that cover the exterior surface of the body and line the body cavities.

Ergosterol   A provitamin form of vitamin D which is converted to vitamin D_2 (calciferol) upon exposure to irradiation or ultraviolet light.

Eructation   The act of belching.

Erythrocyte   A mature red blood cell.

Erythropoiesis   The formation of red blood cells.

Essential amino acid   An amino acid that must be supplied by the diet for tissue growth, repair, and maintenance.

Ethnicity   The part of a person's value system that he learns from his family of origin and his environment. This learning occurs before the person is able to discriminate its usefulness for himself.

Ethnocentric   The belief in one's own way as best and desired.

Etiology   The study of causes of disease.

Exacerbation   An increase in the severity of symptoms.

Exchange lists   Lists that a group together sizes of foods that contain similar quantities of nutrients and/or Calories. There are food exchange lists based on carbohydrate, protein, fat, and Calorie content; sodium content; and protein, sodium, and potassium content.

Excretion   The process of eliminating waste material from the body.

Exogenous   Originating outside the body.

Extracellular fluid   The fluid outside the cell.

Fats   Chemical substances composed of carbon, hydrogen, and oxygen but that contain more hydrogen than carbohydrates. Fats are greasy to the touch and insoluble in water.

Fatty acid   An organic acid composed of carbon, hydrogen, and oxygen. Fatty acids are classified as either saturated or unsaturated.

Febrile   Having a fever.

Feces   The semisolid excrement from the intestines.

Ferritin   An iron-protein complex in the liver, spleen, bone marrow, and reticuloendothelial cells; the main storage form of iron in the body.

Fetus   The developing young in the human uterus from the beginning of the third month until birth.

Fiber   The portions of food that can not be digested in humans.

Fibrinogen   A plasma protein that is converted to fibrin in the blood-clotting process.

Fibrosis   The formation of an abnormal amount of tough, fibrous connective tissue in an organ.

Filariasis   An infectious tropical disease caused by parasitic nematode worms.

Filtration   The selective passage of fluid through a semipermeable membrane under the force of hydrostatic pressure.

Fistula   An abnormal passage between two internal organs or from an internal organ to the surface of the body.

Flatulence   The presence of gas or air in the stomach or intestines.

Flavin adenine dinucleotide (FAD)   A riboflavin coenzyme compound that functions in dehydrogenations. It is a part of many enzyme systems, including D-amino acid oxidase, and results from the condensation of a molecule each of riboflavin 5'-phosphate and adenosine 5'-phosphate.

Flavin mononucleotide (FMN) Riboflavin 5'-phosphate. A riboflavin coenzyme compound that functions in dehydrogenations. It is a part of the L-amino acid oxidase.

Flavoprotein A protein containing a yellow pigment. Two flavoproteins that contain riboflavin are FAD (flavin adenine dinucleotide) and FMN (flavin mononucleotide).

Fluorosis A condition of discolored tooth enamel resulting from the excess ingestion of fluorine.

Folacin (folic acid) A member of the B-complex group of vitamins.

Follicular hyperkeratosis A symptom of vitamin A deficiency in which the skin is dry and scaly and eruptions that resemble goose flesh form around the hair follicles.

Food Any substance that, when ingested, causes an organism to grow and maintain its health.

Food additive Any substance added to a food that affects the functional characteristics of the food or becomes a component of the food.

Foodways Behaviors that influence what people eat.

Fortification The addition of nutrients to a food so that the food contains more nutrients than were present originally.

Fructose A 6-carbon monosaccharide found primarily in fruits and honey or obtained from the hydrolysis of sucrose.

Galactose A monosaccharide that results from the hydrolysis of lactose.

Galactosemia A hereditary disorder characterized by an accumulation of galactose in the blood, resulting from a lack of the enzyme needed to convert galactose to glucose.

Gastrectomy The surgical removal of all or part of the stomach.

Gastric Pertaining to the stomach.

Gastrin A hormone secreted by the pyloric mucosa, and stimulating the parietal cells to secrete hydrochloric acid.

Gastrointestinal Referring to the stomach and intestines.

Gastrostomy The surgical establishment of an opening into the stomach for the purpose of feeding.

Geriatrics A branch of medicine concerned with the diseases and problems of aging.

Gerontology The study of aging and the problems of aging.

Gingival hyperplasia Overgrowth of the gum.

Gingivitis Inflammation of the gums.

Gliadin A protein fraction of the protein gluten.

Glial cells The supporting cells of the central nervous system.

Glomerular filtration rate (GFR) The rate at which blood passes through the glomeruli of the kidney each minute.

Glossitis Inflammation of the tongue.

Glucocorticoid A hormone produced by the adrenal cortex; it increases gluconeogenesis and the level of blood glucose.

Glucogenic Glucose forming.

Gluconeogenesis The formation of glucose from noncarbohydrate sources.

Glucose A 6-carbon monosaccharide occurring in fruit and honey. It is also obtained from hydrolysis of starch, maltose, lactose, and sucrose. Dextrose is another name for glucose.

Gluten The protein in wheat and other cereal grains; it gives an elastic quality to bread dough.

Glyceride A fat formed by combining glycerol and one, two, or three fatty acids.

Glycerol A 3-carbon alcohol resulting from the hydrolysis of fat.

Glycogen A polysaccharide that is the storage form of carbohydrate in humans and animals.

Glycogenesis The formation of glycogen.

Glycogenolysis The breakdown of glycogen to glucose.

Glycolysis The breakdown of glucose or glycogen into simpler compounds, resulting in the release of energy.

Glycosuria The presence of glucose in the urine.

Goiter An enlargement of the thyroid gland.

Golgi complex An organelle concerned with the manufacture and release of substances within the cell. It is connected to the endoplasmic reticulum.

Gustation The sense of taste.

Health A state of physical and psychological well-being; not simply the absence of disease.

Hematemesis Vomiting blood.

Hematocrit The volume percentage of red blood cells in whole blood.

Hematopoietic (hemopoietic)   Concerned with the formation of blood.

Hematuria   Blood in the urine.

Heme   The iron-containing portion of hemoglobin.

Hemicellulose   A type of indigestible carbohydrate in plants.

Hemochromatosis   A genetic disorder of iron metabolism; characterized by deposits of iron in tissues.

Hemodialysis   The removal of certain constituents from the blood by passing the blood through a semipermeable membrane.

Hemoglobin   The iron-protein pigment in red blood cells; it carries oxygen to the tissues

Hemolytic anemia   A type of anemia resulting from an excessive destruction of red blood cells.

Hemoptysis   Coughing and spitting of blood as a result of bleeding from any part of the respiratory tract.

Hemorrhage   An excessive escape of blood from the blood vessels; bleeding.

Hemosiderin   An insoluble form of storage iron.

Hemosiderosis   An increase of the iron stores in the tissues.

Heparin   A mucopolysaccharide that prevents the clotting of blood.

Hepatic   Pertaining to the liver.

Hepatomegaly   Enlargement of the liver.

Homeostasis   The ability of the body to maintain constant physiological conditions.

Hormone   A chemical substance produced in the body by an endocrine gland and released directly into the bloodstream. It has a specific regulatory function on other tissues or organs.

Hunger   The physiological response of the body when energy needs are not being met, accompanied by a drive to secure food to eat.

Hydrogenation   The process of adding hydrogen to an unsaturated fat to make it more saturated, in the process changing the fat from a liquid to a solid.

Hydrolysis   A chemical reaction, occurring in the presence of water, in which compound is split into simpler components.

Hydroxyapatite crystals   The mineral deposits of bone, composed mainly of calcium and phosphorus.

Hyper-   A prefix meaning *elevated* or *excessive*.

Hypercalcemia   An excess level of calcium in the blood.

Hypercalciuria   Abnormal excretion of calcium in the urine.

Hyperchlorhydria   An excessive secretion of hydrochloric acid in the stomach.

Hyperemia   An excess quantity of blood in a part of the body.

Hyperglycemia   An excess amount of glucose in the blood.

Hyperkalemia   An abnormally high level of potassium in the blood.

Hyperlipoproteinemia   Excess levels of lipoproteins in the blood.

Hypernatremia   Excessive levels of sodium in the blood.

Hyperplasia   An increase in the number of cells.

Hypertension   Elevated blood pressure.

Hypertriglyceridemia   Excess levels of triglycerides in the blood.

Hypertrophy   An increase in the size of cells.

Hyperuricemia   An excess quantity of uric acid in the blood.

Hyperventilation   Abnormally prolonged and deep breathing usually associated with anxiety.

Hypervitaminosis   A condition produced by the excess ingestion of vitamins, especially vitamins A and D.

Hypo-   A prefix meaning *lack* or *deficiency*.

Hypoalbuminemia   A decreased level of albumin in the blood.

Hypochlorhydria   A deficiency of hydrochloric acid secreted by the stomach.

Hypochromic   A pale color; usually refers to a decrease in the hemoglobin content of a red blood cell.

Hypogeusesthesia   Decreased taste sensitivity; also called *hypogeusia*.

Hypoglycemia   An abnormally low level of glucose in the blood.

Hypokalemia   An abnormally low level of potassium in the blood.

Hyponatremia   A decreased level of sodium in the blood.

Hyposmia   A decreased sense of smell.

Hypotension   Blood pressure lower than a person's norm; usually less than 100 mmHg systolic and/or 60 mmHg diastolic.

Hypothalamus An area at the base of the brain responsible for regulating a number of physiological functions including the control of appetite and satiety.

Hypovolemia An abnormally decreased volume of circulating fluid (plasma) in the body.

Iatrogenic Physician induced.

Ichthyosis A condition characterized by dry, rough, scaly skin.

Ideal body weight The standard weight at age 25 associated with the most favorable mortality.

Idiopathic Without any known origin or cause.

Ileostomy The establishment of an artificial opening from a region of the ileum to the outside of the body.

Ileum The final portion of the small intestine extending from the jejunum to the colon.

Incontinence The inability to restrain or control the excretion of urine or feces.

Index of Nutritional Quality (INQ) The ratio of the percent standard of a given nutrient to the percent standard of energy (in Calories).

Infarction The death or decay of tissue owing to the obstruction of the flow of blood to that part.

Ingestion The process of taking in food or beverage.

Inorganic Referring to mineral matter; not associated with living things.

Insulin The hormone secreted by the beta cells of the pancreas; it lowers blood glucose.

Integument The skin.

Interstitial fluid Fluid present in the spaces between the tissues.

Intestinal transit time The length of time required for ingested food to travel from the mouth to the anus.

Intracellular fluid Fluid present within the cell.

Intravenous Into or within a vein.

Intrinsic factor A substance present in gastric secretions; required for the absorption of vitamin B_{12}.

Iodopsin The light-sensitive pigment present in the cones; also called *visual violet*.

Ion An atom or group of atoms carrying a positive or negative charge.

Iron-binding capacity The degree of saturation of transferrin with iron.

Ischemia A deficiency of blood in a specific area resulting from constriction or obstruction of a blood vessel.

-Itis A suffix referring to inflammation.

Jaundice Yellowness of the skin and eyes caused by excess of bile pigments.

Jejunum The middle portion of the small intestine between the duodenum and the ileum.

Joule The measurement of energy in the metric system. One joule equals 4.184 calories. *See also* Kilojoule.

Keratin A sulfur-containing protein found in hair, skin, and nails.

Keratomalcia Softening of the cornea a result of a deficiency of vitamin A.

Keto- A prefix referring to the carbonyl (CO) group.

Ketogenesis The formation of ketones.

Ketones Intermediate products of fatty acid breakdown. The three common ketones are acetoacetic acid, β-hydroxybuturic acid, and acetone.

Ketosis A clinical condition in which ketones accumulate in the blood and spill over into the urine because fat is being broken down at an abnormally rapid rate. This may be the result of a disturbance in carbohydrate metabolism (e.g., diabetes mellitus), from starvation, or from a diet very low in carbohydrate content.

Kilocalorie The quantity of heat needed to raise the temperature of 1 kg of water 1 C; also called the large Calorie.

Kilogram A metric unit of weight equivalent to 1,000 mg or 2.2 lb.

Kilojoule The metric unit of energy that is 1,000 times larger than the joule. One kilojoule equals .239 Calories.

Krebs cycle The final common pathway for the release of energy from carbohydrate, protein, and fat; also called the *tricarboxylic acid (TCA) cycle* and the *citric acid cycle.*

Kwashiorkor A nutritional deficiency disease related to inadequate intakes of dietary protein.

Lactalbumin A protein in milk.

Lactic acid 1. An acid produced by the bacterial fermentation of lactose. 2. An acid formed during muscle contraction by anaerobic glycolysis.

Lactose intolerance   A condition caused by a lack of or a deficiency of the enzyme lactase.

Leader nutrient   A term used by the National Dairy Council for the 10 primary nutrients. If adequate amounts of these 10 nutrients are consumed, the other essential nutrients will be consumed in amounts to meet the body needs. The 10 leader nutrients also are the same nutrients that currently appear on the nutritional labeling of foods.

Lecithin   A phospholipid found in many tissues, especially nervous tissue. It is also an emulsifier.

Legume   The pod or fruit of peas or beans.

Lethargy   A condition of drowsiness or sluggishness of mental origin.

Leucocyte   A white blood cell.

Lignin   An indigestible carbohydrate in plants.

Linoleic acid   An essential fatty acid containing 18 carbons and 2 double bonds; a polyunsaturated fatty acid.

Linolenic acid   A polyunsaturated fatty acid containing 18 carbons and 3 double bonds.

Lipase   An enzyme that hydrolyzes fat.

Lipids   A broad classification for fat and fat-related substances.

Lipogenesis   The synthesis of fat.

Lipoic acid   A factor that functions with thiamine pyrophosphate in removing the carboxyl group from alpha keto acids.

Lipolysis   The breakdown of fat.

Lipoprotein   A compound protein that is a combination of a lipid and a protein.

Lipotropic   Pertaining to substances that help prevent accumulation of fat in the liver by mobilizing or transporting the fat.

Lumen   The cavity or channel within a tubular structure such as an artery or the intestine.

Lymph   The colorless fluid circulating in the lymphatic system.

Lymphatic system   The vessels that carry lymph from the tissues to the blood.

Lysosomes   Structures within the cell that contain digestive enzymes.

Macrocyte   An abnormally large red blood cell.

Malaise   A general feeling of uneasiness.

Malignant   Occurring in a severe form often resulting in death; referring to uncontrollable growth of tumors, as in cancer.

Malnutrition   An all-inclusive term referring to bad or poor nutrition. Malnutrition may be the result of an excess or a deficiency of nutrients and/or Calories. It includes both undernutrition and overnutrition.

Maltose   A disaccharide resulting from the hydrolysis of starch.

Mannitol   An alcohol derived from the 6-carbon sugar mannose.

Marasmus   Chronic total undernutrition resulting from inadequate quantities of dietary protein and Calories.

Mastication   The act of chewing food.

Matrix   The intercellular framework of a tissue into which something is deposited, such as mineral salts deposited into the protein bone matrix.

Medium chain triglyceride   Fats composed of fatty acids which are 8–10 carbons in length.

Megaloblast   A large, primitive red blood cell with a large nucleus. An increased number of these are found with deficiencies of vitamin B_{12} and folic acid.

Melanin   A dark pigment found in the hair, skin, and eyes.

Menadione   A synthetic form of vitamin K.

Metabolism   The sum of all the chemical reactions occurring within the body. It includes both anabolism (synthesis) and catabolism (breaking down).

Micelle   The combination of bile salts with a lipid to make it more water soluble.

Microcyte   A small red blood cell.

Microvilli   Microscopic fingerlike projections on the surface of the mucosal epithelium of the intestinal tract; the brush border. These structures aid in absorption.

Micturition   The passage of urine from the body.

Milliequivalent (mEq)   The concentration of a solute per liter of solution; found by dividing the milligrams of the solute by the atomic weight of the solute.

Minerals   Inorganic components of food that remain as an ash when the food is burned. Minerals are part of the composition of the body, and they function in metabolism to perform a wide variety of physiological functions.

Mitochondria   Structures in the cell concerned primarily with the release of energy.

Monoglyceride A fat composed of one fatty acid attached to the glycerol molecule.

Monosaccharide A single sugar that is not changed by hydrolysis.

Monounsaturated fatty acid A fatty acid with only one double bond.

Motility The ability to move spontaneously; commonly used to refer to the movement of substances through the digestive tract.

Mottling A discoloration of the enamel of the teeth caused by excess fluorine intake.

Mucopolysaccharide A complex carbohydrate that contains a small amount of protein.

Mucosa A mucous membrane that serves as a lining, such as the lining of the digestive tract.

Multiparous Having borne many children.

Mutase An enzyme that catalyzes the simultaneous oxidation and reduction of two molecules of the same substrate.

Myelin The insulating material of the nerve fiber.

Myo- A prefix meaning *muscle*.

Myocardium The involuntary muscle of the heart.

Myofibril The contracting unit of muscle.

Myoglobin An iron-protein complex that transports oxygen and gives the red color to muscle.

Myosin One of the two proteins of the muscle fibril. When combined with actin in actomyosin it is involved with muscular contraction and relaxation.

Necrosis Death of tissue.

Neonatal Referring to the newborn.

Nephron The functional unit of the kidney.

Neuron A nerve cell.

Neuropathy A disease of the peripheral nervous system.

Niacin A member of the B-complex group of vitamins.

Niacin equivalent The total niacin available to the diet; composed of preformed niacin and the niacin available from the essential amino acid tryptophan (60 mg of tryptophan = 1 mg niacin).

Nicotinamide adenine dinucleotide (NAD) A coenzyme containing niacin; it is involved with oxidation reduction reactions.

Nicotinic acid The preferred name for niacin, a member of the B-complex group of vitamins.

Nocturia Excessive urination during the night.

Nourish To provide food or other substances necessary to sustain life and growth.

Nucleic acid A complex organic acid composed of purine, pyrimidine bases, ribose or deoxyribose, and phosphoric acid.

Nursing process A problem-solving method for planning and implementing nursing care. It is a cyclic process that involves the steps of assessment, planning, intervention, and evaluation.

Nutrient A chemical substance needed by the body for its proper functioning.

Nutrient density The ratio of the nutrient and caloric content of a food compared to a standard for nutrients and Calories such as the RDA.

Nutrient transport The transport of nutrients and oxygen to the cells by the circulatory and respiratory systems.

Nutrition The study of the physiological and psychological processes by which the living organism receives and uses the nutrients from food for maintenance of its functions and growth of its tissues.

Nutritional status The physical condition of the body resulting from the use of ingested nutrients from food.

Nutritive process The process by which the nutrients contained in food are made available to the body cells for energy, growth, and maintenance. The steps in the nutritive process are ingestion, digestion, absorption, transport, metabolism, and excretion.

Objective data Data gathered directly by the nurse using such senses as touch, smell, hearing, and sight.

Oleic acid An 18-carbon fatty acid containing one double bond.

Olfaction The sense of smell.

Oliguria Low urinary output, usually less than 400 ml in 24 hours.

-ology A suffix meaning *study of*.

Organelles The various structures in the cell.

Organic 1. Pertaining to organs. 2. Dealing with substances containing carbon compounds.

Osmolality The concentration of a solute in a solution per unit of solvent.

Osmolarity The concentration of particles (solute) per unit of total volume of solution.

Osmosis   Passage of a solvent through a selective membrane.

Ossification   Formation of bone.

-Osteo   A prefix meaning *bone.*

Osteoblast   A cell associated with the production of bone.

Osteocyte   An osteoblast that has become imbedded within the bone matrix.

Osteoid   The organic matrix of bone.

Osteomalacia   The adult form of rickets.

Osteoporosis   A disease in which there is a decreased quantity of bone resulting in more porous bones.

Oxaloacetic acid   An intermediate in the tricarboxylic acid cycle.

Oxidation   A chemical reaction that involves the addition of oxygen, the removal of hydrogen, or the loss of electrons.

Oxidative phosphorylation   The formation of an energy-rich phosphate bond when adenosine diphosphate (ADP) reacts with inorganic phosphate to form adenosine triphosphate (ATP).

Pallor   The absence of skin color; paleness.

Palmitic acid   A 16-carbon saturated fatty acid found in many foods.

Palpation   A physical assessment technique done by thumping a body part, usually to determine the presence or absence of fluid or gas.

Pancreozymin   A hormone produced by the intestinal mucosa; it stimulates the secretion of pancreatic enzymes.

Pantothenic acid   A member of the B-complex group of vitamins and a constituent of coenzyme A.

Parathormone   A hormone secreted by the parathyroid gland; it raises blood calcium and lowers blood phosphorus levels.

Parenchyma   The functional elements of an organ.

Parenteral   A route of administration other than by mouth. The route may be subcutaneous, intramuscular, or intravenous.

Paresis   Slight or incomplete paralysis.

Paresthesia   An abnormal sensation such as burning, prickling, tingling, or numbness associated with disorders of the nerves and spinal cord.

Parturition   The process of giving birth to a child.

Pathology   The branch of medicine dealing with the science of disease.

Pellagra   A nutritional deficiency disease caused by inadequate amounts of niacin.

Pepsin   The digestive enzyme secreted in the stomach; it initiates the digestion of protein.

Pepsinogen   The inactive form of the digestive enzyme pepsin.

Peptide bond   The bond between the carboxyl group of one amino acid and the amino group of another.

Perinatal   Pertaining to the fetal period and the first month after birth.

Peristalsis   The rhythmic movement in the digestive tract created by the contraction and relaxation of the muscles for the purpose of moving the food mass.

Petechiae   Small, pin-point hemorrhages into the skin resulting from a deficiency of vitamin C.

pH   A measure of acidity or alkalinity of a solution.

Phenylalanine   One of the essential amino acids.

Phosphorylation   The addition of inorganic phosphorus to adenosine diphosphate (ADP) to form adenosine triphosphate (ATP).

Photosynthesis   The process by which green plants manufacture carbohydrates by combining chlorophyll with carbon dioxide and water in the presence of sunlight.

Pica   Craving for unnatural articles of food such as laundry starch or clay and abnormal appetite.

Pinocytosis   The manner by which cells ingest solution by a "sinking in" of the cell membrane.

Plasma   The fluid portion of the blood before clotting has taken place.

Plaque   A deposit on the surface of the tooth which may serve as a medium for the growth of bacteria in the development of dental caries.

Poly-   A prefix meaning *much* or *many.*

Polydipsia   Increased thirst.

Polyneuritis   The inflammation of many nerves.

Polyneuropathy   The inflammatory degeneration of many nerves.

Polypeptide   A compound consisting of more than three amino acids; an intermediate in protein digestion.

Polyphagia   Ravenous appetite.

Polysaccharide   A class of carbohydrates composed of many single sugar units.

Polyunsaturated fatty acid   A fatty acid that contains two or more double bonds.

Polyuria   Excessive elimination of urine.

Portal blood   The blood in the portal vein, going from the intestine to the liver.

Portal circulation   The flow of blood from the gastrointestinal tract through the portal vein to the liver.

Postpartum   Occurring after childbirth or after delivery.

Precursor   Something that precedes another factor, as carotene is a precursor of vitamin A.

Prenatal   Occurring before birth.

Prognosis   The probable course of a disease and the chances for recovery.

Prophylaxis   Prevention of disease.

Protease   An enzyme that digests protein.

Proteins   Complex chemical substances composed of carbon, hydrogen, oxygen, and nitrogen. Proteins made up of amino acids linked together in a specific number and sequence.

Proteinuria   The excretion of protein in the urine.

Prothrombin   A protein in the blood necessary for blood clotting.

Protoplasm   The essential substance of all living cells.

Provitamin   A precursor of a vitamin.

Pruritis   Itching.

Psychocultural equivalencies   Commonly held beliefs, values, and symbols that exist in the minds of people sharing a similar culture.

Ptyalin   The older name for salivary amylase, the enzyme that initiates starch digestion in the mouth.

Puerperium   The period following birth and until the mother's uterus returns to normal (about 6 weeks after delivery).

Pulp   Connective tissue within the pulp chamber; contains blood vessels and nerve fibers.

Purine   Organic compounds that are components of nucleic acid and that are catabolized to uric acid. Adenine and guanine are the major purine bases.

Purpura   Hemorrhaging into the skin; produces large areas of reddish-purple discoloration; caused by a deficiency of vitamin C.

Pyrexia   Fever or a febrile condition.

Pyridoxine   One of the forms of vitamin B_6, a member of the B complex vitamin group.

Pyrimidine   Organic compounds that are components of nucleic acid. Three pyrimidines are uracil, thymine, and cytosine.

Pyrosis   A burning sensation in the region of the lower esophagus and stomach; heartburn.

Pyruvic acid   An important intermediate compound in the metabolism of carbohydrate, protein, and fat.

Rales   Abnormal respiratory sounds heard in the upper chest during auscultation and indicating a pathological condition.

Rectal   Pertaining to the rectum.

Recommended Dietary Allowances (RDA)   Recommended daily intakes of protein and specific vitamins and minerals for several age and sex categories considered adequate for the maintenance of good nutritional status of people residing in the United States. The RDA is developed by the Food and Nutrition Board of the National Research Council, National Academy of Sciences. These allowances are reevaluated and revised approximately every five years.

Rectum   The lower part of the large intestine from the sigmoid colon to the anal canal.

Regurgitation   The backward flow of food from the stomach to the mouth.

Remission   A decreased severity of symptoms or the temporary cessation of symptoms.

Renal   Pertaining to the kidney.

Renin   An enzyme produced by the kidney.

Rennin   An enzyme present in the stomach; it coagulates milk.

Residue   The material remaining in the colon following the digestion of food.

Respiration   The exchange of oxygen and carbon dioxide through the lungs at the cellular level in the metabolism of the cell. The combining of carbohydrate with oxygen to release energy, carbon dioxide, and water.

Reticuloendothelial   Pertaining to tissues having both reticular and endothelial attributes.

Retinene   The aldehyde form of vitamin A.

Retinol   The alcohol form of vitamin A.

Rhodopsin   A light-sensitive pigment found in the rods of the retina; it is responsible for the ability to see in dim light. It is also known as *visual purple*. Vitamin A is required for the regeneration of rhodopsin.

Rhonchi   A dry, course, abnormal respiratory sound in the bronchial tubes.

Riboflavin   A member of the B-complex group of vitamins.

Ribonucleic acid (RNA)   A nucleic acid present in the cytoplasm and nucleus; it has a role in protein synthesis.

Ribose   A 5-carbon sugar that is a component of nucleic acid.

Ribosomes   The site of protein synthesis within the cell.

Rickets   A disease resulting from a deficiency of vitamin D or a disturbance in calcium-phosphorus metabolism.

Saccharin   An artificial sweetening agent about 500 times as sweet as sugar and that yields no Calories.

Sarcoma   A type of tumor that is often malignant.

Sarcoplasm   The protoplasm between muscle fibers.

Satiety   The feeling of fullness and satisfaction following a meal.

Saturated   Referring to a fatty acid in which all of the bonds are completely filled (i.e., saturated) with hydrogen. A saturated fatty acid contains no double bonds.

Scurvy   A deficiency disease caused by a lack of vitamin C.

Seborrheic dermatitis   A greasy and scaly type of dermatitis seen around the eyes, nose, and ears owing to a deficiency of riboflavin.

Secretin   A hormone secreted by the intestinal mucosa in response to the presence of acid chyme. It stimulates the secretion of pancreatic juice and bile.

Seizure   1. An attack of epilepsy. 2. The sudden attack or recurrence of a symptom or disease.

Self-concept   The total of the beliefs a person has about himself, including his body image and self-esteem.

Sepis   Infection resulting from the spread of bacteria throughout the body.

Serosanguineous   Composed of serum and blood.

Serum   The fluid portion of blood; that which remains after clotting.

Skinfold measurement   Measurement of the thickness of a fold of fatty tissue at selected sites using a caliper.

Sorbitol   An alcohol of glucose or fructose; used as a sweetening agent.

Specific dynamic action (SDA) of food   The energy required for the digestion, absorption, and metabolism of food.

Sphincter   A ringlike muscle that surrounds and closes a body opening.

Sphingomyelin   A phospholipid found primarily in brain and nervous tissue as a component of the myelin sheath.

Stasis   Retardation or stoppage of the flow of blood or other body fluids.

Steatorrhea   The presence of fat in the stool.

Stenosis   Narrowing of a passage.

Steroid   A group of compounds similar in composition to cholesterol, for example, bile acids, sex hormones, and sterols.

Stomatitis   An inflammation of the oral cavity.

Subjective data   Data gathered through the use of communication techniques.

Sucrose   A disaccharide composed of glucose and fructose; cane or beet sugar.

Syncope   A sudden loss of strength.

Syndrome   A set of symptoms that occur together.

Synergism   The combined action of agents with the effect being greater than the algebraic sum of the individual effects.

Synthesis   The combining of two or more substances to form a new material; building up.

Systemic   Pertaining to the body as a whole.

Tachycardia   Rapid heartbeat.

Tetany   Continuous tonic spasm of a muscle.

Thiamine   A member of the B-complex group of vitamins.

Thrombin   An enzyme needed for the conversion of fibrinogen to fibrin in the blood-clotting process.

Thromboembolism   The obstruction of a blood vessel by a thrombus.

Thrombus   A blood clot.

Thyroxine   The iodine-containing hormone from

the thyroid gland that regulates energy metabolism.

Tocopherol The chemical name for vitamin E.

-Tomy A suffix meaning *to cut.*

Toxemia of pregnancy A complication of pregnancy characterized by edema, hypertension, and albuminuria.

Transamination Transfer of a group from one amino acid to another.

Transferase An enzyme that transfers a group from one compound to another.

Transferrin A protein that transports iron in the blood and delivers it to the liver.

Transmethylation The transfer of methyl group (—CH_3) from one compound to another.

Transport The moving of nutrients and oxygen to the cells by the circulatory and respiratory systems.

Trauma A severe wound or injury.

Tricarboxylic acid (TCA) cycle The final common pathway for the release of energy from carbohydrate, protein, and fat.

Triglyceride A compound composed of three fatty acids attached to a glycerol molecule. It is commonly referred to as a *fat.*

Trypsin A digestive enzyme from the pancreas; it hydrolyzes protein.

Trypsinogen The inactive form of the digestive enzyme trypsin.

Tryptophan One of the essential amino acids.

Turgor The normal elasticity of the skin.

Urea The main nitrogenous component of the urine.

Uremia A set of symptoms related to the retention of the end products of protein metabolism in the blood.

Uric acid An end product of purine metabolism excreted in the urine.

US Recommended Daily Allowances (US-RDA) A set of daily quantities of protein, vitamins, and minerals used as the standard for nutritional food labeling. The US-RDA standard was derived from the RDA.

Valence The capacity of an element to combine with another element.

Vasodilation An increase in the diameter of a blood vessel leading to an increased blood supply.

Vegan A person who excludes all animal foods from his diet and eats only foods of plant origin.

Vegetarian A person who excludes one or more groups of animal foods from his diet. All animal products may be excluded, or milk and/or eggs may be excluded.

Venule A minute branch of a vein connected to a capillary.

Vertigo A sensation of rotation or movement of oneself; dizziness.

Villi Fingerlike projections of the inner lining of the small intestine; they greatly enhance the absorptive surface. Each villus is covered with microvilli, which further enhance the absorptive surface.

Visual purple A visual pigment that contains vitamin A and is found in the rods; also called *rhodopsin.*

Visual violet A visual pigment that contains vitamin A and is found in the cones; also called iodopsin.

Vitamins Organic substances present in food in small quantities; their function is regulating metabolism for normal growth and health.

Xerophthalmia A deficiency disease associated with vitamin A deficiency; characterized by dryness of the eye, softening of the cornea, and eventual blindness.

Xerosis Abnormal dryness of the skin or the eye.

Zymogen The inactive form of an enzyme.

INDEX